# OCCUPATIONAL THERAPY FOR CHILDREN

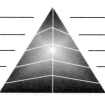

# OCCUPATIONAL THERAPY FOR CHILDREN

*Edited by*

**JANE CASE-SMITH, EdD, OTR**

Associate Professor, Occupational Therapy Division,
The Ohio State University,
Columbus, Ohio

**ANNE S. ALLEN, MA**

Formerly, Assistant Director,
School of Allied Medical Professions,
The Ohio State University,
Columbus, Ohio

**PAT NUSE PRATT, MOT, OTR, FAOTA**

Private Practice,
Gainesville, Georgia

**THIRD EDITION**

*with illustrations by*

**Jeanne Robertson**
**Jody Fulks, MS,** *Medical Illustrator*

*with **40** contributors*
*with **357** illustrations*

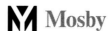 Mosby

St. Louis  Baltimore  Boston  Carlsbad  Chicago  Naples  New York  Philadelphia  Portland
London  Madrid  Mexico City  Singapore  Sydney  Tokyo  Toronto  Wiesbaden

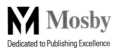

Mosby
Dedicated to Publishing Excellence

A Times Mirror
Company

*Publisher:* Don Ladig
*Editor:* Martha Sasser
*Associate Developmental Editor:* Amy Dubin
*Project Manager:* Patricia Tannian
*Senior Production Editor:* Suzanne C. Fannin
*Book Design Manager:* Gail Morey Hudson
*Manufacturing Supervisor:* Linda Ierardi
*Cover Designer:* Teresa Breckwoldt
*Cover Photos:* Shay McAtee

**THIRD EDITION**
**Copyright © 1996 by Mosby–Year Book, Inc.**

Previous editions copyrighted 1985, 1989

Printed in the United States of America
Composition by Clarinda Company
Printing/binding by Maple-Vail Book Mfg Group

Mosby–Year Book, Inc.
11830 Westline Industrial Drive
St. Louis, Missouri 63146

**Library of Congress Cataloging in Publication Data**

Occupational therapy for children / edited by Jane Case-Smith, Anne S.
   Allen, Pat Nuse Pratt ; with illustrations by Jeanne Robertson, Jody
   Fulks, medical illustrator ; with 40 contributors. — 3rd ed.
       p.    cm.
     Includes bibliographical references and index.
     ISBN 0-8151-1541-5
     1. Occupational therapy for children.   2. Occupational therapy for
children—Practice.   I. Case-Smith, Jane, 1953-   II. Allen, Anne
S., 1923-   .   III. Pratt, Pat Nuse.
     [DNLM:   1. Occupational Therapy—in infancy & childhood.   2. Child,
Exceptional.   3. Child Development Disorders—rehabilitation.   WS
368 015 1996]
RJ53.025022 1992
616.8'515'083—dc20
DNLM/DLC
for Library of Congress                                    95-31362
                                                              CIP

98  99  /  9  8  7  6  5  4

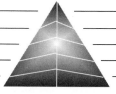

# Contributors

**ANNE S. ALLEN, MA**

Formerly, Assistant Director,
School of Allied Medical Professions,
The Ohio State University,
Columbus, Ohio

**SUSAN J. AMUNDSON, MS, OTR/L**

O.T. Kids,
Homer, Alaska

**JILL ANDERSON, MS, OTR**

Occupational Therapy Supervisor,
Step by Step Infant Development Center,
Brooklyn, New York;
Private Practice,
Rockville Centre, New York

**MARGARET J. BARNSTORFF, BS, MOT, OTR**

Registered Occupational Therapist,
Pediatric Therapy Associates,
Fort Collins, Colorado

**RICARDO C. CARRASCO, PhD, OTR/L, FAOTA**

School of Allied Health Sciences,
Department of Occupational Therapy,
The Medical College of Georgia,
Augusta, Georgia

**JANE CASE-SMITH, EdD, OTR**

Assistant Professor, Occupational Therapy Division,
The Ohio State University,
Columbus, Ohio

**IDA LOU COLEY, OTR**

Formerly, Children's Hospital at Stanford,
Palo Alto, California

**ANNE F. CRONIN, PhD, OTR/L**

AOTA Board Certified Pediatric Occupational Therapist,
Morris Child Development Center,
Gainesville, Florida

**DEBORA A. DAVIDSON, MS, OTR, BCP**

Formerly, Assistant Professor,
Department of Occupational Therapy,
School of Allied Health Sciences,
University of Texas Medical Branch,
Galveston, Texas;
Instructor, Program in Occupational Therapy,
Washington University School of Medicine,
St. Louis, Missouri

**SUE ANN DUBOIS, OTR/L, BCP**

AOTA Board Certified Pediatric Occupational Therapist,
Pediatric and School Consultant,
Porter Corners, New York

**BRIAN J. DUDGEON, MS, OTR**

Lecturer, Division of Occupational Therapy,
Department of Rehabilitation Medicine,
University of Washington,
Seattle, Washington

**SNAEFRIDUR EGILSON, MS, OT**

State Diagnostic and Counseling Center,
Kopavogur, Iceland

**CHARLOTTE E. EXNER, PhD, OTR/L, FAOTA**

Associate Professor and Chairperson,
Occupational Therapy Department,
Towson State University,
Towson, Maryland

**CATHERINE YANEGA GORDON, EdD, OTR/L**

Associate Professor and Chairperson,
Department of Occupational Therapy,
Ithaca College,
Ithaca, New York

**JIM HINOJOSA, PhD, OTR, FAOTA**

Associate Professor,
Director of Postprofessional Graduate Programs,
Department of Occupational Therapy,
New York University,
New York, New York

**RUTH HUMPHRY, PhD, OTR/L**

Associate Professor, Department of Occupational Therapy,
University of North Carolina at Chapel Hill,
Chapel Hill, North Carolina

**JAN G. HUNTER, MA, OTR/L**

Neonatal Clinical Specialist, Children's Hospital;
Assistant Professor, Department of Occupational Therapy,
School of Allied Health,
University of Texas Medical Branch,
Galveston, Texas

**JAN JOHNSON, MS, OTR/L**

Occupational Therapist, Special Education Department,
Columbus Public Schools,
Columbus, Ohio

**KATALIN I. KORANYI, MD**

Associate Professor, Department of Pediatrics,
The Ohio State University,
Columbus, Ohio

**PAULA KRAMER, PhD, OTR, FAOTA**

Professor and Chair, Department of Occupational Therapy,
Kean College of New Jersey,
Union, New Jersey

**ZOE MAILLOUX, MA, OTR, FAOTA**

Director of Administration and Practice,
The Ayres Clinic,
Torrance, California;
Adjunct Instructor,
Department of Occupational Therapy,
The University of Southern California,
Los Angeles, California

**MARY A. McILROY, MD**

Associate Professor of Clinical Pediatrics,
Department of Pediatrics,
College of Medicine,
The Ohio State University,
Columbus, Ohio

**PEGGY METZGER, MS, OTR/L**

Staff Therapist,
Northwestern Illinois Association,
Geneva, Illinois

**CHRISTINE DOYLE MORRISON, MS, OTR/L**

Supervisor, Pediatric Occupational Therapy,
University of Illinois Hospital,
University of Illinois,
Chicago, Illinois

**DEBORAH S. NICHOLS, PhD, PT**

Associate Professor and Director,
Department of Physical Therapy,
The Ohio State University,
Columbus, Ohio

**L. DIANE PARHAM, PhD, OTR, FAOTA**

Associate Professor, Department of Occupational Therapy,
University of Southern California,
Los Angeles, California

**PAT NUSE PRATT, MOT, OTR, FAOTA**

Private Practice,
Gainesville, Georgia

**SUSAN A. PROCTER, OTR**

Private Practice,
Amherst, Ohio

**PAMELA K. RICHARDSON, MS, OTR/L**

Occupational Therapy Consultant,
Private Practice,
Santa Barbara, California

**KAREN E. SCHANZENBACHER, MS, OTR/L**

Occupational Therapist,
Cattaraugus-Allegany Board of Cooperative Education Services,
Olean, New York

**COLLEEN M. SCHNECK, ScD, OTR/L**

Associate Professor, Department of Occupational Therapy,
Eastern Kentucky University,
Richmond, Kentucky

**JOANNE S. SCHOELKOPF, MBA, OTR**

Currently, Easter Seals—Early Intervention Program,
Orlando, Florida
Formerly, Senior Occupational Therapist,
ACLD-Kramer Learning Center,
Bay Shore, New York

**JAYNE SHEPHERD, MS, OTR**

Assistant Professor,
Virginia Commonwealth University,
Richmond, Virginia

**SUSAN DENEGAN SHORTRIDGE, MHS, OTR/L**

Owner,
Developmental Health Care Services, Inc.,
Gainesville, Florida

**ELIZABETH SNOW, MA, OTR**

Assistant Professor and Program Director,
Occupational Therapy Assistant Program,
Mount St. Mary's College,
Los Angeles, California

**KAREN C. SPENCER, PhD, OTR**

Assistant Professor, Department of Occupational Therapy,
Colorado State University,
Fort Collins, Colorado

**LINDA C. STEPHENS, MS, OTR/L, FAOTA**

Owner and Director,
Atlanta Children's Therapy,
Atlanta, Georgia

**KATHERINE B. STEWART, MS, OTR/L, FAOTA**

Clinical Associate Professor,
School of Occupational Therapy and Physical Therapy,
University of Puget Sound,
Tacoma, Washington

**MIRIAM STRUCK, MA, OTR/L**

Itinerant Occupational Therapist,
Services for Physically Challenged Students,
Montgomery County Public Schools,
Bethesda, Maryland

**SUSAN K. TAUBER, MEd, OTR/L**

Executive Director,
The Adaptive Learning Center,
Atlanta, Georgia

**BARBARA BURRIS WAVREK, MHS, OTR/L**

Instructor, Occupational Therapy Division,
College of Medicine,
School of Allied Medical Professions,
The Ohio State University,
Columbus, Ohio

**MARSHA WEIL, MS, OTR/L**

Occupational Therapist, Bellevue School District,
Bellevue, Washington

**CHRISTINE WRIGHT-OTT, MPA, OTR**

Packard Children's Hospital at Stanford,
Rehabilitation Engineering Center,
Palo Alto, California

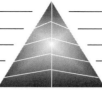

# Foreword

One measure of civilization is the value it places on its children. Case-Smith, Allen, and Pratt, editors of the third edition of *Occupational Therapy for Children,* have combined their expertise with that of colleagues to create a comprehensive introduction to pediatric occupational therapy that reflects this valuing of children. The book, although designed specifically as a pediatric text for entry-level students, is equally useful as a resource book for postprofessional students and practicing therapists.

Strengths of the book include its comprehensiveness, its overall organization, and the study aids included with each chapter. The book starts by laying the foundation for occupational therapy practice and by identifying the broad knowledge base required for this endeavor. Building on this foundation, the book progresses logically from assessment through intervention with specific foci on the performance areas of postural control, hand skills, visual perception, psychosocial and emotional development, feeding and oral-motor skills, self-care and adaptation for independent living, play, handwriting, augmentative communication and computer access, and mobility. Specific strengths in content that merit highlighting are the attention to the psychosocial development and needs of children, the use of technology to increase function, the importance of families and others in the child's system to the continuing process of adaptation, and the legislation that is relevant to children with disabilities and their families.

The book's concluding section on arenas of pediatric occupational therapy practice is addressed from a developmental perspective. This section provides an integrative function facilitating understanding of the therapy process starting in the neonatal intensive care unit; progressing through early intervention, preschool and school programs; and appropriately concluding with transitioning from school to adult life. For pediatric therapists this longitudinal perspective assists with contextualizing a child's program within the child's past and future.

Understanding of the needs of learners when using a text book is reflected in the editor's careful inclusion of study aids within each chapter. Key terms, chapter objectives, and study questions are strategically employed to guide student learning and provide opportunities to apply and integrate knowledge.

The editors have coordinated the efforts of an impressive group of authors reflecting a broad range of expertise in pediatric practice. The diverse and rich contributions of these individuals are organized logically and meaningfully so that this knowledge can be used by students and therapists who work daily to facilitate the potential of children to play, to care for themselves, and to work. The third edition of *Occupational Therapy for Children* is a book that reflects caring, empowering, and respect. It is a treasure for occupational therapists and for children with disabilities and their families.

**Jean Deitz, PhD, OTR, FAOTA**
*Associate Professor*
*Division of Occupational Therapy*
*Department of Rehabilitation Medicine*
*University of Washington*

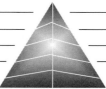

# Preface

Since the first edition of *Occupational Therapy for Children* was published, the practice of occupational therapy has seen tremendous growth and change. Professions grow and evolve, both in philosophy and in practice. The first edition of this book dealt with the roles and functions of the occupational therapist, the core knowledge of the profession, and the process of occupational therapy, as it was in 1983.

Three years later, we began the text revision that was published in 1989, adding some content specific to the treatment of cerebral palsy and hands, changing the assessments presentation, and adding a section on management. Even as we were working on the second edition, occupational therapy for children was rapidly changing. These changes were brought about by external forces, such as new legislation and federal programs, and internal forces, such as research and guidelines published by the profession. Recent amendments to the Individuals with Disabilities Education Act (IDEA, 1990) have had a significant impact on service delivery by increasing services to young children, improving access to assistive technology, encouraging inclusion, and increasing services to the child's family. Other new laws, such as the Americans with Disabilities Act (1990), have increased opportunities for occupational therapists to assume roles as consultants, helping organizations and agencies make accommodations for individuals with disabilities. Maternal Child Health Training Grants have promoted the development of pediatric occupational therapy throughout the 1980s by funding university programs and supporting meetings of national leaders. The purposes of these meetings have been to develop goals and to plan strategies for enhancing occupational therapy practice with children. The written proceedings of these meetings served as a resource for revising this text.

In addition to legislative changes and government supported programs, new professional resources and publications have created new options and models for intervention. Practice guidelines have been published by the American Occupational Therapy Association for Services in School Systems (1987), Early Childhood Programs (1989), and Neonatal Intensive Care Units (1993). Based on extensive surveying of entry level programs and pediatric practice, a task force of occupational therapy leaders developed Guidelines for Curriculum Content in Pediatrics (1992) to help faculty develop the pediatric content of entry level programs.

This third edition reflects many of these changes brought about by the research and legislation of the 1980s and uses the resources developed by our professional organization. The result is substantial change in the content and organization of the text.

The first section of this new edition describes the foundational knowledge required for pediatric practice. This section uses developmental theories as a basis for understanding the child's acquisition of functional skills and social roles. Frames of reference are identified and described as the vital links between theory and practice. The information on physical disabilities and medical problems has been expanded and updated. The chapter on families has also been revised to reflect the great variation in today's family structures and life-styles. In addition, the influence of cultural values on childrearing and on the use of educational and health care systems is described. Family-centered intervention is underscored as a basic element of all practice with children.

The second section of this book includes three chapters on occupational therapy assessment of children. Evaluation is explained as a process, focusing on analysis of functional performance within natural contexts. The section also describes how to administer standardized tests, interpret the findings, and synthesize the assessment information into intervention goals and plans. This section explains the critical nature of occupational therapy evaluation to the family's understanding of the child and the team's ability to establish a comprehensive plan.

The chapters on performance areas in the third section contain detailed and in-depth information based on recently published literature. New chapters on postural development, visual perception, feeding, augmentative communication, handwriting, and mobility have been added. Each chapter has been updated to include information on revised theoretical principles, currently advocated service delivery models, recently developed assessments, innovative intervention strategies, and new technology. Psychosocial aspects of the child's performance are emphasized in several chapters and are covered in detail in Chapter 15. The range of assistive technology is described, as are strategies that enable individuals to integrate technology systems into their daily lives.

This section builds on the problem solving approach defined in the first and second editions. Although identifying developmental problems remains an essential aspect of the occupational therapy process, therapists must also identify and include the individual's coping styles and resources within the system (e.g. family and classroom supports) when formulating intervention plans and strategies. The child's medical, neurologic, or orthopedic problems have more or less impact on functional performance based on the social and physical resources available to him or her. Adapted equipment and assistive technology can enable the child to function without "curing" the problem.

The evolution of our primary theoretical approaches is also explained in this third section. Intervention using sensory integration theory has changed based on new research and the publication of the Sensory Integration and Praxis Tests (Ayres, 1989). The neurodevelopmental treatment approach has also expanded to include dynamic systems and motor control theories, results of efficacy research, and improved understanding of neuromotor impairments, such as cerebral palsy. Our understanding of the use of play in the intervention and the variables that relate to playfulness has increased.

The fourth section is essentially a new addition to the book. This section describes arenas of occupational therapy practice. The section was developed in recognition of the importance of the environment to the child's performance. Current practice has shifted from an emphasis on the individual to the individual within his or her social and physical environments. Therefore the skills and performance areas addressed in therapy must always consider the demands and resources of the child's environment. In many cases, occupational therapy goals shift from changing the individual to modifying the environment so that it supports the child's performance and functional independence.

The section also examines how the work setting affects the occupational therapist's selection of intervention approach and service delivery models. Contrasting examples of therapy in medical, community, private practice, residential, and educational systems clearly illustrate the varying roles of occupational therapists. A developmental framework (birth to adulthood) organizes the section on arenas of practice (that is, neonatal intensive care units (NICUs) through early intervention to school practice). This life-span perspective helps promote understanding of how occupational therapists deal with the functional problems imposed by disabilities at different ages and in different contexts. For example, early intervention services with infants who have neuromotor impairments are essentially different from

school-based services. Neurodevelopmental treatment techniques, although critical for young children, are less important as the child enters school and develops compensatory strategies for functioning in the classroom.

The text also emphasizes cultural competence. The examples and case studies present children of different cultures and emphasize cultural sensitivity in evaluation and intervention. We believe that these case studies, which describe the child's background, history, and family, have greater teaching potential than case studies with clinical emphasis.

We have maintained the primary purpose of the book as an undergraduate text but, at the same time, we recognize that some of the content is beyond entry level. For example, the chapter on NICU practice reflects the more advanced knowledge and skills required to work with preterm infants. Chapters on mobility and augmentative communication also contain information relevant to specialized areas of practice. Reference and resource lists provide helpful information to practitioners who may continue to use the text. In the interest of manageable book size, information on low incidence conditions is presented only when illustrating a frame of reference, intervention approach, or practice setting.

We acknowledge with gratitude the assistance of colleagues—clinicians and curricula faculty—who have commented on ideas, direction, and use of this book. In particular we wish to acknowledge our gratitude to Debora Davidson, Yvonne Swinth, Dr. James Blackman, Jennifer Angelo, and Heather Miller for their review and critique of chapters. We also acknowledge those that have offered inspiration along the way: Barb Hanft, Gordon Williamson, Anne Henderson, and Patti Maurer. Jane would like to thank Greg, David and Stephen Smith, whose love and support made the third edition possible.

**Jane Case-Smith**
**Anne Stevens Allen**
**Pat Nuse Pratt**

## REFERENCES

American Occupational Therapy Association (1987). *Guidelines for occupational therapy services in schools systems.* Rockville, MD: AOTA.

American Occupational Therapy Association (1989). *Guidelines for occupational therapy services in early intervention and preschool services.* Rockville, MD: AOTA.

American Occupational Therapy Association (1992). *Guidelines for curriculum content in pediatrics.* Rockville, MD: AOTA.

American Occupational Therapy Association (1993). Knowledge and skills for occupational therapy practice in the neonatal intensive care units. *American Journal of Occupational Therapy, 47,* (11), 1100-1105.

American Occupational Therapy Association (1994). Uniform Terminology-Third Edition. *American Journal of Occupational Therapy, 48,* 1047-1054.

Ayres, A.J. (1989). *Sensory Integration and Praxis Tests.* Los Angeles: Western Psychological Services.

# Contents

# Knowledge Base of Occupational Therapy in Pediatrics

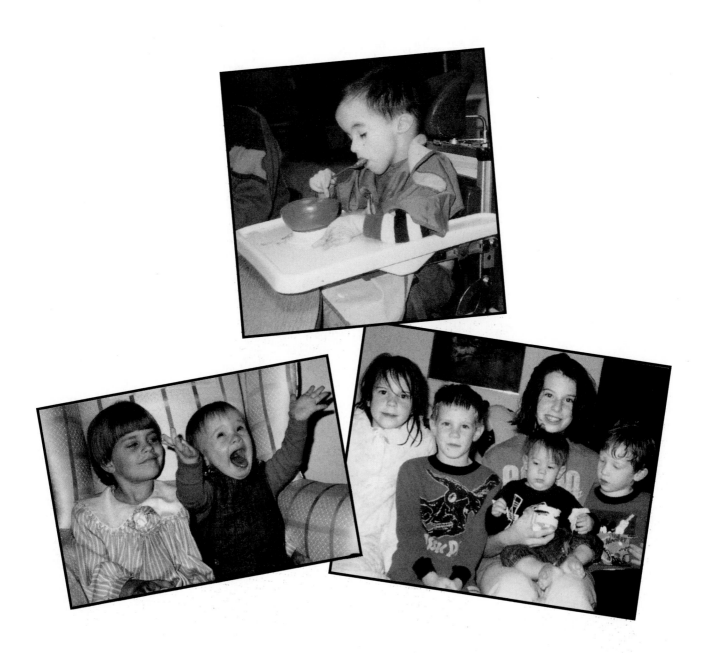

CHAPTER

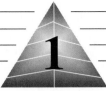

# An Overview of Occupational Therapy with Children

JANE CASE-SMITH

## KEY TERMS

▲ Performance Components and Underlying Skills
▲ Performance Areas and Functional Skills
▲ Performance Context and Physical, Social and Cultural Environments
▲ Social Roles
▲ Impairment, Disability and Handicap
▲ Occupational Therapy Process
▲ Inclusion and Integration of Services
▲ Cost-effectiveness of Service Delivery
▲ Assistive Technology and Trends in Technology

## CHAPTER OBJECTIVES

1. Explain the domains of concern in occupational therapy with children.
2. Define performance components, areas, and context.
3. Explain how performance components and context influence the child's functional performance in daily living, play, and school activities.
4. Apply the goodness-of-fit model to children with disabilities as they influence and are influenced by their environments.
5. Describe the occupational therapy process of screening, evaluation, planning, intervention, and reassessment.
6. Analyze how current themes in health care and education have influenced and will continue to influence occupational therapy practice.
7. Explain how trends in health care and intervention for children with disabilities affect the present-day role of occupational therapists.

Occupational therapists view the child, the child's environment, and the interaction between the child and the environment in a holistic way. The child continually adapts to the environment and influences the environment. The dynamic nature of this interaction is created in part by the child's continual development, maturation, and learning. The environment is also continually evolving and changing; at times in response to the child's needs and actions and at times as a result of external variables. Occupational therapists analyze the child's functional performance within different environments to identify the child's strengths and limitations. They determine whether limitations in performance are attributable to the child's intrinsic skills and characteristics, external factors in the environment, or a combination of intrinsic and external variables. Hence an important role of the occupational therapist is analysis of functional performance to identify the variables to be targeted in intervention. Although functional performance can be analyzed into specific skills and skill components, it is the spirit of a child that holds those components together. The maturation of a child and the complexity of the interrelationships between mind and body and between physical and social development are beyond human analytic ability. This book presents the theories, principles, and strategies that are used in occupational therapy with children. It provides intervention strategies for helping children cope with and overcome their disabilities. Although this technical information is important to occupational therapy practice with children, it is childhood itself that creates meaning for pediatric practice. Childhood is hopeful and joyful and ever new. The spirit, the playfulness, and the joy of childhood creates the context for occupational therapy with children.

3

## OCCUPATIONAL THERAPY DOMAINS OF CONCERN

The occupational therapist is concerned with analyzing the child's ability to perform in everyday contexts. How does the child cope with the dilemmas and problems that confront him or her on a daily basis? Does the child's day have rhythm and order? Can the child influence the environment and master it? Does the child meet the expectations placed on him or her by peers, caregivers, and teachers? Occupational therapists hold two broad goals for the children they serve. These goals are to improve the child's functional performance and to enhance the child's ability to interact within his or her physical and social environments.

The occupational therapist approaches the first goal, that of improving the child's functional performance, from a unique perspective in which performance is analyzed into components of underlying ability and skill. The goal is also viewed from a holistic perspective that considers the supports and constraints of the environment. Occupational therapy begins by examining the child's ability to function in everyday activities. Through observation, testing, and interviewing, information is gathered to elucidate which components of performance are delayed, deficient, or missing. The occupational therapist hypothesizes which performance components appear to interfere with the functional abilities of the child. Postulates about the basis of the delays are often developed from the particular frame of reference that seems to explain the basis of the child's problem (Kramer & Hinojosa, 1993). The frame of reference that seems helpful to understanding the problem is often the frame of reference used in developing solutions to the problems or in defining appropriate intervention strategies.

The second goal of occupational therapy is to improve the reciprocal relationships between the child and the environment. In working toward an optimal *goodness-of-fit* between the child and the environment the therapist recognizes that both the child and the environment are dynamic; therefore the goodness-of-fit is relative to a moment and evolves over time. To promote this interaction, the occupational therapist may emphasize development of underlying skill components (performance components), facilitation of functional performance in everyday activities (performance areas), or adaptation of the environment (performance context) to enable the child to achieve desired and expected social roles.

Christiansen (1991) described a person-environment-performance framework for understanding how each individual is an open system influenced by the environment and how performance should not be isolated from its context. Human performance is the result of intrinsic abilities or underlying performance components and extrinsic factors or variables in the environment. Although underlying skills define the child's ability to master specific activities, the physical and social context enable the child to succeed in and master the tasks associated with the roles defined by culture, age, family, and community. Roles are dynamic as they are acquired and replaced throughout the life span. A child who has delays or deficits in performance areas may be unable to achieve certain social roles or may acquire other delays or deficits particular to his or her disability. The following section describes the categories of performance as defined by occupational therapists (AOTA, 1994).

### Performance Components/Underlying Skills

*Sensorimotor* components include sensory and perceptual processing, neuromuscular abilities, and motor skills. Sensory and perceptual processing (described in Chapters 13 and 14) refers to the ability of the child to take in, assimilate, and interpret sensory information. According to Gilfoyle, Grady, and Moore (1990), to successfully adapt to the environment, a child must assimilate sensory information and accommodate to it with a motor response. Through the developmental process the child also learns to associate the sensory experience with the motor act and to differentiate among sensory experiences.

Perceptual processing refers to the ability to organize sensory information into meaningful patterns. Perceptual skills are often evident in the precision and accuracy of the child's motor responses. They also undergird cognitive development and higher level intellectual skills.

Neuromuscular components are the foundation for development of motor skills. Included are reflexes, muscle tone, strength, endurance, postural alignment and control, and soft tissue integrity. Integrity of these basic components allows for development of motor skills.

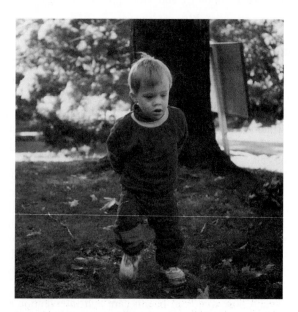

**Figure 1-1**   Play of infants and toddlers is driven by the need to master basic motor skills that enable exploration of the environment.

*Motor* components refer to gross, fine, and oral motor skills. Movement is the first way that a child interacts with the environment (Figure 1-1). It is believed that certain motor skills are genetically programmed (e.g., upright locomotion) and others are learned (e.g., using a writing utensil). Motor skills evolve as a direct response to sensory input from the environment. They reflect the child's ability to adapt to the environment; higher level motor skills support and influence cognitive and social development. Neuromuscular and motor components are described in Chapters 11 and 12.

*Cognitive* components underlie the child's ability to perceive, attend to, and learn from the environment. Cognitive ability is required to learn skills in all performance areas, self-care, play, and school. Understanding of the child's cognitive abilities is critical to establishing intervention goals and to planning activities. The child's cognitive skills determine the amount of cuing and verbal guidance needed to complete an activity, the amount of repetition and reinforcement required for learning, and the degree of assistance required to generalize skills to other contexts.

*Psychosocial* skills refer to the child's underlying abilities to interact with others, to cope with new or difficult situations, and to manage his or her behaviors in socially appropriate ways. Psychosocial skills influence the child's ability to establish friendships and other social relationships (Figure 1-2). Effectively coping with challenging situations and exhibiting socially appropriate actions are aspects of psychosocial skills. As psychosocial components of performance mature, the child develops values, interests, and a self-identify (Llorens, 1977, 1991).

## Performance Areas

The performance areas of the child are self-care, play, and school and work activities. The areas of self-care refer to physical daily living skills. These include feeding and eating, grooming and hygiene, dressing, and functional mobility (AOTA, 1994). Self-care skills, like other performance areas, follow a developmental sequence. In the very young child, self-care focuses on nurturance and feeding. The child learns the oral motor and, later, fine motor competence required for feeding and eating. In early childhood, self-care activities expand to include dressing and bathing. The child may demonstrate independence and helpful participation in dressing. Eating without spillage is achieved. In childhood and adolescence, independence in most self-care skills is achieved, and typically the youth takes pride in his or her appearance and gains satisfaction in maintenance of personal hygiene. Intervention for self-care and daily living skills are described in Chapters 16, 17, and 21.

*Play and leisure* refer to skills and performance of intrinsically motivating activities, spontaneous enjoyment, or self-expression. In early childhood, play activities involve exploration of objects and the environment (Figure 1-3). Play consists of imitating others and repetitive activities. Symbolic play and pretend play demonstrate the child's developing imagination. In childhood, play becomes more social and involves games with groups of children. Play skills evolve from simple play interactions of touch and sounds in infancy to sophisticated construction and art activities in

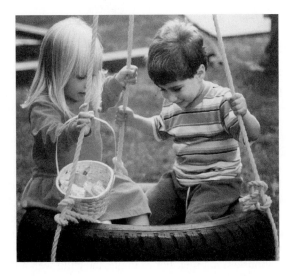

**Figure 1-2**   Social interactions of young children involve participation in the same activities. Interaction may be characterized by physical proximity more than verbal exchange.

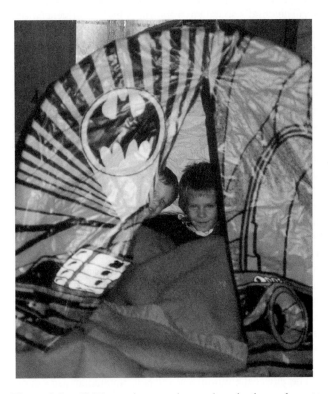

**Figure 1-3**   Children gain great pleasure by selecting and creating their own play space.

adolescence. Increasing levels of structure and rules are applied to play activities as the child reaches adolescence (Llorens, 1991). Play activities and intervention to increase a child's playfulness are described in Chapter 18.

*School* activities do not apply until the child begins preschool. Initially the focus is on social skills, health, and sensorimotor development. At age 6 the child enters school and is expected to master reading, writing, math, and higher level problem solving. The child assumes increasingly greater levels of responsibility for his or her own learning. Socializing within the school environment remains an important focus. The performance area of school activities is described in Chapters 24 and 25. School activities as these relate to work are described in Chapter 32.

## Performance Context

The environment defines a set of extrinsic factors that support the child's functional performance. Physical, social, and cultural dimensions of the environment have great impact on the child's performance. Children and their environments influence each other in a reciprocal way. The environment can help or hinder the child's performance; reciprocally, the child can be a positive or negative influence on his or her environment. The social environment refers to family members, peers, and other significant adults with whom the child interacts (Figure 1-4). The human environment places expectations on the child, supports the child, and provides essential psychosocial interaction opportunities. The child's social environment is highly influenced by the family's socioeconomic status, structure, and composition. For example, the child whose family is of lower socioeconomic status may have fewer toys and incur greater environmental hazards. He may quickly develop independence in self-care because autonomy is expected within his or her social environment. The dynamics of the family support or hinder the development of the child. The mother of a preschool-age child with disabilities may provide a great deal of support for that child in daily care routines. When a second child is born, those routines often change and the preschooler may develop increasing independence or dependence in daily routines. The mother may find she has limited time to devote to the newborn. New routines are established in which the mother can interact with and care for both children at the same time (e.g., feed and bathe them together). Therefore the change in family configuration affects each child's performance. These changes may be positive; for example, the child with disabilities demonstrates increasing levels of independence in certain situations (such as eating), or these changes may be negative; for example, the child regresses to more babylike behaviors (no longer participates in his or her own bathing).

The physical environment refers to nonhuman aspects of the environment, space, objects, and building structures that constitute the child's immediate environment. The materi-

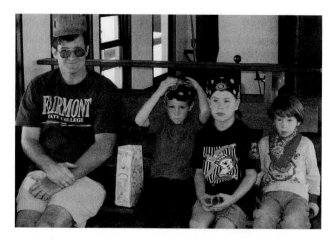

**Figure 1-4** The child's role may include that of son, brother, and friend with prescribed performance expectations on a family's recreational outing, in this case, a train ride.

als and objects of the environment promote the child's curiosity, desire to explore, and interest in play. The physical nature of the environment can motivate the child to attempt higher levels of performance or can create stress and sensory overload, thus inhibiting an adaptive response. Developmentally appropriate environments provide challenging and motivating opportunities, while meeting the child's more basic needs for safety and comfort.

Culture refers to the values, beliefs, customs, and behaviors of the child's family and of others in his or her community. Cultures affect performance by defining the importance and value of certain tasks and prescribing attitudes about such things as child rearing, education, and health care. The values placed on time and personal independence are often determined by cultural norms. The importance of culture as it influences the child's performance is a theme throughout this text.

## Continuum of Function-Dysfunction

The child's ability to perform activities and tasks defines his or her competence in and mastery of social roles. A child's role may be social, for example, as a daughter, sister, or friend, or may be related to specific context, for example, as a student in school or a member of a Sunday school class. According to Christiansen (1991), roles represent the highest level of the occupational performance hierarchy, and role responsibilities define the nature of occupational performance. They form the very nucleus of social interaction. Roles affect development and personality both through strong social approval when roles are enacted successfully and through equally strong sanctions when role expectations are not met. For example, the child with a disability may have a younger brother but never acquire the responsibilities and behaviors associated with the role of an older brother. The child who is frequently ill and in the hos-

▲ Table 1-1  Function-Dysfunction Continuum

| Function | Dysfunction |
|---|---|
| Performance components/underlying skills | Impairments |
| Performance areas/functional activities | Disability |
| Social roles | Handicap |

▲ Table 1-2  Continuum of Performance Function-Dysfunction and Intervention

| Function-Dysfunction Continuum | Intervention Focus (Improve Performance vs. Adapt Environment) |
|---|---|
| Underlying skills and impairments | Remediate and improve performance |
| Performance and disability in functional activities | Improve performance/ adapt activity and environment |
| Social roles and handicaps | Adapt environment/ modify expectations/ adjust perceptions |

pital may acquire a sick role and demonstrate passive and dependent behaviors. Regardless of whether a child has a disability, roles change as a function of the child's increasing skills and the environment's increasing expectations. The child's roles, for example, as student or player, organize his or her performance into specific purposes, define meaning to his or her activities, and create values regarding the importance of those activities (Keilhofner & Burke, 1980).

The terms *impairment, disability,* and *handicap* provide a universal conceptualization of disability as a continuum (World Health Organization, 1980). Table 1-1 shows how different levels of function and dysfunction relate. An *impairment* refers to a performance component deficit, such as a decreased strength, poor kinesthetic awareness, or problems in visual perception. It is the "loss of a psychological, physiological, or anatomical structure or function resulting from any cause" (p. 27). The second level of dysfunction is *disability.* A person with a disability is restricted in or unable to perform daily living activities or expected skills because of an impairment. Therefore a disability affects a performance area. The individual has delayed or deficit performance in self-care activities such as feeding or dressing. The child whose play skills are immature or whose school achievement falls below those of the child's peers experiences disability. The third level of dysfunction is a *handicap.* A handicap refers to the inability to fulfill a social role expected of a typical child in the environment of concern. A handicap results from an impairment or disability. Therefore when the severity of dysfunction is such that it prevents the child from fulfilling a desired social role, it is termed a handicap. The child whose medical problems are such that he or she is unable to attend school is handicapped because he or she is unable to fill the role of student in a classroom, and the child is disadvantaged because he or she does not have an experience valued by society. A child with spastic cerebral palsy who is immobile and unable to feed or dress himself or herself may be called handicapped in that the child does not acquire a role as a family member who independently completes self-care or contributes to the family chores.

## Intervention Based on the Function-Dysfunction Continuum

The person-environment-performance fit is influenced by how underlying impairments seem to affect functional performance and the child's ability to acquire desired social roles. When specific performance components are identified as impaired and seem to interfere with functional performance or coping behaviors, often the focus of intervention is to help the individual remediate those components. Therefore at the first level of this model, the impairment is the focus of intervention. For example, in the child with tightness and limited range of motion in shoulder flexion, the goal of occupational therapy would be elongation of lateral trunk and shoulder muscles to increase the range of the child's reach.

When the impairment prevents the child from accomplishing the daily living and play activities, the therapist intervenes to improve the related impairments and to adapt the performance context to increase the child's success in those activities. Therefore the therapist analyzes which aspects of the child's performance can be remediated and employs strategies to help the child improve performance. Then the therapist also analyzes how the activity can be adapted to improve the child's success. For example, a play activity may be adapted so that the toys are easily reached and manipulated. A dressing activity may be adapted by using clothes of soft stretchable material with Velcro fasteners.

When the child's dysfunction creates a handicap in a life role, substantial adaptations are made to the environment to promote optimal function. Assistive technology is often important to an individual's ability to manage a handicap. Architectural changes may be needed in the home to accommodate a wheelchair or the use of a walker. Thus the intervention focus of the therapist follows a continuum from performance components to functional performance in daily activities to the child's acquisition of desired social roles. Based on the specific goals, the focus of intervention moves from the child to the environment. The intervention focus is always dynamic, with child and environment emphasis shifting as goals and priorities change (Table 1-2).

The concept of handicap is based on the assumption that

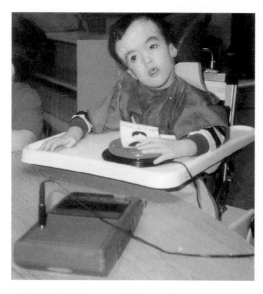

**Figure 1-5** A child uses a switch to activate a tape recorder that plays his favorite song.

certain experiences cannot be adapted for certain levels of disability. Thus it appears that handicaps are created by society when members of society fail to make certain opportunities available to individuals with limited abilities. By adapting and modifying environments, occupational therapists create opportunities for individuals in the community and thereby help eliminate handicaps. Occupational therapists also help reduce a child's handicap by empowering the individual to see new possibilities for achievement and by using a multitude of tools (e.g., Figure 1-5) and models of service delivery to enable the child to function competently within his or her natural environments (Polatajko, 1994).

## OCCUPATIONAL THERAPY PROCESS

*Occupational therapy process* defines how the goals discussed in the previous section are achieved. In this process a sequence of activities is carried out by the occupational therapist with the child, the child's caregivers, and others in the environment who work with or relate to the child. The process involves gathering data and interpreting information, followed by planning and implementing services.

### Screening

Often the first step in the process is screening or determining if the child needs occupational therapy intervention. This step may be omitted if the child has a significant disability, a known diagnosis (e.g., brachial plexus injury), or is referred by a physician for a prescribed purpose.

Through the initial screening the therapist makes an educated decision as to the child's potential needs for service. The therapist uses interview, observation, or standardized assessment to determine the child's needs and potential to benefit from occupational therapy.

At the time of the screening, the therapist also selects a frame of reference and a focus for further assessment of the child. The frame of reference guides the therapist's selection of evaluation instrument and determination of which performance components and activities will become the focus of evaluation. For example, if the screening indicated that behavior was a significant issue, the evaluation tools might emphasize self-esteem, sensory integration, and internal locus of control. If an interview indicated that the child had limited play skills, observation of the child's play would be an appropriate evaluation activity.

Screening involves observation of the child, a chart review, a medical and developmental history, a parent interview, and, when applicable, interviews with others who work with the child. The time of screening might also offer an opportunity to gather initial information about the child's environment. In the screening the therapist gathers essential rather than comprehensive information that allows the therapist to determine whether further evaluation is warranted.

### Evaluation

The goal of comprehensive evaluation is to gather essential information about the child's strengths and limitations in underlying skill components, performance areas, or functional activities and performance context. Each of these interrelates to define the child's occupational performance. The primary focus of occupational therapy is usually the performance areas, that is, self-care and daily living skills, play, and school activities. Evaluation of skill components and performance context emphasizes how these intrinsic and extrinsic factors affect function in self-care, play, and school activities. Typical methods of assessment are described in the following sections.

#### Performance Components

Through structured and naturalistic observation of the child's functional performance in a variety of activities and situations, the therapist gains information about the child's underlying skills and impairments. Standardized observational evaluations may also be used to assess reflexes, righting responses, sensory integration, range of motion, strength, endurance, attention, visual perception, tactile processing, kinesthetic awareness, or other skill components.

#### Performance Areas

The daily activities of the child are evaluated through observation and formal tests. In structured observation the therapist arranges the environment and provides verbal cues to elicit specific responses. These may be recorded and interpreted based on developmental schedules or scales that categorize typical responses. Unstructured observation allows the therapist to gather information of the child's performance in a naturalistic way while identifying typical constraints and enablers in the environment. Through analysis of the child's performance of activities, the therapist identifies the child's qualitative strengths and limitations in performance as these relate to functional skill.

Standardized evaluations allow the therapist to quantify the assessment information. By producing a standard score, the child can be compared with norms and objective baseline information is established for measuring progress. Standardized evaluation gives explicit information about the child's performance on standard items but does not readily generalize it into the context of everyday living.

Interviews are also an important part of the evaluation process. The interview provides important historical information, a perspective of the child at home and in other contexts. An interview with the parents also gives the therapist an assessment of their perception of the problem, their past experiences with medical and educational professionals, and their priorities and concerns. The parents also give important information specific to the child, for example, likes and dislikes, developmental course, general medical history, and unique attributes. It is through interviewing others, using both specific and open-ended questions, that the therapist begins to understand the child's social roles. Their impressions as well as the child's self-assessment provide an important overview of how well the child meets expectations for his or her role as a sibling, play partner, and student. This overall view helps prioritize therapy plans, goals, and activities.

Interviews of other professionals who have worked with the child provide yet another perspective. Other service providers can give important information about the child's behaviors, developmental course, potential for change, and interests.

## Performance Context

In addition to evaluating and defining the child's strengths and limitations in underlying components of skill and in daily activities, the occupational therapist synthesizes how the child's performance is influenced by and influences the environment. The context of performance helps the therapist identify which areas of performance are supported by the environment and which are hindered. What extrinsic factors are critical to the child's performance? What objects, materials, and space are available for play? Is the classroom arranged to promote performance of school activities? The environment includes the curriculum of the educational program, the teacher's expectations for performance, and aspects of the home that may interfere with or promote skill development. In medical settings, assessment may include the expectation of the rehabilitation team and the standards of the rehabilitation program. What opportunities for activity and play are available on the rehabilitation unit? Hospital settings may create an environment in which the child acquires an overly dependent and passive role, typical of a sick patient, or begins to participate in his or her own medical care (e.g., learning to take medicine).

## Summary

Evaluation for purposes of initiating occupational therapy intervention must be comprehensive and should consider the child's assets and limitations at all levels of performance. Priorities about evaluation are decided based on the frame of reference most appropriate for the child's needs, the parents' and child's priorities, and the context of evaluation (e.g., rehabilitation center, school, hospital, or private practice). Not only are specific strengths and limitations in performance components, areas, and contexts identified, but also interrelationships among skill components, activities, and roles are hypothesized. Through this process the occupational therapist gains a comprehensive understanding of the problems to be addressed in therapy and to establish immediate and long-range goals.

## Intervention Planning

From this comprehensive picture of the child's performance, the occupational therapist interprets how the assets and limitations of the child and the environment influence occupational performance. The therapist's analysis of the child's performance and interpretation of how performance components and context affect functional skill result in identifying strategies to guide intervention. Goals should reflect performance areas of daily living, play, and school activities because these are the critical issues in a child's ability to function independently in different contexts. As in evaluation, the frame of reference guides the therapist's thinking. It provides a theory base from which the therapist interprets evaluation results and identifies appropriate goals. How the child will achieve change or accomplish a goal is also determined by the frame of reference. For example, the sensory integration frame of reference helps explain the basis for certain behaviors and identify performance components for emphasis and provides guidelines for goals and activity selection based on the underlying impairments. Through this process the therapist selects specific tools, methods, and activities to enable the child to reach the goals. Christiansen (1991) defined three steps in planning, once the evaluation data have been interpreted.

1. Short-term and long-term goals are established. Often the short-term goals relate to performance components, and long-term goals relate to performance in functional areas of daily living skills, play, and school activities.

2. Intervention plans and methods are selected. Plans reflect the frame of reference and the prognosis for change. Plans include facilitation of the child's development of underlying abilities as these relate to skilled performance. Plans also include methods for adapting

the environment to increase the child's overall function. A balance between skill development and environmental modification is important to enabling the child to successfully participate in appropriate social roles.

3. Throughout the planning process the occupational therapist also recognizes areas where additional information is needed. Plans are made for reevaluation of areas where rapid progress is expected or where the possibility of regression in skills exists.

Throughout the planning process, priorities are made based on the frame of reference, the caregiver's and team's input, and the critical developmental issues that seem to be disrupting the child's ability to perform in functional activities. Assessment, interpretation of results, and planning and implementing services is a continuous process that defines the essence of occupational therapy.

## Intervention

The chapters in the third and fourth sections of this book define intervention with children related to particular performance areas and particular performance contexts (arenas of practice). Those chapters describe the goals of occupational therapy with children. The primary goals are briefly defined in the following section (see box below).

### Improving Performance Components

Once the therapist has identified specific skill components that are delayed, impaired, or absent and that appear related to delays in performance areas, these components become an emphasis of intervention. Examples of performance components that may become a focus for the occupational therapist are grasp and release, reach, and in-hand and bilateral manipulation. Other examples are the child's ability to process sensory information, attend, sequence, and problem solve. The therapist designs activities to improve performance of those targeted components or to remediate specific impairments. For example, poor in-hand manipulation may appear to be related to lack of palmar flexibility, inadequate palmar arch, and reduced strength of the in-

trinsic hand muscles. Increasing flexibility and strength of the hand musculature become the focus of intervention as a means of helping the child improve in-hand manipulation of objects and dynamic grasp of the pencil for writing. The occupational therapist implements specific handling techniques, activities, and exercises aimed at increasing these specific performance components. The occupational therapist also implements activities to help the child generalize newly developed skills into everyday functional activities, for example, the ability to manipulate pencils, coins, or game pieces.

To accomplish change in the child's underlying performance components, occupational therapy may include any of the following:

1. Application of sensory input to inhibit and facilitate muscle tone, flexibility, cocontraction, or balance of muscle activity (Farber, 1982).
2. Application of handling to support and promote postural alignment and control (Boehme, 1988).
3. Activities to elicit higher level adapted responses (Gilfolye, Grady, & Moore, 1990).
4. Use of therapeutic self to encourage, motivate, and reinforce the child's efforts (Mattingly & Fleming, 1994).
5. Teaching others to implement activities that help the child improve component skills (Christiansen, 1991).

### Enhancing Performance of Functional Activities

To improve performance areas, a global approach is needed. The therapist implements strategies to help the child generalize improvements in component skills into daily living, play, and school activities. At the same time, the occupational therapist helps adapt or modify those activities so the child becomes as functional and independent as possible. Because the child performs daily living skills, play, and school activities throughout each day in a variety of contexts, the occupational therapist often uses indirect models of service delivery. The occupational therapist first analyzes how an activity should be adapted and then implements the adapted method to evaluate how well the child can perform the activity using that method (e.g., an adapted method for donning his or her coat and book bag). The therapist then adjusts and refines the adapted technique to ensure the child's success in using it and teaches the adapted method to care providers who typically assist the child during that activity (e.g., parents, nurses, teachers, and classroom aides).

Teaching the child and others is a primary role of the occupational therapist to improve daily living skill, play, and school activities. The occupational therapist may also use consultation to help problem solve why the child exhibits delays or deficits in performance areas, examining both the child's abilities and the factors in the environment that support or interfere with performance. As a consultant the occupational therapist leads a give-and-take interaction to

## Goals of Occupational Therapy Intervention with Children

1. Improve performance components.
2. Enhance performance of functional activities.
3. Modify the performance context.
4. Prevent disability and social role dysfunction.
5. Increase self-esteem and self-actualization.
6. Promote positive interactions and relationships.

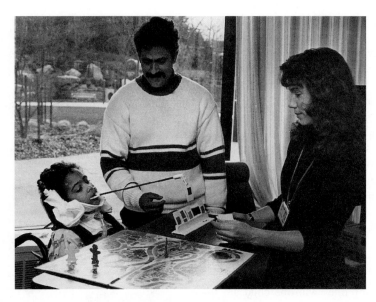

**Figure 1-6**   The occupational therapist designed an adapted method for a child with only face and mouth movement to play a card game with his father.

establish specific goals and strategies. The occupational therapist provides insight as to the underlying impairments and develops recommendations regarding activities for remediation and environmental adaptations that support higher levels of function. The recommendations made by the occupational therapist should be tried, adjusted, and adapted by those who implement them, with ongoing evaluation of their success by the occupational therapist consultant, the team members involved, and the child. Consultation to improve the child's function in everyday activity seems to be an increasingly important role of the occupational therapist as demands for productivity increase and therapists become responsible for serving greater numbers of children. Consultation is also recognized as critical to facilitating the child's ability to generalize emerging skills and function at the highest levels in all environments (Dunn & Campbell, 1990). A combination of teaching and consulting with parents and other team members allows the generalization of skills to occur.

## Modifying the Performance Context

The environment frames the child's ability to perform. The occupational therapist implements or recommends changes in the environment to support or enable the child's performance. Generally, recommendations are made for changing the performance context through problem-solving discussion among team and family members as to what aspects of the environment can and should be modified. Play activities and play objects can easily be modified. Structural changes to a house or building to accommodate the child's functional mobility can substantially affect others in the environment and require financial resources. Environmental adaptations can be quite elaborate, as in helping to design an environmental control system, or may be as

simple as placing toys on lower shelves so that the child can independently obtain them or providing toys that will support imaginative play. Other adaptations involve adapted equipment, for example, a cup and straw holder, utensils with enlarged handles, reachers, and other adapted utensils. A computer word processing program can be used when handwriting is illegible. Figure 1-6 shows a child who recently sustained a spinal cord injury using an adapted mouth stick to play cards with his father. The relative gains to be made through environmental adaptation need to be carefully balanced with the cost to the family, the school, or the agency. The occupational therapist needs to recognize both the advantages and the disadvantages of modifying the environment and to present objective data as to the overall benefits and limitations. Certain aspects of the child's environment, such as cultural values and family routines, need to be respected. The occupational therapist adjusts and adapts the intervention goals and activities to fit within these basic elements of the child's life.

## Preventing Disability and Social Role Dysfunction

The occupational therapist's work with children often involves prevention. For example, delays in sensorimotor performance and lack of mobility may relate to delays in visual-spatial perceptual skills. The occupational therapist may provide perceptual activities on a computer to substitute for lack of manipulative experiences, thereby preventing a secondary disability in visual perceptual skills. Use of battery-operated switch toys can help the child with severe sensory motor limitations learn to control his or her environment and may prevent development of feelings of helplessness and lack of self-efficacy. Dunn, Brown, and McGuigan (1994) suggested another role for the occupational therapists in helping the child both develop as an individual and adapt to the demands of the environment. That role is to create optimal contexts for the child's ability to achieve. An environment that promotes higher levels of performance provides the "just right challenge" (Csikszentmihalyi, 1990). A just right challenge motivates the child to engage in the activities and stresses the child's skills so that higher level performance is elicited. This stress is imposed without creating frustration and with an end goal of success. For example, an environment may entice the child who is immobile to begin to crawl and roll, yet provide a safe environment in which potential hazards are removed. The therapist can provide equipment that entices a child with gravitational insecurity to climb or swing and allows the child to select the posture and position that feels the safest.

### Increasing Self-Esteem and Self-Actualization

These occupational therapy roles with the child are focused on improving and adapting the underlying skills, functional performance, and performance contexts. The occupational therapist also acknowledges the critical nature of certain intrinsic enablers in the child that help the child generalize skills, initiate activity and interaction, and sustain performance over time. Genuine improvement in functional skills implies that the child can independently apply the skill and initiate and sustain the higher level performance. The child's motivation, self-esteem, and locus of control undergird sustained performance and ability to effectively cope with new situations and challenges. Occupational therapists are highly cognizant of the importance of the child's developing self-esteem and sense of control of the environment.

The child's self-esteem and self-image are highly influenced by skill achievement and success in mastering tasks. The occupational therapist artfully uses and adapts activity to promote the child's sense of accomplishment and mastery. By adapting the environment to enable the child to integrate the sensory experience, achieve the motor goal, and successfully complete the task, the child's sense of control and competence increase. Generally, the intrinsic sense of mastery is a much stronger reinforcement to the child than external rewards such as verbal praise or another contingent reward system. The occupational therapist vigilantly attends to the child's performance during an activity to provide precise levels and types of support that enable the child to succeed in the activity. The therapist selects activities that can be easily modified to match the child's skills and interests and to ensure success.

The occupational therapist remains highly sensitive to the child's emerging self-actualization and helps the team and family provide activities and environments that support the child's sense of self as an important efficacious person (Figure 1-7). Self-actualization, as defined by Fidler and Fidler (1978), occurs through successful coping with problems in the everyday environment. It implies more than the ability

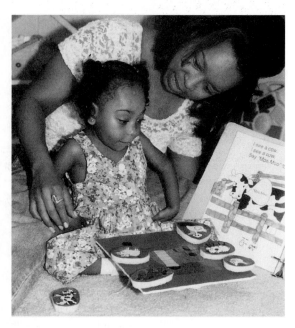

**Figure 1-7** The occupational therapist involves the mother and child in an activity that stimulates the child's imagination and has motor demands adapted to the child's skill level.

to respond to events; it implies that a child is able to manage and control the environment, initiate play activities, investigate problems, and initiate social interactions. The goals of the therapist are that the child demonstrate active and meaningful participation in the environment, independently seek experiences that promote his or her own development, sustain relationships with others, and master activities and tasks important to self-image.

### Promoting Positive Interactions and Relationships

By improving the child's skills and self-esteem and by adapting the environment to meet the child's needs, the interactions between the child and environment are improved so that the child functions successfully in social contexts and social roles. In addition to promoting the child's ability to function within the environment, the occupational therapist helps promote positive relationships between the child and significant others in three ways.

First, the therapist helps the child's parents, caregivers, and peers *understand the disability*. Understanding why a child responds or behaves in a certain way is always important in establishing or improving the relationship. When significant others lack understanding of the child's underlying impairments, they may attribute behaviors to lack of motivation or lack of interest in interaction. Understanding how performance impairments relate to disability, particularly subtle impairments that may not be diagnosed, is an important aspect of accepting the child and supporting his or her development. Understanding the underlying problems is often a first step in developing more positive interactions between the child and the social environment. Thus

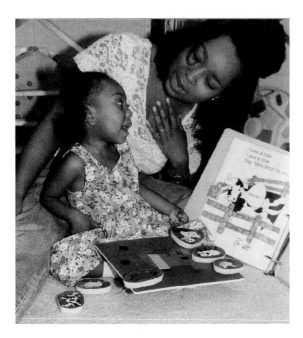

**Figure 1-8**  Physical support and eye contact are important aspects of arranging a play activity for mother and child.

the therapist has a critical role in educating caregivers, peers, and educators about the links between impairments and certain child behaviors that are easily misunderstood.

Second, the occupational therapist helps *improve the child–social environment fit* by giving the caregiver recommendations on how to handle or manage the child so that a more positive interaction ensues. The occupational therapist may provide suggestions of how to improve eye contact or how to position the child during play or caregiving interaction so that the interaction is more successful (Figure 1-8). This role in educating others involves modeling, supporting others in hands-on experiences with the child, and using a variety of verbal and visual instructional methods based on the learning needs of the child's caregivers and teachers.

Third, the occupational therapist can improve the child's fit with the social environment by *improving the child's functional skills* in ways that directly enhance the child's ability to interact with others. By improving manipulative play skills, the child can more successfully interact with peers. Improving feeding skills can enhance interaction at the family mealtime or in the school cafeteria. Helping the child use an augmentative communication device increases the child's ability to interact with peers.

## Reassessment

The intervention process almost always involves reassessment, then refining and adjusting goals and strategies. Objective evaluation is critical to establishing new goals and new priorities. Reassessment may be formal and planned or spontaneous and unplanned. It is critical to the dynamic

nature of intervention, which continually evolves to meet the child's needs and to accommodate to the child's developing repertoire of skills. Reassessment of skill components can regularly occur through observation of the child's performance of activities; reassessment of functional skills may require a formal evaluation using objective standards or criteria. Although changes in isolated skills are important, they should always be related back to the child's ability to function in the everyday environment.

## Summary

The occupational therapy process of evaluation, planning, and implementing intervention is a dynamic process, with the child and family at its center. The occupational therapist's focus on everyday performance in the critical functional areas provides opportunities for the occupational therapist to become involved in the central activities of the child's life. The therapist holds expertise in identifying and helping to remediate impairment in underlying performance components of functional skill. The therapist is also skilled in adapting the context of performance to support the child's functional performance. By using a dynamic balance of intervention activities to remediate, adapt, and modify, the occupational therapist promotes the child's sense of mastery and competence. The selection of goals and activities, while emphasizing the child's functional performance, also focuses on enhancing the child's self-respect and self-actualization by increasing his or her sense of efficacy and mastery.

## PRACTICE ARENAS

Each child functions in a unique set of environments. As described previously, the performance context is critical to the child's ability to successfully perform everyday activities. The occupational therapist also functions within specific environments. Table 1-3 lists typical arenas of practice with children with disabilities. The work settings of the occupational therapist influence the therapist's selected frame of reference, evaluation methods and tools, modalities, activities, and service delivery models. Occupational therapy practice arenas are continually affected by the rapid changes occurring in health care and education administrative structures, payment systems, and technology. To function within the rapidly evolving health care and educational systems, occupational therapists must adapt their strategies and models of service delivery while maintaining the integrity of the profession and high standards for client care. The final chapters of this text describe the constraints and opportunities of present-day practice arenas. Although health and educational settings are characterized by differing purposes and types of services for children, themes described later seem to have global application across practice arenas.

▲ Table 1-3    Arenas of Practice for Pediatric
               Occupational Therapy

| Type of Settings | Examples |
| --- | --- |
| Medical | Neonatal intensive care units |
| | Pediatric units of general hospitals |
| | Children's hospitals |
| | Rehabilitation centers |
| | Outpatient facilities |
| Educational | Early intervention programs |
| | Preschools |
| | Public schools (regular and special education) |
| | Classrooms |
| | Private schools |
| Community | Early intervention programs |
| | Private practice |
| | Homes |
| | Child care centers |
| | Job sites and work settings |
| | Residential settings |

## Trend Toward Integrated Services in the Least Restrictive Environment

That individuals with disabilities should be included in community life is a valued belief of Americans. The civil rights of persons with disabilities are respected and protected through public laws that were enacted in the 1970s and have gained new strength and meaning in the 1990s. These laws recognize that individuals with disabilities are full members of society and should have access to every opportunity in the community. Public laws and policies also recognize that to achieve full inclusion of individuals with disabilities into the community, special programs are needed to support their education and ability to function in the mainstream of society. The first federal civil rights law specifically to protect individuals with disabilities was the Rehabilitation Act of 1973. This law requires nondiscrimination on the basis of disability. Reasonable accommodations must be made in schools and other institutions to assure that the needs of individuals with disabilities are met as adequately as those of nondisabled persons. In 1990 the Americans with Disabilities Act (ADA) was enacted. This law mandates that reasonable accommodations be made for persons with disabilities in all public and private organizations and facilities. These civil rights laws have enabled persons with disabilities to fully participate in the community. Occupational therapists can and do provide consultation to schools, businesses, and agencies as to how accommodations for persons with disabilities can be made. Occupational therapists bring an extensive understanding of disability as it relates to an individual's functional performance to employers and administrators so that environments and programs can be modified to allow the participation of all persons.

The concept of service provision and education in the child's least restrictive environment (LRE) resulted in a strong movement toward inclusion of students with disabilities into their neighborhood preschools and schools. As inclusion becomes more universally implemented, occupational therapists provide more of their service in community day care settings and neighborhood schools. This decentralization of service delivery has resulted in an increase in itinerant services; that is, therapists must travel to multiple schools, sometimes throughout several districts. It has also meant that more services are needed to help teachers without training in special education to work with and adapt the curriculum for students with disabilities. Consultation has become increasingly important in helping teachers accommodate to students with special needs by adapting the classroom arrangement, modifying curricular teaching materials, and individualizing teaching methods. Inclusion also gives occupational therapists opportunities to involve students without disabilities in intervention groups and activities as peer models or peer supports. Helping children have access to and succeed in all environments calls for new strategies and levels of creativity in analyzing the "fit" between the child's performance and the environment. The expertise of the occupational therapist is often called on to help the child gain the skills needed to succeed in regular education in community schools and to modify educational programs to accommodate to the child's unique set of strengths and limitations.

Successful inclusion of children with disabilities into regular education and community activities requires a high level of integration and coordination of educational and rehabilitative services. Integrated services are believed to be most efficacious and beneficial from the child's and family's point of view. In the integrated model, occupational therapy services are coordinated with other disciplines and are provided in the child's natural daily environment. Therefore educational-based services may be provided in the classroom, in the cafeteria, on the playground, or in the home. Medical-based services also seek the environment that is most comfortable and natural for the child, for example, at home or in other settings with typical peers. When the occupational therapist provides services within the child's natural environment, the tasks, materials, and activities of the child's daily life can be adapted to increase functional performance. The adaptations are more likely to increase the child's independence and function when they are made within the natural environment rather than simulated in a clinic. When services are integrated, the occupational therapist enters the child's environment and uses the natural resources that surround the child, for example, a peer's assistance or a brother's help. This allows the therapist the opportunity to test and refine therapeutic solutions. In integrated service delivery the role of the occupational therapist flows from that of direct service provider to that of consultant, teacher-educator, and supervisor. All of those roles are needed to help the child gain new skills and to create adaptations and changes that will become part of the child's everyday life.

## Professional Roles and Models of Service Delivery

In an effort to improve the efficiency of service delivery, new concepts have emerged in transdisciplinary practice that blur the scopes of practice of nursing, allied health, and education disciplines. In transdisciplinary practice the occupational therapist teaches other team members to implement occupational therapy programs. The therapist remains a consultant and provides ongoing input to the child's program. At the same time, the occupational therapist takes on the roles of professionals in other disciplines. The occupational therapist in home health may perform certain nursing functions or may implement the activities recommended by the physical therapist. Redefinition of roles is typical of rural-based practice, where a full array of professionals is not always available. It also occurs in home-based services, where the cost of the program increases exponentially when multiple professionals become involved in direct service delivery and in instances of very young or medically fragile clients when interaction with multiple professionals is not warranted and is potentially harmful. The transdisciplinary model appears to work best when high levels of communication and collaboration exist among team members.

Often occupational therapists help coordinate services for the child and family. Service coordination can involve obtaining additional community resources, ordering equipment, or helping the family find respite care or financial resources. As stated by Polatajko (1994):

> The traditional roles of hands-on clinician, administrator, researcher, and educator are not always adequate to enable occupational competence. Often, particularly when competence requires environment changes, new forms of practice are necessary, such as program designer, consultant, public educator, lobbyist, policy maker, and social critic (p. 593).

These roles are shared across disciplines and are essential to effective intervention.

## Cost-effectiveness and Productivity

The need to deliver cost-effective services has been a strong theme in health care through the 1980s and is a reality of the 1990s. All professionals who work in health care and education settings feel the press for productivity and cost-effective services. Because efficacy studies are few and inconclusive, occupational therapy services are at risk for loss of support from payment sources and administrative structures. Intensive and long-term occupational therapy services have become difficult to justify and often are not fully reimbursed. With the trend toward using the most cost-

effective services, occupational therapists have become responsible for increasing numbers of students and clients. They often supervise high numbers of aides and assistants. The trend toward shorter hospital stays and shorter duration rehabilitation will likely continue. Occupational therapists and other rehabilitation specialists must demonstrate the effects, if any, that reduction in services has on achieving the child's full potential for functional independence.

In pediatric hospitals and rehabilitation centers occupational therapists work with children with complex and often severe medical problems. The time allowed for intensive inpatient treatment has been reduced to the fewest days possible based on the child's medical stability. As a result, extended rehabilitation must take place through outpatient or home-based services. Returning the child to the community as quickly as possible seems to have benefits to the child's reintegration into community life. However, this trend has resulted in new roles for therapists to help coordinate rapid transition between intervention environments, to quickly create environmental modifications that will promote the child's function, and to make recommendations for equipment and assistive technology without an extended time for trial use and evaluation.

Resources are shifting from inpatient to outpatient care. With service decentralized, coordination of services becomes increasingly important. The emphasis of this service coordination will be how to deliver optimal service at the lowest cost. Only cost-effective services will remain in the system. Occupational therapy services have been reduced as administrators have examined and will continue to examine ways that costs can be reduced. For example, the use of occupational therapy aides will likely increase the time and energy that the therapist spends in supervision. Also, when feasible, group sessions will be used (Baum, 1991).

Although solutions for reducing costs are implemented, occupational therapists are under increasing pressure to analyze the cost benefit of their service. Data on the effectiveness of intervention that include the costs of those services need to be produced within individual agencies and institutions and in large-scale research projects. Data collection systems using computers enable occupational therapists to categorize and track service delivery and client outcome are not always able to capture and report data meaningful for analyzing real cost benefit. It is the occupational therapist's responsibility to define what measures best reflect the benefits that occupational therapy brings to clients and to put into place systems that will measure those benefits.

## New and Emerging Technology

Historically, technology and occupational therapists have had a close relationship. Although in the past occupational therapists primarily used low technology, for example, assistive devices such as reachers or rocker knives, today therapists use technology that has become increasingly complex and sophisticated. Present-day technology for persons with disabilities includes computers, robotics, augmentative communication devices, power wheelchairs, electrical stimulation, environmental control systems, and a multitude of other electronic devices and computerized systems. Many technologic devices are available to help the child become more independent and functional. These are devices that the child uses in everyday life to support the child's ability to perform daily living skill or function in play and school environments. Examples of assistive technology for daily living skills are electronic toothbrushes, adapted feeding utensils, electronic page turners, computer software for word processing, and robotic devices to operate switches and retrieve objects (Figure 1-9).

The occupational therapist has several roles in helping the child access and use technology. These roles include assessing the child's need for assistive technology, identifying potential devices that match that need, helping the family obtain the technology, evaluating trial use, adjusting and adapting the device or system, and training the child and family in its use (Smith, 1991). Therefore the occupational therapist has an essential role in the child's functional use of appropriate technology. As more technology becomes available and the level of complexity increases, it becomes increasingly important for the occupational therapist to know what devices and systems are available, how those system work, and how they can most effectively increase the child's daily functional performance. By always evaluating the use of assistive technology from the child's perspective and needs in everyday function, the occupational therapist promotes optimal use of technology and optimal benefit to the child and family. Use of technology to enhance the child's functional performance in daily living ac-

tivities, communication, and mobility is described in Chapters 17, 20, and 21.

## SUMMARY

Trends in service delivery and changes in intervention settings have had profound effects on occupational therapy practice. Because practice is client driven, occupational therapists continually reassess how well services match the child's needs, strengths, interests, dreams, and priorities. The goal of occupational therapy is to promote optimal goodness-of-fit between the child's intrinsic characteristics and the supports and demands of the environment. A goodness-of-fit between the child and the environment has been achieved when the child routinely succeeds in and masters daily living, play, and school activities. Independence in daily routines allows the child to acquire and function in desired social roles.

The occupational therapist is involved in both improving the child's skills and adapting the environment to promote functional performance. Daily activities can best be analyzed and adapted within contexts familiar to the child. Services within the child's environment are most likely to facilitate the child's self-actualization through mastery and control of everyday activities. In addition, child- and family-centered services provided within the child's natural physical, social, and cultural environment enable the

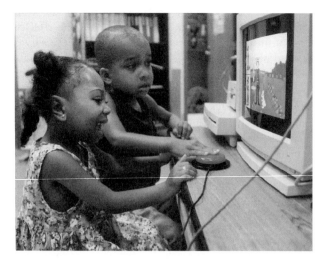

**Figure 1-9**   Use of a switch to activate a computer program that tells a story. Through use of switches, computer play can enhance cognitive, visual, perceptual, and social skills and requires very basic motor skills.

## STUDY QUESTIONS

1. Self-feeding is a functional skill expected of a 2-year-old child. Define one performance component in each of the following areas that is required to self-feed: (a) motor, (b) sensory, (c) social, and (d) cognitive.
2. Cultural background can influence both the physical and social environments. Give an example of a way that culture can influence (a) the child's social environment and (b) the child's physical environment.
3. Explain the concept of goodness-of-fit between the child and the environment. Apply the concept to generate therapy priorities for a child with severe disabilities who is dependent in mobility, manipulation and play, daily living skills, and communication.
4. Explain the meaning of least restrictive environment. Describe two examples of occupational therapy services in the least restrictive environment (a) in the educational system and (b) in the medical system.

child with disabilities to fully participate in the community. Occupational therapists recognize the potential of each child and help the child reach that potential through therapeutic application of activity and adaptation of the environment. This book describes the process, frames of reference, tools, and methods of occupational therapy to promote the child's functional performance and acquisition of meaningful social roles.

## REFERENCES

American Occupational Therapy Association. (1994). Uniform terminology for occupational therapy (3rd edition). *American Journal of Occupational Therapy, 48,* 12.

Americans with Disabilities Act. (1990). (Public Law 101-336) 42 U.S.C. 12101.

Baum, C. (1991). Professional issues in a changing environment. In C. Christiansen & C. Baum (Eds.). *Occupational therapy: overcoming human performance deficits* (pp. 789-804). New York: McGraw-Hill.

Boehme, R. (1988). *Improving upper body control.* Tucson: Therapy Skill Builders.

Christiansen, C. (1991). Occupational therapy: intervention for life performance. In C. Christiansen & C. Baum (Eds.). *Occupational therapy: overcoming human performance deficits* (pp. 3-44). New York: McGraw-Hill.

Csikszentmihalyi, M. (1990). *Flow: the psychology of optimal experience.* New York: Harper Perennial.

Dunn, W., Brown, C., & McGuigan, A. (1994). The ecology of human performance: a framework for considering the effect of context. *American Journal of Occupational Therapy, 48*(7), 595-607.

Dunn, W. & Campbell, P. (1990). The service provision process. In W. Dunn (Ed.). *Pediatric occupational therapy: facilitating service provision.* Thorofare, NJ: Slack.

Farber, S.D. (1982). *Neurorehabilitation: a multisensory approach.* Philadelphia: W.B. Saunders.

Fidler, G.S. & Fidler, J.W. (1978). Doing and becoming: purposeful action and self-actualization. *American Journal of Occupational Therapy, 32,* 305-310.

Gilfoyle, E., Grady, A., & Moore, J. (1990). *Children adapt.* Thorofare, NJ: Slack.

Kielhofner, G. & Burke, J.P. (1980). A model of human occupation, Part 1: Conceptual framework and content. *American Journal of Occupational Therapy, 34,* 572-581.

Kramer, P. & Hinojosa, J. (1993). Domain of concern of occupational therapy relevant to pediatric practice. In P. Kramer & J. Hinojosa (Eds.). *Frames of reference for pediatric occupational therapy.* Philadelphia: Williams & Wilkins.

Llorens, L. (1977). A developmental theory revisited. *The American Journal of Occupational Therapy, 31*(10), 656-657.

Llorens, L. (1991). Performance tasks and roles throughout the life span. In C. Christiansen & C. Baum (Eds.). *Occupational therapy: overcoming human performance deficits* (pp. 45-68). Thorofare, NJ: Slack.

Mattingly, C. & Fleming, M.H. (1994). *Clinical reasoning: forms of inquiry in a therapeutic practice.* Philadelphia: F.A. Davis.

Polatajko, H.J. (1994). Dreams, dilemmas, and decisions for occupational therapy practice in a new millennium: a Canadian perspective. *American Journal of Occupational Therapy, 48*(7), 590-594.

Smith, R.O. (1991). Technological approaches to performance. In C. Christiansen & C. Baum (Eds.). *Occupational therapy: overcoming human performance deficits* (pp. 747-788). Thorofare, NJ: Slack.

World Health Organization. (1980). *International classification of impairments, disabilities and handicaps.* Geneva: World Health Organization.

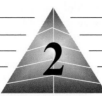

# Relationships with Other Service Providers

ANNE S. ALLEN

## CHAPTER OBJECTIVES

1. Describe the various professionals who provide services for children with disabilities.
2. Describe the different kinds of teams, how they are made up, and how they provide services.
3. Introduce the concept of professional collaboration.

Children with illnesses and emotional, physical, or mental deficiencies must be treated as whole persons within their environments. This is a truism not only in occupational therapy, with its long history of concern for the wholeness of the patient, but also increasingly in the other helping professions where technologic specializations have often divided patient care into units defined by body systems or malfunctioning parts.

Society's concern for the whole person has generated a need for interdisciplinary collaboration. Various specialists must learn to work together as one functioning unit to ensure respect for the patient as a whole person and to treat the person as one complex organism rather than a collection of parts.

Collaborating groups of concerned, helping professionals are usually referred to as teams, and an extensive litera-ture has developed that deals with the formation of teams and their ability to function effectively.*

## CHARACTERISTICS OF TEAMS

Baldwin (1982), one of the leading researchers in team evaluation, has compared teams to traffic on the Los Angeles freeway:

As with teams, cars (read team members) get on and off for different reasons, at different times, at different places, for different destinations, and with different speeds and sizes (read power and prestige).

Occupational therapists must be aware of the potential contributions of each specialist to the well-being of patients and must be able to adapt to the changing team members with their different "destinations . . . speeds and sizes."

Some occupational therapists have a very close relationship with other members of the medical team, and others practice more separately. A therapist on the staff of a children's rehabilitation unit might interact with the majority of the team members several times a day. A therapist in private practice might not make these contacts more than once a week. In both cases, however, and in situations between these two extremes, interprofessional relationships should be collaborative and understanding.

Good team relationships resolve the problems of overlapping roles among the professions. Informed professionals are aware of the areas of overlap and build cooperative relationships. Horwitz (1970) suggests that these relationships can allow practitioners to work at their advanced skill levels for longer periods than can the practitioner who does not have access to team support and consultation.

---

*An excellent source of information on how teams are formed, the essential elements of teamwork, and the developmental stages of a team can be found in Julia and Thompson (1994).

Occupational therapists are trained in skills that sometimes overlap with those of physical therapists, social workers, psychologists, teachers, child developmentalists, and orthotists, to name a few. It is natural to desire autonomy, but this can be counterproductive in professional practice. Keeping open lines of communication; recognizing the skills, overlapping or specific, of other professions; and using those skills to complement one's own are hallmarks of professional competence.

It is the responsibility of each professional to interpret his or her role to others. An occupational therapist can never assume that members of other professions are knowledgeable about the role of occupational therapy in health services for children. A nurse who has experienced occupational therapy as a behaviorally oriented therapy in a clinic for adolescents will be hard pressed to understand the sensory integrative approach used in a school program. A physician who is accustomed to working with child developmentalists in one neonatal nursery must be introduced to the occupational therapist's overlapping expertise in a different neonatal department.

Methods of collaboration among the helping professions have been described as multidisciplinary, interdisciplinary, and transdisciplinary teamwork, transdisciplinary being the most collaborative form. In this book, Stephens and Tauber (see Chapter 23), discuss these methods. Also see Rainforth, York, and MacDonald (1992). Certain aspects of how teams function are determined by the type of setting, for example, hospitals or schools, within which they operate.

## MEDICAL TEAM

The medical team is made up of a variety of persons who are trained in different specialties and who each have different backgrounds, different values, and sometimes different goals. These specialists work together in varying configurations, depending on the needs of the patient. Sometimes the team is made up of a physician and nurse only; sometimes it encompasses the full spectrum of service providers: primary physician, specialist, nurse, social worker, occupational and physical therapists, speech pathologist, and so on. An important aspect of the medical team is its ever-changing nature that reflects the status and needs of the patients.

## EDUCATIONAL TEAM

The educational team is responsible for preparing children with the knowledge and skills essential for productive living in a complex technologic society. It works with children in environments that, unlike the hospital, can be similar to the normal environment of children who have no handicaps or illnesses. This *least restrictive environment (LRE)* was mandated by the Education for All Handicapped Children Act, PL 94-142, 1975, and gives federal funds to programs that place children who have handicaps into "normal" or integrated educational classrooms and extracurricular activities. LRE enables children to practice new skills as they need them and in the appropriate place for that activity. Writing skills are practiced in the classroom; play skills, on the playground during the usual course of the school day. The child's "treatment" becomes an integral part of the school day and is carried out by the member of the educational team who is supervising the children's activities at that particular time. These transdisciplinary educational teams include educational personnel and professionals, such as occupational therapists, who provide "related services." Together they establish goals for the student and assign the oversight of these goals to the professional who is with the child most frequently (or who possesses some other compelling characteristic). The team members instruct the overseeing professional in the techniques of their own disciplines that are specific to the child's goals. This practice is called *role release* and allows all treatments to be carried on in an integrated fashion within the environment most related to the specified goals. The therapists tend to act as consultants to the teachers and special-education personnel when in the school setting.

## COMMUNITY TEAM

The establishment of early intervention programs (EIPs) led to home- and center-based services organized by various community agencies. These programs are designed to stimulate and enhance infant development, prevent the formation of undesirable patterns and behaviors, and increase function. Another goal is to prevent developmental delay in children at risk for such a delay. Parental support and education are concomitant goals.

Occupational therapists, physical therapists, speech-language pathologists, special education teachers, and others make up the community teams and often initiate services as soon as the baby is released from the hospital nursery. These teams also help in the transition from nursery to preschool, working with other teams to develop interagency collaboration. Treatment may be provided in the child's home with active involvement of parents and siblings, or at the agency, where the services of many professionals can be obtained. Often a combination of home- and center-based services is provided.

All team members need to be aware and respectful of the different values and attitudes toward health care that are part of various cultures. Community team members are especially sensitive to these differences because they usually see the child within his or her family and cultural setting. Differing values should be explored and understood by the team to achieve Basuray's (1991) "culturally congruent health care."

# SERVICE PROVIDERS WHO WORK WITH OCCUPATIONAL THERAPISTS

## Physicians

Although occupational therapists can practice without physicians' referrals, in pediatric services the pediatrician is not only a significant source of referrals, but also a source of information about the patient important to joint planning for the patient. The pediatrician is a medical specialist, having completed medical school and several years of specialized study and practice in children's diseases. Specialists in family practice have a similar length of medical preparation, but they work more broadly with conditions affecting the entire human life span and more intensively with family interactions. Both specialties are considered primary care because children may go initially either to a pediatrician or to a family care specialist for checkups or when ill. These physicians' offices, therefore, serve as ports of entry to the medical system. Physicians refer patients to other specialists as the need is perceived.

Consulting physicians are usually specialists to whom the child has been referred by the primary care physician; they include orthopedists, ophthalmologists, neurologists, cardiologists, physiatrists, psychiatrists, and pulmonary specialists. It is not uncommon for a seriously ill child or one with multiple handicaps to have several consulting physicians, some of whom must be integral members of the treatment team; others can be more peripheral.

In reference to Baldwin's (1982) analogy, the consultants represent the large, fast cars on the freeway, entering quickly and moving on. Occupational therapists should be prepared to relate to them by explaining occupational therapy services and establishing or modifying treatment goals to meet the particular condition. In working with all professional colleagues, the occupational therapist's explanations should start with the benefits a particular patient can receive from occupational therapy and the goals to be set and worked toward. From here one can go on to generalities and from generalities to basic theory if the colleague expresses interest. But it is usually desirable to establish interprofessional dialogue by using specific cases.

## Nurses

Nurses often serve a coordinating function in the delivery of patient services and can be directly responsible for referrals to occupational therapy and for making it physically possible for the child to go to treatment sessions. Occupational therapists should acquaint themselves with the nursing staff, explaining the role of occupational therapy in that institution, and cooperating in coordinating programs. It is frequently difficult for a nurse who is caring for several patients to allow exceptions to the necessary floor routine for a patient who needs leniency for specific routines prescribed by the occupational therapist. Whether a child is allowed to practice feeding skills during the very busy breakfast hour in an institution might very well depend on the relationship between the therapist and the nursing staff.

Nursing was the first of the many undergraduate health professions now in practice, and it has the largest number of practitioners. Student nurses can prepare for the certifying examination and become registered nurses through one of the following routes:

1. Hospital schools that are associated with teaching hospitals. Classes and practical experience are offered in a program usually 3 years in length. A diploma is awarded.
2. Community or technical colleges that give classes and laboratory experience and arrange for clinical practice with local hospitals. These programs are 2 years in length and award the associate of arts degree.
3. Four-year colleges and universities that offer undergraduate education along with nursing classes and laboratory experience. Clinical practice is arranged with suitable hospitals. The bachelor of science degree is awarded.

Registered nurses can specialize as pediatric nurses through on-the-job training and experience in pediatric settings. There is also a classification known as pediatric nurse practitioner, which indicates that the nurse has completed advanced education, usually at the master's degree level, and has acquired advanced skills, particularly in physical assessment. These nurses can establish their own practices within a community but generally establish a close working relationship with a specific physician or group of physicians.

*Licensed practical nurses (LPNs)* complete training programs 12 to 16 months in length, usually after high school, and sit for examinations in the state where they will practice. These nurses give bedside care and work under the supervision of registered nurses.

*Nursing aides* are trained in high school vocational programs or on-the-job programs in hospitals. They assist both registered and practical nurses.

The different levels of nurse education make it difficult for newcomers in the health services field to make knowledgeable expectations of nursing staffs. In general, higher levels of education produce nurses with greater theoretical knowledge and therefore higher ability to plan programs, to evaluate patients and systems, and to make changes; the more technically trained nurses develop high skills in bedside care and the techniques of nursing. As with all generalizations, individual exceptions abound.

## Physical Therapists

Occupational and physical therapists work closely together in outpatient clinics, hospitals, special schools, public schools, public health agencies, and private practices. Known together as the rehabilitation therapies, occupational therapy and physical therapy have many common goals in patient treatment, but they usually differ on which goals are emphasized and how the goal is approached (i.e., selection of therapeutic modality).

For example, a common goal for occupational therapy and physical therapy is to establish trunk stability. The physical therapist works toward this goal as a prerequisite to sitting and walking; the occupational therapist works toward the same goal as a prerequisite to sitting and using arms for feeding or other activities. Often the exercises that the physical therapist uses in working toward this goal with children look similar to the activities the occupational therapist uses.

Physical therapy is an undergraduate health profession, as is occupational therapy. Professional education programs for both culminate in the bachelor of science degree, although there are a number of programs that give basic professional education at the master's level. Both professions require extensive clinical experience before certification. Whereas occupational therapists can and do frequently work without physician referrals, physical therapists do not, a situation that tends to lead the physical therapist into the medical model and can present problems when providing educationally based services.

## Speech and Hearing Specialists

Speech and hearing specialists receive their education at the master's or doctoral level and have studied the diagnosis and rehabilitation of speech and hearing disorders, the development of language, the physics of speech, theories and measurements of hearing, communication systems, and other related topics. Depending on their area of specialization, these specialists are referred to as speech and hearing therapists, speech-language pathologists, and audiologists. Specialists within the school system are usually known as speech therapists and are credentialed by the school. All speech-language pathologists and audiologists are credentialed by the American Speech-Language-Hearing Association (1993) and hold the Certificate of Clinical Competence from that organization. These specialists work only with the body systems having to do with verbal communication (talking and listening), and they see many of the same patients that occupational therapists see: primarily children and youth who are developmentally delayed and children and adults who have suffered brain damage from cerebral vascular accidents, head trauma of various origins, and neurologic conditions such as Parkinson's disease and multiple sclerosis.

Frequently occupational therapists collaborate by incorporating procedures initiated by the speech-language pathologist into their own treatment time, for example, using pictures to stimulate proper word sounds as part of educational activities with developmentally delayed children. This is an example of combined treatment time made pos-

sible through careful planning by the two professionals. (See Chapters 24 and 25, role release.)

## Social Workers

Social workers are employed by hospitals, clinics, state and local agencies, and sometimes school systems to assist clients and families in their attempts to adjust financially, socially, and psychologically to the problems besetting them. Occupational therapists have frequent meetings with social workers as they each try to help the patient adjust to handicaps of illness, injury, family loss, and vocational stress. Occupational therapists work through activities, whereas social workers employ counseling sessions and assistive negotiations with financial and social agencies.

There are several levels of social work practice, each capable of different contributions to the care of the client. The levels shown in the box below were established by the National Association of Social Workers, Inc. (1993).

Social workers recognize that social stresses arise from

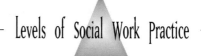

## Levels of Social Work Practice

**SOCIAL WORKER (ACBSW)**

Certification by the Academy of Certified Baccalaureate Social Workers, granted after graduation from a baccalaureate degree program, with a minimum of 2 years postgraduate supervised employment.

**SOCIAL WORKER (ACSW)**

Certification by the Academy of Certified Social Workers, granted after 2 years full-time (or equivalent part-time) paid post-master's or postdoctoral work experience, supervised by a social worker in an organized setting.

**QUALIFIED CLINICAL SOCIAL WORKER**

The National Association of Social Workers (NASW) register recognizes this category of social workers who meet NASW standards for clinical practice: 2 years of full-time (or equivalent part-time) paid post-master's or postdoctoral clinical social work with experience in an organized setting, supervised by a clinical social worker with at least 2 years experience.

**DIPLOMATE IN CLINICAL SOCIAL WORK**

Three additional years of full-time (or equivalent part-time) clinical social work practice.

**SCHOOL SOCIAL WORK SPECIALIST**

At least 2 years of postgraduate supervised school social work experience, after earning the master's degree in social work.

physical and mental illness, and they plan for services to the client that minimize social dysfunction. Knowledge of agencies and how they operate, skills in making interagency referrals to the benefit of the client and family, and understanding of cultural and ethnic differences are all part of what the social workers bring to the health team.

Social workers frequently can assist the occupational therapist by finding resources for needed adaptive equipment, by helping patients accept or psychologically adjust to various aspects of disabling conditions, and by facilitating interagency communications.

## Prosthetists and Orthotists

Prosthetists are the persons who make and fit artificial limbs. Orthotists make and fit permanent splints and braces. Each specialist works closely with the prescribing orthopedist, physiatrist, or pediatrician to ensure the child's benefit and comfort. They also work closely with the occupational therapist, who teaches the child to use the device in the way most effective for that individual.

Occupational therapists have a special relationship with orthotists because fabricating splints and orthotic devices has long been a part of occupational therapy practice. Occupational therapists' knowledge of anatomy, expertise with tools and materials, and dedication to increasing function produced some of the earliest orthotic devices within hospitals and rehabilitation clinics. In some areas, practice is now divided by body part; occupational therapists fabricate orthoses for the upper limbs and face, and the lower limbs and trunk are the province of the orthotist. Service is usually provided by the most accessible qualified person.

Prosthetists and orthotists were at one time apprentice kinds of specialties where the necessary skills were acquired through on-the-job training. Standards were established in the late 1970s, and a national certifying examination was developed. Current requirements to sit for the examination include graduation from an accredited program and 1 year of experience.

## Technical Personnel

Hospitalized children may be alarmed at the array of technical personnel who jab them, prod them, stick things into them, aerate and ventilate them, and perform other incomprehensible and frightening procedures. During planned play periods, which are relatively nonthreatening situations, occupational therapists can often provide comforting interpretations of such treatments and procedures for the child. Cooperation in arranging treatment schedules with laboratory and x-ray personnel, respiratory therapists, and technicians who operate such diagnostic equipment as the electrocardiograph and electroencephalograph can work to the benefit of everyone's schedule by producing a relaxed, unfrightened child at treatment time.

## Certified Occupational Therapy Assistants

The relationship that exists between the registered occupational therapist (OTR) and the certified occupational therapy assistant (COTA) is important and should be defined and nurtured in each setting. Under the supervision of the OTR, the COTA implements intervention activities, monitors progress, and adapts activities based on the goals. COTA educational programs are usually 2 years in length at the associate degree level and incorporate a period of practical experience.

## Teachers

The teaching profession is made up of persons with specific expertise: kindergarten and elementary school teachers, secondary school teachers, special education teachers, guidance counselors, art and music teachers, teachers of industrial arts, home economics teachers, vocational education and automobile driving instructors, coaches and physical education teachers, and administrators. Whatever the specialization of the teacher, all teachers have in common the basic tenets of the profession and the requirements of their particular state regarding certification.

All states require certification for public school teachers, and many require it for teachers in private and parochial schools. Many states require teachers to work toward and achieve master's degrees within specified periods after employment. The education profession has thus mandated the continuing education that all professions encourage as an essential of continuing professional viability. Guidance counselors and teachers in special education are required to have teaching certificates as well as further qualifications in their special areas.

Occupational therapists work closely with special education teachers because both services for children with disabilities are mandated by law (see Chapters 24 and 25). Special education teachers have advanced skills in teaching children who are blind, deaf, emotionally disturbed, mentally retarded, and physically handicapped. They seek the expertise of the occupational therapist in planning for the child's classroom participation through the use of assistive devices, handling techniques, positive self-image and so forth.

The guidance counselor can supplement the prevocational work of the occupational therapist by supplying career information, selected testing services, and counseling with students about vocational, academic, and technical opportunities. The prevocational work that occupational therapists do with handicapped children should be carefully described and demonstrated to the guidance counselor to develop cooperative, effective services for the child. Refer to Chapters 24 and 25 for a thorough presentation of occupational therapy in the school system.

Therapists working outside the school system in clinics or in other agencies should familiarize themselves with the educational program of the particular child to coordinate additional therapy services with the child's educational plan. Teachers can be directly approached for conferences concerning the child.

*Teachers' aides* are trained to assist the professional teacher in the classroom to give the teacher more time to do what he or she is primarily hired to do—teach. Aides grade papers, monitor hallways, help children with outdoor clothing, and, in general, assist in any classroom or area of the school program. Aides often work one-on-one with children with disabilities, assisting them in classroom activities. They are sometimes paid employees of the school system; other times they are volunteers. Because of the assistive nature of their job, aides are often directly involved with helping children adjust to the classroom or to feeding themselves or to doing other self-maintenance activities. Occupational therapists should ensure that the aides as well as the teachers are familiar with prescribed routines and equipment.

## Other Professionals

Others who join the educational team as needed are speech and language teachers, audiologists, and psychologists.

Speech and language teachers have duties that differ from those of the special educators who are specifically trained to teach academic subjects to the deaf. The speech and language teachers teach communication processes and language skills to all needful children, including the deaf, and are qualified in the area of speech and hearing sciences. Similarly, audiologists evaluate the hearing ability of schoolchildren and recommend hearing aids or other treatments to improve hearing.

Psychologists relate to the various teams in two ways: (1) as school psychologists hired by the school system and (2) as consulting or clinical psychologists used on a fee-for-service basis by the individual child and family. Licensure requirements vary from state to state, but in general, psychologists may be prepared at the master's or doctoral levels. They perform services according to their level of qualifications and experience. Most psychologists who serve school systems are prepared to make psychologic evaluations, give treatment, and interpret test results.

## Support Personnel

Bus drivers, maintenance workers, and dietary personnel contribute services to the educational program in their contracted areas and in ways that are not so apparent. The bus driver can have a great influence on the child with a mobility problem, and the dietary worker can influence the child with a feeding problem. All levels of personnel can contribute substantially to the therapeutic and educational programs if the therapists and teachers communicate goals,

elicit suggestions, and instruct them in the use of assistive devices and techniques.

## Administrators

The last decade has produced many regulations for health services and educational programs. Federal, state, and local laws have been enacted that regulate the finances, standards, and environments of most health and educational programs for children. Some laws limit the scope of services, and others mandate extensions of existing services. All of these regulations must be applied and enforced by administrators who are thereby put into the position of setting parameters for the professional programs within their institutions. Their administrative skills and their knowledge of the capabilities of the professions within their departments affect the quality and nature of services delivered.

Administrators come from varied backgrounds. Some are promoted from within the professions whose programs they administer; therefore, they have intimate knowledge of the programs but varying degrees of administrative skill. Others are brought from such backgrounds as public health, business management, educational administration, or hospital administration. These persons have important expertise in the management of personnel, space, and finances but less knowledge of the professional services they administer. It is important, therefore, for the administrators and the service professionals to work together so that administrative goals and service goals are clearly defined and compatible.

The effect of government regulations is felt throughout most service departments; as the variety of services offered and the quality of those services increases, documentation needs to be increased, generating more paperwork. Everyone gains, therefore, from efficiently designed institutional procedures for complying with the many external demands on service personnel.

## SUMMARY

Occupational therapists work with many professionals during their service to children. In health and educational in-

### STUDY QUESTION

Seven-year-old Mary suffered brain injury in an auto accident, has residual motor problems that make it difficult to speak and to write, and has a limited attention span. What professionals would be most likely to work with her? With what sort of team(s) could you expect to be involved?

stitutions, as well as in the community at large, children are best served if the many persons involved in their treatment communicate and collaborate in goal setting and planning. A variety of professional and technical specialties have been introduced in this chapter to acquaint the reader with the level of knowledge and skills of their colleagues in the helping professions.

## REFERENCES

American Speech-Language-Hearing Association. (1993). *Membership and certification handbook 1994.* Rockville, MD: American Speech-Language Hearing Association.

Baldwin, D.C., Jr. (1982). Some conceptual and methodological issues in team research. In J.E. Bachman (Ed.). *Proceedings of the Interdisciplinary Team Care Conference.* Kalamazoo, MI: Center for Human Services, Western Michigan University.

Basuray, J. (1991). Preparing health care professionals for providing culturally congruent care. In J.R. Snyder (Ed.). *Interdisciplinary health care teams: proceedings of the Thirteenth Annual Conference.* Bloomington, IN: School of Allied Health Sciences, Indiana University.

Horwitz, J. (1970). Interprofessional teamwork. *Social Worker, 38,* 5.

Julia, M.C. & Thompson, A. (1994). Group process and interprofessional teamwork. In M. Casto & M.C. Julia (Eds.). *Interprofessional care and collaborative practice.* Pacific Grove, CA: Brooks/Cole.

National Association of Social Workers. (1993). *NASW Professional Credentials.* Washington, DC: National Association of Social Workers.

Rainforth, B., York, J., & MacDonald, C. (1992). *Collaborative teams for students with severe disabilities.* Baltimore: Brookes.

CHAPTER

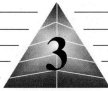

# Foundations of Practice:
## *Developmental Principles, Theories, and Frames of Reference*

JIM HINOJOSA ▲ PAULA KRAMER ▲ PAT NUSE PRATT

## KEY TERMS

- ▲ Developmental Theories
- ▲ Acquisitional Theories
- ▲ Operational Theories
- ▲ Psychosexual Stages of Development
- ▲ Erikson's Stages of Personal-Social Crises
- ▲ Cognitive Theory of Piaget
- ▲ Sociobiology
- ▲ Interactionism
- ▲ Frames of Reference
    Biomechanical
    Coping
    Neurodevelopmental
    Sensory Integration
    Occupational Behavior

## CHAPTER OBJECTIVES

1. Define the parameters of human development that undergird primary occupational therapy theories.
2. Define stress and adaptation.
3. Describe the psychosexual theories of Freud and apply these to the child's development of personality.
4. Explain the personal-social crisis in each of Erikson's developmental stages.
5. Describe cognitive development based on the theories of Piaget.
6. Compare and contrast the acquisition theories of Skinner and Rogers.
7. Identify the developmental tasks that were defined by Havighurst.

8. List and define the sections of a frame of reference.
9. Explain how frames of reference guide the practice of occupational therapists with children.
10. List and briefly describe major frames of reference used in pediatric occupational therapy.

Theory is a reasoned explanation of known facts or phenomena that serves as a basis of action (*Stedman's Medical Dictionary*, 1994). Professional practice should always be based on the use of theoretical information. Theory and practice should be continually linked. Occupational therapists use frames of reference to link theory and practice. Frames of reference enable practitioners to use theory as a basis for their interventions with children. The known facts that precede theoretical speculations are the basic principles of physical and social maturation.

This chapter presents a number of durable concepts and theories that can provide a foundation for occupational therapy practice with children. Some recent trends in the study of child and human development are also considered because these may well affect the direction of theory development and related practice methods.

## BASIC PRINCIPLES
### Maturation and Experience

At the core of most developmental theories is an explanation of the interplay between (1) human biologic capacity and maturation and (2) the influence of the environment of the behavioral experiences of the individual. In fact, theories tend to be distinguished from each other by the specific weighting of these two factors or by an investigator's emphasis on a particular aspect of human biologic function or environment. For example, B.F. Skinner highly valued the influence of the environment on human development, whereas Sigmund Freud emphasized biologic determinants of behavior. In effect, theorists generally agree that human development is both a process and the product of biologic maturation and environmental experiences. *Development* may be defined as the sequential changes in the function of the individual or species. This should be differentiated from the concept of *growth,* which refers to those maturational changes that are physically measurable.

## Parameters of Development

There are three general parameters of development: biologic, psychologic, and social. Each parameter has subcategories that are differentiated later in this section. *Biologic development* is primarily related to enzyme systems that stimulate complex metabolic changes. There are two subcategories of *psychologic development* that generally refer to those functions we consider interactive (or emotional). In the infant, cognitive psychologic function tends to be dominated by neurologic maturation and behavioral motivations for survival. As the child develops, cognitive activity is measured by communication skills and the handling of abstract material. Affective development is characterized by the establishment of bonds of feeling and meaning with human and nonhuman objects in the child's environment. *Social development* provides the child with skills to live in a community of others and is a product of both the child's biologic capacity to learn and the direct influence of the societal environment of the child's maturation. Learning may be equated with acculturation, that is, the acquisition, internalization, and use of skills necessary to function in society.

The parameters of development affect one another. For example, children with cerebral palsy and limited mobility often have immature social skills and fewer friendships than typical children (Werner, 1985; Zeitlin & Williamson, 1994). A number of the physical limitations associated with cerebral palsy seem to relate to delays in social and object play. Fine motor and visual motor delays may prevent the child's participation in games and peer group activities. Studies have shown that young adults with cerebral palsy and other physical disabilities have fewer social opportunities and diminished social skills (Kokkonen, Saukkonen, Timonen, Serlo, & Kinnunen, 1991). All social behavior is mediated by the basic biologic capacities and psychologic needs of the individual and the species and by the changing factors of the environment that influence an individual or group.

## Dimensions of Development

An understanding of development provides the foundational concepts for occupational therapy with children. Three dif-

ferent dimensions of development are the basis of occupational therapy research and practice. One dimension of development is longitudinal. Longitudinal development refers to the chronologic sequence of skills achieved as the child grows and matures. This view of development defines an order of developmental stages that match chronologic ages. Using this longitudinal perspective, specific skills are expected of preschool-age children and more advanced skills are expected of children once they enter school.

Another view of development is that certain prerequisite skills are required to learn higher-level skills. For example, skills in manipulating a writing utensil do not emerge until after the child has achieved fingertip grasp of objects. The skills a child exhibits therefore relate to achievement of more basic foundational skills rather than to chronologic age or stage as defined by age. How quickly the child gains new developmental skills relates to the child's current level of functional skill. Information about the developmental sequence helps determine what skills will likely develop next and whether skills have been missed or development is proceeding in an atypical pattern.

Finally, an understanding of development helps the therapist appreciate skill mastery of specific performance components, for example, hand skills or feeding skills. The developmental sequence applied to specific performance components helps therapists understand how performance components and areas relate to each other. Often the occupational therapist works with children who are developing at different rates in different performance areas. Although a child can develop faster or slower in different areas, function in one developmental area interrelates to function in other areas. This interrelatedness of development across performance areas forms the basis for the holistic approach used by occupational therapists described earlier. In another example, children with high cognitive skills and delayed motor skills often demonstrate rapid improvement in motor performance because of their high level of motivation, curiosity about the environment, and ability to problem solve. Children with limited mobility and difficulty in fine motor skills may have delays in cognitive skills that result from limited opportunities to explore the environment. Therefore although skill mastery of each performance component is often the focus of intervention, the whole or the interaction of all performance components should be considered.

## Gradients of Growth

There are several universal concepts of the directions, or gradients, of growth that have strong implications for treatment. The first principle is that *ontogeny recapitulates phylogeny,* that is, the growth of the individual mirrors the maturational development of the species. This is particularly important to the understanding of the sequential maturation of biologic functions. Second, there is *cephalo-*

*caudal progression* of maturation. For example, the purposeful control of motor activity begins with movements of the head (cephalo) and develops gradually in descending order to the caudal (or tail) region of the body. The change from mass to specific action, as movement becomes more discriminative and refined, is termed *differentiation*. An important more recently developed concept is that the maturation of systems and functions proceeds toward the *integration,* rather than the fragmentation, of the individual (Kaluger & Kaluger, 1984; Sprinthall & Sprinthall, 1981).

## Stress and Adaptation

It is generally agreed that the behavior of living organisms is directed toward maintaining a state of *homeostasis,* or *equilibrium,* that is, a life-maintaining balance of all systems, parts, and forces intrinsic and extrinsic to the individual. *Stress* may be defined as an internal or external force that threatens homeostatic balance. *Adaptation* is the general term for the mechanisms used by the individual to restore homeostasis. The adaptive mechanisms may be physiologic or behavioral and may be used with and without conscious control. The standard example of an unconscious adaptive mechanism is the response of the autonomic nervous system to prepare the body to deal with emergency situations.

Stress has both positive and negative values. The positive result of stress is the initiation of more discriminative, and therefore more mature and adaptive, behavioral responses. This result assumes that the individual has the physiologic capacities and maturity to purposefully deal with a stressful situation and learn from it. The negative influence of stress is most likely to occur when stress is multidimensional or beyond the physiologic capabilities of the individual or when it is continuous to the point that the individual is unable to experience intermittent sensations of equilibrium. Such distress situations eliminate the discriminative learning aspects of adaptation that ordinarily promote development and allow the person to experience a sense of achievement.

Most theories of interest to occupational therapists attempt to explain the processes a child uses to adapt to stress, either of a particular type or at different stages. Theorists often link the healthy resolution of stressful situations to critical periods or events. The term *critical periods* refers to certain times in an individual's life when a particular type of development or learning can take place most readily or spontaneously (Maier, 1969). For example, sometime during the sixth year of life the child's visual and auditory functions, language and social development, and curiosity are at an optimal level for learning to read. This does not mean that the child cannot learn to read 1 year earlier or 10 years later. It simply means that this is developmentally the most opportune period, a time when the overall maturational *readiness* of the individual to engage in a new type of learning or experience is at its peak.

Rigid application of the concept of critical periods does not reflect the variations and individual differences observed in normal development. Research has demonstrated that fixed intervals for learning specific skills are actually quite variable; therefore, the term *sensitive period* has come to replace the stricter term *critical period* (Gardner, 1978). The sensitive period is the developmental stage when certain developmental tasks are commonly addressed and potentially resolved.

Other examples of sensitive periods are found in this chapter in the discussion of various theories and in the developmental sequences presented in Chapter 4.

## THEORIES

It is important to note that occupational therapy practitioners do not develop theories; they apply theoretical material for the purpose of assisting an individual. Occupational therapy, like medicine, is a **science-based profession.** It derives information for its frames of reference from theoretical material that has been developed by scientific disciplines. These **science-based disciplines,** such as biology, physics, chemistry, psychology, and occupational science, are concerned with the development, testing, and refinement, and not the application, of theoretical material. It should be noted that the activities of the professions and disciplines are equally important (Mosey, 1992).

The therapist may select a number of theories to guide intervention with any specific problem. Therapists do not generally use theories as a whole. Instead, they tend to pick and choose sections from a variety of theories and organize this information together to specifically match the individual's needs and abilities. During this process, therapists create a new body of theoretical information, not new theories themselves. This could include elements of biology, physics, or psychology. The therapist would not or could not use all of the theories of biology, but might need to focus on developmental theories and neurologic functioning. Likewise, for physics and psychology, the therapist would use some of this theoretical material, but not all of it. To combine some of these theoretical elements, a therapist selects the information that is relevant to a child's developmental and functional levels and the characteristics of the environment. This selection is based on the general problems and needs of the individual requiring intervention and the knowledge and experience of the therapist and produces a pool of theoretical information from which the therapist works. The therapist must then organize this information in a way that is useful and meaningful. This information will form the foundation for the theoretical base that will substantiate practice decisions.

Occupational therapists draw from a wide range of theoretical information. The possibilities are extensive, but

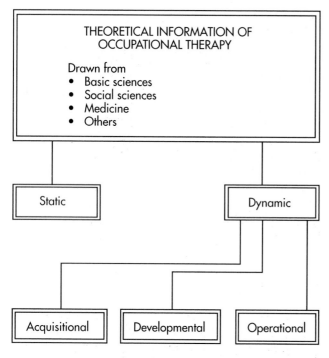

**Figure 3-1** Classification of theories.

occupational therapists tend to draw theoretical information from three broad classifications: basic sciences, social sciences, and medicine. Examples of some basic sciences are anatomy, biology, chemistry, physiology, neurology, kinesiology, physics, and occupation. Although anatomy and neurology may be viewed as subcategories of biology, they have their own bodies of knowledge and may be seen individually as basic sciences. Some examples of social sciences are psychology, sociology, and cultural anthropology. The third category is theoretical information from medicine, which deals with diagnostic categories, treatment, sequelae, prognosis, and therapeutic effects of medications. Medicine may be viewed by some as a subcategory of biology or anatomy, but it encompasses a large body of specific information that health professionals need to understand, and, therefore, should be viewed by occupational therapists as a separate classification (Mosey, 1992).

Theories can be categorized in another way as well. Theories can be static or dynamic. **Static theories** are those theories that describe relationships between phenomena and are not concerned with change. To be useful in a frame of reference, static theories are used in combination with dynamic theories. **Dynamic theories** are those theories that are concerned with change and are of more use to therapists because the profession is ultimately concerned with change. Three subdivisions for dynamic theories are developmental, acquisitional, and operational (Figure 3-1).

**Developmental theories** are based on an understanding of and appreciation for normal development. Developmen-

tal theories are often stage-specific theories because they tend to view the development as moving through a series of stages in which one area of skills is mastered before the child matures to the next level. At each stage the child's behaviors or skills are qualitatively different from the previous stage. Because of this qualitative difference, as growth occurs, the child's behaviors become more complex and richer. Developmental theories also tend to focus on the relationship between chronologic age, level of maturation, and skill mastery. Generally these theories are broad, although they may deal with distinct areas of human development such as motor, psychosocial, and cognitive spheres of development. However, most developmental theories describe a pattern or sequence of development believed to be "universal," or characteristic of all children. All developmental theories describe a sequence of development that includes specific stages.

**Acquisitional theories** are based on changes in learning and behavior. Behavior is shaped by the environment and the individual's interaction with it. Acquisitional theories view learning or change as components of a process and resulting conditional responses. As the child develops, he or she learns new behaviors that are added to or that replace previously acquired behaviors. Each learned behavior is thought to be acquired in its own unique and independent manner. In essence, the child's learning progresses through the continuous acquisition of new and more complex skills, rather than being based on maturation and stages.

**Operational theories** are those theories that explain change relative to improvement in an individual's abilities in a specific area. Change is based on adaptations to the environment that allow the individual to improve performance. These adaptations are generally external to the individual and result in change in the person's functional status. For example, when a child with spasticity in extensor postural tone is given a wheelchair seat insert that increases hip flexion, that child is better able to engage in activities at the table. This functional change is explained by a combination of the theories of physics, physiology, neuroscience, and kinesiology. Another example might be the therapist's use of a splint to reposition a child's hand. It is believed that this method reeducates the muscles, resulting in physiologic changes so that ultimately the child's hand function improves even when the splint is no longer necessary.

Table 3-1 presents the three classifications of theories most commonly used by occupational therapists. These basic theories have been presented in depth elsewhere, and to do so here is beyond the scope of this text. However, the degree to which the practice of occupational therapy is based on developmental theory makes it important that a description of those theories be included in any basic text. Two acquisitional theories are included for the same reason.

▲ Table 3-1    Delineation of the Three Classifications of Theories and Some of the Theories Most Commonly Used by Occupational Therapists

| | Developmental | Acquisitional | Operational |
|---|---|---|---|
| **T H E O R Y** | · Psychosexual (Freud, 1966)<br>· Stage theory of psychosocial development (Erikson, 1963)<br>· Cognitive development (Piaget, 1971)<br>· Moral development (Kohlberg, 1978)<br>· Hierarchy of basic needs (Maslow, 1970)<br>· Developmental schedules (Gesell & Amatruda, 1967)<br>· Developmental tasks (Havighurst, 1972) | · Social learning theory (Bandura, 1977a)<br>· Behaviorism (Skinner, 1974)<br>· Motor learning (Carr & Shepard, 1987)<br>· General systems theory (Boulding, 1968; von Bertalanffy, 1968)<br>· Information processing (Newell & Simon, 1972)<br>· Visual perception (Gibson, 1969) | · Biomechanics (Williams & Lissner, 1962)<br>· Orthopaedic biomechanics (Frankel & Burnstein, 1969)<br>· Schema theory (Schmidt, 1975)<br>· Heterarchical theory (Turvey, 1977) |

## Developmental Theories

### Psychosexual Theories of Freud

Discussion of Freud's theory in this chapter emphasizes his model of personality development. Freud proposed that personality arises from the biologic, instinctual energy of the individual and that this energy is differentiated through typical environmental experiences at different ages.

The initial, motivating part of a person's personality at birth is called the *id*. It represents the psychic energy, the impetus for all behavior. The sole purpose of the id is to rid the person of tension by seeking out pleasurable sensations and avoiding pain. This purpose is called the *pleasure principle*. The id does not think; it only wishes and reacts. If all needs of the id were met, the infant would remain helpless.

The id contains both the life and death instincts of the individual. The *life instincts* include hunger, thirst, and sex drives that ensure the survival of the individual and the species. The source of energy for these drives is called *libido*. The opposing drives, the *death instincts,* are usually subordinate to life instincts but manifest themselves throughout life in the form of destructive energies and aggressive behaviors.

The *ego* is the part of the personality that starts to develop after birth as the infant comes into contact with the mediating influences of the environment. It is the part of the personality that moderates the id's wishes according to environmental constraints.

The ego operates according to the *reality principle*. Nye (1981) stated that the ego "attempts to differentiate between what is desired (by the id) and what is actually available (in the environment)" (p. 13). The *secondary process* used by the ego is called *reality testing*. This involves formulating a plan to see if it works.

The ego modifies libidinal energy through the *displacement process*. This is the transference of energy into alternative actions. The displacement of libidinal energy through

a socially acceptable behavior is called *sublimation.* Freud believed that the world's progress toward civilization was dependent on sublimations. For example, when a person is hungry and has a visitor, he or she does not satisfy the libidinal urges of the id by disappearing into the kitchen and eating alone. Instead, because of the mediating influence of the ego, the person shares the food with the guest.

The third part of the personality is the *superego*. This is the moral component of the personality that reflects the learned values of the culture. Like the id, the superego is not objective. It responds to mental images as well as to personal actions. Only the ego is realistic as it balances the innate needs of the id with the environmentally molded demands of the superego.

*Levels of consciousness.* Freud is best known for his systematic study and organization of concepts related to the unconscious. He constructed a topographic model consisting of the conscious, the preconscious (meaning readily accessible to the conscious), and the unconscious levels. The content of the unconscious realm of the mind is considered to be available at the conscious level with great difficulty. Although only parts of the ego and the superego exist at the unconscious level, all of the id is in the unconscious. Only small aspects of the ego and the superego are at the conscious level at any one time. The major parts of these two components are stored in the preconscious mind and are called on as needed.

The ego acts as a gatekeeper to the unconscious, channeling through those needs of the id that can be met through socially acceptable ways. Libidinal urges that are in conflict with society (and its mirror, the superego) are held back or sidetracked through *defense mechanisms*. There are a variety of defense mechanisms that may collectively be defined as irrational thinking that allow the ego to protect itself from anxiety when rational, adaptive processes are insufficient.

▲ Table 3-2   Contrasted Sequences of Selected Stage Theories

| Age | Freud: Psychosexual Development | Erikson: Ego Adaptation | Piaget: Cognitive Development | Kohlberg: Moral Development |
|-----|-----|-----|-----|-----|
| 6 mo | Pregenital period | Basic trust vs. mistrust | Sensorimotor period | Preconventional morality: punishment and obedience |
| 1 yr | Oral stage | | | |
| 18 mo | Anal stage | Autonomy vs. doubt and shame | | |
| 2 yr | | | Preoperational period: preconceptual phase | |
| 3 yr | Phallic stage | Initiative vs. guilt | Initiative thought phase | |
| 4 yr | | | | |
| 5 yr | | Industry vs. inferiority | | |
| 6 yr | Latency period | | | Instrumental relativism |
| 7 yr | | | Concrete operational period | |
| 8 yr | | | | |
| 9 yr | | | | |
| 10 yr | | | | Conventional morality: social conformity |
| 11 yr | Genital stage | | Formal operational period | |
| 12 yr | | Self-identity vs. role diffusion | | Law and order |
| 13 yr | | | | |
| 14 yr | | | | |
| 15 yr | | | | |
| 16 yr | | | | Postconventional morality: social contracts |
| 17 yr | | | | |
| 18 yr | | Intimacy and solidarity vs. isolation | | Universal ethics |

***Psychosexual stages of development.*** Freud postulated that the impetus for development at different stages of life is centered on obtaining pleasurable sensation in the erogenous zones. Each of his stages is named for the erogenous zone that presumably provided the greatest source of pleasure and contact between the child and environment at that age (Table 3-2).

The *oral stage* is centered on the mouth and lips. Pleasure is derived through sucking, chewing, and feeding. Parent-infant feeding interactions that satiate the infant's need for oral gratification are also important to bonding.

The *anal stage* describes the second and third years of life. Pleasurable sensations are obtained through elimination activities of the anal and perianal sphincter muscles. The most important activity of the anal stage is toilet training.

The *phallic stage,* which covers the period from about 3 to 6 years, was the most controversial part of Freud's theory because of its stress on the child's incestuous feelings toward his or her parents. The centers of sensation here are the external genitalia. In essence, Freud hypothesized that children of this age have sexual drives toward parents of the opposite sex and aggressive drives toward parents of the same sex. This conflict is resolved with the emergence of the superego, which in effect punishes the child for such fantasies. The ego responds to this anxiety-producing situation by suppressing the libidinal urges of the id and promoting identification with the parent of the same sex.

The oral, anal, and phallic stages were collectively considered the *pregenital period.* Freud believed that the personality was essentially formed through this period. The child develops the ability to survive, to form emotional bonds, to delay gratification, to channel energy into socially acceptable behaviors, and to assume a sex role identity.

The *latency period,* which occurs during the elementary school years, is a time of quiescence and recovery from the turbulent conflicts of the phallic stage. The child shifts interest from the self to the outside world and increases the quantity of social skills.

The *genital stage* is characteristic of the teen years, as hormonal changes reawaken the sexual drives of the individual. However, through the socialization process (sublimation and identification), the ego has learned to channel these drives appropriately. The youth seeks heterosexual relationships involving mutual gratification. This emergence of altruistic concerns is characteristic of the adolescent in other areas of life as well. If the ego is successful with sublimation and identification, a healthy adult is the result.

## Ego Psychology of Erikson

Erik Erikson was a student of Freud's, and his theory of development reflects that affiliation. Erikson is viewed as the father of ego psychology and a pioneer of the humanistic school of thought. His work demonstrated a more optimistic view of human nature and focused on the functions of the ego in response to the environment. Whereas Freud saw the id as the most important aspect of the personality, Erikson (1963) gave priority to the adaptive response of the ego in the development of the individual. Much of Erikson's theory crystallized through his studies of the lives of famous people, such as Ghandi and Luther, as he sought to identify what characteristics allow people to go on living in the face of adversity. In addition, he conducted considerable treatment and study with children, including cross-cultural comparisons. He believed that play afforded the best opportunity for observations of adaptive and maladaptive responses of the ego.

Erikson divided the life span into the *eight stages of man*. Each stage is represented by a *personal-social crisis* that gives impetus to ego growth. Erikson accepted Freud's concept of the id as the prime motivator; however, he believed that the ego provided continuity to development. One of Erikson's most important assumptions was that society constitutes itself to provide opportunities for ego growth and identity. The tasks of adulthood direct the individual's attention to facilitating the development of the next generation. All crises recur throughout life, but these particular stages are the critical periods in which crises are best resolved to promote successful living. Erikson viewed development as an autotherapeutic process, that is, the successful resolution of a crisis repairs the wounds of its conflicts and gives the individual a sense of achievement. Erikson prefaced each stage with "a sense of" to refer to the continuing sense of mastery and achievement (Table 3-2). Each stage also results in the acquisition of an abstract personality quality, such as hope or wisdom (Hall & Lindzey, 1978).

***Basic trust versus mistrust.*** The infant, from birth to about 18 months, must develop psychologic trust, the eagerness to approach new experiences without paralyzing fear. Trust develops through the caregiving attentions of the parents, particularly the mother. The initial sense of trust comes from the infant's realization that survival needs will be met and that he or she can exist in a state of comfort. The most difficult task for the infant is to maintain this trust in the absence of the mother. Erikson believed that the parents must provide gradual opportunities for separation that do not provoke excessive anxiety. *Hope* is the acquired characteristic of this stage.

***Autonomy versus doubt and shame.*** Autonomy versus doubt and shame is the stage of the 2- to 4-year old toddler. It is characterized by holding on and letting go and is exemplified by the crisis that occurs through the toilet-training process. Erikson specified the relationship of autonomy to the child's increasing control over his or her body. This permits independent movement into the outer world. Parents must provide opportunities for the child to make choices and develop a sense of self-controlled *will*.

***Initiative versus guilt.*** The newly autonomous preschooler has mastered basic motor skills and must now build a repertoire of social skills to deal with the outer world. Central to this is the achievement of gender (sex) role identity. Erikson's view parallels that of Freud's, but Erikson's view is more broadly concerned with the child's imitation of the variety of role behaviors. Through imitation, children learn to assume responsibility for themselves within the confines of their still-limited environment and develop a sense of *purpose*.

***Industry versus inferiority.*** The elementary school child experiences a period of slow, steady growth. The need for security is transferred from the family to the peer group as the child attempts to master the activities of his or her age-group. The peer group is used as a standard of performance against which the child can measure his or her own skill. The abstract objective of this period is the realization of *competence*.

***Self-identity versus role diffusion.*** Erikson (1963) studied the period of adolescence in great detail, and the scope of his theoretical formulations for this age is therefore much broader than Freud's. The masterful schoolchild is suddenly shaken by the physiologic changes of puberty and must struggle to regain control over body, identity, and future. During adolescence the prolonged childhood draws to a close, and society asks the adolescent to make choices about adult roles. The teenager experiments with patterns of identity until a sense of continuity and control over the ego is regained and a perspective of the future is acquired. In spite of the often turbulent conflicts between adolescents and their elders, Erikson believed that the actions of both were directed to the same end of helping youth clarify their roles as members of society. Through resolution of the identity crisis the individual gains a sense of *fidelity,* the continuity of the past with the future.

***Intimacy and solidarity versus isolation.*** Earlier relationships have helped the young adult define himself or herself. Now the adult seeks to share that identity through the intimate relationships of marriage and family life. In concert with Freud's view, Erikson saw healthy adulthood as a time of love and work. The abstract capacity derived through this period is *love*.

***Generativity versus self-absorption.*** The crisis of middle adulthood is to develop the feeling that one's life is meaningful and productive. The person must find a sense of security in the usefulness of his or her chosen personal, social, and economic roles for the continuity and preservation of society. *Caring* is the abstract phenomenon realized during this time of life.

***Integrity versus despair.*** The stage of integrity versus despair is continuous and largely dependent on a successful sense of generativity. It represents the appraisal of self-worth as the individual faces the physical, economic, and personal losses of old age. It is essentially a case of "it was a very good year" versus "if only." The objective of this stage is the achievement of *wisdom* and the ability to share a satisfying and encouraging philosophy of life with the younger generation.

Erikson began his adult life as an artist, a background that manifested itself in his books through the detailed "life space" portraits he presented in his reports of clinical cases and biographic analyses. His artist's eye as well as his interest in history and anthropology allowed his written work to acquire an insight into and an emphasis on environmental influences, which are lacking in Freud's theories. These factors, as well as the cross-cultural durability of his theories, make Erikson's works especially useful for occupational therapists.

## Cognitive Theory of Piaget

Jean Piaget's concept of the child as a little scientist is remarkably reflective of his own youth. By age 10 he had published his first paper in a biology journal, and at 22 he had completed his doctoral dissertation on mollusks. He attended university at the time that Freud, Adler, and Jung were receiving recognition in Europe, and consequently he was influenced to study a good deal of philosophy and psychology. The academic atmosphere in early twentieth-century Europe was stimulating for the study of human nature, and it produced a number of great theorists such as Piaget, Erikson, and Maslow.

By training, Piaget was a zoologist. By vocation, he became a psychologist. His particular interest was in the genesis and theory of knowledge (genetic epistemology). Piaget's first employment was to assist Binet in the standardization of intelligence tests. What interested Piaget most was not the correct responses made by children during testing but rather the consistency of patterns of incorrect responses at different ages. This interest led him to a research career investigating children's thought patterns. The experimental approach that he developed is called *methode clinique*. This method involved (1) presenting children with familiar objects, such as blocks, pieces of paper, and glasses of water; (2) constructing problem-solving situations with the objects; and (3) asking children to solve the problem *(actions)* and to explain how they had done this *(experience)*. The importance of his method lies in the concern for the processes used by the children regardless of the correctness of their problem solving. Although his initial investigations were conducted with his own children, Piaget's studies have since been replicated with several thousand children.

Piaget's work developed a very elaborate theory of the process of cognition as it matures over the span of life from infancy to adolescence. It is necessary to first examine Piaget's major constructs relating to this process to understand the sequence of cognitive development periods.

***Major constructs.*** Piaget accepted the biologic basis of behavior, but he was more concerned with the developmental *adaptation* of the individual in response to ongoing environmental experiences. He wrote (Piaget, 1971) that "the theory of knowledge is . . . essentially a theory of adaptation of thoughts to reality (resulting from) an inextricable interaction between the subject and objects" (p. 24). He examined adaptation through the child's relationships with human and nonhuman *objects, time, and space.* He said that the child organizes his experiences into *mental schemes* (concepts) through use of mental operations. *Operations* may be defined as the cognitive methods used by the child to organize his or her schemes and experiences and to direct his or her actions. The totality of operational schemes available to the child at a given time constitutes the *adapted intelligence,* or cognitive competence, of the child.

The child's quest is for *equilibrium,* a balance between what the child knows and can act on and what the environment provides. But the child is constantly faced with novel situations and stimuli and in fact would not learn and develop without disequilibrium. Two processes are used by the child to organize novel experiences (and restore equilibrium). *Assimilation* means that the child takes a new situation and mentally changes it to match an existing scheme. This may result in some distortion or reality, but it is typically the first cognitive method used to confront new situations. For example, a young child who sees a furry, small, four-legged animal tends to call it a *dog.* However, if the child's mother is available and corrects the child with the information that the animal is a cat, the child must then use the process of *accommodation.* That is, the child develops a new scheme in response to the reality of the situation. Assimilation tends to result in generalization; accommodation improves discrimination. Both are important to the child's development because although discrimination promotes cognitive maturity, generalization is necessary for organization and continuity.

***Sequence of cognitive periods.*** Piaget also believed that there was an invariant, hierarchic development of cognition that proceeds from the simple to the complex, from the concrete to abstract, and from personal to worldly concerns. At first, thought is *egocentric;* that is, the child relates all experiences to himself or herself. Through cognitive maturations, thought becomes decentered and *relativistic;* that is, relationships among time, objects, and space assume an importance independent of the child's own experiences. Piaget specified four maturational levels, or periods, of cognitive function: (1) sensorimotor, (2) preoperational, (3) concrete operational, and (4) formal operational (Flavell, 1985).

***Sensorimotor period.*** The child from birth to about age 2 responds to and learns about the environment directly through sensations and motor responses. The emphasis is on sensory, movement, and manipulative experiences with objects. This period is characterized by the most egocentric thought. Although it is the shortest period of mental development, it is proportionally the most active.

Piaget differentiated six stages of sensorimotor activity. The *reflexive stage* occurs during the first month. The child's schemes begin in simple biologic reflexes that are primitive, general, and related to survival. Piaget believed that the sucking and palmar reflexes, which modify to promote oral and manipulative exploration, are the most critical to early mental development. The baby assimilates sensory experiences, such as the taste of food, with the kinesthetic sensations derived from the reflexive movements of sucking. Through repetition, the child becomes more proficient in the use of reflexes to satisfy basic needs. There is no differentiation between self and object or between sensation and action.

The next sensorimotor stage, occurring in the second through fourth months, is called *primary circular reactions.* The child repeats reflexive sensorimotor patterns merely for the sake of pleasurable repetition. There is still no separation between sensation and action. Essentially the child is establishing primitive habit patterns as the precursors of voluntary movements that are associated with specific sensations.

The third stage, *secondary circular reactions,* evolves during the fifth through eighth months of life. At this time the child begins to show true voluntary movement patterns based on a coordination of vision and hand function. In effect, the child reaches for and grasps everything that is seen. When the action is rewarded by a pleasurable secondary sensation, such as the sound of a bell inside of a toy, the infant will repeat the action. The child is beginning to have a primitive awareness of cause and effect.

The fourth stage of *coordination of secondary schemata* completes the baby's first year. This marks exciting changes in the child's operations as the child begins to direct movements in response to stimuli that cannot be seen. The child can respond to and then look for a sound and then look for an object that disappears from view. This marks the emergence of *object permanence,* the awareness that something or someone has continuity beyond the child's direct experience with it. In turn, object permanence signals the beginning of decentered thought.

This phenomenon has implications in affective-emotional development as well. The baby now realizes that when the mother leaves the room, she does not cease to exist. The baby can begin to listen for sounds of his or her mother in a nearby room and gradually realizes that sound stimuli can be used to find the missing mother (because locomotor development is also progressing rapidly at this age). As shown in Erikson's theory, this awareness is critical to the child's progress toward independence.

The fifth sensorimotor stage, which lasts until about 18 months, is called *tertiary circular reactions.* The child's mental behavior is characterized by searches for new schemes. This development parallels a motor stage when the child is suddenly able to walk and crawl about freely, and parents are hard pressed to keep their youngsters from getting into everything. Although it happens by chance, one of the most important results of this stage is the beginning of *tool use.* The child discovers that he can get more food into his or her mouth with a spoon or that a distant pull toy can be obtained by pulling on the attached string that previously had no function for the child. Prehension patterns become more refined and precise in the process.

The sixth stage of sensorimotor activity, the transitional stage, is marked by *inventions of new means through mental combinations.* It generally occurs during the last 6 months of the second year. This stage is mentally demonstrated through insight and physically characterized by purposeful tool use. The child is looking for alternate means to solve problems. These changes are in large part aided by the child's increasing motor proficiency in speech production and by an expanding receptive vocabulary. The child can now begin to label or symbolically represent mental schemes. Whereas during the previous stages all schemes were represented as sensorimotor experiences, the child is now beginning to represent concepts without direct manipulation.

***Preoperational period.*** With the emergence of language and symbolic representation of schemes, the child's cognitive patterns undergo significant changes. Through acquisition of verbal schemes, the child is able to expand his or her conceptual repertoire more rapidly. In addition, symbolic representation allows the child to organize knowledge and to call on a scheme at will. During the time from 2 to 7 years of age, children learn to systematically manipulate their environments through development of the organizing operations called classification, seriation, and conservation.

*Classification* is the organization of objects according to similarities and differences. At first, children classify according to one common stimulus characteristic, such as color. Two-year-old children can be seen making little stacks of blocks with each stack a different color. When they have mastered classification according to one common characteristic, children begin to notice other shared characteristics as well as discrete differences. Classification becomes multidimensional. The dog and cat of the example given earlier for assimilation and accommodation become classified as *pets.* Classifications may be made according to sensory characteristics, spatial arrangements, and readily observable cause and effect relationships.

*Seriation* is the relationship of one object, or classification of objects, to another. As with classification, this operation is initially exercised at a unidimensional level. Proximity of objects tends to afford the earliest stimulus for seriation. However, with maturation and increasing vocabulary, the child can rank-order objects in terms of size, weight, color intensity, and other sensory characteristics.

*Conservation* is the end product of the preoperational period. It permits the child to recognize the continuities of an object or class of objects in spite of apparent change. A typical Piagetian example would be to show the child a ball of clay. The clay is flattened or rolled out in front of the child, who is then asked if the amount is the same. A child who is still unable to conserve sees that the physical appearance is different and would say that the amount is not the same.

The most primitive kind of conservation is by the number of objects (in different spatial arrangements). Later the child begins to conserve mass (as in the clay example), area, length, and volume. The ability to conserve is critical to learning to read and to do math, for the child must learn to recognize the sameness of sounds and values in letters and numbers regardless of their arrangements.

The preoperational period is divided into two distinct phases. The 2- to 4-year-old child is considered *preconceptual.* The chief task here is for the child to expand the vocabulary and thus increase the quantity of symbolic representations. Typically classification is the primary operation that develops at this time, although the child is also learning verbal concepts that will promote use of seriation and conservation. Play provides the arena for learning, and the child spends considerable time in verbal play.

The *intuitive thought phase,* from about age 4 to 7, provides the child with substantially more social-environmental contacts. The child uses a tremendous amount of imitation by copying whatever is seen and repeating whatever is heard. Children happily relate all the family secrets in great detail. The child answers questions and solves problems intuitively, not really knowing how conclusions were reached. Seriation and conservation develop during this phase as the child is able to deal with multiple characteristics of objects. Through classification and seriation the child begins to use inductive reasoning to relate parts to the whole. This marks the transition to concrete operations.

***Concrete operational period.*** The concrete operational period, which covers the life span from about age 7 to 11, is important for the acquisition of reversibility, spatial concepts, and rules. During this time the child remains stimulus and experience bound; he or she can think only about things that are at least available for sensory manipulation.

*Reversibility* is an extension of conservation and allows the child to develop more spatial awareness. Children learn

that they not only can add two numbers, but also can subtract. They gain an understanding that the constant features of an object, such as the conservation of the clay mass, permit it to be returned to its previous state.

*Rules* are not new to the concrete operational child, but understanding of rules becomes more realistic and complete, and therefore the child is able to apply them. There are rules of causation that prescribe general cause and effect; rules of attribution, related to social causation, such as custom to outcome or event to event; and moral rules for right, wrong, and situational appropriateness. Mature understanding and application of rules continue to evolve through the formal operations period. For example, the preoperational child knows that he should not hit another child because "it is wrong." At the formal operational level the adolescent can explain that hitting is a form of violence that had an impact on society and that it is justified only under certain conditions.

Classification, seriation, conservation, reversing, and rule use allow the child to develop systematic ways of organizing parts to wholes and determining parts of wholes. The child begins to make combinations and elementary permutations (combinations of combinations). The use of concrete operations constitutes *empirico-inductive thinking;* that is, the child is able to solve problems by use of information that is concretely available.

***Formal operational period.*** The formal operations period, which is the final cognitive period, begins at about 11 years of age and continues through the teen years. It signals the transition to mature thinking. The adolescent begins to think about things that are beyond his or her experience and manipulative control and can begin to use mental, language-based manipulation. A typical characteristic is the developing ability to organize one's time and to relate one's schedule to other people's schedules. The adolescent's thoughts are generally relativistic; that is, the adolescent sees relationships of object to object or event to event as having importance regardless of direct personal experiences. An interest in world events and social problems is manifest. The youth internalizes abstract values.

The ability to perform mental manipulations demonstrates the teenager's proficiencies with permutations and the laws of probability. Because of these, the adolescent is able to conceptualize possibilities. Plans can be made and tried out mentally and changed according to mental judgments regarding the soundness of the plan. This ability to analyze problems and to plan possibilities is called *hypothetico-deductive thinking* and is used by adults in most situations that can be dealt with on a cognitive rather than an emotional basis.

Piaget believed that this sequence of development leads to the cognitive maturity of adulthood. The representative of this is a person with values, goals, plans, and an understanding of one's purpose in society. Piaget and Inhelder

(1969) stated that maturation of cognition is dependent on the following:

1. Organic growth, especially the maturation of the nervous system and endocrine glands
2. Experience in the actions performed on objects
3. Social interaction and transmission
4. A balance of opportunities for both assimilation and accommodation (p. 154)

Knowledge of Piaget's theory is critical to occupational therapists who plan programs for children. Regardless of the psychosocial or neurologic approaches used in treatment, the therapist in an activity-based situation is interacting with a thinking child. The selection and structure of an activity in accordance with the operational skills and concepts of the child are essential.

## Other Developmental Theories
### Kohlberg: Stages of Moral Development

Lawrence Kohlberg (1978) was interested in the relationship between Piaget's concepts of cognitive development and the acquisition of moral value schemes. He designed a series of fascinating experiments that presented moral dilemmas to children and young adults of different ages (Table 3-2). Like Piaget, he did not make judgments about the correctness of children's choices, but instead he collected data about the concepts used by the children to make moral decisions. He described three discrete levels of moral development, each having two complementary stages.

The first level of moral development is called *preconventional morality.* Obedience is the limit to morality until about 8 years of age. Choices are governed by egocentric concerns. The first stage, *punishment and obedience,* is based on the child's desire to avoid punishment from the larger, parental authority figures. The second stage, *instrumental relativism,* is slightly decentered. Decisions are based on personal needs and occasionally on the needs of others when they can be of help to the individual. In other words, you scratch my back, I'll scratch yours.

*Conventional morality,* the second level of moral development, emerges around 9 or 10 years of age (late concrete operations) and is characterized by social conformity. Its appearance indicates some internalization of rules of social causation. The third stage, *social conformity,* demonstrates behavior that is pleasing to others. It is easy to see how this follows the patterns of instrumental relativism. This is the age when children become very serious about their responsibilities to help with classroom chores. Concern with *law and order* marks the fourth stage. Moral behavior is very rule bound in response to emerging notions of social order and fairness. A typical behavior of this stage is concern with cheating and other infractions of honor codes.

The third level of moral development, *postconventional morality,* is marked by relativistic thinking. There is an effort to define moral principles (rather than obedience) that

are flexible for different situations. This is characteristic of the older adolescent with mature formal operations who can consider many variables and possibilities. In the fifth stage, *social contracts,* the young adult makes moral decisions based on social values, with an awareness of the legal implications.

It is interesting to note that Kohlberg's stages are chronologically behind those of Piaget. This indicates that levels of cognition must be fairly mature before an individual can use the higher-level operative methods to examine abstract issues of morality and obedience. Just as adults tend to use concrete and formal operations flexibly according to the merits of a situation, they also use moral thinking in dealing with everyday situations. It appears that when a situation is novel and does not readily lend itself to assimilative use of moral schemes, the individual tends to direct a higher level of moral thinking toward the situation (Kaluger & Kaluger, 1984; Kohlberg, 1978).

### Maslow: Humanistic Psychology

Abraham Maslow is generally considered the father of humanistic psychology in the United States (Hall & Lindzey, 1978). He, like Piaget and Erikson, was profoundly influenced by European philosophic trends during the Age of Enlightenment. He outlined a *hierarchy of basic human needs* that are believed to appear in the following longitudinal sequence: The *physiologic needs,* such as food, water, rest, air, and warmth, are necessary to basic survival. The next level is characterized by the need for *safety,* broadly defined as the need for both physical and physiologic security. The need for *love and belonging* promotes the individual's search for affection, emotional support, and group affiliation. The need for a sense of *self-esteem,* which is defined as the ability to regard one's self as competent and of value to society, is evidenced as persons grow. The need for *self-actualization,* which represents the highest level, is attained through achievement of personal goals.

Maslow proposed that each of these needs serves as a motivator to achieve a higher level of human potential. There is a progression of development that begins with the satisfaction of biologic, egocentric needs, proceeds through needs for social group affiliation; and culminates in the use of intellectual capacities to affect the broader community of the individual.

If the lower-level needs are not met, the individual is not able to direct his or her energies toward higher levels. For example, when a child comes to school hungry, it is difficult to concentrate on the classroom learning activities.

### Gesell: Developmental Schedules

Arnold Gesell was a physician whose work gave impetus to the medical specialty of pediatrics (Knoblock & Pasamanick, 1975). Through his practice, Gesell accumulated data on children's performance of everyday activities, and he was the first to put a timetable on development through a series of developmental schedules. Most of the items on standard developmental evaluations in use today are based on Gesell's findings.

Most of Gesell's work concerns what to look for, how to find it, and at what ages. It would be impossible to list here all of the ages and items that were identified, but a few key definitions should be useful.

Gesell used the term *behavior* to collectively define all kinds of reactions to stimuli, voluntary or involuntary. In contrast, a *behavior pattern* is considered a discrete, voluntarily repeatable response of the neuromotor system to a specific stimulus situation. Developmental schedules help chart key categories of behavior patterns that are critical to determining the progress of the child. *Motor behavior* is directed toward postural control and locomotion. *Adaptive behavior* patterns are used to manipulate the environment. *Language behaviors* include vocabulary, articulation, and social communication skills. The *personal-social behaviors* are learned controls of bodily functions, such as hygiene and grooming. *Maturity stages* are chronologic periods of development in which certain behavior patterns characteristically appear for the first time.

*Adaptation* is the coordination of physical maturation with the skill demands of the environment. In his studies Gesell found that this was not a smooth process. Typically, behaviors become less adaptive when the child is in a period of rapid physical growth. When the growth spurt subsides, the child is able to concentrate on coordinating his or her body in the practice of socially acceptable behavior patterns. This cycle of alternating periods of positive and negative adaptation is called *reciprocal interweaving* (Knoblock & Pasamanick, 1975).

## Havighurst: Developmental Tasks

Robert Havighurst, a renowned American educator, proposed that a person must learn specific groups of skills at different ages to meet social expectations. The acquisition of a particular group of skills enables a person to perform adequately the age-appropriate roles of player, student, worker, or retired person. Havighurst (1972) believed that it was the ability of the person to learn, rather than to merely respond to, situations that differentiated humans from animals.

Havighurst believed that each developmental task had biologic, psychologic, and sociologic bases. Similarly, he proposed that the achievement of each task could be facilitated or inhibited by these three forces. The concept of *sensitive periods* was described as the time at which biologic, psychologic, and sociological conditions were most appropriate to the achievement of a developmental task. These particularly sensitive times often provided a "teachable moment" when the child or adult is most apt to integrate all previous learning to master the skills of a new developmental task with social guidance. Therefore Havighurst (1972) analyzed each task in terms of its biologic, psychologic, and

sociologic bases, as well as its educational implications. He defined the following tasks for each developmental phase:

1. Tasks of infancy and childhood
   a. Learning to walk
   b. Learning to take solid food
   c. Learning to talk
   d. Learning to control the elimination of body wastes
   e. Learning sex differences and sexual modesty
   f. Achieving physiologic stability
   g. Forming simple concepts of social and physical reality
   h. Learning to relate oneself emotionally to parents, siblings, and other people
   i. Learning to distinguish right and wrong and developing a conscience
2. Tasks of middle childhood
   a. Learning physical skills necessary for ordinary games
   b. Building wholesome attitudes toward oneself as a growing organism
   c. Learning to get along with age-mates
   d. Developing fundamental skills in reading, writing, and calculating
   e. Developing concepts necessary for everyday living
   f. Developing a conscience, morality, and a scale of values
   g. Developing attitudes toward social groups and institutions
3. Tasks of adolescence
   a. Achieving new and more mature relations with age-mates of both sexes
   b. Achieving a masculine or feminine social role
   c. Accepting one's physique and using the body effectively
   d. Achieving emotional independence of parents and other adults
   e. Preparing for marriage and family life
   f. Preparing for an economic career
   g. Acquiring a set of values and an ethical system to guide behavior; developing an ideology
   h. Desiring and achieving socially responsible behavior
4. Tasks of early adulthood
   a. Selecting a mate
   b. Learning to live with a marriage partner
   c. Starting a family
   d. Rearing children
   e. Managing a home
   f. Getting started in an occupation
   g. Taking on civic responsibility
   h. Finding a congenial social group
5. Tasks of middle adulthood
   a. Assisting adolescents to become responsible and happy adults
   b. Achieving adult civic and social responsibility

  c. Reaching and maintaining satisfactory performance in one's occupational career
  d. Developing adult leisure-time activities
  e. Relating oneself to one's spouse as a person
  f. Accepting and adjusting to the physiologic changes of middle age
  g. Adjusting to aging parents
6. Tasks of later maturity
  a. Adjusting to decreasing physical strength and health
  b. Adjusting to retirement and reduced income
  c. Adjusting to the death of a spouse
  d. Establishing an explicit affiliation with one's age-group
  e. Adopting and adapting to social roles in a flexible way
  f. Establishing satisfactory physical living arrangements

It is appropriate to conclude this section on developmental theories with Havighurst's sequence. Essentially Havighurst's work is a compilation of concepts developed and studied by the previously discussed theorists. The tasks given are self-explanatory and useful to the therapist to get a quick overview of the social expectations for children at a particular time of life.

## Acquisitional Theories

This section on acquisitional theories is generally limited to Skinner's theory of operant conditioning and Rogers' humanistic theory of the self. This approach was chosen because many useful theories are variations of the work of these two men or of the theorists presented in the section on developmental theories. Skinner's approach is behavioristic and superficially contrasts sharply with Roger's ideas. However, it should be recognized at the start that Skinner and Rogers were equally concerned with the individual's opportunity to achieve maximal potential. The difference between the two lies in the school of thought that gives each man his methodologic orientation. Skinner's view of humanity is considerably less mechanistic than that of other behaviorists.

### Skinner's Theory of Behaviorism

The components of Skinner's work that are presented here constitute a theory of behavioral development and learning. Skinner believed that all human behavior is shaped by the environment and that behaviors may be randomly emitted in response to an environmental stimulus. That is, the organism tries a behavior that worked in a previous situation, or an involuntary, reflexive response is elicited by the environmental stimulus. The behavior is then reinforced in some way by the environmental consequences that follow it. This sequence of (1) stimulus situation, (2) behavioral response, and (3) environmental consequence constitutes a *contingency of behavior.* It is the mechanism through which the environment shapes behavior.

Skinner (1976) clearly stated that through natural occurrences in the environment, the child's adaptive behaviors are reinforced, and those behaviors that are not adaptive are ignored or punished. For example, a young child encounters a dog for the first time. Reaching into his or her behavioral repertoire, the child engages in a reaching-and-touching behavior. If the dog responds by nuzzling and licking the child and providing the child with a generally pleasant sensory experience, it may be said that the child has been positively reinforced (rewarded) by the environmental consequences. If the child comes to associate reaching and touching as a means to obtain a pleasant reaction from dogs, he would tend to repeat that behavior under similar stimulus situations. Thus behavior would be strengthened and maintained as long as it was generally effective in obtaining positive reinforcement. If, on another occasion, the child pets the dog and the dog runs away, the reaching-and-touching behavior might be weakened. In the first instance the behavior was reinforced by the environment. In the latter situation reinforcement was absent, that is, not given and therefore negative. If the dog ran away often enough, it is probable that the child's reaching-and-touching behavior with dogs would be extinguished.

The third type of environmental control, called aversive control, punishment, or *punitive contingency,* is recognized and defined by Skinner. However, he specifically advocates against its use because its effects on behavior are unpredictable and generally do not promote adaptation. Punishment has been a common form of behavioral control throughout the ages and is generally expected to eliminate behaviors. If the child reached and petted the dog and was bitten, that would be a form of punishment. If this resulted in avoidance of all future dog encounters, as sometimes happens in this situation, the contingency would be maladaptive. The child does not learn an effective behavior to use when approaching strange dogs.

Skinner believed that all behavior is a result of the environmental control of the individual, the culture, and the species. He specified that humans, the species, and the culture are part of the environment and therefore control as much as they are controlled. Skinner (1971) described human's influence on their world:

> Man has 'controlled his own destiny'. . . the man that man has made is a product of the culture man has devised. He has emerged from two quite different processes of evolution: the biological evolution responsible for man, the species, and the cultural evolution carried out by that species (p. 198).

Skinner rejected the traditional concept of *autonomous man* who functions with no controls. Skinner provided a number of behavioral explanations for the concepts typically used to support the idea of autonomous man. For example, *aggression* is often said to be part of human nature.

Skinner would say that this behavior resulted from contingencies of survival. He also pointed out that aggressive behaviors are strengthened and maintained by here-and-now contingencies of reinforcement. For example, a father may tell a son that it is wrong to hit another child, but then encourage him to stand up for his rights or to be tough in sports activities.

A traditionally humanistic concept is the capacity for *self-awareness*. Skinner says this is largely dependent on language, which has been acquired and shaped by the verbal community. Small children learn to describe their feelings because they are questioned regarding these. Even a simple "How are you?" helps to shape this behavior.

Another characteristic capacity that has been described as uniquely human is the ability to *think*. Skinner acknowledges that the ability to think is a complex process with a foundation in the genetic endowment of the species (and therefore evolved through contingencies of survival). A behavioral explanation of thinking is that the culture teaches people to make fine discriminations, to solve problems, and to follow rules, including rules for finding rules.

*Self-identity* is readily explained in behavioral terms as a "repertoire of behavior appropriate to a given set of contingencies" (Skinner, 1971; p. 189). Skinner identified a variety of "selfs" that develop according to the specific contingencies of the varied environments of a person's life. Problems arise when an environment changes and becomes inconsistent with prior contingency patterns. For example, children use one set of behaviors with their families and another set with friends. Behaviors that are reinforced by friends may bring complaints or be ignored by parents.

For the purposes of this discussion, the final aspects of human nature to be considered are related to the ability to manipulate the environment. Traditionally, *manipulative ability* has been considered one of the hallmarks of the view of humans as autonomous. Skinner explained this characteristic simply as a result of contingencies of survival. Manipulative ability enabled humans to use tools with skill to change their environment and improved their chances for survival. Because skilled tool use had such a strong impact on the survival of the species, development of manipulation skills came to be highly valued. Skilled manipulation became increasingly accompanied by positive socialcultural reinforcements. Crafts, woodworking, art, and writing are products of skilled manipulation that are highly valued and reinforced across cultures.

### Rogers' Self Theory

Like Maslow, Carl Rogers believed that people have an inborn need for self-actualization. Rogers (1969) took a positive view of human nature that was both deterministic (driven by the actualizing tendency) and epigenetic. Central to Rogers' theory is the individual's *inner experiencing,* that is, how one perceives oneself, one's relationships,

and one's environment. Rogers acknowledged the instrumental influence of the environment in the development of the self, but he believed that the individual has the capacity to choose responses to the environment that maintain a sense of personal control.

Rogers is best known for his formulation of *client-centered therapy.* Like Erikson, Rogers believed that each individual has, and must find within himself or herself, the resources for growth, adaptation, and self-actualization. Client-centered therapy was designed to elicit these resources, and the therapist takes a nondirective role that encourages the client to say what he or she really feels and wants to do. The *nondirective approach* is readily applied in occupational therapy, when the therapist urges the child to "show me what you can do" and "tell me what you think." Child-centered activity is the basis of the sensory integration approach defined by Ayres (1972, 1979) and has recently been described by DeGangi and her colleagues (1991) (see Chapter 10).

***Concepts of the developmental process.*** Rogers conceptualized the infant as being essentially a clean slate for the development of the self. The totality of sensations constitutes reality. Likes and dislikes are clearly demonstrated in response to pleasant and aversive stimuli.

The child grows to want the pleasurable sensations experienced through love and acceptance of *significant others.* Initially these significant others are the child's father and mother. This need for positive regard forces the child to examine what he or she does that pleases and displeases the parents. The child learns to view himself or herself through others' eyes and to suppress feelings and other inner experiences. This is believed to occur because the child receives *conditional positive regard* from the parents; love and acceptance are given under certain conditions according to the child's actions.

Through growth and increased contacts with the outer world, the child slowly loses sight of himself or herself. Externally derived values and feelings of self-worth are internalized. This alienation of the self from the natural organismic (innate) experience is called the *basic estrangement* of humans. The degree to which this prevents the individual from following the self-actualizing tendency is dependent on the amount of *unconditional positive regard* the person receives from significant others.

### Current Trends in Developmental Theory

Current investigators of child development appear to be more concerned with process than were the earlier theorists who have been described thus far. A review of the literature in child development in recent years shows three areas of study that have begun to influence the thinking and practice of occupational therapists: (1) sociobiology, (2) interactionism, and (3) information processing. These terms are from the literature and, although not necessarily parallel, seem to be commonly accepted.

## Sociobiology

Sociobiology is defined as "the application of evolutionary principles to the social behavior of animals . . . and human beings as well" (Barash, 1979, p. 1). According to this theory, much of the behavior of human beings that has heretofore been considered socially derived, and therefore environmentally derived, is actually genetically transmitted. Researchers have sought to identify universal behaviors among species and relate the development of those behaviors through natural selection (Wilson, 1978). They proposed that each species develops a unique behavioral repertoire, over time through the natural selection, of those characteristics that are most adaptive for the species. Their concern was not with the different cultural patterns that are used to refine the behaviors but rather with the species-specific behaviors that are the bases of the cultural patterns. Barash (1979) pointed out that, although there are thousands of language patterns used by different humans, the capacity to speak, develop, and learn a language and communicate with others is biologically derived and shared by the entire species. Again, the critical difference that the sociobiologists make is that these capacities are genetically, rather than socially, transmitted.

The concepts of sociobiology have been rejected by some social scientists on the grounds that the theory does not account for individual differences and that it has an aura of determinism that could conceivably be used to support discriminative practices. Selected review of the literature in sociobiology indicates that individual differences are not overlooked but are deemphasized (Smith, 1978; Wilson, 1978).

In contrast, Thomas (1981) noted that sociobiologic concepts provide considerable explanation for the growing evidence of the complexity of infant behavior. The human capacities for reflexive responses, sensory perception, speech, and learning are recognized as biologically determined. What has been questioned until recently is how well developed these capacities are at birth.

## Interactionism

The concept of interactionism, as defined by Thomas (1981), includes several components. These include the inborn complexity of infant behavior, the plasticity of the human development, and the variable effects of the child's temperament. Simply stated, interactionism postulated that the child is an active social being who contributes to continuity and change in his or her developmental environment.

As was alluded to earlier, research data have demonstrated that infants have definite behavioral patterns at birth, including preferential attention to a variety of auditory, visual, tactile, and gustatory stimuli. Active learning, as evidenced by the rapid manifestation and replication of neurodevelopmental reflexes, begins immediately after birth. Imi-

tative behaviors appear within 2 weeks. These behaviors are now defined as being social rather than reflexive (Thomas, 1981). Whereas it was formerly emphasized that infants learned to respond differentially to their mothers' behaviors, researchers now speak in terms of mothers' increasingly differentiated responses to infants' behaviors (Ainsworth, 1979).

Similarly, it is becoming clearer that the residual effects of early or traumatic experiences are not as permanent as previously thought. Numerous studies of children from varied early environments who later had the opportunity for enriching experiences have led investigators to conclude that the human capacity for change is as important in child development as is the capacity for steady, continuous maturation. Considerable research is now directed toward understanding the influence of multiple attachments and different stages of life (Thomas, 1981). Equally relevant is information about a child's capacity to recover from traumatic experiences, such as separation from parents through divorce or death, as the child develops. Again, the influence of multiple attachments is considered critical, particularly in relation to the need for adequate gender role models. It appears that a child's adaptive development is best facilitated by a balanced combination of continuity and change, rather than overemphasis on either mode.

Finally, interactionism is concerned with the influence of the child's temperament. In a logical extension to the awareness of the strength of the infant's cognitive behaviors and learning, researchers have begun to look at the way the growing child's temperament affects the behaviors and attitudes of others, as well as how the child's temperament affects his or her response to others. A long-term study by Thomas (1981) documented clear-cut patterns of consistency of temperament over time that make important contributions to variations in development. See Chapter 15 for further description of temperament and its influence on development.

## Cognition and Learning

In addition to the concern with physiologic and social foundations of behavior, recent study in child development has been directed toward the examination of cognitive behaviors and learning. Although Piagetian theory had been generally well accepted as an explanation of the developmental maturation of a child's thought content, it left gaps in the understanding of how cognition and learning take place. Researchers have relied heavily on combining concepts from information processing and social learning theories to develop a more sophisticated explanation of the two phenomena (Bornstein & Sigman, 1986).

In essence, *information processing* is actually a conceptual model of how the brain operates from the information it receives. The development of computer technology has provided researchers with terminology for the processes that are involved in cognition. Information processing uses a simple input-operations-output model. The input includes any sensory stimuli that are received through the sensory organs and transmitted to the central nervous system. Therefore input is dependent on attention, curiosity, exploration, sensory awareness, and sensory recognition. The operations (or cognitive functions) include storage in long- and short-term memory, concept formation, association, sorting, and retrieval strategies. These operations are subject to physiologic variations such as age, level of consciousness, and general well-being. The output of cognition is represented by thought or action as the individual makes a choice, moves, or speaks. Output is modified by concurrent operations related to affect and attention.

The information-processing model has been widely adopted in psychology and education, and occupational therapists need to be familiar with its relevance to sensory integrative function (see Chapter 13). It is a useful tool for both research and program design because of its simplicity and well-defined terminology.

One application of the information processing model is shown in Kaluger and Kaluger's (1984) conceptualization of the learning process. Using model components studied by the early social learning theorists, Kaluger and Kaluger proposed that *learning* is the cognitive process through which the individual gathers information and is able to knowledgeably select the appropriate behaviors to reach a desired goal.

The information processing model for learning (Figure 3-2) shows the three main process components and two universal bases involved. The learning processes provide input to the individual. Learning methods are the operational components. Learning outcomes, or outputs, include spe-

cific knowledge and behaviors. Motivation to achieve a goal is essential to the initiation and continuity of learning, as is the development of a repertoire of knowledge and cognitive abilities.

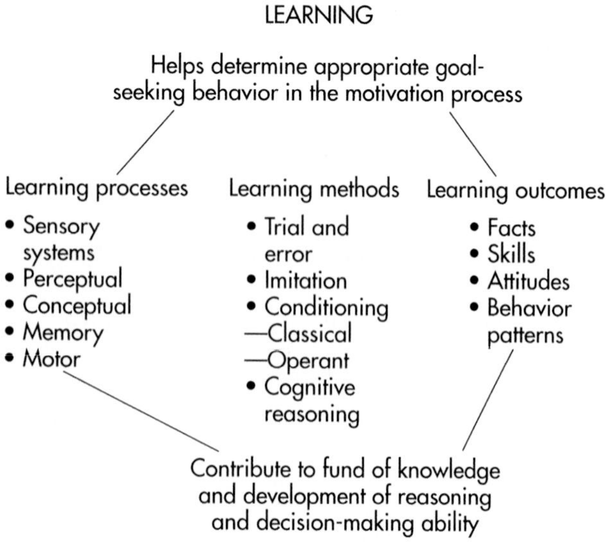

Kaluger and Kaluger (1984) (Figure 3-2) described learning as an active process that does not occur if the goal is not meaningful to the child or if the knowledge and conceptual skills to be attained through the learning situation have no personal relevance. Perhaps it is a sign of maturity when the accumulation of knowledge for its own sake is a goal.

To summarize, the trend toward identification of universal sequences of development that dominated child study through the 1960s has given way to concern with the processes of development and function that underlie such sequences. The purpose of theories is to make predictions about the relationship between sets of events or phenomena. Theories are not designed to deal with practical situations (Mosey, 1986).

Occupational therapists are concerned with integration of these developmental theories to provide an explanation of the process of occupation in purposeful activity. To make theory useful in practice, occupational therapists develop frames of reference to serve as guidelines for intervention. A frame of reference provides an acceptable vehicle for organizing theoretical material and translating it into practice in occupational therapy. Like a blueprint, a frame of reference provides the therapist with guidelines for approaching a child.

## FRAME OF REFERENCE

The frame of reference organizes theoretical material in occupational therapy and translates it into practice through a functional perspective. The therapist's frame of reference is the linkage between theory and practice. It consists of five major sections: theoretical base, function/dysfunction continuum, guidelines for evaluation, postulates regarding change, and application to practice (Mosey, 1986; Kramer & Hinojosa, 1993).

The **theoretical base** is a collection of theoretical information that is organized into a coherent whole. Drawing from one or more theories, the theoretical base provides the foundation of the entire frame of reference. However, it is not just a collection of theoretical information but an organized assembly of information whose purpose is to explain the relationship of theory to practice. If more than one theory is used, the theories must be internally consistent or be operating from the same basic premises (Mosey, 1981, 1986, 1992).

A frame of reference describes the characteristics of the environment that are needed for practice and how the environment will be manipulated to bring about change. The therapist is viewed as a crucial aspect of the environment. Further, the theoretical base includes a dynamic theory that

### LEARNING

Helps determine appropriate goal-seeking behavior in the motivation process

| Learning processes | Learning methods | Learning outcomes |
|---|---|---|
| • Sensory systems | • Trial and error | • Facts |
| • Perceptual | • Imitation | • Skills |
| • Conceptual | • Conditioning | • Attitudes |
| • Memory | —Classical | • Behavior patterns |
| • Motor | —Operant | |
| | • Cognitive reasoning | |

Contribute to fund of knowledge and development of reasoning and decision-making ability

**Figure 3-2**  Component parts of learning process. (From Kaluger, G.A. & Kaluger, M.F. [1984]. *Human development: the span of life,* [3rd ed.]. St. Louis: Mosby.)

explains how change is produced or facilitated by another individual (e.g., the caregiver or therapist) or by an adapted environment.

The next section in a frame of reference is referred to as the **function-dysfunction continua,** which clearly identify those areas of functioning with which the frame of reference is concerned. The specific areas of performance that are important to the child's development of skills or abilities according to the frame of reference are identified in the theoretical base. The continua distinguish what is functional or dysfunctional, consistent with the theoretical base, and therefore determine the areas that the therapist will evaluate. Each function-dysfunction continuum covers one area of performance that is important to the particular frame of reference. One frame of reference usually has several function-dysfunction continua. Although function is at one end of the spectrum and dysfunction is at the other end, there is a range of acceptable abilities and human performance represented on this scale. Ultimately, the theoretical base provides some guidelines as to what is functional and what is dysfunctional.

**Behaviors indicative of function or dysfunction** are a subsection of the function-dysfunction continua. The more behaviors that the child exhibits that are indicative of dysfunction, the closer the child will be to the dysfunction end of the continuum. Likewise, the more characteristics indicative of function that the child exhibits, the closer the child will be to the functional end of the scale.

**Guide for evaluation** suggests possible ways of evaluating for the presence of behaviors indicative of function or dysfunction. The function-dysfunction continua contribute to the guide for evaluation, as they define the areas of the performance that the therapist should assess. The guide for evaluation identifies the behaviors that the therapist assesses to determine if the child is in need of intervention. Through the evaluation the therapist determines the child's status on the function-dysfunction continua. Application of certain frames of reference specifies which evaluations may be used. For example, use of the Sensory Integration and Praxis Test is typical when applying the sensory integration frame of reference. Developmental assessments provide the basis for application of developmental frames of reference.

**Postulates regarding change** are the turning point of the frame of reference. These postulates translate the theoretical base into practical actions. These actions are the methods, techniques, and strategies that the therapist applies to facilitate change in the child. The postulates regarding change give the therapist a mechanism for using the frame of reference to plan the intervention. Postulates regarding change are the guidelines for how the therapists should intervene with the child and must relate back to the important concepts in the theoretical base. The guidelines include ways to adapt the environment to produce change and techniques to promote function. A modification in the child's

behavior or an enhancement of normal growth and development that has been impeded by dysfunction is the expected outcome.

Within the context of a postulate regarding change, environment is much broader than the physical space of the intervention setting. Environment includes the social interaction between the child and the therapist, the various activities to which the child is exposed, and the emotional climate of the intervention. Therapists do not actually create the change in the child, but they create an environment that allows the change to take place (Mosey, 1981, 1986, 1992). The therapist may create an environment that should enhance normal growth and development by providing the child with specific activities in which the child has not engaged previously.

A frame of reference includes information on **application to practice.** How does the therapist effectively put this frame of reference into practice? Application involves the use of certain tools and activities. A specific set of tools or instruments is used by occupational therapists to bring about change. Additionally, the therapist selects appropriate activities and describes how these activities may be graded so that the client may begin to interact and move from a state of dysfunction to function. Appropriate service delivery models for the frame of reference may be proposed in this section as well as environmental factors that should be considered (Kramer & Hinojosa, 1993).

Just as theories can be classified into the three categories acquisitional, developmental, and operational, frames of reference also can be classified. Frames of reference can be categorized in the same manner based on the dynamic theory that explains change that is used in the theoretical base. For example, a frame of reference for intervention with children with visual perceptual deficits would rely on the learning of various skills and therefore would be classified as an acquisitional frame of reference.

## Major Frames of Reference Used in Pediatric Occupational Therapy

There are many frames of reference currently used in pediatric occupational therapy and an infinite number of possibilities for the future. This section briefly presents an overview of nine frames of reference that are frequently employed by therapists when working with children.

### Activities of Daily Living

Many frames of references address specific activities of daily living (ADL) through their focus on feeding, dressing, or toileting. Most therapists approach ADL from an acquisitional perspective, relying on the principles of learning theory to teach specific tasks. ADL are basic and essential concerns of the profession and have always been a major emphasis in practice (Christiansen, 1994). ADL serve as a way to focus and organize evaluation and intervention goals and plans. ADL (self-care and daily living skills) are addressed in Chapters 16, 17, 20, and 21.

### Biomechanical Frame of Reference

The biomechanical frame of reference is categorized as an operational frame of reference. It is used when an individual has neuromuscular or musculoskeletal dysfunction that interferes with his or her ability to maintain adequate posture. Biomechanical principles are employed when artificial supports help the individual compensate for lack of postural control, enabling the body to maintain the most efficient positions for functional activities (Colangelo, 1993). This frame of reference is needed when splints and other adapted equipment, for example, mobile arm support or robotics, are used. The theoretical base of this frame of reference draws from physics, physiology, neuroscience, and kinesiology. The biomechanical frame of reference is further discussed in Chapters 11, 12, and 21.

### Coping Frame of Reference

The coping frame of reference was recently articulated by Zeitlin and Williamson (1994). Coping involves making adaptations so that a person can meet his or her personal needs and respond to the demands of the environment. It also involves the integration and application of developmental skills for functional living. The development and use of coping resources equip the child to deal with current and future challenges and opportunities. This frame of reference is directed at improving a child's coping ability when engaged in all areas of occupational performance. It is somewhat different from other approaches discussed in this section because it is intended to be used in combination with other frames of reference (Williamson, Szczepanski, & Zeitlin, 1993). The theoretical base draws from social learning theory (Bandura, 1977b), and data about the coping process (Antonovsky, 1979; Lazarus & Folkman, 1984). Although this frame of reference uses developmental principles, the dynamic theory involved is social learning theory. It makes the assumption that coping strategies are learned; therefore the frame of reference is considered to be acquisitional. Further description of the coping frame of reference is found in Chapter 10.

### Developmental Frame of Reference

Lela Llorens, an occupational therapist, identified a developmental frame of reference that focused on the physical, social, and psychological aspects of life tasks and relationships (Llorens, 1969). Clearly, this frame of reference would be categorized as a developmental frame of reference. The major premise of this frame of reference is that the child is viewed from two perspectives, the specific period of life, which Llorens (1976) refers to as horizontal development, and the course of time, which is longitudinal development. Both of these perspectives are seen as continua that occur simultaneously. The integration of these two

aspects of life is critical to normal development. Llorens viewed the role of the occupational therapist as facilitating development and assisting in the mastery of life tasks and the ability to cope with life expectations. Her theoretical base draws from Gesell and Amatruda (1967), Erikson (1963), Havighurst (1972), and Freud (1966), all of whom were described in earlier sections of this chapter.

### Neurodevelopmental Treatment

Neurodevelopmental treatment is a frame of reference based on the clinical experiences and personal views of Berta Bobath, a physiotherapist, and her physician husband, Karel Bobath. Since their original conception of the frame of reference, it has been continually revised to reflect the current understanding of sensory and motor development. Neurodevelopmental treatment, a sensorimotor approach, is widely used by occupational therapists to remediate neurologic and developmental motor dysfunction. The goals of neurodevelopmental treatment are to decrease the influence of abnormal postural tone and reactions, to promote functional movement patterns, and to prevent contractures and deformities. This frame of reference draws on theories of normal and abnormal development (Bly, 1980; Illingworth, 1960; Scherzer & Tscharnuter, 1990). This frame of reference is categorized as developmental. Additional explanation and examples of the neurodevelopmental frame of reference are provided in Chapters 11 and 12.

### Occupational Behavior

Mary Reilly originally developed occupational behavior to include those behaviors associated with the roles of being a child, student, worker, and adult. Dr. Reilly's writings were heavily influenced by the works of Adolf Meyer and Eleanor Clarke Slagle (Reed, 1984). Within this frame of reference, Reilly redefined the concept of occupation, identifying occupation as a meaningful need within one's life. She viewed work as providing stability to daily life patterns and routines. Her interventions were based on the use of occupation to learn, relearn, or modify life skills.

In pediatrics she focused on the importance of play. She saw play as the occupation of the child, having an organizing effect on behavior. She believed that play forms the basis for adult competence. One of her central beliefs was that play gives meaning to the daily life of the child. This acquisitional frame of reference is based on two major theoretical orientations, an appreciative system of learning, and play progression. The appreciative system of learning states that learning takes place as one tries to relate external facts to internal values. The learning process is based on personal values, and through these values, a person derives meaning from the external world. The individual's imagination is critical to learning. Play progression relates to the hypothesis that there are three hierarchic levels of play, exploration, competence, and achievement. Through play the child learns different rules, which can then be used in future interactions. Play serves as the foundation for adult competency (Reilly, 1962, 1974) (see Chapter 18).

### Sensory Integration

Sensory integration was developed by A. Jean Ayres (1972) based on her volume of research. Sensory integration is the process of organizing sensory information in the brain to make an adaptive response. Adaptive responses take place when the child is able to successfully meet a challenge within the environment. Inadequate adaptive responses are thought to be caused by poor sensory processing. When these sensory system processing deficits make it difficult for a child to produce an appropriate adaptive response, the sensory integrative frame of reference is used. Adaptive responses are believed to be the foundation of purposeful activity. This frame of reference is strongly based on developmental theory (Ayres, 1972, 1979).

The development of sensory processing for integration occurs in three levels: sensory system modulation, functional support capabilities, and end product abilities. The therapist uses controlled sensory input to facilitate adaptive motor responses. As the child moves through these levels, the input varies and the child is required to make increasingly complex adaptive responses. As the child is able to respond successfully at each level, he or she is able to engage in additional tasks, which are more complex (Ayres, 1979). Chapter 13 describes sensory integration theory, principles, and treatment techniques.

### Spatiotemporal Adaptation

The spatiotemporal adaptation frame of reference was proposed by Gilfoyle, Grady, and Moore (1990). Adaptation is viewed as a continuous process of interaction between the individual and time and space. Development is seen as a spiraling process, moving from simple to complex, where movement and more intricate patterns of adaptation evolve from more primitive behaviors.

The adaptation process involves four components: assimilation, accommodation, association, and differentiation. Assimilation is the reception of sensory stimuli from internal and external environments. Accommodation is the motoric response to those stimuli. Association is the organized process of relating current sensory information with the current motor response and then relating this to past responses. Differentiation is the process of identifying those specific elements in one's situation that are useful and relevant to another situation so as to refine the responsive pattern. Based on prior experience, the child develops a sense of what is useful and what is not useful to motor activity within a current situation. In this view of development, the child is continually modifying older, more primitive behaviors for effective motor responses, rather than continually acquiring new skills (Gilfoyle, Grady, & Moore, 1990).

This frame of reference draws primarily from an understanding of the central nervous system and theoretical material from Piaget (Flavell, 1985) and Gesell and Amatruda (1967). It is the basis for the description of developmental milestones in Chapter 4.

### Visual Perception

There is no one accepted visual perceptual frame of reference; however, many frames of reference deal with aspects of visual perception. Visual perception is the ability to interpret what is seen and to put that interpretation into practical use. Interpretation involves cognition, which helps the child to attach meaning to the stimulus. The continuous interaction of visual experience, intersensory feedback, and cognitive growth enhances the development of visual perceptual abilities. Each influences the others, and the interaction of all three together is necessary for optimal functioning.

Visual perception is highly dependent on the functioning of the central nervous system, especially cortical structures, and therefore is strongly related to the child's maturation. As the child matures, he or she is able to handle greater amounts of visual information, with greater complexity, and to handle both with greater speed. This frame of reference requires active involvement of the child with the environment; it is not based on the passive reception of information.

All visual perceptual frames of reference are acquisitional in nature, positing that learning or information processing is central to the change process. See Chapter 14 for an indepth discussion of visual perception.

Occupational therapists are continually developing frames of reference. Some are new and different from what has been done before, and others are variations on previous frames of reference. The development or refinement of frames of reference requires the use of theoretical information in practice.

## SUMMARY

Each child who is seen in occupational therapy is in the midst of a dynamic process of growth, maturation, and adaptation. Therefore knowledge of the human development process is critical to the foundation of occupational therapy theory and practice. This chapter has reviewed basic principles of growth and development as well as selected systems for classification of theories.

Current trends in developmental theory tend to emphasize process. Scientists are examining the relationships between specialized brain hemisphere functions and human behavior. In addition, they are looking to sociobiology to help differentiate between those human capacities that are derived through the species and those that are environmentally shaped. Current research indicates that many of the social, adaptive, and emotional characteristics of children that were earlier thought to be environmentally shaped may have a greater foundation in inborn capacities.

Learning and cognitive function are explained by information processing theory.

Developmental and acquisitional theories are only useful to occupational therapists if they can be operationalized for practice. This chapter has presented brief descriptions of the work of Reilly, Llorens, Gilfoyle, Grady, Ayres and others. Each of these therapists integrated their studies of developmental and acquisitional theories to formulate an approach to occupational therapy practice in pediatrics. Reilly concentrated on play as the fundamental occupation of the developing child through which the skills that underlie adult competence are shaped. Llorens integrated the developmental theories to propose a model of occupational therapy practice that is related to horizontal and longitudinal aspects of development in the child's life. Gilfoyle, Grady, and Moore (1990) examined the spiraling development of sensory and motor functions of the child as the foundation for purposeful human activity. Ayres studied the role of the brain and its sensory integrative processes that organize and direct observable behavior. No single frame of reference for occupational therapy practice is all inclusive: each must be considered in relation to the others and applied according to the needs of individual children.

The relationship of theory to frame of reference provides a bridge for moving from theory to practice. The methods of choosing a frame of reference and the structure of the frame of reference itself equip the therapist with a way to use theoretical information as the foundation for intervention.

## STUDY QUESTIONS

1. Define what is meant by developmental, acquisitional, and operational theories? How are these categories the same? Different?
2. List the stages of Freud's theory? Of Erikson's personal-social stages? Compare and contrast their descriptions of each developmental stage.
3. Describe one infant behavior that would exemplify the sensorimotor period as defined by Piaget. Describe a behavior of a 5-year-old that would exemplify the preoperational period.
4. According to Piaget's description of cognitive development, how do concrete operations differ from formal operations?
5. What is a frame of reference? List two frames of reference that would be categorized as applications of:
   a. Operational theories
   b. Acquisitional theories
   c. Developmental theories
6. Briefly define the coping frame of reference. Explain how the coping frame of reference is an example of acquisitional theory.

## REFERENCES

Ainsworth, M.D.S (1979). Infant-mother attachment. *American Psychologist, 34,* 932.

Antonovsky, A. (1979). *Health, stress, and coping.* San Francisco: Jossey-Bass.

Ayres, A.J. (1972). *Sensory integration and learning disorders.* Los Angeles: Western Psychological Services.

Ayres, A.J. (1979). *Sensory integration and the child.* Los Angeles: Western Psychological Services.

Bandura, A. (1977a). *Social learning theory.* Englewood Cliffs, NJ: Prentice-Hall.

Bandura, A. (1977b). Self efficacy: toward a unifying theory of behavior change. *Psychological Review, 84,* 191-215.

Barash, D. (1979). *The whispering within.* New York: Harper & Row.

Bly, L. (1980). Abnormal motor development. In D. Slaton (Ed.). *Development of movement in infancy.* University of North Carolina at Chapel Hill, Division of Physical Therapy, May 19-22, 1980.

Bornstein, M.H. & Sigman, M.D. (1986). Continuity in mental development from infancy. *Child Development, 57,* 251-274.

Boulding, K. (1968). General systems theory: the skeleton of sceience. In W. Buckley (Ed.). *Modern systems research for the behavioral scientist* (pp. 3-10). Chicago: Aldine.

Carr, J.H. & Shepherd, R.B. (1987). A motor learning model for rehabilitation. In J.H. Carr, R.B. Shepherd, J. Gordon, A.M. Gentile, & J.N. Held (Eds.). *Movement science: foundations for physical therapy and rehabilitation* (pp. 31-91). Rockville, MD: Aspen.

Christiansen, C. (1994). *Ways of living: self-care strategies for special needs.* Rockville, MD: American Occupational Therapy Association.

Christiansen, C. (1991). Occupational therapy: Intervention for life performance. In C. Christiansen & C. Baum (Eds.). *Occupational therapy: overcoming human performance deficits* (pp. 3-43). Thorofare, NJ: Slack.

Colangelo, C.A. (1993). Biomechanical frame of reference. In P. Kramer & J. Hinojosa. *Frames of reference for pediatric occupational therapy* (pp. 233-305). Baltimore: Williams & Wilkins.

Collier, T. (1991). The screening process. In W. Dunn (Ed.). *Pediatric occupational therapy: facilitating effective service provision* (pp. 11-33). Thorofare, NJ: Slack.

DeGangi, G.A., Craft, P., & Castellan, J. (1991). Treatment of sensory, emotional, and attentional problems in regulatory disordered infants: Part 2. *Infants and Young Children, 3* (3), 9-19.

Erikson, E.H. (1963). *Childhood in society* (2nd ed.). New York: W.W. Norton.

Fisher, A.G, Murray, E.A., & Bundy, A.C. (1991). *Sensory integration: Theory and practice.* Philadelphia: F.A. Davis.

Flavell, J. (1985). *Cognitive development.* Englewood Cliffs, NJ: Prentice-Hall.

Frankel, V.H. & Burnstein, A.H. (1969). *Orthopaedic biomechanics.* Philadelphia: Lea & Febiger.

Freud, S. (1966). *Standard edition of the complete psychological works of Sigmund Freud.* London: Hogarth.

Gardner, H. (1978). *Developmental psychology: an introduction.* Boston: Little, Brown.

Gesell, A. & Amatruda, C. (1967). *Developmental diagnosis.* New York: Harper & Row.

Gibson, E.J. (1969). *Principles of perceptual learning and development.* New York: Appleton, Century, Crofts.

Gilfoyle, E.M., Grady, A.P., & Moore, J.C. (1990). *Children adapt* (2nd ed.). Thorofare, NJ: Slack.

Gilligan, C. (1982). *In a different voice: psychological theory and women's development.* Cambridge, MA: Harvard University.

Hall, C.S. & Lindzey, G. (1978). *Theories of personality* (3rd ed). New York: John Wiley & Sons.

Havighurst, R.J. (1972). *Developmental tasks and education.* New York: David McKay.

Hinojosa, J. & Kramer, K. (in press). Integrating children with disabilities into family play. In D. Parham (Ed.). *Play in pediatric occupational therapy.* Chicago: Mosby.

Illingworth, R.S. (1960). *The development of the infant and the young child, normal and abnormal.* London: E. & S. Livingstone.

Kaluger, G. & Kaluger, M. F. (1984). *Human development: the span of life* (3rd ed.). St. Louis: Mosby.

Keilhofner, G. (1992). *Conceptual foundations of occupational therapy.* Philadelphia: F.A. Davis.

Keilhofner, G. (1985). *A model of human occupation: theory and practice.* Baltimore: Williams & Wilkins.

Keilhofner, G. (1978). General systems theory: implications for theory and action in occupational therapy. *American Journal of Occupational Therapy, 32,* 637-645.

Keilhofner, G. & Burke, J. P. (1980). A model of human occupation. Part I. Conceptual framework and content. *American Journal of Occupational Therapy, 34,* 572-581.

Kimball, J.G. (1993). Sensory integrative frame of reference. In P. Kramer & J. Hinojosa (Eds.). *Frames of reference for pediatric occupational therapy,* (pp. 87-175). Baltimore: Williams & Wilkins.

Knoblock, H. & Pasamanick, D. (Eds.). (1975). *Gesell and Amatruda's developmental diagnosis* (3rd ed.). New York: Harper & Row.

Kohlberg, L. (1978). Revisions in the theory and practice of moral development. *New Directions in Child Development, 2,* 83-87.

Kokkonnen, J., Saukkonen, A. L., Timonen, E., Serlo, W., & Kinnunen, P. (1991). Social outcome of handicapped children as adults. *Developmental Medicine and Child Neurology, 33,* 1095-1100.

Kramer, P. & Hinojosa, J. (1993). *Frames of reference in pediatric occupational therapy.* Baltimore: Williams & Wilkins.

Lazarus R. S. & Folkman, S. (1984). *Stress, appraisal and coping.* New York: Springer-Verlag.

Llorens, L. A. (1976). *Application of developmental theory for health and rehabilitation.* Rockville, MD: American Occupational Therapy Association.

Llorens, L.A. (1969). Facilitating growth and development: the promise of occupational therapy. *American Journal of Occupational Therapy, 24,* 93-101.

Maier, H.W. (1969). *Three theories of child development: the contributions of Erik H. Erikson, Jean Piaget, and Robert R. Sears, and their applications* (rev. ed.). New York: Harper & Row.

Maslow, A.H. (1970). *Motivation and personality.* New York: Harper & Row.

Mosey, A.C. (1992). *Applied scientific inquiry in the health professions: an epistemological orientation.* Rockville, MD: American Occupational Therapy Association.

Mosey, A.C. (1986). *Psychosocial components of occupational therapy.* New York: Raven Press.

Mosey, A.C. (1981). *Occupational therapy: configuration of a profession.* New York: Raven Press.

Mosey, A.C. (1970). *Three frames of reference for mental health.* Thorofare, NJ: Slack.

Newell, A. & Simon, H. A. (1972). *Human problem solving.* Englewood Cliffs, NJ: Prentice-Hall.

Nye, R.D. (1981). *Three psychologies: perspectives from Freud, Skinner, and Rogers* (2nd ed.). Monterey, CA: Brooks/Cole.

Piaget, J. (1971). *Psychology and epistemology: towards a theory of knowledge.* New York: The Viking Press.

Piaget, J. & Inhelder, B. (1969). *The psychology of the child.* New York: Basic Books.

Reed, K.L. (1984). *Models of practice in occupational therapy.* Baltimore: Williams & Wilkins.

Reilly, M. (1974). *Play as exploratory behavior.* Beverly Hills, CA: Sage.

Reilly, M. (1962). Occupational therapy can be one of the great ideas of the 20th century medicine. *American Journal of Occupational Therapy, 16,* 1-9.

Rogers, C.R. (1969). *Freedom to learn.* Columbus, OH: Merrill.

Scherzer, A.L. & Tscharnuter, I. (1990). *Early diagnosis and treatment in cerebral palsy,* (2nd ed.). New York: Marcel Dekker.

Schmidt, R.A. (1975). A schema theory of discreet motor skill learning. *Psychological Review, 82,* 255-261.

Skinner, B.F. (1971) *Beyond freedom and dignity.* New York: Bantam Books.

Skinner, B.F. (1976). *Walden two.* New York: Macmillan.

Smith, J.M. (1978). *The concepts of sociobiology.* In G.S. Stent (Ed.). *Morality as a biological phenomenon.* Berkeley, CA: University of California Press.

Sprinthall, R.C. & Sprinthall, N.A. (1981). *Educational psychology: a developmental approach* (3rd ed.). Reading, MA: Addison Wesley.

*Stedman's Medical Dictionary* (25th ed.). (1994). Baltimore: Williams & Wilkins.

Thomas, A. (1981). Current trends in developmental theory. *American Journal of Orthopsychiatry, 51,* 580.

Turvey, M.T. (1977). Preliminaries to a theory of action with reference to vision. In R. Shaw & J. Bransford (Eds.). *Perceiving, acting and knowing.* Hillsdale, NJ: Lawrence Earlbaum Assoc.

von Bertalanffy, L. (1968). General systems theory: a critical review. *General Systems, 7,* 1-20

Werner, E.E. (1985). Stress and protective factors in children's lives. In A.R. Nichol (Ed.). *Longitudinal studies in child psychology and psychiatry.* New York: John Wiley & Sons.

Williams, M. & Lissner, H.R. (1962). *Biomechanics of human motion.* Philadelphia: W.B. Saunders.

Williamson, G.G., Szczepanski, M., & Zeitlin, S. (1993). In P. Kramer & J. Hinojosa (Eds.). *Frames of reference for pediatric occupational therapy* (pp. 395-436). Baltimore: Williams & Wilkins.

Wilson, E.O. (1978). Introduction: what is sociobiology? In M. Gregory, A. Silvers, & D. Sutch (Eds.). *Sociobiology and human nature.* San Francisco: Jossey-Bass.

Zeitlin, S. & Williamson, G. (1994). *Coping in young children: early intervention practices to enhance adaptive behavior and resilience.* Baltimore: Brookes.

CHAPTER

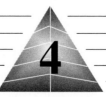

4

# The Developmental Process
## *Prenatal to Adolescence*

JANE CASE-SMITH ▲ SUSAN DENEGAN SHORTRIDGE

## KEY TERMS

▲ Developmental Domains
    Sensorimotor
    Cognitive
    Psychosocial
▲ Developmental Stages
    Neonate
    Infancy
    Early Childhood
    Middle Childhood
    Adolescence

## CHAPTER OBJECTIVES

1. Describe significant physiologic changes that occur at each developmental stage.
2. Identify the sequence of fine motor and gross motor skill development.
3. Using the theories of Piaget, explain the stages of cognitive development.
4. Based on Erikson's model of psychosocial development, describe the issues in each phase of psychosocial development.

Development is a continuous process. It proceeds stage by stage in an orderly sequence, despite individual variations. Increasingly complex behaviors unfold as the nervous system matures. Based on the theories of Gesell (Gesell et al. 1940), DiLeo (1977) characterized development as

    . . .a continuum. It advances upward and forward, not in a linear fashion, but more like a spiral, with its downward as well as upward cycle, yet always a bit more upward and a bit less downward, each stage representing a level of maturity whose features are qualitatively different yet derived from and dependent upon earlier stages (p. 3).

    Childhood is indeed the magic time in the life span when skills blossom. From the moment of conception through the adolescent years, the child passes through many facets of developmental growth. These facets include the physiologic, sensorimotor, cognitive, and psychosocial domains.

## PRENATAL PERIOD

Before birth three distinct phases of development occur in utero. These are the germinal stage, the embryonic stage, and the fetal stage.

    The first prenatal stage, which is the period of the ovum, or the *germinal stage,* lasts approximately 2 weeks. This period is initiated from the moment of fertilization to implantation in the uterus. The major emphasis during this period is in the change from a fertilized egg to a complex structure that will consist of 800 billion cells at birth. The structural changes that occur during cell differentiation are seen in the change from a zygote to a blastocyst. The blastocyst is a free-floating sphere that remains in the uterus for approximately 2 days. During this time cells cluster to one side of the blastocyst to form the embryonic disk from which the fetus will develop. The remaining cells form distinct layers. The upper layer, called the *ectoderm,* will become the infant's epidermis and its derivatives, that is, the sensory organs, brain, and spinal cord. The lower layer, the *endoderm,* will later form the digestive system, as well as the liver, pancreas, salivary glands, and respiratory system. The *mesoderm,* or middle layer, differentiates into the dermis, muscles, skeleton, and excretory and circulatory systems. The outer cells of the blastocyst, called the *trophoblast,* give rise to the protective and nutritive membranes

46

▲ Table 4-1  Prenatal Development During the Fetal Stage

| Stage (Month) | Physical Development | Motor Development |
|---|---|---|
| Third | Length = 3 in<br>Weight = 1 oz<br>Eyelids fused<br>Fingers and toes well formed<br>Fingernails growing<br>Sex differentiation | Kicks, makes fist, turns head; movement not recognizable by mother |
| Fourth | Length = 6 in<br>Weight = 6 oz<br>Most rapid growth | Sucking<br>Pushing with limbs<br>Quickening noted by mother |
| Fifth | Length = 12 in<br>Weight = 1 lb | Sleeps and wakes |
| Sixth | Length = 14 in<br>Weight = 2 lb<br>Red, wrinkled skin<br>Eyes unfused<br>Taste buds form<br>May survive outside womb | Grasp reflex present<br>Slight, irregular breathing<br>Hiccup |
| Seventh | Likely to survive outside the womb<br>Regular sleep and wake cycles | |
| Eighth and ninth | Wrinkled skin fills out with fat<br>Weight gain = ½ lb a week<br>All intrauterine development completed | Startle reflex present<br>Responds to light and sound<br>Motor action limited because of increasingly tight fit of uterus |

Modified from Annis, L.F. (1978). *The child before birth*. London: Cornell University Press.

of the intrauterine environment: the placenta, umbilical cord, and amniotic sac. Once this cell mass is fully implanted in the uterus it is called an embryo.

The second stage of prenatal development, the *embryonic stage,* is swift and lasts from 2 to 8 weeks. Although of short duration, this prenatal period is characterized by rapid growth. The fourth week shows an embryo with a beating heart. Between the fourth and the eighth week the eyes, ears, nose, and mouth become more clearly recognizable. By the end of the first 8 weeks after conception, 95 of the body parts have appeared through the continued process of differentiation. At the end of the prenatal period the embryo is recognizable as a tiny human.

The third prenatal period, the *fetal stage,* lasts from the end of the second month until birth. The appearance of the first bone cells at 8 weeks signals the name change from embryo to fetus. This is the longest of the prenatal stages. At this developmental period almost all of the structures and systems found in the newborn have developed, and many are already functional. These structures are primitive and must be developed further before they can be considered completely functional. This is perhaps most clearly seen in the primitive movements of the fetus. Self-initiated and localized movements are present. A fetus at 20 weeks is about 10 inches long and weighs about 10 ounces.

The primitive movements of the fetus continue to refine over the next 7 months. Milani-Comparetti (1981) described two abilities of the fetus that ready it for birth.

These include *fetal locomotion,* which allows the fetus to move around the fetal chamber to find the correct presentation for physiologic birth, and *fetal propulsion,* which is the active movement of the fetus involving an extension pattern of thrusting. The tremendous growth and development that occur during this fetal state are itemized in Table 4-1.

## Prenatal Influences

The interaction of heredity and environment strongly influences the prenatal period. An ideal environment for the fetus is one that includes an adequate supply of oxygen and nutrients through the functional placenta and umbilical cord, as well as freedom from disease organisms, toxic chemicals, abnormal genes or chromosomes, and maternal stress. Inherited abnormalities make up only a small proportion of birth defects.

Approximately 20% of known birth defects result from specific genetic causes. Another 20% or so are caused by environmental problems that affect the baby while it is developing inside the mother. The remaining 60% are caused by the interaction of hereditary and environmental factors (Howell, 1978).

The internal environment of the uterus is influenced by factors such as maternal nutrition and exposure to infection and bacteria. Pregnancy is also influenced by use of alcohol, coffee, and smoking. Excessive stress during pregnancy can also negatively affect the intrauterine environment (Stechler & Halton, 1982).

Because of the rapid growth during the embryonic period, the unborn child is most vulnerable to environmental insults and disruptions. The effects of many of these prenatal influences depend on the relative stage of development, that is, the point in the developmental sequence when the change in the prenatal environment occurs (Williamsen, 1979). Sensitive periods are times during which a particular influence or stimulus from another part of the environment evokes a specific response.

## INFANCY

### Physiologic Development

The neonate comes into the world looking more like a wrinkled old person than a Gerber baby. Typically the physical appearance of the neonate is characterized by reddish skin covered by vernix caseosa. The vernix caseosa is an oily protection against infection that dries in a few days' time. The head appears larger than the body and is usually elongated and bumpy as a result of molding during birth. In addition, the flat, broad nose that is formed of cartilage is often temporarily pushed out of shape by the birth process. Acrocyanosis, caused by sluggish peripheral circulation and mottling in response to cold, may also be present. The neonate's eyelids are usually puffy, making the eyes appear small. The eyes, smoky blue for the first month or two, change gradually to their permanent color. Hair may be abundant or scanty. Often the permanent hair color is different from that at birth. The external breasts and genitals of both males and females may look enlarged. This appearance is temporary and is caused by female hormones that passed to the baby before birth.

The average weight of the neonate is 7 lb 2 oz. During the first few days of life most neonates lose 5% to 10% of their body weight because of the passage of meconium and urine, as well as delays in feeding. This weight shift is usually regained by 10 days of age. The average length of the neonate is between 19 and 22 inches.

After birth the full-term neonate must make profound adjustments to his or her new life. After 9 months of total dependency on the mother, the neonate must cope with a new environment and must independently master respiration, circulation, digestion, and temperature regulation.

The traditional cry at birth signals a message to the mother that the baby has arrived and is inspiring air for the first time. Breathing is irregular, rapid, and shallow, and marked by abdominal rather than chest movements. During the first few days after birth the neonate experiences periods of coughing and sneezing. This serves to clear the mucus and amniotic fluid from the airways.

The onset of breathing also marks a significant change in the neonate's circulatory system. A change in the vascular resistance alters the blood flow that once passed through the placenta. Closure of a valve between the right and left atrium *(foramen ovale)* and a vessel that leads from the aorta to the pulmonary artery *(ductus arteriosus)* occurs within the first 10 days of life. In addition, the lungs continue to expand.

Before birth the placenta provided nourishment and oxygen for the fetus. After birth the neonate must obtain nourishment from the mother in an external environment. The initial move toward feeding behavior is complemented by hunger contractions, rooting, sucking, and swallowing mechanisms that are present at birth and stimulate physiologic maturation.

The neonate's temperature regulation system also gradually changes. Within the uterus the infant's skin was maintained at a constant temperature. The neonate's subcutaneous fat layer is inadequate for insulation, and the large skin surface area contributes to heat loss. Swaddling is frequently used to maintain temperature.

### Sensorimotor Development

From the moment of birth the neonate shows specific behavioral states of arousal. Brazelton (1973) identified six behavioral states that characterize neonates: (1) deep sleep, (2) light sleep, (3) drowsy, quiet, (4) alert, active, awake, (5) fussy, and (6) crying. The infant typically makes gradual transitions from one state to the next. The infant's response to stimulation is highly influenced by his or her behavioral state.

#### Gross Motor Skills

The neonate's motor responses contribute to his or her organization of the world and to survival within its boundaries. The neonate's gross motor activity is developed from movement patterns that began in the intrauterine environment and from the maturation of reflex behavior that is primarily controlled from the spinal and brainstem level. The neonate is capable of more than reflex behavior. He or she demonstrates orientation, attention, and habituation to visual, auditory, and tactile stimuli.

After the first month of life the neonate is identified as an infant. At this time of life, motor responses in head control, sitting, rolling, and locomotion continue to develop from simple to complex skills (Table 4-2). At 4 weeks the infant can move his or her head side to side. Head lag is noted in the pull to sitting position; however, the infant is able to lift the head long enough to turn it while on the stomach (prone position) to attain a more comfortable cheek-resting posture. By 16 weeks the infant, when prone, is able to lift the head at a 45-degree angle to the supporting surface. Visual stimulation and an increased ability to move against gravity allow the infant to attain a more erect head posture. The infant's progression continues so that the infant is able to support himself or herself propped on the forearms, and, finally, the infant is able to support himself

▲ Table 4-2   Sensorimotor Development: Mobility and Stability

| Age | Gross Motor Skill |
|---|---|
| **PRONE POSITION** | |
| 0-2 mo | Turns head side to side |
| | Lifts head momentarily |
| | Bends hips with bottom in air |
| 3-4 mo | Lifts head and sustains in midline |
| | Rotates head freely when up |
| | Able to bear weight on forearms |
| | Able to tuck chin and gaze at hands in forearm prop |
| | Attempts to shift weight on forearms, resulting in shoulder collapse |
| 5-6 mo | Shifts weight on forearms and reaches forward |
| | Bears weight and shifts weight on extended arms |
| | Legs are closer together and thighs roll inward toward natural alignment |
| | Hips are flat on surface |
| | Equilibrium reactions are present |
| 5-8 mo | Airplane posturing in prone position; chest and thighs lift off surface |
| 7-8 mo | Pivots in prone position |
| | Moves to prone position to sit |
| 9 mo | Begins to dislike prone position |
| **SUPINE POSITION** | |
| 0-3 mo | Head held to one side |
| | Able to turn head side to side |
| 3-4 mo | Holds head in midline |
| | Chin is tucked and neck lengthens in back |
| | Legs come together |
| | Lower back flattens against the floor |
| 4-5 mo | Head lag is gone when pulled to a sitting position |
| | Hands are together in space |
| 5-6 mo | Lifts head independently |
| | Brings feet to mouth |
| | Brings hands to feet |
| | Able to reach for toy with one or both hands |
| | Hands are predominantly open |
| 7-8 mo | Equilibrium reactions are present |
| **ROLLING** | |
| 3-4 mo | Rolls from prone position to side accidentally because of poor control of weight shift |
| | Rolls from supine position to side |
| 5-6 mo | Rolls from prone to supine position |
| | Rolls from supine position to side with right and left leg performing independent movements |
| | Rolls from supine to prone position with right and left leg performing independent movements |
| 6-14 mo | Rolls segmentally with roll initiated by the head, shoulder, or hips |
| **CREEPING** | |
| 7 mo | Crawls forward on belly |
| 7-10 mo | Reciprocal creep |
| 10-11 mo | Creeps on hands and feet |
| 11-12 mo | Creeps well |
| **SITTING** | |
| 0-3 mo (held in sitting) | Head bobs in sitting |
| | Back is rounded |
| | Hips are apart, turned out, and bent |

Modified from Bly, L. (1993). *Normal development in the first year of life*. Tucson: Therapy Skill Builders; Illingworth, R.S. (1991). *The normal child: some problems of the early years and their treatment* (10th ed.). Edinburgh: Churchill-Livingstone; Knobloch, H., Pasamanick, B. (1974). *Gesell and Amatruda's developmental diagnosis: the evaluation and management of normal and abnormal neuropsychological development in infancy and early childhood*. Hagertown, MD: Harper & Row; and Gilfoyle, E., Grady, A., & Moore, J. (1990). *Children adapt*. Thorofare, NJ: Slack.

*Continued.*

| Age | Gross Motor Skill |
| --- | --- |
| **SITTING—cont'd** | |
| 3-4 mo (held in sitting) | Head is steady |
| | Chin tucks; able to gaze at floor |
| | Sits with less support |
| | Hips are bent and shoulders are in front of hips |
| 5-6 mo (supports self in sitting) | Sits alone momentarily |
| | Increased extension in back |
| | Sits by propping forward on arms |
| | Wide base, legs are bent |
| | Periodic use of "high guard" position |
| | Protective responses present when falling to the front |
| 5-10 mo (sits alone) | Sits alone steadily, initially with wide base of support |
| | Able to play with toys in sitting position |
| 6-11 mo | Gets to sitting position from prone position |
| 7-8 mo | Equilibrium reactions are present |
| | Able to rotate upper body while lower body remains stationary |
| | Protective responses are present when falling to the side |
| 8-10 mo | Sits well without support |
| | Legs are closer; full upright position, knees straight |
| | Increased variety of sitting positions, including "w" sit and side sit |
| | Difficult fine motor tasks may prompt return to wide base of support |
| 9-18 mo | Rises from supine position by first rolling over to stomach then pushing up into four-point position |
| 10-12 mo | Protective extension backwards, first with bent elbows then straight elbows |
| | Able to move in and out of sitting position into other positions |
| 11-12 mo | Trunk control and equilibrium responses are fully developed in sitting position |
| | Further increase in variety of positions possible |
| 11-24 mo + | Rises from supine by first rolling to side then pushing up into sitting position |
| **STANDING** | |
| 0-3 mo | When held in standing position, takes some weight on legs |
| 2-3 mo | When held in standing position, legs may give way |
| 3-4 mo | Bears some weight on legs, but must be held proximally |
| | Head is up in midline, no chin tuck |
| | Pelvis and hips are behind shoulders |
| | Legs are apart and turned outward |
| 5-10 mo | Stands while holding on to furniture |
| 5-6 mo | Increased capability to bear weight |
| | Decreased support needed; may be held by arms or hands |
| | Legs are still spread apart and turned outward |
| | Bounces in standing position |
| 6-12 mo | Pulls to standing position at furniture |
| 8-9 mo | Rotates the trunk over the lower extremities |
| | Lower extremities are more active in pulling to a standing position |
| | Pulls to a standing position by kneeling, then half-kneeling |
| 9-13 mo | Pulls to standing position with legs only, no longer needs arms |
| | Stands alone momentarily |
| 12 mo | Equilibrium reactions are present in standing |
| **WALKING** | |
| 8 mo | Cruises sideways |
| 8-18 mo | Walks with two hands held |
| 9-10 mo | Cruises around furniture, turning slightly in intended direction |
| 9-17 mo | Takes independent steps, falls easily |
| 10-14 mo | Walking: stoops and recovers in play |
| 11 mo | Walks with one hand held |
| | Reaches for furniture out of reach when cruising |
| | Cruises in either direction, no hesitation |
| 15 mo | Able to start and stop in walking |
| 18 mo | Seldom falls |
| | Runs stiffly with eyes on ground |

or herself by extending the arms and resting on the palms of his hands. This developmental sequence of head and trunk control is assisted by the emerging righting reactions and maturing postural control.

Rolling is usually the infant's first method of mobility. The body righting on head reactions enable trunk movement to follow head movement. Usually the infant develops the ability to roll first from the back (supine position) to the side, then from the stomach to the side, and then from the stomach to the back. By 7 months the infant is able to roll voluntarily from stomach to back and back to stomach.

The neonate of 4 weeks of age sits with a rounded back and a head that is erect only momentarily. In the infant, however, more muscle extension exists, and the infant's ability to control the head and trunk results in a more upright sitting posture. The 7-month-old can sit with back support provided by a chair or a pillow or with the infant's arms propped forward in a tripod posture. By 8 to 9 months the infant can sit erect and unsupported for several minutes and soon progresses from a sitting to prone posture. By 12 months the infant can rotate and pivot when sitting without losing his or her balance. The infant can attain a creeping position from sitting.

Creeping refers to four-point mobility with only the hands and knees on the floor. This reciprocal limb motion requires coordination of the two sides of the body, good shoulder and pelvic stability, and control of trunk rotation. Mature creeping ability is an excellent example of the development of controlled mobility imposed on postural stability. Further description of postural control is found in Chapter 11. Through practice of creeping the child develops trunk flexibility and rotation (Figure 4-1). The emergence of equilibrium and protective reactions assists the 10- to 12-month-old infant in creeping as fast as others can walk.

The ability to stand is influenced by the emergence of postural stability. When the infant's weight bearing is secure, a 7-month-old baby bounces in delight at the new skill and practices the freedom of movement from flexion to extension. The infant begins to prepare for the upright posture by first attaining a kneel-standing posture, then progressing to a half-kneel, and finally to a full-standing position. A 10-month-old baby practices rising and lowering postures by supporting himself or herself on furniture. At this time the infant becomes interested in objects denied him or her. This interest stimulates an even stronger desire to stand when the objects are moved out of reach. Cruising at 12 months of age first occurs when the infant learns to shift his or her weight onto one leg and step to the side with the other. The infant soon takes small forward steps while holding onto furniture or the parent's finger.

The infant's first efforts of unsupported forward movement are often seen in short, erratic steps, unnecessary lifting of the legs, and uncontrollable excitement. By 18 months the infant moves throughout the world with the help of a relatively immature balance system, a high protective guard of the upper extremities, and a wide-based gait. When hurried, the infant may select to use the more reliable creeping pattern. However, with maturational changes in the infant's body proportions and the development of strength and coordination, walking soon becomes the primary means of mobility. Walking brings forth new avenues of exploration and a sense of autonomy (Figure 4-2). The parent must now protect this moving, explorative infant more than previously.

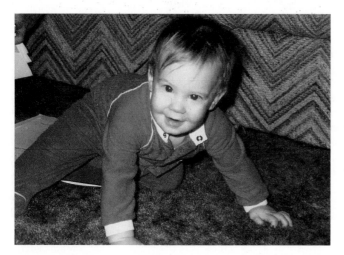

**Figure 4-1** Creeping allows the child to develop trunk rotation and transitional movements.

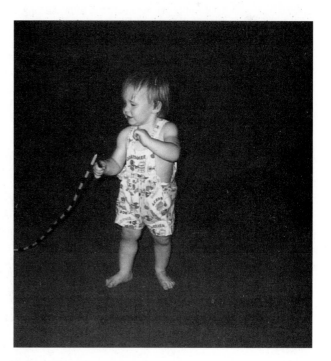

**Figure 4-2** Infant's first stance is characterized by a wide base and high guard arm position.

▲ Table 4-3   Sensorimotor Development

| Age | Motor Skill |
| --- | --- |
| **REACHING** | |
| 0-2 mo | Visual regard of objects |
| 1-3 mo | Swipes at objects |
| 1-4½ mo | Alternating glance from hand to object |
| 1-5 mo | Alternating gaze from one hand to the other |
| 2-6 mo | Inspects own hands |
| | Reaches for, but may not contact, object |
| 3½-4½ mo | Visually directed reaching |
| 3½-6 mo | Hands are oriented to object |
| | Rapid reach for object without contact |
| 3½-12 mo | Circuitous reach out to side |
| | Straight approach in reach |
| 4 mo | Shoulders come down to natural level |
| | Hands are together in space |
| | Sitting: bilateral backhand approach with wrist turned so thumb is down |
| 5 mo | Prone: bilateral approach, hands slide forward |
| | Two-handed corralling of object |
| 5-6 mo | Elbow is in front of shoulder joint |
| | Developing isolated voluntary control of forearm rotation |
| 6 mo | Prone: reaches with one hand while weight bearing on the other forearm |
| | Elbow is extended, wrist is straight, midway between supination and pronation |
| 7 mo | Prone: reaches with one hand while weight bearing on the other extended arm |
| 7-8 mo | Experiments with forearm rotation by stabilizing against rib cage |
| 8-9 mo | Unilateral direct approach, reach and grasp single continuous movement |
| 9 mo | Controls supination with upper arm in any position, if trunk is stable |
| 10 mo | Wrist extended, appropriate finger extension |
| 11-12 mo | Voluntary supination, upper arm in any position |
| **GRASP** | |
| 0-3 mo | Hands are predominantly closed |
| 2-7 mo | Object is clutched between little and ring fingers and palm |
| 3-3½ mo | Hands clasped together often |
| 3-7 mo | Able to hold a small object in each hand |
| 4 mo | Hands are partly open |
| 4-4½ mo | Hands are open in anticipation of contact |
| 4-6 mo | Hands are predominantly open |
| 4-8 mo | Partial thumb opposition on a cube |
| | Attempts to secure minute objects |
| | Picks up cube with ease |
| 5-9 mo | Rakes or scoops minute objects |
| 6-7 mo | Objects held in palm by fingers and opposed thumb (radial palmar grasp) |
| 6-10 mo | Picks up minute objects with several fingers and thumb |
| 7-12 mo | Precisely picks up minute objects |
| 8 mo | Minute objects are held between the side of index finger and thumb (lateral scissors) |
| 8-9 mo | Objects are held with opposed thumb and fingertips; space is visible between palm and object |
| 9-10 mo | Small objects are held between the thumb and index finger, first near middle of index (inferior pincer) finger and later between pads of thumb and index finger with thumb opposed (pincer) |
| 10 mo | Pokes with index finger |
| 12 mo | Small objects are held between the thumb and index finger, near tips, thumbs opposed (fine pincer) |
| 12-18 mo | Crayon is held in the fist with the thumb up |
| 2 yr | Crayon is held with fingers, hand on top of tool, forearm turned so thumb is directed downward (digital pronate) |

▲ Table 4-3   Sensorimotor Development—cont'd

| Age | Motor Skill |
|---|---|
| **RELEASE** | |
| 0-1 mo | No release; grasp reflex is strong |
| 1-4 mo | Involuntary release |
| 4 mo | Mutual fingering in midline |
| 4-8 mo | Transfers object from hand to hand |
| 5-6 mo | Two-stage transfer; taking hand grasps before releasing hand lets go |
| 6-7 mo | One-stage transfer; taking hand and releasing hand perform actions simultaneously |
| 7-9 mo | Volitional release |
| 7-10 mo | Presses down on surface to release |
| 8 mo | Releases above a surface with wrist flexion |
| 9-10 mo | Releases into a container with wrist straight |
| 10-14 mo | Clumsy release into small container; hand rests on edge of container |
| 12-15 mo | Precise, controlled release into small container with wrist extended |

Modified from Halverson, H.M. (1931). An experimental study of prehension in infants by means of systematic cinema records. *Genetic Psychology Monographs, 10,* 107-286; Gesell, A. & Amatruda, C.S. (1947). *Developmental diagnosis.* New York: Harper & Row; Knobloch, H. & Pasamanick, B. (1974). *Gesell and Amatruda's developmental diagnosis: the evaluation and management of normal and abnormal neuropsychological development in infancy and early childhood.* Hagertown, MD: Harper & Row; and Case-Smith (1995). Grasp, release, and bimanual skills in the first two years of life. In A. Henderson & C. Pihoski (Eds.). *Hand function in the child: foundation for remediation* (pp. 113-135). St. Louis: Mosby.

## Fine Motor Skills

The infant's hands provide a means to reach out to the world and discover it. As in all development, sequences of motor development do not occur independent of each other. The development of mobility and hand function occurs simultaneously, each progressing chronologically toward maturation (Table 4-3).

The grasping reflex is present at birth and allows the infant to have automatic contact with anything placed in the palm. The first 12 weeks involve contacting objects more with the eyes than with the hands. Infants look, stare, and track objects within their visual fields. By the fourth month infants develop more voluntary control of hand and arm movement. The first voluntary, physical, prehensile activity is swiping at objects. By 5 months the accuracy of reaching toward objects increases, although the grasping skill is limited to a precarious ulnar palmar grasp in which the fifth and fourth fingers press the object (Figure 4-3). By 6 months a direct unilateral reach (with one arm) is observed. The development of grasp follows a sequence from primitive grasp within the palm to more precise grasp using the fingertips. The 3- to 4- month-old infant grasps an object within his palm using a primitive squeeze in which the fingers move as a unit to squeeze the object into the palm. This grasp includes no active thumb involvement. At 4 to 5 months a palmar grasp is displayed. The fingers press the object against the palm and an adducted thumb. At 6 months the infant uses a radial palmar grasping patterns in which the first two fingers hold the object against the thumb (Figure 4-3). At this time the infant secures small objects using a raking motion of the fingers.

Grasp rapidly changes between 7 and 12 months. A radial digital grasp emerges in which the thumb opposes the index and middle fingertips. At about 9 months the wrist extends while grasping a small object such as a cube, and the mature grasping pattern is demonstrated. With this ability the infant also learns to use a pincer grasp in which the distal pad of the index finger opposes the distal pad of the thumb. The first pincer grasp pattern is termed an *inferior pincer* and is characterized by the thumb opposing the side of the index finger. By 12 months the infant grasps a raisin with a mature pincer grasp in which the thumb opposes the index finger and the wrist extends.

Voluntary release develops at about 8 months. The first release is awkward and is characterized by full extension of all fingers. The infant becomes interested in dropping objects, and cognitive development of object permanence reinforces the infant's desire to practice release. By 10 months the infant releases an object into a container, and by 12 months he or she consistently places objects in containers. A favorite game of the 1-year-old child is placing objects into a container, dumping them out, and then beginning the activity again.

Voluntary reach, grasp, and release expand the horizons of the infant's exploration and promote bilateral hand coordination. The fine motor play of the infant in the first year of life includes mouthing, banging, and shaking objects. By 12 months the infant is interested in combining objects and in exploring their functional use. Practice in combining objects is enhanced by the development of controlled and well-graded release, which occurs between 12 and 15 months. Between 15 and 18 months the infant demonstrates release of a raisin into a small bottle and the ability to stack

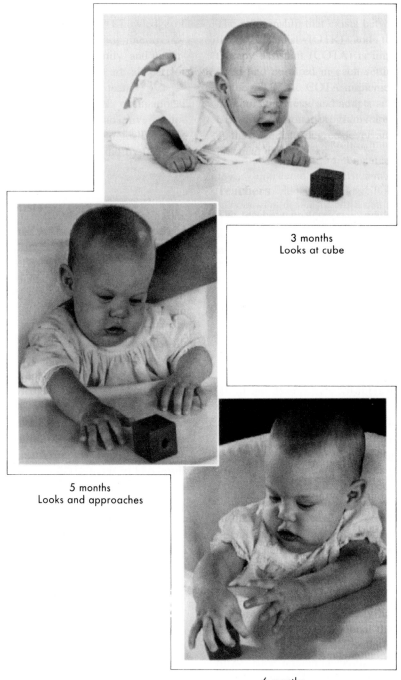

3 months
Looks at cube

5 months
Looks and approaches

6 months
Looks and crudely grasps with whole hand

**Figure 4-3** Developmental progression of prehensile behavior. (From Ingalls, A.J. & Salerno, M.C. [1983]. *Maternal and child health nursing* [3rd ed.]. St. Louis: Mosby.)

two cubes. The infant can place large, simple puzzle pieces and pegs. As the infant approaches 2 years, he or she acquires the ability to discriminate simple forms and shapes. Stacking blocks is enjoyed and contributes to the development of arm control in space, precision grasp without support, controlled release, spatial relations, and depth percep-

tion. For a detailed discussion of the development of fine motor skills, see Chapter 12. Chapter 14 provides additional information about the development of visual perception. A detailed description of the development of oral motor skills is found in Chapter 16.

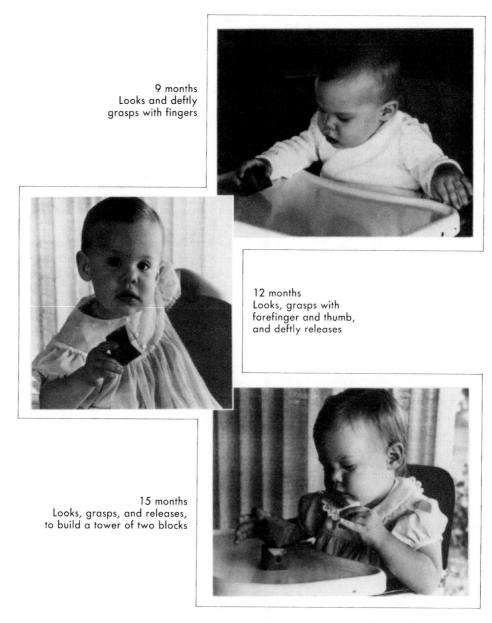

9 months
Looks and deftly
grasps with fingers

12 months
Looks, grasps with
forefinger and thumb,
and deftly releases

15 months
Looks, grasps, and releases,
to build a tower of two blocks

**Figure 4-3, cont'd.**    Developmental progression of prehensile behavior.

## Cognitive Development

The cognitive development of the infant, as described through Piaget's sensorimotor period, has already been discussed in Chapter 3. The cognitive process in this period is first initiated through reflexive reactions to stimuli and later becomes more purposeful as the infant accidentally discovers behaviors that affect the environment. The infant's attention is gradually directed away from his or her own body as the infant becomes aware of the results of his or her activity. This process proceeds to experimentation as the infant tries to produce new events. The infant's developing cognitive repertoire includes schemata for the actions of his or her own body and the concept that objects in the environment are influenced by his or her body's actions. The infant does not yet understand the effects of other persons on objects. Table 4-4 lists the major milestones in cognitive development in the first 2 years of life.

Although most cognitive development is expressed through sensorimotor exploration, the development of communication is also highly related to the infant's cognitive abilities. Prelinguistic speech is a central theme and proceeds through distinct stages. The major stages of prespeech that progress from undifferentiated crying to expressive jargon are listed in Table 4-5.

Physiologic maturation is central to the development of

▲ Table 4-4    Major Milestones in Cognitive Development

| Age | Developments |
|---|---|
| **EARLY OBJECT USE** | |
| 3-6 mo | Focuses on action performed by objects (banging, shaking) |
| 6-9 mo | Begins to explore characteristics of objects |
| | Range of schemes expands (e.g., pulling, turning, poking, tearing) |
| 8-9 mo | Begins to combine objects in relational play (e.g., objects in a container) |
| 9-12 mo | Begins to see the relation between complex actions and consequences (opening doors, putting lids on containers) |
| | Differential use of schemes according to the toy played with, functional use of toys (e.g., pushes cars, throws ball) |
| 12 mo + | Acts on objects with a variety of schemes |
| 12-15 mo | Links schemes in simple combinations (puts person in car and pushes car) |
| **PROBLEM-SOLVING SKILLS** | |
| 6-9 mo | Finds object after watching it disappear |
| | Uses movement as a means to attain an end |
| | Anticipates movement of objects in space |
| | Attends to environmental consequences of actions |
| | Repeats actions to repeat consequences |
| 9-12 mo | Demonstrates tool use after demonstration |
| | Uses goal-directed behavior |
| | Performs an action to produce a result |
| 12-15 mo | Uses an adult to achieve a goal |
| | Attempts to activate simple mechanisms |
| | Rotates and examines three-dimensional aspects of an object |
| | Uses nonsystematic trial-and-error problem-solving |
| 18-21 mo | Attends to shapes of things and uses them appropriately |
| | Uses some foresight before acting |
| **SYMBOLIC PLAY** | |
| 12-16 mo | Simple pretend play directed toward self (eating, sleeping) |
| 12-18 mo | Can focus pretend play on animate and inanimate objects and others |
| | Combines simple schemes in acting out familiar activity |
| 18-24 mo | Increased use of nonrealistic objects in pretending (similar to real) |
| | Can have inanimate objects perform actions (doll washes self) |

Modified from Cohen, M.A. & Gross, P.J. (1979). *The developmental resource: behavioral sequences for assessment and program planning.* New York: Basic Books; Fewell, R.R. (1983). *Play assessment scale* (research ed.). Seattle: University of Washington; Nicholich, L. (1977). Beyond sensorimotor intelligence: assessment of symbolic maturity through analysis of pretend play. *Merril-Palmer Quarterly, 16,* 136-141; and Linder, T. (1990). *Transdisciplinary play-based assessment: a functional approach to working with young children.* Baltimore: Brookes.

▲ Table 4-5    Stages of Prespeech

| Stage | Speech Development |
|---|---|
| 1 | Undifferentiated crying: reflexive, produced by expiration of breath |
| 2 | Differentiated crying: varied patterns and intensities; pitches signal hunger, sleep, anger, or pain |
| 3 | Cooing: chance movement of vocal cords produces simple sounds; first sounds are vowels; first consonant is b (6 weeks) |
| 4 | Babbling: repetition of simple vowel and consonant sounds (3 to 4 months) |
| 5 | Lallation: accidental repetition of what has been heard (6 to 12 months) |
| 6 | Echolalia: conscious imitation of sounds (9 to 10 months) |
| 7 | Expressive jargon: meaningful utterances that sound like sentences with pauses, inflections, and rhythms (18 months) |

Modified from Lennenberg, E.H. (1967). *Biological functions of language.* New York: John Wiley & Sons.

expressive speech. The pseudo-cry and cooing are made possible by changes in the infant's vocal equipment. The larynx, which contains the vocal cords, changes as the child grows, allowing the infant to produce a greater variety of sounds. Because the ability to produce different sounds is evidenced in crying, lack of crying ability in the infant may indicate neurologic impairment.

## Psychosocial Development

The infant's emotional transition from the protective, neutral womb is dramatically changed at the moment of birth. The sense of basic trust or mistrust becomes a primary theme in the child's affective development. The primary concern of the infant is to maintain body functions of the cardiovascular, respiratory, and gastrointestinal systems. As the infant matures, the focus then moves to increasing competence in interacting with the environment through his or her body functions. According to Erikson (1963) "the first demonstration of social trust in the baby is in the ease of his feeding, the depth of sleep, the relaxation of his bowels." The infant's development of trust is highly dependent on his or her relationship with primary caregivers.

The basic trust relationship has varying degrees of involvement. Feelings of maternal love are not endowed but are acquired over time within experiences between the mother and child. This is seen in the progression of physical contact between the parent and infant. Klaus and Kennell (1976) discussed the importance of the en face position and stressed the importance of this early eye-to-eye contact between parents and the infant in the attachment process.

The importance of the quality of maternal relationships was demonstrated earlier by Harlow and Zimmerman (1959) in their studies of infant attachment relationships among rhesus monkeys. Their research demonstrated that it was not the mere provision of nutrients but rather the close body contact that was essential to the attachment process.

Ainsworth (1973) discussed the attachment process in terms of four stages of attachment. These include undiscriminating social responses (2 to 3 months), discriminating social responses (4 to 6 months), active initiative in seeking proximity and contact (7 months), and goal-corrected partnership or the ability to alter mother's plans to better fit the infant's. Precursors of attachment affect the first two stages of the development of attachment and include both reflexive and early sensorimotor behaviors such as rooting-sucking, looking, listening, smiling, vocalizing, crying, grasping, and clinging.

Fathers are increasingly participating in the birth process and in the caregiving roles. Greenberg and Morris (1974) identified strong evidence of paternal feelings and involvement with the neonate by new fathers. The father-neonate bond was characterized by engrossment, suggesting that fathers develop feelings of preoccupation, absorption, and interest in their neonate within the first 3 days after birth. Some studies have found differences between early mother-infant and father-infant interactions. Fathers tend to engage in more physical, vigorous types of play, whereas mothers tend to engage in more verbal and toy-mediated play (Power, 1985). Table 4-6 lists the sequence of development of early social skills.

## EARLY CHILDHOOD
### Physiological Development

Preschoolers are much more mobile than infants. The preschool period is marked by the development of autonomy, the beginning of expressive language, and sphincter control. The growth rate of the preschooler is less dramatic than that of the infant. The child at this age is still top heavy, with a large cranium and small lower jaw, similar to the cupids in Renaissance paintings. The abdomen sticks out because a relatively short trunk must accommodate the internal organs. The posture may appear lordotic.

Physiologic differences from the mature adult are noted in the characteristic shape, position, and structure of the middle ear. The eustachian tube, which is shorter, more horizontal, and wider than that of the adult, allows free passage to invading organisms and thus increased susceptibility to ear infections in the younger child. The digestive tract also shows lack of full maturation. The shape of the stomach is straight and has less than half the capacity of the average adult stomach. This structural disparity results in frequent stomach upsets in the preschooler.

The special senses demonstrate noteworthy differences as well. The taste buds are more numerous and are located on

▲ Table 4-6　Psychosocial Skill Development

| Age | Skill |
|---|---|
| **ATTACHMENT, SEPARATION, AND INDIVIDUATION** | |
| 5-8 mo | Shows active differentiation of strangers |
| 6-8 mo | Recognizes self in mirror |
| 7-8 mo | Shows special dependence on mother—wants food, attention, stimulation, and approval from her, even when others are available |
| | As long as child sees parent, he or she plays contentedly. As parent leaves the room, child cries and tries to follow |
| 5-8 mo | Shows mild to severe anxiety of separation |
| 10-12 mo | Shy period passes, eager to go out into the world |
| 12+ mo | Distinguishes self from others |
| | Reacts sharply to separation from parent |
| | Reacts to emotions expressed by parents and others |
| 12-15 mo | Uses mother for emotional "refueling" |
| 15-18 mo | Moves away from parent as home base into widening world |
| | Brings toys to share with parent |
| 18-24 mo | Demands proximity of familiar adult |
| | Alternates between clinging and resistance to familiar adult |
| | Refers to self by name |
| | Conscious of own acts as they are related to adult approval or disapproval |
| **SOCIAL RELATIONS WITH PEERS** | |
| 6-8 mo | Infant-to-infant interactions increase |
| 9-12 mo | Responds differently to children and adults |
| 12+ mo | Begins to prefer interactions with peers |
| 12-15 mo | Contacts with peers center around an object |
| 15-18 mo | Simple actions and contingent responses between peers |
| 18-24 mo | Spends most group time in solitary activity, watching other children |
| | Interactive sequences become longer until role sharing and turn taking are evident |
| 24+ mo | Intense watchfulness of peers |
| | Child imitates peers |
| | Child watches, points at, takes toys of other child |
| | Parallel, noninteractive play predominates |

Modified from Cohen, M.A. & Gross, P.J. (1979). *The developmental resource: behavioral sequences for assessment and program planning.* New York: Basic Books; and Linder, T. (1990). *Transdisciplinary play-based assessment: a functional approach to working with young children.* Baltimore: Brookes.

the side of the cheeks and the throat as well as on the tongue. Because of the immaturity of the macula of the retina, the young child is farsighted.

Significant physiologic changes occur in the physiologic pathways necessary for sphincter control. Thus the preschooler is capable of entering and successfully complet-

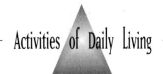

## Activities of Daily Living

### DRESSING

2 years: Puts on shoes, socks, and shorts. Takes off shoes and socks.

3 years: Dresses and undresses fully; needs help with buttons, back and front, left and right shoe.

4 years: Can manage buttons completely.

5 years: Can dress completely and often ties shoelaces, but cannot tie a necktie.

### SELF-FEEDING

2 years: Can use a spoon well enough to feed self without accidentally inverting it.

3 years: Can feed self with little or no spilling. Drinks from a cup with one hand. Can pour from a pitcher into cup if not too heavy. Feeding skills are now learned and become part and parcel of social skills in accordance with family standards of table manners.

4 years: Holds fork in fingers. Can spoon soup without spilling.

5 years: Uses knife for spreading. Uses blunt knife to cut soft foods.

Modified from Gesell, A. & Amatruda, C.S. (1954). *Developmental diagnosis* (2nd ed.). New York: Harper & Row.

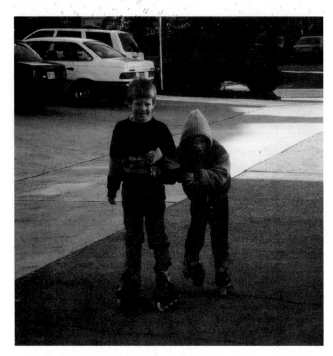

**Figure 4-4** Preschool children demonstrate sufficient equilibrium for roller skating.

ing toilet training. This is evidenced in the change from bulky diapers to training pants.

## Sensorimotor Development

Preschoolers are amazingly competent individuals. They initially walk with a wide stance and body sway; however, as they physically mature, preschoolers' repertoire of motor activity steadily advances. Coordination and manipulation refine as evidenced by increasing skills in activities of daily living (see box above).

### Gross Motor Skills

By age 2, the toddler walks with an increased stride length and increased control of weight shift in the anterior-posterior direction. The 4-year-old child demonstrates a walking pattern similar to that of an adult. Running, which requires greater strength and balance than walking, emerges between 3 and 4 years of age. Running is also characterized by trunk rotation and arm swing. By 5 to 6 years of age the mature running pattern develops.

Walking upstairs precedes walking downstairs. One reason for skills emerging in this order is that walking down-

stairs requires graded control of knee flexion. By 2 years of age the child climbs stairs without holding onto the rail or a hand, and by 2½ the child climbs downstairs without support. The 3½-year-old child walks up and down stairs alternating feet and without support.

Running and stair climbing become possible in part because of the child's increasing balance. Emerging balance can be observed as the 2-year-old stands on one foot for 1 second. By 5 years of age the child can maintain a one-foot stance with hands on his hips for 10 seconds; he can also walk forward and backward across a balance beam. Figure 4-4 shows two preschoolers in their first pairs of skates, additional evidence of the maturation of bipedal equilibrium reactions.

Jumping is first observed in the 2-year-old child. This skill requires both strength and balance. By 3 years the child can jump easily from a step and between 3 and 6 years learns to jump forward. Hopping requires greater strength and balance than jumping and is first observed at 3½ years. Skipping is the most difficult gross motor pattern; it involves sequencing a rhythmic pattern that includes a step and a hop. This step-hop pattern is first observed in galloping (in the 3- to 4-year-old child). A coordinated skipping pattern is not observed until 5 years of age. Table 4-7 lists the sequence of development of stair climbing and jumping/hopping skills.

***Ball skills.*** The first ball skills develop in early childhood. The first pattern of throwing to emerge involves a pushing motion, with the greatest movement occur-

▲ Table 4-7   Development of Stair Climbing and Jumping/Hopping Skills

| Age | Skill |
|---|---|
| **STAIR CLIMBING** | |
| 15 mo | Creeps up stairs |
| 18-24 mo | Walks up stairs while holding on |
| | Walks down stairs while holding on |
| 18-23 mo | Creeps backwards down stairs |
| 2-2½+ yr | Walks up stairs without support, marking time |
| | Walks down stairs without support, marking time |
| 2½-3 yr | Walks up stairs, alternating feet |
| 3-3½ yr | Walks down stairs, alternating feet |
| **JUMPING AND HOPPING** | |
| 2 yr | Jumps down from step |
| 2½+ yr | Hops on one foot, few steps |
| 3 yr | Jumps off floor with both feet |
| 3-5 yr | Jumps over objects |
| 3½-5 yr | Hops on one foot |
| 3-4 yr | Gallops, leading with one foot and transferring weight smoothly and evenly |
| 5 yr | Hops in straight line |
| 5-6 yr | Skips on alternating feet, maintaining balance |

Modified from Gesell, A. & Amatruda, C.S. (1947). *Developmental diagnosis.* New York: Harper & Row; Bayley, N. (1993). *Bayley scales of infant development* (revised ed.). New York: Psyhological Corporation; and Knobloch, H. & Pasamanick, B. (1974). *Gesell and Amatruda's developmental diagnosis: the evaluation and management of normal and abnormal neuropsychological development in infancy and early childhood.* Hagertown, MD: Harper & Row.

▲ Table 4-8   Fine Motor Skills

| Age | Skill |
|---|---|
| 2½-3 yr | Strings large beads |
| | Rolls clay into snake shape |
| | Cuts paper with scissors |
| 3-3½ yr | Puts together simple puzzles |
| | Builds tower of nine blocks or more |
| 3½-4 yr | Places small pegs in holes on board |
| | Strings small beads |
| 4-5 yr | Cuts across paper following straight and curved lines |
| 4½-5 yr | Folds paper in half with edges meeting |
| | Places key in lock and opens lock |
| 5 yr | Cuts out small square, triangle, and circle with scissors |
| | Strings small beads, reproducing color and shape sequence |
| | Cuts out pictures, following general shape |
| 5½-6 yr | Cuts out complex pictures following outlines |
| | Builds five-block bridge |
| | Copies from models of letters and numbers in correct sequence |
| 6 yr | Puts together complex puzzles |

Modified from Gesell, A., Halverson, H.M., Thompson, H., Ilg, F.L., Castner, B.M., Ames, L.B., & Amatruda, C.S. (1940). *The first five years of life.* New York: Harper & Row; Illingworth, R.S. (1991). *The normal child: some problems of the early years and their treatment* (10th ed.). Edinburgh: Churchill-Livingstone; and Knobloch, H. & Pasamanick, B. (1974). *Gesell and Amatruda's developmental diagnosis: the evaluation and management of normal and abnormal neuropsychological development in infancy and early childhood.* Hagertown, MD: Harper & Row.

ring at the elbow. By 4 years the child demonstrates more forward weight shift with throwing. Catching requires rapid eye-hand coordination. By 2½ years most children can catch a 10-inch ball. This pattern matures such that by 4 years of age the child succeeds in catching a small ball (e.g., a tennis ball). At this time the child follows the ball with the eyes and brings the arms together with the hands cupped to catch the ball. Kicking a ball requires a one-foot stance and sufficient balance to swing the lifted leg. Kicking emerges in the 2- to 3-year-old, with accurate kicking to a target exhibited by 6 years of age.

*Fine motor skills.* The preschool child learns functional use of drawing and cutting tools. Grasping of a pencil refines from a pronated palmar grasp to a tripod grasp. Between 3 and 4 years the child holds a pencil with a tripod grasp and uses forearm and wrist movements to draw. A mature dynamic tripod develops by 5 years. In this grasping pattern the pencil is held in the tips of the radial fingers and is moved using finger movements. The development of prewriting skills is described in Chapter 19. Drawing skills progress in the following sequence: a vertical line

(2 years), a horizontal line (3 years), a cross (4 years), and a diagonal line (5 years).

The development of scissors skills follows other tool use. Mature use of scissors is not achieved until 5 to 6 years because it requires isolated finger use (intrinsic muscles), control of two hands together, and eye-hand coordination. The first cutting skill, observed at 3 years, is snipping with alternating full-finger extension and flexion. Between 4 and 6 years, bilateral hand coordination is refined and the child learns to cut out simple shapes.

Early childhood is an important time for learning fine motor skills that require new levels of dexterity, bilateral coordination, and eye-hand coordination (Table 4-8). Daily living skills that require two-hand coordination are practiced, for example, lacing, typing, pouring liquids, buttoning, and fastening. Development of daily living skills is described in Chapter 17.

## Cognitive Development

Symbolic representations of the preschooler, particularly in language, are the hallmarks of what Piaget (1952) termed the *preoperational stage* of cognitive development from 2 to 7 years of age. The child is now able to represent people, objects, and places through the use of words as symbols. Symbols used by children have personal reference for them.

The child's egocentrism, or the belief that everyone perceives and interprets the world in exactly the same way, inhibits the development of such desirable behavior as acceptance of another person's point of view. Preschoolers relish their interactions with the environment through imaginative play; however, they are still not able to share or adhere to "fair play." They act as though they are the center of the universe.

Preschool children exhibit deferred imitation; that is, they can create and hold mental images. Play becomes more complex and symbolic. Although play is sophisticated and imaginative, the child remains centered on his or her activity; that is, the child concentrates his or her attention on one idea or one aspect of an event. As a result, often children with preoperational thought appear illogical in a problem-solving task.

This cognitive period is divided into two parts: the preconceptual stage, ages 2 to 4, and the intuitive stage, ages 5 to 7. The ability of the child to handle multiple characteristics marks the preconceptual stage. Children's reasoning skills are simple. Their experiences are not broad enough to allow them to understand the relationships between representatives of a class and the class itself. Between the ages of 4 and 7 years, children appear to cope intuitively with the physical world, but they continue to be dominated by egocentrism and illogical reasoning. They approach logical thinking but are constantly distracted by surface appearances. Play skills for ages 2 to 5 years are listed in Table 4-9.

## Psychosocial Development

Erikson (1963) defined the early psychosocial phase of early childhood as autonomy versus shame and doubt. Autonomy dominates the early part of the preschooler's psychosocial development from 2 to 4 years. The preschooler is adamant about making his or her own decisions. The development of trust in the environment and the improvement in language bring forth control over self and the corresponding strengthening of the preschooler's autonomous nature.

The discovery of the body and how to control it promotes independence in feeding, dressing, and toileting. The success in doing things for himself or herself instills a sense of confidence and self-control in the preschooler. The negative side of autonomy is a sense of shame or doubt. If the child fails continuously and is labeled messy, inadequate, or bad, shame and self-doubt are learned.

This stage, therefore, becomes decisive for the ratio of love and hate, cooperation and willfulness, freedom of self-expression, and its suppression. From a sense of self-control without loss of self-esteem comes a lasting sense of good will and pride; from a sense of loss of control comes a lasting propensity for doubt and shame (Erikson, 1963, p. 254).

▲ Table 4-9   Play Skill Development

| Age | Skill |
|---|---|
| **OBJECT PLAY AND IMITATION** | |
| 18-24 mo | Recognizes ways to activate toys in imitation of adult |
| | Deferred imitation |
| 2 yr | Uses nonrealistic objects in pretending |
| | Uses objects to perform actions (teddy bear climbs onto bed) |
| 21-24 mo | Varies own imitation creatively from that of model |
| 2-3 yr | Can use more abstract representation of object in play |
| | Uses multischeme combinations (feed doll with bottle, pat it on the back, put it to bed) |
| 3-4 yr | Plans out pretend situations in advance, organizing who and what are needed for role play |
| | Events in play are sequenced into a scenario that tells a story |
| 3-3½ yr | Can use imaginary objects in play |
| | Acts out sequences with miniature dolls (in house, garage, airport) |
| 3-5 yr | Demonstrates increasingly complex role imitation |
| 3½+ yr | Can make dolls carry out several activities or roles |
| | Creates imaginary characters |
| | Can direct actions of two dolls, making them interact within two roles |
| 4-5 yr | Imitates scenes from different aspects of life; pieces together into new script |
| 5+ yr | Organizes other children and props for role play |
| | Can direct actions of three dolls, making them interact |

Modified from Fewel, R.R. (1983). *Play assessment scale* (research ed.). Seattle: University of Washington; Nicholich, L. (1977). Beyond sensori-motor intelligence: assessment of symbolic maturity through analysis of pretend play. *Merrill-Palmer Quarterly, 16,* 136-141; Watson, N.W. (1981). The development of social roles: a sequence of social-cognitive development. In K. Fischer (Ed.). *Cognitive development: new directions for child development* (Vol. 12) (pp. 33-42). San Francisco: Josey-Bass; and Linder, T. (1990). *Transdisciplinary play-based assessment: a functional approach to working with young children.* Baltimore: Brookes.

Erikson described the latter part of the psychosocial period as initiative versus guilt. Children aged 4 or 5 explore beyond themselves. They seek new experiences for the pleasure of knowing, understanding, and getting projects started. The child's world entails real and imaginary people and things. If the child's seeking activities are successful, effective, and meet with parental approval, a sense of initiative is developed. This provides a foundation for learning to deal with people and things in a constructive way and provides a method for looking for new solutions, answers, and reasons. Children need a balance between the initiative to carry out activities and the sense of responsibility for their own actions.

Peer play becomes an important avenue for the preschooler's social development. The preschooler is now able to combine motor, language, and cognitive abilities to become an active participant. Play is essential to the child's continued development in these areas. Although adult-child relationships represent different social interactions, early home experiences are said to influence later peer relations. Evidence supports the fact that children whose attachments to their mothers are rated as secure tend to be more responsive to other children in nursery school (Moore, 1967).

The development of autonomy provides a foundation for the preschooler's imagination. Now the young child explores the world not only through use of the senses but also through the use of thinking and reasoning to imagine future situations. Play includes fantasy and motor activities that are complemented by words, rhymes, or noises. The power of symbolic thought enables the child to go beyond the immediate perception of objects and react to them in a manner that can be wishful rather than real.

The preschooler's progression to games with rules requires a stronger component of social skills (Rubin, Maioni, & Hornung, 1976). The child must now conform to established guidelines, and the rule now replaces the symbol. The game presents a real-life situation during which the preschooler tests his or her newfound social graces.

## MIDDLE CHILDHOOD
### Physiologic Development

With the continued development of initiative, the school-aged child is seen playing throughout neighborhoods and schoolyards. The middle, or school-age, years, as they are sometimes referred to, stress the relative tranquility between the turmoil of autonomous growth of the preschool years and the identity crisis of the adolescent years (Stone & Church, 1973). Striking physical differences are noted in growth patterns. Physical development is characterized by slow but steady advances in height and weight that continue until puberty. The basic pattern of body build, which shows such great variation, also affects motor skills. Problems sometimes arise because the school-aged child wants to copy new things done by friends but physical limitations prevent success (Brophy, 1977). A wide span of physical abilities is observed; skills, dexterity, and coordination differ widely based on innate ability and practice. The period of slow growth ends with the onset of the pubescent growth spurt. Although this is generally associated with adolescents, some school-aged children begin this phase of development. Growth increases at about age 9 in girls and age 11 in boys. These physical growth differences result in the disparity of height between the

sexes. The older elementary school female child is larger than her male counterparts, whereas the younger female child does not show as much variation.

The facial features of the school-aged child become more distinct and individual. The successive losses of baby teeth and the appearance of permanent teeth distinguish the changing face to a greater degree. Organ systems show continued maturation, specifically in the development of keener vision. The digestive system shows added maturity with longer food retention. Middle ear infections are less likely to occur because of changes in the eustachian tube location.

### Sensorimotor Development

Gross motor development during the elementary school years continues to focus on refinement of previously acquired skills. With this refinement, hours of repetition of activity to attain mastery of common interests are seen. Motor capabilities are very diverse for this age group. The skills of the average 8- to 9-year-old child include swinging a hammer well, using garden tools, sewing, drawing in good proportion, writing or printing accurately and neatly, cutting fingernails, riding bicycles, scaling fences, swimming, diving, skating, jumping rope, and playing ball (Knobloch & Pasamanick, 1974; Stone & Church, 1973). Research indicates that children who master a physical skill tend to think better of themselves (Short-DeGraff, 1988). Not only does self-esteem improve, but also children who have attained mastery of a skill enjoy greater acceptance by other children (Clark & Green, 1963).

Writing is an example of a skill that continues to be refined through childhood. Achievement of skilled writing involves refinement of grasp and coordination of hand movements to make smooth strokes, form smaller letters, reduce space between letters, and increase speed.

Factors involved in learning of skilled movements include motivation, instruction, and practice. Motor learning during this period is characterized by the child achieving (1) speed, strength, and precision, and (2) balance and coordination.

### Cognitive Development

The cognitive period of concrete operations (7 to 11 years) gives the child an opportunity to grasp concepts and relationships in the physical world (Piaget, 1952). The child understands space and time and can think in terms of future and past. The middle school child uses reasoning as a primary basis for conceptualizing the world. Older children are now able to weigh several pertinent factors at one time, but their thinking is limited in flexibility. They are still not able to see abstracts, but they deal with concrete objects. The period of concrete operations is highlighted by the addition of two mental operations:

reversibility and decentration. Reversibility enables the school-aged child to try out different courses of action mentally rather than relying on sensorimotor aspects of the situation. In addition, this mental process results in quicker problem-solving capabilities. The child is also able to decenter or pay attention to more than one physical characteristic at a time. These add to the systematic, logical, concrete thinking of the school-aged child.

Three other abilities emerge in the stage of concrete operations. These mental abilities are associated with increased problem-solving skills in the school-aged child. They are conservation, seriation and understanding relations, and class inclusion. When the child has conservation, he or she understands that volume, number, or mass of objects do not change when some apparent perceptual alteration occurs. Seriation is the ability to order objects by size and implies that the child understands the relationships among objects. Class inclusion is the ability to reason about the whole and its parts. To imagine objects or pieces as parts of a whole requires symbolism or representing actions in the mind. At this time the child becomes able to give instructions and tell simple stories.

## Psychosocial Development

During the middle years the child is busy with basic school subjects, perfecting motor skills, and participating in activities with like-sex peer groups. The time of industry versus inferiority is highlighted by building new skills and refining old ones. Middle school children focus on meeting challenges in themselves as well as those presented by the environment. Industry, meaning to build, is evidenced in the child's exploration of the inner workings of things and not just physical appearance. The child now learns to win recognition by producing things, and he or she experiences a sense of finality when projects are completed.

Comparison with peers is increasingly important during this time. A negative evaluation of a child's self compared with others or an inability to attain mastery of industrial achievements can result in a sense of inferiority (Clark & Green, 1963).

The school-aged child is beginning the quest for independence of identity. School-aged children are less egocentric and able to view themselves more objectively. Children at this age have a definite subculture that includes magical rituals and gangs and is exclusively limited to children. This separate subculture is quick to criticize the different sizes and shapes of its members, and it is common for membership to entail a nickname related to these differences as a rite of passage (Stone & Church, 1973).

Rejection by the child's peers may result from lack of conformity in dressing or physical appearance. Data suggest that social skills are also important determinants of peer acceptance. Children who rarely praised their peers, who had difficulty communicating, and who did not know how to initiate a new friendship were found to be unlikely candidates as friends (Newman, 1982).

Middle school children may aspire to be teenagers, emulating teenage dress and current slang; however, questions of masculinity and femininity are prominent. Boys associate with boys, and girls associate with girls, each sex pursuing its own separate interests and identities with little communication between them.

Age becomes psychologically important to the middle school child. Both boys and girls tend to associate primarily with peers of the same age. It is not uncommon to add halves or "almost" to age description.

During this age, children are disinterested in adults and their parents and unite to form a society of children. Values from peers become significantly more important than those of adults. One of the major functions of the peer group involves changing the child's attitudes. The peer group may strengthen existing attitudes, weaken those in conflict with peer group values, or establish new ones (Hartop, 1970). Data indicate that children between 7 and 10 years of age are highly compliant; they shift consistently in the direction of the peer consensus. Children tend to be less compliant as they approach the adolescent age-group (Kaluger & Kaluger, 1984).

This society of school-aged children dominates neighborhood streets and backyards with bicycle races, clubhouses, and endless exploration of woods, trash cans, and rain-swept streets. Large numbers of school-aged children are seen congregating in group activity, which includes such popular games as hide-and-seek, tag, hopscotch, and dodge-ball. Many of the middle school child's games are accompanied by ritualistic chants. The words are often empty of any literal meaning; however, the sense of participation in group ways aids in this repetition (Stone & Church, 1973).

The child's progression from structured ritualistic games to participation in competitive games with scores is seen in his or her perception of rules. Piaget (1955) identified stages of moral development including rules. Early in the child's thinking (ages 4 to 7), rules are viewed as absolute, sacred, and untouchable. Later, children (ages 7 to 10) recognize that rules come from somewhere and they accept what these rule-maker authorities say. Finally, late in the elementary school years (ages 10 to 11), children cast aside their belief in the absolute infallibility of rules because they have gained the knowledge that humans are the creators of such rules. Children now no longer accept adult authority, rules, or society without questioning them.

## ADOLESCENCE
### Physiologic Development

Adolescents are surely identified by the unique circles with which they symbolically identify. However, no formal rite of passage exists for the adolescent in the United States. Various cultural expectations within our society highly influence this adolescent period.

There is great discussion regarding distinction between physical maturation and culturally defined roles. *Pubescence* refers to the period encompassing the physical changes that lead to puberty. These include the physiologic growth of reproductive functions and maturation of primary sex organs resulting in secondary sex characteristics. Pubescence lasts an average of 2 years and ends in puberty. According to Ausubel (1977), the normal sequence of development during pubescence is as shown in Table 4-10.

In the male these characteristics include the regular production of sperm by the testes, the development of the penis, growth of pubic and axillary hair, and marked voice changes. The deepening of the voice in the male is a result of the growth of the larynx in ventrodorsal diameter (Brophy, 1977). Female secondary sex characteristics become obvious in the emergence of breasts, a change in bodily proportions, as well as the onset of menstrual periods and the hormonal reactions that accompany them. *Puberty* is the resolution of all morphologic and physiologic changes in the growing boy or girl while the gonads mature. The adult state refers to sexual maturation and the ability to reproduce.

The adolescent growth spurt is perhaps the most outstanding physical change that occurs. Within a year's time the growth rate can almost double. A typical year's growth during adolescence is between 2.5 and 4.5 inches; however, growth of 5 to 6 inches in a year is not rare. The average age onset of the adolescent growth spurt is approximately 14½ years for boys and 12½ years for girls (Tanner, 1970). Much of the growth occurs in the long bones of the legs and arms and is stimulated by the increased output of sex hormones (testosterone in the male and estrogen in the female).

▲ Table 4-10  Sequence of Development During Pubescence

| Girls | Boys |
|---|---|
| Initial enlargement of breasts | Growth of testes |
| Straight, pigmented pubic hair | Straight, pigmented pubic hair |
| Kinky, pigmented pubic hair | Early voice change |
| Age of maximal growth | First ejaculation of semen |
| Menarche | Kinky pubic hair |
| Growth of axillary hair | Age of maximal growth |
| | Growth of axillary hair |
| | Marked voice changes |
| | Development of the beard |

Modified from Ausubel, D.P. (1977). *Theory and problems of adolescent development* (2nd ed.). New York: Grune & Stratton.

The process of sexual maturation brings forth many complex social and emotional problems. It is a period of relative sexual maturity in contrast to relative immaturity of social and mental development, and the result of these newfound hormonal changes is confusing. Personal appearance becomes a source of conflict. There is greater emphasis on the good looks of physical attractiveness and physique than at any other time. The culture's current definition of attractiveness serves as the established norm for bodily proportions and facial features. Marked deviations from idealized norms and cultural stereotypes of masculinity and femininity may adversely influence the adolescent's self-concept and treatment by others (Mahon, 1983). With experience and maturation, some changes in this overwhelming concern about appearance may be expected.

## Cognitive Development

The development of formal operational thought is a highlight of adolescence. Complex written material can now be comprehended without reliance on concrete schemata. The ability to imagine an infinite variety of options establishes the presence of hypothetic reasoning. Formal thought involves the ability to generate hypotheses, to mentally consider all of the possible ways a problem may be solved, and to be able to examine and evaluate one's thought processes. The adolescent may become interested in abstract games such as computer simulation, where all possible combinations of problems are considered and high-level logic is required.

The addition of reasoning permits mature understanding of such subjects as mathematics and philosophy. The adolescent's ability to think about his or her own thinking signifies complex mental operations. The mature teenager can now consider all possible relationships that might exist and evaluate these relationships one by one to eliminate falsity and to arrive at the truth.

## Psychosocial Development

Erikson (1963) emphasized the role of identity in the adolescent's psychosocial development. During this period society begins to ask the youth to define his or her own role and career aspirations. Erikson believed that to solve one's identity crisis, one must be committed to a role, which in turn means showing commitment to an ideology. The adolescent must define a personal ideology and confirm beliefs, values, and ideals (Erikson, 1964). This commitment, or fidelity, should coincide with prerequisites for the adolescent's desired occupation. The acting out of behaviors, experimentation with new roles, fantasy, self-doubts, and rebellion are seen as the adolescent attempts to establish a firm identity and role that will be most suited to him or her. If a youth fails to integrate a central identity or cannot resolve conflicts between roles and a value system, ego diffusion is the result.

Elaborating on Erikson's theory, Marcia and Freidman (1970) evaluated adolescents' levels of crisis and commitment in relationship to occupational choice, religion, and political ideology. They described four identity statuses or modes of resolving the identity issue characteristic of adolescents. Those classified by these modes were defined in terms of the presence or absence of a decision-making period (crisis) and the extent of personal investment (commitment) in two areas: occupation and ideology.

*Identity achievers* are individuals who have shown a commitment to an occupation and to an ideology. They have experienced a decision-making period. *Foreclosures* are adolescents who have never experienced a crisis. They are committed to occupational and ideologic positions but have adopted identities that have been parentally chosen with little or no question. *Identity diffusions* are young people who have no set occupational ideologic direction. They may or may not have experienced crisis, but their defining characteristic is their lack of concern regarding lack of commitment. *Moratoriums* are individuals who are currently in crisis. They have a vague commitment to an occupation or ideology but are in a state of search.

The establishment of ego identity, including occupational identity, is often complex and potentially confusing for the adolescent. Even at the age of 25, one young adult in four is still uncertain what vocation he or she should choose. Decisions concerning occupations interact with other choices in development so that when commitment to the occupational choice is firm, the individual has, to some extent, fitted himself or herself for it.

A multitude of theories of vocational choice and development exists. Ginzberg (1972) presented a developmental theory proposing movement through three primary psychologic periods: a fantasy period, a tentative period, and a realistic period.

Because the central theme of adolescence focuses on identity, the adolescent is in conflict between the emerging responsibility of being an adult and the past of adult society's expectations. The peer group serves as a support system for the young person who is trying to make this transition from childhood to adulthood. As adolescents are faced with this pressure, aggressive rebellion may result. This rebellion is often displayed in increased social contact outside of the home. A desire to escape from the demands of parents and community and to retreat to an environment where one's views are appreciated is seen in group attachment (Stone & Church, 1973). The heightened importance of the peer group increases the adolescent's desire to conform to the values, customs, and fads of the peer culture. This culture often proclaims its differences through symbolism in manners of dress, language, or food fads.

Although the rise of peer attachment introduces an important source of social control into the life of the young person, both peers and parents are important. Data suggest that, depending on the meaning and context of the social relationship, parents or peers may be more important. A vast majority of young people report considerable respect for their parents as individuals, and almost half desire more parental support of their own political and social opinions (Smart & Smart, 1973; Tanner, 1973). These differences in opinion tended to be on finer points of policy rather than on the overall issue. Lerner and Knapp (1974) assessed the comparability of parents' and adolescents' attitudes toward societal issues. Their results indicate that although both groups were able to successfully assess the attitudes of each other, "there was a tendency for parents to minimize discrepancies between themselves and their children and a tendency for adolescents to magnify such discrepancies" (p. 35).

## SUMMARY

An overview of growth and development from conception through adolescence clearly indicates that children are complex individuals. Although the sequences described offer some guidelines for typical development, the characteristics of physiologic, sensorimotor, cognitive, and psychoso-

---

### STUDY QUESTIONS

1. Describe key milestones of sensorimotor development in infancy (0 to 3 months). Define the cognitive skills of the infant. Describe how the sensorimotor skills allow the infant to engage in activity that promotes cognitive skill development. Describe how the infant's cognitive level promotes maturation of sensorimotor skills.

2. During the preschool years, fine motor skills are refined through maturation and experience. List three bilateral manipulation skills that are first accomplished in early childhood. What are two prerequisite sensorimotor skills that enable the preschool-age child to accomplish these skills?

3. In middle childhood, peer relationships become important. Define two possible advantages and two disadvantages for a child's psychosocial development related to the increasing importance of peer relationships.

4. The adolescent seeks an identity and a vocational choice. Identify two primary factors that influence an adolescence's development of self-concept and two that influence vocational choice.

cial domains are variable for each child. Understanding of typical development provides a framework for evaluation and a basis for establishing intervention goals. Horowitz (1981) provides her wisdom for using the developmental continuum as a basis for predicting an infant's potential. She explained that an evaluation of an infant:

. . .will never net us an understanding of human development, which is probably the most complex phenomenon on this planet. An accurate model of development must include variables associated with the organism as well as variables assioacted with the environment, and it should depict developmental outcome as resulting form interactions within and across these domains. (p. 32)

## REFERENCES

Ainsworth, M.D.S. (1973). The development of infant-mother attachment. In B.M. Caldwell (Ed.). *Review of child development,* (Vol 3). Chicago: University of Chicago Press.

Ausubel, D.P. (1977). *Theory and problems of adolescent development,* (2nd ed.). New York: Grune & Stratton.

Bayley, N. (1993). *Bayley scales of infant development* (revised ed.). New York: Psychological Corporation.

Berenda, R.W. (1950). *The influence of the group on the judgement of children: an experimental investigation.* New York: King's Crown Press.

Bly, L. (1993). *Normal development in the first year of life.* Tucson: Therapy Skill Builders.

Brazelton, T.B. (1973). *Neonatal behavioral assessment scale.* Philadelphia: J.B. Lippincott.

Brophy, J.E. (1977). *Child development and socialization.* Chicago: Science Research Associates.

Clarke, H.H. & Greene, W.H. (1963). Relationship between personal-social measures applied to 10 year-old boys. *Research Quarterly, 34,* 288-302.

Cohen, M.A. & Gross, P.J. (1979). *The developmental resource: behavioral sequences for assessment and program planning.* New York: Basic Books.

DiLeo, J.H. (1977). *Child development: analysis and synthesis.* New York: Bruner/Mazel.

Erikson, E.H. (1963). *Childhood and society* (2nd ed.). New York: W.W. Norton.

Erikson, E.H. (1964). *Insight and responsibility.* New York: W.W. Norton.

Fewell, R.R. (1983). *Play assessment scaled* (research ed.). Seattle: University of Washington.

Gesell, A. & Amatruda, C.S. (1954). *Developmental diagnosis* (2nd ed.). New York: Harper & Row.

Gesell, A., Halverson, H.M., Thompson, H., Ilg, F.L., Castner, B.M., Ames, L.B., & Amatruda, C.S. (1940). *The first five years of life.* New York: Harper & Row.

Gilfolye, E., Grady, A., & Moore, J. (1990). *Children adapt.* Thorofare, NJ: Slack.

Ginzberg, E. (1972). Toward a theory of occupational choice: a restatement. *Vocational Guide Quarterly, 20,* 169-175.

Greenberg, M. & Morris, N. (1974). Engrossment: the newborn's impact upon the father. *American Journal of Orthopsychiatry, 44(4),* 520-526.

Halverson, H.M. (1931). An experimental study of prehension in infants by means of systematic cinema records. *Genetic Psychology Monographs, 10,* 107-286.

Harlow, H.F. & Zimmerman, P.R. (1959). Affectional responses in the infant monkey, *Science, 130,* 421-430.

Hartop, W.W. (1970). Peer interaction and social organization. In P.H. Mussen (Ed.). *Carmichael's manual of child psychology* (3rd ed.) (Vol. 2). New York: John Wiley & Sons.

Horowitz, F.D. (1981). Toward a model of early infant development. In C.C. Brown (Ed.). *Infants at risk: assessment and intervention: an update for health care professionals and parents.* Skillman, NJ: Johnson & Johnson.

Howell, L. (1978). Birth defects, genetic counseling. A. Disabling birth defects. In R.M. Goldenson (Ed.). *Disability and rehabilitation handbook.* New York: McGraw-Hill.

Illingworth, R.S. (1991). *The normal child: some problems of the early years and their treatment.* (10th ed.). Edinburgh: Churchill-Livingstone.

Kaluger, G. & Kaluger, M.F. (1984). *Human development: the span of life* (3rd ed.). St. Louis: Mosby.

Klaus, M.H. & Kennel, J.H. (1976). *Maternal-infant bonding.* St. Louis: Mosby.

Knoblock, H. & Pasamanick, B. (1974). *Gesell & Amatruda's Developmental Diagnosis* (3rd ed.). New York: Harper & Row.

Lerner, R.M. & Knapp, J.R. (1974). Actual and perceived intrafamilial attitudes of late adolescents and their parents. *Journal of Youth and Adolescents, 4,* 17-25.

Linder T. (1990). *Transdisciplinary play-based assessment: a functional approach to working with young children.* Baltimore: Brookes.

Mahon, N.E. (1983). Developmental changes and loneliness during adolescence. *Topics in Clinical Nursing, 5,* 66-76.

Marcia, J.E. & Freidman, M.L. (1970). Ego identity status in college women. *Journal of Personality, 38(2),* 249-260.

Milani-Comparetti, A. (1981). Pattern analysis of normal and abnormal development: the fetus, the newborn, and the child. In D.S. Slaton (Ed.). *Development of movement in infancy.* Chapel Hill, NC: Division of Physical Therapy, The University of North Carolina.

Moore, S.B. (1967). Correlates of peer acceptance in nursery school children. *Young Children, 22,* 281-286.

Newman, P.R. (1982). The peer group. In B.B. Wolman (Ed.). *Handbook of developmental psychology.* Englewood Cliffs, NJ: Prentice-Hall.

Nicholich, L. (1977). Beyond sensorimotor intelligence: assessment of symbolic maturity through analysis of pretend play. *Merrill-Palmer Quarterly, 16,* 136-141.

Piaget, J. (1952). *The origins of intelligence in children.* Translated by M. Cook. New York: International Universities Press.

Piaget, J. (1955). *The moral judgment of the child.* New York: MacMillan.

Power, T.G. (1985). Mother and father play: a developmental analysis. *Child Development, 56,* 1514-1524.

Rubin, K.H., Maioni, T.L., & Hornung, M. (1976). Free play behaviors in middle and lower class preschoolers: Parten and Piaget revisited. *Child Development, 47,* 414-421.

Short-DeGraff, P. (1988). *Human development for occupational and physical therapists.* Baltimore: Williams & Wilkins.

Smart, M.S. & Smart, R.C. (1973). *Adolescents: development and relationships.* New York: MacMillan.

Stechler, G. & Halton, A. (1982). Prenatal influences on human development. In B.B. Wolman (Ed.). *Handbook of developmental psychology.* Englewook Cliffs, NJ: Prentice-Hall.

Stone, J.L. & Church, J. (1973). *Childhood and adolescence: a psychology of the growing person,* (3rd ed.). New York: Random House.

Tanner, J.M. (1970). Physical growth. In P.H. Mussen (Ed.). *Carmichael's manual of child psychology,* (3rd ed.) (Vol. 1). New York: John Wiley & Sons.

Tanner, J.M. (1973). Growing up. *Scientific American, 229,* 34-43.

Watson, M.W. (1981). The development of social roles: a sequence of social-cognitive development. In K. Fischer (Ed.). *Cognitive development: new directions for child development* (Vol. 12) (pp. 33-42). San Francisco: Jossey-Bass.

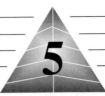

# Working with Families

RUTH HUMPHRY ▲ JANE CASE-SMITH

## KEY TERMS

- ▲ Family Systems and Subsystems
- ▲ Structure, Boundaries
- ▲ Family Traditions and Rituals
- ▲ Determinants of the Parenting Role
- ▲ Cultural Diversity
- ▲ Family Functions
- ▲ Life Cycle
- ▲ Family Resources and Strengths
- ▲ Coping and Adaptation
- ▲ Parent-Professional Partnerships
- ▲ Communication Strategies
- ▲ Families with Special Needs

## CHAPTER OBJECTIVES

1. Apply the terms about families to describe your own family.
2. Discuss the nature of diversity in family structure.
3. Analyze a family system and discuss the implication of intervention for each family member.
4. Identify family functions and analyze the impact of a child with special needs.
5. Synthesize information about family life cycle and transitions to identify times of potential stress for families.
6. Develop a description of the roles of the occupational therapists in working with families.
7. Plan strategies to establish and maintain collaborative relationships with a family.
8. Describe methods of communication that promote family-therapist partnerships.
9. Describe the range of ways families may participate in intervention services.
10. Explain strategies for working with families who have special needs.

## UNDERSTANDING FAMILIES

### Why Work with Families?

Occupational therapists have traditionally recognized the importance of environmental influences on different aspects of a child's development and skill acquisition. Research has demonstrated that when the child's development is challenged by a medical condition, disease, or disability, the ultimate outcome is highly influenced by the caregiving environment (Sameroff & Chandler, 1975). Once service providers understand that a young child's developmental status is intimately related to transactions between the child and his or her caregivers, they recog-nize the critical importance of interventions that are family centered (Sameroff & Fiese, 1990). Occupational therapists work with families to plan and create experiences that promote each child's progress. As the care-givers in the child's environment help the child compensate for threats to development, the long-term outcome improves.

From an occupational performance perspective, the social and cultural context influences the rate and pattern of development. The child's family is a complex network of relationships that forms a large part of his or her occupational context. After birth, meaningful contact with people starts with family members. Family characteristics determine the range of experiences the child receives. Children become part of a variety of social groups at day care centers, schools, neighborhoods, clubs, and after-school jobs. Over the years the family represents the most enduring set of relationships in the child's life.

During the course of his or her lifetime, an individual with a disability interacts with and relates to a multitude of professionals. These relationships may be short-term or they may endure for several years; however, they always change as the child moves into new systems and new life stages. The child's family represents a source of continuity. Family members with their unique emotional involvement and everyday contact have gathered insight into the child's abilities and needs. The occupational therapist recognizes the family's position as the expert on the child.

The critical perspective families bring to services for children who have special needs is reflected in federal legislation. The role of the child's parent or guardian is ensured by requiring their input and permission on any assessment, intervention plan, and placement decision. In the early period of the child's life (birth until 3 years old) the importance of the family is reflected by the emphasis on family-centered services in Part H of the Individuals with Disabilities Education Act (IDEA; P.L. 101-476). By placing the family at the heart of the intervention process, professionals are guided to support the people most influential in the developmental process. The Individual Family Service Plan (IFSP) is developed through dialogue with the parents regarding what resources the family needs to help promote the child's development. The IFSP and early intervention legislation are further described in Chapter 23.

After 3 years of age the child's program may become more child focused, but input from parents on the Individual Educational Plan (IEP) is an important element of the process. Although a specific parent role in IEP development is defined in IDEA, the parent's role does not stop with planning the child's educational program. The expectation of development is that the young person will leave home and live in the community. Acquisition of independent living and prevocational skills enables the student with special needs to move from school to community participation. In services for young adolescents with special needs, IDEA recognizes the importance of family's input to and approval of transition plans. The law confirms that parents are in the best position to guide the adolescent's transition planning process.

## What is a Family?

Given the powerful role families play in their children's health, development, and education, it is important that the clinician understands how families work. Who and what constitutes a child's family? Given the diversity of different cultures and every family's changing membership, a single answer to "Who is your family?" may not be possible. Does family include people not living in the household? Is the great aunt who watches the children after school a part of their family? If a mother's children call the man she lives with "Uncle John," is he part of their family? An outsider cannot decide what people or relationships constitute a family (Levin & Trost, 1992).

Families do have *boundaries* that determine if an individual is in or out of the unit. Membership in the family may change with many life events. For example, a person may be added to the family unit by birth, adoption, or marriage. At times the boundary may be porous, and a nonrelated individual may become part of the family. Families also lose members because of divorce, death, or decreased

contact and emotional commitment. "Tell me about your family" is one way an occupational therapist can learn about membership without suggesting any preconceived status.

Another way to define a family is by what families do. The family unit includes individuals that have an interdependent relationship with an enduring emotional commitment. Regardless of membership and cultural background, all families must address particular issues and accomplish certain functions. *Family functions* are to nurture and provide emotional support, socialize, recreate, and promote health and development of each member. To accomplish these tasks, families have to acquire and maintain physical resources such as shelter, food, and clothing. Energy and time are intangible resources that families also need to accomplish their tasks. Physical, financial, and emotional resources have to be shared among the members. As a result, another task is to set priorities and allocate resources. Frequently families are organized in a hierarchy so one or two members have more power than others to determine how the family resources are allocated.

## Family as a System

To understand how families fulfill their tasks, occupational therapists have learned from social scientists in anthropology, developmental psychology, and sociology. A common theoretical approach is to view the family as a dynamic, interacting system (Minuchin, 1985). Each aspect or principle of a family system is discussed in some depth (see box below).

Through a systems model the family can be seen as a *group of individuals with interrelated lives* such that changes in one family member affect all other members. For example, when a baby brother starts to walk, his new skill affects all other members in the family. His parent acquires a new role as a disciplinarian because he or she has to restrict the toddler's behavior. The big sister's activities

## Key Concepts of a Family System Model

1. A family system is composed of individuals that are interdependent with reciprocal influences.
2. Within the family, subsystems are defined with their own patterns of interaction and recurrent behaviors.
3. Families must be understood as a whole, and they are more than the sum of the abilities of each member.
4. The family system works to achieve homeostasis on a day-to-day basis and to be part of a larger community.
5. Change and evolution are inherent in a family.
6. Families, as open systems, are influenced by their environments.

may also change now that her brother can explore her room and toys. The toddler's grandmother, who watches him during the day, may experience more physical fatigue and have less energy to pursue leisure interests. From a family system's perspective a new developmental milestone or life transition for one individual results in adjustments for the whole family.

There are reciprocal dynamic effects within family systems as each member reacts to how the others change. The grandmother's decreased energy is the direct effect of her grandson's new gross motor abilities. Increased fatigue directly influences her responsiveness to the toddler's bids for attention. An indirect effect of the toddler's walking might be a change in the grandmother's activity on weekends, as the grandmother finds she has less energy to take her granddaughter shopping.

Family members come together and form *interactive subsystems* with their own boundaries and roles. Families with two adults and more than one child are composed of a marital subsystem, a sibling subsystem, and parent-child subsystems. Family members belong to several subsystems at a time, and consequently they often feel stretched between different role demands. For example, a mother and wife feels the need to balance those two roles, giving adequate attention to both her son and her husband. In pediatric practice the occupational therapist may primarily interact with the mother and child subsystem. At the same time the clinician recognizes that not all family tasks are accomplished by the mother-child subsystem and may include other family members. For example, a session that involves a sibling may effectively enhance occupational performance in play because play opportunities occur most frequently in the sibling subsystem.

A third principle of family systems theory is that a family cannot be completely understood by gathering information about each individual. The quality of family function is a product of a *whole interacting unit.* For example, knowing that all the children are old enough to get dressed for school without physical assistance does not mean the therapist can assume that mornings run smoothly for parents and that each child leaves home relaxed and ready to start learning at school. The clinician cannot directly observe all aspects of family function that may affect the child with special needs. However, interviewing the primary care providers and collaborating with the family in program development increases the probability that any intervention ideas consider the interactive functioning of the whole family.

Another principle is that a family system works to stabilize how it functions or strives for *homeostasis.* To maintain itself, meet needs of members, and maintain relationships with others in the community, the family establishes rituals or symbolic forms of communications (Wolin & Bennett, 1984). Rituals include interactive routines, unique family traditions, and celebrations shared with others in the community. Families who report that they have established rituals that are important to them tend to demonstrate higher levels of family function (Fiese, Hooker, Kotary, & Schwagler, 1993).

*Interactive routines* within families form in the context of daily lives and help define role responsibilities (Fiese et al., 1993). Besides helping the family function effectively and anticipate members' behaviors, routines have symbolic and emotional meaning. Families develop their own interactive routines that have special meaning around daily events such as meals, saying goodbye, or getting ready for bed. Interactive routines may be difficult for families to articulate (Sameroff & Fiese, 1990). A therapist who asks about *how* something is done at home may hear about the activity but not the meaning it holds. For example, a parent and child with severe motor involvement have an established bath-time routine in which the mother sits supporting her 10-year-old daughter in the bathtub. The occupational therapist learned about how the child was bathed and ordered a bath chair so that the child could be well supported and bathed with minimal supervision. However, because the interactive routine of the bath held special meaning to the mother and daughter, the bath chair remained unused. If the occupational therapist had involved the mother and child in the decision to purchase the bath chair, a more appropriate recommendation, if any, could have been made. If an interactive routine is valued as a time of interaction, the family members may not wish to change or adapt an activity despite the time and effort required.

In addition to rituals for daily activities, families also have traditions and celebrations. *Family traditions,* such as special food for birthday celebrations or leisure activities on Sunday afternoons, help families develop a sense of group cohesion and make each family feel unique. These traditions are another way families maintain a predictable pattern in their lives. Families may decide to maintain their tradition rather than address an individual member's needs. For example, a family who traditionally visits the grandparents for several weeks in the summer may experience family-therapist conflict if the occupational therapist assumes their first choice would be weekly treatment sessions for the child during the summer. When the occupational therapist asks the family to set priorities for treatment, the family should consider all their traditions and determine how they want occupational therapy to fit into their lives.

Events and behaviors that are shared with a community are *celebrations,* a third form of family ritual. Religious or community celebrations also guide family conduct, contributing to homeostasis. Behaviors that form family celebrations are common with other families who share the same background. Special events, such as religious holidays, involve celebration with the shared rituals and give the family a sense of belonging to a larger group. Participation of the child with special needs in family celebrations is one

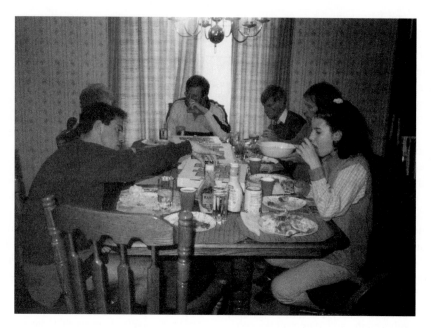

**Figure 5-1**   Family meals on the holidays are often an important part of family celebrations.

way a family confirms that their child is like other children (Figure 5-1).

Families may resist change by trying to maintain homeostasis, but another principle is that family systems *experience metamorphosis and adaptation.* Although families develop and grow even when there are no children in the family, most models of family development are linked to the ages of their children. At the different stages of family development there are common developmental tasks the family must address. These are described in a later section on the family life cycle. The service provider needs to consider changing characteristics of the disability, individual family members' development, and the developmental status of the family system (Rolland, 1987).

With each new stage of family development, members need to change. The degree families can share roles and adapt routines to normal developmental changes and unexpected circumstances varies. During times of transition to a new stage, a flexible family may experience shifts with slight confusion and no interruption in meeting family tasks. The more fixed family roles, the more disruption the family experiences when developmental changes or unexpected events occur. For example, the husband who believes that his roles are employment outside the home and yardwork has difficulty taking on new roles in caregiving when a child requires extra attention in feeding and dressing tasks.

The final principle of a systems model is that families, as *open systems,* are influenced by outside forces. For example, if a father's employing agency downsizes and the father is unexpectedly unemployed, the family experiences loss of income and may need to subsist at a different economic level. This circumstance may result in changes in the

family's recreational and leisurely pursuits. A lengthy period of unemployment may affect family roles, for example, the mother may begin employment outside the home, and the father may have more time to devote to caregiving and play interactions with the children. Neighborhoods are another source of influence on families. Families living in an inner city housing project may not have access to well-constructed, safe playgrounds and may be restricted in the number and types of outdoor play areas available.

Families are also influenced by societal attitudes and community services (e.g., programs for children with special needs). The education laws discussed earlier have had a direct impact on families, making it easier for them to voice their wishes and express concerns. Each community varies in support services for families who provide care for special children. For example, a research study by Crowe (1993) demonstrated that parents of children with physical handicaps spend more time in physical caregiving activities and may need respite services. The availability of respite care services influences parents' abilities to cope and to continue in caregiving roles.

The degree the family is open to external influences varies. At times of transition and change, the family's boundaries may be especially closed to external influence. Families with a new baby may find all their energies focused on the new member and changing roles. A need to exclude external influences and become a family may be why some parents wait months before following through with a referral to an early intervention program (Calhoun, Calhoun, & Rose, 1989). At other times, families may be very open to external forces. For example, families with adolescents might be greatly affected by the adolescent's friends and peers.

## Sources of Diversity in Families

Families with children who need occupational therapy services come in many different forms. A clinician working with children has the opportunity to learn about many different types of families and is challenged to help each family feel accepted and respected for who they are. When a family has a child with special needs and does not conform to the image in the dominant culture, the family may feel especially alienated from mainstream services (Lynch & Hanson, 1992). A frequently recommended step to increasing sensitivity to diversity is to become familiar with one's own culture and values. With self-knowledge, the therapist is better prepared to recognize how his or her own background influences attitudes, values, and behaviors and to appreciate families of different backgrounds.

Families can vary according to their structure, life-style choices, socioeconomic status, and ethnic backgrounds. Much of the diversity is translated into different dynamics in family rituals and parenting styles. Individual families have characteristics, beliefs, and values that relate to their cultural background in unique ways. Therefore generalizations about cultural values are rarely appropriate, and sensitivity to cultural differences is always needed. Family diversity and cultural values are discussed in a later section of this chapter.

### Family Structure

Family *structure* is determined by relationships among family members and the roles they fulfill. An important consideration in family structure is to determine who is the head of the household. Families can be headed by a married man and woman, a single parent, grandparents, or other adults who fulfill the roles associated with being full-time caregivers to the children.

In 1988 more than 25% of all children lived with a single parent (U.S. Bureau of Census, 1989). A larger percentage (nearly 40%) lived in a single-parent household at least some of the time during their childhood. In a study of adults who became single parents, several strengths and problems were identified in single parenting (Richards & Schmiege, 1993). The family strengths included better parent-child communications, personal growth, and enhanced skills in managing a family. Without another adult to share the parenting role, children in single-parent families may be given more household chores, which may possibly enhance the child's sense of responsibility. The problem most frequently identified by mothers and fathers who were single parents was role overload. Concerns over money occur most often when the single parent is a woman; 80% of the women who became single parents identified this issue (Acock & Kiecolt, 1989). Men who were single fathers were more likely to experience continued problems with the former spouse who might share custody of the children (Richards & Schmiege, 1993).

Another type of family structure includes the extended family. These families may be large and chaotic with shifting membership; however, in general, an extended or augmented family has more resources to help promote the child's development (Slaughter-Defoe, 1993). The members of the extended family may directly care for the child or they may serve as resources for information on child care and may provide emotional support to the parents. Today's families often combine nuclear and extended family members into a single household. Aunts, uncles, grandparents, or other members may be primary caregivers. In working with families the service provider needs to encourage all family members who participate as care providers to have input.

### Adult Life-Style

Another variation of families might be created by the life-style of their parents. Children can be born or adopted into families headed by gay or lesbian partners. Mothers who have lesbian partners express many of the same needs and stresses as heterosexual couples with children, but they also experience some unique needs (Hare, 1994). A primary concern is that not everyone recognizes them as a family. Clinicians working with children parented by lesbian or gay couples can communicate that they recognize the partners as co-parents by naming both parents in invitations to IFSP or IEP meetings.

### Ethnic Background

Ethnic variations can contribute to cultural differences between families (Lynch & Hanson, 1992) and differences between roles of fathers and mothers within families (Julian, McKenry, & McKelvey, 1994). Julian and her colleagues (1994) contrasted responses of parents with African American, Asian American, Hispanic, and Caucasian backgrounds. They concluded that parents of all ethnic groups use similar techniques for socializing their children (modeling reinforcement and identification) but place different emphasis on independence, doing well in school, and having the child control his or her temper. How the family values independence versus interdependence is of particular importance to the occupational therapist. One example may be when a team recommends working on community travel skills of an adolescent with Down syndrome. If the parents do not place a high priority on independence, the team's suggestions may be rejected as not worth the effort. Learning about and respecting the value systems of ethnic groups is discussed in a later section.

Parents of minority ethnic groups are faced with the double task of socializing children to their own culture and helping them to interact with members of the dominant culture. What the parent selects to pass on to the children is influenced by the values and experiences of each culture. For example, African American mothers who place a high priority on the children's independence and ability to control his or her temper may do so to prepare children to deal with negative impact of racism encountered in the dominant culture (Julian et al., 1994). To understand a family's cultural background, therapists should consider the interrelationship between an ethnic group's culture of origin, history of economic concerns, and experience with racism.

### Socioeconomic Background

For a family, financial resources, educational background of adults, and social status of the occupation of the primary income providers influence how others describe their socioeconomic status (SES). The family's SES can be viewed as an index for the types of experiences and opportunities that are part of the social and cultural context of children's occupations. Financial resources are used to buy material goods and services that contribute to differences in how families function. Children in a family where finances are limited may be expected to contribute to household activities by performing home management activities such as laundry or yard maintenance. Household duties enable the child to contribute to the well-being of the families and may be the foundation for practicing prevocational skills. For other families with more financial resources, these same occupations may be performed by hired help, allowing adults and children time and energy for other activities. In occupational therapy the family's financial status may determine whether a child is covered by insurance or whether a parent can afford to take time away from work to bring the child to therapy or attend an IEP meeting during regular school hours.

The impact of SES on family function is not a simple issue of whether a family has financial resources (Bronfenbrenner & Crouter, 1982). Poverty creates a complex environment for providing services designed to help families (Halpern, 1993). Society has negative attitudes about poverty; families may be blamed for their circumstances or viewed as victims. Whatever their circumstances, parents must "qualify" to receive financial support from the government. This process can be frustrating, depersonalizing, and degrading.

Families living in poverty have multiple challenges that make them at greater risk for poor parenting. Lack of parental education and concerns about income create a stressful environment. A sense of emotional support often promotes better parenting. Low income influences the parents' sense of well-being and psychologic health and the quality of interactions in the parenting subsystem (Brody et al., 1994). Working with families in poverty is discussed in a later section of this chapter.

The socioeconomic background of the parents tends to influence goals and characteristics that are valued for their children (Luster, Rhodes, & Haas, 1989). The adult's perspective of how the world works and what characteristics are needed for success can be strongly influenced by what he or she needs to succeed in his or her job or career. Par-

ents with less education and less-skilled jobs are thought to value traits that would help their children follow directions and work cooperatively with a team. For these parents, obedience and good manners in their children are important. For parents with higher socioeconomic status, their success in jobs requires more problem-solving and independent work. As a result, higher SES groups tend to have goals that encourage self-direction and curiosity.

### Parenting Style

What makes a good parent? In addition to the ethnic and socioeconomic background, parenting style is a product of complex interactions of the adult's personality and own history of being parented (Vondra & Belsky, 1993). Two broad dimensions of parenting style are the extent the adult works to nurture or support the child and the degree of control the parent exerts over the child (Peterson & Leigh, 1990). Although parents most often feel warm and committed to their children, they may hold different ideas regarding the traits that are important. The different values lead to alternative caregiving strategies to help their children acquire the valued traits.

For example, parents that value independence and self-direction may encourage their children to explore the house and give the children few restrictions (Luster et al., 1989). Conversely, parents who believe that conformity to rules is important to their children's later success may restrict their children's access to parts of the house and have high expectations for obedience.

An important aspect of working with families with diverse backgrounds is to recognize the variation in parenting styles and realize that a parent's style may not be consistent with the therapist's own internal model of a good parent. The therapist working from a family systems perspective realizes that the parenting style that is observed is a product of reciprocal interactions between the characteristics of the child and the traits of the parent. A hyperactive child with a difficult temperament may elicit a different type of parenting than her sister who is relaxed and easygoing.

## What Does It Mean to Have a Child with a Disability?

As explained earlier, any significant family event has an effect on all family members. To understand the family dynamics when a child with a disability is born, it is useful to return to the family systems theory. Again this theory helps define the individual family subunits and explain how the family functions as a whole.

### Parent-Child Relationship

The relationship between the *parent and child* is highly influenced by characteristics of the child, including those associated with the disability. Several studies have found that additional caregiving time is required when the child has a disability (Brotherson & Goldstein, 1992; Crowe, 1993). The time required relates to the severity and type of disability. Disabilities that seem to create more stress and time for the family include autism, severe and multiple disabilities, behavior disorders, and medical problems that require frequent hospitalization and in-home medical care. Greater time demands may be placed on the mother, who is typically the primary care provider. The mother may become "enmeshed" with the child, focused on his or her care, and may lack the time and energy to give needed attention to her husband and other offspring. When the mother does not work outside the home, she may begin to feel that she has all of the responsibility for the child with special needs. This happens when the mother is the sole family member to interact with the physicians, therapists, and teachers and therefore becomes the primary parent to give and receive essential information about the child.

Fathers may want to become more involved but may not have time for the same caregiving activities. Young and Roopnarine (1994) found that fathers spend about one-third the time in child care that mothers spend. Often the father may be interested in "play" with his child, but may become discouraged when the child does not respond or responds in unexpected ways, making interaction difficult.

Gallagher, Beckman, and Cross (1983) described typical role differences between mothers and fathers. Mothers have expressive roles, that is, they are concerned with affection, physical care, and self definition. Fathers fill instrumental roles; they are more concerned with the family's finances and with the child's achievement in education and vocation. Although these roles seem to be changing as more mothers work outside the home and more fathers are involved in daily caregiving, the concept that mothers perform expressive roles and fathers instrumental remains valid. Several implications follow:

1. Because fathers are more concerned with the child's relationship to the external world, a father can also be more concerned with the social stigma that may result from the disability.
2. A father may be more concerned with physical appearance.
3. A father may have fewer ways to interact with the child whose physical or mental delays limit the child's ability to participate in recreational activities such as sports. Interaction may be most limited when the child is male and has a physical disability.
4. A mother may have additional demands on her role of caregiving for a child who continues to require assistance in feeding, bathing, hygiene, and dressing.
5. A mother may feel needed and competent and gain more satisfaction from her role as caregiver.
6. A father's employment may support his adaptation. Employment offers the father a chance to "get away"

and to distance himself from the strain of child care (May, 1990; Sparling, Berger, & Biller, 1992).

These statements do not apply to all families. Mothers have described the positive roles that they perceive their husbands have:

I always think that [my child] likes [his father] more than he likes me because I have to do all the things that he doesn't like . . . make him take a bath . . . and when [his father] comes home his savior has arrived. Dad takes over in the evening and allows me to cook dinner and take care of the house (Nastro, 1992, p. 43).

Fathers are often masterful playmates and can produce positive effects on the child's self-esteem, sexual identity, cognitive growth, and social skills.

Fathers are not always included in intervention programs. One father reported a recurring situation when his son's teachers and therapists phoned his home:

Whenever they called about Tim, they immediately asked for my wife. Why don't the therapists want to talk with me? Do they feel I will not understand the information? Will I not answer their questions? Do they think that I don't care to learn about what is happening at school? I used to feel hurt and hand the phone to my wife, but now I reply that if they have information or a question about Tim they can talk with me. (Ballard, D., personal communication, 1991).

Ninio and Rinott (1988) recommended a number of strategies for encouraging the father's participation. The programs that seem to best support the father's involvement include the following components:

1. Involve the father in program planning.
2. Offer convenient scheduling, for example, evenings and Saturdays.
3. Focus on providing information about the disability and community resources.
4. Provide opportunities for the father to enjoy activities with his child.

Meyer developed a model for father support groups (Meyer, 1986; Vadasy, Fewell, & Meyer, 1986). The programs were based on support, education, and involvement of fathers. Support was generated from their peers, other men in similar situations. Discussion revolved around common joys and concerns, the impact of the disability, and the changing role of the father in today's society. The education components included information about the nature of the child's disability, resources and materials available, and the medical and educational system. Fathers also learned positive ways to interact with their children and effective strategies for advocating for their children.

Sparling, Berger, and Biller (1992) explained the importance of involving fathers. As the family's primary decision makers, fathers often decide how the family's resources are spent. For the father to support ongoing therapy, new equipment, and other resources for the child, he must thoroughly understand the benefits and advantages. Fathers need on-going information to understand the course of intervention and to participate in decision making. When many options for their involvement are presented, their ongoing involvement is more likely (Sparling et al., 1992).

### Siblings

*Siblings* are affected by a child with a disability in many different ways. The factors that contribute to the sibling relationship include the severity of the disability, the time frame and birth order (Was the child with a disability born before or after the sibling?), and the family's attitude toward the disability. Many times the siblings keep their emotions to themselves or have difficulty expressing their negative feelings for a brother or sister. A comprehensive study of college-age siblings indicated that more than half believed they had benefited from having a brother or sister with an exceptionality. Grossman (1972) and Meyer (1993) reported that benefits perceived by siblings included (1) increased understanding of others, (2) increased tolerance and compassion, and (3) greater appreciation of health and ability. Comments made by siblings show the importance of growing up with disability in the family:

Stacy [my sister] has taught me to never judge people without understanding them first. A hasty judgment of Stacy does not reveal her acute perceptiveness . . . As a result I hesitate to classify other people too quickly (Levitt, 1988, p. 5).

My experience with my sister has been one of the most important in my life . . . it has definitely shaped my life and channeled my interests (Itzkowitz, 1990, p. 4).

Parents have indicated that siblings, particularly older siblings, are of great help in managing child care and the extra needs of the child with a disability. Siblings usually take on the extra responsibility willingly. Older sisters are most often expected to take responsibility for caretaking (Cleveland & Miller, 1977). Siblings are often willing to help with caregiving or teaching while living with their family of origin but express concern and anxiety about their future responsibilities for their brother or sister with an exceptionality.

The needs and the importance of siblings can be addressed in intervention programs. Many centers and some schools run sibling workshops. These vary in format from educational, information workshops to sibling support groups (Meyer, 1993). The workshops are typically designed to help siblings learn more about the disability, how to handle situations that may occur with their siblings, and ways to be helpful to their siblings. In peer support groups, siblings meet in a relaxed and recreational atmosphere. These groups generally have open-ended discussions about what it means to have siblings with disabilities and about some of their joys and concerns.

When possible, siblings should be involved in occupational therapy sessions. As mentioned previously, siblings

are likely to be the best playmates and can often elicit efforts and motivation in the child with a disability that others cannot. They can be models for teaching new skills and can provide the needed support in a natural context, for example, help with a puzzle or game.

### Extended Family

*Extended family,* particularly *grandparents* may experience the same emotions that the parents experience: grief, anger, and disappointment (Meyer, Vadasy, & Fewell, 1986). Grandparents may feel intense grief because they believe they cannot help or control the situation.

Grandparents need accurate information about the disability. Because grandparents often receive information secondhand and do not share in the day-to-day experiences with the child, they may not have a clear understanding of the child's problems. As a result the grandparents may lack understanding of the child's needs and of the parents' needs. They may benefit from the support of other grandparents in similar situations.

Grandparents should be welcomed to therapy sessions. When they express interest in participating, these interests should be encouraged. A grandfather may take delight in building a piece of adapted equipment or a toy as his contribution to the child's ability to play and function. Grandparents and other extended family can be enormously helpful by providing child care, giving advice, and offering emotional support. Parents should be encouraged to include the grandparents and to rely on them for caregiving and support.

### Influence of a Child with Disabilities on Family Function

In addition to understanding the subsystems of the family and how the subsystems can be addressed in intervention, therapists must appreciate the family's ability to perform necessary *functions*. As a whole, each family must accomplish certain functions. The importance of each function and the time and energy devoted to each function is based on the priorities and resources of the family. They are also determined by where in the life cycle the family is positioned. Each is influenced when the family has a child with a disability. Although certain functions may have a low priority for a certain time (e.g., recreation); the priorities continually shift.

All of the functions require family members' time and energy, therefore an emphasis on one function takes time and energy from other functions. For example, a mother who has a full-time job (vocation and economic function) and spends 4 hours a day feeding her child with a severe disability (daily care) has almost no time remaining for socialization and recreation. Children who need 2 hours of extra help each night on their homework (education) also have little recreation and socialization time remaining. Brotherson and Goldstein (1992) discussed how, in families with disability, time is controlled externally by people, institutions, and events that impose expectations and requirements on the family. The possible effects of a child with a disability on the family's time and function are briefly described in the following sections.

## Economic Status

General factors that influence the family's economic status were discussed earlier. In addition, the child with a disability almost always has a direct impact on the family's economics. First, their expenditures can increase because the child requires additional medical care, therapy, and equipment. Second, income may decrease because one parent may need to stay home to provide caregiving that is not otherwise available. Often the mother finds she cannot manage full-time employment and devote the time required for therapy visits, pediatrician appointments, and educational programming. Parents with children with disabilities have many hidden and ongoing expenses (Patterson, 1993). Expenses such as transportation, phone, child care, meals, and motels are incurred when children are hospitalized. These are added to the hospital costs that are not covered by insurance. Children who require extensive medical treatment can bring devastation to a family's economics, especially when their insurance coverage is inadequate. Although financial problems create added stress, therapists are often reluctant to discuss finances, especially costs associated with their own services. In a sample of mothers with children with cerebral palsy, Nastro (1992) found that insurance coverage was inadequate to meet their needs. One mother reported her experiences:

. . . each piece of equipment has a big price tag. Even the smallest piece has a couple hundred dollar price tag . . . most insurance companies do not cover it, Medicaid does not cover everything (p. 52).

Another mother explained how her family managed:

. . .the insurance covers 15 OT [occupational therapy] visits, 15 PT [physical therapy] visits, and 15 speech each year, so we pay for Martin's therapy ourselves. We took out a home equity loan to pay for it. . . . There isn't anything free if you have a middle income status. Insurance would not pay for Pedisure, which is $35 a case. . . . We did access Respite services (p. 52).

Another mother reported that therapy cost $11,000 for her twins with cerebral palsy in the first year of life. This mother also explained that she and her husband took vacation time and leave without pay during periods that their children were in the hospital for surgical procedures and illness (Nastro, 1992).

Therapists can provide information about financial resources that parents might be able to access. Information about or applications for financial assistance should be made available at the intervention programs.

## Daily Care Needs

Children with disabilities often have extra daily care needs that extend for many years. The amount of time spent in daily living tasks can be wearing and frustrating for family members. The mother who spends hours feeding a child with severe oral motor problems has less time to spend with her other children, less energy to give to her husband, and probably less satisfaction with her daily accomplishments. When a child requires range of motion in the bath tub or extra support during bathing, an enjoyable task may become one of drudgery. A child with a pervasive developmental disability who needs constant verbal direction and supervision during mealtimes is draining to all family members. Parents' stress is highly related to the caregiving demands of the child (Seligman & Darling, 1989; Gallagher, Beckman, & Cross, 1983). When parents spend all of their day caring for their children's needs, they sometimes overlook their own needs.

Occupational therapists have important roles in helping parents manage the daily living tasks with their children. After observing the parent feeding or dressing the child, the occupational therapist can offer recommendations that help the child perform daily living activities with greater skill and independence (Figure 5-2). They also offer suggestions to the parents on how to perform the tasks more efficiently, how to conserve energy during the task, and how to turn the task into a positive interaction. Any suggestions made to the parent regarding daily living activities should be weighed by their cost and benefit. Does the recommended adapted procedure require more time? Is it too difficult or

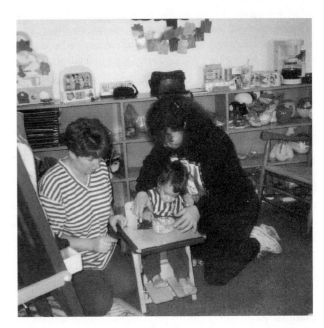

**Figure 5-2** Therapist gives the mother recommendations to increase the child's skills in self-feeding. Supportive positioning equipment and adapted feeding utensils make the task easier for the child and the mother.

complicated? If performed incorrectly, may it injure the child?

Because daily living skills such as feeding and dressing are routine activities, a mechanism for ongoing communication about the child's performance among the occupational therapist, teacher, parents, and others is essential. A notebook that the child carries between school and home might serve this purpose. Any extra time that the therapist asks the parent to spend on feeding, toothbrushing, bathing, or other daily living tasks should be well justified and should bring immediate change. Alternative suggestions should be quickly made when an adapted technique does not work. For example, the therapist may implement a program to reduce tactile defensiveness by organized brushing of the child's extremities and back. If the brushing program does not increase the child's tolerance of clothing, the occupational therapist might suggest that the mother purchase soft-lined clothing, remove tags, and use laundry softener. The goal of occupational therapy recommendations should be increased independence at minimal energy and time cost, thus benefiting the child and the family.

## Recreation and Leisure Activities

Healthy families are able to relax and enjoy recreational activities together. Often this function is diminished when a family member has a disability. Recreation may not have the priority of other areas of function, and therefore time for leisure activities is replaced by educational or therapeutic tasks. Yet leisure and recreation are critical areas of family function. Diamond (1981) explained this need when he related the experiences he had as a young child:

Something happens in a parent when relating to his disabled child: [she] forgets [he] is a kid first. I used to think about that a lot when I was a kid. I would be off in a euphoric state, drawing or coloring or cutting out paper dolls, and as often as not the activity would be turned into an occupational therapy session. "You're not holding the scissors right," or "sit up straight so your curvature doesn't get worse." The era was ended when I finally let loose a long and exhaustive tirade. "I'm just a kid! You can't therapize me all the time! I get enough therapy in school every day! I don't think about my handicap all the time like you do (Diamond, 1981, p. 30)!

Occupational therapists should encourage recreation and show flexibility in scheduling therapy and education programs to enable families to engage in recreational activities. They can also provide suggestions of adapted equipment to make recreational activities possible (see Chapters 17 and 18). With the passage of the Americans with Disabilities Act (1990), more recreational opportunities are available to individuals with disabilities. Information about community recreational activities are typically available in local newsletters. Therapists can note which are accessible and appropriate for children with disabilities.

## Socialization

Socialization is a vital aspect of life. The social relationships of all family members often change when a child with a disability enters the family. Although inclusion has increased the child's social opportunities, peer relations can remain problematic. Children with disabilities engage in fewer social interactions and have less mature social behaviors than their peers without disabilities (Odom, McConnell, & McEvoy, 1992). Delayed social skills may relate to language or cognitive delays or to the negative attitudes of peers. Children with disabilities may be in more adult-directed situations and may lack social interaction skills with peers or siblings.

The child may also create barriers to the parents' opportunities to socialize. Children with behavior problems who act out or demonstrate disruptive behaviors may be particularly difficult to take into social situations. The therapist can give the parent ideas of ways to manage difficult child behaviors in a social situation.

Persons who lack experience and understanding of disability may feel awkward in social interaction with the family who has a child with special needs. One mother explained why she no longer went to neighborhood gatherings:

Before Peter, we had many good friends in our neighborhood. I used to walk Peter in his stroller, however, each time we ran into neighbors they would ask how he was doing and ask if he was walking yet. I would always reply that he was doing well and that he wasn't walking yet. Then they were silent; like they did not know what to say next. I don't seem to have anything in common with my old friends now that I have Peter (Young N, personal communication, 1992).

Therapists can suggest responses for the parent to give when others make inappropriate or awkward comments about the disability.

Often parents develop new friendships with other parents who are experiencing similar circumstances. Parents should be encouraged to participate in other social situations. Vincent (1988, p. 4) described the importance of an informal social support system:

Parents are most likely to rely upon family members, friends, neighbors or coworkers for support when confronting problems in raising their children. Only as a last resort do they consult professionals. The implication of this finding for us is that we need to focus more of our attention in helping families develop and strengthen their own support networks. We need to emphasize to families that they are the ones best able to solve their own problems (p. 4).

The family's social life is important to the child's social life and social skills development. Because social skill development is almost always delayed in children with disabilities, opportunities to observe and imitate family members socializing can be critical to acquiring and enhancing social interaction skills.

## Self-Identity and Self-Esteem

All family members may have problems in self-esteem and feelings of worth when a member has a disability. When a child is difficult to manage or handle, the parents may feel incompetent. Siblings may overidentify with the child with a disability and may suffer from low self-esteem. The sibling may believe he or she will also acquire the disability and may be unable to differentiate his or her abilities from those of the disabled sibling. When parents give the child with a disability extra attention, the sibling may feel ignored or less important (Kronick, 1976).

Siblings need specific information about the disability and to be helped to understand that they are both related to and yet separate from their disabled sibling. Siblings who assist in caring for the disabled child may gain feelings of competence and self-esteem from the role as a helper. When other children make unkind comments about the disability, the sibling should be given positive strategies for managing the situation. Turnbull and Turnbull (1990) suggested that all members should develop self-identity in areas other than the exceptionality by pursuing their own interests, hobbies, and personal goals.

## Affection Needs

The family is the first place that a child experiences affection. Affection is the bond that creates and sustains the family (Figure 5-3). A child with a disability can have both a negative and a positive effect on the family's expression of affection for each other. Often the child has a positive influence and draws the family members closer together.

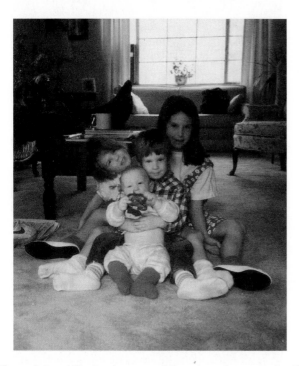

**Figure 5-3** Affection between siblings is an important family function.

The sister of Billy, who had Down syndrome, described her appreciation of her brother:

. . . Billy has a deep concern for the feelings of other people. He has a kind nature, and I cannot remember ever hearing a malicious word leave his mouth. When anyone in the family travels, Billy calls to be sure we arrived safely. And when someone has a problem, is ill, or has died, Billy's sincere sympathy is heartwarming (Schulz, 1993, p. 38).

Like other areas of function, affection may become an issue when the child with a disability becomes an adolescent with sexual desires that he or she either does not understand or is not able to express. When affection for peers of the opposite sex is not reciprocated or is not understood, self-esteem can be affected. The issues of expressing sexuality and affection among adolescents can be a difficult and challenging situation for the family. Once again, information on making this transition is needed. The therapist might suggest positive ways to express affection to peers.

## Educational and Vocational Needs

Every child attends school and spends great amounts of time in academic learning, ultimately to prepare for a vocation. When a child has a disability, often educational and vocational activities require more time and receive greater emphasis. Parents and family members of children with disabilities express appreciation of the educational system, but they also report being overwhelmed by the demands of the educational program (Brotherson & Goldstein, 1992). Parents are asked to attend meetings, to visit the school, and to work on school activities at home. The parents may believe that extra help and attention needs to be given to the child so that he or she can maintain the same pace of learning as his or her classmates. The amount of homework and therapy performed in the evening can increase by small increments; then suddenly the parents realize that all evening, every evening, is spent in therapy or school-related tasks.

Both parents and therapists need to strive toward a balance of educational activities with other family functions. Parents should always be given choices regarding their level of participation (Gartner, Lipsky, & Turnbull, 1990; McBride, Brotherson, Joanning, Whiddon, & Dermitt, 1993). A balance of activities—recreational, social, educational, and daily care—helps the family maintain their equilibrium and should remain a priority of the intervention team (Turnbull & Winton, 1984).

## Family Life Cycle

Perhaps the most predominant characteristic of families is change. As described earlier, the family is always a dynamic unit in which roles, functions, and interactions change. Families that are cohesive and adaptable thrive well with the transitions that each must make when children enter school, when husbands change jobs, or when the family relocates. Families that have more rigid structure and less positive interactions often struggle through periods of transition. All families need coping skills during periods of transition; these are described in the next section.

All families go through developmental stages; however, these stages have particular meaning for families who have children with disabilities. Parents have told their stories of experiences throughout the life cycle (Turnbull & Turnbull, 1985; Turnbull & Turnbull, 1990).

In discussing the family's life cycle, a few points of emphasis are particularly important to the occupational therapist. An understanding of the entire family life cycle helps a therapist recognize that the family cares and provides for the child always, during all developmental stages, often extending through adulthood. In contrast to this commitment, the therapist enters the family's life cycle for relatively brief periods. As critical as therapy may seem to the parent or to the professional, it is likely to be a relatively small part of the family's life.

Second, occupational therapists provide the most meaningful services when they consider all the life span events that occurred before and that may occur after the services currently provided. Therapists who work in early childhood should think about and discuss with families the issues that may arise in adolescence. The purpose of this forward thinking is not to crush hopes or discourage parents but to help them realistically plan and help the team develop goals that are important over time to the child's future.

A third aspect of the family life cycle is recognition that families often experience the greatest challenge and stress during the transitions between stages rather than in any one stage. The stress is created when family roles become redefined (Figure 5-4) and family functions may shift in unexpected ways. The child's stress in beginning a new program or undergoing rapid physiologic changes (e.g., puberty) compound the family's stress as they learn to work with new programs and new professionals and deal with role changes.

For example, parents are often unprepared for the differences between early intervention and preschool programs or preschool and school programs. They express concern that their children are also unprepared to cope with the new expectations. For these reasons more emphasis has been placed on helping families make the transitions from one program to another by planning for them throughout the program and implementing transitional activities to prepare the child and family (IDEA, 1991; P.L. 102-119).

A fourth point relates to the uniqueness of each family. Although the life cycle consists of predictable events, the individuality of each family must always be acknowledged. The characteristics and issues at each life stage are highly variable, and each family moves through the stages at different rates. A family may experience and resolve their grief when they first learn about their child's diagnosis, generally in infancy, but the family experiences cycles of grief

and acceptance within and between life stages. Therefore assumptions about whether a family has achieved a stage of acceptance or has worked through the grief cycle cannot be made. Issues that the family seemed to resolve and accept when the child was an infant, for example, a diagnosis, may occur again when the child reaches school age and an "educational diagnosis" is made or a learning problem is identified. Other stage-related events, for example, the child's developing friendships when first entering grade school, may become an issue again when the child enters high school.

Finally the child's development and transition through the life cycle stages cannot be assumed to always be congruent with the family's life cycle. The interaction between the family's stages and the child's phase of development must always be considered. A young couple may have more energy and resources to cope with the birth of a child with special needs than an older couple with four other children. The older parents may have more established resources; however, with four children participating in school activities, regular attendance in an early intervention program would be difficult. A young adult who requires close supervision may become an increasing burden to parents who retire and desire to travel. Caregiving activities for a child with exceptional needs become increasingly challenging to perform when a second child is born. Although families and children move through the life cycle together, it is impor-

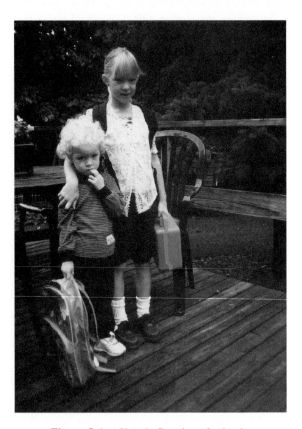

**Figure 5-4**   Sister's first day of school.

tant to recognize that not all members make transitions at the same time in the same way.

Turnbull and Turnbull (1990) described the tasks that families undertake at key stages of the life cycle. Although each stage emphasizes different activities, precise distinctions between stages cannot be made because developmental events occur at different times. Families from different cultures may experience different life cycles that may include longer periods of dependency and may not include community living apart from the family of origin. Therefore the following brief descriptions of developmental stages are general and unproven, but they give occupational therapists a framework for exploring where and how family members view the life cycle.

### Early Childhood

The first tasks of any family at the birth of a child are loving and nurturing that child. The new child generally brings great joy and results in pulling family members together around their new responsibility (Figure 5-5). When a child is born with a disability or given a medical diagnosis soon after birth, the family often enters a grief cycle that has been described by parents (Helsel, 1985; Akerley, 1985; Featherstone, 1980; Ziskin, 1985) and professionals (Seligman & Darling, 1989). The grief cycle has three stages: (1) feelings of shock, denial, and disbelief; (2) feelings of anger, guilt, and depression; and (3) acceptance or reframing, acknowledgement of tasks that must be done for the child's special needs. Generalizations cannot be made about how quickly parents move through these stages. Occupational therapists who work with very young infants are often among the first professionals whom the family encounters and inevitably interact with families who are grieving.

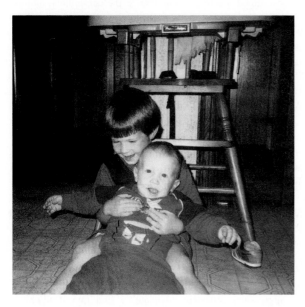

**Figure 5-5**  Brotherly affection.

The parents' stage of grief may be critical to their acceptance of intervention. Families in denial may retreat from or reject the initial offering of services. Also if parents express their anger to the therapist, the therapist should evaluate if the anger is a result of grieving or of an actual injustice that has occurred. The grief cycle is further described in the section on coping. An understanding of this process helps the occupational therapist realize that grieving about a disability is a natural, normal process and that parents find the ability to cope and accept the problem by working through their grief. Parents may mourn again at expected times, for example, the child's birthdays, entry into school, or a required surgery. They may also grieve at unexpected times for reasons not apparent to the professional, for example, when the neighbor's child first walks or learns to ride a bike.

The other tasks of early childhood are those of obtaining intervention services. The parents probably have minimal prior knowledge of early intervention programs. To successfully enter early childhood systems, parents must learn about legal issues, parental rights, therapy and educational services, available programs, and community resources. When parents participate in early childhood programs they often take on new roles, becoming their child's therapist and teacher, becoming advocates, and coordinating services.

The extent to which parents desire to take on any or all of these roles is discussed in Chapter 23. Parents often seek as much information as possible during this stage. The issue of what lies ahead becomes very important. Often parents of young children ask questions of therapists, which may include: Do you think he can go into a regular classroom? Do you think he will be able to live on his own some day? Responding to these questions is seldom easy. Although honest and realistic statements are important, parents have often expressed the importance of optimism and hope. Even therapists with years of experience and extensive knowledge about disability and development cannot make definitive statements about the future. Long-range prediction of when the child will achieve certain milestones is always speculative. However, it is frustrating for parents to be told that the future cannot be predicted. To respond to parents' questions about the future, the occupational therapist might describe the developmental course of a child with a similar disability or might explain the options in services for older children. When appropriate the therapist should refer the family to the physician for additional prognostic information.

Sometimes the parents' questions about the future reflect their desire to express and discuss their anxiety about the future. The occupational therapist might ask the parents about concerns, dreams, and hopes for the future, emphasizing the importance of those dreams and encouraging the parents to share their vision with other professionals who work with the child. As one parent expressed (Schulz, 1985):

The greatest anxiety for parents of handicapped children is uncertainty of the future. The services established for [our children] have only been stopgaps. With the exception of rare, lifelong institutional placements, we don't have plans for the future (p. 17).

## School Age

When the child enters school, the typical family is excited about the new opportunities for learning and the child's new demonstration of independence. Entry into school is not always a positive event for families with children with disabilities. If the family received early intervention services, they may be disappointed to find fewer family services and less family support offered by the school. They are no longer openly invited to attend each class and therapy session. Many parents view this change as an opportunity to be less involved and as a sign of their child's maturation. However, for some, the loss of communication with the intervention team is difficult. Also, as part of the transition, the parent needs to learn about the school's programs, schedules, rules, and policies.

For children with mild learning disabilities, entry into school may be the first time that a disability is identified. Therefore the first year of school marks the time that some parents experience the initial reactions and the issues other parents faced in early childhood.

To the school-aged child, making friends and maintaining friendships becomes critically important. Many parents report great sorrow that their children appear lonely, isolated, and friendless. In certain situations social stigma may be an issue. Much emphasis has been placed on methods that teachers and therapists can use to promote friendships in inclusive environments. Peer relations can be promoted when the disability is explained to the other children in the classroom and when activities are designed to promote cooperation and positive interaction. Inclusive models of education seem to have successfully increased social opportunities for children with disabilities and, by extension, their ability to enjoy friendships (Odom & Brown, 1993; Odom & McEvoy, 1988). Increased accessibility of playgrounds, theaters, and children's recreation areas promotes more opportunities for friends to participate in community activities, although this is not always true:

Because we live in a rural area, there are few social activities designed for handicapped people. . . . As a result, Billy has learned to enjoy his own company and the solitude of his home (Schulz, 1985, p. 17).

## Adolescence

Adolescence is a challenging and potentially stressful time for all families. Several issues emerge in the lives of children with disabilities when they reach adolescence. Parents may need to prepare the child to handle his or her growing sexual needs. In certain cases parents face decisions about their child's use of birth control and protection from sexually transmitted diseases. With adolescence clearly comes new concerns about a son or daughter's new vulnerability.

Although the child usually is well accepted by family members, the social stigma with peers and others may increase during adolescence. As one mother expressed:

The community accepts our children much more easily when they are small and cute. Babyish mannerisms are no longer acceptable . . . [Our son] has had real problems with his social relationships. He simply does not know how to initiate a friendship. He has difficulty maintaining a sensible conversation with his peers. He doesn't handle teasing well, so he is teased unmercifully (Anderson, 1983, p. 90).

The cute toddler with unusual behaviors may become a not-so-cute adolescent with socially unacceptable behaviors. As one parent explains why her son was not invited to a Christmas party:

Everyone in the family was invited except Billy. I thought it must be an oversight, but the friend later explained apologetically, "I thought Billy's presence might make the other guests uncomfortable." This kind of attitude is difficult to accept, particularly when he had been included very successfully in a similar party. I find myself crying at the unfairness (Schulz, 1985, p. 16).

Others have expressed difficulty in caring for their child's growing physical needs. As the child reaches adulthood, parents' strength and energy may decline.

The sapping of energy occurs gradually. The isolation it imposes does too. As I work professionally with young mothers, I see them coping energetically with the demands of everyday life. They are good parents, caring ones, doing everything possible to help their retarded child reach full potential, sometimes doing more than they have to; and if they have other children, they are doing the same for them. Most of these mothers even get out, see friends, attend meetings, volunteer in the community, and do all the things their friends and families expect them to do. All this is at least possible when one's child is little, though it demands enormous energy. But to look at the mothers of children who have turned into teenagers is to see the beginnings of the ravages. Their life-style is changing. They go out less, see fewer people, do less for their children. They are stripping their living to the essentials (Morton, 1985, p. 144).

The parents may face the possibility of institutionalization of the child for the first time, as they begin to wonder whether they can continue to provide the necessary care of their adolescent. Schulz (1993) wrote:

There are serious issues in the future. There is the age-old question of who will care for him if something happens to me. We have planned the best we can; we have provided for Billy financially; he has skills that with supervision, should enable him to continue his contented life. But who will supervise him? Who will provide his transportation? What if he loses his job? Who will be his aggressive, persistent advocate? I find myself thinking, as many parents of persons with disabilities have thought before me, that it would be easier if I outlive him. These are issues that we can't laugh about, or shrug off (Schulz, 1993, pp. 38-39).

### Working with Families Throughout the Life Cycle

Occupational therapists who appreciate the balance of family systems between stability and change will be in the best position to work with each family. When a child has special needs, the family may experience stress because they do not fit into the same developmental stages as other families.

For example, parents of infants with special needs find it difficult to consider enrolling their babies in an early intervention program (Calhoun et al., 1989) because other parents with infants do not use educational programs until the child is older. Other parents may feel tension about the transition of their adolescents with disabilities into the adult world and want to postpone this stage of family development. Yet, a family with adult children living at home may also seem out of phase with other families in a similar life stage.

## FAMILY COPING AND ADAPTATION

An important philosophic shift has occurred in the last decade in how families of children with special needs are viewed by professionals. The original assumption among professionals was that the presence of a disabled member led to family dysfunction and a life of recurring sorrow (Summers, Behr, & Turnbull, 1989). Parents of children with special needs have explained that their children bring growth-producing challenges, a sense of pride, fulfillment, and joy to their families (Turnbull, Guess, & Turnbull, 1988). The strength and resilience of many families that meet life events and achieve a level of happiness and life satisfaction can be a source of inspiration to clinicians.

The fact that most families successfully adjust to disabilities should not lead occupational therapists to ignore the challenges that families face. After the diagnostic period, when the child's problems are identified, the family must go about the process of living a normal life under unusual circumstances. A family's ability to cope with unanticipated news, life events, and new roles has been widely studied. No one model completely explains how the family adapts to the presence of a child with special needs. In the following section, three models with different perspectives are examined.

### Stages of Adjustment

A frequently used model for understanding how families respond has been used to describe developmental stages of adjustment (Rape, Bush, & Slavin, 1992). This model fits into the family life cycle that was previously described. Typically there are four stages, of which, the first begins with initial shock. When the family first learns that the child

has a problem, they may respond with confusion, anger, and concern during the early period. In the case of injury or sudden illness, this stage may have a sudden onset in which the child's life is also threatened. When the stage model is applied to children with developmental disabilities, the stage may last over several months. Many developmental problems are not immediately diagnosed and require a variety of tests that may include input by occupational therapists. When conflicting information is given about the diagnosis, the family's anger and disorganization heightens.

The second general stage includes a sense of relief that the uncertainty is over and denial that the family member is as disabled as professionals may think. During this period of adjustment family members may surprise professionals with what appears to be unrealistic expectations for the child's future. For example, parents of a baby with Down syndrome may talk about when their son learns to drive, goes out on dates, and leaves for college. It is important for therapists to appreciate that a family's expression of unrealistic expectations may not mean that the parents do not accept the diagnosis. The expectations that the professional believes are unacceptable goals may reflect the family's need for hope. An image of a different future for their child gradually occurs as the family moves into the next stage and acknowledges that the child has health problems or developmental challenges. Another factor contributing to unrealistic expectations during this stage may be the lack of visible evidence. When a young child has problems but no visible sign of a disability, parents may anticipate a life like every other child and entry into regular educational programs (Kraus-Mars & Lachman, 1994). Families in this period may find excuses such as "he is just lazy" or "his teacher does not explain things the right way," to explain why the child does not do well.

The next stage in most developmental models of adjustment is described as one of mourning or "working through it." This stage can be thought of as the process of giving up the image of the child as a healthy, typical individual and developing a new image for the child's future. Although this is a commonly discussed stage in adjustment, it is not clear that all families experience the sorrow and mourning process (Rape et al., 1992). The lack of a period of mourning may be especially true when the child has been born with the disability so the parents know very early that their child will be different. Parents of children with congenital conditions such as mental retardation appear less likely than parents of children with closed head injury to express regret about the child's condition (Batten & Cutler, 1990).

The final stage in most developmental models of adjustment is one of acceptance and restructuring the family (Rape et al., 1992). This stage can be described as getting on with the business of living. The restructuring of the family may occur only when the child's disabilities are caused by an accident or illness experienced after infancy. All families experience a process of reorganization when a new member joins the family. So when a child has been born with a disabling condition, the reorganization may be partly integrated with the typically occurring developmental transition of the family. Families in this stage may not believe that they are too different from any other family in the neighborhood.

The developmental stage model for describing family adjustment has several limitations. First, many of the stages are based on clinical observation and become shared theories among professionals, but the stages have not been confirmed through research (Rape et al., 1992). A second limitation is that not all families go through all stages of development, and some families adapt better than others. A third issue to a developmental approach is that the family may return to a stage of denial or unrealistic expectations in times of stress or transition. Another limitation is that individual family members may be at different stages at the same time. For example, after joining a parent support group one parent may appear to return to denial while the partner appears to accept the child's condition and becomes active in the group.

A developmental stage theory of adjustment can act as a general model to organize and understand some families, especially those that are confronted with an accident or sudden illness that threatens the well-being of a child. The model is less helpful in understanding the day-to-day family adjustments if the child's condition is chronic. Families have to adjust to new demands with each stage of family development.

## Family Adjustment and Adaptation Model

When a child continues to have special needs, it may be more effective to think of the family's adaptation in a way that helps the therapist focus on family strengths, resources, and needs. Hill (1958) proposed a model that has become a classic way of framing the family adjustment process. He recognized that the extent an event can disrupt a family and create a crisis depends on several interacting elements. Several of the elements can vary between families. By using this model, the occupational therapist recognizes how each family may be different from any other family. As a result, an event that may require extensive adaptations in one family could lead to minor adjustments in another. Table 5-1 applies the ABC=X Family Crisis Model to a family who is dealing with the potential crisis of losing services when an adolescent graduates from high school.

A family attempts to adjust to the demands of the event while maintaining homeostasis. With repeated demands or an event that leads to disequilibrium, the family works to restore homeostasis by (1) getting more resources and learning new skills, (2) reducing the number of demands that they have to deal with, or (3) redefining the situation (Patterson, 1988). The occupational therapist can support the family in their adaptation process (Table 5-1). The clinician may first address resources by providing additional information about what programs are available or training the parents on how to practice community living skills development. Or the therapist may reduce some of the stress on the family by identifying some of the skills the therapist will help the young adult develop and relieve the family's sense of total responsibility. Finally the therapist can help the family develop a positive, confident attitude about their child's graduation and transition into the adult world and help them access community resources and services outside the educational system.

Anticipated and unanticipated stressful events can require a family to adjust or adapt. As discussed earlier, families of children with special needs share certain life events with all families. Typically occurring life events may have special meaning for the family with a child who has special

▲ **Table 5-1**  Interactive Elements That Influence How a Family Adjusts to a Critical Event (X) in Their Child's Life

| Element of the Model | Example |
| --- | --- |
| Stress event (A) | Son will graduate from high school next month but has yet to achieve the skills needed for employment and community travel<br><br>Family is notified that their son will not be eligible for services through the schools |
| Family's resources for meeting the crisis (B) | Formal resources may be the school's team that has identified the skills the adolescent needs to learn and an appropriate job in the community<br><br>Informal resources are friends who have had a daughter graduate from the high school's special education program 2 years earlier<br><br>Family resources are time and role flexibility so all members work together, practicing community living |
| Meaning the family makes of the event (C) | Family worries that their son is not ready to graduate. They recognize that additional resources are needed to prepare him. They identify that their son has perseverance and has taken risks in the past |
| Family adapts to the stressful event (X) | Family contacts a social services agency to obtain a part-time coach for their son |

needs. For example, the birth of a second child without medical or developmental problems may be the first time the family is confronted with how delayed their first child really is. Unique stresses may also occur. For example, when children have recurring or degenerative medical conditions that require repeated hospitalization, the family must continually reorganize how they accomplish their daily routines.

One advantage of a model that examines the adaptation process is that it helps the clinician understand why families respond differently to similar events. The family's ability to meet multiple demands depends on both family resources and their coping behaviors (Patterson, 1988). Stress can accumulate and deplete resources. For example, an event such as having the child catch a new bus in the morning may require adjustments in the family routine. Most families could organize their lives to get the child to the bus on time. The same demand may appear insurmountable to a family dealing with unemployment and neighbors that keep them awake at night. By using this model the therapist recognizes that additional resources are needed before the family can adjust their schedule to get the child up and ready for the bus to the new program.

## Cognitive Adaptation

The family's appraisal of a situation is important in determining the amount of stress they experience. Taylor (1983) proposed three strategies that individuals use to frame the problem and potentially reduce their stress.

One strategy is to find a meaning behind the crisis or event (Taylor, 1983). Parents of children with special needs may ask the question, "why did this happen to me?" Based on their cultural background, families may have different explanations for the causes of an illness or congenital problem (Krefting & Krefting, 1991). Religious explanations are frequently given for the birth of a child with special needs. The event can take on special meaning because it helps the family focus on what is important to them. Until a crisis event requires decisions about changing the distribution of family resources, family members may not have coherent priorities. Career, trips, material possessions, or having a neat house may not be as important as they once were. The reflection on what is important to family members may lead them to new commitments to each other and what they believe is most important. When positive attitudes are developed through finding meaning behind the event, the presence of a child with special needs can become a positive asset in other members' psychologic lives.

The second strategy used to adapt to a stressful situation is to find a way to believe they have some mastery and personal control over events (Taylor, 1983). One way that parents of children with special needs gain control of the situation is to gather information about the disability and how to help their child develop (Gowen, Christy, & Sparling,

1993). Sometimes their search for more information leads the parents to pursue further testing and to visit numerous "experts" and specialists. The therapist should appreciate the potential reasons the parents need to "shop around" and recognize that it does not necessarily mean that they do not accept the child's problems.

Parents searching for control over their child's problem may develop their own therapy routines. For example, a parent may decide that practicing standing will make the child stronger and able to walk. The therapist, seeing the child standing on his or her toes because of spasticity needs to encourage the coping strategy (independent problem solving) while helping the parent find other ways to reach his or her goal.

Another strategy in cognitive coping is to think about the problem in a way that enhances self-esteem (Taylor, 1983). The parent may identify an admired role model with similar challenges. Knowledge of celebrities who have a child with special needs or finding another parent who has gone through it can enhance the parent's coping process. An alternative strategy to improving self-esteem is to imagine how the problem or disability might have been worse. The parent may specifically find another parent who has a child with greater problems as a way of feeling better about his or her own child's problems. This comparison might be seen when a parent says "Well, at least my child has autism and not mental retardation." The clinician should not only realize that the comparisons are not accurate or fair but also recognize that cognitive coping strategies are important to parents (Summers, Behr, & Turnbull, 1989)

## DEFINING FAMILY-CENTERED SERVICES

Parents have reported what services are most appreciated from therapists and other professionals (Summers et al., 1990; Mahoney, O'Sullivan, & Denebaum, 1990, McBride et al., 1993). Although parents' needs change developmentally as the child grows and as they adapt to the disability, a number of themes consistently occur when parents are surveyed or asked about the services they value.

## Parents Want Information First

Summers et al. (1990) interviewed nine consumer focus groups of families receiving early intervention service to determine what families expected from professionals. The expected outcome mentioned most by respondents was to gain needed information. Parents strongly desired information about (1) disability, (2) services for the child, (3) the future, (4) services for the parents, (5) general child development, and (6) services for the siblings (Summers et al., 1990). Suggested formats ranged from written materials to videotapes and verbal explanations. Parents wanted informational materials not only for themselves, but also for their other children and for extended family members to help explain the child's needs. Participants agreed that early intervention programs should be prepared to repeat information in several formats, if necessary, as family members' changing emotional states allow them to attend to the information.

Mahoney and his colleagues (1990) surveyed 503 mothers of children who received intervention services to gather descriptive data about the types of services they received in early childhood programs. The mothers reported that the family services most often involved provided information about (1) the intervention system, (2) the child, and (3) specific family instruction. The information therapists provide to families about the intervention system prepares the families to work with existing systems, to use resources available, and to understand their rights as consumers. This information enables the family members to become informed decision makers and to choose their level of participation in the intervention program.

The child-related information that may be of benefit to parents includes information about the child's development, the disability, the child's health, and test results. The information that therapists typically provide includes instruction on ways to play, position, handle, and interact with the child, a weekly plan of therapy activities, and ways to use toys and household items in those activities.

The need for information appears to be greatest when the family is first coping with the disability, although the need increases at times of program transition or when unexpected health problems arise. Once informational needs are satisfied, parents often report a need for support. Social support can give the family a sense of normalcy and help them place the problems in perspective.

## Principles of Family-Centered Practice

Families have also described the principles that should undergird intervention programs. Professionals have reached consensus on important principles of family-centered, early intervention services that seem to generalize across education programs.

### Respect and Accept Family Diversity

The types of family diversity that constitute today's society were discussed in the first part of this chapter. Respecting and accepting family diversity is demonstrated when professionals acknowledge that all families have strengths and resources. The positive aspects of families are recognized and used as the foundation for the intervention program. This principle becomes particularly relevant when families are of different racial, ethnic, cultural, and socioeconomic status.

Families from different cultures often have different perspectives on child rearing, health care, and disabilities. Table 5-2 lists cultural characteristics, examples, and the possible consequences for intervention programs.

## Suggestions for Trust Building with Culturally Diverse Families

1. Invite an interpreter or bilingual family members to meetings or therapy.
2. Provide written materials in the family's native language.
3. Use community representatives and peers to develop initial relationships.
4. Be sensitive to the logistical constraints and be flexible in working with the family to find viable solutions that are comfortable for the family.
5. Encourage families to share with you their view of their situation. Listening to the family's story and perspective can reinforce to the family your genuine interest and concern.
6. To the greatest extent possible, take the "shoes test" and try to assume the family's point of view.

Modified from Seligman, M. & Darling, R.B. (1989). *Ordinary families, special children: a systems approach to childhood disability.* New York: The Guilford Press.

The occupational therapist needs to recognize the balance of family roles and responsibilities and how much emphasis is placed on nurturing the child versus promoting the child's independence. The family may appear to be overprotective of the child when they are simply behaving according to their cultural norm. In some families autonomy is valued, and in others, the child is expected to obey rules and not question authority.

Therapists need to be sensitive to the implications of these subtle differences in child rearing. For example, in one family all of the children slept in the parents' bed for their first 12 years. This tradition made it difficult to increase the independence and self-sufficiency of a 10-year-old boy with myelomeningocele. Although the therapist was concerned about the child's dependence in bedtime routines, the parents were not. If the therapist gave the family recommendations for increasing independence that included sleeping in his own bed, the parents' responses may have been negative. Choosing to change a family routine is entirely a parental decision. The parents may indicate that they prefer that the occupational therapist focus on activities other than those that challenge the family's values.

Seligman and Darling (1989) proposed five principles for building trust when working with families who are culturally diverse. These are presented in the box above.

Wayman, Lynch, & Hanson (1990) presented a number of strategies for working with families of different cultures. As suggested earlier, professionals can begin by learning

▲ Table 5-2   Suggestions for Cultural Considerations

| Cultural Considerations | Examples | May Determine |
|---|---|---|
| Meaning of the disability | Disability within a family may be viewed as shameful and disgraceful or as a positive contribution to the family | Level of acceptance of the disability and the need for services |
| Attitudes about professionals | Professionals may be viewed as persons of authority or as equals | Level of family members' participation; may be only minimal in the partnership out of respect and fear |
| Attitudes about children | Children may be highly valued | Willingness of the family to make many sacrifices on behalf of the child |
| Attitudes about seeking and receiving help | Problems within the family may be viewed as being strictly a family affair or may be easily shared with others | Level of denial; may work against acknowledging and talking about the problem |
| Family roles | Roles may be sex specific and traditional or flexible. Age and sex hierarchies of authority may exist | Family preferences; may exist for the family member who takes the leadership role in the family-professional partnership |
| Family interactions | Boundaries between family subsystems may be strong and inflexible or relaxed and fluid | Level of problem sharing/solving in families; family members may keep to themselves and deal with problems in isolation, or they may problem solve as a unit |
| Time orientation | Family may be present or future oriented | Family's willingness to consider future goals and future planning |
| Role of the extended family | Extended family members may be close or far, physically and emotionally | Who is involved in the family-professional partnership |
| Support networks | Family may rely solely on nuclear family members, on extended family member, or on nonrelated persons. Importance of godparents | Who can be called on in time of need |
| Attitude toward achievement | Family may have a relaxed attitude or high expectations for achievement | Goals and expectations of the family for the family member with the disability |
| Religion | Religion and the religious community may be a strong or neutral factor in some aspects of family life | Family's values, beliefs, and traditions as sources of comfort |
| Language | Family may be non–English speaking, bilingual, or English speaking | Need for translators |
| Number of generations removed from country of origin | Family may have just emigrated or be several generations removed from the country of origin | Strength and importance of the cultural ties |
| Reasons for leaving country of origin | Family may be emigrants from countries at war | Family's readiness for involvement with external world |

From Turnbull, A.P. & Turnbull, H.R. (1990). *Families, professionals and exceptionality: a special partnership* (pp. 156-157). Columbus, OH: Merrill.

about their own culture and acknowledging how their culture might differ from families with whom they work.

One important way to understand a family's culture is to visit their home. The parents are often most comfortable in their own home. Also, viewing the home environment gives the occupational therapist an opportunity to better understand the cultural traditions and family values. With this understanding the therapist can adjust his or her expectations and strategies to fit into the family's routines. If the home is very simply and sparsely furnished, recommending state-of-the-art electronic equipment will not be well received. The therapist can learn more about family rituals and celebrations that need to be considered in the therapy schedule and program.

### Be Flexible, Accessible, and Responsive

Because each family is different and has individualized needs, services must be flexible and adaptable. The occupational therapist should continually adapt the intervention activities as the family's interests and priorities change. Although therapists are often flexible and responsive to the child's immediate needs and the parent's concerns, often the range of possible services is limited by the structure of the system. When a parent desires additional services, a change in location (e.g., home-based versus center-based), or services to be held at a different time, the therapist may or may not be able to accommodate the parent because of the therapist's own tight schedule. Often the agency or school system enforces policies regarding the therapists' caseloads and scope of services. Practitioners are caught in the middle between the system's structure and individualized family needs. A ready solution does not exist for the therapist who acknowledges a family's needs, yet who is constrained by limitations in his or her time and the demands of a large caseload.

Much of the time the therapist recognizes that he or she cannot change the structure of the system and must work as efficiently as possible within the system. At the same time the therapist should inform the family regarding the program's rules and policies so that they are aware of the constraints of the system. The therapist may recommend additional services through other agencies or similar activities that can complement the effect of therapy (e.g., swimming lessons, gymnastics, or horseback riding). The occupational therapist can also take initiative to work toward change in the system that allows more flexibility in meeting family needs. When a therapist has a caseload of 40 children each week, can he or she provide services that are responsive to family priority concerns for each of those children? Large caseloads and tight schedules are reality for therapists that limit the degree to which services can be flexible in meeting family needs.

Parents have offered advice on providing flexible and responsive services (Turnbull & Turnbull, 1990):

1. Listen with empathy to understand family concerns and needs.
2. Verbally acknowledge family priorities.
3. Make adaptations to services based on parents' input.
4. Explain the constraints of the system when the parents' request cannot be met.
5. Suggest alternative resources to parents when their requests cannot be met within the system.
6. Discuss parents' suggestions and requests with administrators to increase the possibilities that policies and agency structure can change to benefit families.

### Encourage Partnerships and Collaboration

Collaboration means working together toward a common goal, and partnership means the pooling of resources that can be used toward some joint interest. In a parent-therapist partnership, the family and a therapist function collaboratively using agreed on roles in pursuit of agreed on goals for the child (Dunst, 1991). Therapists and parents develop partnerships to promote the child's functional skills. Partnerships imply a solid working relationship with open communication that is built on mutual respect for each other. Parent-therapist partnerships may seem easy to accomplish, but a number of barriers have traditionally prevented strong collaborative models of service delivery. Often when ob-

taining services, parents have reported feeling "intimidated, unheard, or dismissed by the professionals who are trying to help them" (Singer & Irvin, 1989, p. 17).

Wood (1989) explained:

[Professionals] will have to be prepared to alter structures to make room for parental choice, control, and evaluation. They will have to work in more open situations which involve sharing with and supporting other professionals, as well as parents (p. 204).

Both the parent and the therapist bring certain perspectives and have certain responsibilities in the partnership. Dunst (1991) indicated that the therapist must assume greater responsibility for ensuring the success of the family/professional relationship.

It is incumbent upon them to share all information openly and honestly right from the start and to treat families with respect and dignity. Families, however, may choose to withhold information, understanding, and support until such time as they feel a trusting relationship has been established (p. 69).

The goal is not for parents to become quasi-professionals. Parents and therapists have different relationships to the child. The parents' relationship with the child is individual, intimate, lifelong, and subjective. The professional's involvement with the child is time limited and objective. As with most partnerships, it is in bringing together persons with differing skills and expertise that a successful relationship emerges (Gartner et al., 1990). Parents have indicated that professionals who work with a family over time can build better communication and can better observe the progress of their child. Many parents have reported that "starting over" with new therapists is stressful and disruptive to the intervention process (Brotherson & Goldstein, 1992; Case-Smith & Nastro, 1993).

Healy, Keesee, and Smith (1988, p. 63) provided guidelines for establishing partnerships with parents. Their wisdom included the following key points:

1. Although parents with at-risk and disabled children may at times be parents in crisis, they are not disabled parents. They have capacities for creative problem solving and coping that professionals need to respect, promote, and encourage.
2. Parents and involved professionals may have widely differing perspectives, experiences, and goals for a particular at-risk or disabled child. The difficult process of sharing and learning to understand these differing perspectives is an important part of care for the child.
3. Finding the professional balance between promoting competence and independence in families and providing needed expertise and emotional support are part of a developmental process. A particular kind of support at one time may at a later time promote inappropriate dependence.
4. The professional needs to share large amounts of in-

formation, often of a technical nature, with the parents of special needs children. This process can be aided by appropriate translation of technical language, the provision of relevant written materials, open acknowledgement of unknowns, and direction to other service providers.

## Family Roles in Decision Making

Parents should be the primary decision makers in intervention for their child. Although professionals tend to readily acknowledge the role of the parents as decision makers, they do not always give parents choices or explain options in ways that enable parents to make good decisions. Parents are involved in decision making about their child in the following ways:

1. They can defer decision making to the therapist. Deferring to the therapist may reflect confidence in the therapist's judgment and may be an easy way for parents to make a decision about an issue that they do not completely understand.

2. Parents have veto power. It is important that parents know that they have the power to veto any decision made or goal chosen by the team. Awareness of the legitimacy of this role gives parents assurance that they have an important voice on the team and can make changes should they desire them. This role appears to be quite satisfying to parents (McBride et al., 1993).

3. Parents share in decision making. As described in the previous section, when parent-professional partnerships have been established, the parents fully participate in team discussions that lead to decisions about the intervention plan. Service options and alternatives are made clear, and parents have the information needed to make final decisions. Requests of parents are honored (within the limitations of the program).

In a qualitative study in which families were interviewed, McBride et al. (1993) found that although family members assumed limited roles in decision making and were provided few meaningful choices, most families reported satisfaction with these practices. Families cannot always be given a wide range of choices about who will provide services and when and where these services will be provided; however, their role in decision making should be emphasized. Families who are empowered early to make decisions will be better prepared for that role throughout the course of the child's development. In most cases assessment of choices and good decision making will be a skill that parents promote in their children as they approach adulthood.

## COMMUNICATION STRATEGIES

As previously discussed, a priority of parents is to receive information regarding typical child development, the diagnosis of disability, therapeutic activities to enhance the child's skills development, and methods to cope with the disability within the family's routine. A key role of the occupational therapist is to provide this information. As mentioned earlier, therapists have tremendous amounts of information to impart to parents. Effective helping is most likely to occur when the information given is requested or sought by the parent (Dunst, Trivette, & Deal, 1988). Effective communication is built on trust and respect. A number of resources are available in learning interpersonal communication skill; it is recommended that the reader become familiar with these resources (Turnbull & Turnbull, 1990; Johnson & Johnson, 1986).

Occupational therapists communicate with parents using a variety of methods, formal and informal, written, verbal, and nonverbal. The following section describes communication strategies consistent with the principles described earlier. The strategies are based primarily on feedback from parents regarding what they have found as effective helping from occupational therapists (Hinojosa, 1990; Case-Smith & Nastro, 1993).

## Formal Team Meetings with Families

Sometimes the therapist's first meeting with a family is a formal team meeting to develop the IEP. To increase the parents' participation and comfort level in such a meeting, it is important to provide them with specific information about the purpose, structure, and logistics of the meeting. They should be provided with specific information about their role and questions the team members may ask. In an IFSP or IEP meeting the parents should receive assessment results before the meeting. Therapists might contact the parents by phone to express their concerns and to suggest possible goals. As a result, parents have an opportunity to think about the assessment and goals and to be prepared to discuss them in the team meeting. A phone call before the meeting also gives the therapist an opportunity to ask about the parents' concerns and to prepare options for meeting those concerns in the child's educational or intervention plan.

Turnbull and Turnbull (1990) use the work of Stephens and Wolfe (1980) to describe the components of a parent-professional conference. They suggested that each conference have four components.

### Building a Rapport

Family members need to feel comfortable and connected to the other team members. All members should be introduced, and the purpose of the meeting should be reviewed. Parents should be encouraged to ask questions, express opinions, or take notes.

### Obtaining Information

Family members should be encouraged to share information, using open-ended questions. All team members should respectfully attend to what the parents say, ask for clarification when needed, and indicate understanding by paraphrasing or summarizing their information. Summer et al. (1990) found that families appreciated an "unhurried atmosphere [that conveyed] the sense that family concerns and needs are important to practitioners (p. 85)."

### Sharing Information

Jargon-free language should be used, avoiding technical terms. When technical terms are used, they should be explained in ways that everyone understands. Professionals should begin with positive points and then explain problems and deficits. In describing the problems, anecdotes or real examples of the child's performance should be given. When giving information, the occupational therapist should be sensitive to the parent's response and provide opportunities for questions.

### Summarizing and Follow-up

After plans and decisions about goals are made, they should be summarized. Plans should be specific and include dates, tasks, and names of those who are responsible for the plans. The meeting should end on a positive note with plans made for another meeting or the next mode of communication.

### Informal Meetings

Many parents prefer informal individual meetings with the occupational therapist over a structured, more formal meeting. When parents are interested in a one-on-one conference, they should be given a list of times that the therapist has open. Meetings during or after the child's therapy, although convenient, are not always ideal. The therapist needs to be organized and prepared for parent encounters. Often the answer to a casual question such as, "How is Sherry doing in OT?" holds great importance to the parent. Casual or general responses are not adequate. The therapist should either describe specific examples of recent performance or state when reevaluation will occur and how those results will be reported.

When unplanned meetings occur, the therapist needs to listen to and acknowledge the parent's concerns. When the parent asks for specific information about intervention or intervention goals, the therapist should indicate that he or she prefers to respond after review of his or her daily notes and charts on the child. The therapists can later make a phone call to the parent with the child's chart in front of him or her, thus avoiding giving the parent erroneous or misleading information.

### Written Communication

In many intervention settings, particularly in the schools, parents are not physically present, and regular communication with family members relies on written strategies. Because written communication does not require the sender and recipient to be in the same place at the same time, it is a practical and important way to maintain communication with parents.

### Notebooks

Notebooks shared between therapists and parents seem to be a highly valued and successful way for parents to keep important information and to have a regular, reliable method for expressing concerns to the therapist and other team members. The notebook is usually used by all team members. The information may include a new skill the child demonstrated that day, an action by the child that delighted the class, an upcoming school event, materials requested of the parent, or snack information. It might also include a new strategy for working on self-feeding or dressing. The parents can share their perception of the child's feelings, new accomplishments at home, or new concerns. Notebooks are important regardless of whether the therapist and parent have face-to-face contact. Home-based therapists may initiate a notebook for the parent to record significant child behaviors and for the therapist to make weekly suggestions for activities. In the neonatal intensive care unit, notebooks are sometimes kept at the infant's bedside. The notebooks provide a method for the parents and therapists to communicate to all nursing staff on the likes and dislikes of the infant and successful strategies for feeding and handling.

### Handouts

When judiciously used and appropriate to the child, handouts can be helpful and valued by the parents. Handouts should be individualized and applicable to the family's daily routine. Handouts copied from books and manuals are appropriate if they are individualized. Many parents prefer pictures and diagrams. One mother expressed her appreciation of handouts:

> The home-based therapist who came out would not only show me and do things, she would watch me handle Martin and correct me if I did it wrong. She brought me pictures and diagrams and explained what each meant. . . . I still go back to them at times (Nastro, 1992, p. 70).

Other mothers indicated that photographs were helpful. In the hospital, occupational therapists often take photographs of the child in a good position for feeding or other caregiving tasks to serve as a reminder to parents and staff of how to improve postural alignment.

### Progress Reports

An occasional progress report is important to parents. A simple report of a few areas of performance might be more meaningful to the parents than a lengthy, complicated report. As mentioned previously, a report of specific performance is more important than global and general remarks.

## Other Methods of Communication

Many options are available for communication between parents and therapists. Telephone calls and simple notes sent home are good ways to maintain communication regarding issues in which both parties have common understanding. Informal communication methods are not appropriate when the therapist has concerns or issues about the child. If the therapist expects a lengthy discussion, the telephone is not the method of choice, although a call might be used to set up a meeting.

Some therapists use videotapes as a method of conveying information about handling or feeding methods. The videotape might be an effective way to teach the parent handling and positioning skills. In selecting videotaping as a method of conveying information, it should be recognized that parents must invest time in watching the tape; short clips of direct relevance to current goals are most efficient.

## Home Programs

Throughout this text authors have made recommendations for ways to implement therapeutic activities into the daily lives of children with the clear recognition that learning occurs best in the child's natural environment. Skills demonstrated in therapy translate into meaningful functional change only when the child can generalize the skill to other settings and demonstrate the skill within his or her daily routine.

Therapists often recommend home programs for the parents to implement helping the child demonstrate new skills at home. A number of studies have supported the importance of home programs and have helped define what type of home programs are most beneficial to parents.

Rainforth and Salisbury (1988) described an approach for developing home programs that fit into the family's daily routine. Before making specific recommendations for home activities, the parents were asked to chart the typical flow of family activities during the week. They were also asked when, where, and how they typically interact with the child. Together the therapist and parents discussed those interactions and whether therapeutic goals could be addressed at those times. With the parents' help, the therapist identified naturally occurring opportunities to teach the child new skills. The result of this close examination of the typical week enabled the therapist and parent to embed goals and activities into naturally occurring family routines.

Hinojosa (1990) and Case-Smith and Nastro (1993) examined how mothers use home programs and the characteristics of home programs that parents value and implement. Hinojosa completed a qualitative study in which eight mothers of preschool children with cerebral palsy were interviewed. Most of the mothers did not carry out the prescribed home programs. The mothers reported that they did not have the time, energy, or confidence to effectively follow the programs. Hinojosa (1990) suggested that it is inappropriate to expect mothers to follow a strict home program. Instead, therapists should assist mothers in adaptive ways to meet their children's needs with minimal disruptions to their lives. He described the resultant home intervention as "mother directed," meaning that the mothers made the decision as to how therapy might be implemented at home.

Case-Smith and Nastro (1993) replicated Hinojosa's study using a sample of mothers from Ohio who had young children with cerebral palsy. Each had accessed private therapy as well as public-funded therapy. Initially, when their children were infants, these mothers had participated extensively in home programs. The mothers believed that the activities performed at home were self-motivated efforts to help their children. They also indicated that specific home programs were not "an imposed expectation" on the part of the therapists. As the children reached preschool age, the mothers no longer implemented specific home programs with their children. Reasons for discontinuing home programs included lack of time and increased resistance on the part of their children. Lyon (1989) expressed a mother's perspective on implementing therapy at home:

I've come to terms with being "only human." If I could ensure that Zak could go through the day always moving in appropriate ways, flexing when he should flex, straightening when he should straighten, and play and learn and experience and appreciate . . . I would. But that is not possible. I do have a responsibility to help Zachary develop his motor skills, but I also have a responsibility to help him learn about life. So on those days when we have so much fun together or are so busy that bedtime comes before therapy time, I finally feel comfortable that I have given him something just as vital to his development—a real mom (p. 4).

Although mothers tend not to implement specific prescribed strategies, they have reported appreciating the therapists' suggestions and ideas about home activities that promoted the child development or made caregiving easier. Case-Smith and Nastro (1993) found that the mothers in their sample frequently used the written handouts with specific activities and recommendations long after they had been given to them. Summers et al. (1990, p. 91) explained that parents found written materials and videotapes helpful because they were "not always ready to hear, understand, or accept some information, but that it could be available for later use."

## Summary

Positive relationships with families seem to develop when open and honest communication is established, and parents are encouraged to participate in their child's program to the extent that they desire. When asked to give advice to therapists, parents stated that they appreciated (1) specific objective information, (2) flexibility in service delivery, (3) sensitivity and responsivity to their concerns, and (4) positive, optimistic attitudes (Case-Smith & Nastro, 1993). One mother expressed that hope and optimism are always best:

> Given a choice, I would want my therapist to be an optimist and perhaps to strive for goals that might be a bit too optimistic, keeping in mind that we might not come to that (Nastro, 1992, p. 64).

## WORKING WITH CHALLENGING FAMILIES

As discussed earlier, families are characterized by diversity. The principles just presented become critically important and more challenging to implement when working with families with atypical structures or from different cultural groups. Other significant variables that affect family function include poverty, mental retardation (MR) and mental illness (MI), poor physical health, and parental drug addiction. Family situations that encompass problems such as these are particularly challenging for occupational therapists. These problems require new definition of family centeredness and new strategies that include additional flexibility and sensitivity by therapists.

### Families in Poverty

An important variable that affects how the family functions and how they participate in therapy is socioeconomic status. Families who live in poverty may be crisis oriented and may have chaotic lives in which daily survival drives the parents' actions. These families often have transportation problems and may have difficulty with regular attendance because of the current crisis.

If the family is worried about basic food and shelter needs, recommending that they purchase toys and equipment is inappropriate. Use of toy libraries and of household objects as toys would be more appropriate ways to promote the child's play skills.

When families are crisis oriented, they tend to focus their attention on the present and on providing for their children today. The current crisis consumes the parents' energy, for example, a stove in need of repair and finding a reliable method of transportation. Brinker (1992) described a model program that was developed to increase the involvement of families who received public aid and early intervention services. Brinker and his colleagues were concerned about the sporadic attendance and dropout rate of their families who lived in poverty. The program gave a selected group tangible incentives for attendance. The incentives included boxes of food, clothing, and toys based on the parents' request. The intervention program consisted of weekly therapy and parent discussion groups. Despite the incentives, attendance in the program was between 40% and 50%. The parents who received formula, clothing, and toys attended no more often than parents in similar conditions who did not. This attendance rate was markedly below the 75% rate for families with middle incomes. Brinker suggested that families in poverty have individualized needs, and a standard program that provides certain incentives may not meet those needs. Even a program logically based on Maslow's hierarchy of needs is not effective if it becomes a standard approach rather than an individualized one.

The importance of informal support networks that are family generated has been documented in numerous research studies (Dunst, 1985; Werner & Smith, 1989). For families in chaotic and discordant homes, the support of professionals seems to be critical to the child's development (Werner, 1990). Formal systems of professional intervention play a crucial role for children who are in a nonoptimal home situation and for families whose members are at the greatest risk because of abusive or neglectful situations.

### Parents with Special Needs

Parents themselves may have special needs that require an emphasis on supportive services. Parents who struggle with drug addiction or mental illness often require counseling, mental health services, and opportunities to participate in support groups. When parents have special needs that strongly influence their caregiving ability, often their needs become the first emphasis of intervention.

Parents with MR, MI, or drug addiction are at risk for having children with developmental disabilities. Professionals have questioned the competency of parents with MR. Parents at risk because of MR or MI appear to be more successful in caring for young children when they are married, have few children, have adequate financial support, and have other sources of support (Tymchuk, Anrom, & Unger, 1987).

In providing support to parents with MR, Espe-Sherwindt and Kerlin (1990) recommended that professionals focus on the parents' internal and external control, self-esteem, social skills, and problem-solving skills. Therapists can help empower parents to make their own decisions, thus increasing their sense of self-control. Often individuals with MR or drug addiction have low self-esteem and lack confidence in their ability to make decisions. Because self-esteem is important in interactions with children, this aspect of interaction should be considered.

One task of parenting a child with a disability is accessing and using community resources. Social skills are needed to ask questions and develop relations with professionals and others who can provide supportive services. Social skills and roles are also important to model for their children. Many social skills are learned in the context of the home.

Professionals should also focus on helping parents with

MR and MI build problem-solving skills. Everyday care for children requires constant problem solving. Many times professionals give advice or recommendations without encouraging the parents to independently solve the problem or to first try their own actions. When parents are directed by others, they become more dependent. When parents successfully solve a problem, they become empowered to act independently in daily decision making. Problem solving can be taught and modeled. Espe-Sherwindt and Kerlin (1990) suggested that teaching problem-solving skills in daily caregiving can be critical to parents' development of caregiving competence.

When occupational therapists work with parents with MR or MI, it becomes essential to know their learning styles and abilities. Many times instructions need to be repeated and reinforced. Therapists must use good judgment in what techniques are taught to these parents, with emphasis on safe and simple methods. The occupational therapist should also recognize the need for additional supports to help parents with MR access those supports. Regular visits in the home by aides, nurses, or teaching assistants can meet the level of support needed. If the occupational therapist communicates his or her goals and strategies with the visiting aide, therapy activities are more likely to be implemented by the parents and other professionals who work with the family.

Working with parents who are MR or MI can be frustrating when appointments are missed or requests are not followed. An understanding of the parents' needs is essential. Development of simple, repetitive routines and systems that the parents can learn and follow enables them to become competent caregivers. With support they can offer the child a positive and loving environment that fosters both health and development.

## Summary

Professionals use a variety of strategies to deal with chalenging families. When families have continual stress and problems, it is important for therapists to begin slowly, to first build trust, to share observations and concerns, and to accept parents' choices (DeGangi, Wietlisbach, Poisson, Stein, & Royeen, 1994). When parents do not seem to understand the intervention process, professionals can attempt to establish rapport by using concrete, simple terms, providing both written and verbal information, and providing ideas that would immediately help the child. Professionals also have reported that parents could better articulate their concerns when services were home based, when lay terminology was used, and when services were presented in a slow, nonjudgmental way (DeGangi et al., 1994). Focusing on the child's strengths and developing trust and responsiveness were also believed to be important when parents had difficulty articulating concerns.

## SUMMARY

Working with families is one of the most challenging and rewarding aspects of pediatric occupational therapy. The family's participation in intervention is of critical importance to how much the child can benefit. The family's contributions to therapy goals and activities determine how well they match the family's priorities and whether they will result in meaningful outcomes.

This chapter described families as systems with unique structures and interaction patterns. The potential effects of a child with a disability on family function were related to implications for the occupational therapist's role. Issues that arise during different stages of the family's life cycle were described. In the final section, principles and strategies for working with families were discussed. The strategies included communication methods to inform and involve parents in the intervention program. Of critical importance is the occupational therapist's sensitivity to the family's values and interests, respect for those interests, provision of information, and consistent support of family members.

## STUDY QUESTIONS

1. Take a random selection of 10 friends and five people of different ages. Ask them to write down the names of everyone in their family. If asked if they should include a stepparent or deceased sister, reply, "it is up to you," and ask them to include anyone they want. Can you write a definition of "the family" that would include all the characteristics of the families described by your subjects? (Idea adapted from Levin and Trost, 1992.)

2. Use Table 5-2 to identify your own cultural characteristics. What would you want an occupational therapist to be aware of if he or she were giving services to your family?

3. The priorities of parents change over the life cycle. When a family includes a low-functioning child with severe and multiple disabilities, what might be two priorities of the parents in infancy? During school ages? In adolescence? For each priority, describe the role of the occupational therapist in meeting that priority need.

4. List three strategies that the occupational therapist might employ in working with a family of low SES in which the father is of normal intelligence and the mother has moderate mental retardation. Neither parent works outside the home. They have a 2-year-old daughter with moderate delays in language and fine motor skills.

**REFERENCES**

Acock, A.C. & Kiecolt, K.J. (1989). Is it family structure or socio-economic status? Family structure during adolescence and adult adjustment. *Social Forces, 68,* 553-571.

Akerley, M.S. (1985). False goads and angry prophets. In H.R. Turnbull & A. Turnbull (Eds.). *Parents speak out: then and now* (pp. 23-38). Columbus, OH: Merrill.

American with Disabilities Act (1990).

Anderson, D. (1983). He's not "cute" anymore. In T. Dougan, L. Isbell, & P. Vyas (Eds.). *We have been there* (pp. 90-91). Nashville, TN: Abington Press.

Batten, B. & Cutler, P. (1990). *A comparison of coping strategies used by families with children with special needs based upon the time of onset of the disability.* Unpublished student research project, University of North Carolina, Chapel Hill, NC.

Brinker, R.P. (1992). Family involvement in early intervention: accepting the unchangeable, changing the changeable, and knowing the difference. *Topics in Early Childhood Special Education, 12*(3), 307-332.

Brody, G.H., Stoneman, Z., Flor, D., McCrary C., Hastings, L., & Conyers, O. (1994). Financial resources, parent psychological functioning, parent co-caregiving, and early adolescent competence in rural two-parent African American families. *Child Development, 65,* 590-605.

Bronfenbrenner, U. & Crouter, A.C. (1982). Work and family through time and space. In S. Kamerman & C.S. Hayes (Eds.). *Families that work: children in a changing world.* Washington, DC: National Academy Press.

Brotherson, M.J. & Goldstein, B.L. (1992). Time as a resource and constraint for parents of young children with disabilities: implications for early intervention services. *Topics in Early Childhood Special Education, 12*(4), 508-527.

Calhoun, M.L., Calhoun, L.G., & Rose, T.L. (1989). Parents of babies with severe handicaps: concerns about early intervention. *Journal of Early Intervention, 13,* 146-152.

Case-Smith, J. & Nastro, M. (1993). The effect of occupational therapy intervention on mothers of children with cerebral palsy. *American Journal of Occupational Therapy, 46,* 811-817.

Cleveland, D.W. & Miller, N. (1977). Attitudes and life commitments of older siblings of mentally retarded adults: an exploratory study. *Mental Retardation, 15*(2), 38-41.

Crowe, T.K. (1993). Time use of mothers with young children: the impact of a child's disability. *Developmental Medicine and Child Neurology, 35,* 612-630.

DeGangi, G.A., Wietlisback, S., Poisson, S. Stein, E., & Royeen, C. (1994). The impact of culture and socioeconomic status on family-professional collaboration: challenges and solutions. *Topics in Early Childhood Special Education, 14*(4), 503-520.

Diamond, S. (1981). Growing up with parents of a handicapped child: a handicapped person's perspective. In J.L. Paul (Ed.). *Understanding and working with parents of children with special needs* (pp. 23-59). New York: Holt, Rinehart & Winston.

Dunst, C.J. (1985). Rethinking early intervention. *Analysis and Intervention in Developmental Disabilities, 5,* 165-201.

Dunst, C.J. (1991). Implementation of the Individualized Family Service Plan. In M.J. McGonigel, R.K. Kaufmann, B.H. Johnson (Eds.). *Guidelines and recommended practices for the Individualized Family Service Plan.* Bethesda, MD: Association for the Care of Children's Health.

Dunst C.J., Trivette, C., & Deal, A. (1988). *Enabling and empowering families: principles and guidelines for practice.* Cambridge, MA: Brookline Books.

Espe-Sherwindt, M. & Kerlin, S.L. (1990). Early intervention with parents with mental retardation: do we empower or impair? *Infants and Young Children, 2*(4), 21-28.

Featherstone, H. (1980). *A difference in the family: living with a disabled child.* New York: Basic Books.

Fiese, B.H., Hooker, K.A., Kotary, L., & Schwagler, J. (1993). Family rituals in the early stages of parenthood. *Journal of Marriage and the Family, 55,* 633-642.

Gallagher, J., Beckman, P., & Cross, A. (1983). Families of handicapped children: sources of stress and its amelioration. *Exceptional Children, 50*(1), 10-19.

Gartner, A., Lipsky, D.K., & Turnbull, A.P. (1990). *Supporting families with a child with a disability: an international outlook.* Baltimore: Brookes.

Gowen, J.W., Christy, D.S., & Sparling, J. (1993). Informational needs of parents of young children with special needs. *Journal of Early Intervention, 17,* 194-210.

Grossman, F.K. (1972). *Brothers and sisters of retarded children: an exploratory study.* Syracuse, NY: Syracuse University Press.

Halpern, R. (1993). The societal context of home visiting and related services for families in poverty. In B.E. Behrman (Ed.). *The future of children: home visiting* (pp. 158-171). Los Altos, CA: Center for the Future of Children.

Hare, J. (1994). Concerns and issues faced by families headed by a lesbian couple. *Families in Society: The Journal of Contemporary Human Services, 75,* 27-35.

Healy, A., Keesee, P.D., & Smith, B.S. (1989). *Early services for children with special needs: transactions for family support* (2nd ed.). Baltimore: Brookes.

Helsel, E. (1985). The Helsels' story of Robin. In H.R. Turnbull & A. Turnbull. *Parents speak out: then and now* (pp. 81-108). Columbus, OH: Merrill.

Hill, R. (1958). Generic features of families under stress. *Social Casework, 49,* 139-150.

Hinojosa, J. (1990). How mothers of preschool children with cerebral palsy perceive occupational and physical therapists and their influence on family life. *Occupational Therapy Journal of Research, 10*(3), 144-162.

Individuals with Disabilities Education Act of 1990 (P.L. 102-119), 20 U.S.C. Secs. 1400-1485.

Itzkowitz, J. (1990). Siblings' perceptions of their needs for programs, services and support: a national study. *Sibling Information Network Newsletter, 7*(1), 1-4.

Johnson, D.W. & Johnson, R.T. (1986). Mainstreaming and cooperative learning strategies. *Exceptional Children 52*(6), 553-561.

Julian, T.W., McKenry, P.C., & McKelvey, M.W. (1994). Cultural variations in parenting: Perceptions of Caucasian, African American, Hispanic, and Asian-American parents. *Family Relations, 43,* 30-37.

Kraus-Mars, A.H. & Lachman, P. (1994). Breaking bad news to parents with disabled children: a cross-cultural study. *Child: Care, Health and Development, 20,* 101-113.

Krefting L.H. & Krefting, V. (1991). Cultural influences on performance. In C. Christiansen & C. Baum (Eds.). *Occupational therapy: overcoming human performance deficits* (pp. 101-122). Thorofare, NJ: Slack.

Kronick, D. (1976). *Three families: the effect of family dynamics on social and conceptual learning.* San Rafael, CA: Academic Therapy Publications.

Levin, I. & Trost, J. (1992). Understanding the concept of family. *Family Relations, 41,* 348-351.

Levitt, M. (1988). Away from home for the first time. *The Exceptional Parent, 18*(5), 55.

Luster, T., Rhoades, K., & Haas, B. (1989). The relationship between parental values and parenting behavior: a test of the Kohn hypothesis. *Journal of Marriage and the Family, 51,* 139-147.

Lynch, E.Q. & Hanson, M.J. (1992). (Eds.). *Developing crosscultural competence: a guide for working with young children and their families.* Baltimore: Brookes.

Lyon, J. (1989). I want to be Zak's Mom, not his therapist. *Developmental Disabilities Special Interest Section Newsletter, 12*(1), 4.

Mahoney, G., O'Sullivan, P., & Dennebaum, J. (1990). Maternal perceptions of early intervention services: a scale for assessing family focused intervention. *Topics in Early Childhood Special Education, 10,* 1-15.

May, J. (1990). *Fathers of children with special needs: new horizons.* Bethesda, MD: Association for the Care of Children's Health.

McBride, S. L., Brotherson, M.J., Joanning, H., Whiddon, D., & Dermitt, A. (1993). Implementation of family-centered services: perceptions of families and professionals. *Journal of Early Intervention, 17*(4), 414-430.

Meyer, D.J. (1986). Fathers of children with special needs. In M.E. Lamb (Ed.). *The father's role: applied perspectives* (pp. 227-254). New York: John Wiley & Sons.

Meyer, D.J. (1993). Lessons learned: cognitive coping strategies of overlooked family members. In A.P. Turnbull, J.M. Patterson, S.K. Behr, D.L. Murphy, J.G. Marquis, M.J. Blue-Banning. (Eds.). *Cognitive coping, families, and disability* (pp. 81-94). Baltimore: Brookes.

Meyer, D.J. & Vadasy, P.F., & Fewell, R.R.(1986) *Sibshops: a handbook for implementing workshops for siblings of children with special needs.* Seattle: University of Wahington Press.

Minuchin, P. (1985). Families and individual development: povocations from the field of family therapy. *Child Development 56,* 289-302.

Nastro, M. (1992). An ethnographic study of mothers of children with cerebral palsy and the effect of occupational therapy intervention on their lives. Master's thesis, the Ohio State University, Columbus, Ohio.

Ninio, A. & Rinott, N. (1988). Fathers' involvement in the care of their infants and their attributions of cognitive competence to infants. *Child Development, 59,* 652-663.

Odom, S.L. & Brown, W.H. (1993). Social interaction skills interventions for young children with disabilities in integrated settings. In C.A. Peck, S.L. Odom, & D.D. Bricker (Eds.). *Integrating young children with disabilities into community programs.* Baltimore: Brookes.

Odom, S.L., McConnell, S.R., & McEvoy, M.A. (1992). Peer-related social competence and its significance for young children with disabilities. In S.L. Odom, S.R. McConnell, & M.A. McEvoy (Eds.). *Social competence of young children with disabilities: nature, development and intervention* (pp. 3-35). Baltimore: Brookes.

Odom, S.L. & McEvoy, M.A. (1988). Social integration of young children with handicaps and normally developing children. In S.L. Odom & M.B. Karnes (Eds.). *Early intervention for infants and children with handicaps: an empirical base* (pp. 241-268). Baltimore: Brookes.

Patterson, J.M. (1988). Families experiencing stress. *Family Systems Medicine, 6,* 202-237.

Patterson, J.M. (1993). The role of family meanings in adaptation to chronic illness and disability, In A.P. Turnbull, J.M. Patterson, S.K. Behr, D.L. Murphy, J.G. Marquis, M.J. Blue-Banning (Eds.). *Cognitive coping, families, and disability* (pp. 221-238). Baltimore: Brookes.

Peterson, G.W. & Leigh, G.K. (1990). The family and social competence in adolescence. In T.P. Gullotta, G.R. Adams, R. Montemayer (Eds.). *Developing social competency in adolescence* (pp. 97-138). Newbury Park, CA: Sage.

Rainforth, B. & Salisbury, C. (1988). Functional home programs: a model for therapists. *Topics in Early Childhood Special Education, 7*(4), 33-45.

Rape, R.N., Bush, J.P., & Slavin, L.A. (1992). Toward a conceptualization of the family's adaptation to a member's head injury: a critique of developmental stage models. *Rehabilitation Psychology, 37,* 3-22.

Richards, L.N. & Schmiege, C.J. (1993). Problems and strengths of single-parent families: implications for practice and policy. *Family Relations, 42,* 277-285.

Rolland, J.S. (1987). Chronic illness and the life cycle: a conceptual framework. *Family Process, 26,* 203-221.

Sameroff, A.J. & Chandler, M.J. (1975). Reproductive risk and the continuum of caretaking causality. In F. Horowitz (Ed.). *Review of child development research,* (Vol. 4). Chicago: University of Chicago Press.

Sameroff, A.J. & Fiese, B.H. (1990). Transactional regulation and early intervention. In S.J. Meisels & J.P. Shonkoff (Eds.). *Handbook of early childhood intervention* (pp. 119-149). New York: Cambridge University Press.

Schulz, J.B. (1985). The parent-professional conflict. In H.R. Turnbull & A.P. Turnbull (Eds.). *Parents speak out: now and then.* (pp. 3-22). Columbus, OH: Merrill.

Schulz, J.B. (1993). Heroes in disguise. In A.P. Turnbull, J.M. Patterson, S.K. Behr, D.L. Murphy, J.G. Marquis, M.J. Blue-Banning (Eds.). *Cognitive coping, families, and disability* (pp. 31-42). Baltimore: Brookes.

Seligman, M. & Darling, R.B. (1989). *Ordinary families, special children: a systems approach to childhood disability.* New York: The Guilford Press.

Singer, G.H.S. & Irvin, L.K. (1989). Family caregiving, stress, and support. In G.H.S. Singer & L.K. Irvin (Eds.). *Support for caregiving families: enabling positive adaptation to disabilities* (pp. 3-26). Baltimore: Brookes.

Slaughter-Defoe, D.T. (1993). Home visiting with families in poverty: Introducing the concept of culture. *The future of children: home visiting* (pp. 173-183). Los Altos, CA: Center for the Future of Children.

Sparling, J.W., Berger, R.G., & Biller, M.E. (1992). Fathers: myth, reality, and public Law 99-457. *Infants and Young Children, 4*(3), 9-19.

Stephens, T.M. & Wolf, J.S. (1980). *Effective skills in parent/teacher conferencing.* Columbus: Ohio State University, National Center for Educational Material and Media for the Handicapped.

Summers, J.A., Behr, S.K., & Turnbull, A.P. (1989). Positive adaptations and coping strengths of families who have children with disabilities. In G.H.Q. Singer & L.K. Irvin (Eds.). *Support for caregiving families* (pp. 27-40). Baltimore: Brookes.

Summers, J.A., Dell'Oliver, C., Turnbull, A.P., Benson, H., Santelli, E., Campbell, M., & Siegel-Causey, E. (1990). Examining the individualized family service plan process: what are family and practitioner preferences? *Topics in Early Childhood Special Education, 10*(1), 78-99.

Taylor, S.E. (1983). Adjustment to threatening events: a theory of cognitive adaptation. *American Psychologist, 38,* 1161-1173.

Turnbull, A.P. & Turnbull, H.R. (1990). *Families, professionals and exceptionality: a special partnership* (2nd ed.). Columbus, OH: Merrill.

Turnbull, A.P. & Winton, P.J. (1984). Parent involvement policy and practice: current research and implications for families of young severely handicapped children. In J. Balcher (Ed.). *Severely handicapped children and their families: research in review* (pp. 377-397). New York: Academic Press.

Turnbull, H.R., Guess, D., & Turnbull, A.P. (1988). Vox Pouli and Baby Doe. *Mental Retardation 26,* 127-132.

Turnbull, H.R. & Turnbull, A.P. (1985). *Parents speak out: then & now* (2nd ed.). Columbus, OH: Merrill.

Tymchuk, A.J., Andron, L., & Unger, O. (1987). Parents with mental handicaps and adequate child care: a review. *Mental Handicap, 15,* 49-54.

U.S. Bureau of Census (1989) Changes in American Family Life. (Current Population Reports, Series P-23, No. 165).

Vadasy, R.F., Fewell, R.R., & Meyer, D.J. (1986). Grandparents of children with special needs: insights into their experiences and concerns. *Journal of the Division of Early Childhood, 10*(1), 36-44.

Vincent, L.J. (1988). What we have learned from families. *Family Support Bulletin,* (Fall), 3.

Vondra, J. & Belsky, J. (1993). Developmental origins of parenting: personality and relationship factors. In T. Luster & L. Kodak (Eds.). *Parenting: an ecological perspective* (pp. 1-34). Hillsdale, NJ: Lawrence Erlbaum & Associates.

Wayman, K.I., Lynch, E.W., & Hanson, M.J. (1990). Home-based early childhood services: cultural sensitivity in a family systems approach. *Topics in Early Childhood Special Education, 10*(4), 56-75.

Werner, E. (1990). Protective factors and individual resilience. In S.J. Meisels & J.P. Shonkoff (Eds.). *Handbook of early childhood intervention* (pp. 97-116). Cambridge, MA: Cambridge University Press.

Werner, E. & Smith, R.S. (1989). *Vulnerable but invincible: a longitudinal study of resilient children and youth.* New York: Adams Bannister Cox.

Wolin, S.J. & Bennett, L.A. (1984). Family rituals. *Family Process, 23,* 401-420.

Young, D.M. & Roopnarine, J.L. (1994). Fathers' childcare involvement with children with and without disabilities. *Topics in Early Childhood Special Education, 14*(4), 488-502.

Ziskin, L. (1985). The story of Jennie. In H.R. Turnbull & A.P. Turnbull (Eds.). *Parents speak out: now and then* (pp. 65-80). Columbus, OH: Merrill.

## SUGGESTED READINGS

Bronfenbrenner, U. (1979). *The ecology of human development: experiments by nature and design.* Cambridge, MA: Harvard University Press.

Christiansen, C. (1991). Occupational therapy: intervention of life performance. In C. Christiansen & C. Baum (Eds.). *Occupational therapy: overcoming human performance deficits* (pp. 1-44). Thorofare, NJ: Slack.

Dallos, R. (1991). *Family belief systems, therapy and change: a constructional approach.* Bristol, PA: Open University Press.

Hinojosa, J. & Anderson, J. (1991). Mothers' perceptions of home treatment programs for their preschool children with cerebral palsy. *American Journal of Occupational Therapy, 45,* 273-297.

Horowitz, F.D. (1985). Making a model of development and its implications for working with young infants. *Zero to Three, 6*(2), 1-6.

Kraus, M.W. & Jacobs, F. (1990). Family assessment: purposes and techniques. In S.J. Meisels & J.P. Shonkoff (Eds.). *Handbook of early childhood intervention* (pp. 303-325). New York: Cambridge University Press.

McAdoo, H. (1988). *Black families* (2nd ed.). Newbury Park, CA: Sage.

Morton, K. (1985). Identifying the enemy: a parent's complaint. In H.R. Turnbull & A. Turnbull (Eds.). *Parents speak out: now and then* (pp. 143-148). Columbus, OH: Merrill.

Richards, M.H. & Duckett, E. (1994). The relationship of maternal employment to early adolescence daily experiences with and without parents. *Child Development, 65,* 225-236.

Scott, M.M. (1993). Recent changes in family structure in the United States: a developmental systems perspective. *Journal of Applied Developmental Psychology, 14,* 213-230.

Vadasy, P.F., Fewell, R.R., Meyer, D.J., & Greenberg, M.T. (1984). Supporting fathers of handicapped young children: preliminary findings of program effects. *Analysis and Intervention in Developmental Disabilities, 5,* 151-163.

Winton, P.J. & Turnbull, A.P. (1981). Parent involvement as viewed by parents of preschool handicapped children. *Topics in Early Childhood Special Education, 1*(3), 11-19.

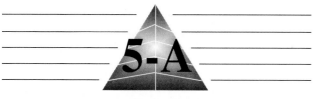

## A Parent's Perspective
### Beth Ball

When I was first asked to contribute to this chapter on parents and families of children with disabilities, I thought about the myriad of experiences and feelings that have come as a result of having children with disabilities. It seemed too vast a topic to be captured in a few typed pages The following discussion is a brief glimpse into the thoughts and feelings about my life with my three children who have disabilities. There is more than facts or history. There are, of course, feelings—deep and undeniable—and there is poetry. It is the first shed tear of realization that this child of mine will have a life that is difficult. It is the happy smile of childhood with supportive therapists and teachers, and it is the frustrated panic of adolescence when things are hard and troublesome and the phone does not ring on Saturday night.

## INITIAL RESPONSE

Learning about the disabilities of each of my children came at different times in their lives, and the impact that it had varied as a result of that and, of course, of the disability that was presented. Benjamin was born on a warm June day in 1971. The nurse turned the mirror away, and I complained that I could not see the baby. Everything seemed to happen in slow motion. The doctor held him up and announced that he was a boy but there was a small problem. He only had one thumblike digit for a right hand, and his left was a modified claw hand, having four fingers with syndactyl and a center cleft. The nurses placed him on my tummy and he peed a fountain all over the sterile drapes. They said, "That works," which was comforting but scary because I had not considered that other things could be wrong also.

It was not until that night when I had him to myself in the privacy of my own room that I felt the bifed femur on his right side, the block at his knee that refused to let it extend, the very thin lower leg, which turned out to be missing the tibia, and the club foot. The very sick feeling in my stomach was guilt. There must have been something that I had done wrong to have caused this. Even though I had fol-

lowed all the doctor's instructions, I must have missed something, and what would others think of me? I was not good enough to have a child.

Mick and I were lucky to have a wonderful pediatrician whose first advise was exactly what we needed to hear. He told us not to withdraw from our family and friends, alluding to the feelings of shame and guilt that were not overtly expressed. He told us to be open to them supporting us—that they would only want to help. The unspoken message that they would not judge us was very important.

And so we started on our journey of new experiences with orthopedic surgeons, prosthetists, genetic counselors, neurologists, internists, pediatricians, urologists, physical therapists, occupational therapists, and eyes, nose, and throat (ENT) specialists; and from the other side, special education teachers, psychologists, insurance companies, and vision therapists. We searched for answers to "why?" We searched for options to deal with the problems. We searched for resolution to our own feelings. But we were lucky because, as husband and wife, we never blamed each other.

Mick and I started the journey together, and we have had each other's support through the hard times and the joyous ones. Part of the reason that we have been able to deal with the problems and have come out on top is that we have a commitment to each other and deep faith in God and His support. This statement is much too simplistic for the deep feelings of need, grace, and oneness that we have that allow us to go forward to meet challenges. The other reason is that each of our children is a gift. They are grace without gracefulness. They are charm without all the social skills. They are fun with a sometimes struggling sense of humor. They are individuals who have enriched our lives and given us humility, wonder, and awe at their commitment to living, loving, and succeeding.

## ACCESSING SERVICES AND RESOURCES

Gaining services and resources for our children has not come without pain, questioning, depression, or anger. It has been a constant struggle. A first barrier started with finding the money to supply the prosthetics and the medical care necessary. One of the first things that the orthopedic surgeon told us was that we had better find a source of funding because prosthetics would cost more than a house by the time Benjamin was 16. I will not go into all the details but will give you a few insights that parents must face when they do not know where to turn or who has the funds that may help. The doctors have a few ideas, but they are not the source of information. Agencies such as hospitals may have more information, but getting connected to the right person to get the information is not an easy task. Also, we dealt with feelings of begging and not being good enough to supply the needs of the child that we brought into the world who is our responsibility.

In the search for money to cover the cost of prosthetics,

---

**Editor's note:** Beth Ball is the mother of three children with disabilities. She is also an occupational therapist and has worked in the school system a number of years.

we approached a well-known agency because we knew that they worked with individuals who had physical disabilities. After being told that prosthetics were not covered among their services, and because this was the third or fourth rejection that we had encountered, Mick broke down and joined me with some tears. We were then informed that we had better pull ourselves together—that this was *our* child and *our* responsibility and we had better face it. Shame turned to anger as we left, and seeking any other service with that agency was carefully avoided. Luckily, the Shriners accepted our application and they provided most of the cost of Benjy's prosthetics until he turned 18. I do not want to think of what might have been if we had not had their help. Dealing with financial issues created a new level of trauma from the outside that was added to the earlier inside pain.

What we discovered in this process was the necessary and valuable process of networking. It was through work and friends and family that we made contact with the Shriners. It was through people at school that we came in touch with the Parent Advisory Council at the local Special Education Regional Resource Center, where we continue to receive information and support. It was through many of the parents that we met in these places that we learned about the Ohio Coalition for Children with Disabilities. If it had not been for these people and agencies, we would not have received the personal, educational, and emotional support that we have greatly appreciated.

## WHOSE GRIEF, WHOSE STRUGGLE?

Many people have described the feelings that occur in families when there is a child with a disability. Many have used the same cycle that occurs with death—the grief cycle. When my children were small, the path of feelings about the disability could be set aside for the new dream of having the brightest, cutest, most wonderful amputee or visually impaired child—the well-spoken poster child. These dreams also may have been called denial. The opportunity to focus on the strengths can lead others to believe that you are unaware of the problems; and, in truth, it may be so.

The feelings do not come from the big picture of the disability. They come from all the little incidents. When Benjy was 12 to 13 months old, I was taking him out of a nice warm tub of sudsy water and I stood his chubby, slippery little body next to the tub so that he could hold on while I toweled him dry. He stood straight and tall on his left leg but as I watched, he tried to bear weight on that useless dangling right leg. He kept bending his left leg so that the right toes touched the floor and even turned a little to try to see what the problem was. It was a moment of revelation for me. Until that moment, I think all the focus had been on me, my inadequacy, my problem, my pain. This was harder. This was too deep even for tears. This was Benjy's life, *his* surgeries, *his* pain, *his* inability to run swiftly through life. My only involvement was help and support.

Of course every now and then I have my own private pity party, but it is not my pain that is the issue—it is his.

Somehow for me there is a deeper pain in watching someone I love struggle than the pain in struggling myself.

In our minds, Jessica, our second, had no disabilities through her first five years of life. She did have four eye surgeries by age 5. During those preschool years she attended a church-related preschool. At parent conference times, when the teacher would point out problems or ask pointed questions about behavior at home, I would justify her performance by telling myself or Mick that every surgery sets a child back about 3 months. When she was supposed to go on to kindergarten, we were called in to a special conference where they carefully told us that she was not ready. I did not hear anything else that day. The impact of that statement and the carefully worded explanations was that of an icy shower. It was almost as if I had awakened from a dream with clear vision of how disabled and delayed she really was. I felt guilty and ashamed. I am an OT. I know developmental milestones. I had let my doctor and others calm my fears about delays in walking, slight ataxia, and fine-motor challenges because I did not want to believe that this second child of mine could have more than just the visual impairments. I was in denial for 5 years—helped by well-meaning people who did not want to hurt me.

## IT'S OK TO BE THIS WAY

One night soon after Jessica's conference, I received an answer to my prayer of, "Where do I go from here?" I attended a presentation by Ken Moses, a psychologist and counselor who writes and speaks about parenting children with disabilities, and I experienced a new step on my journey. His talk was about the grief cycle and how we were grieving for a lost dream. He gave permission to be in denial. He emphasized how important denial is for helping to deal with life-affecting decisions. He pointed out that denial buys us time to gather our resources so that we can deal straight on with the problems.

He also talked about how important it is to recognize that anger can be productive . . . . that anger gives us the energy to take action to make that call or that appointment for our child. Unless anger is turned inward or used on others, it can help. I came away with a sense of relief. To have these feelings were normal, and I was not a bad person, mom, or therapist.

## WHERE DO WE GO FROM HERE?

Decisions are forced on parents. There are medical decisions, therapy decisions, educational decisions, second opinion decisions, decisions made with fevers in the middle of the night and in emergency rooms, and decisions that are avoided until the last possible moment. They start immediately with diagnosis or with searching for a diagnosis. What doctor should we use? What hospital? What about insurance? How much intervention do we need—do we want?

What will they think if we say no to this thing that they think is important for our family? Is it important?

Sitting on our staircase landing, waiting for the bus in the morning, Jessica and I spent 20 minutes every morning doing "eye exercises." Some days it was easier. Other days Jessica would complain and resist and attempt to divert my attention from the task. One day when she was 7 or 8 years old, about 10 minutes into the session, we were discussing her braces and eye surgery and an OT session for that afternoon. She suddenly looked up at me and asked, "Mom, is there anything about me that you don't have to fix?" Of course I quickly named all of her gifts and attributes that I treasured. As the bus, with Jessica on it, turned the street corner, I was left sitting on the steps with feelings of emptiness and guilt and a new insight into the impact of much therapy, surgeries, and home programs.

It also made me face the other aspect of denial . . . the unavoidable fact that there are some aspects of disability that cannot be fixed. I became an occupational therapist so that I could help people and make things better for them. I truly believed that I could help eliminate some problems . . . that I could help heal hurts . . . that I could provide training so that people could be more independent. I guess that once I "saw" Jessica's problems, I wanted to make up for lost time and joined the mother-on-a-mission society. There were no stones unturned if I thought that something would help her "get better." So there have been several forms of denial that I have used within my life: denial that there is a problem, denial that the problem is not going to be cured with a lot of intervention, denial that I am upset about the problem, denial that if we just provide the same experiences as others our children will function the same, and denial that they can do well in some things and they do not need intervention in those.

## AND THEN THERE WAS SCHOOL

Physical disabilities are very apparent—not so learning disabilities. When attention turned to education instead of medicine, the challenges were not just medical, and the challenges were not just developmental. Our priorities turned to cognition and classroom-skill building. After two real and implied rejections at parochial and neighborhood schools, Benjamin attended kindergarten through third grade in a school that had an orthopedic handicapped program. He was in a self-contained classroom until third grade, when we requested that he receive most of his instruction in a regular classroom. My, what a response! I think I still have a "severe reputational disorder." That year was a struggle for all of us as we decided to change priorities to allow the learning disabled program to meet his needs. The most intimidating place in the world is a room with educators, including heads of programs and psychologists, teachers, OTs, and PTs, and the only ones that really believe that you are doing the right thing are you and your husband. It turned out to be just fine. But I still get stomach cramps when it is time for an IEP meeting, even those for which I am the OT.

When we find ourselves making judgments about families, a red flag needs to go up. As was pointed out in the first part of this chapter, each family has a different structure and different values. Decision making in each family is complicated and sacred. When we decided to have a third child, I know many people thought that we were crazy. Some were even brave enough to tell us so. Service providers held their breath, and educators looked for another Ball child in their classroom.

Alexander was born on a cold February day in 1981. He had no physical problems, but he was just as colicky as the other two. He walked at 9 months without a problem. In preschool meetings I was the one to point out small discrepancies. The teacher complimented me on being accepting. I carefully informed her that I had been through this twice before and that I had *not* been accepting the first time, but that was OK too—that my children had not fallen off the face of the earth because I could not accept their delays. They were doing just fine, and parents need to be allowed to feel the way that they do. It does not mean, however, that professionals should not be honest.

Sympathetic honesty is the only way to know that you have all the facts before you make a decision. Honesty is the gift that you give parents. It does not mean that parents will follow your suggestions or even that your opinions are always right, but your honesty gives a piece of the picture that parents are trying to build to help their child succeed. It helps if you take the time to listen to those parents' dreams or if you help parents put words to their dreams. Many of my dreams were not even able to be expressed because fear of not achieving them would cut them off. There were and still are weeks that I cannot deal with the long term. I can only take it one crisis at a time. There are days that I do not even know that I have a dream for my children. But there are days that I see clearly the life that I think my children may achieve, and that is where I like to be.

Qualifying for special education is one of the hardest things that a parent deals with, besides the medical issues. It is obvious that Benjy has an orthopedic handicap, but to "qualify," we had to attend an intake meeting. Benjy had to be tested. When Jessica was tested, we requested the testing and the school said that it was too early but we pursued it. A discrepancy was found, and she did qualify for the learning disabled program. Then we spent the next 5 years adjusting to Jessica's resource room, changing schools each year. Each year we were told that it was in her best interest because the room would then be stable. In the fourth grade we were told to take her for counseling because she was withdrawn and had no friends on the playground. Guess why! In the sixth grade we moved to another district because it had neighborhood schools with special education resources available in each. There, too, the resource room for learning disabilities was in a different school from that of everyone else in the neighborhood. Can't win!

Alexander has turned out to be a borderline gifted, learning disabled (LD), attention deficit disorder (ADD), dyslexic child, and at 14, he continues to reverse letters and numbers. He once wrote out in bold letters on a T-shirt, a commitment to avoid drugs: "Lust say on." Classic notes left for me on the kitchen counter often tell me that his "homework is bone" or "bog has ben out." He was identified between kindergarten and first grade at our insistence. Most school districts want to wait to see if the delays that are seen in the earlier grades will disappear as the child matures. Because of family history, it was agreed that he be tested. Like Jessica, a discrepancy was found.

Alexander's disability has been no less difficult for us than the other two. The feelings of loss and sadness that accompanied the identification and the knowledge that we somehow had failed again resurfaced. I had fought for a label of learning disabilities so that he could receive services. He has received assistance in a resource room for some of his academic subjects from first grade. Luckily his resource room only moved once during the last 8 years.

## GIFTS AND DREAMS

Recently, I heard someone use that old saying, "I'm playing the hand I've been dealt." I think that applies to all of us. It seems to me that everyone has many sources of grief in their lives. We, as parents of children with disabilities, can focus on the delays and the fears and the "poor me" or "poor them" attitudes, and we should be allowed to feel the feelings that are associated with this. However, most of us are proud of the accomplishments of our children . . . learning to put on his prosthesis by himself, learning to turn a somersault at age 7, or hitting the right key on the keyboard to match what is on the screen.

There are some things that our children will never be able to do, activities they choose not to attempt. Jessica has chosen not to pursue bike riding. Ben has chosen not to run a marathon, and Alex has chosen not to read piano music. All of these things would be next to impossible for them to do, but I never told them that they couldn't. Parents are always in the position of encouraging the impossible. Help givers that are more objective think that parents are denying reality, but the reality is that it is the child that will ultimately determine what they can and cannot do. We have made and still make many mistakes in parenting our children with disabilities, but we have not allowed their disabilities to limit the possibilities. to see.

I remember tears over *The Velveteen Rabbit* when I read it to the kids. It seemed that the problems of my children prohibited them from being "real" too. But I knew that all the love that I was showering on them would not change their physical makeup. I knew also that all that love might help them cope with their "realness." Benjy has told me that he will run in heaven and I believe that, but I also know that they all run in their hearts every day here, and others seeing them are challenged to be more.

## BOTTOM LINE

Benjy is now 23 years old and is doing well in his fifth year at Miami University, studying to be a special education teacher. Jessica has just started at the University of Toledo, and she also has chosen to be a special education teacher. Alexander just turned 14 and is always on the go. He is into art and wrestling. He has an eclectic outlook on life. There is not a day without real or imagined trauma, but there is also not a day without pride. My dream for them now is the same that I had when they were small . . . that they will be as independent as they can be, that they will be happy, and that they will always have someone who loves them.

If you take your time to hear a parent's dream, you may hear the sound of laughter and tears. You may hear the strong heartbeat of anger or the resistance to life that is nothingness. You are the gift to each parent as you touch their lives. You have a key to a piece of that dream. You have a solution to some of that frustration. You have the opportunity to be as honest as you can and provide those pieces of information that a parent needs to make decisions. You are an answer to some parent's question. Thank you.

CHAPTER

6

# General Pediatric Health Care

MARY A. McILROY ▲ KATALIN I. KORANYI

## DELIVERY OF HEALTH CARE SERVICES

### General Aspects

Quality pediatric health care strives toward one primary objective: to enable each individual to pursue childhood and enter adulthood at his or her optimal state, physically, intellectually, and emotionally. Occupational therapists share this objective. In striving toward this goal, occupational therapists must collaborate with parents, physicians, and other resource personnel and therefore understand the various components of pediatric health care and their effective use.

Children receive pediatric health care in various settings, including private offices of pediatricians and family physicians, hospital or community clinics, health department stations, and hospital emergency rooms. Despite differences in

locations, staffing, costs, and other amenities, each program offering pediatric care should share the common aim just stated.

Health care needs of children vary over time. Most of the physician's effort in pediatrics is involved in the delivery of health promotion services and acute episodic care. Smaller amounts of time are given to rehabilitation, the coordination of home health care, and the establishment of educational programs. This chapter presents a description of each of these types of care and details more thoroughly the most important aspects of preventive care and acute episodic care.

### Health Promotion

Prevention of illness, screening for disease, and monitoring health through well child checks are accepted goals of pediatrics and are essential in standard practice. Health promotion extends beyond prevention and maintenance and attempts to teach patients and families the importance of healthy life-styles.

Health promotion is a long-term process through which patients and families are assisted in accepting the responsibility for health care. It encourages them to take an active role in determining their own health, rather than relying on curative medicine in the future. The development of a mutually satisfying physician-patient-family relationship is important for the success of this process. A constructive relationship allows for better care during acute problems and crises, whether physical or psychosocial, and permits more effective counseling and teaching at routine visits (Figure 6-1). An effective relationship should also help patients and parents develop self-esteem and self-help skills to deal with routine daily problems. The desired result of such efforts in health promotion is to have patients and families establish lifetime goals and patterns that will be beneficial to good health and that will encourage appropriate use of health services.

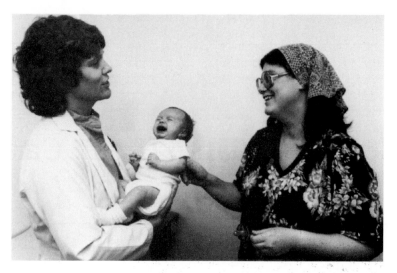

**Figure 6-1**   Effective and constructive physician-family relationships permit better care and counseling and help parents develop self-confidence in dealing with problems.

Preventive and screening services, which are vital parts of pediatric health care and health promotion, are discussed in detail later in this chapter. The aim of such services is the prevention of mortality and the minimization of morbidity from the many illnesses that afflict children. Early intervention is a necessary part of preventing mortality and morbidity and requires caregivers who are skilled in effective interviewing and the detection of problems. Routine checkups with thorough physical examinations may aid in the early identification of physical problems. Opening the lines of communication about behavior, development, school performance, sex education, and family relationships assists in early diagnosis and treatment of many of the most common problems in childhood. Parents are often reluctant to begin the discussion about a child's behavior and, in fact, may not recognize a developing pattern of difficulty unless physicians use a developmental approach to health promotion. By using basic knowledge of the stages of development in childhood, the physician can question parents about the most common problems occurring in the child's age-group. If the answers indicate that abnormalities exist, treatment programs can be instituted. Often the discussion indicates that the parents need education to increase their understanding of the normal childhood stages. The parents' understanding of normal child development can promote positive interactions and can decrease the potential for psychosocial disorders.

## Acute Episodic Care

Many visits to pediatric health caregivers are for diagnosis and treatment of acute problems, such as infections, minor trauma, or other physical complaints. Upper respiratory tract diseases, otitis media, and diarrheal illnesses account for a large proportion of these visits. In general, acute ill-

nesses are most common between 6 months and 4 years of age. A small peak is often seen in the first 2 years of school, but otherwise the frequency decreases with increasing age. Data from the *National Health Survey,* collected by household interview, indicate that children younger than age 6 have about 3.8 acute illnesses each year, whereas children aged 6 to 16 have 2.8 acute illnesses each year.

Many of the acute illnesses of childhood are mild and self-limited, yet they account for a large part of the demand for physician's time. Patients with acute illnesses seek care from private offices, community clinics, urgent care centers, and hospital clinics and emergency rooms. The use of scattered services occurs frequently but interrupts continuity of care. The education of children and families to deal with minor symptoms by themselves and to use health care services wisely may have great impact on the cost and delivery of health care. All encounters with health care professionals should be used as opportunities to provide preventive services, update immunizations, and educate patients and families.

## Habilitation and Rehabilitation

Children with disabilities have various needs that can best be met through comprehensive care programs. The physician often serves as a coordinator for the various agents of the child's program. More importantly, the physician should be an advocate for the child so that the child and family can live more comfortably with long-term disabilities. Children with disabilities need a great variety of experiences that are appropriate for their ages. The physician assists the family in ensuring that the appropriate programs and opportunities for learning, social interaction, and physical habilitation are provided for the child. Encouraging the family to help the child with special needs lead a fulfilling life, where self-discipline rather than overindulgence prevails, is an important aspect of chronic care (see Chapter 5).

The physician serves as a referral source for specialists and services available in the community, such as occupational and physical therapists, psychologists, relief caretakers, public health nurses, and special education programs. The physician also serves as an advisor for decisions about the child's education and residence plans, such as placing a previously institutionalized child into alternative living arrangements.

Unfortunately, some children with disabilities do not have a primary care physician directing their overall care. These children may be seen by multiple subspecialists, each dealing effectively, but specifically, with isolated aspects of a child's problems. Despite many visits to these specialists, the patient's general health care, developmental needs, behavioral changes, and family relationships may be overlooked or ignored.

Many reasons exist to explain the lack of follow-up care by the primary care physician. Some patients may not recognize the need for such services or may expect that the physician subspecialists or other health care personnel will tell them when to see the general physician. They may resent the involvement of so many subspecialists, who indeed may be superficial in their relationships with the family and may offer differing opinions about a concern. Family members may believe the primary care physician has relinquished caring for them by virtue of referrals to subspecialists who manage some aspects of the child's care. Financial constraints and transportation problems are among other stated reasons for lack of continuity with the primary care physician.

The impact may be great in situations in which children with disabilities are not cared for by a primary care physician. Even such important aspects of health promotion as immunizations and screening tests may be neglected because subspecialists do not perform or monitor such procedures. Developmental, behavioral, and psychosocial issues may be inadequately addressed, if discussed at all. Parents are often unsure to whom they should direct their questioning. If they seek answers about behavioral or emotional issues from a subspecialist who is untrained in that area, their concerns may be ignored or minimized. The parents may view this lack of discussion or action by the subspecialist as an indication that the matter is insignificant and of no concern. Or they may believe they were foolish to mention the issue and then may be reluctant to raise other concerns later.

Occupational therapists can play a beneficial role for their clients by identifying children who are not receiving primary care and then assisting those families in finding a primary care physician. If a previous relationship with a primary care provider was satisfactory for the family, then it may be sufficient to suggest the family seek input from that physician regarding general health issues. Because of temperament, interest, or training, some physicians are better suited than others to provide ongoing care to children with disabilities and their families. If a family's previous experience with a primary care physician was unsatisfactory, they can be encouraged to seek care from another primary physician who has been recognized by other community professionals and families for providing comprehensive care to children with disabling conditions.

## Home Health Care

The length of stay during hospitalizations has decreased significantly in recent years. Many services previously provided in the hospital can be provided at home at less expense and greater comfort for the patient and family.

Continuing health care in the home for a high-risk child, such as an infant with low birth weight, a child who fails to thrive, or a child with multiple disabilities, may be provided by home health care nursing services or visiting public health nurses. They serve as a liaison between the family and the physician or medical facility. Hospice care for the terminally ill child permits patients to receive medical care in familiar surroundings with their families.

## Educational Programs

Health education of children and families is provided by a variety of health care professionals in hospital-based and community programs. There is little research showing how this is most effectively accomplished. In providing routine care the pediatrician has an excellent opportunity to discuss various health problems, preventive care, anticipatory guidance, and child safety. In addition, teaching materials (videotapes and booklets) can be made available in patient waiting areas. Other individuals responsible for the care of children, such as nurses, social workers, nutritionists, and teachers, can offer discussion programs regarding health care through organizations such as schools, parents' groups, and churches. Occupational therapists may be called on to participate in this role in community education. Informing the general public regarding important health issues, such as immunizations, health hazards, and safety, can be done through the news media.

## PREVENTIVE PEDIATRICS
### General Aspects

One important part of health promotion, as mentioned previously, is preventive care. Three aspects of preventive care can be identified. First is the prevention of specific childhood illnesses through immunizations. Second is the attempt to prevent disability from asymptomatic diseases by use of screening tests. Early detection of asymptomatic diseases, such as hypothyroidism and phenylketonuria, permits treatment before the disease impairs its victim. Screening of development is also essential because early recognition of developmental delays and dysfunctions permits earlier intervention.

A third aspect of service in preventive care is the promotion of good health through the teaching of healthy life habits and counseling concerning proper diet, exercise, and accident prevention, among other things.

In addition, preventive care is provided in other ways. Health care personnel try to detect and treat symptomatic diseases as early as possible to prevent secondary complications or sequelae. Habilitative and rehabilitative services are sought to prevent physical and emotional dysfunction from chronic disabling conditions. Both of these aspects are discussed in other chapters of this book.

## Well Child Care

Regularly scheduled health supervision visits for children are important for the assessment of general health, growth, and development. They permit effective administration of immunizations and allow for important screening tests to be performed. These practices are discussed later in this chapter.

Routine visits also allow for anticipatory guidance in preparing parents for both the certainties and uncertainties of the future. (Chamberlin, 1982; Christopherson, 1982) (For a more detailed discussion of this topic, see Suggested Readings: Cataldo; Green & Haggerty; and Behrman & Vaughan.) For example, when a baby is 2 to 3 months old, parents should be informed that the ability to roll over will be developing in the following 2 or 3 months. This knowledge prepares the parent so that the infant is not left unguarded on a surface where he or she might roll off the edge and fall to the floor. Similarly, because most infants undergo a decrease in appetite at around 1 year of age, parents need to be aware of this change so that they avoid unnecessary conflicts concerning feeding. Uncertainties, for example, a child's reaction at times of stress or crisis, should also be discussed to aid the parent in being prepared to handle such situations.

At these visits the physician can assess the mental and emotional well-being of the patient and the family unit. Although this is not strictly preventive care, it does allow for, if necessary, the early intervention for problems such as behavior abnormalities, discipline difficulties, parental anxieties about normal variations, and toilet training (Chamberlin 1982; Christopherson, 1982; Metz, Allen, Barr, & Shinefield, 1976). These problems, although not causing physical illnesses, lead to psychosocial disorders and may have effects throughout an individual's life (Starfield, 1982).

Health care visits for preventive services must be sufficient in number and frequency to meet the individual needs of the child. Determining the optimal number of visits or procedures for all children or parents is impossible. But guidelines and recommendations have been published by the American Academy of Pediatrics (Recommendations for Preventive Care, 1992) "for the care of well children who receive competent parenting, who have not manifested any important health problems and who are growing and developing satisfactorily."

Clearly, many circumstances or conditions may indicate a need for additional visits, and the physician will recommend a schedule. More frequent visits are indicated for children with low birth weight or with congenital problems that cause no serious difficulties but result in parental anxiety. Also at risk and generally requiring increased professional contact are families with a previous child with an abnormality, those who have lost a child, adoptive or foster parents, and parents who are found to be in greater need of education and guidance, such as teenage mothers.

The current American Academy of Pediatrics' recommendations (Recommendations for Preventive Care, 1992) reflect this emphasis on meeting individual needs. They suggest that each health supervision visit should include initial or interval history, measurements of growth, physical examination, sensory screening, and developmental appraisal as indicated by age, immunizations, and diagnostic tests according to age, discussion of findings, and counseling that concerns problems or anticipatory guidance.

The timing of health supervision visits in the first 2 years has previously been scheduled around the immunization needs of the child, rather than out of concern for the developmental needs of the child and parents. The need for immunizations at certain ages still holds true, but the intervals can be more flexible in an attempt to avoid rigid adherence to providing well child care at specific ages. This attitude also allows for completing a health supervision visit with a visit initiated by a minor acute problem whenever possible.

Six well child visits are recommended as a minimum in the first year, generally by 4 weeks, at 2 months, 4 months, 6 months, 9 months, and 12 months. In the second year three health supervision appointments are encouraged, at 15 months, 18 months, and 24 months. Each of these visits is important for documenting satisfactory growth and development, discussing dietary and feeding practices, and assessing parental needs for guidance or reassurance. Immunizations are also provided during several of these visits. The immunization schedule is discussed later.

Beyond 2 years of age the need for routine health promotion visits is generally diminished, but it will vary according to the health of the particular child and the family conditions. Yearly visits are encouraged from 3 to 6 years of age (Figure 6-2). The American Academy of Pediatrics (Recommendations for Preventive Care, 1992) recommends six routine visits in alternate years for school-aged children 8 to 18 years of age. For the older child and adolescent these visits serve a much different purpose. Very few abnormal conditions will be discovered in asymptomatic children in these groups. Although documentation of normality and the updating of immunizations is important, more pertinent topics for these visits include behavioral concerns, school performance, family and peer relationships, psychomotor development, and sexual development. With adolescents, counseling about drug and alcohol use and about sexual behavior is valuable. (For further reading on this subject, see Suggested Readings: Felice and Friedman and Mercer.)

## Screening Tests and Procedures

Screening procedures are one of the major thrusts of health promotion and are a part of all the routine visits described previously. Various tests are performed at different visits according to age and are discussed individually in this section. The purpose of the screening tests is to identify illnesses or abnormalities in specific functions that are more likely to respond to corrective treatment while being asymptomatic and that may be more difficult to correct after symptoms are evident or when secondary problems appear. Extremely important, then, to the success of screening for disease is the assurance that programs exist for the treatment of children with abnormalities identified through screening.

Some screening procedures detect diseases that are asymptomatic in early infancy but will lead to damage if left untreated. For example, infants with hypothyroidism appear normal at birth. Over the first few months characteristic physical signs may occur, but they may be subtle. Mental retardation will occur unless treatment with thyroid replacement is instituted within the first 2 months. A screening test to detect hypothyroidism at birth is now in use and is valuable in preventing this avoidable retardation.

Developmental screening may help identify treatable diseases and is beneficial for recognizing delays so that appropriate counseling of parents and attempts at remediation can occur. Early therapeutic intervention for the primary developmental problem often leads to a more successful outcome. In addition, the occurrence of secondary developmental difficulties may be prevented by early recognition and treatment programs. Especially responsive to early attempts at correction are those developmental delays and dysfunctions that result from a patient's major health and environmental problems, such as burns, diabetes, or neglect.

The prevention of secondary problems is important. Aiding a child to develop appropriate adaptive maneuvers or mechanisms to compensate for a primary disability may prevent a later need for extensive rehabilitation.

Most physicians recommend some caution in the use and application of screening tests results. The importance of appropriate identification of a child at risk and the provision of needed services has already been stated. But evidence has shown that children who are labeled as having problems or as being at risk for developing problems have an increased chance of later dysfunction. This effect seems to be related to a child's change in self-image and his or her expectations as a result of being labeled abnormal.

Occupational therapists should be cognizant of such effects and should be extremely careful in discussing with parents and patients the results of developmental testing and their implications. Significant discrepancies must be communicated to the primary care physician, and questions of causative factors and prognosis should be referred back to the physician for discussion with the family.

### Monitoring Growth

Growth parameters of height, weight, and head circumference aid in screening infants and children for problems that result in abnormal growth. Abnormalities can be either insufficient rate of growth or excessive rate of growth, and either variation may be seen in height, weight, and head

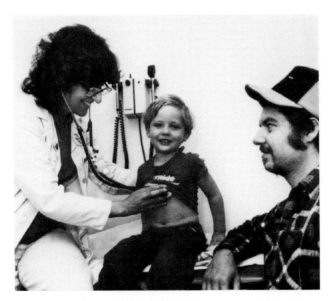

**Figure 6-2** Routine visits for healthy children document normalcy and allow for discussions of parental concerns about behavior, development, peer relationships, and school performance.

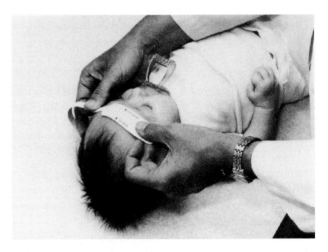

**Figure 6-3** Occipitofrontal head circumference measures the largest diameter of an infant's head and is vital to detect insufficient or excessive head growth.

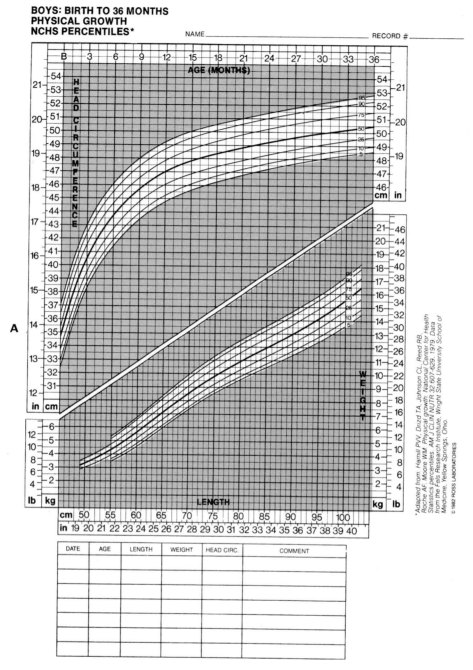

**Figure 6-4** **A,** Standard growth for plotting head circumference and weight for length measurements for boys from birth to 36 months. (Modified from Hamill, P.V.V., Drizd, T.A., Reed, R.B., Roche, A.F., & Moore, W.M. [1979]. Physical growth: national Center for Health Statistics percentiles. *American Journal of Clinical Nutrition, 32,* 607-629.)

circumference. In fact, knowing whether there is an abnormality in only one parameter or in two or all three measurements is important because that knowledge often suggests different causative explanations.

Measurements of weight and height (supine length in infants) should be recorded accurately at every visit to the physician or caregiver. Head circumference (Figure 6-3) is most valuable during the first 3 years, when the rate of head growth is the greatest. It is generally not recorded beyond that age. Standard curves or growth charts are available to delineate the percentile ranking of any measurement according to age (Figure 6-4). The data obtained from the patient should be plotted on such a graph at each visit. This process provides a visual display of the data and quickly alerts the physician to abnormalities that otherwise might be overlooked.

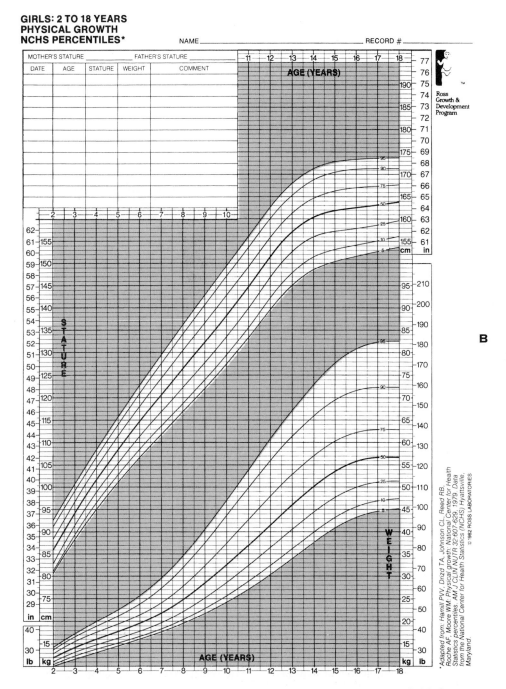

**Figure 6-4, cont'd.** **B,** Standard growth curve for plotting heights and weights of girls from age 2 to 18 years.

Single measurements provide little valuable information in most cases, unless they deviate markedly from normal or demonstrate a significant discrepancy between simultaneously obtained percentiles for height, weight, and head circumference. For example, if the baby's length and weight at a single examination are at the 50th percentile, but the head circumference is less than the 10th percentile, abnormalities of the skull or central nervous system should be suspected. The subsequent measurement and recording of

growth parameters at each visit allow comparison over time, and a change of two or more percentile lines (for example, from 50th to 10th) signifies a need for explanation.

Among the most common abnormal occurrences is one in which an infant or toddler shows significantly less weight gain than expected while continuing to grow normally in length and head circumference. Generally this reflects a nutritional basis for inadequate growth. The physician must then try to delineate whether there is a problem in acquiring adequate intake, in losing excessive quantities of calories, or in the utilization of food delivered to the body. Insufficient intake may result from poor feeding practices, maternal ignorance or neglect, poverty, or birth defects, such as cleft palate, which may hinder the mechanics of feeding. Excessive loss of calories may be caused by recurrent vomiting or losses in stool from diarrhea or malabsorption. Improper utilization of food may be seen in metabolic disorders such as diabetes, glycogen storage diseases, or cystic fibrosis.

Other patterns of abnormalities should indicate different concerns. Lack of adequate growth in length or height may be seen in metabolic disorders such as renal disease, hypothyroidism, or hypopituitarism. Early excessive growth in height may signify precocious puberty. In severe central nervous system disorders with brain damage, growth curves often show markedly low values in height, weight, and head circumference. An infant whose head growth is more rapid than expected shows a change toward higher percentiles or may have a head circumference greater than the 95th percentile for his or her age and would likely be evaluated for hydrocephalus.

Accurate and repeated measurements of height, weight, and head circumference are an exceptionally good screening tool for detection of many illnesses and problems. Routine use of these statistics may aid the physician in early detection of diseases, and it provides other health personnel involved in a patient's care some objective data that may be reassuring with regard to the patient's general health or that may arouse concern, resulting in consultation with or referral back to the physician.

### Sensory Evaluation

Sensory screening for vision and hearing is mandatory to detect major defects early, to enable development to progress as normally as possible, and to permit maximal rehabilitation before school age for those in whom normal development has been altered.

Children's eyes must be examined for screening purposes in early infancy, before beginning school, and at intervals during the school years. Examination of the infant's eyes should be done several times during the first 6 months. At birth this may consist of only a determination of light perception (blinking in avoidance when a bright light is presented) and visualization of a red reflex by funduscopy. By 3 or 4 months of age the infant should be able to follow a light 180 degrees and therefore demonstrate both visual perception of the light and conjugate movements of the eyes. The eyes should be assessed for alignment by checking to see if light reflects from the same location in both eyes when the patient looks at the light. Further screening procedures can also be done to detect intermittent changes in alignment. This testing is performed by interrupting a patient's conjugate gaze at an object by covering one eye (Figure 6-5). The examiner observes for deviation of that eye away from the object of gaze. Such deviation is readily

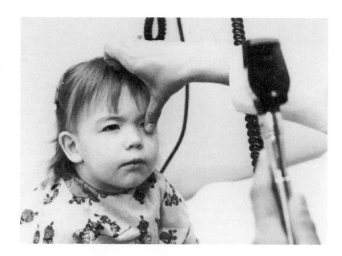

**Figure 6-5** Screening for intermittent abnormalities in ocular alignment is performed by blocking the vision of one eye and then observing for correction of alignment to return the eye to conjugate gaze when vision is no longer blocked.

detected as the interrupted eye moves back into conjugate alignment when vision is no longer blocked.

Visual acuity and muscle alignment should be screened between 3 and 5 years of age and again at other visits during the school years. Acuity can be checked by using standard eye charts or small projection machines. Because this screening is simple and requires minimal equipment, schools and communities often provide large screening programs. Children with abnormalities of acuity or alignment should be referred for appropriate and thorough evaluation by their physician.

Hearing and language are informally assessed at each visit as the physician interacts with the patient or observes patient-parent communications. Screening of hearing is now routinely performed in many hospital settings for high-risk newborns, and appropriate referrals are made if problems are detected. The newborn or young infant should respond to a loud noise or clap with blinking of the eyes or a Moro response (Figure 6-6). Normal hearing is demonstrated in 6- to 9-month-old infants by their attempts to locate a familiar sound. A bell or rattle can be used to produce sound, and older infants should turn their heads to locate it. The older infant should also be making babbling sounds. At 12 months hearing is indicated by the following of simple directions and the use of two or three meaningful words. Vocabulary continues to expand, and the complexity of language increases so that by 3 years of age the child should be able to speak in simple sentences.

Screening of hearing should be done again before the beginning of school so that any loss that might impair classroom work can be dealt with before academic problems are created. Many communities and schools provide hearing screening programs to be certain this service is provided to all children, not just to those who seek professional health care.

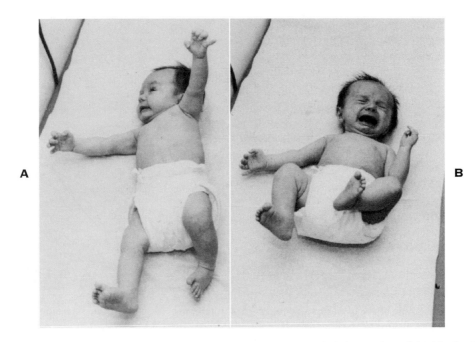

**Figure 6-6**  Moro reflex is a normal neurologic response in early infancy, often elicited by loud noises or a sudden change in position. **A,** Initial phase involves stiffened extension of arms and legs. **B,** Second phase is flexion and abduction of extremities and, often, crying.

Abnormalities in vision or hearing, if detected by occupational therapists in the course of patient evaluation or therapy, should most certainly be communicated to the referring physician to assure that adequate evaluation has been or will be done.

### Developmental Assessment

Developmental appraisal should occur at every contact between patient and caregiver and is an important aspect of each visit. Initially, simple observation of the infant's motor and social development suffices. As the infant develops, more motor and social skills become obvious and language and cognitive abilities appear. These capabilities become progressively more complex with age, and the physician must not only observe but also must interact with the patient to determine developmental level. Through informal assessment, the physician should identify the infant or child likely to benefit from more formal evaluation, whether performed in the office situation or in a referral system by occupational therapists or other trained personnel.

For screening purposes the Revised Denver Developmental Screening Test (DDST II) (Frankenberg, Fandal, Sciarillo, & Burgess, 1981) is widely used. It allows establishment of a baseline for an infant's development and can be used repeatedly up to age 6 to help measure progress. It is a brief sampling of abilities and is limited in items tested at very early ages, but it can provide an estimation of a child's developmental course. Concerns noted by informal evaluation or deficiencies noted on the DDST II assessment should receive more extensive evaluation by personnel trained in standardized developmental appraisals. The occupational therapist often serves as a resource for evaluation and therapy of noted delays, and the therapist can assist in the establishment of home programs, occupational therapy sessions, or referrals to community programs. In this role the occupational therapist can support the physician-patient relationship and enhance the care given to the child and family.

### Metabolic Screening

Several specific screening tests are used routinely in pediatric health supervision. Blood tests are used to screen neonates for the presence of metabolic diseases such as phenylketonuria, hypothyroidism, galactosemia, and sickle-cell anemia. The benefits of early detection of these diseases, which is discussed in Chapter 7, are obvious because, in many cases, early treatment can prevent or minimize mental retardation or other pathologic consequences of the disease.

### Hematology Testing

Hemoglobin or hematocrit testing is a valuable screen for anemia and is usually performed in infants at 9 to 12 months of age. Nutritional anemia from iron deficiency occurs at this age among disadvantaged populations. The Women, Infants and Children program, funded by the federal government, has been successful in decreasing the incidence of iron-deficiency anemia by providing iron-fortified formulas during the first year of life. If anemia is detected on testing, treatment with iron preparations is fairly simple and prevents the complications of anemia. Parents of children with anemia also need counseling about proper diet and nutrition for children. The American Academy of Pediatrics suggests hemoglobin or hematocrit testing again at 2 to 4 years of age, during late childhood, and in adolescence.

Identification of sickle-cell disease or trait cannot change its presence. Patients identified as having sickle-cell anemia should receive preventive care and counseling. Genetic counseling can also be provided for families of patients with sickle-cell trait or sickle-cell anemia.

Also at 9 to 12 months of age, a lead level should be measured if indicated, especially in infants living in older homes. The presence of lead overload should be diagnosed so that any necessary treatment is provided and recurrence is prevented.

### Tuberculosis Screening

Recommendations concerning the use of routine tuberculosis screening tests have changed. The risk of tuberculosis infection is extremely low for most children in the United States. For this reason, nonselective testing of children is not believed to be an efficient public health practice. The American Academy of Pediatrics has indicated that routine annual skin testing for tuberculosis (Mantoux) in children with no risk factors in low-prevalence communities is not indicated (Report of the Committee on Infectious Diseases, 1994). Children at high risk should be tested annually, using Mantoux tests. Some of the risk factors for tuberculosis include contact with adults with infectious tuberculosis, abnormalities on chest roentgenogram suggestive of tuberculosis, HIV seropositivity, and immunosuppressive conditions.

### Urine Testing

The benefit of routine urinalysis and urine culture in healthy children is controversial. During preschool and early school years urine cultures of asymptomatic girls may yield positive results in 1% to 2%. But it is unclear what relationship this finding has to the development of chronic renal disease and whether treatment of asymptomatic bacteriuria prevents such complications.

### Blood Pressure Screening

Blood pressure screening is recommended (Report of the Second Task Force on Blood Pressure Control in Children, 1986, 1987) for all children 3 years of age and older (Figure 6-7). Previously most childhood hypertension was thought to be secondary to renal disease, metabolic abnormalities, or other pathologic causes, and extensive evaluation was warranted. Essential or primary hypertension is becoming increasingly recognized in children, although debate still exists as to what blood pressure levels actually constitute hypertension and at what point treatment is indicated (Report of the Second Task Force on Blood Pressure

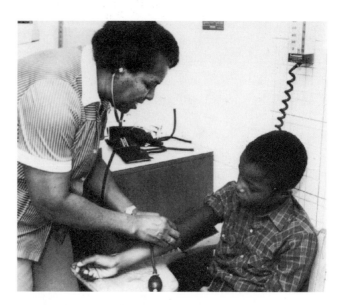

**Figure 6-7**   Blood pressure screening should be performed in all children over 3 years old.

Control in Children, 1986, 1987). Prevention of the adult complications of hypertension (heart disease and stroke) seems to be a logical aim and might be aided by the detection of elevated blood pressure during childhood, by effective therapy, where appropriate, and by development of healthy eating habits.

### Immunizations

Prevention of childhood illnesses and their morbidity and mortality is one of the proven benefits of pediatric health supervision. Death and disability from poliomyelitis and measles are almost unknown today. Tetanus occurs uncommonly, and deaths and brain damage from pertussis have decreased remarkably.

Immunizations against diphtheria, tetanus, pertussis, poliomyelitis, measles, mumps, rubella, hepatitis B, and *Haemophilus influenzae* type b infections are given routinely during infancy and early childhood. Recommended schedules have been established to provide early and effective protection from these diseases. Table 6-1 displays the schedule as currently recommended (Report of the Committee on Infectious Diseases, 1994).

Known risks and side effects do occur from these immunizations, but most are mild (fever, irritability, and soreness at the site) and are to be expected. Severe reactions to pertussis vaccine are rare, and even rarer are documented cases of vaccine-related poliomyelitis. The use of the acellular pertussis vaccine (DTaP) at 15 months of age decreases the incidence of fever and adverse local reactions. The details of these complications have been well described in other texts (Feigin, 1992). Despite these risks, it is a major concern for the public's and individual's health and welfare that children receive the recommended immunizations.

▲ Table 6-1  Recommended Immunizations and Ages
for Their Administration

| Recommended Age | Immunizations |
|---|---|
| Birth | Hepatitis B virus vaccine |
| 1-2 mo | Hepatitis B virus vaccine |
| 2 mo | Diphtheria and tetanus toxoids and pertussis vaccine, *Haemophilus influenzae* type b conjugate vaccine, oral poliovirus vaccine (containing attenuated poliovirus types 1, 2, and 3) |
| 4 mo | Diphtheria and tetanus toxoids and pertussis vaccine, *Haemophilus influenzae* type b conjugate vaccine, oral poliovirus vaccine (containing attenuated poliovirus types 1, 2, and 3) |
| 6 mo | Diphtheria and tetanus toxoids and pertussis vaccine (*Haemophilus influenzae* type b conjugate vaccine*) |
| 6-18 mo | Hepatitis B virus vaccine, oral poliovirus vaccine (containing attenuated poliovirus types 1, 2, and 3) |
| 12-15 mo | *Haemophilus influenzae* type b conjugate vaccine, live measles, mumps, and rubella viruses vaccine |
| 15-18 mo | Diphtheria and tetanus toxoids and acellular pertussis vaccine or diphtheria and tetanus toxoids and pertussis vaccine |
| 4-6 yr | Diphtheria and tetanus toxoids and acellular pertussis vaccine or diphtheria and tetanus toxoids and pertussis vaccine, oral poliovirus vaccine (containing attenuated poliovirus types 1, 2, and 3), live measles, mumps, and rubella viruses vaccine |
| 11-12 yr | Live measles, mumps, and rubella viruses vaccine (if not given at 4 to 6 wks) |
| 14-16 yr | Adult tetanus toxoid (full dose) and diphtheria toxoid (reduced dose) for children ≥7 years and adults |

Modified from American Academy of Pediatrics. (1994). *Report of the Committee on Infectious Diseases.* Elk Grove, IL: American Academy of Pediatrics.

*Dose 3 of *Haemophilus influenzae* type b conjugate vaccine is not indicated if product for doses 1 and 2 was PRP-OMP form.

## Nutrition

The importance of nutrition counseling has been increasingly recognized as people realize that good health is a result of good health practices, not just good medical care. The converse is also true: bad health may develop from unhealthy life-styles, not just as a result of poor medical care.

Health promotion for children includes the encouragement of better feeding habits and sound nutrition. The trend toward breastfeeding is increasing and should be supported by individuals responsible for child health care. Nutritious

and complex infant formulas are available when babies are not nursed, and they are recommended in preference to whole cow's milk or skim milk. Cow's milk products are a potential cause of microscopic blood loss from the gastrointestinal tract. Cow's milk has insufficient iron to meet an infant's needs, and it has higher sodium and renal solute content than human milk or commercial formulas. Whole cow's milk is acceptable after 1 year of age. Reduced-fat milk does not contain sufficient fat for infant brain development and should not be fed to children under 2 years of age.

Introduction of solid foods should be delayed until 4 to 6 months of age. Changes in prepared infant foods have markedly decreased the content of salt and sugar, both of which had been added for adult tastes. In addition, attention must be given to supplementation of the diet with vitamins, iron, or fluoride when conditions warrant.

The importance of nutrition extends far beyond the feeding of infants. As pediatric practice moves more into the role of health promotion, increased attention is being given to prevention of illnesses in adulthood. Heart disease, stroke, and cancer cause the majority of deaths in American adults. Many of the habits that contribute to adult morbidity from these problems begin in childhood.

The prevention of obesity in adulthood can probably be aided by the discouragement of obesity in childhood. Advice to parents is important to change the idea that a happy baby has to be a fat baby and to encourage proper nutrition (but not overnutrition) throughout childhood.

Sodium intake is believed to play a role in adult hypertension. It is unclear if control of sodium intake in infancy and childhood contributes to decreasing the incidence of hypertension. Although the answer to that question is being sought, prudent eating practices might include the avoidance of excessive salt.

Obesity and salt intake have been mentioned as contributors to heart disease. Lack of exercise also contributes to heart disease, and continuing exercise programs should be encouraged by those who provide health care to children.

Smoking is associated with the development of lung cancer, and the use of alcohol and drugs contributes to the number of accidental deaths. The prevention of such problems through education of children and families has not been sufficiently researched to determine effectiveness, but such programs deserve a trial. The aim of health promotion in pediatrics is to keep an individual healthy throughout childhood and his or her entire life.

## ACUTE EPISODIC CARE
### General Considerations in Outpatient Care of Sick Children

Ambulatory care services provide for both emergency and nonemergency care of sick children. In recent years there has been a growth of ambulatory services for children. This increase has resulted from several factors, such as the rising cost of inpatient care and the recent advances in diagnostic and therapeutic procedures by which children can now be treated in an outpatient setting.

Acute care cannot be scheduled in advance, so health care facilities must be prepared for urgent calls. Ideally the same physician or group of physicians provide acute and ongoing care for the child. If the child has been examined periodically at the same office or clinic, it is assumed that a complete personal and family history is available; thus the physician can concentrate on the acute visit. If the child is being seen for the first time by the physician, a brief history regarding factors that may influence the present illness (for example, allergies and chronic illness) must be obtained. A follow-up appointment for a complete history and examination can be arranged. For those children who usually receive only episodic or crisis care, it is important to provide preventive health care during the visit for the acute illness. If a child does not have an established source of continuing health care, it is important to emphasize and encourage the benefits of such service.

The emotional aspects of an illness also deserve consideration. Children seldom understand illness. They often view sickness as a punishment for bad behavior. The physician needs to keep in mind the various ages and levels of understanding of children and direct all explanations in a way that is meaningful to the patient. The child deserves simple but honest explanations regarding the illness, procedures, and expected degree of discomfort. Parents may worsen the situation because they often feel guilty, anxious, and tired, and they may ventilate their frustrations on the child or the health care personnel.

## Hospitalized Children

Many children are hospitalized at least once during childhood. Because of the emotional stress for the child and the family and the significant expense, hospital admissions should occur only when diagnostic and treatment procedures cannot be performed on an ambulatory basis.

If it is at all possible, the family should be prepared for the hospital admission so that potential problems can be addressed before they arise and anxieties can be diminished. When children are admitted to the hospital, they often feel that they are being punished; they feel abandoned by their parents, and they are afraid. In many hospitals, preadmission visits are arranged for the child and the parents to develop a sense of familiarity with the setting, the procedures, and the personnel. Showing one child a patient who is happily eating ice cream after a tonsillectomy could allay that child's fears regarding his or her own surgery. In addition to the hospital tours, materials such as coloring books, pamphlets, or videotapes can be made available to families.

A child should be allowed to express his fears, whether real or fantasized. Preparation at home and in the hospital by playing out fears (for example, giving a shot to the doll) and by role-playing games (for example, as doctor or nurse) may provide insight to the child's fantasies and help alleviate some of the fear. In case of an emergency admission, many of the preparations cannot take place, and the event is often confusing and hectic. Nevertheless, the physician and the nurse should try to answer questions of the parents and the child.

Children should be admitted to a pediatric unit and, if possible, matched with children of similar ages. A realistic and fair statement as to the estimated length of the hospitalization is important. All personnel need to be aware that children are not little adults and that they have special needs. Before any kind of procedure, the physician should talk with the patient and explain what will be done and why it is necessary. For children, terms such as *mend a break, fix up,* or *make well* are preferred over more threatening and confusing medical terms. When it benefits the patient, a support person (parent, nurse, or occupational therapist) should be permitted to accompany the child for procedures, such as radiographs, venipuncture, and even minor surgical procedures.

Care should be taken that children do not witness very agitated or very sick patients; tubes, machines, and bandages can be frightening to them. In the event a child is exposed to a very ill or dying patient, he or she deserves a sensitive and careful explanation.

Parental attitudes help to allay a child's fears, so parents and hospital personnel need to cooperate and understand each other. The child may view the hospitalization as a rejection or lack of love by the parents. The parents and hospital personnel need to become aware of possible changes in the behavior of a child during or after hospitalization, such as regressive behavior, increased clinging, antagonism, or aggressiveness. Parents should be encouraged to bring to the hospital some familiar object (for example, a favorite toy or blanket) that suggests a tie to the security of home. Frequent visits by parents should be encouraged.

Pediatric units should have age-appropriate playrooms or recreational areas for the children. School-aged children staying for an extended period (over 2 weeks) should continue their education through homework or hospital-based teachers. Whenever it is possible, hospitalized children should be allowed to get out of their rooms, go to other hospital areas, or receive passes to leave the hospital for a few hours.

## Childhood Disability

Most childhood illnesses are minor traumatic injuries and acute infectious diseases that leave no sequelae. However, a portion of these problems leads to chronic conditions or results in psychosocial difficulties.

The incidence of various illnesses has changed tremendously over the past decades. Diseases that were once prevalent, such as poliomyelitis, measles, tuberculosis, and diphtheria, have disappeared as the leading causes of mortality and morbidity. After the age of 1 year, accidents (in particular, motor vehicle accidents) are the leading cause of mortality in childhood. The second cause before 4 years of age is congenital malformations, whereas malignancies are the second cause of mortality from 4 to 18 years of age. Infection with human immunodeficiency virus is now increasing in frequency and is the eighth ranking cause of death among children younger than 4 years of age.

The *new morbidity* is a term frequently used now. In pediatric health care, this refers to the recently noted increase in care provided for behavior problems, school difficulties, and family social problems. The incidence of severe illness in childhood has decreased as a result of better technology, the prevention of many childhood diseases, and improved treatment of illness. Concurrently, changes in society require increased emphasis on dealing with problems resulting from violence, drug and alcohol abuse, and family dysfunction. Childhood health care personnel must keep pace with changing causes of morbidity and mortality, and their efforts must be directed toward prevention and treatment of these problems.

## SUMMARY

Occupational therapists are called on to direct or participate in efforts to facilitate a child's development of age-appropriate abilities and to help that child respond to the environment with whatever adaptations are necessary. It is important, therefore, that significant health concerns be identified and properly addressed before treatment is initiated or whenever they appear during the course of therapy.

When appropriate pediatric health care services are effectively delivered, as described in this chapter, the child in need of occupational therapy should be readily identifiable. The careful monitoring of physical, mental, and psychosocial development through the use of routine health promotion visits and screening procedures provides the physician with the necessary understanding of the child's primary developmental problem and level of abilities and aid recognition of other health problems. Such background information is of great importance for the occupational therapist designing treatment plans, along with determinations of whether the problems are temporary or permanent, what the expected outcomes and prognoses are, and what influence any health problems may have on both the child's development and therapy. Obvious, then, is the need for maintaining effective communications between occupational therapists and the primary physician to meet the changing needs of the child.

## REFERENCES

American Academy of Pediatrics. (1994). *Report of the Committee on Infectious Diseases* (23rd ed.). Elk Grove Village, IL: American Academy of Pediatrics.

Chamberlin, R.W. (1982). Prevention of behavioral problems in young children. *Pediatric Clinics of North America, 29,* 239.

Christopherson, E.R. (1982). Incorporating behavioral pediatrics into primary care. *Pediatric Clinics of North America, 29,* 261.

Feigin R.D. & Cherry, J.D. (1992). *Textbook of pediatric infectious diseases.* Philadelphia: W.B. Saunders.

Frankenburg, W.K., Fandal, A.W., Sciarillo, W., & Burgess, D. (1981). The newly abbreviated and revised Denver Developmental Screening Test. *Pediatrics, 99,* 995-999.

Metz, J.R., Allen, C.M., Barr, G., & Shinefield, H. (1976). A pediatric screening examination for psychosocial problems. *Pediatrics, 58*(4), 595-606.

*National health survey,* Series 10, No. 141, Washington, DC, 1981, U.S. Department of Health and Human Services.

Recommendations for Preventive Care. *American Academy of Pediatrics News,* July 1992, American Academy of Pediatrics.

Report of the Second Task Force on Blood Pressure Control in Children—1986. (1987). *Pediatrics, 79,* 1.

Starfield, B. (1982). Behavioral pediatrics and primary health care. *Pediatric Clinics of North America, 29,* 377.

## ▲ STUDY QUESTIONS

1. Identify three problems that may occur when a child with a disability is cared for only by subspecialists. Describe how an occupational therapist might help the family recognize the need for and obtain ongoing health supervision by a primary care physician.
2. Identify the parameters of growth that should be monitored in children and discuss why these aspects should be carefully recorded and evaluated.
3. Describe how the parents and the health care professionals can prepare a child emotionally for an elective hospital admission.
4. Name five illnesses that can be prevented by adequate childhood immunization.

## SUGGESTED READINGS

American Academy of Pediatrics. (1986). *Hospital care of children and youth.* Evanston, IL: American Academy of Pediatrics.

Behrman, R.E. & Vaughan, V.C. (Eds.). (1992). *Nelson textbook of pediatrics.* Philadelphia: W.B. Saunders.

Cataldo, M.F. (1982). The scientific basis for a behavioral approach to pediatrics. *Pediatric Clinics of North America, 29,* 415.

Feldman, K.W. (1980). Prevention of childhood accidents: recent progress. *Pediatric Review, 2,* 75.

Felice, M.E. & Friedman, S.B. (1982). Behavioral considerations in the health care of adolescents. *Pediatric Clinics of North America, 29,* 399.

Green, M. & Haggerty, R.J. (Eds.). (1990). *Ambulatory pediatrics III,* Philadelphia: W.B. Saunders.

Mercer, R.T. (1979). *Perspectives on adolescent health care,* Philadelphia: J.B. Lippincott.

North, A.F. (1974). Screening in child health care, *Pediatrics, 54*(5), 631-640.

Paulson, J.A. (1981). Patient education. *Pediatric Clinics of North America, 28,* 627.

Rudolph, A.M. (Ed.). (1991). *Pediatrics.* Norwalk, CT: Appleton-Century-Crofts.

Strasburger, V.C. & Brown, R.T. (1991). *Adolescent medicine: a practical guide.* Boston: Little, Brown.

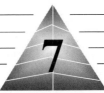

CHAPTER

7

# Diagnostic Problems in Pediatrics

CATHERINE YANEGA GORDON ▲ KAREN E. SCHANZENBACHER
JANE CASE-SMITH ▲ RICARDO C. CARRASCO

## KEY TERMS

- ▲ Cardiopulmonary Dysfunction
- ▲ Musculoskeletal Conditions
- ▲ Neuromuscular Conditions
- ▲ Traumatic Brain Injury
- ▲ Developmental Disabilities
- ▲ Autism
- ▲ Toxic Agents
- ▲ Infectious Conditions
- ▲ Neoplastic Disorders
- ▲ Burns

## CHAPTER OBJECTIVES

1. Describe the incidence, signs and symptoms, causes, and pathology of common medical diagnoses in children.
2. Describe the primary medical conditions associated with developmental disabilities.
3. Explain how functional performance is affected by various medical and pathologic conditions.
4. Explain precautions and special considerations for working with children who have specific medical conditions.

This chapter is intended to familiarize the occupational therapist with some of the major medical conditions and diseases found in pediatric occupational therapy practice. Pediatric conditions can be viewed in a number of ways: as congenital and acquired, occurring at different stages of development, acute or chronic, stable or aggressive, discrete or pervasive, or by systems affected. None of these alone is totally satisfactory. However, the body systems approach tends to be the simplest and most useful for educational and reference purposes.

This chapter is therefore organized in a body systems format, including a section with pervasive, mixed, and developmental disorders. The chapter provides information on the incidence and prevalence, signs and symptoms, cause, pathology, general medical treatment, and prognosis of the conditions included. Functional performance and treatment issues are also introduced. Pediatric psychiatric conditions are reviewed in Chapter 15, and neonatal medical conditions are described in Chapter 22. No single chapter can provide complete information about all conditions that may affect children. A list of key medical texts is provided at the end of the chapter.

## CARDIOPULMONARY DYSFUNCTIONS

This section addresses the conditions affecting the cardiac and respiratory systems of the infant and child. Included are congenital and acquired conditions that affect the child's health and ability to participate fully in life's occupations and roles.

### Congenital Cardiac Defects

Most cardiac problems in children are congenital in nature or secondary to other conditions. When they occur, they are serious, frightening, and can be life threatening. The section below discusses several of the major anomalies found in the heart and major vessels.

Congenital heart disease is the major cause of death in the first year (other than prematurity) (Wong, 1993). Three major cardiovascular changes must take place at birth. The foramen ovale, the hole between the right and left atria, must close. Also the ductus arteriosus and ductus venosus must close to allow blood to flow to the lungs and to the liver, respectively. Many complications can arise when these changes do not occur. One of the most common conditions found in premature newborns with respiratory distress syndrome is *patent ductus arteriosus (PDA)*. In this condition the ductus arteriosus does not constrict, and this can lead to eventual heart failure and inadequate oxygenation of the brain. Treatment includes the administration of the drug indomethacin, which often triggers closure of the arterial wall. Surgery follows if the drug does not work (Clark, 1992).

Another cardiovascular complication that may occur during the perinatal period is *intracranial hemorrhage*. This may occur prenatally, during the birth process, or postnatally. The site and the extent of the bleeding affect the prognosis. For example, extracranial bleeding, or cephalhematomas, are usually considered minor and usually cause no permanent damage. Conversely, subdural, subarachnoid, and intraventricular hemorrhages are much more serious and, depending on the extent of damage, may cause seizures, brain damage, cerebral palsy, and even death.

The other major congenital malformities are *atrial septal defects (ASDs), ventricular septal defects (VSDs), tetralogy of Fallot (TOF)*, and *transposition* of the great vessels (TGV). When an opening in the septum between the right and left atrial chambers occurs, it is called an ASD (Figure 7-1). This opening may be of any size and can occur anywhere along the septum. As a result, when the left atrium contracts, blood is sent into the right atrium. This is called a left-to-right shunt and causes more blood than normal to be sent to the lungs, resulting in "wet lungs," a condition that makes the lungs more susceptible to upper respiratory infections. This also causes the right atrium, and especially the right ventricle, to work much harder, and it can eventually cause heart failure in the older child. Symptoms include poor exercise tolerance and the appearance of being thin and small for age. Information for diagnosis is gathered from listening to the characteristic heart murmur,

evaluating chest x-ray films and electrocardiograms, and performing echocardiograms or heart catheterization.

Surgical procedures are done if the child is in distress. The surgery may be done early, or it may be postponed until the child is 4 or 5 years old. Until that time the child is closely watched for complications, especially for signs of heart failure (Malinowski & Yablonski, 1986).

VSDs are the most common type of congenital cardiac malformations and are often more serious than ASDs. This type of defect consists of a hole or opening in the muscular or membranous portions of the ventricular septum (Figure 7-2).

In these defects the blood flows from the left ventricle to the right ventricle, a left-to-right shunt, and, as in an ASD, an increased amount of blood is pumped to the lungs. The defect is considered less serious if the opening is in the membranous section of the septum and more serious if there are multiple muscular holes (Collins, Calder, Rose, Kidd, & Keith, 1972).

Symptoms associated with this defect include feeding problems, shortness of breath and increased perspiration, fatigue during physical activity, increased incidences of respiratory infections, and delayed growth. Causative factors are often idiopathic, but congenital infections, various teratogenic agents, and genetic predisposition may contribute to the cause (Clark, 1992; Monnett & Moynihan, 1991).

As in ASDs, the diagnosis is based on the murmur, chest x-ray film results, electrocardiograms, echocardiograms, and heart catheterization. In these defects improvement often occurs after 6 months of age, and more than 50% of the cases correct themselves by the age of 5 years (Clark, 1992). However, if the extent of damage is great or if the hole does not repair itself, surgical procedures to close the defect may need to be undertaken early in the child's life

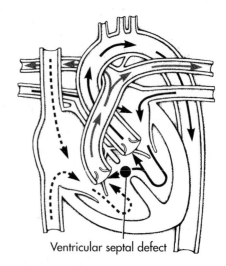

**Figure 7-1** Atrial septal defect. (From Whaley, L. & Wong, D. [1991]. *Nursing care of infants and children.* [4th ed.]. St. Louis: Mosby.)

**Figure 7-2** Ventricular septal defect. (From Whaley, L. & Wong, D. [1991]. *Nursing care of infants and children.* [4th ed.]. St. Louis: Mosby.)

Careful monitoring of these children must occur to prevent the life-threatening situation known as Eisenmenger's complex. In this situation pulmonary vascular obstruction has occurred as a result of prolonged exposure to increased blood flow and high pressure. Eventually the heart is no longer capable of pumping against the increased pulmonary pressure, the child goes into congestive heart failure, and blood pools in the right ventricle. This poses a medical emergency, requiring immediate surgical intervention.

The prognosis for infants with VSDs continues to improve as both surgical techniques and management of heart failure progress. These children are at risk for several serious complications, including cardiovascular accident (CVA), embolism, brain abscess, growth retardation, seizures, and death during an anoxic attack (Collins et al., 1972).

As its name implies, TOF is associated with four different problems: (1) pulmonary valve or artery stenosis with (2) ventricular septal defect present prenatally, causing (3) a right ventricular hypertrophy, and (4) overriding of the ventricular septum by the aorta (Figure 7-3). Physiologically the unoxygenated blood that is returning from the body cannot easily exit to the lungs because of the pulmonary stenosis. Instead it takes two paths of least resistance: the defect, creating a right-to-left shunt, and the aorta (Clark, 1992; Monnett & Moynihan, 1991).

Symptoms include central cyanosis, coagulation defects, clubbing of fingers and toes, feeding difficulties, failure to thrive, and dyspnea (Wong, 1993). The cause of TOF is probably similar to that of VSD. It is believed that the insult to the developing fetus occurs in the early weeks of fetal development when the right ventricle is at a critical stage (De La Cruz, Gomez, & Cayre, 1991).

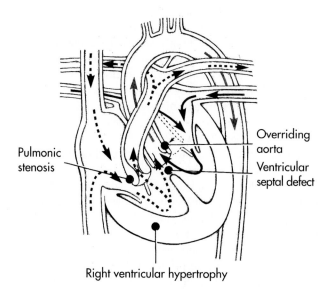

Pulmonic stenosis

Overriding aorta

Ventricular septal defect

Right ventricular hypertrophy

**Figure 7-3**   Tetralogy of Fallot. (From Whaley, L. & Wong, D. [1991]. *Nursing care of infants and children.* [4th ed.]. St. Louis: Mosby.)

Diagnosis is usually based on cyanosis, analysis of the heart murmur, right ventricular hypertrophy and right axis deviation demonstrated on the electrocardiogram, a chest x-ray film showing the characteristic "boot-shaped heart," and echocardiography demonstrating the overriding aorta (Clark, 1992; Wong, 1993).

Initial management consists of medication; surgery is delayed as long as possible. In severe cases a temporary shunt may be put in to bypass the stenosis. Usually, the Blalock-Taussig surgical procedure is used until "total corrective surgery" can be done, in which the pulmonary outflow obstruction is removed, the VSD is closed, and the aorta may be enlarged.

As with VSD, prognosis is improving as techniques and maintenance improve. Operative mortality has been reduced to 5% to 10%, but surgery is still a dangerous and complicated procedure (Wong, 1993).

TGV involves the anatomic transfer of the great arteries. Severity depends on the amount of circulatory mixing between the two sides. This can be accomplished by coexisting congenital cardiac defects, such as a VSD, or a pulmonary stenosis, or congenital transposition of the ventricles, called corrected transposition (Malinowski & Elixson, 1985). The severity of the symptoms varies, but cyanosis, congestive heart failure, and respiratory distress are common.

Diagnosis may be helped by the use of echocardiography, which can help identify the transposition, and by heart catheterization. Surgical treatment techniques include enlarging the foramen ovale by inserting a catheter with a balloon tip through the foramen ovale and into the left atrium. Next the catheter is pulled back through the foramen ovale to enlarge it, thus increasing the flow of oxygenated blood to the right atrium (Malinowski & Elixson, 1985). Another procedure involves excising the atrial septum and inserting a patch that redirects the blood flow. A third technique that is very new involves severing the great vessels at their bases and reattaching them to the proper ventricles. Operative mortality for TGV is 5% to 10%, regardless of the surgical procedure used. In later life these children have been known to develop arrhythmias and ventricular dysfunctions.

The child with congenital cardiac defects that have not yet been repaired can be expected to have reduced endurance for exertion but may be normal in other ways. This child will want to participate in a wide range of self-care and play activities. Pacing and selecting activities that are appropriate may be essential to the child's health and ability to participate in family and peer activities.

The involvement of the occupational therapist in congenital cardiac defects may be direct or indirect. For example, congenital heart defects are often found as secondary diagnoses in children with genetic syndromes. Children with Down syndrome or other types of mental retardation and multiply handicapped children may have histories of congenital heart problems. In these cases occupational therapists must be aware of the associated signs, symptoms, treatment procedures, complications of medications to watch for, and the effect of these conditions on the child's functioning.

Direct involvement might include participation on a pediatric rehabilitation team. In this instance the occupational therapist is concerned with physical restoration as well as the monitoring of various developmental and functional skills.

## Rheumatic Heart Disease

*Rheumatic heart disease (RHD)* is the sequela of rheumatic fever, a childhood infection. Acute rheumatic fever occurs from 2 to 4 weeks after an acute infection of streptococcal pharyngitis. The incidence of rheumatic fever has been greatly reduced in the past century but should still be considered a potentially dangerous condition.

School-aged children are most frequently affected, especially after a streptococcal pharyngitis epidemic. Rheumatic fever usually begins with one of the following serious symptoms: carditis, polyarthritis, or chorea (Griffiths, 1992).

Treatment consists of prescribing bed rest and administering antibiotics (usually penicillin) and antiinflammatory agents. Most patients take penicillin or erythromycin from the time of diagnosis for at least another 5 years as a preventive measure. It appears that a high percentage of children who experienced carditis during the first phase of rheumatic fever experience future heart problems (Wong, 1993).

The chorea that is associated with rheumatic fever may occur some time after the illness. This pattern appears gradually and presents as clumsiness and behavioral or learning changes. As it becomes more severe, this condition may impair the child's ability to perform functional activities and may be quite frightening to the child and family. Fortunately, this condition is transient and abates in time.

The child who has repeated infections is at increased risk for developing chronic RHD. Mitral valve insufficiency and stenosis and aortic insufficiency and stenosis may occur secondary to RHD. These problems may develop between 6 months and 10 years after infection. Changes in the affected valve may continue for an extended period and can lead to left ventricular hypertrophy, right ventricular hypertrophy, and mitral valve fibrosis. The individual experiences a progressive increase in symptoms and reduction in function. Rest and activity restrictions, antibacterial and antiinflammatory agents, dietary changes, and valve replacement surgery may be required (Walker, 1980).

## Dysrhythmias

Irregular cardiac rhythms, *dysrhythmias,* are not as common in children as in adults. However, the incidence of these problems is increasing, possibly because more of the chil-

dren with congenital heart defects are surviving surgery. This may leave them with a residual dysrhythmia. Three classes exist: bradydysrhythmia, tachydysrhythmia, and conduction disturbances. Diagnosis is primarily based on standard and 24-hour electrocardiogram monitoring.

*Bradydysrhythmia* is marked by an abnormally slow heart rate. The most common is a complete heart block, or atrioventricular (AV) block. This is not uncommon after surgery or myocardial infarcts and may occasionally require a pacemaker. Sinus bradycardia can be caused by anoxia or autonomic nervous system disorder. In this condition the child's heart rate may be reduced to less than 60 beats per minute and may have extra beats and slow nodal rhythms (Curley, 1985).

*Tachydysrhythmia* is an abnormally fast heart rate. Sinus tachycardia may be a symptom of a number of other conditions, including fever, anxiety, anemia, and pain, or it may be pathologic. Supraventricular tachycardia (SVT) involves a rapid heart beat of 200 to 300 beats per minute and is among the most common disturbances in children. This is a serious condition that can lead to congestive heart failure. The child with SVT is irritable, eats poorly, and is pale. In some cases a vagal maneuver, such as the Valsalva maneuver, can reverse the SVT, but in others the child may require hospitalization, esophageal overdrive pacing, or synchronized cardioversion (Wong, 1993).

*Conduction disturbances* are common after surgery and may be temporary. Premature contractions may be atrial, ventricular, or junctional. These can sometimes be handled with interim or permanent pacing, depending on the nature and severity of the disturbance.

## Neonatal Respiratory Problems

Respiratory problems are common in neonates and can be dangerous. Some of these problems are acute, and others are considered chronic lung diseases. Respiratory distress problems may be caused by prematurity, the aspiration of amniotic fluid or meconium, malformations or tumors of the respiratory organs, neurologic diseases, central nervous system damage, use of drugs, air trapped in the chest or pericardium (the sac surrounding the chest), and pulmonary hemorrhages (see Chapter 22).

One of the acute respiratory problems often found in any neonate, especially preterm babies, is *respiratory distress syndrome.* This disease is caused by a deficiency of surfactant, the chemical that prevents the alveoli from collapsing during expiration. Because this chemical is not produced until about the 34th to the 36th week of gestation, many premature infants are born with this deficiency. As the air sacs collapse, oxygen absorption and carbon dioxide elimination are hindered. Treatment includes administration of surfactant and supplemental oxygen. Ventilator support may be needed. After 3 to 4 days of treatment, most infants begin to recover as surfactant begins to be produced by the baby's body. Some infants develop chronic lung problems after respiratory distress syndrome.

Chronic lung disease implies a long-term need for supplemental oxygen. The chronic lung disease often seen in neonatal centers is *bronchopulmonary dysplasia (BPD)*. Initially, these neonates would have had some type of acute respiratory problem that precipitated the prolonged use of mechanical ventilation and other types of necessary, but perhaps traumatic, interventions. Because of the ventilation, airways begin to thicken, excess mucus forms, and alveolar growth is retarded. As a result, babies who develop BPD are often susceptible to respiratory infections and other respiratory problems until they are 5 or 6 years old. Problems such as BPD that are a result of the techniques used to save neonates' lives are called *iatrogenic disorders*.

The artificial respirators that are currently used are sophisticated and allow careful control of the oxygen mixtures. In addition, they are designed to maintain a constant pressure on the alveoli, thus keeping them open in the absence of surfactant. This is known as positive end-expiratory pressure (PEEP), which has significantly lowered the rate of fetal death and overall risk of severe developmental delays.

## Asthma

*Asthma* is an obstructive disorder characterized by bronchial, smooth-muscle hyperreactivity that causes airway constriction in the lower respiratory tract, difficulty in breathing, and bouts of wheezing. It is one of the most common long-term respiratory disorders of childhood. Most children who contract asthma have their first symptoms in early childhood, before the age of 5 (Behran & Vaughn, 1987). It appears to be an inherited trait and is often associated with familial patterns of allergy.

Asthma attacks may be triggered by allergen exposure, smoking, cold air, exercise, inhalant irritants, or viral infection (Behran & Vaughn, 1987; Wong, 1993). Asthma attacks are characterized by smooth muscle spasm of the bronchi and bronchioles and inflammation and edema of the mucous membranes with accumulations of mucus secretions. The child has difficulty breathing, particularly in expiration. The forceful expiration through the narrowed bronchial lumen creates the characteristic wheezing. The child also has a hacking, nonproductive cough. This experience can be frightening for the child, and the symptoms may become more severe in response to this panic. The effort of breathing may also leave the child's ribs sore and the child exhausted. Status asthmaticus is a serious asthmatic condition in which normal outpatient assistance does not improve the condition and emergency medical intervention is needed.

Treatment for asthma may include environmental control measures, skin testing, immunotherapy for allergies, emotional support, and a combination of pharmacologic agents, usually beta-adrenergic agonists and methylxanthine (Wong, 1993). These drugs may be related to school performance problems and in some cases can cause dependencies. Monitoring the child's schoolwork and educating him or her regarding the use and abuse of the medications should minimize difficulties in this area.

Children with asthma may be fearful of overexertion and may be concerned about contact with triggering allergens. This may result in a self-limited life-style. Assisting the child to manage the condition, respond calmly to stress, and pace activities can be essential to maintaining a normal childhood pattern. Structured peer group activities can also be useful in preventing social isolation. Breathing exercises, stretching, and controlled breathing can assist in managing the attacks.

## Cystic Fibrosis

The most common serious pulmonary and gastrointestinal problem of childhood is *cystic fibrosis (CF)*. This condition is an inherited disorder related to a gene located on chromosome 7. The condition is found in 1 in 1600 births among white children and 1 in 17,000 births among black children in the United States (Wong, 1993; Doershuk & Boat, 1987). CF is a multisystem disease that appears to be related to an impermeability of epithelial cells to chloride, causing the exocrine, or mucus-producing glands, to malfunction and their secretions to be thick, viscous, and lacking in water (Doershuk & Boat, 1987). These thick secretions block the pancreatic ducts, bronchial tree, and digestive tract.

One of the earliest signs of CF occurs in the newborn. In *meconium ileus* the small intestine is blocked by a thickened, puttylike substance that cannot be eliminated (Wong, 1993). The abdomen becomes extended, and the child is unable to pass stools, with vomiting and dehydration occurring in the absence of treatment (Doershuk & Boat, 1987).

Chronic pulmonary disease is the most serious complication of CF. A chronic cough, wheezing, lower respiratory infections, abscesses and cysts, hemoptysis, and recurrent pneumothorax are examples of the serious pulmonary complications that develop in CF. Other complications often result from hypoxemia, nasal polyps, and enlargement of the right side of the heart (right ventricular hypertrophy), which may eventually cause heart failure (Wong, 1993).

Also in patients with CF the sodium absorption-inhibiting factor is affected, which causes excessive amounts of sodium chloride to be secreted from the sweat glands onto the skin. Mothers may detect that their children taste salty when they kiss them. This alerts the physician, who will perform the simple diagnostic test known as the "sweat test." In this test an electrode is placed on the skin, causing the child to sweat at the contact site. A sample of the sweat is taken. If excessive levels of sodium chloride are detected, the diagnosis is made.

Pancreatic insufficiency causes characteristic foul-smelling and greasy stools. Associated problems include malabsorption; clinical diabetes; deficiencies of vitamins A, E, and K; and gastrointestinal obstruction. In the liver, bile ducts also become blocked, resulting in destruction of cells behind the blocked ducts. Although this is a serious problem, a positive point is that children's livers are often capable of regeneration.

Medical management consists of vigorous antibiotic, enzyme, and vitamin therapy and sound nutritional counseling. In an effort to keep the lungs as free as possible, the following physical or respiratory therapy techniques may be employed: mist tent therapy, intermittent positive pressure breathing, aerosol therapy, and postural drainage techniques (Tizzano & Buchwald, 1992).

The child with CF frequently spends time in and out of hospitals with various complications and for various treatments. These children may have a series of crises alternating with periods of comparative health, although there is a general degeneration that occurs. Children who primarily have gastric symptoms have a better prognosis than those whose first problems were respiratory related. All require a careful balance of nutrition, fluid intake, and exercise. Boys generally have a longer life span than girls, but degeneration of body functions and death occur for many in their teens and early twenties (Wong, 1993). Early detection and treatment has been shown to prolong life. The child and family may need assistance in dealing with grief and impending death.

Medical, nursing, dietary, and respiratory therapy staff are central to the treatment of this child. Respiratory therapists may have a key role in providing postural drainage, clapping, and chest expansion exercises. The occupational therapist may be concerned with energy conservation (activities that promote efficient breathing) and prevocational, recreational, and psychosocial support groups. Social, psychologic, and pastoral staff may provide essential family supports.

## HEMATOLOGIC DISORDERS

A number of hematologic disorders affect child development and function. This section addresses some of those most commonly seen by occupational therapists as primary or secondary diagnoses.

### Iron-Deficiency Anemia

*Iron-deficiency anemia* is the most frequently encountered blood condition in infancy and childhood. Iron is an essential part of the hemoglobin module, and when it is deficient, problems may occur. Children with this condition are most often asymptomatic but may be pale, irritable, and listless and may have some growth delays and feeding difficulties. The primary cause of iron-deficiency anemia is diet related.

The diagnosis is usually made easily with office screening procedures that are routinely conducted because of the high incidence of this condition in children.

In the infant and young child, treatment consists of giving the child iron-enriched cereals and formulas. Breast milk contains easily absorbed iron, but whole milk has insufficient iron and must be supplemented. The older child should be given a diet rich in foods containing a high amount of iron such as liver, beans, peas, and whole-grain cereals.

Older children whose diet is too heavy in milk may also suffer from this anemia and may require dietary changes as well as medication. In teenagers, this problem is often caused by their uneven eating habits and is therefore hard to control.

### Sickle Cell Anemia

More correctly called homozygous sickle cell disease, *sickle cell anemia* (SCA) is a hereditary, chronic form of anemia in which abnormal sickle, or crescent-shaped, erythrocytes are present that contain an abnormal type of hemoglobin called hemoglobin S (Milne, 1990). In the United States most cases occur in African Americans; the incidence is about 8% among black infants. SCA is rare in caucasians but can be found in people of Hispanic, Middle Eastern, and Mediterranean ancestry (Wong, 1993). It is now possible to determine this condition in the newborn. A few states already require sickle cell screening for all neonates, and more states are considering this course of action.

The clinical course of children with SCA is interspersed with episodes of severe worsening called sickle cell crises, which can be grouped into four types (Evans & Rogers, 1990). Aplastic and hyperhemolytic crises are characterized by imbalances in the production and premature destruction of red blood cells. These may cause the hemoglobin to decrease by 50%, necessitating immediate transfusions. Sequestration crises consist of the sudden and rapid enlargement of the spleen. This type of SCA traps much of the blood volume and can possibly cause shock or death. Painful, or vasoocclusive, crises are characterized by pain in the hands, feet, toes, and abdomen.

SCA affects other organs as well. Lungs may become infected, and hypoxemia is common; liver and kidney involvement causes urine problems and hematuria; CVAs may occur; the legs develop ulcers; and spleen damage can leave the child defenseless against major infections (Evans & Rogers, 1990). Additionally, children with SCA also experience chronic anemia, growth retardation, increased risk of septic infection, and delayed sexual maturation (Figure 7-4).

Sickle cell symptoms do not usually appear until the fourth month of life. However, screening can be done on the newborn with a blood test, the *Sickledex*. This test is followed by hemoglobin electrophoresis, which can provide a definitive diagnosis. This allows for early identification

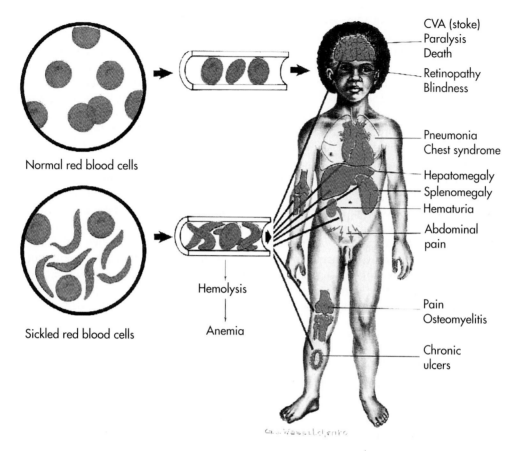

CVA (stoke)
Paralysis
Death

Retinopathy
Blindness

Pneumonia
Chest syndrome

Hepatomegaly
Splenomegaly
Hematuria

Abdominal
pain

Pain
Osteomyelitis

Chronic
ulcers

Normal red blood cells

Sickled red blood cells

Hemolysis

Anemia

**Figure 7-4** Differences between normal and sickled blood cells. (From Wong, D. [1993]. *Whaley and Wong's essentials of pediatric nursing.* [4th ed.]. St. Louis: Mosby.)

and treatment (Wong, 1993). There is no cure for sickle cell disease. Treatment focuses on reducing the sickling phenomena and treating the medical emergencies and their sequelae. Medical management includes bed rest, hydration and electrolyte replacement, oxygen therapy, analgesics, antibiotics, periodic exchange transfusions, and, sometimes, splenectomy (Wong, 1993). Bone marrow transplantation is being used in some cases and holds promise for a cure, but it is a painful and high-risk procedure.

Even with medical treatment, children with SCA may experience anoxia, CVAs, seizures, and cardiac failure. Disability and death are not uncommon (Milne, 1990). Rehabilitation and school-based professionals may provide treatment for the functional deficits created by these serious complications. Supportive counseling, activity adaptation, family support, and monitoring of the child's day-to-day functions are also important potential roles for occupational therapists.

## Hemophilia

The *hemophilias* are a group of conditions characterized by prolonged clotting (coagulation) times and abnormal and excessive bleeding. This bleeding occurs any place in the body, after serious or minor traumas, or spontaneously. There are two major types of hemophilia. Hemophilia A, or classic hemophilia, is caused by a deficiency of a factor in plasma necessary for blood coagulation. This factor has been called factor VIII, antihemophilic globulin, and antihemophilic factor. Hemophilia B (Christmas disease) results from a deficiency of clotting factor IX. They are sex-linked hereditary disorders and occur almost exclusively in boys (Wong, 1993).

Symptoms are not usually noticeable or bothersome until near the end of the first year of life, then soft tissue hemorrhages begin to occur. Soft tissue hemorrhages and hemarthroses are treated at home by replacing the missing factor to a level that will again control the bleeding. This is called replacement therapy, and most children can be trained to administer their own infusions.

Bleeding into joints (hemarthrosis) can cause severe musculoskeletal problems that can lead to joint deterioration if untreated. Consequently, the child may have increasing difficulty with ambulation and functional activities. The following procedures can be used to protect the joints: blood can be drained from a joint; chemical agents can be injected into the joint; and specific preventive range-of-motion activities can be initiated. Surgical procedures, such as joint replacements or synovectomies, contain some element of risk for hemophiliac patients (Lusher, 1989). Also, recreational activities must be carefully chosen to avoid trauma. For boys this can be frustrating and limit social interaction. These children may frequently miss school during crisis periods.

Prognosis for these young men depends largely on the management of the condition and on the avoidance of "bleeds" in critical organs. Intracranial hemorrhage is one of the most dreaded and serious complications of hemophilia. For older hemophiliacs, acquired immunodeficiency syndrome (AIDS) is also a significant risk. It is estimated that 60% of the hemophiliacs transfused before the 1980s when human immunodeficiency virus (HIV) screening programs were initiated will acquire the disease. As they reach the age when they become sexually active, patient education related to safe sex is essential. With this exception the treatment of hemophilia has improved sufficiently over the last 20 years to make a normal life expectancy possible (Lusher, 1989; Wong, 1993).

## MUSCULOSKELETAL DISORDERS

Bone tissue is one of the few body tissues that actively regenerates itself. The skeletal system is malleable; it deposits or resorbs bone based on the stresses it receives. Elements of the skeletal system include the bones, joints, cartilage, and ligaments. The muscular system includes the muscle fibers and their covering of fascia; it is activated by the nerves and moves the bones to create functional motion. Connecting the muscular and skeletal system at the origins and insertions of the muscles are the tendons.

Bone is mesenchymal tissue. As the child develops, the bone is first laid down as either membranous or cartilaginous and gradually becomes ossified through a calcium deposition process. The bones are formed, initially, early in fetal development. The growth and ossification processes generally occur at the epiphyseal plates, which are located at the ends of the bones. This process continues until the age of 25, at which time the epiphyses fuse (Brashear & Raney, 1986).

The musculoskeletal system can be affected by genetic and congenital disorders, trauma, infection, and metabolic, endocrine, circulatory, and neurologic disorders (Brashear & Raney, 1986). This section addresses some of the major disorders that affect primarily the musculoskeletal system.

### Congenital Anomalies and Disorders

A relatively large number of conditions affecting the musculoskeletal system have a genetic or congenital cause. These conditions often affect the child throughout life, causing disability, deformity, and sometimes death.

*Osteogenesis imperfecta (OI)* also called brittle bones or fragilitas ossium, is a disorder characterized by decreased

bone deposition probably because of the inability to form collagen. OI is believed to be transmitted by an autosomal dominant gene in most cases. However, the most severe, fetal type appears to have an autosomal recessive inheritance pattern (Brashear & Raney, 1986; Wong, 1993). This condition can run several different courses, from mild to severe, with most individuals having a milder form of the disease.

In all cases, however, the bones are unusually fragile, causing the child to fracture bones on minor traumas. The severity of the disorder varies greatly, depending on the time of onset (Table 7-1). Multiple fractures or repeated fractures to the same bone may cause a limb to become misshapen and eventually muscularly underdeveloped because of the long periods of immobilization and disuse. Prevention must be attempted through, at least, the use of padded arm and leg protectors, splints, and, in severe cases, long leg braces and crutches (Salter, 1983). To provide internal support and to correct deformities that may develop, surgical procedures using metal rods and segmental osteotomies may be helpful. Unfortunately, as the child grows, the rods must be replaced to accommodate the growth.

Medications are of little use, and over time these children can be expected to develop progressive deformities. Additionally, their activity patterns are affected by caution and time spent in casts. In the fetal and infantile types of this disorder, maternal education on handling and positioning is essential to prevent fractures during child care activities. These children need to be involved in movement activity, however, so that muscle strength and the postural effects of weight-bearing and exercise can be achieved. Children with less severe forms of the condition may participate in many normal activities, including some sports.

*Osteopetrosis,* also called marble bones or Albers-Schönberg disease, is an autosomal recessive disorder characterized by defective bone resorption that results in in-

▲ Table 7-1   Effect of Onset of Osteogenesis Imperfecta

| Type | Severity | Effect |
|---|---|---|
| Fetal | Most severe | Fractures occur in utero and during birth. Mortality is high. |
| Infantile | Moderately severe | Many fractures occur in early childhood. Severe limb deformities and growth disturbances occur also. |
| Juvenile | Least severe | Fractures begin in late childhood. By puberty, bones often begin to harden and fewer fractures occur. Dental problems may be present. |

creased bone thickness and narrowing of the foramina (Brashear & Raney, 1986; Salter, 1983). Gradually the bones become dense, and the hemopoietic marrow spaces are infiltrated with bony deposits, causing aplastic anemia. Other local complications may include pathologic fractures of the neck of the femur, nerve deafness or blindness as the nerve foramina begin to close because of bony encroachment, and enlargement of the liver and spleen. In severe cases hydrocephalus and mental retardation may be present. Prognosis is poor, and many children die in childhood. Treatment includes the administration of steroids and aggressive treatment of the anemia (Salter, 1983; Brashear & Raney, 1986).

Habilitation of these children is often symptomatic and addresses their deficits in mobility, vision, cognition, and perception. The focus is on developing self-help, school performance, and in some cases, prevocational skills.

*Marfan's syndrome,* arachnodactyly, is attributed to an autosomal dominant trait and produces excessive growth at the epiphyseal plates, as well as skull asymmetry and changes in the joints, eyes, heart, and aorta. Joints are lax and hypermobile, and striated muscles are poorly developed. Visual problems are often present because of the dislocation of the lens (Brashear & Raney, 1986). Symptoms include increased height and decreased weight for age, excessively long extremities, scoliosis, coxa vara, depressed sternum, stooped shoulders, elastic skin, and fragility of the blood vessels. A child with Marfan's syndrome may begin walking later than usual because of decreased postural stability, but the child need not have developmental delays. Treatment is symptomatic, addressing any skeletal deformities such as scoliosis that interfere with function.

*Achondroplasia,* or chondrodystrophia, is the most common cause of dwarfism. It is caused by stunted epiphyseal plate growth and cartilage formation. It is an autosomal dominant trait; fairly frequent spontaneous mutations are known to occur. The limb bones continue to grow to appropriate widths but are abnormally short. It is rare for these individuals to grow to more than 4 feet in height. Additionally, although skull size is normal, face size may be small, with a prominent forehead and jaw and a small nose. Trunk growth is nearly normal. Skeletal abnormalities include lumbar lordosis, coxa vara, and cubitus varus. There is no known cure for achondroplasia. Adults may experience back pain and, occasionally, paralysis caused by spinal stenosis. Surgical treatment may occasionally be necessary to relieve neurologic complications, improve functional movement, or correct extreme deformities (Brashear & Raney, 1986; Salter, 1983).

*Arthrogryposis multiplex congenita* is characterized by incomplete fibrous ankylosis of many or all of the child's joints. Its cause is unknown, and it is probably not hereditary. The child presents with stiff, spindly, and deformed joints and may also have clubfoot, hip dislocation, and characteristic posturing. Knee and elbow joints may appear thickened. Muscles may be absent or incompletely formed. The anterior horn cells of the spinal cord may be absent. If so, the child may also experience paralysis. Treatment focuses on maintaining and increasing functional range of motion and strength. Splints, casts, surgery, and daily stretching may be included in this regimen (Brashear & Raney, 1986). Adapted equipment and training for activities of daily living (ADL), school, play, and work performance may also assist this child.

A common abnormality of the foot is *congenital clubfoot,* or *talipes equinovarus.* The incidence of congenital clubfoot is high (1 to 2 per 1000) and much higher in cases where a sibling has clubfoot (1 in 35). Boys are affected twice as frequently as girls (Adams, 1981). The condition may be unilateral or bilateral, with the major clinical features consisting of forefoot adduction and supination, heel varus, equinus of the ankle and medial deviation of the foot (Figure 7-5). Some of the bones involved may be malformed, and the muscles of the lower leg are often underdeveloped. In a small number of cases a paralysis and permanent deformity may be present.

In some cases clubfoot is associated with other congenital problems and conditions, but the exact cause or causes of clubfoot are unclear; during fetal development something adversely affects the development of the muscles on the me-

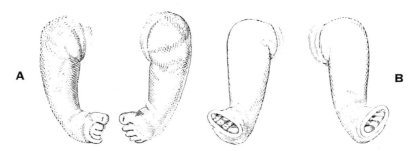

**Figure 7-5**    Bilateral congenital talipes equinovarus. **A,** Before correction. **B,** Undergoing correction in plaster casts. (From Brashear, H.R. & Raney, R.B. [1986]. *Handbook of orthopedic surgery.* [10th ed.] [p. 39]. St. Louis: Mosby.)

dial and posterior aspects of the legs, causing them to be shorter than normal (Adams, 1981). These contractions, in turn, lead to the bone and joint problems.

Complete correction of clubfoot is difficult to attain. Many times the deformity is corrected in infancy only to recur during periods of rapid growth (Salter, 1983). Initial treatment consists of manually correcting the deformity with gentle pressure and then using one of the following methods for holding the foot in the correct position: casting, metal splints of the Denis Browne type, adhesive strapping, and special boots. Gradually the amount of time the child spends in the piece of equipment is decreased until the child is only in it at night. If progress has not been noted in 2 to 3 months, soft tissue operations such as tendon lengthenings, tendon transfers, and capsulotomies may be performed. Salter (1983) stated that these early operations can greatly decrease recurrence of the problem.

In older children and in neglected cases of recurrent cases, treatment may have to be geared toward the creation of a plantigrade foot so that the child can walk on the sole of his or her foot. The soft tissue surgeries mentioned earlier may be used, as well as bony operations such as arthrodesis of joints, osteotomies, and the insertion of a bone wedge on the medial side of the calcaneus to correct the line of weight bearing (Adams, 1981). This treatment reduces foot mobility but increases function and stability. These children, too, will require ongoing monitoring. In general, prognosis is best for children when treatment is initiated early.

The analogous condition in the upper extremity, *congenital clubhand,* is far less common and is associated with partial or full absence of the radius and bowing of the ulnar shaft. Radial musculature, nerves, and arteries may be absent or underdeveloped as well. Often the hand remains functional. Treatment includes progressive casting and range of motion, static or dynamic splinting, or surgery. These procedures provide more cosmetic than functional benefit, however. This child may occasionally require some training or adaptations for school or daily living activities.

*Congenital dislocation of the hip* is almost as common as clubfoot, occurring in 1.5 per 1000 live births (Salter, 1983). It is often bilateral and occurs five times more commonly in girls than boys (Brashear & Raney, 1986). The causes of congenital hip dislocation (head out of socket) and subluxation (head partially out of socket) are both genetic and environmental. Hip laxity may be genetically inherited or may be a result of a hormonal secretion of the uterus. Environmental factors related to hip dislocation include birth complications from uterine pressure or poor presenting positions. Also, dislocation or subluxation of the unstable hip may be caused by sudden, passive extension or by positioning that maintains the legs extended and adducted.

Early diagnosis of this abnormality is critical because delay can cause serious and permanent disabilities. Three clinical observations that may be used in diagnosing congenital hip dislocation in infants are the Ortolani test, Galeazzi's sign, and Barlow's test. The Ortolani test consists of flexing the infant's knees and hips and then alternately adducting and pressing the femur downward and then abducting and lifting the femur. If the hip is unstable, it will dislocate when it is adducted but can reduce back into the socket as it is abducted. The evaluator feels and often hears a "click" as this happens. Galeazzi's sign consists of one knee being lower than the other when the child is placed in the supine position on a table with knees flexed to 90 degrees. This results from the dislocated femur lying posteriorly to the acetabulum. A positive Barlow's test occurs when the unstable hip clicks out of the acetabulum when the leg is abducted and pressure is placed on the medial thigh (Brashear & Raney, 1986).

In the older child with congenital hip dislocation, a Trendelenburg's sign is seen. Trendelenburg's sign consists of the hips dropping to the opposite side of the dislocation and the trunk shifting toward the dislocated hip when the child is asked to stand on the foot of the affected side.

If treatment is begun within the first few weeks of life, normal development of the hip can nearly always be assured. The longer it goes unresolved, the poorer the prognosis. Specific treatment techniques vary according to the age of the patient when treatment is initiated, but generally the techniques, ranging from those used on the younger child to those used on the older child, include stabilizing the hip in an abducted and flexed position to facilitate femoral and acetabular development. This may be accomplished with the use of splints, traction, the hip spica plaster cast, or the pillow splint (Adams, 1981). If these methods do not correct the problem, a number of surgical procedures may be used to correct bony and soft tissue problems. In severe cases, arthrodesis or total replacement arthroplasty may be performed. Again, it should be emphasized that every infant should be examined for this deformity in the first weeks of life to prevent the complications this defect can cause.

*Hypoplasias or aplasias* are relatively rare but do occur in the fibula, tibia, and femur, limiting gait and stability, or in the clavicles and the radius. Other congenital defects occasionally seen are *Sprengel's deformity* (congenital high scapula), recurvatum of the knee, congenital dislocations, and alignment deformities. Surgical revision or amputation is often performed in these cases to improve function (Salter, 1983).

## Limb Deficiencies

Limb deficiencies in children are most commonly attributable to congenital malformations. A small number occur also because of accidents, or electively, to prevent the spread of cancer such as Ewing's sarcoma. Congenital limb deficiencies occur more frequently in the upper extremities. Limb deficiencies and malformations may be familial or they may result from early fetal insult, or, rarely, from congenital constricting bands. In the latter case the soft tissue and overlying skin on a small body part fail to grow in circumference. If this is severe enough, the band stops distal limb circulation, causing gangrene and intrauterine amputation (Salter, 1983; Brashear & Raney, 1986). Traumatic amputations are becoming less common because of better emergency care and the improved ability of surgeons to re-attach a traumatically removed body part.

Congenital malformations of the hands or feet occur in 1 of every 600 live births, usually in the fingers and toes (Brashear & Raney, 1986). *Polydactyly* is an excess of fingers or toes. This is relatively common and may consist of one or more extra complete digits or duplication of only part of a digit. There may be bony changes or just extra soft tissue. In most cases surgical amputation or reconstruction are completed early in childhood, particularly if the hand is involved. *Syndactyly,* or webbing between the fingers or toes, occurs frequently. It is most common in the upper extremity and in boys. It sometimes coexists with polydactyly, which makes repair more complicated. In simple cases the fingers are surgically separated in early childhood (Salter, 1983; Brashear & Raney, 1986). Extensive hand therapy is usually unnecessary, although splinting and scar reduction may be helpful in some cases. *Bradydactyly* and *microdactyly* are overly large or small digits, respectively. Plastic surgical techniques may be used if the digits involved are unsightly or impair function.

Congenital limb deficiencies include amelia, phocomelia, paraxial deficiency, and transverse hemimelia (Figure 7-6). *Amelia* is the absence of a limb or the distal segments of a limb. In *phocomelia* the child may have a full or partially formed distal extremity but is missing one or more proximal segments of the limb. In *paraxial deficiencies* the proximal part of the limb is correctly developed, but either the medial or lateral side of the rest of the limb may be missing. *Transverse hemimelia* is a term used when the amputation occurs across the central area of a limb segment. It is not uncommon for a child with malformation of one body part to have bilateral or hemilateral problems.

Children with congenital limb deficiencies may require surgery for removal of skin flaps or "nuisance" parts if they interfere with function. It is not unusual for children to have some shoulder, trunk, and rib asymmetries, as well. These children are fitted with prostheses as early as 2 months but usually by 6 months. This allows the child to incorporate the prosthesis into his or her body image, promotes balance, prevents scoliosis, facilitates bilateral function, and reduces dependence on the residual limb for tactile input (NYU Staff, 1982). The child is often followed by a multidisciplinary prosthetic clinic or team, who follows the child and his or her family into adolescence.

Initial prostheses often have fixed knees or elbows to simplify prosthetic operation. Young infants with upper extremity amputations are often given a passive mitt, or a ter-

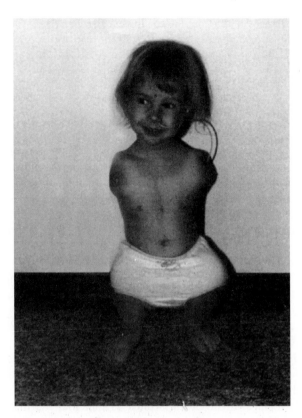

**Figure 7-6** Child with multiple congenital limb deficiencies including bilateral transverse upper arm deficiency and bilateral proximal femoral focal deficiency. (From Stanger, M. [1994]. Limb deficiencies and amputations. In S. Campbell [Ed.]. *Physical therapy for children.* New York: W.B. Saunders.)

minal device (TD) without cabling. This allows the child to hold objects placed in the hand by the parent and to develop early eye-hand skills. As the child grows and matures, new prostheses are fabricated that reflect the child's increased size and skills. Active TD use is instituted between 15 and 24 months; elbow operation, if necessary, is not introduced until the child is developmentally able to operate the mechanism (NYU Staff, 1982). As expected, this process is more complex for upper extremity than for lower extremity amputees and for children with multiple amputations.

Acquired limb deficiencies are treated much like those of adults, except that tasks must be developmentally structured and sequenced. Bimanual activities for play, school, and self-care are emphasized. Independent donning, doffing, and care of the prosthesis are also part of the treatment process for school-aged children. The child needs to be taught ADL skills, with and without the prosthesis, and may require assistance and adaptations for some school, work, and play tasks. Occasionally, children experience overgrowth of the long bones, causing pain, and if severe enough, skin penetration and infection. Conservative skin stretching and surgical revision may be necessary (Brashear & Raney, 1986). Psychosocial, self-concept, and social play experiences may assist these children, particularly as they approach puberty.

## Juvenile Rheumatoid Arthritis

Rheumatoid arthritis is a systemic disease that affects every aspect of an individual's life. It is characterized primarily by inflammatory changes and destruction to the synovial joints (Figure 7-7). Largely a disease of adults, it can also affect children (Melvin, 1989). *Juvenile rheumatoid arthritis (JRA)* is a major cause of physical disability in children younger than 16 years old. It is estimated that approximately 250,000 children in the United States suffer from some form of this disease (Adams, 1981). This disease usually begins between the ages of 2 and 4 years and is more common in girls (Salter, 1983; Wallace & Levinson, 1991).

The exact cause of JRA is unknown, but the following factors are believed to play undefined roles in its cause: genetics, emotional trauma, histocompatibility antigens, viruses, and antigen-antibody immune complexes (Adams, 1981).

JRA is usually described as taking three different forms: (1) pauciarticular, (2) polyarticular, and (3) systemic, or Still's disease. The pauciarticular form usually affects only a few joints. Involvement is often asymmetric, and there are few or no systemic manifestations. The joints most often affected are the knee, hip, ankle, and elbow. Many times overgrowth in the long bones surrounding the inflamed joint causes gait problems and flexion contractures. Many children suffering from pauciarticular JRA develop iridocyclitis, an inflamed condition of the iris and ciliary body of the eye that can lead to blindness if early treatment is not begun.

In the polyarticular form, onset is often abrupt and painful, with symmetric involvement of the wrist, hands, feet, knees, ankles, and sometimes the cervical area of the spine.

Other symptoms include a low-grade fever, malaise, anorexia, listlessness, and irritability.

Systemic JRA, or Still's disease, consists of polyarticular symptomatology plus involvement in other organs such as the spleen and lymph nodes (Adams, 1981). Signs and symptoms include a high fever, rash, anorexia, enlargement of the liver and spleen, and an elevated white blood cell count. Epiphyseal plates adjacent to an affected joint may initially show an acceleration of growth but later may be destroyed, causing local growth retardation.

Medical management primarily centers on the use of the following therapeutic drugs (in order of preference): salicylates; nonsteroidal antiinflammatory analgesic drugs; gold salt injections; and adrenocorticosteroids (Rennebohm & Correll, 1984; Salter, 1983). Surgical repair and reconstruction are seldom recommended for children. Other forms of treatment may include splinting, active and passive range of motion of the joints, and monitoring each joint to maintain maximal function and prevent deformity.

The prognosis for JRA varies, depending on a number of factors, but it is important to remember that the largest percentage of children (with the pauciarticular type) often recover completely within 1 to 2 years. Only about 15% of all children with the disease will have permanent disabilities (Wallace & Levinson, 1991).

Children with JRA may be in pain at times, may show signs of fatigue, and may have reduced range of motion in one or more joints. As a result they may have difficulty performing ADLs and certain school tasks. Adaptive equipment such as pen and pencil grips, dressing aids, and built-up handles on utensils or other adaptations to feeding equipment often improve functioning and reduce fatigue and stress on joints. Seating needs must be monitored to help reduce fatigue and prevent undue pressure on joints as well.

Play and recreational activities may be adapted to allow

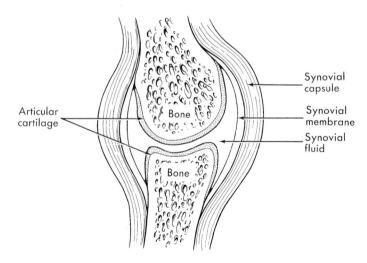

**Figure 7-7**   Components of a typical synovial joint.

full participation and to maintain strength and range of motion. Children with severe deficits also may require prevocational evaluation and treatment. Patient and parent education in joint protection and energy conservation techniques are essential for JRA at all ages and stages.

## Soft Tissue Injury

Children, being active and busy, are frequently subject to traumatic injury, particularly soft tissue injury. *Contusions* include damage and tears to the soft tissue, skin, muscles, and subcutaneous tissue. When they occur, an inflammatory response occurs and the child experiences pain, swelling, and hemorrhagic responses. These are usually not serious in the normal child but can be difficult for children with disordered response to trauma, such as hemophilia. *Crush injuries* are common—fingers caught in doors, for example. These can also involve bone and nails and may swell and be painful.

A *dislocation* occurs when forces on the joint pull or push the joint out of its socket. This creates obvious problems in alignment, deformity, and immobility. Dislocations should be reduced as soon as possible so that inflammation does not increase the pain and difficulty of this procedure. After reduction the child's extremity is usually immobilized for some time to allow healing. If the forces exerted on the ligaments are strong enough to tear them, the injury is called a *sprain*. Muscles, nerves, tendon, and blood vessels in the area also may be damaged by these forces. There are a number of "special tests" for joint laxity that are used for sprain evaluation. Pain may or may not be severe, but swelling and favoring the extremity usually occur. Sprains must be positioned and immobilized for an extended period, and in severe cases, may be casted or splinted for 3 to 6 weeks.

## Fractures

*Fractures* are extremely common in children. Fractures can occur prenatally and perinatally in children with other pathologic conditions but are uncommon in normal infants. As the child grows older, however, and as independence and activity levels increase, children may be injured in automobile, skateboard, and bicycle accidents, falls, and sports. Childhood fractures can also be caused by child abuse. Any child with an unusually large number of fractures may trigger an investigation into the possibility that abuse has occurred.

Fractures may be classified in many ways. An open, or compound, fracture refers to the fact that there is an open wound or penetration caused by an object outside the body or caused by the bone penetrating from within the body. A *closed* fracture indicates that no penetration has occurred. Open fractures present added complications because the wound must be closed in addition to treating the fracture. The risks of infection and soft tissue and nerve damage are higher with the open fracture, and complications are more common.

Traumatic fractures are often complicated by the fact that bones are displaced and malaligned. Figure 7-8 shows some of the most common types of malalignment caused by serious fractures.

Children's fracture patterns are not identical to those of adults. Their bones may buckle or bend rather than break because their bones are thinner and less solid. *Greenstick* fractures occur when the bone is not completely separated on one side, much as a twig breaks when bent. Sometimes the bone breaks completely, but the periosteal covering remains partially intact, holding the fragments together. This *periosteal hinge* may assist or complicate fracture reduction. *Comminuted* fractures occur

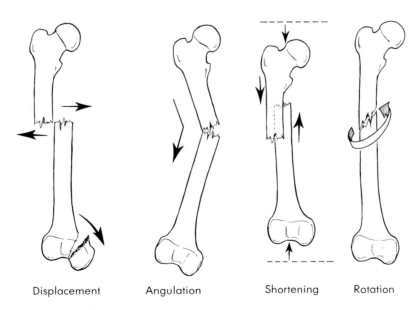

Displacement     Angulation     Shortening     Rotation

**Figure 7-8**   Types of malalignment caused by fractures.

when multiple fragments are created by the injury (Mc-Cullough, 1989).

Children's ligaments are often stronger than their epiphyseal plates. Therefore when stress is applied, it is more common to find a fracture than a dislocation or sprain. Fractures involving the epiphyseal growth plate, which account for 15% of childhood fractures, are of particular concern because they may affect the growth and alignment of the bone and the integrity of the joint in later life. The type of problem and its severity depends on the location and extent of the injury in relation to the growth plate. Figure 7-9 illustrates the Salter-Harris classification system (Salter, 1983). Under this system the more severe injuries are given higher numbers. Injuries that cross the joint surface are generally the most serious because they may result in uneven growth on the joint surface and therefore impair the normal slide, glide, and alignment of the joint in adolescence and adulthood.

Treatment of fractures requires open or closed reduction, or realignment, of the bony fragments and immobilization until the bone heals. Open surgical reduction is rare in children but may be performed for injuries to the growth plate and serious compound or comminuted fractures (Salter, 1983). Fractures in children heal more quickly than those in adults. Young children and infants may heal in 2 to 4 weeks and school-age-children in 6 weeks. Adolescents require immobilization for the same 8 to 10 weeks required by adults with similar injuries (Hansell, 1988).

Immobilization is usually by means of a cast, although in severe cases, pins, traction, and external fixation may be used. The advent of synthetic, fiberglass, and polyurethane resin casting materials are a boon for children because these materials are waterproof and come in bright colors. Casted children should be checked to assure that circulation and skin integrity are maintained under the cast and that the cast is not breaking down from active use. The child in traction may need adapted devices and activities to maintain independence while he or she is immobilized. Prevention of skin breakdown is also a concern for any individual on bed rest.

## Torsion Deformities

Particularly in children, prolonged twisting forces may cause changes in epiphyseal plate growth, causing the long bones to twist in the direction of the abnormal force. These are known as *internal, external, or combinational torsional deformities.* For example, "toeing out" is common in young children. This deformity is characterized by externally rotated feet and knees and by limited internal rotation of the femur. It is often seen in infants who habitually sleep in the prone position with their legs externally rotated, causing external femoral torsion. Conversely, children who spend a great deal of time sitting on the floor with knees in front, feet out to the side, and femors internally rotated (the "television position" or "W-sitting"), may begin to "toe in," resulting from the internal femoral tension.

Bow legs, or genu varum, is an example of a deformity caused by combinational torsional forces, that is, prolonged internal torsion to the tibia and external torsion to the fe-

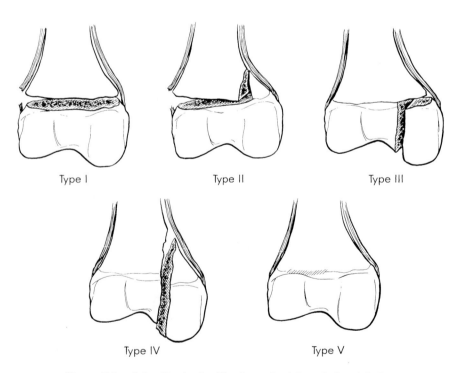

**Figure 7-9**    Salter-Harris classifications of epiphyseal plate injuries.

mur. This deformity is often present at birth because of prenatal posturing, but it usually corrects itself unless compounded by specific neuromuscular problems or unusual sleeping and sitting postures that continue to apply the abnormal torsions.

## Legg-Calvé-Perthes Disease

Sometimes called coxa plana, *Legg-Calvé-Perthes disease* is an acquired skeletal disease that most commonly affects white boys between the ages of 4 and 8 years. The condition is usually unilateral, resulting from an idiopathic ischemic aseptic necrosis of the femoral head. The condition appears to have four stages, through which the child passes in a period from 18 months to several years. Pathologically, the epiphysis of the femoral head becomes necrotic, then is slowly reabsorbed, sometimes causing the collapse of the femoral head. The bone then is replaced and regenerated over the next 2 years or so (Brashear & Raney, 1986).

Clinically, the child may acquire symptoms gradually, including intermittent limping and discomfort. Pain is most common at the end of the day. Over time these periods increase, and joint limitations, tenderness over the hip, and external rotation appear. Conservative therapy includes rest, abduction bracing to position the hip, crutches, and non–weight-bearing harnesses. Prognosis is generally good if the child complies well, particularly in younger children. These children do experience an extended period of functional disability, however, because the treatment limits mobility and participation in many of the normal activities of school-aged boys.

## Curvature of the Spine

*Scoliosis, lordosis,* and *kyphosis* are the terms used to describe the three major deformities of the spine. These conditions may occur functionally, posturally, and structurally; they may be secondary to muscle imbalance, bony deformities, or other pathologic conditions such as cerebral palsy; or they may occur idiopathically. They may be congenital or acquired. In most cases the cause of these disorders is unknown; however, some familial patterns do exist.

*Lordosis* is an anteroposterior curvature in which the concavity is directed posteriorly. Also called hollow back, this condition is often secondary to other spinal deformities or anterior pelvic tilt. It is usually predominantly in the lumbar area of the back and is occasionally painful. It can also be secondary to extreme obesity, hip flexion contractures, or conditions such as muscular dystrophy. It also may occur during the adolescent growth spurt experienced by many girls. Treatment focuses on correcting the underlying conditions, stretching tight hip flexors, and strengthening abdominal musculature. Postural training and occasionally, in severe cases, back bracing is included.

The opposite anteroposterior curvature, with the convexity posterior, is called *kyphosis*. Also called round back, and in adolescents, Scheuermann's disease, the curvature is usually primarily in the upper back. This deformity is common in children and adolescents and is usually secondary to faulty posture. This is particularly true as the teenage girl's skeletal growth outpaces her muscular growth and may relate to her self-confidence. The deformity may occur in children with spina bifida cystica, arthritis, and tuberculosis. Treatment depends on the cause and severity of the problem. In mild cases, postural training and strengthening activities such as weight training, swimming, and dance are often useful. In severe cases, bracing or Harrington rods may be used to guide and support the spine (Brashear & Raney, 1986).

*Scoliosis* is the most common and serious of the spinal curvature disorders. Treatment is considered when a lateral curvature of more than 10 degrees is present. Lateral curvature of the spine is often accompanied by rotation of the vertebral bodies. Functional scoliosis is flexible and can be caused by poor posture, leg length discrepancy, poor postural tone, hip contractures, or pain. Congenital scoliosis is usually structural in nature, caused by abnormal spinal or spinal cord structure. Diseases of the nervous system or spine also may create a scoliosis. However, most scoliosis has no known cause.

Scoliosis is rarely painful. About 85% of the cases occur in girls. Diagnosis is based on careful examination and history. If preliminary evaluation and palpation suggest the condition, radiographic analysis is also done. Structural scoliosis often progresses over time; the vertebral bodies may become wedge shaped and rotate toward the convex part of the curve, and the intervertebral disk may shift and deform (Brashear & Raney, 1986). Curves of less than 20 degrees are considered mild. Those of more than 40 degrees may result in permanent deformity, and those of 65 to 80 degrees may result in reduced cardiopulmonary function. Skin breakdown between the ribs and pelvis may also develop in some cases.

Treatment is usually begun early, and focuses on postural exercises, maintaining range of motion, and strengthening of abdominal and spinal musculature. These have been found to be of limited value in most cases. If the curvature progresses, bracing with a Milwaukee or similar brace and electrical stimulation may be added to the regimen. The brace is large, cumbersome, and unsightly and is worn 23 hours a day. It allows the child to continue normal activities, with minimal adaptations. If the condition continues unchanged or worsens, surgery and internal fixation of the spine are the usual course of treatment. Common fixation systems are Harrington, Luque, or Cotrel-Dubousset rods, Dwyer cable, or combinations thereof. After surgery the child is casted or braced for 6 months to a year. Postoperative physical therapy and adapted ADL are sometimes needed; in general, children and adolescents progress well after surgery and maintain a normal life-style into adulthood.

## NEUROMUSCULAR DISORDERS

Children with neuromotor disorders constitute a large percentage of the clients of occupational therapy practice. A variety of conditions exist in which the neurologic system is impaired, interfering with the child's ability to interact effectively with the environment. The site of damage may be the brain, spinal cord, peripheral nerves, neuromotor junction, or the muscle itself. It may interfere with the reception and processing of sensory input, the ability to act effectively on the environment, or a combination thereof. These deficits may occur before, at, or after birth. This section addresses several of the major conditions in this category.

### Cerebral Palsy

*Cerebral palsy (CP)* is the name given to a group of conditions characterized by brain damage that creates neurologic and motor deficits in the developing child. Intellectual, seizure, and behavioral disorders may coexist with these motor deficits. Although CP is usually the result of injury or disease at or before birth, children injured in early childhood display similar symptoms and are also classified as having CP (Bobath, 1980; Wong, 1993).

CP can be defined as a disorder of movement and posture that is caused by a nonprogressive brain lesion that occurs in utero, during, or shortly after birth and is expressed through variable impairments in the coordination of muscle action and sensation (Bobath, 1980).

CP is estimated to occur in 0.6 to 2.4 of 1000 live births. This incidence dropped during the middle of the century, and has remained steady since the 1970s (Batshaw, Perret, & Kurtz, 1992; Wong, 1993). The exact number of cases is difficult to estimate because there is a continuum of dysfunction from mild to severe and profound.

In recent years the incidence of certain types of CP seems to have shifted. The incidence of spastic diplegia, often associated with prematurity and low birth weight, has increased, and that of athetosis, often attributed to fetal anoxia and hyperbilirubinemia, has decreased (Batshaw, Perret, & Kurtz, 1992). Causes of CP include perinatal asphyxia and trauma, intracranial hemorrhage, developmental brain anomalies, toxicosis, infections, trauma, near drowning, hypoxia, and metabolic disorders. Sickle cell disease, uncontrolled hydrocephalus, and familial inheritance have also been associated with CP.

Characteristically, the child with CP shows impaired ability to maintain normal postures because of a lack of muscle coactivation and the development of abnormal movement compensations. These compensatory patterns develop over time as disruptions to the child's center of gravity as well as other sensory stimuli and result in impaired motor and postural responses. For example, the child's poor head control, resulting from poor coactivation of cervical flexors and extensors, causes the center of gravity to move anteriorly; this results in compensatory reactions in the thoracic and lumbar spine as the child attempts to stay upright. Likewise, hyperreactive responses to tactile, visual, or auditory stimuli may result in fluctuations of muscle tone that often adversely affect postural control and further diminish participation in meaningful activities.

Through regulation of reflexes and reactions the child's central nervous system matures and begins to regulate the "degree, strength, balance, and distribution of muscle tone" (Fiorentino, 1981, p. 26). Without this regulation the child experiences difficulty in performing automatic movements. Critical to optimal development of postural behavior is the sequential interaction and coordination of the postural reflexes. Eventually the integration of reflexes into higher level righting, protective, and equilibrium reactions forms a solid foundation for skilled and coordinated movements in work, self-care, and play or leisure.

During normal movements the brain registers sensory feedback from weight-bearing and weight-shifting experiences. The child develops a stable base for performing cognitive and interactive tasks without having to think consciously about maintaining a particular position. This process is reversed when experienced by a child with CP. The sensory feedback from compensatory movements feeds into more compensations. Inaccurate feedback leads to further distortions of movements and sensation, contractures, and deformities, together with adverse influences on the psychologic and prevocational development of the child.

#### Classification of Cerebral Palsy

The locale of the lesion affects the development and quality of movement patterns present in the child with CP. For example, CP with spasticity indicates a fixed lesion in the motor cortex. Lesions in the basal ganglia typically cause fluctuations in muscle tone that are described as diakinesis, dystonia, or athetosis. Cerebellar damage tends to produce the unstable movements characteristic of the ataxic child.

The variability of the movement and postural disorder may be classified according to which limbs are affected. Involvement of one extremity is commonly referred to as monoplegia, upper and lower extremities on one side as hemiplegia, both lower extremities as paraplegia, and all limbs as quadriplegia. When the child demonstrates quadriplegia with mild upper extremity involvement and more significant impairment in lower extremity function, this is called diplegia.

Several classifications of cerebral palsy have been developed according to quality of tone, disorder distribution, and even locale of brain lesions. A combination of these classifications is featured in Table 7-2. Characteristics are described according to quality and distribution of muscle tone, range of motion, quality of movement, presence of reflexes and reactions, oral motor problems, associated problems, and personality characteristics.

Although CP is considered to be nonprogressive, abnormal movement patterns, muscle tone, and sensory function, combined with the effects of gravity and normal growth, may cause the child to develop contractures and deformities over time. Function may become more limited as the child grows to adulthood. Further, the effects of normal aging may result in decreased function, physical discomfort, and arthritic responses over time.

Antispasticity drugs are occasionally effective, and muscle relaxants can reduce discomfort in older children for short periods. In cases where spasticity is severe, neural blocks may be done to disrupt the reflex arc (Batshaw & Perret, 1992). Active and passive range of motion activities, positioning and handling to normalize postural tone, and orthotics may be used alone or in combination to minimize these effects (Bobath, 1980; Bobath & Bobath, 1972). Orthopedic surgery may be performed to balance uneven muscular action, reduce contractures, and facilitate ambulation and functional movement. Orthotic management in support of surgery, or to reduce tone, prevent contractures, or stabilize or position often improves and increases functional activity. Tone-reducing or inhibitive casts made for the lower extremity can gently strengthen and lengthen spastic muscles. Often a series of casts are applied to gradually increase range of motion. When range of motion within normal limits has been achieved, the cast is worn intermittently to maintain the increased muscle length.

Language and intellectual deficits often coexist with CP. Delays in cognitive development with below-average intelligence have been seen in between 50% and 75% of children with CP. This impairment may range from mild to profound (Batshaw & Perret, 1992). Speech disturbances occur in approximately 30% of this population. Articulation problems may be associated with impairment of tongue and lip movements. Speech and language problems may be receptive or expressive, relating to central processing impairment. Limitations in communication tend to isolate the child, may create stress and frustration for the child and parent, and can negatively affect the development of psychosocial skills. Use of augmentative communication equipment can prevent some of these consequences of speech impairment and is critically important for increasing the communication abilities of some children with CP.

Seizure disorders occur in approximately 50% of individuals with CP (Roberts, 1979). When they occur, the impairments range in intensity from occasional petit mal episodes to serious, almost continuous grand mal seizures. The incidence appears to be higher among children with spastic disorders (Roberts, 1979). In children with severe seizures, some degeneration may continue after birth. Anticonvulsant drugs are commonly used to control the seizure activity. These drugs must be carefully monitored and may affect the state of the child's digestion and gums, requiring feeding adjustments and good dental care.

Feeding problems are associated with the abnormal oral movements, tone, and sensation. The child may be hypersensitive or hyposensitive to touch around and in the mouth; sucking, chewing, and swallowing may be difficult to initiate or control (Batshaw & Perret, 1992; Wong, 1993). Diet may need to be adjusted and special feeding techniques employed. These children also may require medication to maintain regularity of elimination. Positioning helps improve postural stability for feeding and toileting.

A variety of sensory deficits may be present. A wide continuum of problems with the visual system may include impaired vision, blindness, limitations in eye movements and eye tracking, squinting, strabismus, eye muscle weaknesses, and eye incoordination. In addition, children with CP may have visual perception problems that can interfere with school progress. It is estimated that 40% to 50% of children with CP have visual defects of some type (Batshaw & Perret, 1992). Auditory disturbances include hearing (acuity) problems that can range from slight hearing loss to total deafness. Auditory perceptual problems and agnosia are also common. An estimated 25% of children with CP have some type of auditory disturbance.

Children with CP often require glasses, low vision or visual perceptual training, or hearing aids. Sensorimotor integration approaches may be used to assist in interpreting and interacting with the environment.

Finally, children with CP must be monitored for signs of behavioral problems and psychosocial delays that can become serious problems if not found early and corrected. Evaluation of these areas, emotional support, normalizing social experiences, and behavior management programs should be integral parts of the total assessment and treatment regimen for these special children.

It is important to remember that each child with CP has a unique set of problems. Comprehensive medical assessment is necessary in children with CP because of the multiple problems that may exist. The physician usually bases the diagnosis on abnormal delays in development that have been observed during physical examinations and on what the parents have reported over a period of months or years. Types of problems that should alert the physician that something may be wrong include the retention of primitive reflexes, variable tone, hyperresponsive tendon reflexes, asymmetry in the use of extremities, clonus, poor sucking or tongue control, and involuntary movements. Another clue might be a large discrepancy between motor and intellectual areas of development.

Although prognosis varies for each type of CP, most children with CP live to adulthood, but their life expectancy is less than that of the normal population. Functional prognosis varies greatly from type to type, with hemiplegia and spastic diplegia having a better prognosis than the more severe, rigid types. Children with CP may have limitations in

▲ Table 7-2  Cerebral Palsy Classifications

| | Severe Spasticity | Moderate Spasticity | Mild Spasticity | Pure Athetosis |
|---|---|---|---|---|
| Quality of tone | Severely increased tone; flexor and extensor cocontraction are constant; tone is high at rest, asleep, or awake; tone pattern is more proximal than distal. | Moderately increased tone; near normal at rest but increases with excitement, movement attempts, effort, emotion, speech, sudden stretch; agonists and distal muscles more spastic. | Mildly increased or normal tone at rest; increases with effort or attempts to move or attempts at quicker movements. | Fluctuation of tone from low to normal; no or little spasticity; no coactivation of flexors and extensors. |
| Distribution of tone | Quadriplegia, but can also be diplegia or paraplegia. | Same as severe spasticity. | Same as severe spasticity, but more diplegia and hemiplegia. | Quadriplegia with occasional hemiplegia. |
| Range of motion | Abnormal patterns can lead to scoliosis, kyphosis, hip/knee/finger deformity; forearm pronation contracture, hip subluxation, heel cord subluxation with equinovarus or equinovalgus; decreased trunk, shoulder, and pelvic girdle mobility; limited midrange control where cocontraction is least balanced. | More available movement and more flexor/extensor imbalance can lead to kyphosis, lordosis, hip subluxations or dislocations, hip and knee flexion contractures; tight hip internal rotators and adductors; heel cord shortening and foot rotation. | Limitations more distally; minimal deformities. | Transient subluxation of joints such as shoulders and fingers; may have valgus on feet or knees; rarely any deformities. |
| Quality of movement | Decreased midrange, voluntary and involuntary movements; slow and labored stereotypical movements. | May be able to walk; stereotypical, asymmetrical, more associated reactions, total movement synergies. | Often able to walk; seems driven to move; has increased variety of other movements, some stereotypical. | Writhing involuntary movements, more distal than proximal; no change with intention to move; many fixation attempts caused by decreased ability to stabilize. |
| Reflexes and reactions | Obligatory primitive reflexes (positive support, ATNR, STNR, neck righting); protective, righting, and equilibrium reactions are often absent. | Strong primitive reflexes—Moro, startle, TNR, TLR, positive support prominent; decreased neck righting; associated reactions strong; righting may be present, but equilibrium reaction develops to sitting and kneeling. | Primitive reflexes used for functional purposes and not obligatory; righting, protective, and equilibrium reactions delayed, but not established; may not get higher-level reactions. | Primitive reflexes not usually obligatory or evoked; protective and equilibrium reactions usually present but involuntary movements affect grading. |

Modified from Bobath, B. (1978). *Classification of types of cerebral palsy based on the quality of postural tone.* London: The Bobath Centre.
*ATNR,* Asymmetric tonic neck reflex; *STNR,* symmetric tonic neck reflex; *TNR,* tonic neck reflex; *TLR,* tonic labyrinthine; *MR,* mental retardation.

| Athetosis with Spasticity | Athetosis with Tonic Spasms | Choreoathetosis | Flaccid | Ataxia |
|---|---|---|---|---|
| Fluctuates from normal to high; some ability to stabilize proximally; moderate proximal spasticity and distal athetosis. | Unpredictable tone changes from low to very high; either all flexion or extension of extremities. | Constant fluctuations from low to high with no cocontraction; jerky involuntary movements more proximal than distal. | Fluctuating, markedly low muscle tone; seen at birth or toddler initially as flaccid; later classified as spastic, athetoid, or ataxic. | Ranges from near normal to normal; when increased tone is present, usually involves lower extremity flexion. |
| Same as athetosis. | Quadriplegia, hemiplegia, or monoplegia. | Quadriplegia. | Quadriplegia. | Quadriplegia. |
| Incidence of scoliosis; some flexion deformities at hips, elbows, and knees; usually full range of motion proximally/hypermobile distally. | More pronounced scoliosis; more dislocation of arm because of flailing spasm; possible kyphoscoliosis, hip dislocation on skull side, flexion contracture on hips/knees, subluxation of hips, fingers, or lower jaw. | Many involuntary movements with extreme ranges but no control at midrange; deformities rare, but tendency for shoulder and finger subluxation. | Hypermobile joints tend to sublux; flat chest; later range limitations due to limited movement. | Range is usually not a problem; when present, decreased range is in flexion. |
| Decreased ability to grade movements; decreased midline control and selective movement; proximal stability and distal choreoathetosis; varies with case. | Extreme tonic spasm without voluntary control; some involuntary movement, distal more than proximal. | Wide movement ranges with no gradation; jerky movements more proximal than distal; no selective movement or fixation of movement; weak hands and fingers. | Ungraded movements; slow movements difficult; many static postures as if hanging on to anatomic structures instead of active control. | Lack point of stability so coactivation is difficult; use primitive rather than abnormal patterns, hence gross, total patterns; incoordination, thus dysmetria disdiadochokinesia, tremors at rest, symmetric problems. |
| TNR/TLR strong but intermittent and modified by involuntary movements; equilibrium reactions when present are unreliable and may or may not be used. | Strong ATNR, STNR, TLR; protective and equilibrium reactions absent during spasm, otherwise present, unreliable, or absent. | Intermittent TNR; righting and equilibrium reactions present to some extent, but abnormal coordination. Abnormal upper extremity protective extension but often absent. | Usually less reactive because of decreased tone; righting is delayed; delayed protective extension more available than equilibrium reaction. | May develop righting reactions but uncoordinated, exaggerated, and poorly used; equilibrium reactions when developed are not coordinated; needs wide base of support because of poor weight shift. |

*Continued.*

▲ Table 7-2   Cerebral Palsy Classifications—cont'd

| | Severe Spasticity | Moderate Spasticity | Mild Spasticity | Pure Athetosis |
|---|---|---|---|---|
| Oral motor | Immobile, rigid chest; shallow respiration and forced expiration; lip retraction with decreased lip closure and tongue thrust; communication through forced expiration. | Not as involved as severe spasticity. | Increased mobility, thus more respiratory function for phonation; shortness of breath limits sentence length; better ability to dissociate mouth parts, but poor lip closure causes drooling. | Fluctuations adversely affect gross and fine motor performance; volume of speech may go up or down with breath; feeding may be decreased due to instability and tongue/jaw/swallow incoordination. |
| Associated problems | Seizures; cortical blindness; deafness; mental retardation; prone to upper respiratory tract infection (URTI); malnutrition. | Seizures; MR; perceptual motor problems; imbalance of eye musculature. | Seizures; less MR; perceptual problems. | Hearing loss; less mental retardation. |
| Personality characteristics | Passive, dependent; resistant and adapts poorly to change; anxious and fearful of being moved; generally less frustrated than athetoid. | A lesser picture of severe spasticity. | More frustrated and critical about self because of awareness of better performance; more patient than children of same age. | Emotional lability; less fearful of movement; more outgoing, but tends to be frustrated. |

all areas of human occupation to some degree. Functional performance in self-care and independent living, school and work performance, play, and recreation may all need to be addressed at some point in the child's life. Parents may require support and respite, as well as education, to handle this child and meet the needs of the family as a whole (Scherzer & Tscharnuter, 1990).

## Epilepsy

*Epilepsy* is a group of neuromuscular conditions whose center of dysfunction is in the brain. A *seizure* may be defined as a temporary, involuntary change of consciousness, behavior, motor activity, sensation, or automatic functioning (Menkes, 1990). Individuals are considered to have epilepsy if they have recurring seizures.

A *seizure* starts with an excessive rate and hypersynchrony of discharges from a group of cerebral neurons that spreads to the adjoining cells, called the *epileptogenic focus* (Wong, 1993). Some seizures may be directly attributed to the factor or factors that trigger the seizure. For example, acute factors often described are hypoglycemia, fever, trauma, hemorrhages, tumors, infections, and anoxia. Other seizures may be attributed to previous scarring and structural damage or to hormonal changes. Many seizures, especially in children, have no discernible underlying disease and are, therefore, idiopathic in nature (Menkes, 1990).

Many authors classify seizures by their clinical characteristics or symptoms. With this form of categorization there are four major types of seizures: (1) grand mal seizures that account for 40% to 50% of the total incidence, (2) petit mal seizures that occur 12% to 15% of the time, (3) focal or psychomotor seizures that occur 5% of the time, and (4) mixed-type seizures that account for the remainder of time.

A child having a *grand mal seizure* may have an aura, or sensation, that the seizure is about to begin. This is usually followed by a loss of consciousness during which the body becomes rigid or tonic, and then rhythmic clonic contractions of all the extremities occur. Incontinence is frequent. The seizure may last for 5 minutes, followed by a postictal period that may last from 1 to 2 hours in which the child is drowsy or in a deep sleep (Batshaw & Perret, 1992; Roberts, 1979).

*Petit mal seizures* are characterized by a momentary loss of awareness and no motor activity except eye blinking or rolling. There is no aura, the seizures usually last only 5 to 10 seconds, and there is no postictal period. One important factor to remember with this type of seizure is that it is frequently mistaken for daydreaming. Petit mal seizures are common in children and early adolescents, but they are seldom seen after the age of 15.

| Athetosis with Spasticity | Athetosis with Tonic Spasms | Choreoathetosis | Flaccid | Ataxia |
|---|---|---|---|---|
| Difficulty with head control, thus decreased oral motor, strained speech; decreased coordination of suck/swallow, resulting in decreased feeding and speech. | Feeding may be difficult because aspiration is unpredictable; severe language and speech impairment caused by decreased control. | Facial grimaces; dysarthria; irregular breathing; difficulty in sustaining phonation; poor intraoral and extraoral surfaces. | Quiet soft voice because of decreased respiration; delayed speech; increased drooling; often expressionless face. | Speech is monotone, very slow; uses teeth to stabilize tongue or hold cup to mouth when drinking; decreased articulation. |
| Same as athetosis. | Same as athetosis. | Same as athetosis. | Obesity; sensory impairment; URTI. | Nystagmus; mental retardation; sensory problems; uses vision for righting and as reference point for movement. |
| Same as athetosis. | Same as athetosis. | Same as athetosis. | Visually attentive; cannot move; therefore, is a "good" baby; decreased motivation. | Does not like to move. |

*Psychomotor seizures,* or temporal lobe seizures, may consist of tonic-clonic movements, but they also show automatic reactions such as lip smacking, chewing, and buttoning and unbuttoning clothing. In addition, the individual may appear to be confused and disorganized and may have sensory experiences such as smelling and tasting items not in the environment and hearing sounds of various types.

*Minor motor seizures* include those found in infancy. The most common type of seizure in infancy is the febrile seizure. This is often a single, brief episode that is precipitated by fever and usually is unassociated with either prior or residual neurologic signs or with an abnormal electroencephalogram (EEG).

*Infantile spasms* pose a serious threat to development. They typically begin at 6 months and disappear by 24 months. During this time development appears to stop, and skills may be lost. Early treatment with adrenocorticotropic hormone can inhibit the seizure activity; however, the effects on development are almost inevitable. More than 90% of children with known causes for their seizures have mental retardation (Batshaw & Perret, 1992).

Two other mild forms of seizures are (1) myoclonic seizures that consist of contractions by single or small groups of muscles and (2) akinetic seizures in which the primary problem is a loss of muscle tone. Children rarely have serious seizures for an extended period (30 minutes or more).

This condition is called *status epilepticus,* and requires medical management to maintain body functions and hydration. Intravenous anticonvulsant medication is also indicated at this time.

The incidence and prevalence of seizures are difficult to estimate. Generalized seizures, including grand mal, petit mal, and myoclonic seizures, have been reported in approximately 2.5 in 1000 children. Partial seizures have been reported in between 1.7 and 3.6 in 1000 children, with unclassified and mixed seizures accounting for another 2 in 1000 (Menkes, 1990). In young children the most common seizure is associated with the presence of illness or fever. Many of these may occur infrequently and cease as the child matures.

A child who has a seizure must undergo a thorough evaluation so that the factors causing the seizure can be determined. A family history, medical history, and developmental history must be completed, as well as an EEG to help determine the type of seizure.

Anticonvulsive medications are administered in an attempt to control the seizures. In theory these medications increase the intensity required to trigger the seizure or eliminate the recruitment of surrounding cells. Batshaw and Perret (1992) and Roberts (1979) have described some of the common side effects from these anticonvulsive medications: cataracts, weight gain, high blood pressure, pathologic fractures, drowsiness, hair loss or gain, nausea, liver damage, vomiting, gum enlargement, hyperactivity, anorexia, and lymphoma-like syndrome (Eadie, 1984). Commonly prescribed medications include valproic acid (Depakene, Abbott, North Chicago, IL), phenytoin (Dilantin, Parke-Davis, Morris Plains, NJ), phenobarbital, ethosuximide (Zarontin, Parke-Davis), and carbamazepine (Tegretol, Geigy, Ardsley, NY).

Balancing the dosage of anticonvulsant medications can be a difficult process and is often repeated at various times as the child grows and matures. Antiepileptic medication is often withdrawn or reduced if the child has been seizure free with a normal EEG for at least 2 years. This is done slowly and with caution, and health care workers are often asked to monitor the child closely during this period (Dodson, 1989).

Even with optimal care, only about 50% to 75% of children can be controlled completely on medication. Having a seizure can be frightening to the child and those around him or her. When a child has a seizure, staff must remain calm, move spectators away, and protect the child. The box at right outlines the emergency treatment procedures of seizures.

## Muscular Dystrophies

The muscular dystrophies are the most common muscle diseases of childhood. They include a group of conditions, most of them believed to be genetic in origin, causing changes in the biochemistry and structure of the surface and internal membranes of the muscle cells and resulting in progressive degeneration and weakness of various muscle groups, disability, deformity, and sometimes, death.

Types of muscular dystrophy include *limb-girdle, facioscapulohumeral, congenital,* and *Duchenne's* (pseudohypertrophic) *muscular dystrophy.* Figure 7-10 graphically demonstrates the differential distribution of paralysis with these dystrophies.

A somewhat debated type of muscular dystrophy is congenital muscular dystrophy (CMD). Although the literature dates back to the mid-1960s, it does not appear to provide definitive data on incidence, essential features, or long-term follow-up. The disease is transmitted by autosomal recessive inheritance. Essential features reported in various studies include hypotonia and multiple joint contractures from birth, general muscle weakness and atrophy, and normal intelligence. Associated problems include clubfoot, torticollis, diaphragmatic involvement, congenital heart defects, and spinal defects. Often little to no progression of the disease is seen after childhood, and some functional improvement may be seen around this time (Thomas & Dubowitz, 1989).

Diagnosis is made from the presence of high serum levels of the muscle enzyme creatine kinase, by electromyography analysis, and by examination of muscle tissue taken during biopsy. Clinical examination often reveals a "floppy" child with muscle weakness in the face, neck, trunk, and

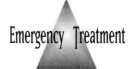

## Emergency Treatment

### Seizure

Protect child during seizure:
   Do not attempt to restrain child or use force
   If child is standing or sitting in wheelchair at beginning of attack, ease child down so that he or she will not fall; when possible, place cushion or blanket under child
   Do not put anything in child's mouth
   Loosen restrictive clothing
   Prevent child from hitting hard or sharp objects that might cause injury during uncontrolled movements
      Remove object(s)
      Pad object(s)
      Move furniture out of way
   Allow seizure to end without interference
When seizure has stopped, check for breathing; if not present, use mouth-to-mouth resuscitation
Check around mouth for evidence of burns or suspicious substances that might indicate poisoning
Remain with child
When child is able to move, seek help

From Wong, D. (1993). *Whaley and Wong's essentials of pediatric nursing* (4th ed.) (p. 973). St. Louis: Mosby.

limbs; decreased muscle mass; and absent deep tendon reflexes (Thomas & Dubowitz, 1989).

In *limb-girdle* muscular dystrophy the initial muscles affected are the proximal muscles of the pelvis and shoulder girdles. Onset may begin anywhere from the first to the third decade of life, with progression usually slow, but sometimes moderately rapid. Its hereditary pattern is autosomal recessive like the congenital form.

*Facioscapulohumeral muscular dystrophy* is autosomal dominant, and onset usually occurs in early adolescence. Although severity varies greatly among patients, involvement is primarily in the face, upper arms, and scapular region, as the name implies. Clinical manifestations include a slope to the shoulders, decreased ability to raise arms above shoulder height, and decreased mobility in the facial muscles that gives a "masked" appearance.

The most common and the most severe form of muscular dystrophy is called Duchenne's dystrophy. It is inherited in a sex-linked recessive manner, affects males, and has an incidence of 1 per 3500 live male births (Wong, 1993).

Symptoms usually begin between the second and sixth year of life. Parents describe their child as having increasing difficulty climbing stairs and rising from a sitting or lying position. The child stumbles and falls excessively and tires easily. A distinctive characteristic of this form is the

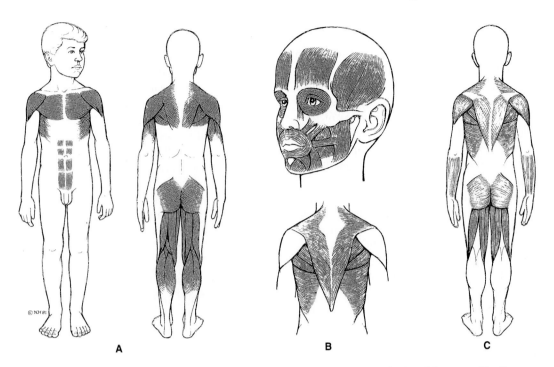

**Figure 7-10**   Initial muscle groups involved in muscular dystrophies. **A,** Pseudohypertrophic. **B,** Facioscapulohumeral. **C,** Limb-girdle. (From Wong, D.L. [1993]. *Whaley and Wong's essentials of pediatric nursing.* [4th ed.] [p. 1126]. St. Louis: Mosby.)

enlargement of calf muscles and sometimes of forearm and thigh muscles, giving the appearance of strong, healthy muscles. However, this enlargement is caused by extensive fibrosis and proliferation of adipose tissue, which, when combined with the other pathologic changes in the muscle tissue, actually causes muscle weakness. This phenomenon is referred to as pseudohypertrophy of muscles.

Involvement begins in the proximal musculature of the pelvic girdle, proceeds to the shoulder girdle, and finally affects all muscle groups. As leg and pelvic muscles weaken, the child often uses his arms to "crawl" up his thighs into a standing position from a kneeling position. This is known as Gower's sign and is diagnostically significant (Figure 7-11). Independent ambulation is one of the first functions to be lost, and wheelchair dependence is common by 9 years of age. Gradually the simplest ADLs become difficult and then impossible. In the advanced stages of the disease, lordosis and kyphosis are common, as are contractures at various joints. Death, usually as a result of infection, respiratory problems, or cardiovascular complications, often occurs before the early twenties (Carroll, 1985).

At this time there is no treatment that arrests or reverses the dystrophic process, but antibiotic therapy and other advances in dealing with pulmonary complications have helped to extend life expectancy. Steroids can help, but their use remains controversial because of their side effects. Myoblast transfer is used on a trial basis. Gene therapy holds promise as an effective treatment. The use of ortho-

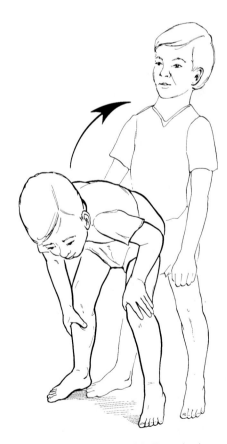

**Figure 7-11**   Child with Gower's sign.

pedic devices and adaptive equipment and activity can increase mobility, minimize contractures, delay spinal curvatures, and maximize independence in daily activities and thus in role functioning. Maintaining the child's independent mobility for as long as possible is a major goal. These children appear to degenerate more rapidly once in a wheelchair. Because these children are generally aware of their situation, the therapist working with this child should also be prepared to work with the issues of death and dying. Genetic counseling for parents and female siblings and family support programs are also of value.

All other disorders of muscles are usually called *myopathies.* Congenital myopathies are rare in infants; however, when they occur they are usually caused by autosomal dominant patterns of inheritance but may also be caused by prolonged treatment with certain drugs such as steroids. Clinically, the children present similarly to the dystrophies with proximal muscle weakness of the face, neck, and limbs. Congenital dislocation of the hip, scoliosis, seizures, and reduced cognitive skills may also be present. Diagnosis is made by muscle biopsy. Unlike the dystrophies, progression of the condition is slow and nonexistent, making the prognosis much better (Pryse-Phillips & Murray, 1982).

## Spina Bifida

*Spina bifida* is the term most commonly used to describe a congenital defect of the vertebral arches and the spinal column. This defect may be mild, with the laminae of only 1 or 2 vertebrae affected and no malformation of the spinal cord, or it may involve extensive spinal opening with an exposed pouch made up of cerebrospinal fluid (CSF) and the meninges *(meningocele)* or CSF, meninges, and nerve roots *(myelomeningocele).* These latter conditions are also called *spina bifida cystica,* as opposed to *spina bifida occulta,* where no pouch is evident (Brashear & Raney, 1986; Menkes, 1990) (Figure 7-12). This deficit appears to occur in the fourth week of prenatal development and can be identified by amniocentesis. Heredity, intrauterine, and environmental factors have been associated with these conditions (Brashear & Raney, 1986). Recently the research suggests that a combination of heredity and a folic acid deficiency may account for up to 50% of cases. Spina bifida cystica is believed to occur from 0.2 to 4.2 times per 1000 live births (Wong, 1993).

The degree of impairment depends on the level and degree of spinal cord involvement. This continuum of impairment ranges from no functional impairment, to mild muscle imbalances and sensory losses, to paraplegia, and even to death in severe cases.

Many times in spina bifida occulta there are no external manifestations visible, or the skin overlying the defect may be dimpled, pigmented, or covered with hair. Internally the spinal cord may be divided by a bony spur or congenital neoplasm, or there may be a slight bony malformation of one or more vertebrae (Charney, 1992). Occasionally, this area is slightly unstable, and some neuromuscular impairments may occur, including mild gait deficits and bowel or bladder problems.

Spina bifida cystica is more serious and complex. In the neonatal period, great care must be taken not to rupture the sac and to prevent infection. Surgical skin closure is usually done soon after birth to protect the cyst. In some cases part or all of the sac is removed.

Spina bifida with meningocele is characterized by a sac, or meningocele, that is visible above the bony defect. This sac is covered with skin and subcutaneous tissue, contains CSF, and while the meninges extend into the sac, the spinal cord remains confined to the spinal canal.

Spina bifida with myelomeningocele is the most severe form of spina bifida. In this form the sac may be covered with only a thin layer of skin, or the meninges and the spinal cord or nerve roots protrude into the meningocele.

Complications with these forms of spina bifida include meningitis and hydrocephalus. Infection is easily contracted because of environmental exposure of the meninges and spinal cord. Hydrocephalus is a common secondary complication that may be caused by either a developmental defect in the brain, such as aqueduct stenosis, or by the lower portion of the brain (and part of the cerebellum) slipping through the foramen magnum, a condition known as Arnold-Chiari syndrome (Charney, 1992; Menkes, 1990).

Children with myelomeningocele usually display sensory and motor disturbances below the level of the lesion. Most lesions are in the thoracic or lumbar spine, resulting in lower extremity paralysis. Sensory dysfunction is variable. Some children also demonstrate hip, spinal, or foot deformities. Bowel and bladder incontinence is often a problem. Medication, bowel training, and intermittent catheterization may assist significantly in this area.

Many children with myelomeningocele function well within normal educational and social environments. Those with hydrocephalus or significant motor deficits may also demonstrate sensory processing and perceptual problems. Often they exhibit fine motor delays in association with visual perceptual impairment or dyspraxia. Medical management of these children includes surgery for repair of deformities or for shunt implantation and urologic management. Orthotic interventions include lightweight bracing, casting, orthopedic shoes, and assistive devices for ambulation. Patient education in the areas of skin care, urology, and diet enhances the child's independence, as does ADL training. Special education, recreation, and vocational training may also be necessary, depending on the nature and extent of the child's abilities and disabilities.

## Hydrocephalus

*Hydrocephalus* occurs when CSF builds up in the ventricles of the brain. This occurs when there is an imbalance between the amount of CSF produced and absorbed. Noncom-

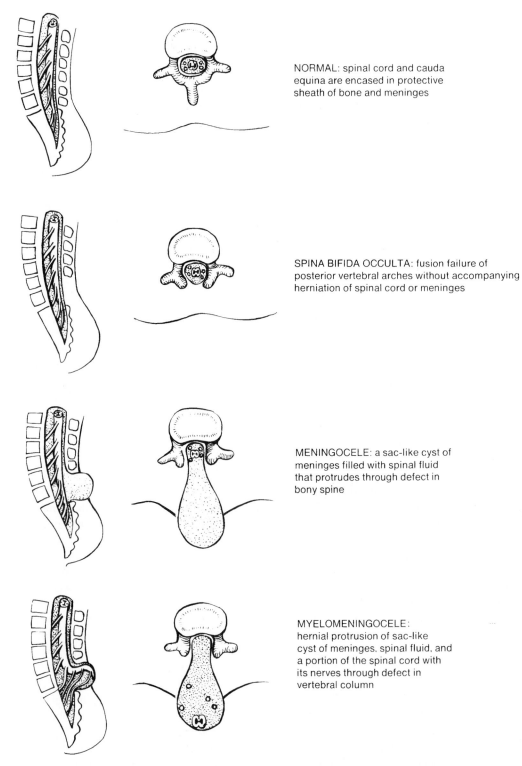

NORMAL: spinal cord and cauda equina are encased in protective sheath of bone and meninges

SPINA BIFIDA OCCULTA: fusion failure of posterior vertebral arches without accompanying herniation of spinal cord or meninges

MENINGOCELE: a sac-like cyst of meninges filled with spinal fluid that protrudes through defect in bony spine

MYELOMENINGOCELE: hernial protrusion of sac-like cyst of meninges, spinal fluid, and a portion of the spinal cord with its nerves through defect in vertebral column

**Figure 7-12**    Three forms of spina bifida. (From Whaley, L. & Wong, D. [1983]. *Nursing care of infants and children.* [2nd ed.]. St. Louis: Mosby.)

municating ventricles, obstructed outflow of CSF from the ventricles, Arnold-Chiari malformation, or, occasionally, a tumor may produce this phenomenon. This imbalance results in enlargement of the ventricles, pressure on the brain, and enlargement of the infant's head.

This dysfunction occurs in 5.8 per 10,000 live births and is often associated with spina bifida. In infants an early sign of the condition is an enlarged head size. In older children, where the head cannot grow, intracranial pressure is increased. Definitive diagnosis may be made by sonography,

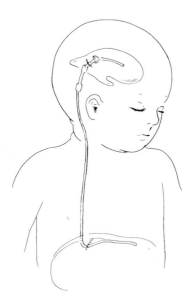

**Figure 7-13** Ventriculoperitoneal shunt. Catheter is threaded subcutaneously from small incisions at the sites of ventricular and peritoneal insertions. (From Wong, D.L. [1993]. *Whaley and Wong's essentials of pediatric nursing.* [4th ed.]. St. Louis: Mosby.)

computed tomography (CT), or magnetic resonance imaging (MRI) scans (Batshaw & Perret, 1992; Charney, 1992).

Clinical signs of hydrocephalus in infants include abnormal head growth with bulging fontanels, dilated scalp veins, and separated sutures; eyes that appear to deviate downward, producing a "sunsetting" appearance of the iris and visible sclera; and, after time, lethargy and irritability and problems with reflexes, feeding, and tone. In older children, headache, irritability, development of strabismus or nystagmus, and cognitive changes may occur (Page, 1992).

Left untreated this pressure can result in an extremely large head size, visual and perceptual deficits, mental retardation, seizures, and death. If the hydrocephalus is caused by an obstruction, its removal may alleviate the condition. The usual medical treatment for idiopathic hydrocephalus is the placement of a ventriculoperitoneal (VP) shunt. Shown in Figure 7-13, this procedure reduces the CSF pressure by means of a catheter that runs under the skin from one of the ventricles to the abdominal cavity, where the fluid can be safely absorbed. These shunts are usually effective but must be monitored regularly for signs of infection, clogging, kinking, or migration of the tube. Even with shunting, however, many of these children have cognitive, perceptual, visual, or other neurologic problems (Wong, 1993).

## Guillain-Barré Syndrome

*Guillain-Barré Syndrome* is an acute polyneuropathy. It is caused by a virus that attacks the nerve roots. The body then interprets the infected roots as foreign bodies and destroys them with an autoimmune response. The result is a progressive, flaccid muscle paralysis similar to that seen in poliomyelitis. This condition has been associated with the swine flu vaccination but can also be idiopathic in origin (Menkes, 1990). Children are affected by this condition less often than adults. Among children it is most common in middle childhood.

Illness typically begins with an upper respiratory infection and progresses through a period with muscle tenderness, symmetric muscle weakness, and, occasionally, paresthesias. Paralysis usually begins peripherally and in the lower extremities, ascending to the upper extremities, diaphragm, and occasionally facial area. At this time respiration and feeding may be compromised, and the child may require technologic support (Eisen & Humphreys, 1974). The child may experience discomfort and some sensory loss, and incontinence is not uncommon (Ropper, 1992).

Muscle function begins to return a few days to a few months after onset. During the early stages of the illness, adaptive devices and palliative care may be provided. In most cases a full recovery can be attained, particularly with physical rehabilitation. Physical and occupational therapy activities to maintain range of motion, regain strength and coordination, and reacquire independent living skills are essential components of the rehabilitation program.

## Peripheral Nerve Injuries
### Birth Injuries

Infants and children occasionally suffer traumatic injuries, perinatally and postnatally, that temporarily or permanently cause peripheral nerve impairment. For example, breech deliveries with after-coming arms can cause brachial plexus lesions. These babies might demonstrate weakness or wasting of the small muscles of the hands and sensory diminution in the area of the hand and arm served by this plexus (Pryse-Phillips & Murray, 1982).

This condition, called *Erb-Duchenne palsy,* is usually unilateral and related to the upper brachial plexus only. It is usually a result of stretching the shoulder in extreme shoulder flexion (with the hand over head). Paralysis of the arm results and is often more pronounced in the shoulder musculature than the hand. The child often holds his or her arm in a characteristic posture, with shoulder adducted and internally rotated, elbow extended, forearm pronated, and wrist flexed. Prognosis depends on the extent of the damage to the nerves but can be good with early treatment and positioning. In *Klumpke's palsy,* or lower brachial plexus paralysis, the stretching injury is generally more severe. Klumpke's palsy results in paralysis of the hand and wrist muscles. A brachial palsy injury may be so severe that the entire arm is paralyzed.

Therapy often involves fabrication of a sling (that fits proximally around the humerus) and passive and active-assistive exercises. Later in infancy, resistive exercises may be recommended for development of optimal strength in the affected arm.

### Traumatic Injury of Peripheral Nerves

In older children, injury to a peripheral nerve is usually caused by an accident, either through severing of the nerve or secondary to fractures, dislocations, excessive exercise, or, occasionally, medical treatments such as injections. Injuries of this type are common to the radial, ulnar, and median nerves and the brachial plexus, lumbar plexus, peroneal, or sciatic nerves.

Diagnosis is made using a combination of techniques such as family and medical histories, nerve conduction studies, observations of sensory and motor involvements, muscle biopsies, electromyograms (EMGs), and in more serious accidents, surgical exploration. Specific treatment depends on the extent, progression, location, and especially the cause of the nerve damage. In general, treatment techniques include rest, splinting, nerve and local anesthetic injections, and surgical intervention to relieve nerve compression.

## TRAUMATIC BRAIN INJURIES

Head injuries during childhood constitute a major medical and public health problem. Approximately 4000 children per year die of head injuries in the United States. Three to four times that number are seriously injured and must endure prolonged hospitalizations and lifelong complications of some degree. Common causes of head injuries in young children are falls and child abuse. In older children most head injuries are caused by motor vehicle accidents. Sports-related injuries increase as children reach adolescence.

Head traumas may be classified as closed or open. A closed head trauma indicates a blow to the head that has not caused an open or penetrating wound. An open head trauma denotes a penetration or laceration. Open wounds often require additional treatment such as debridement, removal of bone fragments or other foreign bodies, surgical repair of blood vessels, and closure of the wound (Jennett & Teasdale, 1981).

Damage to nervous system tissue may occur at the time of impact or penetration. However, secondary damage may occur resulting from brain swelling, intracranial pressure, hematomas, emboli, and hypoxic brain conditions (Ylvisaker, 1985). It is these secondary causes of nervous system damage that must be prevented or at least minimized through early medical intervention.

Two distinct clinical patterns in unconscious children with head injuries have been described. In the first type the child goes into unconsciousness or coma immediately after the trauma. In the second type, known as the pediatric concussion syndrome, the child may become unconscious right after the injury but then becomes lucid before showing progressive signs of involvement. These may include drowsiness, vomiting, loss of consciousness, and even more serious indicators such as Babinski's sign, decerebrate posturing, and even brain death. This pediatric concussion syndrome may resolve at any stage of its continuum or complete its full course (Michaud & Duhaime, 1992).

Once the child's condition is stabilized, level of consciousness is determined. One scale that is often used is the Glasgow Coma Scale (Jennett & Teasdale, 1981). This system ranks children according to their ability to elicit sounds or words, to demonstrate tendon reflex and motor responsiveness in general; and to voluntarily or involuntarily open their eyes. Next, a neurologic assessment of brainstem reflexes is conducted. Additional diagnostic procedures may involve MRI, CT scan, EEG, angiography, and radiography to determine the extent and location of fractures (Raphaely, Swedlow, Downes, & Bruce, 1980).

Treatment includes the close monitoring and control of cerebral circulation and of intracranial pressure through the use of sophisticated devices and control systems. When intracranial pressure cannot be controlled by use of traditional means, a large dose of barbiturate, such as phenobarbital, may be administered. If this attempt fails to control the pressure, lowering the body temperature may help. Withdrawal from the latter two forms of treatment is difficult and may cause sleep disturbances, behavioral problems, apnea, and some decreased intellectual functioning (Raphaely et al., 1980).

The prognosis for children who receive the type of treatment previously described is good. Most children with head trauma make a good recovery, have only moderate impairments, and are able to return to a regular school setting. The milder effects include auditory and visual perceptual deficits, body image problems, minimal difficulties with some gross and fine motor skills, a slowing of response, and moderate problems with some types of academic performance.

Children who have shown decerebrate posturing, flaccidity, scores of less than 5 on the Glasgow Coma Scale, or prolonged coma are considered to have a guarded prognosis (Jaffe & Hays, 1986). These children often require rehabilitation for ambulation, motor skills, self-help skills, language skills, cognitive skills, and the previously mentioned problems. In addition, some children demonstrate severe emotional disturbances that require professional help (Jaffe & Hays, 1986; Ylvisaker, 1985).

## DEVELOPMENTAL DISABILITIES

This section addresses those disorders found in childhood that are not specifically associated with one body system and that delay the developmental progress of the child. In general, developmental disabilities are characterized by prenatal, perinatal, or early childhood onset. Each developmental disability has the potential to affect multiple areas of the child's development and to impair the child's performance of multiple functional skills and tasks.

## Mental Retardation

*Mental retardation* (MR) is the most common of developmental disabilities, affecting between 0.8% and 3% of the population, depending on the definition used (Batshaw, Perret, & Shapiro, 1992). These definitions have three key factors: significantly impaired intellectual ability, usually measured on standardized psychoeducational tests; onset before the age of 18; and impairment of the adaptive abilities necessary for independent living.

Diagnosis of mental retardation is usually made by formal testing and history. Testing usually includes intelligence quotient (IQ) testing and tests of adaptive behavior (basic reasoning, environmental knowledge, and developmentally appropriate daily living and self-maintenance skills). A child is usually considered to have MR if he or she scores more than two standard deviations below the norms for age. MR is usually classified by severity—*mild, moderate, severe,* and *profound.* Although this classification has changed over the years and is somewhat artificial, it is commonly used to describe these children (Figure 7-14).

Children with mild mental retardation have an IQ range of 55 to 69. Characteristics include the ability to learn academic skills at the third to seventh grade level and the usual achievement of social and vocational skills adequate to minimal self-support (80% are employed and 80% are married) (Batshaw, Perret, & Shapiro, 1992).

Children with moderate mental retardation have an IQ range of 40 to 54. This group is unlikely to progress past the second grade level in academics; they can usually handle routine daily functions and do unskilled or semiskilled work in sheltered workshop conditions. Some type of group home or supervised housing situation is usually the best placement for these individuals.

Children with severe retardation have an IQ range of 25 to 39. These individuals can usually learn to communicate, they can be trained in basic health habits, and they require supervision to accomplish most tasks.

Children with profound retardation have IQs below 25. These children need caregiver assistance for basic survival skills. Usually they have minimal capacity for sensorimotor or self-care functioning. Individuals with profound retardation also often have interrelated neuromuscular, orthopedic, or behavioral deficits.

Mental retardation is actually a functional deficit that describes a number of disabilities. It can occur secondarily to another condition or without apparent cause. It has been estimated that there are more than 300 causes of mental retardation (Moser, 1985). These causes are usually categorized into the following headings: problems acquired in childhood (toxins, trauma, infection); problems of fetal development and birth; chromosomal problems; central nervous system malformations; congenital anomalies; and neurocutaneous, metabolic, and endocrine disorders.

Approximately 80% of children with MR have additional problems. For example, it is estimated that approximately 50% have speech problems, 50% have ambulation problems, 20% have seizures, 25% have visual problems, and 40% have chronic conditions such as heart disease, diabetes, anemia, obesity, and dental problems (Shapiro & Batshaw, 1993).

The physician's role begins with a history that focuses on gestation, neonatal events, illnesses, and developmental progress. During the physical examination, all major and minor abnormalities must be identified to detect the possibility of a syndrome. In addition, laboratory tests such as chromosomal analysis, metabolic tests, and EEGs may be ordered. Referrals for psychologic, education, developmental, and speech and hearing evaluation may be made and then interpreted for the parents. Services must be determined, and parents, siblings, and other family members must be given support and advice.

Today the emphasis in the field of MR is toward deinsti-

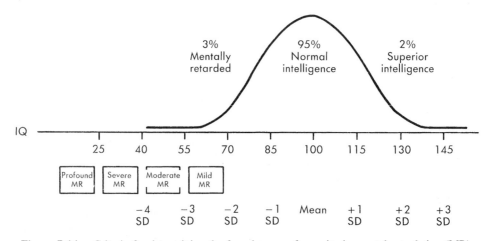

**Figure 7-14** Criteria for determining the four degrees of severity in mental retardation (MR).

tutionalization, normalization, and providing individuals with every opportunity to be able to reach their maximal level of functioning in the least restrictive environment. Although MR cannot usually be cured, early identification and intervention are essential to increasing the child's ability to grow and develop to his or her maximal potential.

Early signs of developmental delays are often seen by parents, physicians, and allied health professionals involved in well baby care and screening. Early signs of cognitive impairment include delays in meeting motor and speech milestones, nonresponsiveness to handling and physical contact, reduced alertness or spontaneous play, feeding difficulties, and "soft neurologic signs." Actual diagnosis of MR is generally made when the child reaches school age.

Early programming for children with retardation or delays is usually focused on facilitating the attainment of developmental milestones and normal experiences, enriching the environment, developing self-help and motor skills, and educating and supporting the parents. As the child grows, specific deficits may be addressed in special education programs. For the adolescent with MR, the development of vocational interests and skills, social skills and sex education, and community mobility skills are essential.

## Pervasive Developmental Disabilities

*Autism* is a pervasive developmental disability (PDD) characterized by severe, complex, and permanent behavioral and cognitive disabilities. Clinically defined by the child's behavior and performance, this condition affects all areas of performance (Rapin, 1991). Particularly associated with autism are the inability to relate to others and the display of ritualistic, repetitive behaviors. It may exist in isolation or in combination with other disorders and probably has many causes.

Autism is one of the most devastating of the chronic developmental disabilities because of the unusual combinations of sensorimotor and behavioral characteristics displayed by these children. In the almost 40 years since Leo Kanner first identified 11 children as having "extreme autistic aloneness," many theories have been suggested for autism. At first it was hypothesized that the parents' inability to provide appropriate nurture because of their extreme personality types and traits or because of their psychopathies caused the child to withdraw socially and to become autistic. Next came the theorists who proposed that various hereditary and biologic factors were present but that the parents were still at least partially responsible for causing the syndrome. These theorists were followed by ones who focused on the psychologic problem of the child. During this period autistic children were described under the term *childhood schizophrenia.* Today there is general agreement among most researchers that autism is caused by organic brain pathology. However, at this time neither the location of the exact affected site or sites in the central nervous system is certain, nor the factors that cause this organic pathologic condition.

Onset can occur at either of two times, at birth and any time up to the age of 30 months. It can occur in children with normal or impaired intellectual function.

The National Society for Autistic Children estimates that approximately four to five children with autism are born per 10,000 live births and that four times as many boys as girls are afflicted with the disorder (NSAC, 1980). Children with autism are found in families in all racial, ethnic, intellectual, and socioeconomic backgrounds. There are some familial patterns of autism, however. Parents of one child with autism are at a small increased risk of having a second child with this condition (Batshaw, Perret, & Reber, 1992).

The behavioral characteristics of autism are critical to its diagnosis. They can be categorized into the following five subclusters of disturbances (Ornitz, 1973):

1. Disturbances in relating to persons and things
2. Disturbances in communication
3. Disturbances in motility
4. Disturbances of developmental rate
5. Disturbances of sensory processing and perception

*Disturbances in relating to persons and things* affect the child's ability to establish meaningful relationships with people and inanimate objects. Although abnormalities in this area vary with age and degree of severity, they directly involve interactions that require initiative or reciprocal behavior from the child. Specific behaviors that are observed are poor or deviant eye contact, delayed or total lack of a social smile, apparent aversion to physical contact, delayed or absent anticipatory response to being picked up, and an apparent preference for being alone. Disturbances in relating to inanimate objects are often observed during the play of these children. Many times a toy or an object is not used in the manner that it was intended but instead is twirled, spun, flicked, tapped, or in other ways manipulated, arranged or rearranged. In addition, the child's use of play materials is often rigid and inflexible; these children seldom demonstrate cooperative and imaginative play (Wing, 1988).

*Disturbances in communication* may be thought of as being on a continuum from severe to mild. At the severe end of the continuum appears a complete lack of speech, or mutism. At the other end of the continuum normal language accompanied by only slight articulation or tonal deficits may be seen. Many other communication problems have been described at points along the continuum. For instance, much of the speech of children with autism is repetitive, or echolalic, in nature. Classic echolalia consists of parrotlike repetitions of phrases immediately after the child has been exposed to them, and delayed or deferred echolalia consists of the repetition of phrases at a later time. Echolalic speech occurs out of social context and appears to have little or no communicative value. Other types of speech and language problems include syntax problems, atonal and arrhythmic speech, pronoun reversals, and a lack of inflection and emotion during communication (Rutter, 1985).

Regardless of the time of onset, most children with autism display *disturbances of their developmental rate.* Specifically, they show deviations and discontinuities in the normal sequence of motor, language, and social milestones (Minshew & Payton, 1988). For example, the child may demonstrate the ability to perform one task precociously, such as sitting up, but another motor task, such as pulling to the standing position, may be delayed well past the normal time. Or the child may walk on time but not learn to speak until many years later.

*Disturbances of motility* are considered to be indicative of central nervous system dysfunction in autistic children (Damasio & Maurer, 1978; Howlin & Rutter, 1987). Deviant motility may involve the arms, hands, trunk, lower extremities, or entire body. Motor patterns in the upper extremities are common and include wiggling and flicking of fingers, alternating flexion and extension of the fingers, and alternating pronation and supination of the forearm. Other motility patterns often seen include head rolling and banging, body rocking and swaying, lunging and darting movements, toe walking, dystonia of the extremities, involuntary synergies of the head and proximal segments of the limbs, and an inability to perform two motor acts at the same time (Damasio & Maurer, 1978; Howlin & Rutter, 1987).

*Disturbances of sensory processing and perception* have been reported in autistic children for almost 30 years. These include abnormal responses to various visual, vestibular, and auditory stimuli. A. Jean Ayres describes two types of sensory processing problems in children with autistic behaviors. The first deals with the registration of, or orientation to, sensory input. It appears that in these children the neurophysiologic processes that decide that sensory stimuli will be brought to their attention are working correctly at some times but not at others (Ayres & Tickle, 1980). Therefore they react normally to sensory stimuli one minute, and the next minute (hour or day) they may overreact or underreact to the same stimuli.

The second sensory processing disturbance described by Ayres involves the control or modulation of a stimulus once it has entered the system. Again, the child with autistic behavior is believed to be capable of exerting control at some times but not at others, resulting in a child who processes tactile information normally at times and who, at other times, appears to be the victim of uncontrolled overstimulation—the tactilely defensive child.

Although most children with autism have normal life expectancies, the functional prognosis is often severely limited. Only about 50% of children with autism develop socially useful speech. Overall about 15% have a good outcome, 15% a fair outcome, and 70% a poor outcome in terms of functioning independently in society. Most persons with autism live at home or in supervised living situations (Rumsey, Rapoport, & Sceery, 1985). These prognostic figures may be accurate indicators of the overall potential of these children, or they may simply reflect that society has not yet developed the support systems and interventions needed to increase independence in these individuals.

Autism is complicated by the fact that it often coexists with other problems such as MR, seizure disorders, and a number of diseases associated with organic brain damage. The fact that a large percentage of children with autism also suffer from cognitive deficiencies has been a controversial but relatively accepted issue. The cognitive deficiencies exhibited by children with autism are as disabling as in those in children with MR, with the same long-term consequences.

Also considered a pervasive developmental disorder, *Rett's syndrome* appears similar to autism. This condition appears to be caused by an inborn error in metabolism (Kyllerman, 1986). Damage to the X chromosome is believed to be the mode of transmission and occurs exclusively in girls. The defining characteristics are cerebral atrophy, progressive dementia, and loss of motor skills.

Development appears normal in these children until about 6 months of age; thereafter the child demonstrates regression in cognition, praxis, and behavior. Microcephaly, spasticity, and seizures develop, and the child develops autistic-like behaviors such as hand mouthing, flapping, or wringing. Functional hand use disappears, and waking hyperventilation is characteristic. These girls can survive for some time, but are usually nonambulatory and nonverbal by late childhood. This is an incurable condition, but carbamazepine may be helpful in reducing symptoms and improving alertness (Menkes, 1990).

Pervasive developmental disability is also often seen in conjunction with conditions that are associated with brain damage, including fragile X syndrome, phenylketonuria, Addison's disease, celiac disease, and infantile spasms. Seizure disorders occur in high incidence in children with autism. Both tonic-clonic and partial-complex seizures have been reported in this population.

Because no one method of treatment has yet proved to be totally effective in treating autism, an interdisciplinary approach is usually selected. The role of the physician on the interdisciplinary team is to make appropriate referrals, offer support to the parents, monitor the child's progress, and, often, prescribe medications. The medications used with these children are varied: sedatives, stimulants, major and minor tranquilizers, antihistamines, antidepressants, and psychotomimetics. It is believed that these medications work best when used in conjunction with an interdisciplinary special education program.

The use of sensory integrative techniques is showing promise with children with autistic behaviors. New research is also being done with a technology-based technique called facilitated communication, although the research on this approach is in its infancy and has had equivocal results (Graley, 1994; Hutton, 1994). Other intervention programs provide intensive training in activities of daily living and vocational readiness. Vocational and housing options for adolescents and adults may be essential to their successful integration in the community. Support and education of parents are also critical.

## Learning Disabilities

The term *learning disabilities (LD)* describes a group of problems that affect the ability of a child to master school tasks, process information, and communicate effectively. These disabilities are often not associated with a specific neurologic insult and may or may not be accompanied by MR (Gallico & Lewis, 1992). Learning disabilities are associated with a variety of other neurologic problems, for example, attention deficit disorder (ADD) and attention deficit/hyperactivity disorder (ADHD). Specific learning disabilities include auditory processing, language disabilities, and perceptual impairments. The definition for learning disabilities has changed over the years, primarily in response to the changing political and philosophic positions of parental and political groups and service agencies. Over the years the focus of attention has shifted from the medical and psychiatric arenas to education and psychology. The National Joint Committee on Learning Disabilities defines learning disability:

a generic term that refers to a heterogeneous group of disorders manifested by significant difficulties in the acquisition and use of listening, speaking, reading, writing, reasoning, or mathematical abilities (Hammill, 1990, pp. 77-78).

The following definition taken from Public Law 101-476, the Individual with Disabilities Education Act, has perhaps been the most influential:

A disorder in one of the more basic psychological processes involved in understanding or in using language, spoken or written, which may manifest itself in an imperfect ability to listen, think, speak, read, write or do mathematical calculations.

Most children with LD have average or above average intelligence, have adequate sensory acuity (are not blind or deaf), and have been provided with appropriate learning opportunities. In spite of all these positive features, there is a significant discrepancy between the child's academic potential and the child's educational performance.

Although different studies and agencies report varying incidence figures, the figure most often given is approximately 10% of the school population. As with autism, more boys than girls are affected; in this instance a 4:1 ratio exists (Gallico & Lewis, 1992; Shaywitz & Shaywitz, 1987).

A child with LD may display any number of the behaviors listed under the following eight categories. Disorders of motor function include both motor skills and motor activity level. Motor skills dysfunctions may range from clumsiness to poor performance in gross or fine motor skills, to problems planning new tasks (dyspraxia), to equilibrium deficits, to sensorimotor problems in a number of areas. Occasionally tics, grimaces, and choreoathetoid movements in the hands may be seen. The child may be described as always being in motion (hyperactive) or being slow and lethargic (hypoactive).

Educational disorders can occur in one or more academic subjects. Related educational skills that are often limited or delayed are copying from the blackboard, printing and cursive writing, the organization of time and materials, understanding written and oral directions, symbolic confusion (reversal of letters), cutting, coloring, drawing, and keeping place on the page.

Disorders of attention and concentration include short attention span and other attention deficits, restlessness, impulsivity, and motor and verbal perseveration.

Characteristics included under disorders of thinking and memory are poor ability for abstract reasoning, difficulty with concept formation, and poor short- and long-term memory.

Difficulties with speech and communication may include difficulty shifting topics of conversation and difficulty with "small talk," the sequencing of words, sentences, or sounds, slurred words, and articulation.

Auditory difficulties associated with LD often stem from auditory perceptual and auditory memory problems and not acuity (hearing) problems. Children with these types of problems are often the ones who cannot remember the oral directions just given to them (auditory memory), cannot sound words out or blend sounds into words (phonemic synthesis), cannot block out background noise (speech-in-noise), and cannot remember the sequencing of sounds, words, or numbers (auditory sequencing). These types of problems often affect school performance and should be explored by an audiologist who is familiar with the specific instruments and programs that are available to assess and to treat these auditory perceptual (central auditory processing) problems. The high incidence of allergies and ear infections in learning disabled children puts them at risk for auditory perceptual problems.

Children with LD often have various sensory integrative and perceptual disorders. Many of these children have difficulty with laterality and directionality concepts and tasks that require visual perception skills (Hammill, 1990).

Last but not least, children with LD may have psychosocial problems; for example, they may demonstrate temper tantrums or antisocial behavior. Their social competencies may be delayed when compared with chronologic age and mental age. Many of these children are sensitive and decidedly at risk for poor self-esteem and for self-concept problems because they have the intelligence to know when they are being teased and to know the frustration of being good at some things and not at others.

It appears that a number of factors can cause LD. In some cases heredity appears to be a possibility, allergies are another factor, sensory integrative dysfunction has been found in others, and all the prenatal, perinatal, and early childhood factors that have been mentioned earlier are potential contributors.

The role of the physician in the management of learning disabilities includes making referrals when special evaluations and services are needed, documenting the child's progress, monitoring parental support and guidance, and, when needed, prescribing medications to control agitation and hyperactivity.

Most children with LD retain some degree of disability as adults; however, most are contributing members of society. As with all disorders, prognosis is affected by the severity of the disability. Therefore individuals with limited impairment should not be limited in their life and career skills. But those with severe LD may need vocational planning; counseling; and adaptations to ensure as high a level of social, emotional, and vocational functioning as possible.

The therapist's role in an intervention program for the child with LD may change as the child develops, and it depends on the nature and extent of each child's specific disability. With young children, sensory integration, play, and basic socialization and self-help skills may be addressed through early intervention and parent education. As the child progresses into school, sensory integration may continue but additional intervention to promote social play, perceptual motor integration, and writing skills is indicated. By early adolescence the focus of evaluation and treatment may shift to independent living skills, development of compensatory and adaptive techniques, and development of vocational skills, interests, and habits.

## Tourette's Syndrome

*Tourette's syndrome* (TS) is a pervasive disorder affecting neurologic and behavioral function. This condition is believed to be an autosomal dominant trait linked to a gene on chromosome 18. Dopamine dysfunction may be present. Prevalence of the condition varies geographically, but the condition is rare in African Americans and occurs more frequently in boys than in girls. Symptoms of the condition appear in middle childhood, worsen for about 10 years, and then lessen somewhat. However, they usually continue through the child's lifetime, although there are periods of remission (Menkes, 1990).

Most characteristic of TS are involuntary vocal and motor tics. Tics are sudden, nonrhythmic, rapid, and recurrent. At some time or another the child with TS has both vocal and motor tics. The child may also display obsessive behavior and significant dysfunction in social, academic, or occupational skills. Usually tics begin with simple motor movements of the head, including eye movements, grimacing, and shoulder shrugging. Vocal tics may begin with

throat clearing, grunting, barking, sneezing, and coughing. As the disease progresses, complex behavioral tics and compulsive echolalia and cursing may occur. In severe cases self-mutilation may occur at times. Specific tics tend to appear, recur frequently for a period, and then fade to be replaced by others (Menkes, 1990).

Tics may be suppressed voluntarily at some times, leading to problems in diagnosis and behavioral management; complex tics may be misinterpreted as emotional or behavioral disorders. Children who suppress tics may experience an "explosion" of tics in the latter part of the day. These may be accompanied by behavioral disturbances as well. Stress, anxiety, and even anticipation of pleasant events can increase the frequency and intensity of tics and behaviors. A large proportion of these children may also demonstrate ADD, obsessive-compulsive disorders, or LD. These factors combine to impair social, school, and work functions, which must be addressed.

Treatment includes clonidine and neuroleptic medication, such as haloperidol. These drugs have significant side effects, however, which also may cause functional deficits. Children who have obsessive-compulsive symptoms may also receive antidepressants. School- and play-based interventions may be necessary to address problems in writing, attention, and perceptual skills. Children may benefit from social skills and stress reduction programming, as well as understanding and empathetic interactions with staff. Additional time for testing may also assist in school performance.

## Genetic and Chromosomal Abnormalities

Human beings normally have 23 pairs of chromosomes in each cell of the body. Smaller or larger numbers of chromosomes can cause significant developmental disabilities. These syndromes may present characteristic symptom patterns and can often be identified by chromosomal analysis of the child's body tissues. For purposes of prevention, analysis of the amniotic fluid may identify these children before they are born (Batshaw & Perret, 1992).

Genetic diseases are inherited abnormalities caused by abnormal genes that have had a negative effect on development. There are four different patterns of gene inheritance. The first, autosomal dominant inheritance, indicates that an abnormal gene is present on one of the non–sex chromosomes. Usually this gene has been directly passed from one of the parents to the child. On rare occasions the gene is not present in either the mother or father, and it is then known as a new or "fresh" mutation. There is no carrier state; if the gene is present the baby will have the abnormal characteristics. An example of an autosomal dominant illness is von Recklinghausen's disease (neurofibromatosis).

The second pattern, autosomal recessive inheritance, indicates that an abnormal gene must be in a paired condition because it is less potent. This condition exists, as with the first pattern, on non–sex chromosomes. Commonly, both parents are carriers but have no symptoms of the illness. Examples of common autosomal recessive illnesses are cystic fibrosis, phenylketonuria, and diabetes. Many of the inherited diseases and illnesses have this pattern of inheritance, and in many instances the carrier states can be detected using various diagnostic procedures.

A third inheritance pattern is x-linked inheritance. In this case the abnormal gene sits on the female sex chromosome, the x chromosome. Because this gene is recessive, in females, the normal gene on the second sex chromosome prevents expression of the disease. However, males who inherit the abnormal gene on their mother's X chromosome will be affected. Duchenne-type muscular dystrophy and hemophilia (factor VIII deficiency) are examples of diseases inherited through this pattern.

The last type of pattern is the polygenic or multifactorial inheritance. The trait is a result of the interaction of heredity and the environment. Some congenital heart problems, cleft lip and palate, and meningomyelocele are examples of polygenic inheritance problems.

Excess chromosomal material is evidenced in the trisomy syndromes. The most common trisomy syndrome is *trisomy 21,* or *Down syndrome,* which is characterized by one additional chromosome 21. This syndrome, found in approximately 1 in 660 neonates, causes specific mental and physical problems. Although a wide range of physical characteristics may be associated with Down syndrome, a few are common to the majority of the children. Most of the children have a short and stocky stature with a protruding abdomen. The heads are often small and flattened at the back, with upward slanting eyes that have abnormal epicanthal folds. Other common facial features include low-set ears, a flat nose, and often the mouth is held slightly open with the tip of the tongue protruding. Extremities are shorter than normal, and fingers and toes are usually broad and short. The palms of the hands usually have a single crease known as the "simian" crease (Batshaw, Perret, & Shapiro, 1992).

Related health problems often include: cardiovascular abnormalities, obesity, increased respiratory and other infections caused by immune system inefficiency, thyroid deficiencies, gastrointestinal problems, and an apparent increase in the risk of leukemia (Batshaw, Perret, & Shapiro, 1992; Ensher & Clark, 1986). Often visual acuity is poor and requires correction. One problem that is potentially dangerous to the child is the atlantoaxial dislocation. This condition results in a tendency for dislocation to occur between the first and second cervical vertebrae. If this dislocation is severe enough it could result in spinal cord damage. If this dislocation is found through radiographs, surgery may be performed and precautions may be given to the family about roughhouse play or participation in activities that put stress on this joint.

Life expectancy for children with Down syndrome has improved greatly over the last several years. Those without cardiac anomalies can be expected to live into late adulthood. It is not uncommon, however, for these older individuals to develop an Alzheimer's-like syndrome (Pueschel & Pueschel, 1992).

Children with Down syndrome are usually recognized at birth by their facial characteristics. They frequently also present with low body tone, hypermobile joints, and problems in sucking. Medical examination is done to assure that none of the related congenital cardiac and medical problems are present. These problems may extend the hospitalization of the child. As the child grows, developmental delays in all areas of function are noted, although the degree can vary greatly among individual cases. Motor planning skills and gait, speech, and learning can be expected to develop slowly. Parent support and education, early intervention, and special education assist this child to achieve his or her optimal function.

There are many other trisomies possible, but most are uncommon and many children who suffer from these problems are stillborn or aborted as fetuses. *Trisomy 18, Edwards' syndrome,* occurs in about 1 in 3000 births (Menkes, 1990). These children have long, narrow skulls; low-set, malformed ears; prominent occiput; a weak cry and small mouths; syndactyly and webbed neck; congenital heart and kidney malformations; severe mental retardation; failure to thrive, and early death (Menkes, 1990). Survival rate beyond infancy is only about 10% (Ensher & Clark, 1986).

*Trisomy 13, Patau's syndrome,* occurs in 1 in 5000 births (Menkes, 1990). Children with this trisomy have multiple anomalies including eye, ear, and nasal anomalies; cleft lip and palate; polydactyly and syndactyly; and microcephaly and neural tube defects (Menkes, 1990). Of the 20% of these children who survive, most are severely retarded and suffer from seizures (Ensher & Clark, 1986; Menkes, 1990).

A decrease in the number of chromosomes (45 or less) also causes problems. Many of the fetuses who have this type of genetic abnormality die early in gestation. One exception to this statement is children born with *Turner's syndrome.* This syndrome is found in approximately 1 in 5000 females (only) and is caused by one missing sex chromosome. These babies may be born with webbing of the neck or congenital edema of the extremities and may have cardiac problems. Small stature, obesity, and underdeveloped ovaries that cause infertility and absence of secondary sexual characteristics are symptoms that must be dealt with in the school-aged child and adolescent with Turner's syndrome. Although visual perception problems are common, most of these children do not have mental retardation, which certainly improves their functional prognoses.

There are many other chromosomal abnormalities caused by a missing portion of an individual chromosome (deletion) or by a portion of a chromosome breaking off and reattaching to another chromosome (translocation). The incidence of these events is more rare than the chromosomal problems described, and because the amount of chromosomal material that is missing or duplicated is variable, the resulting conditions are expressed differently. Problems common in these types of conditions are MR, abnormal brain development, and facial abnormalities.

*Cri du chat* syndrome is rare (1 in 20,000 live births) and is caused by deletion of part of chromosome 5. This condition is so named because this baby has a weak, mewing cry. These children have a small head and widely spaced, downslanting eyes; cardiac abnormalities; failure to thrive; and profound MR. These babies also have hypotonia and feeding and respiratory problems (Batshaw & Perret, 1992).

*Klinefelter's syndrome* is caused by an XXY sex chromosome pattern. This condition occurs in approximately 1 in 500 live male births and results in a mild disorders that may not be recognized until adulthood. LD and emotional and behavioral problems are characteristic of Klinefelter's syndrome. These boys appear tall and slim, with small genitalia, and are infertile. The XYY pattern also is that of tall stature and occurs in 4 in 1000 males. These individuals may be expected to have mildly depressed IQ scores, tremors, reduced coordination, radioulnar synostosis, and increased incidence of temper tantrums, impulsiveness, and inability to plan or to handle frustration and aggression.

*Fragile X syndrome* is somewhat controversial in that it has been associated and disassociated with several other developmental disabilities. This condition is most evident in males, who have only one X chromosome. It occurs in 1 in 2000 live male births (Batshaw, Perret, & Shapiro, 1992) but does occur in girls as well. In addition to MR, fragile X children have hyperactivity, seizures, sensorimotor deficits, prominent jaws and large ears, high foreheads, and epicanthal folds. Hypotonia is common.

*Prader-Willi syndrome* is associated with a defect in chromosome 15. This condition causes severe obesity, short stature, decreased muscle tone, a long face and slanted eyes, poor thermal regulation, and underdeveloped sexual organs. Moderate MR and extreme food-seeking behaviors are classic signs. This condition occurs in 1 in 15,000 live births (Menkes, 1990).

*Neurofibromatosis,* or von Recklinghausen's disease, has two forms with different genetic patterns. The condition can be called peripheral or type 1 neurofibromatosis, which is the more common form; or central neurofibromatosis, type 2. Incidence is estimated at between 1 in 3000 and 1 in 5000 live births, occuring more commonly in boys, and the condition is associated with a dominant trait (Menkes, 1990). This condition causes multiple tumors, usually neurofibromas, on the central and peripheral nerves, cafe-au-lait spots on the skin, and vascular and visceral lesions. If these tumors occur in critical areas, they may cause death. Mild MR and LD are associated with the condition, as are speech dis-

orders. Hypertension, optic gliomas (type 1), auditory tumors (type 2), skeletal anomalies, and short stature are also associated with the disease.

Treatment for the condition may include surgical removal of dangerous or disfiguring lesions, reduction of symptoms, special education, and monitoring for cerebral tumors.

## Inborn Errors of Metabolism

Several genetic problems produce errors in metabolism of environmental and internal substances. Untreated, they may cause serious disability and, sometimes, death. For some, early diagnosis allows treatment or prevention of these consequences, but for others, no known treatment has yet been found. For these individuals, prenatal diagnosis and genetic counseling may be the only options.

*Tay-Sachs disease* is a degenerative nervous system disorder caused by the absence of an enzyme, called *hexosaminidase A,* that is usually found in the blood and major organs. This enzyme converts $GM_2$ ganglioside, a product of nerve cell metabolism, into a nontoxic substance. Because this conversion is not happening in patients with Tay-Sachs disease, the toxic substance builds up in the brain and other body organs and leads to brain damage.

This disorder is common in Jewish persons whose ancestry can be traced to the Mediterranean region. Today nearly 1 of every 27 American Jews carry the Tay-Sachs gene (Menkes, 1990). Because Tay-Sachs is an autosomal recessive trait, both parents must be carriers of the abnormal gene for the disease to be passed to the child.

Carriers of Tay-Sachs disease can be detected by a simple blood test. In addition, through amniocentesis, the disease can be detected in the fetus by examining the amniotic fluid for the presence of hexosaminidase A. These tests, in addition to the relatively small and well-defined population in which the disease is primarily found, make Tay-Sachs disease hypothetically a preventable condition.

Prevention is particularly important because Tay-Sachs disease is a devastating and fatal condition. Children with Tay-Sachs disease usually appear healthy at birth and develop normally for about 6 to 10 months. The child then becomes listless and regresses cognitively and motorically. A cherry red spot appears in both macular areas. Vision, hearing, loss of voluntary motor control, and seizures appear, leading to death by the age of 3 in most cases. There is no effective treatment for Tay-Sachs disease; medical and therapeutic efforts are essentially palliative and supportive.

Research efforts are focusing on a number of treatment approaches that may someday offer help for these children. For example, the search continues for a substance that could substitute for the hexosaminidase A or for a procedure to graft healthy cells into Tay-Sachs disease patients so that the transplanted cells could produce hexosaminidase A. Research is also progressing on gene transplantation from normal into defective cells. Until an effective treatment is found, the best strategy is prevention through genetic counseling (Menkes, 1990).

*Phenylketonuria* (PKU), is an inborn error in the metabolism of phenylalanine, an amino acid commonly found in some proteins. This condition affects 1 in 15,000 children but is rarer in individuals of Jewish origin and African Americans. Untreated, children usually develop blond hair, blue eyes, and severe cognitive and behavioral disabilities, sometimes mimicking autism. Diagnosis can be made at birth with the Guthrie test. Treatment, which is effective, is dietary: withholding foods having the precursors of phenylalanine. The new food-labeling regulations are helpful.

A similar condition, *galactosemia,* involves the inability of the child to convert galactose, a milk sugar, into glucose. Galactose then builds up in the blood and causes hepatic and splenic dysfunction (Menkes, 1990). Consequences of this condition when untreated include jaundice, vomiting and diarrhea, drowsiness and lethargy, cataracts, systemic infections, and death. Urine testing can detect this condition and is required for newborns in many states. Treatment involves a diet without galactose, including milk, milk products, and breast milk, and is usually effective in compliant children. In poorly controlled cases, some intellectual dulling, perceptual problems, tremors, choreoathetosis, and ataxia may be present (Menkes, 1990).

*Lesch-Nyhan syndrome* is a progressive neuromuscular disease that is limited to boys and involves the inability to metabolize purines. Children suffering from this condition appear normal for the first year but then experience significant MR, neuromotor degeneration and spasticity, and the compulsive need to bite their lips and fingers and rub their faces. This behavior is involuntary and becomes self-mutilating if unchecked. Vocal tics may also occur. Arthritis, anemia, and renal calculi are also frequent. Treatment usually includes protecting the child from self-mutilation, developmentally focused therapies, and medication to prevent secondary problems and to reduce mutilation. Naltrexone, an opioid antagonist, has provided some relief in this area (Menkes, 1990).

### Fetal and Neonatal Threats to Development

Each mother hopes for an uneventful pregnancy and delivery of a normal baby. In addition to the conditions mentioned already, several prenatal and perinatal factors may threaten the child's health and development. The *general health and nutrition* of the mother and sometimes of the father can either enhance or limit conception or the status of the infant. For example, exposure of the father to extremes of temperature or certain chemicals, maternal underweight (under 120 pounds) or overweight (over 180), age of the parents, drug and substance abuse, and abnormalities of maternal or paternal genital tracts are but a few of the factors that might affect conception. In addition to these

physical factors, a multitude of psychosocial and socioeconomic factors can affect conception.

Once conception has taken place, the intact mental and physical well-being of the fetus is critically linked to the well-being of the mother. Chronic health problems or chronic diseases can also cause spontaneous abortions, fetal malformations, premature births, or fetal growth problems or can present other problems to the mother or the fetus. Diabetes, high blood pressure, severe anemia, transplacental or ascending infections, heart disease, cancer, toxemia, and various surgical procedures are examples of conditions that can present these kinds of problems.

Chronic stress is also believed to have the potential to cause birth defects because it reduces the blood flow to the uterus, thus limiting the amount of nutrients and oxygen to the fetus. In addition, stress causes the release of hormones, such as cortisone, that in turn can have a teratogenic effect on the fetus.

Maternal nutrition is important before conception as well as throughout the pregnancy. Maternal malnutrition during periods of fetal growth may be detrimental to the health of the baby. For example, a reduction in protein and caloric intake between 26 and 32 weeks of gestation can permanently reduce the number of brain cells. Continued poor maternal diet is believed to result in low birth weight, neuromuscular disorders, and, later in life, LD.

The period just before, during, and immediately after birth is known as the *perinatal period.* Many factors can affect the birth process and also that critical period immediately after birth when the neonate must make so many biophysical adjustments to extrauterine life. Labor and delivery are critical times in the pregnancy. Some of the factors that negatively affect these processes are maternal in origin, and others are caused by infant complications. Neonatal medical conditions associated with maternal complications and lifestyle are described in Chapter 22. Chapter 22 also discusses medical factors during and immediately after birth that place the infant at risk for long-term disability.

## TOXIC AGENTS
### Prenatal Toxins

A variety of birth defects may be caused by adverse changes within the fetal environment. Substances and factors that negatively affect the developing fetus are called *teratogens.* Drugs, radiation, and chemicals are the most common teratogens known to affect fetal development. Table 7-3 lists some common teratogens and their possible effects on the developing fetus. It is important to remember that a number of factors determine whether a teratogen will affect the fetus. The dosage, the gestational stage of the infant, and the specific sensitivity of the developing organs at the time of exposure to the teratogen are all factors that contribute to the outcome (Kennard, 1990; Schuster & Ashburn, 1986).

▲ Table 7-3    Effects of Common Teratogens on the Developing Fetus

| Substance or Factor | Effect on Fetus |
| --- | --- |
| **DRUGS** | |
| Alcohol | Intrauterine growth retardation, mental deficiency, stillbirth. Babies born to chronic alcoholics may have fetal alcohol syndrome or withdrawal symptoms, hyperactivity, learning disabilities. |
| Aspirin | In large amounts may be fatal or cause hemorrhagic manifestations. |
| Cortisone | Possible relation to cleft palate. |
| Caffeine | Increased incidence of miscarriage; limb and skeletal malformations. |
| Dilantin | Fetal hydantoin syndrome (growth and mental deficiency, abnormalities of the face, anomalies of the hands). |
| Heroin, codeine, morphine | Hyperirritability, shrill cry, vomiting and withdrawal symptoms, decreased alertness and responsiveness to visual and auditory stimuli; can be fatal. |
| Lysergic acid diethylmide (LSD) | Spontaneous abortions, chromosomal changes, suspected anomalies. |
| Lead | Spontaneous abortion, intrauterine growth retardation, congenital anomalies, anemia; can be fatal. |
| Tetracycline | Stains teeth, inhibits bone growth. |
| Thalidomide | Phocomelia, hearing loss, cardiac anomalies; can be fatal. |
| Tobacco | Intrauterine growth retardation. |
| Tranquilizers | All may cause withdrawal symptoms during the neonatal period. |
| **HORMONES** | |
| Diethylstilbestrol (DES) | Cancer of reproductive system in females (20 years later), reproductive anomalies in males. |
| **CHEMICALS** | |
| Methylmercury | Congenital abnormalities, growth retardation; can cause abortions. |
| Pesticides (some types) | Congenital anomalies. |
| **SOCIAL FACTORS** | |
| Maternal stress | Increased fetal anomalies, premature labor. |
| Poor nutrition | Prematurity; toxemia, anemia, intrauterine growth retardation; lower levels of intellectual performance. |
| **RADIATION THERAPY** | Congenital anomalies, growth retardation, chromosomal damages, mental deficiency, stillbirth. |

Modified from Klaus, M.H. & Farnaroff, A.A. (1979). *Care of the high-risk neonate.* Philadelphia: W.B. Saunders; and Schuster, C.S. & Ashburn, S.S. (1986). *The process of human development: a holistic approach,* (2nd ed.). Boston: Little, Brown.

## Fetal Alcohol Syndrome

One of the most serious examples of a fetal syndrome caused by maternal exposure to a teratogen is *fetal alcohol syndrome* (FAS). FAS is a specific pattern of altered growth structure and function seen in babies of women who consume alcohol during pregnancy (Jones, 1986). FAS is the third leading cause of birth defects and mental retardation and has been reported to occur in 1 in 600 to 1000 live births in the United States. It occurs in approximately 30% to 45% of infants born to chronic, heavy daily drinkers and in approximately 11% of babies born to mothers who drink moderately (Abel & Sokol, 1987).

Alcohol, like other teratogens, causes a spectrum of defects that vary from severe physical and mental problems that are readily detectable at birth to more subtle learning problems that may not be detected until school age (Day, 1992; Jones, 1986). The principle features of FAS include prenatal and postnatal growth deficiencies, with weight and head circumference being most affected. Typical craniofacial features include ptosis, a long philtrum, short palpebral fissures, maxillary hypoplasia, and a thin vermilion of the upper lip. Musculoskeletal problems include congenital dislocations, foot positional defects, cervical spine abnormalities, specific joint alterations, flexion contractures at the elbows, and tapering of the terminal phalanges. Many of these craniofacial and skeletal defects are secondary to the effect of the alcohol on brain development. Another result of alcohol's effect on brain development is the impaired intellectual performance displayed by these children. This can range from LD to profound mental retardation, with an average IQ of 63 reported (Jones, 1986). Functionally, these children often have speech problems, otitis media that causes hearing and auditory perceptual problems, poor attention spans, and fine motor dysfunction demonstrated by weak grasp and poor eye-hand coordination (Streissguth, Clarren, & Jones, 1985).

Children with alcohol-related birth defects (ARBD) usually have decreased intellectual capacities, disturbances in sleep and behavior patterns, lack of motor coordination, and any of the physical anomalies associated with FAS. The nature and extent of fetal injuries produced by alcohol depends on a number of factors, including the amount of alcohol consumed per day, the time during the pregnancy that the alcohol was taken, whether food was eaten near the time of alcohol consumption, whether other substance abuse occurred during the pregnancy, and the general health of the mother.

The prognosis for FAS children varies with the extent and severity of the various malformations and growth deficiencies. Two other important factors to consider are the severity of the maternal alcoholism and the quality and stability of the home environment (Jones, 1986). Studies of the long-term effect of FAS are just beginning to inform us about the influence of growth and development on the affected child. Size delays appear to continue for some time, with head circumference remaining smaller into middle childhood. The developmental performance of FAS children is delayed in cognitive (IQ and achievement), fine and gross motor, and behavioral (attention and self-monitoring) areas, particularly for those children whose mothers binged or drank heavily.

Hypothetically, FAS could be completely preventable if the public were educated to the deleterious effects of alcohol on unborn babies and changed its behavior accordingly. It seems that the best that can be hoped for is a reduction in the number of babies born with FAS and ARBD.

## Cocaine and Opiates

The effects of cocaine, crack and opiates on infants are of increasing concern to developmental specialists. The use of these drugs has increased markedly in the 1980s and 1990s, particularly the use of cocaine and "crack," a relatively cheap cocaine derivative. Maternal drug use is also complicated by the tendency of abusers to abuse other substances, such as alcohol and tobacco. Additionally, many of these mothers have been poorly nourished and received less than adequate prenatal care. At this time it is estimated that more than 100,000 infants per year are born of mothers who used drugs during pregnancy, although accurate counts are made difficult by the social and legal implications of reporting drug use (Conlon, 1992; Zuckerman & Frank, 1992).

Cocaine is extremely addicting, causing ecstatic "highs," and significant and prolonged "lows." Addiction to crack-cocaine is said to be possible after one or two uses (Conlon, 1992). It increases the levels of norepinephrine, serotonin, and dopamine and has strong vasoconstrictive effects. Cocaine crosses the placenta and causes similar effects in the fetus. It is this vasoconstriction that is believed to be damaging to the fetus. Use of opiates, heroin, or methadone by the mother results in an addicted infant who experiences drug withdrawal at birth.

The extent to which cocaine and drug abuse cause developmental problems is still in question (Zuckerman & Frank, 1992). Research in the area continues; however, controlled studies are difficult to accomplish. Several general patterns are emerging. Babies born of addicted mothers have often presented as SGA, with reduced head size and irritability and hypersensitivity to stimuli (Wong, 1993). Babies whose mothers smoke marijuana tend to be more irritable than those who used cocaine (Zuckerman & Frank, 1992). Cocaine has been associated with congenital anomalies, limb deficiencies, cerebral hemorrhage, increased muscle tone, necrotizing enterocolitis, and rapid shifts of arousal state (Conlon, 1992). Neonates who are exposed to narcotics intrauterine go through active withdrawal, during which time they are irritable, hypertonic, and poor feeders. Often they profusely and frantically suck on their hands. Motor coordination is reduced, and activity level may be high. Respiratory distress has also been noted (Wong, 1993). These babies tend to require quiet, low-stimulus environments and may respond positively to swaddling (Conlon, 1992). Parenting these children can be difficult for several months.

Long-term effects are unclear. Some studies have found that by school age these children perform up to expectations. However, others have reported longer-term problems, including hyperactivity and organizational problems, subtle learning and cognitive deficits, and play deficits. Further, the mothers of these children often have few social supports and may be young, homeless, or remain addicted. Children may also be placed in foster care. Early intervention programs and school intervention programs may be necessary to identify, prevent, or minimize the long-term effects of the maternal substance abuse.

## Heavy Metals

Heavy-metals poisoning is a serious health concern. Because small children often put everything in their mouths, they are at particular risk for poisoning by these substances (Menkes, 1990). *Mercury poisoning,* which can cause tremors and memory loss, anorexia, weight loss, diarrhea, and acrodynia (painful extremities), enters the body through inhalation. Liquid mercury evaporates quickly and should be cleaned up immediately to prevent this problem.

*Lead poisoning* is usually caused by ingestion of environmental lead, such as the lead paint in buildings built and painted before World War II. This has been a significant problem in some inner city communities and in older houses that have been renovated (Batshaw & Perret, 1992; Menkes, 1990). Lead water piping and some ceramic glazes have also been associated with lead poisoning.

A child may be acutely or chronically affected. Lead affects three body systems in particular—renal, blood, and nervous. Renal damage occurs in the proximal tubules of the kidneys, resulting in abnormal excretion of important nutrients and impairment of vitamin D synthesis. Lead severely limits the body's ability to synthesize heme, leading to accumulation of alternate metabolites in the body and, ultimately, anemia (Wong, 1993). The most significant and irreversible effects of lead poisoning on the body occur in the nervous system. Fluid builds up in the brain, and intracranial pressure can reach life-threatening levels (Menkes, 1990). Cortical atrophy and lead encephalitis are almost always associated with high blood lead levels. This can lead to MR, paralysis, blindness, and convulsions. Low-level exposure has been associated with LD, ADHD, hearing impairment, and milder intellectual deficits. Other lead poisoning symptoms include cramping, digestive difficulty, lethargy, headache, and fever (Menkes, 1990).

## INFECTIOUS CONDITIONS
### Maternal Infections

The fetus may be infected by a variety of organisms. Some of the infections are passed from the mother to the fetus during pregnancy (transplacental infections), and others are present in the vagina and are passed to the baby at birth (ascending infections). These infections invade the fetus at a time when it has a limited capacity to ward off disease and, in the case of transplacental infections, at a time when they can have a profound effect on growth and development or the formation of tissues and organs (Ensher & Clark, 1986).

The most common maternal infections are the *STORCH infections,* also called TORCH or TORCHS. Each of these conditions is caused by a specific virus or bacterium and possesses a different set of characteristics. Table 7-4 summarizes these five infections and their effects on the fetus. *Congenital syphilis,* the incidence of which is increasing rapidly, may be transmitted in the late stages of pregnancy or during delivery. It is the most virulent form of syphilis and requires isolation of the infected infant. the usual treatment is penicillin. Early-stage congenital syphilis is characterized by hepatitis, failure to thrive, neurologic involvement, fever, anemia, restlessness, irritability, and syphilitic rhinitis. Characteristic lesions may be present; hair and nails may be damaged. Osteochondritis at the joints and other bone abnormalities are relatively common. Late-stage congenital syphilis, because of residual damage from the infection, is marked by bony and dental anomalies and visual and auditory deficits (Behran & Vaughan, 1987).

*Toxoplasmosis,* transmitted at any point throughout pregnancy, may be contracted by the mother through ingestion of raw meat or contact with the feces of newly infected cats. It is also an increasingly common opportunistic infection in AIDS (Feldman & Remington, 1987; Siegel, 1990a). In the United States the incidence of the condition is about 1.3 in 1000 live births (Siegel, 1990a). Stillbirth and death are common. Children born with this condition are often severely mentally handicapped. Hydrocephaly, cerebral calcification, and chorioretinitis are classic symptoms. CP, seizures, cardiac and liver damage, and gastrointestinal problems are also found. Treatment with sulphonomides and pyrimethamine is usually initiated in infected mothers and children. The neurologic deficits related to the disease may be reduced by maternal treatment but, once acquired, will not be reversed by this treatment (Feldman & Remington, 1987; Siegel, 1990a). These children may therefore require extensive rehabilitation for a variety of developmental delays.

*Rubella,* a common and fairly mild disease in children, can be devastating when contracted by a newly pregnant woman. With the advent of a preventive vaccine, congenital rubella syndrome has declined 99% in the last 25 years; however, the dangers to unvaccinated mothers are significant (Behran & Vaughn, 1987; Siegel, 1990b). Congenital defects, spontaneous abortion, and stillbirth may occur. Central processing hearing loss, MR, microcephaly, and seizures are possible outcomes. Congenital heart defects, including patent ductus arteriosus, are characteristic, as are visual deficits, hepatomegaly, and splenomegaly (Behran & Vaughn, 1987; Wong, 1993). These children may be SGA and may suffer from numerous respiratory infections in infancy. Late-occurring symptoms include diabetes, encephalitis, hearing loss, and thyroid problems. Functionally,

▲ Table 7-4   Intrauterine Infections (STORCH)

| Name | Cause | Type* | Effects on Fetus |
|---|---|---|---|
| Syphilis | Parabacterial infection | A; T | Large liver and spleen; jaundice; anemia; rash; rhinorrhea |
| Toxoplasmosis | Parasitic infection | T | Deafness; blindness; mental retardation; seizures; pneumonia; large liver and spleen |
| Rubella | Virus | T | Meningitis; hearing loss; cataracts; cardiac problems; mental retardation; retinal defects |
| Cytomegalovirus | Virus | T | Hearing loss; in severe form, problems are similar to rubella |
| Herpes | Virus | A | Localized form: lethargy, rash, respiratory distress, jaundice, enlarged liver and spleen. Generalized form: attacks CNS, causing MR, seizures, and other problems |

*A, Ascending; T, transplacental.

children with congenital rubella symptoms may be expected to have mixed developmental delays and hearing and vestibular deficits. Adjustments to the child's therapy program may be necessary to accommodate cardiorespiratory effects.

*Cytomegalovirus,* or cytomegalic inclusion disease, has transmission and effects that are similar to rubella. It may be transmitted before, during, or after birth and is a herpes-type viral infection. This infection may also be active or latent in the newborn so that infection control precautions are appropriate when working with this child. Clinical manifestations include low birth weight, sensorineural hearing loss, microcephaly, hepatomegaly, splenomegaly, and purpuric rash. Jaundice and hepatitis may also be present. Children may be asymptomatic at birth. Symptomatic newborns have a poor prognosis related to neurologic deficits. LD and diminished intellectual development may necessitate habilitative intervention.

The final STORCH infection is *congenital herpes.* The neonate most often contracts this condition during or after delivery by a mother with herpes simplex, often genital herpes (Wong, 1993). The infected child often develops skin, mouth, or eye lesions within 6 to 10 days of contact, but this is not always the case. Some children do not develop overt symptoms. In the disseminated form, a sepsislike picture presents itself and the child may develop internal organ lesions and encephalitis with central nervous system involvement. Infusion of antiviral agents may reduce the severity of this condition markedly and has been known to prevent serious brain damage.

*Gonorrhea* and *chlamydia* are both transmitted to the infant late in fetal development or during delivery. Both may result in eye infections. Gonococcal arthritis, septicemia, and meningitis may also occur. Fortunately both respond well to antibiotic therapy if discovered early. Other maternal infections known to affect neonatal health include varicella (chicken pox), coxsackie, parvovirus, hepatitis B, listeriosis, Lyme disease, and AIDS.

## Acquired Immunodeficiency Syndrome

AIDS has become a major health concern for all Americans, including infants, children, and adolescents. In 1994 the cumulative total of AIDS cases was estimated at about 500,000 in the United States. The first pediatric AIDS case was reported in 1982; in the subsequent 10 years more than 4000 cases have been reported (Stephenson, 1994).

AIDS is believed to be transmitted exclusively through blood and body fluid exposure, particularly semen (Ammann, Cowan, & Wara, 1983). Most adults and adolescents who contract the disease do so through sexual contact with an infected individual or the sharing of contaminated syringes in drug use. Before blood bank screening, some individuals also contracted the disease through medical blood products administration, as in surgery or hemophilia treatment. Most infants and children contract AIDS from their

mothers before or during the birth process. Not all babies born to infected mothers develop AIDS, however. The second most common cause is through transfusion or hemophilia treatment. Some evidence exists for transmission through breast feeding, sexual exposure, or assault (Stephenson, 1994; Ammann et al., 1983).

AIDS is a disease that infects and damages cells of the immune system, thus making the child vulnerable to life-threatening illnesses that do not affect children with normal immunity. The virus that causes AIDS and AIDS-related complex (ARC) has had several different names, including human T-lymphotrophic virus (HTLV), lymph-adenopathy-associated virus (LAV), and, commonly, HIV.

T4 lymphocytes are the type of white blood cells primarily affected by the AIDS virus. This type of lymphocyte is primarily made up of helper cells and inducer cells that, when diminished, lessen the body's abilities to carry out normal immune responses. Once the AIDS virus has infected some cells, it appears to lie dormant for weeks to years while the infected person remains healthy and apparently free of symptoms. At this stage the person is designated as HIV positive and might not enter the acute phase of AIDS for years, if ever.

AIDS is nearly always fatal. It is currently one of the leading causes of death among children, particularly in large urban areas (Cohen, 1992). The period between exposure and the development of AIDS symptoms varies markedly. In adults it is typically about 3 years, but in children the incubation period varies with the method of transmission and age of the child (Butler & Pizzo, 1992; Simonds & Rogers, 1992). Children infected perinatally typically have a shortened incubation period, and the course of the disease may progress quickly. Most of these children will have symptoms by 15 to 18 months of age (Stephenson, 1994) and may be expected to survive less than 3 to 5 years (Simonds & Rogers, 1992). In children infected because of hemophilia treatment, however, the child's life expectancy may be up to twice as long as an adult's and inversely relates to the age of infection (Butler & Pizzo, 1992). For teenagers who are affected through sexual contact or by sharing contaminated syringes, the course may be expected to fall between that of hemophiliacs and that of adults with similar modes of infection (Butler & Pizzo, 1992).

Some persons infected with AIDS develop ARC, which includes symptoms such as swollen glands, fever, chills, diarrhea, weight loss, fatigue, dizziness, night sweats, dry cough, unexplained bleeding from any body opening or from growths on the skin or mucous membranes, and signs of unexplained confusion and disorientation. It is unknown at this time what percentage of persons with ARC will develop AIDS.

Persons with the AIDS disease itself have symptoms similar to those with ARC. In addition, they often develop other problems such as rare, fatal diseases. For example, the HIV virus may attack the central nervous system, causing severe motor problems such as ataxia and paraplegia. Many AIDS patients develop bacterial infections as well as a parasitic infection of the lungs called *Pneumocystis carinii* pneumonia (PCP). This infection is almost never seen outside of patients with immune disorders. Early in the disease, PCP shows a good response to antibiotic treatment, but the patient often must stay on the antibiotics for long periods to prevent relapses. Herpes complex and cytomegalovirus are two other serious viruses commonly found in AIDS patients (Conlon, 1992).

The specific AIDS symptomatology found in infants and young children varies slightly from that of adults. Symptoms of congenitally infected children often begin to appear at about 5 months of age but may be more nonspecific than those of adults, making early diagnosis difficult (Rubenstein, 1986). Also, antibody testing may not be revealing in young children (Butler & Pizzo, 1992). By far the most common symptom in children is PCP, followed by lymphoid pneumonia or pulmonary hyperplasia, HIV wasting syndrome, encephalopathy, and recurrent bacterial infections. Candidiasis, impetigo, and microencephaly and atrophy may also be found (Stephenson, 1994). Karposi's sarcoma, common in adults with AIDS, is rarely seen in children.

Medical treatment regimens include intravenous gamma globulin, which appears to assist in resisting infections. The importance of childhood vaccinations for these children cannot be exaggerated. Infections may be treated with antibiotics and sulfonomides, often with the same medications that are used for non–HIV-infected children. Antiretroviral agents may also be used. Azidothymidine (AZT), interferon-alpha, and sulfated polysaccharides are used to slow the progress of the disease and may be effective. These treatments are fairly toxic, however, and produce a variety of negative side effects. AZT treatment of infected mothers is being explored to prevent the occurrence of the disease in newborns (Pizzo & Wilfert, 1991).

As the disease progresses, these children often become noticeably weakened by chronic respiratory illness, skin and other infections, and diarrhea. These conditions often respond to treatment slowly (Simonds & Rogers, 1992). Developmental delays and degeneration may result in delayed or lost motor, speech, and independent living skills, and neurologic deficits including ataxia, spasticity, rigidity, tremor, and seizures may be expected as the disease progresses (Diamond & Cohen, 1992; Stephenson, 1994). Early intervention, rehabilitative, and educational services are often indicated.

Additionally, both the child and the family may be socially isolated. Drug-dependent mothers, particularly, require training in the care and parenting skills needed to work with HIV-infected children. Older children may require opportunities for normal play, social, and prevocational activities. The interactions between children with AIDS, their families, and health care workers need to be positive, accepting, and supportive. The risk of HIV infection from patients to occupational therapists is extremely small. Few health care workers of any kind have contracted AIDS from their patients, and nearly all of these did so through prolonged or open skin contact with infected blood products (Lyons & Valentine, 1994). Use of correct universal precautions with all patients should allow any occupational therapist to work safely with patients. Further, the role of preventing HIV infection through patient and family education of children with developmental delays and learning and emotional disabilities belongs to all health professionals, including occupational therapists.

## Hepatitis

*Hepatitis* may be contracted congenitally or directly. Five major types of hepatitis have been identified at this time: hepatitis A, B, C, D, and E. Hepatitis may also be caused by cytomegalovirus (CMV), Epstein-Barr virus, and herpes. The most common types are A, B, and C. *Hepatitis A* (HAV) is an acute, highly contagious condition. Direct contact with contaminated individuals or foods is ordinarily responsible. For children it may be fairly mild, and it is characterized by fever, fatigue, nausea, and decreased appetite. Jaundice occurs only occasionally. This condition is usually treated with bed rest and nutritional restrictions. Complete recovery is common, although 3% to 5% develop chronic hepatitis. HAV has rarely been associated with congenital hepatitis (Brunell, 1987).

The pattern of *Hepatitis B* (HBV) is somewhat different. Its onset may be slower and less obvious, and the acute symptoms are less common. This disease may be mild or very severe. Rash, jaundice, and arthralgia are common. Chronic hepatitis and liver cancer are long-term effects of the condition. Transmission is usually through the exchange of body fluids, including the sharing of needles, blood transfusion, congenitally from mother to child, and through bites, spitting, and ingested fluids (Novak, Suchy, & Balestreri, 1990). Asymptomatic individuals may be carriers of this disease, and it is not uncommon to find large numbers of infected individuals in centers for the developmentally disabled (Novak et al., 1990). Blood and body fluid precautions are appropriate when treating children suspected of having or carrying this condition, particularly when engaged in feeding and oral-motor treatments. Vaccines have been developed for this condition, greatly reducing the risk for peers and health care workers, and the American Academy of Pediatrics is now encouraging the immunization of all children and adolescents.

*Hepatitis C* is commonly called non-A, non-B hepatitis (NANB). This condition also begins insidiously and produces mild to severe symptoms. Jaundice is common, and nausea and vomiting are not uncommon. Epidemics of NANB have been documented, and chronic sequelae similar to those of HBV are of concern. Immune globulin administration may not be as effective in preventing NANB as for HAV and HBV (Novak et al., 1990).

## Tuberculosis

*Tuberculosis* (TB) of the lungs is one of the oldest diseases reported to be found in humans. It is an infectious disease caused when the tubercle bacillus is inhaled into the lungs. For years this condition has been well controlled in the United States and other developed countries, but it is experiencing a resurgence, particularly in urban and overcrowded areas. It is often associated with poor living conditions and has been a particular problem for the Native American, immigrant, and AIDS populations (McIntosh & Lauer, 1987). TB is most common in the young children, who are probably infected through contact with infected adults, and in adolescent girls. It is particularly dangerous in very young children.

This condition may not produce any symptoms at all, and some individuals come into contact with the bacillus without ever contracting active TB. Signs and symptoms can vary greatly in children. Fever, fatigue, persistent cough, anorexia, and chest pain may occur. As the disease progresses, the child may display listlessness, weight loss, reduced respiratory function, and hemoptysis. Pulmonic lesions of one or more lobes of the lungs may spread to other body areas (Brooks, 1987). Meningitis, hepatitis, infection of the kidneys, osteomyelitis, enteritis, arthritis, and TB of the bone may occur. These lesions may heal by calcification, and the disease may become inactive.

A number of different tuberculin tests may be performed that indicate whether an individual has ever been infected or exposed to tubercle bacillus. However, these tests do not indicate whether the infection is currently active or inactive. These tests consist of applying tuberculin to the skin directly or intradermally and then watching for a local inflammatory reaction within 48 to 72 hours or 48 to 96 hours, depending on the test administered. Diagnosis may also be done through the examination of sputum samples and through chest x-ray films.

Treatment consists of chemotherapy using medications such as ethambutol, isoniazid (INH), rifampin paraaminosalicylic acid (PAS), or streptomycin. Bed rest and nutritional counseling may also be recommended. In advanced cases various surgical procedures may be required. Medications must be taken for an extended period, often up to a year, and treatment requires excellent medication compliance on the part of the child and family. If the disease is not completely healed and requires retreatment, the prognosis becomes much poorer (McIntosh & Laurer, 1987).

On occasion TB of the bone (tuberculous osteomyelitis) occurs as an isolated lesion, but it usually forms from infection at a primary lesion in another part of the body or from an adjoining joint. The most common sites for TB of the bone are the long bones, synovial joints, and vertebrae. The joints most often affected are the hips and the knees. Initially, swelling of the soft tissue around the joint is noted. Then the synovial membrane changes, and articular cartilage necrosis occurs. Finally the adjacent bones may begin to collapse.

TB of the spine, or Pott's disease, usually begins with pain, tenderness, and muscle spasms in the back. As the disease progresses, the anterior sections of the vertebral bodies begin to collapse, causing the spine to tilt anteriorly. Infection may spread to adjacent disks and vertebrae or to the spinal cord. Pott's paraplegia may be a direct result of spinal cord involvement or a result of pressure on the cord. Functional or structural kyphotic deformity is often present in spinal TB; a limp is apparent if the hip is affected. Treatment includes antibiotic therapy, bed rest, and immobilization. In rare cases hip or spinal fusion may be performed. Rehabilitation effort focuses on increasing strength, range of motion, and endurance, as well as functional adaptations.

## Lyme Disease

Caused by a spirochete infection secondary to a bite from a tick of the genus Ixodes, *Lyme disease* has grown to epidemic proportions in recent years (Speck, 1987; Hollister, 1987). The disease is often mistaken for JRA in children, and differential diagnosis may be done serologically. The condition may be seen as having three stages, with early treatment often valuable in preventing the disabling effects of the latter stages.

Stage 1 is the actual tick bite, usually from a deer tick. In Stage 2 the individual develops a distinctive, red, target-shaped lesion, often at the site of the tick bite. This usually occurs 3 to 30 days after infection (McIntosh & Lauer, 1987). These lesions may be present for 1 to 3 weeks and may foster secondary lesions in some children (Wong, 1993). The individual may also develop flulike symptoms, including fever, pain, and fatigue. Several weeks or months later, in Stage 3, the child may develop cardiac, neurologic, muscular, or joint disorders. The intensity and duration of the condition may vary considerably. In severe cases they can be debilitating.

Neurologic involvement includes cranial nerve palsies, meningitis, and radiculoneuropathy, causing pain, nausea, lability, and sensory disturbances. Arthritis-like symptoms are among the most common indications of the syndrome, usually occurring in the large joints. These symptoms are often of sudden onset and affect single joints, although they may be migratory. Attacks may be of short or long duration. Cardiac symptoms are less common and are usually brief in duration. These may include myocarditis or ventricular dysfunctions.

Treatment includes rest and antibiotic therapy, usually penicillin, erythromycin, or, in older children, tetracycline (Speck, 1987). Intravenous, high-dose penicillin has had some effect. Sequelae of this condition are often treated symptomatically, including pain relief, support, mobilization, and assistance in self-care activities. This child may also demonstrate reduced endurance, general malaise, and depression if symptoms continue over an extended period.

## Polio

*Polio,* or poliomyelitis, is a viral disease that affects the anterior horn cells of the spinal cord. In less severe forms of the disease, symptoms may last a few days or weeks and consist of flulike symptoms with no clinically detectable neurologic deficit. The paralytic form of polio, however, progresses quickly to meningitis and muscle weakness, followed by some degree of paralysis. Often, for example, the anterior horn cells of the cervical and lumbar regions are involved, causing quadriplegia and interfering with innervation to the diaphragm and intercostal muscles, thus hampering or completely eliminating the person's ability to breathe independently (Levy & Pilmer, 1992).

Before 1955, thousands of infants and children contracted poliomyelitis each year, but fewer than 50 cases have been reported in the United States in the last decade. The reason for this is the highly successful oral polio immunization program recommended for infants between 2 and 4 months of age (see Chapter 6). In developing nations, including Mexico and Central America, polio is still a significant health problem. Pediatric therapists working with immigrants may still encounter children with the condition.

There is no specific treatment for polio in the acute stages. The child is often sick and in pain. Bed rest and palliative care are indicated at this stage. For the child who has paralytic polio, the damage is considered permanent. Rehabilitative services include positioning and orthoses to support affected body parts and prevent deformity. Many classical pediatric rehabilitative approaches were developed to meet the needs of individuals and are still relevant today. Technology advances in respiratory and environmental control should provide these individuals with opportunities for increased independence in the future.

## Encephalitis and Meningitis

Encephalitis and meningitis, infections of the brain and its coverings, are frightening and sometimes dangerous. *Encephalitis* is an inflammation of the brain, which may be caused by bacteria, spirochetes, and other organisms, but usually is caused by a viral infection (Weil, 1990). The specific cause of the infection is often not identified clinically. The condition may be localized or may also include the spinal cord or meninges. Infection of the brain may be direct or secondary to another infection. Several of its viral forms are spread by mosquitos; therefore summer onset is common. Herpes simplex has also been associated disproportionately with encephalitis in young children.

The severity of these conditions varies with the cause. Onset may be sudden or gradual, and it is often difficult to distinguish from other infections. Symptoms include fever, headache, dizziness, stiff neck, nausea and vomiting, tremors, and ataxia. In severe cases, stupor, seizures, disorientation, coma, and death may occur. Diagnosis is based on environmental patterns of infection, clinical findings, EEG, and MRI, as well as laboratory examination of blood, brain tissue, or CSF. Treatment may include antibiotics if bacterial infection is suggested but is primarily supportive while the acute disease runs its course (Wong, 1993).

Unfortunately, this condition may be expected to leave severe to mild residual brain damage. How much damage depends on the age of the child, type of infection, and care. Young children are at increased risks for neurologic complications. Health care staff must monitor the child's progress and neurologic status after the infection. MR, LDs, behavior disorders, seizures, and neuromotor deficits are not uncommon. Neurorehabilitation techniques may be applied to limit the disability, and compensatory equipment and training may assist this child in school, play, and, later, prework activities (Powell, 1992).

*Meningitis* is an infection of the meninges, the tissue covering the brain and spinal cord. Meningitis, like encephalitis, may have several causes: tubercular, fungal, protozoan, viral, and, most commonly, bacterial. Clinical manifestations of meningitis vary slightly from neonates to infants to children to adolescents, but the clinical picture is not unlike encephalitis. Headache, fever, and rigidity in the neck are classic signs. These may be accompanied by seizures, vomiting, spasticity, behavioral and arousal state changes, and, in young children, bulging fontanels. In neonates, jaundice, cyanosis, hypothermia, and respiratory distress may also be present (Weil, 1990).

Diagnostic evaluation may include lumbar puncture, analysis of CSF, and blood, throat, and nasal cultures. Treatment includes management of the underlying infection with antibiotics, hydration, maintenance of intracranial pressure, and treatment of symptoms and complications. Because many forms of the disease are highly contagious, the acutely ill patient may be isolated. The child may be monitored for apnea and cardiac function. As with encephalitis, neuromotor, visual, auditory, seizure, and learning disorders may remain after the acute infection abates. Anticonvulsant and rehabilitative therapy is necessary to manage and overcome these sequelae.

## Osteomyelitis

*Osteomyelitis* is an inflammation of the bone marrow that may be caused by puncture wounds, infection adjacent to the bone, or microorganisms that travel in the blood (Roberts, 1979). Initially the organisms settle in the distal end of the metaphysis. As the disease progresses, the infection spreads throughout the bone and outward to the periosteum. Initial symptoms include pain, tenderness, and unwillingness to use or bear weight on the involved limb. Osteomyelitis occurs most commonly in boys between the ages of 5 and 14 (Wong, 1993). These symptoms are followed by fever, soft tissue swelling, and, often, anorexia. The child is often ill and experiences pain on movement.

Treatment must be initiated as soon as possible because prolonged infection may cause bone destruction, pathologic fractures, septic arthritis, and, eventually, growth disturbances (Salter, 1983). Diagnosis is usually made based on clinical signs, and confirmation is made from specimen aspiration test results, blood cell counts, and positive radiographic evidence (Salter, 1983; Scoles, 1982). Initial treatment usually consists of oral or intravenous antibiotic therapy for at least 3 weeks and bed rest and immobility of the affected body part, including splinting. If improvement is not seen, surgery is done, which includes drilling into the bone to remove the pus and damaged tissue and putting in place drainage tubes and intravenous tubes that are used to infuse the site with a saline and antibiotic solution (Salter, 1983). After these procedures, splinting of the extremity or traction helps prevent the spread of infection, reduces pain, and prevents contractures. Relapses can lead to chronic osteomyelitis that may involve continued discharge of pus from a sinus over the infected area, pain, or the formation of an abscess cavity in the bone itself. Bed rest and antibiotics may clear the problem, or surgical procedures may have to be repeated. Chronic untreated osteomyelitis presents serious medical problems that can be minimized by early detection and prolonged antibiotic therapy.

### Otitis Media

*Otitis media* is one of the most common infections in children. Approximately 30% of all children in the age range of 6 to 36 months show evidence of middle ear problems (Bluestone, 1989). In otitis media the eustachian tube usually becomes blocked, and fluid collects in the middle ear. One of the following organisms is usually found: pneumococcus, *Haemophilus influenzae,* or streptococcus. Milder cases of otitis media may go undetected. However, pain, a sense of fullness in the ear, and low-grade fever, vertigo, nausea, and loss of balance are symptoms that often accompany this condition (Roberts, 1979).

Investigators studying the long-term effects of otitis media have suggested possible language and cognitive delays, hearing loss, and central auditory processing problems (Zincus, Gottleib, & Shapiro, 1978). Of special interest to occupational therapists is the possible relationship between otitis media and vestibular disorders. Although further research is necessary to verify this relationship, initial data warrant considering vestibular dysfunctions as possible contributors to some of the developmental delays found in children with chronic otitis media.

The goal of medical treatment is to eradicate the organisms, clear the fluids, and prevent chronic serous otitis media. This is accompanied by the administration of antibiot-

ics such as penicillin, ampicillin, amoxicillin, or sulfonamides (Bluestone, 1989). The insertion of tympanotomy, pressure equalizer tubes may be necessary in more chronic cases of otitis media.

## NEOPLASTIC DISORDERS

Cancer is devastating for anyone, but it seems somehow even more insidious when it attacks children. The pain, fear, and life disruption it causes is chronic and affects the child, the child's family, and all of those around the child. This section discusses some of the major neoplasms that attack children and adults.

### Leukemia

*Leukemia* is a cancer of the blood-forming tissues. It is the most common form of cancer found in children, occurring in 6 to 7 children per 100,000. It occurs in boys more frequently than girls, almost always in white children, and most frequently in children with Down syndrome. It has a peak incidence between ages 2 and 5. Two forms of leukemia recognized in children are acute lymphoid leukemia (ALL) and acute nonlymphoid or acute myelogenous leukemia (ANLL or AML) (Wong, 1993). The symptoms of these two forms of cancer are similar, but they react differently to treatment, with ALL having the more favorable response. The causes of this condition are unknown, but immunologic and chromosomal factors have been associated with the condition.

Leukemia is characterized by the uncontrolled multiplication of immature white blood cells, which prevents the bone marrow from producing normal blood cells (Champlin, 1988). Symptoms include loss of weight, night sweats, chronic fatigue, paleness, a high fever; repeated infections; purpura; and enlarged lymph nodes, spleen, and liver. Diagnosis is usually made by examining a specimen of bone marrow for lymphoblasts. Blood counts are also taken.

The goal of medical management is the achievement of complete "cure" by inducing remission, eliminating cells in "sanctuaries" like the central nervous system, and maintaining the remission. Specifically, treatment is conducted in three phases. The first phase is called induction therapy and is designed to rid the bone marrow and the rest of the body of the leukemia cells. The second phase is called central nervous system prophylaxis and is aimed at killing cells in the brain and spinal cord. The third phase of treatment is called maintenance therapy in which chemotherapy is administered to treat small deposits of cells that remain after remission (Hockenberry & Coody, 1986).

Prognosis is much improved over previous years, with the majority of patients with ALL experiencing remission for at least 5 years. Many go long periods with no recurrent signs. Prognosis for children with central nervous system involvement and ANLL is poorer but still hopeful, particularly with bone marrow transplantation. Still these children undergo long courses of treatment that can be painful and frightening, and recurrence of the disease and death remain possibilities that must be handled emotionally.

## Brain Tumors

Tumors of the brain and spinal cord are the most common tumors of solid tissues in children. Most of these tumors occur in the cerebellum and brainstem, with *medulloblastomas* and *astrocytomas* accounting for 30% of all childhood tumors. *Gliomas* and *ependymomas,* ventricular tumors, are also relatively common. The cause of brain tumors is unknown but is believed to be developmental or chromosomal in nature. Tumors may not become evident early in life because they are usually related to increases in intracranial pressure. In the young child the skull is soft enough to provide some accommodation for this phenomenon. Diagnosis is based first on clinical signs and then confirmed with CT scans, MRIs, EEGs and lumbar puncture.

Symptoms of brain tumors include recurrent and progressive headaches, vomiting (particularly in the morning), loss of coordination or strength, increased reflex activity, changes in behavior, seizures, and vital sign disturbances. Specific symptoms may relate to the location of the tumor. Treatment includes surgical removal of the tumor, radiation therapy, and chemotherapy. Prognosis varies with the type, size, and location of the tumor. The survival rate for astrocytomas (75%) is better than that for medulloblastomas (25% to 35%), which is better than glial cell tumors (20% to 30%). Survival with ependymomas varies from 15% to 60%, depending on the study (Maul-Mellott & Adams, 1987). Recurrence of brain tumors is not uncommon, and surgery, chemotherapy, and radiation therapy may cause permanent brain damage. Children recovering from these tumors may require a broad spectrum of central nervous system-based rehabilitation to improve residual sensorimotor and cognitive function.

## Hodgkin's Disease

*Hodgkin's disease* and other *lymphomas* are far less common than leukemia (15 in 1,000,000 people) but are still significant. The condition is uncommon under the age of 5 and among younger children, is more common among boys than girls. It is more commonly a disease of later childhood and adolescence. This cancer of the lymphatic system is marked by painless adenopathy in the cervical region, with or without fever. The child may also experience chills and night sweats, anorexia and weight loss, and general malaise. Diagnosis is made by histologic examination of the node. Blood studies may also show characteristic abnormalities. Four stages of the disease have been identified. In stage I only one node is involved. Stage II demonstrates involvement on only one side of the diaphragm. In stages III and IV progressively more organs are involved.

Treatment consists of radiation therapy, chemotherapy, or splenectomy. Prognosis is excellent for children in stages I, II and III, but patients with widespread disease have only a 50% survival rate (Maul-Mellott & Adams, 1987).

*Non-Hodgkin's lymphomas* (NHLs) occur primarily in school-aged children. They are more common in boys and are a significant problem for African Americans. They may also occur as a second malignancy after Hodgkin's disease. Onset is acute, and progression is rapid; most children have disseminated disease at diagnosis. Symptoms include abdominal pain, vomiting, anorexia, diarrhea, ascites, and distention of the abdomen. Fever, a palpable mass, and paraplegia may also be present. Diagnosis is made through physical examination and analysis of laboratory results. Radiation therapy, chemotherapy, and surgery may be initiated to treat these conditions. Prognosis varies with the degree of bone marrow and CNS involvement and with the number and size of tumors present. Between 50% and 80% of those diagnosed survive beyond 3 years (Maul-Mellott & Adams, 1987).

## Wilms' Tumor

*Wilms' tumor,* or nephroblastoma, is a neoplasm of the kidney and is the most common abdominal cancer of children (7.8 in 1,000,000). It is a highly malignant cancer but may be encapsulated for some time and responds well to chemotherapy and surgery. Clinical signs of this tumor include a firm, palpable mass on one side of the body, fatigue and malaise, fever, and, occasionally, hematuria and hypertension. It can metastasize to the lung, which may produce respiratory symptoms as well. Surgery is performed as soon as the diagnosis is suggested and includes full or partial nephrectomy, with great care taken to maintain the tumor capsule (Wong, 1993). Survival rates are excellent and improving for most cases, even in some children who experience a recurrence.

## Bone Tumors

The two major tumors of the bone, osteosarcoma and Ewing's sarcoma, are relatively uncommon, but result in physical disability, and, not infrequently, death. Most of these tumors occur in adolescence, more frequently in boys; Ewing's sarcoma rarely occurs in African American children. Survival for both cancers is dependent on early diagnosis, before metastatic disease appears. Diagnosis is made by radiologic analysis, with each tumor having a characteristic pattern. Clinical signs include localized pain that may be relieved by change in position, lumps, and reduction in activity level.

*Osteosarcoma* usually occurs at the end of the long bones, particularly the femur. Large spindle cells and malignant osteoid bone is formed next to the growth plate. A painful mass develops. Frequently a secondary trauma at the site of the tumor brings it to attention. Because this condition is resistant to radiation therapy, amputation is performed if possible. This is followed by a course of chemotherapy. If metastases occur, they are usually located in the bones or lungs. In their absence the chance of survival is good, up to 50%, but not certain. This child also requires prosthetic equipment and training after surgery (Pizzo & Poplack, 1989; Simon, 1988).

*Ewing's sarcoma* occurs more frequently in the bones of the trunk but also in the long bones and skull. It does not form osteoid tissue but rather small, round groups of cells. This condition spreads its metastases hematologically, particularly to the bones and lungs. Surgery is not performed routinely and often is done only late in treatment. This tumor responds well to radiation therapy, however. Chemotherapy is also routinely prescribed. In the absence of metastases and for distal lesions, survival rates are good, up to 60%. However, if there are metastases, the prognosis is poor (Pizzo & Poplack, 1989).

## BURNS

Serious burn injury accounts for a large number of children who must undergo prolonged painful and restrictive hospitalizations. Additionally, countless other children suffer from less serious burns. Burns can be caused by thermal, electrical, chemical, and radioactive sources, but thermal burns are by far the most common. Most burns can be attributed to accidents, but 10% of hospital admissions for burns may be attributed to child abuse. Among small children, hot water and hot beverage scalds are the most common causes. Older children more commonly present with flame (match, gasoline, or firecracker) or chemical burns. Short periods of high heat or long periods of low heat both can cause significant burns. Chemical burns can cause serious injury, but their effect can often be stopped with prompt emergency treatment. Electrical burns, however, may damage not only the skin, but also underlying bone, muscle, and nerve tissue along the conduction path. Damage can also be caused by smoke inhalation, respiratory failure, shock, and posttraumatic infection (Wong, 1993).

The prognosis for survival of a child with a burn is determined by the size of the area burned and the depth of the burn. The area is assessed according to percent of surface area involved, and depth, according to the number of layers of tissue involved (Clark, 1983). *First-degree* or *superficial burns* demonstrate minimal tissue damage, although they can be painful. In these burns the skin is red and dry, and complete healing usually occurs. *Partial-thickness,* or *second-degree, burns* can be further classified into deep and superficial burns. Second-degree burns involve the epidermis and sometimes dermal tissues as well. They are characterized by blistered, reddened, and moist wounds. These are the most painful of burns and may result in some scarring, although they may heal spontane-

ously. In *full-thickness,* or *third-degree, burns,* all layers of the skin are destroyed, as may be some of the underlying subcutaneous tissue. Some systems include a *fourth-degree burn* classification when the damage extends to underlying muscle, bone, and fascia. These burns may be charred, brown, or red; nerve endings and blood vessels may be damaged, and pain may not be present in the central area. Most third- and fourth-degree burns also have borders of second-degree burns that are painful (Wong, 1993).

When significant burns occur, emergency medical care focuses on prevention of infection and burn shock, early skin coverage, correction of cosmetic damage, restoration of function, and integration back into the environment. Because burned tissue provides a fertile bed for infection, many types of intervention procedures must be used to minimize the possibility of sepsis. Environmental bacteria must be minimized. Surface bacteria must be reduced by using medicated ointments, administering antibiotics, removing dead tissue early, and covering the areas with skin grafts. Burn shock is prevented by administering various intravenous solutions that help replace lost body fluids. Nutrition may be maintained through tube feedings, oral feedings, and intravenous feedings, if indicated (Deitch, 1990).

Full-thickness, partial-thickness, or meshed skin grafts, may be used to cover large burned areas. Debridement of necrotic tissue is also essential to recovery. These procedures may need to be repeated if the grafts do not "take," and as healing progresses. During the acute period, positioning, hydrotherapy, splinting, range of motion, and daily living activities are essential for rehabilitation. Many of these procedures are painful, and infection is a continued threat until all burned areas are closed. During this period the child also experiences malaise and may be heavily sedated.

After the acute period, deformities, contractures, and loss of motion must be prevented by early intervention. Exercise programs, splinting, proper positioning, use of pressure garments, and reconstructive surgery are all methods used to limit the long-term effects of burn injuries. A child who faces a long hospital stay needs to have academic assistance to prevent any educational delays. The family and the child may need counseling in adjusting to any disfigurements or any limiting physical conditions. Without this help the emotional handicap may be as great as the physical one. The family and child require patient education, support, and assistance for a prolonged period. Burn scar can hypertrophy and contract for up to 2 years after the acute period, and the child needs to continue with exercises and use of pressure garments and splints daily, until this period is completed (Clark, 1983).

## DIABETES

*Diabetes mellitus* is a metabolic disorder of the pancreas in which the hormone insulin is secreted in insufficient amounts. Increased concentrations of glucose are found in the blood, and several systemic problems occur. The causes of diabetes are unknown, but it is familial in pattern and is now thought to be an autoimmune response to a viral infection in some cases. There are two major types of diabetes. Type I, or *insulin-dependent diabetes mellitus (IDDM)*, usually begins in childhood. This form of the disease tends to be more acute and requires the administration of insulin, carefully balanced with food intake and exercise, to provide adequate metabolic balance. Type II, or *non–insulin-dependent diabetes mellitus (NIDDM),* occurs more frequently in adults older than 40 years of age, is characterized by a resistance to insulin action, and may sometimes be controlled by diet, exercise, or oral medications. Insulin may also be required in some stages of NIDDM.

Virtually all childhood diabetes is insulin dependent. Onset is usually around age 10 but may occur earlier or later. Early symptoms include polyuria, increased thirst, weight loss, and dehydration. Later symptoms may include acidosis, vomiting, hyperventilation, and coma (Drash, 1989). Overdose of insulin may cause insulin shock or hypoglycemia.

Over the long term, microvascular lesions may result in retinopathy that leads to blindness, nephropathy, and peripheral nerve damage. Sensory loss and increased infection, especially in the extremities, may occur. Individuals with diabetes are at increased risk for heart disease, and diabetic women are at increased risk for complications in pregnancy (Wong, 1993). Because this is a lifelong condition, the child and parents must be taught to administer insulin injections and to adjust and monitor blood glucose and life and dietary patterns. These children must also adjust to being drug dependent. In adolescence this adjustment is often particularly difficult.

The general goals of treatment are to ensure satisfactory growth, ensure emotional development, help the child acquire some degree of normal life, resolve the symptoms, prevent ketoacidosis, and prevent long-term sequelae, such as renal and cardiac damage and eye disease (Drash, 1989). The achievement of these goals is difficult because it depends on maintaining a delicate balance between so many factors: exercise, nutritional intake, hormones, emotions, and many other internal and external influences on blood sugar levels.

## RENAL FAILURE

Renal failure occurs when the kidneys are unable to operate efficiently to excrete waste and general proper urine and to maintain electrolyte balance for the child. Toxins build up in the body, affecting all body systems. *Acute renal failure (ARF)* occurs when the kidneys suddenly shut down because of trauma, toxins, obstructions, dehydration, or as the end stage of chronic renal failure. When this occurs, glomerular filtration is reduced and blood urea nitrogen (BUN) increases sharply. Symptoms of ARF include reduction or cessation of urine production, edema, nausea and vomiting, and hypertension. Treatment is aimed at reversing the phenomenon by treating the underlying cause, providing supportive therapy and minimizing the complications of the disease. Fluid intake and output are monitored and managed carefully, and efforts are made to prevent hyperkalemia, hypertension, anemia, seizures, and cardiac failure. Prognosis depends on the underlying cause (Wong, 1993).

*Chronic renal failure (CRF)* is a permanent, progressive reduction in renal function. CRF may be caused by renal diseases such as glomerular nephrosis, membranoproliferative nephritis, lupus erythematosis, vasculitis, and hereditary disorders. The kidneys can maintain fluid and electrolyte balance even when they are able to function at only 50% capacity. When this is no longer possible the child develops uremia, causing acidosis, growth failure, deformities of the bones and teeth, bleeding and anemia, increased infections, gastrointestinal deficits, hypertension, and central nervous system involvement (Foreman & Chan, 1988).

Because CRF is progressive, it may not be detected until late in the course of the disease. Early signs of the condition include lethargy and fatigue, pallor, and, sometimes, hypertension. As the disease progresses, the skin becomes paler and muddy, urine output changes, nausea and vomiting may cause decreased appetite, and lethargy increases. Weight loss and changes in skin, growth, and sensorimotor functions may also occur. If the child is still untreated, becomes uremic, and is in end-stage renal disease, he or she develops additional gastrointestinal problems, bleeding, characteristic changes in skin and breath smell, and serious neurologic and cardiorespiratory deficits. This is a very sick and debilitated child.

Treatment of CRF is focused on treating the underlying causes, managing diet and fluid balance, treating systemic problems and maintaining the child's life-style as long as possible (Wong, 1993). If failure is evident, dialysis and transplantation may be necessary. Transplantation is preferred but not always possible. Although 75% of kidney transplants in children function well for extended periods, it is difficult to identify and obtain donor organs (Weiss, 1988).

Dialysis may take three forms: hemodialysis, in which the blood is circulated through external, artificial membranes; peritoneal dialysis, in which fluid exchange is done in the abdominal cavity and the peritoneum is used for filtration; and hemofiltration, in which a blood filtrate is pumped out of the body while a replacement solution flows in. Peritoneal dialysis is preferred because it can be done at home by family members and requires the least disruption of the child's life. Hemodialysis is preferred if there is no one at home who can do peritoneal dialysis and for children who live near a dialysis center. The child's health often improves markedly when dialysis is instituted, but this does not reestablish renal function and is a long and stressful process for the child and family.

## INFLAMMATORY BOWEL DISEASE

There are two major inflammatory bowel diseases of childhood: Crohn's disease and ulcerative colitis. *Crohn's disease* is the more common of the two among children, is considered more serious, and is less responsive to treatment. The disease involves all layers and the full length of the bowel but, particularly, the terminal ileum. It is characterized by edema, inflammation, granulomas, fistulas, and deep, long ulcerations. Pain, bloody diarrhea, anorexia, growth retardation, and weight loss are common. Treatment consists of antiinflammatory medications, steroids, antispasmodics, bowel management programs, diet, and psychologic support. Surgery does not reverse the damage, and recurrence is virtually assured. Colostomy or ileostomy surgery may be necessary when extensive damage has been done to the intestine. Cancer of the colon is a frequent complication of the disease (Wong, 1993).

*Ulcerative colitis* is an inflammation of the colon and rectum, with the mucosa distal portions most commonly affected. Bowel scarring, narrowing, and smoothing occur as the disease progresses. The child experiences less pain than in Crohn's disease, but rectal bleeding and diarrhea occur. Antiinflammatory drugs, steroids, diet modifications, and surgery are included in the treatment regimens. As with Crohn's disease, colon cancer is a risk, but this risk is eliminated if a colectomy is performed, which also cures the disease. Children with these conditions require psychologic support, patient education in ostomy care, and diet management, as well as activities to improve self-image.

## METABOLIC GROWTH DISORDERS

After stimulation by the hypothalamus, the pituitary gland secretes the thyroid-stimulating hormone into the bloodstream. This hormone stimulates the thyroid gland to produce thyroxine, a hormone that affects body growth, metabolism, and brain growth. If the thyroid gland secretes too little thyroxine, brain development may be hampered during the critical prenatal and infant periods of life. Later in development body growth may decrease or stop, and the child may develop dry skin, become constipated, and show a decreased heart rate.

To prevent, or at least minimize, the effects of thyroid deficiency, early diagnosis is critical. Today many states have mandated screening for this deficiency during the first few days of life. Once the deficiency is found, the children are given daily dosages of thyroxine for as long as they continue to show a deficiency (Wong, 1993).

Conversely, an overproduction of thyroxine can cause sleeplessness, diarrhea, a slight tremor in the upper extremities, and an increase in appetite with no weight gain. Growth is usually unaffected in this condition. Treatment consists of the administration of a medication that blocks the production of thyroxine. In extreme cases surgery may be used to remove part or all of the thyroid gland, thus reducing the production of thyroxine. The child can then be given correct dosages of thyroxine on a daily basis.

Also influencing the growth of the child is a growth hormone that is produced in the pituitary gland. If this hormone is deficient or absent, growth is slowed or stopped and deviations appear on growth charts.

The hypothalamus stimulates the pituitary gland, which in turn stimulates the testes to produce testosterone and the ovaries to produce estrogen. Both of these hormones accelerate growth of the bones, assist in the fusion of the growth plate, and contribute to the development of secondary sex characteristics. These hormones can be deficient or exces-

---

### STUDY QUESTIONS

1. Describe the pathologic condition of cystic fibrosis. How does this disease affect the child's daily living function?
2. Describe osteogenesis imperfecta. What are precautions in working with a child with this diagnosis?
3. Name two general goals in intervention with children with juvenile rheumatoid arthritis. What is the typical course of this disease?
4. Describe the pathology of two different neuromuscular conditions. Explain how impairment in functional performance results from the pathologic condition.
5. List four functional performance consequences for children with cerebral palsy. Explain the difficulties that might be incurred in self-feeding in the child with (a) upper extremity spasticity and (b) upper extremity athetosis.
6. What are three impairments associated with myelomeningocele? Explain why a child with this diagnosis might have difficulty achieving independence in dressing.
7. Define autism and describe the primary problems that affect the child's ability to engage in social play with peers.
8. *Learning disabilities* is a term used to categorize a multitude of learning problems. Name two types of impairments that are categorized as learning disabilities.
9. The common infections that a mother can transmit to the fetus are called (S)TORCH infections. What are these five infections? Briefly describe each.
10. List three types of cancer common to children. Define the prognosis for each.

sive. A balance can be achieved through medication and hormone administration (Usala & Blumer, 1989).

## SUMMARY

This chapter has provided an overview of commonly oc-curing medical diagnoses in children who often receive oc-cupational therapy services. Knowledge about the child's medical condition is important for developing appropriate intervention plans and for communicating with family and team members. Application of this information should take into consideration that each child's presentation of the di-agnosis is unique and that the effect of the disease or dis-ability on the child's function is highly influenced by envi-ronmental and developmental variables. The field of medi-cine is in continual flux, and the occupational therapist must attempt to stay abreast of new developments and current information. Best practice requires thorough research of each diagnosis incurred. To assist in researching the impli-cation of the medical diagnoses discussed in this chapter, key references for each of the diagnoses have been cited and should be accessed to obtain additional information.

## REFERENCES

Abel, E.L. & Sokol, R.J. (1987). Incidence of fetal alcohol syndrome and economic impact of FAS-related anomalies. *Drug and Alcohol Dependence, 19,* 51-70.

Adams, J.C. (1981). *Outline of orthopedics* (9th ed.). New York: Churchill Livingstone.

Ammann, A.J., Cowan, M.J, & Wara, D.W. (1983). Acquired immu-nodeficiency in an infant: possible transmission by means of blood products. *Lancet, 1,* 956.

Ayres, A.J. & Tickle, L. (1980). Hyperresponsivity to touch and ves-tibular stimuli as a predictor of positive response to sensory inte-gration procedures in autistic children. *American Journal of Occu-pational Therapy, 34,* 375-340.

Batshaw, M.L., & Perret, Y.M. (Eds.). (1992). *Children with disabili-ties: a medical primer* (3rd ed.). Baltimore: Brookes.

Batshaw, M.L., Perret, Y.M. & Kurtz, L.A. (1992). Cerebral palsy. In M.L. Batshaw, & Y.M. Perret (Eds.). *Children with disabilities: a medical primer* (3rd ed.). Baltimore: Brookes.

Batshaw, M.L., Perret, Y.M. & Reber, M. (1992). Autism. In M.L. Bat-shaw & Y.M. Perret (Eds.). *Children with disabilities: a medical primer* (3rd ed.). Baltimore: Brookes.

Batshaw, M.L., Perret, Y.M. & Shapiro, B.K. (1992). Normal and ab-normal development: mental retardation. In M.L. Batshaw & Y.M. Perret (Eds.). *Children with disabilities: a medical primer* (3rd ed.). Baltimore: Brookes.

Behran, R.E. & Vaughan, V.C. (1987). *Nelson textbook of pediatrics.* (13th ed.). Philadelphia: W.B. Saunders.

Bluestone, C.D. (1989). Modern management of otitis media. *Pediat-ric Clinics of North America, 21,* 379.

Bobath, K. (1980). *A neurophysiological basis for the treatment of ce-rebral palsy.* Philadelphia: J.B. Lippincott.

Bobath, K. & Bobath, B. (1972). Cerebral palsy. In P.H. Pearson & C.E. Williams (Eds.). *Physical therapy services in the developmen-tal disabilities.* Springfield, IL: Charles C. Thomas.

Brashear, H.R. & Raney, R.B. (1986). *Handbook of orthopedic sur-gery* (10th ed.). St. Louis: Mosby.

Brooks, J.G. (1987) Respiratory tract and mediastinum. In C.H. Kempe, D. O'Brien, & H.K. Silver (Eds.). *Current pediatric diag-nosis and treatment* (9th ed.). Norwalk, CT: Appleton & Lange.

Brunell, P.A. (1987). Hepatitis. In R.E. Behran & V.C. Vaughan (Eds.). *Nelson textbook of pediatrics* (13th ed.). Philadelphia: W.B. Saun-ders.

Butler, K.M. & Pizzo, P.A. (1992). HIV infection in children. In V.T. DeVita, S. Hellman, & S.A. Rosenberg (Eds.). *AIDS: etiology, di-agnosis, treatment, and prevention* (3rd ed.). Philadelphia: J.B. Lip-pincott.

Carroll, J.E. (1985). Diagnosis and management of Duchenne muscu-lar dystrophy. *Pediatric Review, 6,* 195-200.

Champlin, R. (1988). Acute myelogenous leukemia: biology and treat-ment, *Mediguide to Oncology, 8*(4), 1-4, 6, 9.

Charney, E. (1992). Neural tube defects: spina bifida and myelomenin-gocele. In M.L. Batshaw & Y.M. Perret (Eds.). *Children with disabil-ities: a medical primer* (3rd ed.) (pp. 471-488). Baltimore: Brookes.

Clark, A.M. (1983). Burns in childhood. *World Journal of Surgery, 2,* 175.

Clark, E.B. (1992). Congenital heart disease. In R.A. Hockelman, B. Stanford, B. Friedman, N.M. Nelson, H.M. Seidel (Eds.). *Primary pediatric care* (2nd ed.). St. Louis: Mosby.

Cohen, H.J. (1992). Child and family. In A.C. Crocker, H.J. Cohen, & T.A. Kastner (Eds.). *HIV infection and developmental disabili-ties.* Baltimore: Brookes.

Collins, G., Calder, L., Rose, V., Kidd, L., & Keith, J. (1972). Ven-tricular septal defect: clinical and hemodynamic changes in the first five years of life. *American Heart Journal, 84,*(5), 695-705.

Conlon, C.J. (1992) New threats to development: alcohol, cocaine and AIDS. In M.L. Batshaw & Y.M. Perret (Eds.). *Children with dis-abilities: a medical primer* (3rd ed.). Baltimore: Brookes.

Curley, M.A. (1985) *Pediatric cardiac dysrhythmias.* Bowie, MD: Brady Communications.

Damasio, A.R. & Maurer, R.G. (1978). A neurological model for child-hood autism. *Archives of General Psychiatry, 35,* 777.

Day, N.L. (1992). Effects of prenatal alcohol exposure. In I.S. Zagon & T.A. Slotkin (Eds.). *Maternal substance abuse and the develop-ing nervous system.* San Diego: Academic Press.

Deitch, E.A. (1990). Management of burns. *New England Journal of Medicine, 323*(18), 1249-1253.

De La Cruz, M.V., Gomez, C.S. & Cayre, R. (1991). The devel-opmental components of the ventricles: their significance in con-genital heart malformations. *Cardiology with the Young, 1*(2), 123-128.

Diamond, G.W. & Cohen, H.J. (1992). Developmental disabilities in children with HIV infection. In A.C. Crocker, H.J. Cohen, & T.A. Kastner (Eds.). *HIV infection and developmental disabilities.* Bal-timore: Brookes.

Dodson, W.E. (1989). Medical treatment and pharmacology of anti-epileptic drugs. *Pediatric Clinics of North America, 36,* 421-433.

Doershuk, C.F. & Boat, T.F. (1987). Cystic fibrosis. In R.E. Behran & V.C. Vaughan (Eds.). *Nelson textbook of pediatrics* (13th ed.). Philadelphia: W.B. Saunders.

Drash, A. (1989). Insulin-dependent diabetes mellitus. *Nursing Clin-ics of North America, 20,* 191-198.

Eadie, M.J. (1984). Anticonvulsant drugs: an update. *Drugs, 27,* 328-363.

Eisen, A. & Humphreys, P. (1974). Guillian-Barré syndrome. *Archives of Neurology, 30,* 438.

Engle, M.A. (1972). Ventricular septal defects: status report for the seventies. *Cardiovascular Clinics, 4,* 282.

Evans, J.P.M. & Rogers, D.W. (1990). Sickle cell disease and thalassemia. *Current Opinion in Pediatrics, 2*(1), 121-123.

Feldman, H.A. & Remington, J.S. (1987). Toxoplasmosis. In R.E. Behran & V.C. Vaughan (Eds.). *Nelson textbook of pediatrics* (13th ed.). Philadelphia: W.B. Saunders.

Fils, D.H. (1978). *The developmental disabilities handbook.* Los Angeles: Western Psychological Services.

Fiorentino, M.R. (1981). *A basis for sensorimotor development: normal and abnormal.* Springfield, IL: Charles C. Thomas.

Foreman, J. & Chan, J. (1988). Chronic renal failure in infants and children. *Journal of Pediatrics, 113,* 793-800.

Gallico, R. & Lewis, M.E.B. (1992). Learning disabilities. In M.L. Batshaw & Y.M. Perret (Eds.). *Children with disabilities: a medical primer* (3rd ed.). (pp. 365-385). Baltimore: Brookes.

Graley, J. (1994). A path to the mainstream of life: facilitated communication/behavior/inclusion: three interacting ingredients. *Proceedings of the 1994 Autism Society of America Conference.* Arlington, TX: Future Education.

Griffiths, S.P. (1992). Rheumatic fever. In R.A. Hoekelman B. Stanford, B. Friedman, N.M. Nelson, & H.M. Seidel (Eds.). *Primary pediatric care* (2nd ed.). St. Louis: Mosby.

Hammill, D.D. (1990). On defining learning disabilities: an emerging consensus. *Journal of Learning Disabilities, 23*(2), 74-84.

Hansell, M.J. (1988). Fractures and the healing process. *Orthopedic Nursing, 7*(1), 43-49.

Hockenberry, M.J. & Coody, D.K. (1986). *Pediatric oncology and hematology: perspectives on care,* St. Louis: Mosby.

Hollister, J.R. (1987). Rheumatic diseases. In C.H. Kempe, D. O-brien, & H.K. Silver (Eds.). *Current pediatric diagnosis and treatment* (9th ed.). Norwalk, CT: Appleton & Lange.

Howlin, P. & Rutter, M. (1987). *Treatment of autistic children.* New York: John Wiley & Sons.

Hutton, C. (1994). Awakening of autism: facilitated communication and sensory integration as dual tools to reach the autistic. *Proceedings of the 1994 Autism Society of America Conference.* Arlington, TX: Future Education.

Jaffe, K.M. & Hays, R.M. (1986). Pediatric head injury: rehabilitative medical management. *Journal of Head Trauma Rehabilitation, 1,* 30-40.

Jennett, B. & Teasdale, G. (1981). *Management of head injuries.* Philadelphia: F.A. Davis.

Jones, K.L. (1986). Fetal alcohol syndrome. *Pediatrics in Review, 18,* 122.

Kennard, M.J. (1990). Cocaine use during pregnancy: fetal and neonatal effects. *Journal of Perinatal and Neonatal Nursing, 3*(4), 53-63.

Kyllerman, M. (1986). The epidemiology of chronic neurologic diseases in children in Sweden. In J.H. Rench, S. Harel, & P. Casaer (Eds.). *Child neurology and developmental disabilities.* Baltimore: Brookes.

Levy, S.E. & Pilmer, S.L. (1992). The technology assisted child. In M.L. Batshaw & Y.M. Perret (Eds.). *Children with disabilities: a medical primer* (3rd ed.) (pp. 137-157). Baltimore: Brookes.

Lusher, J.M. (1989). Management of hemophilia. In R.G. Westphal & D.M. Smith, (Eds.). *Treatment of hemophilia and von Willebrand's disease: new developments.* Arlington, VA: American Association of Blood Banks.

Lyons, B.A. & Valentine, P. (1994) Prevention. In R.D. Muma, B.A. Lyons, M.J. Borucki, & E.B. Pollard (Eds.). *HIV: manual for health care professionals.* Norwalk, CT: Appleton & Lange.

McCullough, F.L. (1989). Sketetal trauma in children. *Orthopedic Nursing, 8*(2), 41-50.

McIntosh, K. & Lauer, B.A. (1987). Infections: bacterial and spirochetal. In C.H. Kempe, D. O'Brien & H.K. Silver (Eds.). *Current pediatric diagnosis and treatment* (9th ed.). Norwalk, CT: Appleton & Lange.

Malinowski, P. & Elixson, E.M. (1985). Transposition of the great arteries. *Critical Care Nurse, 5*(3), 35-48.

Malinowski, P. & Yablonski, D. (1986). Congenital heart disease in infants: nursing assessment. *Critical Care Quarterly, 9*(2), 6-23.

Maul-Mellott, S.K. & Adams, J.N. (1987). *Childhood cancer: a nursing overview.* Boston: Jones and Bartlett.

Melvin, J.L. (1989). *Rheumatic disease in the child and adult: Occupational therapy and rehabilitation* (3rd ed.). Philadelphia: F.A. Davis.

Menkes, J.H. (1990). *Textbook of child neurology* (4th ed.). Philadelphia: Lea & Febiger.

Michaud, L.J. & Duhaime, A.C. (1992). Traumatic brain injury. In M.L. Batshaw & Y.M. Perret (Eds.). *Children with disabilities: a medical primer* (3rd ed.) (pp. 525-546). Baltimore: Brookes.

Milne, R.I.G. (1990). Assessment of care of children with sickle cell disease: implications for neonatal screening programs. *British Medical Journal, 300,* 371-374.

Minshew, N.J. & Payton, J.B. (1988). New perspectives in autism. Part I. The clinical spectrum of autism. Part II. The differential diagnosis and neurobiology of autism. *Current Problems in Pediatrics, 18,* 561-694.

Monett, Z. & Moynihan, P. (1991). Cardiovascular assessment of the neonatal heart. *Journal of Perinatal Neonatal Nursing, 5*(2), 50-59.

Moser, H.M. (1985). *Prenatal/perinatal factors associated with brain disorders* (NIH Publication T5-1149). Washington, DC: U.S. Government Printing Office.

National Society for Autistic Children. (1980). *Autism fact sheet.* Washington, DC: National Society for Autistic Children.

New York University Staff. (1982). *Upper limb prosthetics.* New York: New York University Post-Graduate Medical School.

Novak, D.A, Suchy, F.J., & Balistreri, W.F. (1990). Disorders of the liver and biliary system relevant to clinical practice. In F.A. Oski, C.D. DeAngelis, R.D. Feigin, J.B. Warshaw (Eds.). *Principles and practice in pediatrics.* Philadelphia: J.B. Lippincott.

Ornitz, E. (1973). Childhood autism: a review of the clinical and experimental literature. *California Medicine, 118,* 21.

Page, R.B. (1992). Hydrocephalus. In R.A. Hoekelman et al. (Eds.). *Primary pediatric care* (2nd ed.). St. Louis: Mosby.

Pizzo, P.A. & Poplack, D.G. (1989). *Principles and practice of pediatric oncology.* Philadeplphia: J.B. Lippincott.

Pizzo, P.A. & Wilfert, C. (Eds.). (1991). *Pediatric AIDS: the challenge of HIV infection in infants, children and adolescents.* Baltimore: Williams & Wilkins.

Pollard, R.B. (1994) Introduction. In R.D. Muma, B.A. Lyons, M.J. Borucki, & R.B. Pollard (Eds.). *HIV: manual for health care professionals.* Norwalk, CT: Appleton & Lange.

Powell, K.R. (1992). Meningitis. In R.A. Hoekelman, B. Stanford, B. Friedman, N.M. Nelson, & H.M. Seidel (Eds.). *Primary pediatric care* (2nd ed.). St. Louis: Mosby.

Pryse-Phillips, W. & Murray, T.J. (1982). *Essential neurology* (2nd ed.). Garden City, NY: Medical Examination.

Pueschel, S.M. & Pueschel, J.K. (1992). *Biomedical concerns in persons with Down Syndrome.* Baltimore: Brookes.

Raphaely, R.C., Swedlow, D.B., Downes, J.J., & Bruce, C.A. (1980). Management of severe pediatric head trauma. *Pediatric Clinics of North America, 27,* 715.

Rapin, I. (1991). Autistic children: diagnosis and clinical features. *Pediatrics, 87,* 761-766.

Rennebohm R. & Correll, J.K. (1984). Comprehensive management of juvenile rheumatoid arthritis. *Nursing Clinics of North America, 19,* 647-662.

Roberts, K.B. (1979). *Manual of clinical problems in pediatrics.* Boston: Little, Brown.

Ropper, A.H. (1992). The Guillain-Barré syndrome. *New England ournal of Medicine, 326*(17), 1130-1136.

Rubenstein, A. (1986). Schooling for children with acquired immunodeficiency syndrome. *Journal of Pediatrics, 109,* 242.

Rumsey, J.M., Rapoport, J.L., & Sceery, W.R. (1985). Autistic children as adults: psychiatric, social and behavioral outcomes. *Journal of the American Academy of Child Psychiatry, 24,* 465-473.

Rutter, M. (1985). The treatment of autistic children. *Journal of Child Psychology and Psychiatry and Allied Disciplines, 26,* 193-214.

Salter, R.B. (1983). *Textbook of disorders and injuries of the musculoskeletal system* (2nd ed.). Baltimore: Williams & Wilkins.

Scherzer, A.L. & Tscharnuter, I. (1990). *Early diagnosis and treatment in cerebral palsy: a primer on infant developmental problems.* New York: Marcel Dekker.

Scoles, P.V. (1982). *Pediatric orthopedics in clinical practice.* Chicago: Year Book Medical Publishers.

Shapiro, B.K. & Batshaw, M.L. (1993). Mental retardation. In F.D. Burg (Ed.). *Current pediatric therapy* (14th ed.). Philadelphia: W.B. Saunders.

Shaywitz, S.E. & Shaywitz, B.A. (1987). Attention deficit disorder: current perspectives. *Pediatric Neurology, 3,* 129-135.

Siegel, J.D. (1990a). Toxoplasmosis. In F.A. Oski, C.D. DeAngelis, R.D. Feigin, & J.B. Warshaw (Eds.). *Principles and practice in pediatrics.* Philadelphia: J.B. Lippincott.

Siegel, J.D. (1990b). Rubella. In F.A. Oski, C.D. DeAngelis, R.D. Feigin, & J.B. Warshaw. (Eds.). *Principles and practice in pediatrics.* Philadelphia: J.B. Lippincott.

Simon, M.A. (1988). Limb salvage for osteosarcoma, *Journal of Bone and Joint Surgery, 70A,* 307-310.

Simonds, R.J. & Rogers, M.F. (1992). Epidemiology of HIV infection in children and other populations. In A.C. Crocker, H.J. Cohen, & T.A. Kastner (Eds.). *HIV infection and developmental disabilities.* Baltimore: Brookes.

Speck, W.T. (1987). Lyme disease. In R.E. Behran & V.C. Vaughan (Eds.). *Nelson textbook of pediatrics* (13th ed.). Philadelphia: W.B. Saunders.

Stephenson, K.S. (1994). Pediatric HIV infection. In R.D. Muma, B.A. Lyons, M.J. Borucki, & R.B. Pollard (Eds.). *HIV: manual for health care professionals.* Norwalk, CT: Appleton & Lange.

Streissguth, A.P., Clarren, S.K., & Jones, K.L. (1985). Natural history of the fetal alcohol syndrome: a 10 year follow-up of 11 patients. *Lancet, 2,* 89.

Teberg, A.J., Walther, F.J., & Pena, I.C. (1988). Mortality, morbidity, and outcome of the small-for-gestational age infant. *Seminars in Perinatology, 12,* 84-94.

Thomas, N.H. & Dubowitz, V. (1989). Muscular dystrophy and other muscle disorders. *Current Opinion in Pediatrics, 1,* 296-300.

Tizzano, E.F. & Buchwald, M. (1992). Cystic fibrosis: beyond the gene to therapy, *Journal of Pediatrics, 120*(3), 337-349.

Travis, L.B., Brouhard, B.H., & Scheiener, B. (1987). *Diabetes mellitus in children.* Philadeplphia: W.B. Saunders.

Usala, A. & Blumer, J.L. (1989). Pharmacology of new hormonal therapists in the treatment of pediatric endocrine disorders. *Pediatric Clinics of North America, 36,* 1157-1182.

Walker, C.H.M. (1980). Rheumatic fever and rheumatic heart disease. In G. Graham & E. Rossi (Eds.). *Heart disease in infants and children.* London: Edward Arnold.

Wallace, C.A. & Levinson, J.E. (1991). Juvenile rheumatoid arthritis: outcome and treatment for the 1990s. *Rheumatic Diseases Clinics of North America, 17,* 891-905.

Weil, M.L. (1990). Infections of the nervous system. In J.H. Menkes (Ed.). *Textbook of child neurology.* (4th ed.). Philadelphia: Lea & Febiger.

Weiss, R. (1988). Management of chronic renal failure, *Pediatric Annuals, 17,* 584-589.

Wing, L. (1988). The continuum of autistic characteristics. In E. Schopler & G.B. Mesibov (Eds.). *Diagnosis and assessment in autism* (pp. 91-110). New York: Plenum Press.

Wong, D.L. (1993). *Whaley and Wong's essentials of pediatric nursing* (4th ed.). St. Louis: Mosby.

Ylvisaker, M. (Ed.). (1985). *Head injury rehabilitation: children and adolescents.* San Diego: College-Hill Press.

Zinkus, P.W., Gottleib, M.L., & Shapiro, M. (1978). Developmental psychoeducational sequelae of chronic otitis media. *American Journal of Diseases of Children, 132,* 1100.

Zuckerman, B. & Frank, D.A. (1992). Prenatal cocaine and marijuana exposure: research and clinical implications. In I.S. Zagon & T.A. Slotkin (Eds.). *Maternal substance abuse and the developing nervous system.* San Diego: Academic Press.

## SUGGESTED READINGS

Batshaw, M.L. & Perret, Y.M. (Eds.). (1992). *Children with disabilities: a medical primer* (3rd ed.). Baltimore: Brookes.

Behran, R.E., & Vaughan, V.C. (1987). *Nelson textbook of pediatrics* (13th ed.). Philadelphia: W.B. Saunders.

Brashear, H.R. & Raney, R.B. (1986). *Handbook of orthopedic surgery* (10th ed.). St. Louis: Mosby.

Menkes, J.H. (1990). *Textbook of child neurology* (4th ed.). Philadelphia: Lea & Febiger.

Thomas, C.L. (1981). *Taber's cyclopedic medical dictionary.* Philadelphia: F.A. Davis.

Wong, D.L. (Ed.). (1993). *Whaley and Wong's essentials of pediatric nursing* (4th ed.). St. Louis: Mosby.

# Occupational Therapy Assessment in Pediatrics

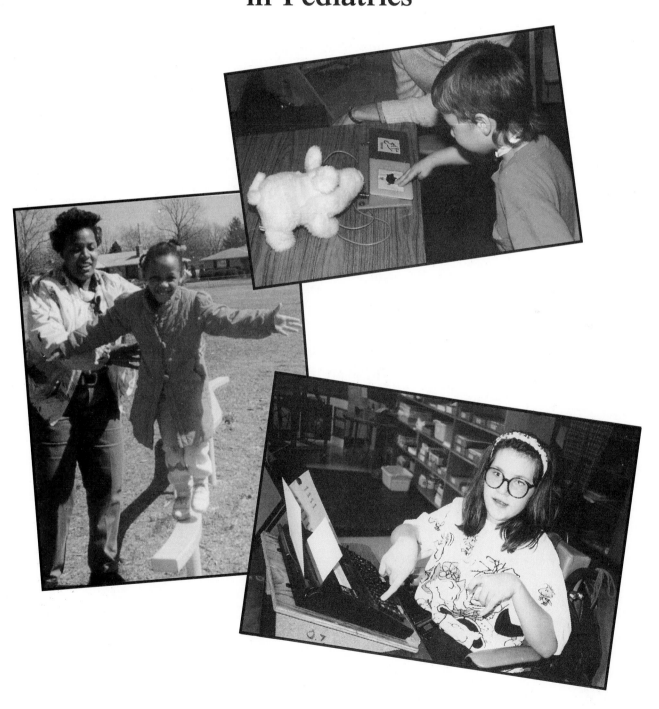

# Occupational Therapy Assessment in Pediatrics

## *Purposes, Process, and Methods of Evaluation*

KATHERINE B. STEWART

▲ Assessment
▲ Functional Assessments
▲ Screening
▲ Comprehensive Evaluation
▲ Reevaluation
▲ Clinical Research
▲ Standardized Tests
▲ Clinical Observations
▲ Developmental Quotient
▲ Referral
▲ Evaluation Plan
▲ Norm-Referenced Measures
▲ Criterion-Referenced Measures
▲ Ecologic Assessments
▲ Skilled Observation
▲ Interviews with Caregivers
▲ Arena Assessments

## CHAPTER OBJECTIVES

1. Recognize the general domains of the pediatric occupational therapy assessment.
2. Define the key terms used in pediatric occupational therapy assessments.
3. List four primary reasons assessments are conducted, and discuss the variety of decisions pediatric occupational therapists make throughout the assessment process.
4. Describe the specific steps pediatric occupational therapists follow in the process of assessing children.

5. Describe the primary evaluation methods commonly used in pediatric occupational therapy.
6. Discuss the major factors that therapists should consider when selecting evaluation methods and measures.
7. Apply the knowledge gained in this chapter to specific case situations of children at risk for or with disabilities.

Those who observe human behavior must be vigilant when examining the details of the behavior and at the same time relate those details to each other within the context of that behavior. Pediatric occupational therapists involved in the assessment of and intervention with children are faced with this challenge. Inherent in assessing occupational performance in children is viewing the child within the context of his or her environment. While carefully evaluating the performance components of sensorimotor, cognitive, psychosocial, and psychologic aspects of the child's development, the occupational therapist determines the functional abilities of that child in performance areas such as activities of daily living (ADL), school-related activities, and play or leisure. To do this fully, the therapist must also consider the sociocultural and physical characteristics of the child's natural environments (e.g., home, classroom, and playground).

The assessment process is one of the most fundamental, yet complex, aspects of occupational therapy services. Bailey and Wolery (1989) defined *assessment* as the "process of gathering information for the purpose of making a decision" (p. 2). How the occupational therapist views this assessment process, whether the therapist is open to new ways of understanding the child, which methods and measures the therapist selects to evaluate the child, and how the therapist interprets and documents the assessment data, all contribute to the important decisions concerning which occupational therapy services will be provided for the child and the family.

The purpose of this chapter is to describe the occupational therapy assessment process with children. The first section of the chapter defines the domains of practice and provides a conceptual framework for assessing children. The second section outlines the purposes of assessment and includes specific examples common in pediatric occupational therapy practice. The third section of the chapter describes the assessment process and provides clinical examples. The fourth section of the chapter explains the general methods, measures, and principles used in selecting and administering pediatric occupational therapy assessments.

Four primary concepts are reinforced throughout this chapter: (1) the assessment of a child is an ongoing, dynamic process that begins with the initial referral for therapy and continues throughout the intervention and discharge phases of occupational therapy services; (2) assessments should be ecologically and culturally valid; (3) the views and priorities of the child's primary caregiver should be held central throughout the assessment process; and (4) the outcome of the assessment should be an in-depth understanding of the child's functional abilities in performance components and occupational performance areas.

## DOMAINS

The American Occupational Therapy Association's (AOTA's) document on *Uniform Terminology for Occupational Therapy,* 3rd ed. (AOTA, 1994) outlines the basic domains of occupational therapy assessment (see Appendix 8-A). Performance areas, performance components, and performance context are the three main categories all occupational therapists consider in assessment.

An essential responsibility of the therapist is to provide *functional assessments* and interventions for children with special needs. Bundy (1991) recommended that pediatric occupational therapists write functional outcome goals that have obvious relevance to the child's performance in day-to-day tasks. To write functional goals, the therapist evaluates the child's performance areas and asks meaningful questions to the caregivers regarding the child's functional performance (Figure 8-1).

Although the assessment of performance areas is of primary concern for the occupational therapist, most of the evaluation tools used currently by therapists measure children's performance components. Performance components are the sensorimotor, cognitive, psychosocial, and psychologic skills essential for the attainment of function in performance areas. Sensorimotor components in children include sensory, neuromuscular, and motor skills. Standard-

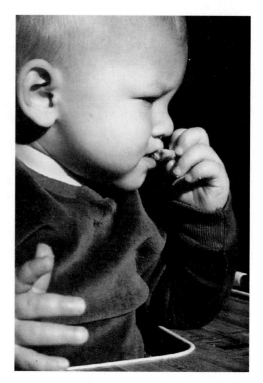

**Figure 8-1**    Infant learning to finger-feed.

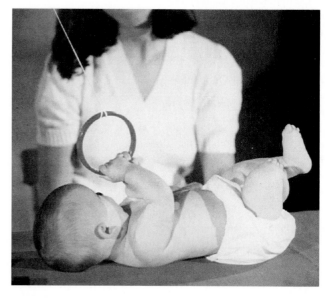

**Figure 8-2**    Movement Assessment of Infants test item: posture in supine.

ized instruments commonly used by pediatric occupational therapists to evaluate neuromuscular and motor components of performance include the Movement Assessment of Infants (Chandler, Andrews, & Swanson, 1980) (Figure 8-2), the Peabody Developmental Motor Scales (PDMS; Folio & Fewell, 1983), the Miller Assessment for Preschoolers

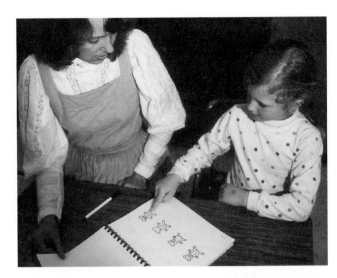

**Figure 8-3**    Administration of the Motor Free Visual Perception Test.

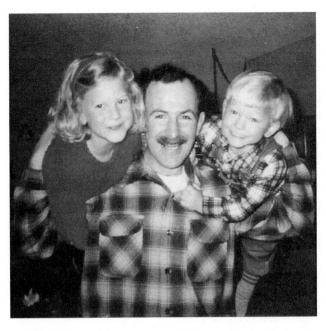

**Figure 8-4**    Family environment: father playing with his two children.

(Miller, 1982), and the Bruininks-Oseretsky Test of Motor Proficiency (Bruininks, 1978). The Sensory Integration and Praxis Tests (Ayres, 1989) and the Motor Free Visual Perception Test (Colarusso & Hammill, 1972) are examples of tests that measure sensory processing and perceptual skill components (Figure 8-3).

Cognitive integration (e.g., orientation, recognition, attention span, memory, and problem solving) and psychosocial (e.g., psychologic, social, and self-management skills) performance components are often assessed by the occupational therapist through direct observations of the child during everyday tasks within the child's natural environments. An example of this is recording attention span while the child is in the classroom, observing the child's social behavior on the playground, and watching the child problem-solve a new task at home. The Early Coping Inventory (Zeitlin, Williamson, & Szczepanski, 1988) and the Coping Inventory (Zeitlin, 1985) are observational instruments that assess a child's coping effectiveness across various environments. Williamson, Szczepanski, and Zeitlin (1993) describe a theoretical model of the coping frame of reference useful for occupational therapists when assessing the adaptive process or coping in children. According to Williamson et al. (1993), function or dysfunction is determined by the goodness-of-fit between the demands of the environment and the child's available coping resources. The box on p. 168 lists examples of measures used to assess performance areas and components in children.

When assessing performance components in the cognitive and psychosocial domains, the pediatric occupational therapist works in conjunction with parents and professionals from other disciplines, including psychology, social work, nursing, education and special education, speech pathology, and pediatrics. The interdisciplinary nature of assessment in the cognitive and psychosocial domains is essential for a comprehensive, accurate understanding of a child's abilities and limitations.

To gain a more in-depth understanding of the child's abilities and limitations, the occupational therapist must also assess the features of the environments in which the child performs the tasks. The performance context, outlined as the third domain of concern in *Uniform Terminology for Occupational Therapy*, 3rd ed. (AOTA, 1994), refers to the physical, temporal, and sociocultural features of the child's environments. Considering the context of the child's environments (e.g., home, classroom, and playground) is a critical process in occupational therapy assessments. Children and their families (Figure 8-4) are embedded in a network of social system including extended family, friends, neighbors, day care, schools, medical and religious institutions, and cultural groups (Bronfenbrenner, Moen & Garbarino, 1984). To thoroughly understand a child and his or her development, therapists must view the child within the context of these social environments. Dunn, Brown, and McGuigan (1994, p. 595) reported the following:

... occupational therapy has many assessments that examine muscle strength, social skills, vestibular function, dressing, or use of leisure time. However, contextual features such as the physical qualities of an environment, the cultural background of the person, or the effect of friendships on performance are often missing from assessment tools typically used in occupational therapy.

The therapist should consider the nonhuman (e.g., space, objects, and time) and the human (e.g., relationships with peers and caregivers and cultural and societal values) demands and supports within the child's environment.

## Examples of Evaluations Categorized by Performance Areas, Components, and Context

### PERFORMANCE AREAS

Pediatric Evaluation of Disability Inventory (Haley, Coster, Ludlow, Haltiwanger, & Andrellos, 1992)

Developmental Checklist for Pre-Dressing Skills (Dunn-Klein, 1983)

Pediatric Assessment of Self-Care Activities (Coley, 1978)

Preschool Play Scale (Knox, 1974; Bledsoe & Shepherd, 1982)

Play Skills Inventory (Takata, 1974)

Play Assessment Scale (Fewell, 1986)

Adolescent Role Assessment (Black, 1976)

Transdisciplinary Play-Based Assessment: A Functional Approach to Working With Children (Linder, 1990)

Children's Handwriting Evaluation Scale (Phelps & Stempel, 1987)

Test of Legible Handwriting (Larsen & Hammill, 1989)

### PERFORMANCE COMPONENTS
#### Developmental Screening Tools

First STEP (Miller, 1993)

Miller Assessment for Preschoolers (Miller, 1982)

Denver Developmental Screening Test—Revised (Frankenburg et al., 1990)

Infant Monitoring System (Bricker & Squires, 1989)

#### Developmental Comprehensive Evaluations

Assessment of Preterm Infant Behavior (Als, Lester, Tronick, & Brazelton, 1982)

Brazelton Neonatal Behavioral Assessment Scale (Brazelton, 1984)

Bayley Scales of Infant Development (Bayley, 1993)

Gesell Developmental Schedules (Knobloch, Stephens, & Malone, 1980)

Developmental Programming for Infants and Young Children (Schafer & Moersch, 1981)

Early Intervention Developmental Profile (Rogers, D'Eugenio, Brown, Donovan, & Lynch, 1981)

Vulpe Assessment Battery—Revised (Vulpe, 1994)

Brigance Diagnostic Inventories (Brigance, 1978)

Battelle Developmental Inventory (Newborg, Stock, Wneck, Guidubaldi, & Svinicki, 1984)

Hawaii Early Learning Profile (Furuno et al., 1979)

Vineland Adaptive Behavior Scales (Sparrow, Balla, & Cicchetti, 1984)

Carolina Curriculum for Handicapped Infants (Johnson-Martin, Jens, & Attemeier, 1986)

#### Sensory/Sensory Integration

Test of Sensory Functions in Infants (DeGangi & Greenspan, 1989)

DeGangi-Berk Sensory Integration Test (Berk & DeGangi, 1983)

Sensory Integration and Praxis Tests (Ayres, 1989)

Erhardt Developmental Vision Assessment (Erhardt, 1988)

Test of Visual Perceptual Skills (Gardner, 1988)

Motor Free Visual Perception Test (Colarusso & Hammill, 1972)

#### Neuromuscular

Movement Assessment of Infants (Chandler, Andrews, & Swanson, 1980)

Alberta Infant Motor Scale (Piper & Darrah, 1994)

Toddler and Infant Motor Evaluation (Miller & Roid, 1994)

Test of Infant Motor Performance (Campbell et al., 1993)

Quick Neurological Screening Test (Mutti, Sterling, & Spalding, 1978)

#### Motor

Peabody Developmental Motor Scales (Folio & Fewell, 1983)

Bruininks-Oseretsky Test of Motor Proficiency (Bruininks, 1978)

Gross Motor Function Test (Russell et al., 1989)

Milani-Comparetti Motor Development Screening Test (Milani-Comparetti & Gidoni, 1967)

Test of Visual-Motor Skills (Gardner, 1986)

Erhardt Developmental Prehension Assessment (Erhardt, 1982)

Exner's In-Hand Manipulation Test (Exner, 1993)

#### Cognitive Integration and Cognitive Components

Learning Accomplishment Profile (Sanford & Zelman, 1981)

Carolina Record of Infant Behavior (Simeonsson, 1979)

#### Psychosocial Skills and Psychologic Components

Uzgiris-Hunt Ordinal Scales of Psychological Development (Uzgiris & Hunt, 1975)

Piers-Harris Children's Self-Concept Scale (Piers, 1984)

Carey Infant Temperament Scale (Carey & McDevitt, 1978)

Early Coping Inventory (Zeitlin et al., 1988)

Coping Inventory (Zeitlin, 1985)

### PERFORMANCE CONTEXT

NCAST Caregiver/Parent-Child Interaction: Feeding Manual (Barnard, 1993)

NCAST Caregiver/Parent-Child Interaction: Teaching Manual (Barnard, 1993)

Parent and Caregiver Involvement Scale (Farran, Kasari, & Jay, 1984)

Home Observation and Measurement of the Environment (Caldwell & Bradley, 1978)

Parent Behavior Progression (Bromwich, 1981)

To comprehensively assess a child with special needs, the occupational therapist must understand the interface between the child's abilities and the environmental demands. Sameroff and Chandler (1975) conceptualized an intervention model that described the transactional effects of familial, social, and environmental factors on human development. Longitudinal research in this area supports the notion that a child's social and family environments act to foster or impede the continuing positive developmental course of the child (Sameroff, 1986; Werner & Smith, 1982). Sameroff and Fiese (1990) suggested that intervention programs cannot be successful if changes are made only in the individual child. In the transactional model the child's developmental outcomes are neither a function of the individual child alone nor of the child's environment alone. Outcomes are a product of the combination of the individual and his or her experience. Therefore occupational therapists must recognize the importance of the reciprocal, transactional nature of the child and his or her environment.

Primarily informal methods are needed to evaluate the environment. Observation of the child at home or in the classroom provides this information. An understanding of the variety of contexts in which the child functions must be gained through observation over time and at different times during the day and week. Often this information is gained through interview with the child's primary caregivers and teachers.

## Application of Domains of Concern

The following case study highlights how specific evaluation measures were selected within the domains of concern

of occupational therapy for a child with developmental delay.

### Description of Child

Kevin is a 6-year-old boy with developmental delay and an attention deficit disorder. Specific deficits that limit Kevin's occupational performance at school and at home include his extreme hyperactivity, fine and gross motor coordination problems, possible visual perceptual deficits, and difficulties in peer interaction.

### Description of Classroom Environment

Kevin attends a developmental preschool classroom that consists of 14 children ranging in age from 3 years to 6 years. Four of the children are nondisabled, and 10 of the children exhibit mild to moderate developmental delays in speech and language, behavior, or motor skills.

### Description of the Home Environment

Kevin lives with his mother, father, and 3- and 4-year-old younger brothers. The family recently moved to a two-bedroom, one-bath home with a kitchen and living room. Financial resources are limited. The father, who describes himself as having a learning disability, works part-time as a gardener. The home is situated on a busy urban street in a lower socioeconomic neighborhood. The mother, who does not work outside the home, reported that she attended special education classes throughout her childhood. When asked what they hoped Kevin could accomplish at school in the next year, the parents said they wanted him to become independent in toileting, to print his first name, and to make friends with other children (Figure 8-5).

Given this information, the evaluation measures listed in Table 8-1 would be appropriate options for the occupational therapist to consider when assessing Kevin's performance areas, performance

▲ Table 8-1   Appropriate Measures for Kevin's Assessment

| Assessment Categories | Evaluation Measures | Rationale |
| --- | --- | --- |
| Performance areas | Pediatric Evaluation of Disability Inventory | To assess functional status in activities of daily living |
| | Functional Behavior Assessment for Children with Sensory Integrative Dysfunction | To objectively rate child's behavior on specific functional life tasks |
| Performance components | Peabody Developmental Motor Scales | To assess gross and fine motor skills |
| | Transdisciplinary Play-Based Assessment | To assess development in context of play |
| | Clinical observations of neuromotor status | To assess child's muscle tone, range of motion, presence of primitive reflexes, automatic reactions, posture, and quality of movement |
| | Test of Visual Perceptual Skills | To assess child's visual perception |
| | Informal observations of cognitive and psychosocial skills | To gain insight into child's performance on everyday tasks |
| | Coping Inventory (preschool version) | To assess child's overall coping style and identify adaptive coping attributes |
| Performance context | Home Observation for Measurement of the Environment | To assess home characteristics related to child's development |
| | Interviews with parents, teachers, and other caregivers | To gain insight into perceptions of child's caregivers regarding child's performance on functional tasks |

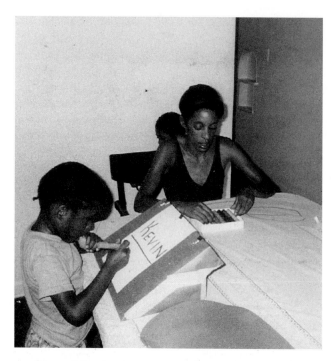

**Figure 8-5**   Kevin learning to print his name at home.

components, and performance context. However, the reader must understand that assessments of this child would occur over time and would be ongoing with the initiation of occupational therapy services. Refer to the section on the process of evaluation for more specific guidance on the sequence of the assessment process.

In summary, the occupational therapy assessment plan should stem from the theoretical base of occupational therapy and include measures of the child's occupational performance areas, specific performance component skills, and the performance context in which the child performs daily functional tasks. With this theoretic foundation in mind, the therapist must then consider the many different purposes of an assessment.

## PURPOSES

Pediatric occupational therapy assessments are multifaceted, with a focus on obtaining information about the child's developmental and functional status. As mentioned previously, the definition of assessment is the process of gathering information for the purpose of making a decision. The following section discusses the decisions occupational therapists make through various steps of careful screening and comprehensive evaluation of children at risk for or with disabilities.

The six primary purposes for occupational therapy assessment include (1) to decide if the child should be further assessed, using more comprehensive evaluations; (2) to decide if the child is eligible for occupational therapy services; (3) to assist in the diagnostic process; (4) to develop an intervention plan; (5) to evaluate the child's progress in therapy and decide if further therapy is war-

ranted; and (6) to research the efficacy of intervention services or to describe patterns of development and functional changes in children with specific diagnoses.

## Screening

The primary reason to screen children is to determine if they warrant further, more comprehensive evaluations. There are two levels of *screening* in which pediatric occupational therapists may participate. The first level (type I) is a basic screening in which children's general health (e.g., vision and hearing), growth (e.g., weight and height), and development (physical, social, language, and personal and adaptive skills) are checked. In some settings, such as public school programs, occupational therapists may participate in screening large numbers of children to determine which children should receive further testing. Public policies, including the Individuals with Disabilities Education Act (IDEA), Head Start, and Medicaid programs for children, mandate early screening activities to identify those children at risk for disabilities. Some examples of developmental screening tools useful for basic screening of children include the Infant Monitoring System (Bricker & Squires, 1989), the Denver Developmental Screening Test—Revised (Frankenburg et al., 1990) and the First STEP (Miller, 1993). The pediatric therapist can refer to several resources for an overview of developmental screening tools (Bailey & Wolery, 1989; Collier, 1991; Gibbs & Teti, 1990; Glascoe, Martin & Humphrey, 1990).

More frequently, pediatric therapists are involved in the second level of screening children (type II). This type of screening usually occurs after the child has been identified by a health or educational professional as being at risk for developmental or functional deficits. The child is then referred to the pediatric occupational therapist to obtain a more focused screen of the child's development. At this point in the screening process the therapist, oftentimes with other interdisciplinary team members, determines whether the child is a candidate for more comprehensive testing and, if so, what developmental or functional areas need further assessment. For example, a kindergarten teacher may observe a child's clumsiness in the classroom and refer the child to the occupational or physical therapist to determine if the child needs a comprehensive motor assessment. In this case the therapist may choose the Quick Neurological Screening Test (Mutti, Sterling, & Spalding, 1978) or the Bruininks-Oseretsky Test of Motor Proficiency—Short Form (Bruininks, 1978) (Figures 8-6 and 8-7).

In addition to administering a standardized screening tool, the therapist gathers pertinent information from the child's parents and teachers as well as from informal observations of the child's performance in his or her natural environments (e.g., classroom, playground, and home).

Regardless of the setting and the level of screening (type I or type II), the therapist should consider the following

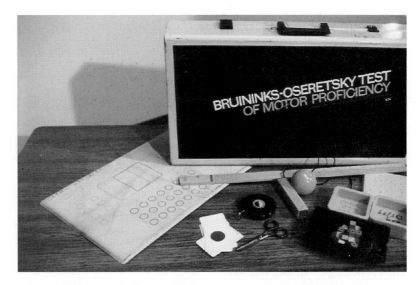

**Figure 8-6**    Bruininks-Oseretsky Test of Motor Proficiency.

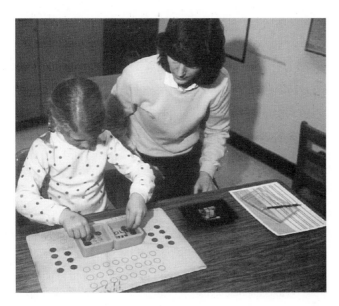

**Figure 8-7**    Child completing a Bruininks-Oseretsky Test of Motor Proficiency item.

points when screening children to determine if they warrant further, more comprehensive assessment:

1. Standardized screening tools should be implemented whenever possible to ensure that results of the screening are reliable and valid. *Standardized tests* require uniform procedures for administration and scoring. Refer to Chapter 9 for more specific information on using standardized instruments.
2. In addition to standardized screening tools, the therapist should gather relevant information from the child's teacher, parents, or other caregivers.
3. Information gathered during the screening process should include the child's performance across a vari-

ety of developmental domains and in different environments to substantiate the need for further assessment.
4. Screening tools should be carefully evaluated for their cultural validity, and the results should be interpreted cautiously when administered to children from diverse cultural backgrounds. A few instruments, such as the Miller Assessment for Preschoolers (Miller, 1982) have established norms for different ethnic populations.

## Comprehensive Evaluations

The primary role of occupational therapists in the assessment process is *comprehensive evaluation* of the children they serve. It is important for the therapist to keep clearly in mind the purpose of comprehensive assessment because, depending on the purpose, the therapist may select different methods and measures for the assessment. The primary evaluations used by occupational therapists with children are listed in Appendix 8-B.

### Eligibility Purposes

When assessing children for eligibility or placement, standardized, norm-referenced measures should be used to ensure that the test results are reliable and valid. Many public school systems mandate the use of norm-referenced tests by special educators and related service providers, including occupational therapists, when qualifying students for special services. For a specific example, in Washington state, children between 3 and 6 years old must perform at least 2 standard deviations below the norm on a standardized test in one or more of the specific developmental areas to qualify for related services in the public school setting (Washington Administrative Code, 1990).

Standardized, norm-referenced instruments are helpful in determining how the individual child's performance compares with that of the children in the normative sample. However, Bailey and Wolery (1989, p. 36) alerted professionals who participate in making decisions regarding a child's placement in intervention programs:

When determining placement, the primary question should be 'Which placement option will best meet a child's needs?' rather than 'Which placement option does the child qualify for according to test scores.'

Caution must be taken when interpreting a child's performance on most standardized developmental instruments. Often these instruments have not been standardized on disabled populations (Farran, 1990). For example, a child with Down syndrome may score more than 2 standard deviations below the mean for his or her chronologic age, but this does not tell us how he or she performs relative to other children with Down syndrome.

The Individuals with Disabilities Education Act, mandates

. . . procedures to assure that testing and evaluation materials and procedures utilized for the purposes of evaluation and placement of children with disabilities will be selected and administered so as not to be racially or culturally discriminatory (Sec. 1412).

Unfortunately, many tools standardized on the U.S. population have limited cultural validity for children who have recently immigrated from other countries or for children from ethnic groups not fully represented in the U.S. norms.

In summary, standardized tools have an important but specific purpose in the occupational therapy assessment process. Some service systems may require their use for determining eligibility of the child. However, standard scores, when used alone, do not provide complete data on a child and may be misleading, particularly for children with established disabilities. In addition, therapists should carefully interpret standard scores when evaluating children from diverse cultural or ethnic backgrounds.

## Diagnostic Purposes

Often a child is referred to occupational therapy by another health care provider or educator to gain more information about why a child may be delayed or exhibits performance deficits. This calls for a comprehensive assessment by the occupational therapist. To assist in the diagnostic process, the therapist should consider a combination of norm-referenced tools and clinical observations. *Clinical observations* (Figure 8-8) are nonstandardized measures that have been developed by therapists to objectively gather data on critical performance components or performance areas. The quality, frequency, and duration of performance are assessed. Refer to the fourth section in this chapter for more specific information regarding the use of skilled observation. The box on p. 173 provides a sample form for clinical

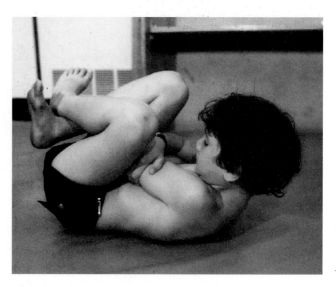

**Figure 8-8** Clinical observations of child in supine flexion.

observations of children's neuromotor status. A norm-referenced tool may provide the "anchor" regarding the child's developmental status relative to typically developing children, whereas clinical observations of child's performance provide rich information on the quality of performance and possible reasons for reduced performance on quantitative tests. To illustrate how norm-referenced measures are used in combination with nonstandardized clinical observations, the following case example is provided.

Jason is an 8-year-old boy with mild motor coordination deficits. The therapist administers a norm-referenced tool such as the Sensory Integration and Praxis Tests (Ayres, 1989) to obtain standard scores on his sensory and motor performance. Figure 8-9 shows the materials provided in the test kit. In addition, the therapist obtains qualitative data regarding Jason's muscle tone, primitive reflexes, righting and equilibrium reactions, posture, and gait through clinical observations. This information is combined to gain an understanding of Jason's sensory processing and sensory integration. It is also used to determine whether direct occupational therapy services are needed.

## Treatment Planning Purposes

Another reason why an occupational therapist may conduct a comprehensive assessment of a child is to determine the most appropriate intervention plan. When this is the primary reason for assessment, the therapist should consider evaluation methods that include in-depth observations of the child's performance within his or her natural environments. Interviews with parents and other adults working with the child are another primary source of data regarding the

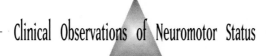

# Clinical Observations of Neuromotor Status

## Checklist for Clinical Observation of Neuromotor Status

***General instructions:*** First observe as many of the functional gross and fine motor skills as possible while the child spontaneously plays or moves. Note the child's posture, coordination, and transitional movement patterns during this time. When there is a question or concern regarding the quality of movement or posture during functional gross and fine motor skills, examine the child's muscle tone, primitive reflexes, and automatic reactions through direct testing and physical handling.

### FUNCTIONAL GROSS MOTOR SKILLS

Sit
Pivot in prone
Crawl (on stomach? in quadruped?)
Stand (with or without support?)
Cruise along furniture
Walk (with or without support?)
Ascend and descend stairs (with or without support? alternating feet?)
Jump with both feet (in place? forward?)
Run

### TRANSITIONAL MOVEMENT PATTERNS

Rolling (prone-to-supine, supine-to-prone) with rotation?
Sit-to-prone with rotation?
Prone-to-sit with rotation?
Supine-to-sit with rotation?
Pull to stand from half-kneel?
Stand to sit with control?

### FUNCTIONAL FINE MOTOR SKILLS

Reach (bilateral? unilateral? arm preference?)
Prehension patterns (whole hand grasp? partial hand grasp? digital grasp? pincer grasp?)
Release of objects (support of hand? well-controlled?)
Transfer of objects between hands
Manipulation of objects within the hand
Crossing midline of body
Bilateral hand use
Hand preference (hand dominance established?)
Use of scissors (previous experience?)
Use of writing utensil (crayon, marker, and pencil) (Note type and amount of pressure of grasp)
Ability to button and use other fasteners on clothing
Ability to use eating utensils

### POSTURE (Observe symmetry and alignment)

Supine
Prone
Sit
Stand
Prone extension
Supine flexion

### MUSCLE TONE

At rest? During movement?
Hypertonia? Hypotonia? Fluctuating?
Abnormal tone in extremities? In trunk?
Exaggerated stretch reflex (clonus?)
Asymmetries?

### RANGE OF MOTION

Limitations in upper extremity joints?
Limitations in lower extremity joints?
Limitations from bone or soft tissue contractures?
Asymmetries?

### PRIMITIVE REFLEXES

Asymmetric tonic neck reflex
Symmetric tonic neck reflex
Tonic labyrinthine reflex (prone? supine?)
Walking reflex
Neonatal positive support reflex in standing
Grasp reflex
Plantar reflex

### AUTOMATIC REACTIONS

Equilibrium reactions (head righting? trunk incurvation? extremity counterbalancing?)
Protective arm extension reactions (forward? sideways? backwards?)
Asymmetries?

### OCULAR-MOTOR SKILLS

Ability to visually focus on object
Ability to visually track a moving object
Esotropia? exotropia? nystagmus?
Peripheral vision

### PHYSICAL AND STRENGTH ENDURANCE

Physical strength to complete functional tasks
Physical endurance to complete functional tasks

### RESPONSE TO PHYSICAL HANDLING AND MOVEMENT ACTIVITIES

Response to examiner's or caregiver's touch
Response to activities that require movement through space (e.g., being carried or moved in different positions)

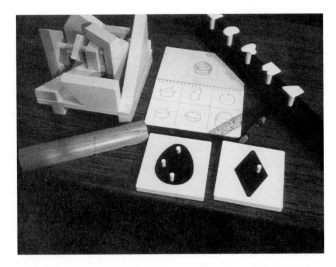

**Figure 8-9** Sensory Integration and Praxis Tests materials.

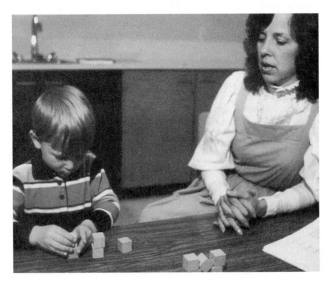

**Figure 8-10** Child completing a fine motor item on the Peabody Developmental Motor Scales.

child's performance. For the purpose of treatment planning, norm-referenced instruments may have limited value. Norm-referenced developmental assessments measure skills that are commonly seen in a typically developing population, but they do not necessarily measure what is critical for functional performance in children with disabilities. Figure 8-10 shows administration of a fine motor item from the PDMS. For example, most children by 6 years old can stand on either foot for at least 10 seconds (Folio & Fewell, 1983). However, is this a critical skill for the child's everyday function? A common mistake of occupational therapists is to design treatment goals and activities directly from items on norm-referenced assessment tools. Unfortunately this approach not only misses the mark with regard to functional outcomes, but it also invalidates the use of

these standardized tests to document the progress of the child and the efficacy of therapy intervention because of the practice effect on the child.

The following examples illustrate how treatment goals can be written in more functional terms for children.

***Assessment finding.*** Because of poor fine motor release of objects, Jill was unable to stack 1-inch cubes on the PDMS.

***Inadequate treatment goal.*** Jill will stack two 1-inch cubes, three out of four trials, by June 15, 1997.

***Functional goal.*** Jill will demonstrate release of small toys into a small container, three out of four trials, by June 15, 1997.

***Assessment finding.*** Because of increased muscle tone and poor reciprocal movements in the lower extremities, Ryan was unable to assume standing from the half-kneel position on either leg, an item on the Gross Motor Function Test (Gross Motor Measures Group, 1990).

***Inadequate treatment goal.*** Ryan will maintain the half-kneel position for 30 seconds, three times over two consecutive therapy sessions, by June 15, 1997.

***Functional goal.*** Ryan will step up on a 6-inch stool to use the classroom toilet without losing his balance, three out of four times, by June 15, 1997.

Therapists often use criterion-referenced and curriculum-based measures when the primary assessment purpose is treatment planning. These measures provide information regarding specific skills important to daily living or school performance. Some examples of criterion-referenced measures used by pediatric occupational therapists include the Hawaii Early Learning Profile (HELP; Furuno et al., 1979), the Carolina Curriculum for Handicapped and At-Risk Infants (Johnson, Jens, & Attermeier, 1986), and the Developmental Programming for Infants and Young Children (Schafer & Moersch, 1981) (see Appendix 8-B for ordering information).

### Reevaluation Purposes

The fourth primary reason an occupational therapist conducts comprehensive assessments is to reevaluate children's performance so that progress can be measured and the need for continued therapy can be determined. The content and structure of the *reevaluation* vary depending on the specific purpose of the reassessment. If a decision needs to be made regarding whether the child continues to qualify for therapy, the reevaluation will likely include a standardized, norm-referenced measure to ensure reliable results. However, if the primary purpose of reevaluation is to determine whether the child is making progress as a result of therapy, other measures, such as the specific functional goals and objectives written by the therapist during the initial phase of intervention, would be more appropriate and probably more sensitive to developmental and functional changes in the child.

For example, an infant with Down syndrome may show a drop in scores on a standardized test over the course of the intervention year. These standard scores only indicate that the infant with Down syndrome is developing at a slower rate compared with the test's normative group. More sensitive measures of progress in these infants may be the specific goals and objectives written by the early interventionists for each individual child. These short-term objectives are developed by therapists through task analysis, a process that lists child behaviors that sequentially lead to more advanced behavior in the long-term goals.

It is important to reemphasize here that the process of reevaluation of children is an ongoing, dynamic process. Every time a therapist works with a child, the therapist makes clinical judgments regarding the child's response to therapy and functional performance on tasks. The data gathered during each therapy session are analyzed and interpreted by the therapist to determine whether the therapy plan needs to be adjusted.

In summary, although a formal reevaluation is conducted at specific times during therapy intervention, the occupational therapist engages in an ongoing reassessment of the child and the therapy environment throughout each and every therapy session.

### Clinical Research

Instruments used in clinical research are carefully selected to measure the subject's performance and behavior. Although a more complete discussion on standardized tests used for *clinical research* is offered in Chapter 9, a few major points are introduced here. First, whether the research design is a large group or a single subject, the instruments used must be reliable and valid measures of the dependent variable. Second, the measures used depend on the research design and may vary from standardized, norm-referenced instruments often used in large-group designs to criterion-referenced instruments or therapy objectives that are operationally defined for single-subject research. Third, one of the most challenging aspects in designing clinical research is finding an appropriate and accurate measure to document change in the subjects. Palisano, Haley, and Brown (1992) described a research method called goal attainment scaling (GAS) as an alternative to norm-referenced scales to document change as a result of therapy intervention. GAS is an individualized criterion-referenced measure of change that appears to be

. . . advantageous in measuring qualitative change and small, but clinically important, improvement in motor development of children receiving physical therapy (p. 433).

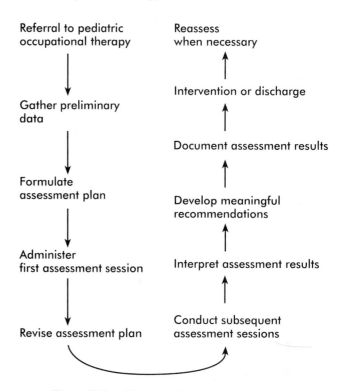

**Figure 8-11**    Flow chart for assessment process.

This section discussed the many purposes for assessment. The following section, discusses the process, including the sequential steps of assessment.

## PROCESS

The purpose of this section is to provide a logical sequence of steps that pediatric occupational therapists follow in the process of assessing children. Kevin's case, introduced earlier in the chapter, is a good illustration. After reviewing the numerous tools listed as appropriate for Kevin's occupational therapy assessment, the occupational therapist may wonder where to begin. Do all nine evaluations need to be completed before occupational therapy can commence for this child? The answer is no. To reiterate, the process of assessment in occupational therapy starts with the initial referral and is ongoing throughout the duration of therapy services. The family and the rest of the team, including the occupational therapist, select specific assessment areas that have priority for completion before developing a service plan and initiating therapy. Other areas of assessment are completed as the child and family become better known to the therapist. Therefore the therapist must continually consider the new challenges that the child must meet and other priorities that will become clear to the family.

To conduct thorough assessments and provide accurate interpretation and documentation of evaluation results, therapists follow logical steps in the assessment process. Figure 8-11 illustrates a flow chart of the assessment sequence.

**PEDIATRIC OCCUPATIONAL THERAPY REFERRAL**

CHILD'S NAME: <u>Kevin</u>    M X F __ DATE OF REFERRAL: <u>9/15/94</u>
DATE OF BIRTH: <u>7/15/88</u>    AGE OF CHILD: <u>6 years 2 months</u>
DIAGNOSIS/RELEVANT MEDICAL HISTORY: <u>Developmental delay and attention deficit disorder. Family history with learning disorders in both parents and developmental delay in siblings</u>
PRECAUTIONS/SPECIAL CONSIDERATIONS: <u>on medication (Ritalin) to reduce hyperactivity.</u>
BRIEF HISTORY REGARDING PREVIOUS OR CURRENT SPECIAL SERVICES: <u>Received early physical therapy as an infant. Has participated in a developmental special education preschool since age 3. Public health nurse reports parents need education & support in child management.</u>
PARTICIPATION IN COMMUNITY PROGRAMS: <u>Limited play experiences in neighborhood due to safety concerns. No participation in community programs.</u>

REASON(S) FOR REFERRAL TO OCCUPATIONAL THERAPY:
    Performance Tasks
__ activities of daily living (eating, bathing, dressing,
    toileting, functional mobility)
✓ school/work activities (classroom, playground, home)
✓ play/leisure activities (school, home, community)
    Performance Components
✓ sensorimotor skills (sensory processing, perceptual skills)
✓ neuromuscular status (muscle tone, ROM, posture, balance)
✓ motor skills (functional gross, fine, oral-motor skills)
✓ cognitive skills (orientation, attention, problem-solving)
✓ psychosocial skills (self-concept, self-management)
    Performance Context
__ physical environment (e.g. need for adaptation)
✓ social environment (e.g. need for caregiver information)

COMMENTS: <u>School records indicate that some of Kevin's behavior difficulties may be due to environmental stressors of poverty and parental disabilities (learning disorders)</u>

<u>Julie White</u>    <u>Developmental Preschool — 206-1234</u>
Signature of referring person    Address and phone number

**Figure 8-12**    Sample form for pediatric occupational therapy referral.

## Referral

Children at risk for or with disabilities are referred to occupational therapists for the assessment of and intervention for performance deficits. Often the child's diagnosis or deficits in specific developmental areas are listed on the referral form. To assist in identification of appropriate referrals, it is critical that the occupational therapist be involved in the development of the referral format used in a particular setting. This format may use *Uniform Terminology for Occupational Therapy,* 3rd ed. (AOTA, 1994) (Appendix 8-A) to elicit explicit descriptions of problems in performance areas or components that indicate the need for an occupational therapy referral (Figure 8-12).

## Evaluation Plan

Once a referral for therapy has been received, the therapist should consult with parents, other caregivers, and professionals from other disciplines to determine which measures to use, the evaluation setting, and the schedule for the occupational therapy evaluation activities. Most therapists find it helpful to formulate a written *evaluation plan* that is based on the child's chronologic age, presenting problems, parent's priorities regarding reasons for referral, availability of evaluation tools, type of service delivery model, and amount of time available for initial evaluation activities. Refer to Table 8-2 for an example of Kevin's initial evaluation plan. Note how the

▲ Table 8-2   Initial Evaluation Plan for Kevin: Part I

## PEDIATRIC OCCUPATIONAL THERAPY INITIAL EVALUATION PLAN

Child's name: Kevin

Child's age: 6 yrs 2 mos

Diagnosis: Developmental delay and attention deficit disorder

| **Reason(s) for referral** | **Source of referral** |
|---|---|
| 1. Fine motor deficits | Teacher |
| 2. Hyperactivity and distractibility | Physician |
| 3. Poor peer interaction | Teacher |
| 4. Possible visual perceptual deficits | Teacher |
| 5. Gross motor incoordination | Teacher |
| 6. Delay in some self-help skills | Parent |

|  | **Difficulty Developing Friendships** | **Unable to Print Name** | **Unsafe on Playground Equipment** | **Needs Assistance in Toileting and Dressing** |
|---|---|---|---|---|
| **SENSORIMOTOR** | | | | |
| Sensory processing | | | | |
| Sensory awareness | | X | X | |
| Perceptual skills | | X | | |
| **NEUROMUSCULAR** | | | | |
| Muscle tone | | | | |
| Reflex integration | | | X | |
| Postural control | | X | | |
| Range of motion | | | | |
| Strength | | | | |
| Endurance | | | X | |
| **MOTOR** | | | | |
| Gross motor skills | | | | |
| Bilateral | | | X | |
| Coordination | | | X | |
| Motor planning | | | X | |
| Fine motor skills | | X | | |
| Visual-motor | | X | | X |
| Integration | | X | | X |
| Oral-motor control | | | | |
| **COGNITIVE INTEGRATION** | | | | |
| Attention span | X | X | | X |
| Sequencing | | X | | X |
| Problem-solving | X | | | X |
| **PSYCHOLOGIC SKILLS** | | | | |
| Psychologic | X | | | |
| Social | X | | | |
| Self-management | X | | | X |

therapist lists the major performance areas of concern and checks those performance component deficits that may interfere with the child's achievement in those functional areas. As shown in Table 8-3, the therapist then lists those evaluation methods and measures selected to assess the child's performance. The column on the right side of the form (Table 8-3) is reserved for comments the therapist may have regarding adaptations of or deviations from standard procedures and contingency plans.

As mentioned previously, the complete assessment process takes place over time. Given the complexity of problems in children referred to pediatric occupational therapists, it may be difficult to formulate a comprehensive evaluation plan based on the limited referral information. Therefore it is expected that the therapist will revise the ini-

▲ Table 8-3   Initial Evaluation Plan for Kevin: Part II

| Functional Concerns | Evaluation Methods and Measures | Comments |
|---|---|---|
| Difficulty making friends | Coping Inventory<br>Parent interview<br>Teacher interview | Observe Kevin in classroom and at home |
| Unable to print | Peabody Developmental Motor Scales (PDMS)<br>Test of Visual Perception Skills | May need to adapt standard procedures because of attention deficits |
| Safety on playground | PDMS<br>Clinical observations of neuromotor status | |
| *Delay in self-help* | *Home observation*<br>*Self-help developmental checklist* | *Parent interview* |

Note: Information added after initial evaluation visit printed in italics.

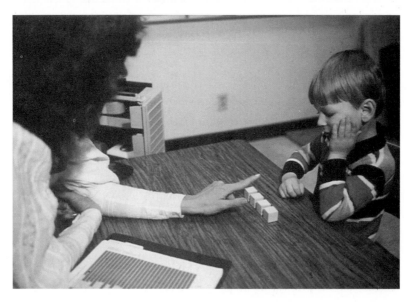

**Figure 8-13**   Administration of a standardized test (Miller Assessment for Preschoolers).

tial evaluation plan after the child has been seen at least once by the therapist and more information is gained regarding the caregiver's priorities and the child's developmental status. In the instance of Kevin, the therapist learned from the parent interview during the first evaluation session that Kevin's mother is most concerned about his delayed toileting skills. Table 8-3 illustrates how Kevin's evaluation plan was altered based on additional data obtained after the referral was received.

## Administration of Evaluation Measures

Once the evaluation plan has been revised, administration of the various measures selected can proceed. For most entry-level therapists in pediatrics, one of the most challenging aspects of the assessment process is the management of the child's behavior during the administration of the evaluation measures, particularly when the measures are more formal, structured, and standardized. Testing infants

and young children in a structured situation can be enormously demanding on the children, the parents, and the therapist (Figure 8-13). However, much can be done in the preparation for and during the occupational therapy evaluation to reduce potential behavior problems during testing. The box on p. 179 outlines several effective strategies for managing young children's behavior during structured, standardized evaluations.

Chapter 9 offers a more in-depth discussion on competent administration of standardized tests and also outlines some important ethical considerations for therapists when using standardized tests.

The administration of nonstandardized tools, clinical observations, environmental assessments, and interviews with the child's caregivers should receive the same careful attention and preparation by the occupational therapist as standardized measures require. For some children a combination of standardized tests and nonstandardized measures is appropriate. But for many children who are severely dis-

## Behavior Management Strategies for Testing Young Children

1. Be prepared! Know your testing procedures so well that you can focus on the child's behavior and performance, not on the test manual or your paperwork.

2. Be sensitive to the child's and parents' physical and emotional needs. Whenever possible, adjust the pace of the examination to match the child's style and acknowledge any concerns the parents may express.

3. Be purposeful in carrying out the examination. Keep the situation friendly, interesting for the child, and informative for the parent.

4. Be sure the testing room supports the child's optimal performance. Chair and table should be the appropriate size. Lighting should be sufficient. Remove all auditory and visual distractions. Use test materials that are attractive to children.

5. Build a rapport with the child before physically interacting with or handling the child. Some children may do better when they start with table-top tasks in which the child sits across from the examiner and observes the situation before being handled physically for motor testing. Other children may do better with a spontaneous play situation while the examiner focuses on the parent interview before directly testing the child. Be flexible and follow the child's lead, whenever possible.

6. Use positive reinforcement that is meaningful to the child (e.g., praise, stickers, or a fun activity). Be sure to reinforce the child's effort rather than success.

7. Start and end with some easy items. This helps the child feel more comfortable at the beginning and leaves a good feeling for both the child and parents at the end.

8. Watch the complexity of your language. Be clear and concise in your instructions to the child. Consider using the parents' level of language complexity as a guide to what the child can understand.

9. Be organized! Keep the test materials arranged neatly in an area that is easily accessible to you but not to the child. It is sometimes helpful to have an attractive toy (not from the test kit) on the table or nearby for the child to play with while you are not directly testing the child.

10. Try to develop reciprocal interactions with the child. When you first show the child a test object, allow him or her to briefly explore it in his or her own way before you give the test instructions. This time provides an excellent opportunity for clinical observations. Then give the child the test instructions and allow him or her to demonstrate his or her skill. If the child continues to be actively engaged with the object when you want to present a new item, it is often effective to present the new test object as you remove the old one.

---

abled, norm-referenced tests are neither valid nor meaningful. In these cases data gathered from nonstandardized measures provide the essential information for planning intervention. These evaluation methods, including naturalistic observation, clinical observations, criterion-referenced measures, and interviews with child's caregivers (e.g., teachers, parents, and day care providers), are more fully described in a subsequent section on evaluation methods.

## Interpretation of Results

Once all the initial assessment information has been gathered on a child's performance areas, performance components, and performance context, the therapist then analyzes these quantitative and qualitative data from standardized test results, clinical observations of the child's performance, caregiver interviews, and environmental assessments. When a standardized test is used, the therapist must carefully follow procedures outlined in the test manual regarding the interpretation of test results. When nonstandardized measures are used, the therapist must skillfully look for patterns of strength and areas of concern across all measures. Of-

tentimes data obtained from nonstandardized measures can be instrumental in understanding the possible underlying reasons for a child's specific performance on standardized tests. To further illustrate this point, consider Joey, a 3-year-old boy with motor delays. The quantitative data on the PDMS confirmed that he was functioning below age expectations. The qualitative data from the clinical observations of his neuromotor status indicated possible reasons for his motor delay, including low muscle tone and delayed righting and equilibrium reactions.

Accurate and complete interpretation of all the accumulated data is one of the most important and demanding tasks of the assessment process. Again, the occupational therapist must be thorough in examining the details of a child's performance, yet at the same time view the child's behaviors within the context of environmental demands and supports. Accurate and complete interpretation of assessment data allows therapists to make sound clinical decisions, including whether the child is a candidate for occupational therapy, and if so, the frequency, duration, and type of therapeutic intervention. Once assessment data have been analyzed, the therapist then turns to the task of developing recommendations for the child.

## Development of Recommendations Based on Results

To develop meaningful recommendations based on assessment results, the therapist must keep in mind several factors. First, and foremost, the *priorities of the child's caregivers* should be considered. Hanft (1994) suggested that every recommendation from an occupational therapist to a parent of a child with special needs should be followed up with the question to the caregiver, "How will this work for you?" For example, during a feeding evaluation in the child's home, a therapist observes a mother and her child with athetoid cerebral palsy and failure to thrive. The therapist notes that the mother has placed the child in an infant walker at mealtime. Because infant walkers have been declared unsafe by the American Academy of Pediatrics, and this particular child would benefit from a more stable seating device that provides trunk and head support needed for optimal oral-motor skills, the therapist might recommend that the infant walker be discontinued and that a special feeding seat be ordered. However, unless the therapist asks the caregiver what the implications of this recommendation may be for the child and the family, this important recommendation may not be implemented by family members. In this case additional history taking showed that the child refused to be fed in any position other than in the walker, and the mother was concerned about her child receiving adequate nutrition for growth. Based on the mother's input the intervention goal became that the child continue to demonstrate oral-motor skills adequate for weight gain and growth. The therapist added a short-term recommendation to provide the parents with information regarding the safety of infant walkers and the importance of proper positioning when eating.

Another factor therapists must consider when developing recommendations from assessment findings is the *type of service delivery model* in which they are working. Dunn and Campbell (1991) described the wide range of service delivery models in which pediatric occupational therapists work, including direct treatment, monitoring, and consultation. Depending on the service delivery model or combination of models, the therapist's recommendations should be consistent with the primary service delivery model. For example, if the therapist's only role with the child is consultation, recommendations from the initial assessment would center around how the primary caregiver and other adults working with the child can adapt the child's environment. Recommendations for direct service in which the therapist provides hands-on intervention for this child may conflict with the service delivery model.

The third factor the therapist should consider when developing recommendations based on assessment results is the *functionality* of the recommendations. Functionality refers to the relevance of the recommendation to the child's daily life (Notari & Bricker, 1990). When developing recommendations for a child, the therapist must always ask, "Does this recommendation relate to the child's occupa-

tional performance?" and "Is this recommendation relevant to the child's everyday function?"

How does a therapist reconcile these three, sometimes conflicting factors when developing recommendations? Certainly years of experience can teach a therapist to skillfully negotiate through the maze of issues regarding the child, family, team, environments, and service delivery systems! However, entry-level therapists can use several basic strategies early in their careers that help them become more competent in assessing children:

1. Find a mentor who is well experienced in working with children of varying diagnoses and families from diverse backgrounds.
2. Be willing to continually search for new knowledge and resources that are relevant to working with children with special needs.
3. Be open to new ways of viewing children and families.
4. Learn to build effective communication skills and collaboration skills with team members, including the child's primary caregiver.

## Documentation of Evaluation Results and Recommendations

The next step in the assessment process is to provide written and oral reports of the assessment findings and recommendations. The primary purpose of documenting the results of the pediatric occupational therapy assessment is to describe to caregivers, physicians, teachers, and other individuals working with the child what the child's current abilities and limitations are on various functional tasks. McClain (1991) suggested the following:

Effective documentation is telling a true story with a particular style. It calls for the ordinary tasks of day-to-day experience to be succinctly stated in writing. The true story about any child who has a disability is not a simple tale (p. 213).

When providing written documentation, the therapist must first consider for whom the reports are intended and then carefully construct reports that are understandable and useful to those individuals. The format and content of evaluation reports may vary significantly, depending on the referral concern, the complexity of the child's problem, and the regulations of the service delivery system in which the child is served (e.g., public school setting, hospital, or home health agency). In some situations, for eligibility purposes, written evaluation reports must also include specific standardized scores documenting developmental delay. In all occupational therapy practice settings, documentation stands as a legal record (AOTA, 1986).

Therapists should recognize that their words have great power. Words should be carefully chosen when documenting a child's assessment results. Hanft (1989) cautioned pediatric therapists that "words convey powerful personal images that can be positive and supportive, or negative and destructive" (pp. 2-77). Pediatric occupational therapists should use words that reflect positive attitudes toward children with disabilities. Unfortunately, daily therapy language is filled with technical terms that may not convey our intended message, but often may confuse or alienate parents. Therapists should always refer to the child first and the disability as one characteristic of the child (i.e., a child with cerebral palsy, not a cerebral palsy child). Table 8-4 shows how words have either negative or positive attitudes toward children with disabilities.

The box on pp. 182 and 183 provides a written example illustrating how a therapist documented Kevin's assessment findings and recommendations. One important aspect of the report is how the therapist carefully worded it so that the information was helpful to Kevin's parents as well as to his teacher. The format of the report structures the description of Kevin's occupational performance, including his functional abilities and limitations.

To summarize the major points discussed in the previous sections, occupational therapists must ask themselves the following questions as they assess children. Did the assessment process:

1. Address the caregiver's concerns?
2. Use evaluation instruments that measure occupational therapy domains including the child's performance areas, performance components, and performance context?
3. Use multiple methods of evaluation, including clinical observations, caregiver interview, direct observation of child in natural environment, and standardized tools?
4. Fully recognize the influence of the child's cultural background on his or her evaluation performance and consider these cultural influences when developing an intervention plan for the child?
5. Adhere properly to the administration procedures and ethical considerations when using standardized tests?
6. Recognize and acknowledge the child's strengths as well as areas of concern?
7. Result in a summary that contributes meaningful, user-friendly information regarding the child's functional abilities and disabilities?

This section described the process. It included important sequential steps for conducting accurate, thorough evaluations of children and communicating assessment findings to caregivers and other professionals working with the child. The next, and last, section of this chapter, provides the reader with the methods or the "what" of pediatric occupational therapy assessments.

## EVALUATION METHODS

A variety of evaluation methods are available to pediatric occupational therapists. The challenge for therapists is to know which evaluation methods should be selected for a particular child or group of children. The purpose of this section is to describe each of the primary evaluation methods commonly used in pediatric occupational therapy prac-

▲ Table 8-4    Preferred Terms for Documentation

| Inaccurate or Negative Terms | Preferred or Positive Terms |
|---|---|
| Afflicted | Children with disabilities |
| Defective, deformed | Child with a physical disability |
| Retarded | Child with developmental delay |
| Wheelchair-bound | Wheelchair-user |
| Deaf | Hearing impaired |
| Blind child | Child with visual impairment |
| Normal child | Nondisabled child |

▲ Table 8-5    Selection of Appropriate Evaluation Methods

| Purpose of Assessment | Evaluation Methods | | | | |
|---|---|---|---|---|---|
| | Norm Referenced | Criterion Referenced | Skilled Observation | Interview | Checklists |
| **Screening** to determine need for further assessment | X | | X | X | X |
| **Comprehensive assessment** to determine eligibility | X | | | | |
| **Comprehensive assessment** to assist in diagnosis | X | X | | X | |
| **Comprehensive assessment** to determine intervention plan | X | X | | X | X |
| **Reevaluation** to monitor child's progress and determine need to continue therapy | X | X | X | X | X |
| **Research** to investigate clinical populations | X | | | | |

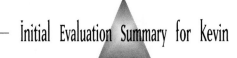

## Initial Evaluation Summary for Kevin

### University of Puget Sound School of Occupational Therapy Pediatric Clinic

Name:   Kevin
School:  Newport Elementary
Grade:  Kindergarten

Evaluation Date:   September 18, 1994
Date of Birth:      July 15, 1988
Chronologic Age:   6 years 2 months

### Occupational Therapy Initial Evaluation

#### REASON FOR REFERRAL

Kevin was referred to the Occupational Therapy Pediatric Clinic at the University of Puget Sound by his special education teacher, Mrs. Julie White. He has a history of developmental delay and a diagnosis of attention deficit disorder. Approximately 6 months ago Kevin's pediatrician, Dr. Mark Walker, placed him on Ritalin to control his extreme hyperactivity. Primary reasons for referral to occupational therapy include his fine motor delay, possible visual perceptual deficits, poor socialization skills, and gross motor incoordination.

Kevin attends a developmental preschool program five half-days per week. His classroom consists of some nondisabled children and several children who exhibit mild to moderate developmental delays in speech and language, behavior, or motor skills.

Kevin is the firstborn of three children in an African-American family. He lives with both of his parents and his two younger brothers in a small home located in inner city Tacoma.

#### FORMAL AND INFORMAL ASSESSMENTS ADMINISTERED

Peabody Developmental Motor Scales (PDMS)
Clinical observations of neuromotor status
Coping Inventory
Test of Visual Perceptual Skills (TVPS)
Parent interview and home observations
Classroom and playground observations

#### BEHAVIOR DURING FORMAL (STANDARDIZED) ASSESSMENTS

Kevin was a friendly child who easily engaged in conversation with the examiner. He had significant difficulty attending to the structured test items, but when provided frequent social reinforcement and tangible rewards (e.g., stickers), he was able to complete most of the items presented. Kevin's hyperactivity and attention deficit limited his performance on some of the items. Therefore his standard scores on the PDMS and the TVPS may underestimate his actual abilities.

#### ASSESSMENT RESULTS

The following section describes Kevin's performance on functional tasks within his school and home environments and then provides results of Kevin's performance components on specific measures of motor and visual perception and psychosocial abilities.

#### Performance Areas

*Functional areas at school.* Based on teacher interview and classroom observation, Kevin is experiencing difficulties in learning to print, making friends, and playing safely on playground equipment. In general, he enjoys school and wants to do well on his classroom activities.

*Functional areas at home.* Based on parent interview and home observation, Kevin is experiencing difficulties on specific self-help tasks of dressing and toileting. Parents describe him as "difficult to manage" and report he often requires physical punishment. Home observation showed few toys and no space to play outdoors.

#### Performance Components

*Fine motor performance.* On the Peabody Developmental Fine Motor Scale, Kevin scored solidly through the 30- to 35-month level and successfully completed some items up to the 42-month level. His performance on this scale was more than 2 standard deviations below the mean and was reflective of functional fine motor skills in the approximate 38- to 40-month age range. Kevin preferred his right hand for most tasks that required the skilled use of a tool (e.g., crayons and scissors). He demonstrated hand tremors when attempting various fine motor tasks, but these tremors were not observed at rest. He moved impulsively and, even with verbal cues from the examiner, was unable to slow his movements down.

Initial Evaluation Summary for Kevin—cont'd

*Gross motor performance.* On the Peabody Developmental Gross Motor Scale, Kevin scored solidly through the 48- to 52-month level and successfully completed some items up to the 60-month level. His overall performance on this scale was 1.5 standard deviations below the mean and was reflective of functional gross motor skills in the approximate 56- to 58-month age range. Kevin scored within age expectations on tasks requiring speed and agility, but significantly below his age on tasks that required static balance (e.g., standing on one foot) and gross motor tasks that required more precise coordination (e.g., throwing a ball at a target).

*Neuromuscular status.* Clinical observations showed muscle tone, range of motion, integration of primitive reflexes, and development of automatic reactions (righting and equilibrium responses and protective extension reactions) within the normal range. Posture and gait also appeared normal. His frequent falls and clumsiness on the playground may be more related to his motor impulsivity and his inattentiveness than to delayed balance responses.

*Visual perceptual skills.* On the TVPS Kevin obtained a percentile rank of 21, indicating an overall performance in the low normal range (−0.8 standard deviation from the mean). His performance on each of the subtests varied significantly, suggesting relative strengths and weaknesses in visual perception. Specific results were as folows:

| | Raw Scores | Perceptual Ages | Scaled Scores | Percentile Ranks |
|---|---|---|---|---|
| Visual discrimination | 6 | 6-9 | 11 | 63 |
| Visual memory | 2 | 4-8 | 6 | 9 |
| Visual spatial | 6 | 5-2 | 8 | 25 |
| Visual form constancy | 5 | 5-11 | 10 | 50 |
| Visual sequence memory | 1 | 4-1 | 5 | 5 |
| Visual figure-ground | 2 | 4-5 | 6 | 9 |
| Visual closure | 7 | 7-6 | 12 | 75 |

*Social skills.* As measured by the Coping Inventory, Kevin lacked the necessary internal and external resources to meet the demands of his home environment and the unstructured playground environment at school. He demonstrated a minimally effective coping style in these settings, including erratic mood swings and aggressiveness toward others. However, within his classroom environment when the activities were scheduled, structured, and predictable, Kevin could regulate his activity level, and he interacted with peers and adults more successfully.

## SUMMARY

Kevin is a 6-year 2-month-old boy with attention deficits and developmental delays. He is currently enrolled in a developmental preschool program. This initial assessment shows that he is functioning almost 2 years below age expectations on the fine motor scale and almost 6 months below on the gross motor scale of the PDMS. Clinical observations of neuromotor status were within normal limits. Kevin's relative strengths and weaknesses in visual perception were substantial, although his overall performance on the TVPS was within the low normal range.

Kevin is a friendly, charming boy, but his extreme hyperactivity and distractibility limit his physical and social performance in both his home and school environments. Kevin's coping effectiveness varied depending on the degree of structure in his environment.

## RECOMMENDATIONS

Based on this initial assesment, the following recommendations are suggested:
1. Direct occupational therapy to improve his performance on functional fine motor tasks, particularly learning to print his name.
2. Consult with parents and teachers regarding modifications to his home and school environments to optimize his coping effectiveness.
3. Consult with parents regarding strategies to help teach Kevin self-help skills and behavior management at home.
   If there are any questions regarding this report, please contact this therapist at 123-4567.

_____

Occupational Therapist

tice and discuss the major factors that therapists should consider when selecting these methods. The starting point in the selection process is to first clearly identify the purpose of the assessment and then to match appropriate evaluation methods with the identified purpose. Table 8-5 offers a list of the common purposes of assessment, described earlier in this chapter, and matches evaluation methods appropriate for those purposes. For example, if the only purpose for the assessment is to determine the child's eligibility for occupational therapy in a public school setting, then the primary evaluation method is most likely be a norm-referenced, standardized test. However, if the primary purpose of the assessment is to gain information useful for planning an intervention program for the child, the evaluation measures should also include skilled clinical observations and interviews with the child's caregivers. Often the initial assessment of a child serves more than one purpose. Therefore therapists frequently use multiple measures and methods when conducting child assessments.

The following subsections describe each of the evaluation methods commonly used in pediatric occupational therapy.

## Norm-Referenced Tests

*Norm-referenced measures* are tests that have been developed by administering the test items to a sample of children (in a normative group) who are representative of the population to be tested. The child's score can then be compared with those of the normative group. To evaluate the usefulness of a norm-referenced measure, the pediatric occupational therapist should carefully read in the test manual how the norm-referenced scores were derived and the characteristics of the normative sample. The therapist using norm-referenced tests must also know how to accurately interpret an individual child's scores, including the developmental quotient, the standard score, and the percentile rank. Refer to Chapter 9 for a more in-depth discussion on the use of standardized tests, including norm-referenced and criterion-referenced measures.

## Criterion-Referenced Tests

*Criterion-referenced measures* are tests that consist of a series of skills in functional or developmental areas, usually grouped by age level. These tests compare the child's performance on each test item with a standard or criterion that must be met if the child is to receive credit for that item. Criterion-referenced tests are made up of items selected because of their importance to the child's school performance or daily living. Because of their importance to everyday function, the items often become intervention targets when the child exhibits difficulty in successfully completing the items. The primary advantage in using criterion-referenced tests is that the examiner obtains important information regarding the child's strengths and weaknesses on critical skills. Some examples of criterion-referenced measures

used in pediatric occupational therapy include HELP (Furuno et al., 1984), the Erhardt Developmental Prehension Assessment (Erhardt, 1982), the Evaluation and Programming System for Infants and Young Children (Bricker, Bailey, Gumerlock, Buhl, & Slentz, 1986), and the Developmental Programming for Infants and Young Children (Schafer & Moersch, 1981) (see Appendix 8-B). Information gained from criterion-referenced tests is particularly helpful when determining the child's specific skills and when planning appropriate intervention activities to enhance those skills.

## Ecological Assessments

Neisworth and Bagnato (1988) defined *ecological assessments* as "the examination and recording of the physical, social, and psychological features of a child's developmental context" (p. 39). Consistent with the transactional approach (Chandler & Sameroff, 1975), ecological assessments are also concerned with the interaction between the individual child and the child's environments (Figure 8-14).

Pediatric occupational therapists are particularly interested in ecological measures because these tools are a primary mechanism for obtaining data relevant to the child's performance context. Ecological assessments employ techniques that consider the cultural influences, socioeconomic status, and value system of the family. Some of these techniques include naturalistic observations, interviews, and rating scales. Ecological measures familiar to pediatric occupational therapists include the Home Observation for Measurement of the Environment (HOME) Inven-

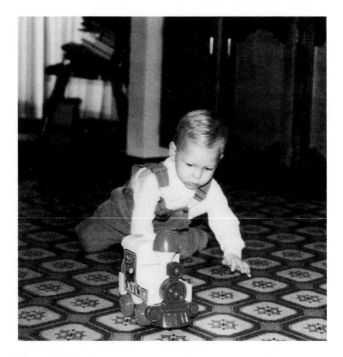

**Figure 8-14**   Observing a child playing in his natural environment.

tory (Caldwell & Bradley, 1972) and the Transdisciplinary Play-Based Assessment (Linder, 1990).

## Skilled Observations

An essential skill of the pediatric occupational therapist is the ability to keenly and accurately observe and record children's behavior in an objective manner. Although formal, standardized assessments are highly valued in pediatric practice, *skilled observation* of a child performing a functional task offers different but equally important information about the child's performance.

Bailey and Wolery (1989) suggested the following:

Observation of children in familiar settings and routines allows more characteristic views of their abilities and may be actually more reflective of how children can be expected to perform even under the most optimal learning opportunities (p. 256).

For example, skilled observations of a child's performance on functional tasks add important information not gained on standardized motor assessments (Figure 8-15).

Cook (1991) described the important components of skilled observations to include the setting, the behavior of the child, the quality of the behavior, and the frequency and duration of the behavior. When skilled observations are used in the assessment process, therapists must select a systematic, objective recording procedure so that data collected are accurate and reliable. Bailey and Wolery (1989) outlined the following important steps in using direct observations of children:

1. Define the behaviors and identify the relevant dimensions of that behavior.
2. Select appropriate data collection systems and data sheets.
3. Select appropriate times and situations for observation.
4. Check the accuracy of data collection.
5. Use the results for decision making.

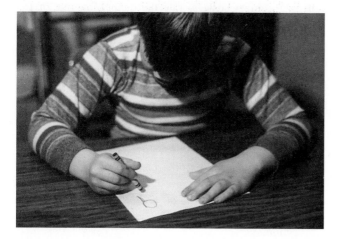

**Figure 8-15** Skilled observation of child performing a functional task at school.

Huber and King-Thomas (1987) proposed that there are at least three different methods, or data collection systems, for recording direct observations. These include (1) recording the rate of behavior (frequency or duration), (2) using a checklist or rating scale, and (3) reporting a specific behavioral event in an anecdotal fashion.

Although direct observations within the child's natural environment provide valuable information, some disadvantages to this method must be noted. First, the examiner loses some control over assessment conditions. Second, if the examiner is not skilled, he or she may not recognize key behaviors and their meaning when they are couched within the context of self-care, play, or other daily activities.

## Interviews

Another primary method used in pediatric occupational therapy assessment is the *interview* with the child's primary caregiver, teacher, or other adults working with the child. Caregiver interviews regarding their child's development can serve several functions: (1) to collect information about the child's skills from the parents' perceptions; (2) to validate information collected through direct observations or testing by the professional; and (3) to provide an opportunity for the parents to identify their values and priorities about the skills being assesed by the therapist (Bailey & Wolery, 1989).

Interviews are best used in conjunction with other evaluation methods that employ direct observation of the child. An important outcome of the interview is the accurate, meaningful exchange of information between the professional and the parent or other caregiver. Interviews, when done well, can provide an opportunity to build rapport between the therapist and caregivers. Interviews provide a unique opportunity for families to identify and discuss issues that are important to them. Therefore interviews are particularly useful when therapists are interested in family perceptions of children's abilities, the impact of events such as transitions in services on the family, and the family's priorities for services. When interviews are conducted in a flexible manner, parents and therapists are able to explore areas of concern as they arise.

Interviews may include closed- or open-ended questions or a combination of both. Specific questions, which are often closed-ended, allow the therapist to gather a predetermined set of information from a caregiver in a relatively short amount of time. Unstructured interviews using open-ended questions allow caregivers to take the lead and set the priorities within the discussion. Open-ended questions invite the caregiver to elaborate on a topic and provide critical information about their child. Conducting an effective interview requires experience and sensitivity.

Several investigators have analyzed and described effective interview skills (Brammer, 1988; Carkhuff & Anthony,

## Basic Strategies for Conducting Effective Caregiver Interviews

1. At the beginning, clarify the purpose of the interview with the caregiver in terms that are meaningful to him or her.
2. Be sensitive to the caregiver's physical and emotional needs throughout the assessment.
3. Promote interaction by asking open-ended questions, and guide caregivers to where they may sit to participate fully in the conversation.
4. Through careful questioning, attempt to understand what is typical for the family regarding their values and cultural influences in raising their child.
5. Carefully plan when to take notes, preferably after the interview or when the caregiver is busy tending to the child.
6. Remain positive and realistic in your approach with caregivers and the information you provide.
7. Be flexible throughout the interview, responding sensitively to the caregivers' questions and need for information. If you cannot answer their question, let them know and then figure out a plan with them to begin to find the needed information.
8. Use effective verbal and nonverbal communication skills. Often, nonverbal communication can override verbal information.
9. Avoid the use of therapy and medical jargon. If technical terms are used, be sure they are adequately explained.

1979; Ivey, 1971). Refer to the basic strategies for conducting effective interviews shown in the box above.

For more in-depth information on interviewing caregivers, the reader is referred to Winton (1988).

In summary, a skilled therapist conducts interviews with caregivers by carefully selecting questions and sensitively listening to their responses. Interviews offer a unique opportunity for exchange of information between caregivers and therapists. During the interview, therapists must reciprocate by providing caregivers with accurate, relevant information about their child's functional abilities, the intervention services, and community resources.

## Inventories and Scales

A variety of inventories and scales are used to gather data on a child's development, the caregiver-child interactions, or the child's environments. Some published inventories, checklists, and scales are well developed. One example is the Early Intervention Developmental Profile (Rogers et al., 1981). This tool assesses a small sample of the child's skills across several developmental domains, which makes the

tool useful as a screening measure and for intervention planning. However, the test items were derived from other developmental measures, and the tool itself is not norm-referenced. Therefore therapists are cautioned against using this instrument if the primary assessment purpose is to determine eligibility of a child for services.

The Pediatric Evaluation of Disability Inventory (PEDI) is an assessment of functional capabilities and performance in children aged 6 months to 7.5 years. It stands as one of the few inventories that has been normed and standardized. The PEDI is administered through structured interview of the parents or by professional judgment of clinicians and educators who are familiar with the child. It measures both capability and performance of functional activities in (1) self-care, (2) mobility, and (3) social function. The inventory consists of 197 functional skills items; the child is scored either 1 (has capability) or 0 (has not yet demonstrated capability, unable) on each item. Twenty additional items rate the amount of caregiver assistance required to complete key functional tasks.

The PEDI was designed for use with young children who have a variety of disabling conditions, although the test authors were primarily concerned with designing an instrument to be used with children who have physical disabilities. The test authors completed a series of reliability and validity studies and developed standard scores using Rasch Analysis techniques (Haley et al., 1992). As a result, the PEDI stands as a well-developed and well-researched assessment tool for evaluating the child's functional performance and capabilities.

Some measures used in pediatric occupational therapy assessment are therapist-made checklists. For example, Wilbarger's (1973) Sensorimotor History checklist describes specific behaviors that may indicate sensorimotor problems in children. This tool is intended to be used with other, more formal measures to assess children's sensory processing abilities.

Rating scales are similar to checklists but may provide more complete qualitative data. A rating system usually involves a number scale to rate the quality, degree, or frequency of a behavior. For example, the Observational Scale for Mother-Infant Interaction During Feeding (Chatoor et al., 1988) is designed to assess feeding problems during infancy by observing interactions of mothers and their children ranging in age from birth to 3 years. The following item illustrates the type of qualitative data obtained using the scale's rating system.

**Item 1: Positions Infant for Reciprocal Exchange**

None (0): The mother places the infant in a position that precludes or makes difficult face-to-face interaction during feeding.

A little (1): The mother places the infant in a position that neither precludes nor facilitates face-to-face interaction.

Pretty much (2): The mother places the infant in a position in which face-to-face interaction is facilitated but in a position that is not optimal.

Very much (3): The mother places the infant in a position that is optimal for face-to-face interaction.

Some checklists and rating scales can be completed by a parent, teacher, or other caregiver. For example, the Infant Monitoring System (Bricker & Squires, 1989) relies exclusively on parent report. On this scale the items are clearly described, and many are illustrated so that parents can elicit specific behaviors from their children. After each item parents check the appropriate box: yes, sometimes, or not yet. The Developmental Profile II (DP-II) (Alpern, Boll, & Shearer, 1986) may be given by parent interview exclusively or by direct testing. The Developmental Checklist for Pre-Dressing Skills (Dunn-Klein, 1983) can be administered by a classroom teacher or parent.

## Transdisciplinary Arena Assessments

Federal legislation states that assessments for infants and young children with disabilities be conducted by a multi-disciplinary team (IDEA, Part H, Sec. 1477). The implementation of multidisciplinary assessments in various intervention programs differs significantly with regard to the scope and form of the assessment process. For example, in some settings each professional provides an individual assessment of the child or family, then meets with the other team members to discusss evaluation findings and recommendations. Sometimes little or no communication occurs between team members before and during the administration of the evaluation measures. In contrast, a team in another setting may use the transdisciplinary approach in which one primary discipline team member conducts the assessment with the child and family, and other key discipline team members provide their expertise to the assessment process through consultation.

One concept in transdisciplinary assessments that appears to be gaining recognition is the *arena assessment*. An arena assessment is one in which the child interacts with one professional throughout the evaluation visit, and other professionals observe, on occasion, directly testing the child. While observing the assessment, other team members interview the parents. An excellent example of an arena assessment is Linder's (1990) Transdisciplinary Play-Based Assessment (TPBA). This model places a major emphasis on a team approach to assessment of young children. The purpose of the TPBA is to obtain developmental information on the child using multidimensional, functional observations of the child during a play session. Parents and professionals together plan, observe, and analyze the child's play session.

Arena assessment of feeding difficulties in children can also be effective in gathering relevant information without overtesting children or requiring the caregiver to participate in repeated interviews with different professionals.

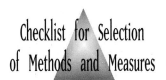

## Checklist for Selection of Methods and Measures

- ▲ Start with reasons for referral.
- ▲ Gather relevant medical, educational, and family histories (e.g., note precautions for testing, need for interpretor, and previous tests given).
- ▲ Consider the caregiver's priorities regarding the child's functional skills.
- ▲ Consider the developmental and chronologic age of the child.
- ▲ Determine the theoretical frames of reference most appropriate for the assessment of the child.
- ▲ Consider the purpose of the evaluation, and select the most appropriate methods for the assessment (refer to chart that matches purpose with methods).
- ▲ Consider the requirements of the testing agency.
- ▲ Identify available resources (e.g., child's caregiver, other professionals, instruments and test materials, time, and space).

For example, an arena feeding assessment for a child with cerebral palsy and failure to thrive may include an occupational therapist, nurse, and nutritionist. One professional is designated as the lead examiner, depending on the primary referral concern. The occupational therapist may take the lead if the child has oral-motor deficits such as chewing or swallowing difficulties, postural difficulties that create the need for external support of mealtime posture, or fine motor difficulties that limit self-feeding skills. The nurse may take the lead in the assessment process if the child exhibits behavioral difficulties, if the parent's caregiving skills seem to be limited, or if parent-child interaction appears strained. The nutritionist may take the lead if the child's diet needs careful analysis and if the family would benefit from specific information on types and amounts of food the child should eat. The benefit of an arena assessment of feeding is that the child and caregiver are subjected to the mealtime evaluation only once, rather than three different times. The arena assessment allows the opportunity for collaboration among the parents and professionals to observe, discuss, and problem-solve critical areas together.

## Selecting Appropriate Evaluation Measures and Methods

Before appropriate assessment methods and measures can be selected for a child, the therapist must consider several factors. The box above outlines each of the important steps for the therapist to take in the process of selecting appropriate methods and measures.

# STUDY QUESTIONS

## Case Study #1

Chelsea is an 8-month-old (corrected age) infant who was born at 32 weeks' gestation. Primary problems in the Neonatal Intensive Care Unit (NICU) included infant respiratory distress syndrome and neonatal abstinence syndrome secondary to maternal drug use. Cranial ultrasounds in the NICU indicated intraventricular hemorrhage. Chelsea is living with her mother, who is single, and her 2-year-old brother in a one-room studio apartment. Her mother is concerned because Chelsea is irritable throughout the day. She does not like her bath, nor does she enjoy being cuddled. Chelsea's pediatrician referred her for a therapy assessment because she has some increased tone in her legs and has not yet achieved independent sitting.

1. Discuss the purpose of the therapy assessment for Chelsea.
2. Using the Uniform Terminology III (Appendix 8-A), list the primary performance areas and performance components the occupational therapist might use to assess Chelsea.
3. Describe what evaluation methods would be appropriate for an initial assessment of Chelsea and her family, and list two to three specific instruments.
4. What other professionals might be involved with Chelsea?

## Case Study #2

Tin is a 2-year-old toddler with developmental delay of unknown cause. He is the firstborn of a newly immigrated South Vietnamese family. The public health nurse administered the Denver Developmental Screening Test–II, which showed that Tin was functioning around the 18-month-old level in gross motor skills, near the 12-month-old level in fine motor and adaptive skills, and at the 10-month-old level in language skills. Tin and his family were referred to a community-based early intervention program. The occupational therapist working in the early intervention program serves on a team that includes a physical therapist, a speech pathologist, and an early childhood special educator. The team is preparing to meet with the family to develop the Individual Family Service Plan.

1. What are some of the major points the early intervention team should consider when assessing this child and reporting assessment information to the family?

2. Discuss the advantages and disadvantages of an arena assessment for this child.

## Case Study #3

Eva is a 6-year-old girl with mild cerebral palsy who has participated in early intervention and preschool programs since she was 2 years old. Her cognitive abilities appear to be within the normal range. The early intervention staff report that Eva has some difficulty following adult-directed activities and playing with her peers. Her parents are interested in enrolling her in a regular kindergarten class this year. She is currently being evaluated by the public school occupational therapist to determine if she is eligible for therapy in the school setting. Eva's previous therapist at the early intervention program administered the Peabody Developmental Motor Scales last year.

1. Given the primary purpose of the school occupational therapy assessment, what methods and measures would be most appropriate for Eva's assessment?
2. Explain why a norm-referenced test should be used in this situation rather than a criterion-referenced test.
3. Discuss some important behavioral strategies effective in assessing young children when using standardized tests.
4. In which natural environments should the therapist observe Eva to gain a better understanding of her occupational performance skills?

## Case Study #4

Michael is a 9-year-old boy with sensory processing deficits and a learning disability. His mother reports Michael has difficulty making friends in the neighborhood and following through with simple chores at home. Michael's teacher indicates that Michael continues to have difficulty in completing his written assignments and frequently disrupts his classmates while they are working. He has recently been referred to the school's occupational therapist to determine if he would benefit from therapy.

1. What are the occupational performance areas that the therapist should assess in this case, and which performance components may be underlying his performance area deficits?
2. Write two functional, measureable therapy goals for Michael for this school year.
3. Which measurements would be most appropriate for Michael's initial assessment?

# SUMMARY

The provision of accurate, reliable assessments of children is one of the most challenging and rewarding services a pediatric occupational therapist can offer. This chapter described the purposes, process, and methods of assessment in pedatric occupational therapy. The domains of occupational therapy practice, including the children's performance areas, performance components, and performance contexts, provide a comprehensive base on which meaningful, functional assessments of children can be created. Understanding the many purposes of assessment and carefully matching appropriate methods and measures to those purposes are critical skills of the pediatric occupational therapist. Observing the details of children's performance on tasks and recognizing the importance of the context in which the child performs those tasks are also essential assessment skills. Equally important assessment skills that therapists learn to develop over time include working collaboratively with the child's caregiver and other team members to gain an in-depth understanding of children and their environments. This understanding, shared among team members, leads to the development of relevant, appropriate intervention plans and effective intervention strategies.

# REFERENCES

Achenbach, T.M. & Edelbrock, C.S. (1983). *Manual for the Child Behavior Checklist and Revised Child Behavior Profile.* Burlington: University of Vermont, Department of Psychiatry.

Alpern, G., Boll, T., & Shearer, M. (1986). *Developmental Profile II.* Los Angeles: Western Psychological Services.

Als, H., Lester, B.M., Tronick, E.Z., & Brazelton, T.B. (1982). Toward a research instrument for the Assessment of Preterm Infants' Behavior (APIB). In H. Fitzgerald, B.M. Lester, & M.S. Yogman (Eds.). *Theory and research in behavioral pediatrics* (Vol. 1) (pp. 35-132). New York: Plenum.

American Occupational Therapy Association. (1986). Guidelines for occupational therapy documentation. *American Journal of Occupational Therapy, 40,* 830-832.

American Occupational Therapy Association. (1987). *Guidelines for occupational therapy services in school systems.* Rockville, MD: American Occupational Therapy Association.

American Occupational Therapy Association. (1992). Standards of practice for occupational therapy. *American Journal of Occupational Therapy, 46,* 1082-1083.

American Occupational Therapy Association (1994). Uniform terminology for occupational therapy, third edition. *American Journal of Occupational Therapy, 48,* 1047-1054.

Ayres, A.J. (1989). *Sensory Integration and Praxis Tests.* Los Angeles: Western Psychological Services.

Bailey, D.B. & Wolery, M. (1989). *Assessing infants and preschoolers with handicaps.* Columbus, OH: Merrill.

Barnard, K.E. (Ed.) (1993). *Nursing Child Assessment Satellite Training: parent/infant interaction manual.* Seattle: Nursing Child Assessment Training Publications.

Bayley, N. (1993). *Bayley Scales of Infant Development* (2nd ed.). San Antonio, TX: The Psychological Corporation.

Berk, R.A. & DeGangi, G.A. (1983). *Degangi-Berk Test of Sensory Integration.* Los Angeles: Western Psychological Services.

Black, M.M. (1976). Adolescent role assessment. *American Journal of Occupational Therapy, 30*(2), 73-79.

Bledsoe, N.P. & Shepherd, J.T. (1982). A study of reliability and validity of a preschool play scale. *American Journal of Occupational Therapy, 36,* 783-788.

Brammer, L.M. (1988). *The helping relationship: process and skills.* Englewood Cliffs, NJ: Prentice Hall.

Brazelton, T.B. (1984). *Neonatal Behavioral Assessment Scale: clinics in developmental medicine.* (2nd ed.). Philadelphia: J.B. Lippincott.

Bricker, D. & Squires, J. (1989). *Infant monitoring system.* Eugene: University of Oregon.

Bricker, D., Bailey, E.J., Gumerlock, S., Buhl, M., & Slentz, K. (1986). *Evaluation and Programming Systems for Infants and Young Children.* Eugene, OR: Center on Human Development.

Brigance, A.H. (1978). *Brigance Diagnostic Inventory of Early Development.* Woburn, MA: Curriculum Associates.

Bromwich, R. (1981). *Working with parents and infants: an interactional approach.* Baltimore: University Park Press.

Bronfenbrenner, V., Moen, P., & Garbarino, J. (1984). Child, family, and community. In R.D. Parke (Ed.). *Review of child development research* (Vol. 7) (pp. 283-328). Chicago: University of Chicago Press.

Bruininks, R. (1978). *Bruininks-Oseretsky Test of Motor Proficiency.* Circle Pines, MN: American Guidance Service.

Bundy, A. (1991). Writing functional goals for evaluation. In C.B. Royeen (Ed.). *AOTA self-study series: school-based practice for related services* (pp. 7-30). Rockville, MD: American Occupational Therapy Association.

Caldwell, B.M. & Bradley, R.H. (1972). *Home Observation and Measurement of the Environment Inventory.* Little Rock, AR: Center for Child Development and Education, University of Arkansas.

Campbell, S.K., Osten, E.T., Kolobe, T.H.A., & Fisher, A.G. (1993). Development of the Test of Infant Motor Performance. In C.V. Granger & G.E. Gresham (Eds.). *New developments in functional assessments in rehabilitation medicine.* Philadelphia: W.B. Saunders.

Carey, W.B. & McDevitt, S.C. (1978). Revision of the infant temperament questionnaire. *Pediatrics, 61*(5), 735-738.

Carkhuff, R.R. & Anthony, W.A. (1979). *The skills of helping.* Amherst, MA: Human Resource Development Press.

Chandler, L., Andrews, M., & Swanson, M. (1980). *The Movement Assessment of Infants: a manual.* Rolling Bay, WA: Infant Movement Research.

Chatoor, I, Menvielle, E., Getson, P., & O'Donnell, R. (1988). *Occupational scale for mother-infant interaction during feeding.* Washington, D.C.: Children's Hospital Medical Center.

Colarusso, R.P. & Hammill, D.D. (1972). Motor Free Visual Perception Test. Novato, CA: Academic Therapy Publications.

Coley, I.L. (1978). *Pediatric assessment of self-care activities.* St. Louis: Mosby.

Collier, T. (1991). The screening process. In W. Dunn (Ed.). *Pediatric occupational therapy: facilitating effective service provision* (pp. 11-33). Thorofare, NJ: Slack.

Cook, D.G. (1991). The assessment process. In W. Dunn (Ed.). *Pediatric occupational therapy: facilitating effective service provision* (pp. 35-72). Thorofare, NJ: Slack.

DeGangi, G.A. & Greenspan, S.I. (1989). *Test of Sensory Functions in Infants*. Los Angeles: Western Psychological Services.

Dunn, W., Brown, C., & McGuigan, A. (1994). The ecology of human performance: a framework for considering the effect of context. *American Journal of Occupational Therapy, 48*(7), 595-607.

Dunn, W. & Campbell, P.H. (1991). Designing pediatric service provision. In W. Dunn (Ed.). *Pediatric occupational therapy: facilitating effective service provision* (pp. 139-159). Thorofare, NJ: Slack.

Dunn-Klein, M. (1983). *The developmental checklist for pre-dressing skills*. Tucson: Therapy Skill Builders.

Erhardt, R.P. (1982). *Erhardt Developmental Prehension Assessment*. Tucson: Therapy Skill Builders.

Erhardt, R.P. (1988). *Erhardt Developmental Vision Assessment*. Tucson: Therapy Skill Builders.

Exner, L.E. (1993). Content validity of the In-Hand Manipulation Test. *American Journal of Occupational Therapy, 47*, 505-513.

Farran, D.C. (1990). Effects of intervention with disadvantaged and disabled children: a decade review. In S.J. Meisels & J.P. Shonkoff (Eds.). *Handbook of early childhood intervention* (pp. 501-539). Cambridge, MA: Cambridge University Press.

Farran, D., Kasari, C., & Jay, S. (1984). *Parent-caregiver interaction scales: training manual*. Chapel Hill, NC: Frank Porter Graham Child Development Center.

Fewell, R.R. (1986). *Play Asessment Sale*. Seattle: College of Education, University of Washington, Seattle.

Folio, M.R. & Fewell, R.R. (1983). *Peabody Developmental Motor Scales*. Chicago: Riverside Publishers.

Frankenburg, W., Dodds, J., Archer, P., Bresnick, B., Maschka, P., Edelman, N., & Shapiro, H. (1990). *Denver Developmental Screening Test (revised)*. Denver: Ladoca Publishing Foundation.

Furuno, S. et al (1979). *The Hawaii Early Learning Profile*. Palo Alto, CA: VORT.

Gardner, M.F. (1988). *Test of Visual-Perceptual Skills (non-motor)*. Seattle: Special Child Publications.

Gardner, M.F. (1986). *Test of Visual-Motor Skills*. East Aurora, NY: Slossman Educational Publications.

Gibbs, E.D. & Teti, D.M. (1990). *Interdisciplinary assessment of infants: a guide for early intervention professionals*. Baltimore: Brookes.

Glascoe, F.P., Martin, E.D., & Humphrey, S. (1990). A comparative review of developmental screening tests. *Pediatrics, 86*(4), 547-554.

Haley, S.M., Coster, W.J., Ludlow, L.H., Haltiwanger, M.A., & Andrellos, P.J. (1992). *Pediatric Evaluation of Disability Inventory*. Boston: New England Medical Center Hospitals and PEDI Research Group.

Hanft, B. (1989). How words create images. In B. Hanft (Ed.). *Family-centered care: an early intervention resource manual* (Unit 2) (pp. 77-78). Rockville, MD: American Occupational Therapy Association.

Hanft, B. (1994). The good parent: a label by any other name would not smell as sweet. *Developmental Disabilities Special Interest Section Newsletter, 17*(2), 5.

Huber, C.J. & King-Thomas, L. (1987). The assessment process. In L. King-Thomas & B. Hacker (Eds.). *A therapist's guide to pediatric assessment*. Boston: Little, Brown.

*Individuals with Disabilities Act of 1990*. (Public Law 101-476). 20 U.S.C. Sec. 1400-1465.

Ivey, A. (1971). *Microcounseling: innovations in interview training*. Springfield, IL: Charles C. Thomas.

Johnson, N., Jens, K.G., & Attermeier, S.M. (1986). *The Carolina Curriculum for Handicapped Infants and Infants at Risk*. Baltimore: Brookes.

Knobloch, H., Stevens, F., & Malone, A.F. (1980). *Manual of Developmental Diagnosis*. New York: Harper & Row.

Knox, S.H. (1974). A play scale. In Reilly, M. (Ed.). *Play as exploratory learning* (pp. 247-266). Beverly Hills, CA: Sage Publications.

Larsen, S.C. & Hammill, D.D. (1989). *Test of Legible Handwriting*. Austin, TX: Pro-Ed.

Linder, T.W. (1990). *Transdisciplinary play-based assessment: a functional approach to working with young children*. Baltimore: Brookes.

Mardell-Czudnoswki, C. & Goldenberg, D. (1983). *Developmental indicators for assessment of learning—revised*. Edison, NJ: Childcraft Educational Corporation.

McClain, L.H. (1991). Documentation. In W. Dunn (Ed.). *Pediatric occupational therapy: facilitating effective service Provision* (pp. 35-72). Thorofare, NJ: Slack.

Milani-Comparetti, A. & Gidoni, E.A. (1967). Routine developmental examination in normal and retarded children. *Developmental Medicine and Child Neurology, 9*, 631-638.

Miller, L.J. (1982). *Miller Assessment for Preschoolers*. Littleton, CO: Foundation for Knowledge in Development.

Miller, L.J. (1993). *First STEP screening tool*. San Antonio, TX: Psychological Corporation.

Miller, L.J. & Roid, G.H. (1994). *Toddler and Infant Motor Evaluation*. Tucson: Therapy Skill Builders.

Mutti, M., Sterling, H.M., & Spalding, N.V. (1978). *Quick Neurological Screening Test*. Novato, CA: Academic Therapy Publications.

Neisworth, J.T. & Bagnato, S.J. (1988). Assessment in early childhood special education: a typology of dependent measures. In S. L. Odom & M.B. Karnes (Eds.). *Early intervention for infants and children with handicaps: an empirical base* (pp. 23-49). Baltimore: Brookes.

Newborg, J., Stock, J., Wneck, L., Guidubaldi, J., & Svinicki, J. (1984). *Battelle developmental inventory*. Chicago: Riverside Publishing.

Notari, A. & Bricker, D. (1990). The utility of a curriculum-based assessment instrument in the development of individualized education plans for infants and young children. *Journal of Early Intervention, 14*, 117-132.

Palisano, R.J, Haley, S.M., & Brown, D.A. (1992). Goal attainment scaling as a measure of change in infants with motor delays. *Physical Therapy, 72*(6), 432-437.

Phelps, J. & Stempel, L. (1987). *The Cildren's Handwriting Evaluation Scale for Manuscript Writing*. Dallas: Texas Scottish Rite Hospital for Crippled Children.

Piers, E. (1984). *The Piers-Harris Children's Self-Concept Scale*. (revised manual) Los Angeles: Western Psychological Services.

Piper, M.C., & Darrah, J. (1994). *Motor assessment of the developing infant*. Philadelphia: W.B. Saunders.

Public Law 102-119. Individuals with Disabilities Education Act of 1991. Washington, DC: U.S. Government Printing Office.

Rogers, S.J., D'Eugenio, D.B., Brown, S.L., Donovan, C.M., & Lynch, E.W. (1981). *Early Intervention Developmental Profile*. Ann Arbor: University of Michigan Press.

Russell, D.J., Rosenbaum, P.L., Cadman, D.T., Gowland, C., Hardy, S., Jarvis, S. (1989). The Gross Motor Function Measure: a means to evaluate the effects of physical therapy. *Developmental Medicine and Child Neurology, 31*, 341-352.

Sameroff, A.J. & Chandler, M.J. (1975). Reproductive risk and the continuum of caretaking casualty. In F.D. Horowitz, M. Hetherington, S. Scarr-Salapatek, & G. Siegel (Eds.). *Review of child development research* (Vol. 4) (pp. 187-244). Chicago: University of Chicago Press.

Sameroff, A.J. (1986). Environmental context of child development. *Journal of Pediatrics, 109,* 192-200.

Sameroff, A.J. & Fiese, B.H. (1990). Transactional regulation and early intervention. In S.J. Meisels & J.P. Shonkoff (Eds.). *Handbook of early childhood intervention* (pp. 119-145). Cambridge, MA: University of Cambridge Press.

Sanford, A.R. & Zelman, J.G. (1981). *Learning Accomplishment Profile.* Winston-Salem, NC: Kaplan.

Schafer, D.S. & Moersch, M. (1981). *Developmental Programming for Infants and Young Children.* Ann Arbor: University of Michigan Press.

Simeonsson, R.J. (1979). *Carolina Record of Individual Behavior.* Chapel Hill, NC: University of North Carolina, Frank Porter Graham Child Development Center.

Sparrow, S.S., Balla, D.A., & Cicchetti, D.V. (1984). *Vineland adaptive behavior scales.* Circle Pines, MN: American Guidance Service.

Takata, N. (1974). Play as a prescription. In Reilly, M. (Ed.). *Play as exploratory learning* (pp. 209-246). Beverly Hills, CA: Sage Publications.

Uzgiris, I. & Hunt, J.M. (1975). *Assessment in Infancy: ordinal scales of psychological development.* Urbana: University of Illinois.

Vulpe, S.G. (1994). *Vulpe Assessment Battery—revised.* East Aurora, NY: Slosson Educational Publications.

Washington Administrative Code. (1990). *Rules and regulations for programs providing services to children with handicapping conditions.* W.A.C. 392-171, Section 381. Olympia, WA: Office of Superintendent of Public Instruction.

Werner E.E. & Smith, R.S. (1982). *Vulnerable but invincible: a longitudinal study of resilient children and youth.* New York: McGraw-Hill.

Wilbarger, P. (1973). *Sensorimotor history.* St. Paul: Special education workshop, St. Paul Public Schools.

Williamson, G.G., Szczepanski, M., & Zeitlin, S. (1993). Coping frame of reference. In P. Kramer & J. Hinojosa (Eds.). *Frames of reference for pediatric occupational therapy* (pp. 395-436). Baltimore: Williams & Wilkins.

Winton, P.J. (1988). The family-focused interview: an assessment measure and goal setting mechanism. In D.B. Bailey & R.J. Simeonsson (Eds.). *Family assessment in early intervention* (pp. 185-205). Columbus, OH: Merrill.

Zeitlin, S., Williamson, G.G., & Szczepanski, M. (1988). *Early Coping Inventory.* Bensenville, IL: Scholastic Testing Service.

## SUGGESTED READINGS

American Occupational Therapy Association. (1994). *Pediatric Resource Guide.* Rockville, MD: American Occupaitonal Therapy Association.

Asher, I. (1989). *An annotated index of occupational therapy evaluation tools.* Rockville, MD: American Occupational Therapy Association.

Clancy, H. & Clark, M.J. (1990). *Occupational therapy with children.* Melbourne, Australia: Churchill Livingstone.

King-Thomas, L. & Hacker, B. (1987). *A therapist's guide to pediatric assessment.* Boston: Little, Brown.

# APPENDIX

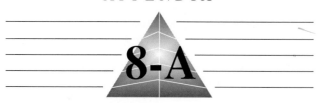

## 8-A

## Uniform Terminology for Occupational Therapy, Third Edition*

*Occupational therapy* is the use of purposeful activity or interventions to promote health and achieve functional outcomes. *Achieving functional outcomes* means to develop, improve, or restore the highest possible level of independence of any individual who is limited by a physical injury or illness, a dysfunctional condition, a cognitive impairment, a psychosocial dysfunction, a mental illness, a developmental or learning disability, or an adverse environmental condition. Assessment means the use of skilled observation or evaluation by the administration and interpretation of standardized or nonstandardized tests and measurements to identify areas for occupational therapy services.

Occupational therapy services include, but are not limited to the following:

1. The assessment, treatment, and education of or consultation with the individual, family, or other persons.
2. Interventions directed toward developing, improving, or restoring daily living skills, work readiness or work performance, play skills or leisure capacities, or enhancing educational performances skills.
3. Providing for the development, improvement, or restoration of sensorimotor, oral-motor, perceptual or neuromuscular functioning; or emotional, motivational, cognitive, or psychosocial components of performance.

These services may require assessment of the need for and use of interventions such as the design, development, adaptation, application, or training in the use of assistive technology devices; the design, fabrication, or application of rehabilitative technology such as selected orthotic devices; training in the use of assistive technology and orthotic or prosthetic devices; the application of physical agent modalities as an adjunct to or in preparation for purposeful activity; the use of ergonomic principles; the adaptation of environments and processes to enhance functional performance; or the promotion of health and wellness (AOTA, 1993, p. 1117).

I. Performance areas—Throughout this document, activities have been described as if individuals performed the tasks themselves. Occupational therapy also recognizes that individuals arrange for tasks to be done through others. The profession views independence as the ability to self-determine activity performance, regardless of who actually performs the activity.

A. *Activities of daily living—self-maintenance tasks*
1. *Grooming*—Obtaining and using supplies; removing body hair (use of razors, tweezers, and lotions); applying and removing cosmetics; washing, drying, combing, styling, and brushing hair; caring for nails (hands and feet), skin, ears, and eyes; and applying deodorant.
2. *Oral hygiene*—Obtaining and using supplies; cleaning mouth; brushing and flossing teeth; and removing, cleaning, and reinserting dental orthotics and prosthetics.
3. *Bathing and showering*—Obtaining and using supplies; soaping, rinsing, and drying body parts; maintaining bathing position; and transferring to and from bathing positions.
4. *Toilet hygiene*—Obtaining and using supplies; clothing management; maintaining toileting position; transferring to and from toileting position; cleaning body; and caring for menstrual and continence needs (including catheters, colostomies, and suppository management).
5. *Personal device care*—Cleaning and maintaining personal care items such as hearing aids, contact lenses, glasses, orthotics, prosthetics, adaptive equipment, and contraceptive and sexual devices.
6. *Dressing*—Selecting clothing and accessories appropriate to the time of day, weather, and occasion; obtaining clothing from storage area; dressing and undressing in a sequential fashion; fastening and adjusting clothing and shoes; and applying and removing personal devices, prostheses, or orthoses.
7. *Feeding and eating*—Setting up food; selecting and using appropriate utensils and tableware; bringing food or drink to mouth; cleaning face, hands, and clothing; sucking, masticating, coughing, and swallowing; and management of alternative methods of nourishment.
8. *Medication routine*—Obtaining medication, opening and closing containers, following prescribed schedules, taking correct quantities, reporting problems and adverse effects, and administering correct quantities using prescribed methods.
9. *Health maintenance*—Developing and maintaining routines for illness prevention and wellness promotion, such as physical fitness, nutrition, and decreasing health risk behaviors.
10. *Socialization*—Accessing opportunities and interacting with other people in appropriate contextual and cultural ways to meet emotional and physical needs.

*From the American Occupational Therapy Association, Inc. (1994). *American Journal of Occupational Therapy, 48,* 1047-1054.

11. *Functional communication*—Using equipment or systems to send and receive information, such as writing equipment, telephones, typewriters, computers, communication boards, call lights, emergency systems, Braille writers, telecommunication devices for the deaf, and augmentative communication systems.

12. *Functional mobility*—Moving from one position or place to another, such as in in-bed mobility, wheelchair mobility, and transfers (wheelchair, bed, car, tub, toilet, tub or shower, chair, and floor), performing functional ambulation, and transporting objects.

13. *Community mobility*—Moving self in the community and using public or private transportation, such as driving, or accessing buses, taxi cabs, or other public transportation systems.

14. *Emergency response*—Recognizing sudden, unexpected hazardous situations and initiating action to reduce the threat to health and safety.

15. *Sexual expression*—Engaging in desired sexual and intimate activities.

B. *Work and productive activities*—Purposeful activities for self-development, social contribution, and livelihood.

   1. *Home management*—Obtaining and maintaining personal and household possessions and environment.

      a. *Clothing care*—Obtaining and using supplies and sorting, laundering (hand, machine, and dry clean), folding, ironing, storing, and mending clothes.

      b. *Cleaning*—Obtaining and using supplies, picking up, putting away, vacuuming, sweeping and mopping floors, dusting, polishing, scrubbing, washing windows, cleaning mirrors, making beds, and removing trash and recyclables.

      c. *Meal preparation and cleanup*—Planning nutritious meals; preparing and serving food; opening and closing containers, cabinets, and drawers; using kitchen utensils and appliances; cleaning up and storing food safely.

      d. *Shopping*—Preparing shopping lists (grocery and other), selecting and purchasing items, selecting method of payment, and completing money transactions.

      e. *Money management*—Budgeting, paying bills, and using bank systems.

      f. *Household maintenance*—Maintaining home, yard, garden, appliances, vehicles, and household items.

      g. *Safety procedures*—Knowing and performing preventive and emergency procedures to maintain a safe environment and to prevent injuries.

   2. *Care of others*—Providing for children, spouse, parents, pets, or others, such as giving physical care, nurturing, communicating, and using age-appropriate activities.

   3. *Educational activities*—Participating in a learning environment through school, community, or work-sponsored activities, such as exploring educational interests, attending to instruction, managing assignments, and contributing to group experiences.

   4. *Vocational activities*—Participating in work-related activities.

      a. *Vocational exploration*—Determining aptitudes, developing interests and skills, and selecting appropriate vocational pursuits.

      b. *Job acquisition*—Identifying and selecting work opportunities and completing application and interview processes.

      c. *Work or job performance*—Performing job tasks in a timely and effective manner and incorporating necessary work behaviors.

      d. *Retirement planning*—Determining aptitudes, developing interests and skills, and selecting appropriate avocational pursuits.

      e. *Volunteer participation*—Performing unpaid activities for the benefit of selected individuals, groups, or causes.

C. *Play or leisure activities*—Intrinsically motivating activities for amusement, relaxation, spontaneous enjoyment, or self-expression.

   1. *Play or leisure exploration*—Identifying interests, skills, opportunities, and appropriate play or leisure activities.

   2. *Play or leisure performance*—Planning and participating in play or leisure activities; maintaining a balance of play or leisure activities with work, productive activities, and activities of daily living; obtaining, using, and maintaining equipment and supplies.

II. Performance components

A. *Sensorimotor component*—The ability to receive input, process information, and produce output.

   1. *Sensory*

      a. *Sensory awareness*—Receiving and differentiating sensory stimuli.

      b. *Sensory processing*—Interpreting sensory stimuli.

         (1) *Tactile*—Interpreting light touch, pressure, temperature, pain, and vibration through skin contact and receptors.

         (2) *Proprioceptive*—Interpreting stimuli originating in muscles, joints, and other internal tissues that give informa-

tion about the position of one body part in relation to another.

(3) *Vestibular*—Interpreting stimuli from the inner ear receptors regarding head position and movement.

(4) *Visual*—Interpreting stimuli through the eyes, including peripheral vision and acuity, and awareness of color and pattern.

(5) *Auditory*—Interpreting and localizing sounds and discriminating background sounds.

(6) *Gustatory*—Interpreting tastes.

(7) *Olfactory*—Interpreting odors.

c. *Perceptual processing*—Organizing sensory input into meaningful patterns.

(1) *Stereognosis*—Identifying objects through proprioception, cognition, and the sense of touch.

(2) *Kinesthesia*—Identifying the excursion and direction of joint movement.

(3) *Pain response*—Interpreting noxious stimuli.

(4) *Body scheme*—Acquiring an internal awareness of the body and the relationship of body parts to each other.

(5) *Right-left discrimination*—Differentiating one side from the other.

(6) *Form constancy*—Recognizing forms and objects as the same in various environments, positions, and sizes.

(7) *Position in space*—Determining the spatial relationship of figures and objects to self or other forms and objects.

(8) *Visual closure*—Identifying forms or objects from incomplete presentations.

(9) *Figure-ground*—Differentiating between foreground and background forms and objects.

(10) *Depth perception*—Determining the relative distance between objects, figures, or landmarks and the observer and changes in planes of surfaces.

(11) *Spatial relations*—Determining the position of objects relative to each other.

(12) *Topographic orientation*—Determining the location of objects and settings and the route to the location.

2. *Neuromusculoskeletal*

a. *Reflex*—Eliciting an involuntary muscle response by sensory input.

b. *Range of motion*—Moving body parts through an arc.

c. *Muscle tone*—Demonstrating a degree of tension or resistance in a muscle at rest and in response to stretch.

d. *Strength*—Demonstrating a degree of muscle power when movement is resisted, as with objects or gravity.

e. *Endurance*—Sustaining cardiac, pulmonary, and musculoskeletal exertion over time.

f. *Postural control*—Using righting and equilibrium adjustments to maintain balance during functional movements.

g. *Postural alignment*—Maintaining biomechanical integrity among body parts.

h. *Soft tissue integrity*—Maintaining anatomic and physiologic condition of interstitial tissue and skin.

3. *Motor*

a. *Gross coordination*—Using large muscle groups for controlled, goal-directed movements.

b. *Crossing the midline*—Moving limbs and eyes across the midsagittal plane of the body.

c. *Laterality*—Using a preferred unilateral body part for activities requiring a high level of skill.

d. *Bilateral integration*—Coordinating both body sides during activity.

e. *Motor control*—Using the body in functional and versatile movement patterns.

f. *Praxis*—Conceiving and planning a new motor act in response to an environmental demand.

g. *Fine coordination and dexterity*—Using small muscle groups for controlled movements, particularly in object manipulation.

h. *Visual-motor integration*—Coordinating the interaction of information from the eyes with body movement during activity.

i. *Oral-motor control*—Coordinating oropharyngeal musculature for controlled movements.

B. *Cognitive integration and cognitive components*—The ability to use higher brain functions.

1. *Level of arousal*—Demonstrating alertness and responsiveness to environmental stimuli.

2. *Orientation*—Identifying a person, place, time, and situation.

3. *Recognition*—Identifying familiar faces, objects, and other previously presented materials.

4. *Attention span*—Focusing on a task over time.

5. *Initiation of activity*—Starting a physical or mental activity.

6. *Termination of activity*—Stopping an activity at an appropriate time.

7. *Memory*—Recalling information after brief or long periods of time.
8. *Sequencing*—Placing information, concepts, and actions in order.
9. *Categorization*—Identifying similarities of and differences among pieces of environmental information.
10. *Concept formation*—Organizing a variety of information to form thoughts and ideas.
11. *Spatial operations*—Mentally manipulating the position of objects in various relationships.
12. *Problem solving*—Recognizing a problem, defining a problem, identifying alternative plans, selecting a plan, organizing steps in a plan, implementing a plan, and evaluating the outcome.
13. *Learning*—Acquiring new concepts and behaviors.
14. *Generalization*—Applying previously learned concepts and behaviors to a variety of new situations.

C. *Psychosocial skills and psychologic components*—The ability to interact in society and to process emotions.
  1. *Psychological*
    a. *Values*—Identifying ideas or beliefs that are important to self and others.
    b. *Interests*—Identifying mental or physical activities that create pleasure and maintain attention.
    c. *Self-concept*—Developing the value of the physical, emotional, and sexual self.
  2. *Social*
    a. *Role performance*—Identifying, maintaining, and balancing functions one assumes or acquires in society (e.g., worker, student, parent, friend, or religious participant).
    b. *Social conduct*—Interacting by using manners, personal space, eye contact, gestures, active listening, and self-expression appropriate to the environment.
    c. *Interpersonal skills*—Using verbal and nonverbal communication to interact in a variety of settings.
    d. *Self-expression*—Using a variety of styles and skills to express thoughts, feelings, and needs.
  3. *Self-management*
    a. *Coping skills*—Identifying and managing stress and related factors.
    b. *Time management*—Planning and participating in a balance of self-care, work, leisure, and rest activities to promote satisfaction and health.
    c. *Self-control*—Modifying one's own behavior in response to environmental needs, demands, constraints, personal aspirations, and feedback from others.

III. *Performance contexts*—Assessment of function in performance areas is greatly influenced by the contexts in which the individual must perform. Occupational therapy practitioners consider performance contexts when determining feasibility and appropriateness of interventions. Occupational therapy practitioners may choose interventions based on an understanding of contexts or may choose interventions directly aimed at altering the contexts to improve performance.
A. *Temporal Aspects*
  1. *Chronologic*—Individual's age.
  2. *Developmental*—Stage or phase of maturation.
  3. *Life cycle*—Place in important life phases, such as career cycle, parenting cycle, or educational process.
  4. *Disability status*—Place in continuum of disability, such as acuteness of injury, chronicity of disability, or terminal nature of illness.
B. *Environment*
  1. *Physical*—Nonhuman aspects of contexts. Includes the accessibility to and performance within environments having natural terrain, plants, animals, buildings, furniture, objects, tools, or devices.
  2. *Social*—Availability and expectations of significant individuals, such as spouse, friends, and caregivers. Also includes larger social groups, which are influential in establishing norms, role expectations, and social routines.
  3. *Cultural*—Customs, beliefs, activity patterns, behavior standards, and expectations accepted by the society of which the individual is a member. Includes political aspects, such as laws that affect access to resources and affirm personal rights. Also includes opportunities for education, employment, and economic support.

## REFERENCES

American Occupational Therapy Association. (1979). *Occupational therapy product output reporting system and uniform terminology for reporting occupational therapy services.* Rockville, MD: AOTA.

American Occupational Therapy Association. (1989). Uniform terminology for occupational therapy (2nd ed.). *American Journal of Occupational Therapy, 43,* 808-815.

American Occupational Therapy Association. (1993). Definition of occupational therapy practice for state regulation (Policy 5.3.1). *American Journal of Occupational Therapy, 47,* 1117-1121.

## AUTHORS

The Terminology Task Force:
Winifred Dunn, PhD, OTR, FAOTA, Chairperson
Mary Foto, OTR, FAOTA

Jim Hinojosa, PhD, OTR, FAOTA
Barbara Schell, PhD, OTR/L, FAOTA
Linda Kohlman Thomson, MOT, OTR, FAOTA
Sarah D. Hertfelder, MEd, MOT, OTR/L, Staff Liaison

for

The Commission on Practice, 1994
Jim Hinojosa, PhD, OTR, FAOTA, Chairperson

Adopted by the Representative Assembly July, 1994

NOTE: This document replaces the following documents, all of which were rescinded by the 1994 Representative Assembly:

*Occupational Therapy Product Output Reporting System* (1979)
*Uniform Terminology for Reporting Occupational Therapy Services,* ed. 1 (1979)
*Uniform Occupational Therapy Evaluation Checklist* (1981)
*Uniform Terminology for Occupational Therapy,* ed. 2 (1989)

## Common Pediatric Evaluation Tools

### Alberta Infant Motor Scales (AIMS)

Piper, M.C., & Darrah, J. (1994)
Motor Assessment of the Developing Infant
W.B. Saunders Company
Philadelphia, PA 19106

### Battelle Developmental Inventory

Newborg, J., Stock, J.R., Wnek, L., Guidubaldi, J., & Svinicki, A. (1988)
Riverside Publishing
8420 West Bryn Mawr Avenue
Chicago, IL 60631
(800) 767-8378

### Bayley Scales of Infant Development, 2nd ed.

Bayley, N. (1994)
The Psychological Corporation
555 Academic Court
San Antonio, TX 78204
(210) 299-1061

### Beery Developmental Test of Visual Motor Integration (3rd rev)

Beery, K.E. (1989)
Modern Curriculum Press
13900 Prospect Road
Cleveland, OH 44136
(216) 572-0690

### Brigance Diagnostic Inventories

Brigance, A.H. (1978)
Curriculum Associates
5 Esquire Road, N
Billerica, MA 01862

### Bruininks-Oseretsky Test of Motor Proficiency

Bruininks, R. (1978)
American Guidance Service
4201 Woodland Road
Circle Pines, MN 55014
(612) 786-4343

### Coping Inventory

Zeitlin, S. (1991)
Scholastic Testing Service
Bensenville, IL 60106-8056

### DeGangi-Berk Test of Sensory Integration

Berk, R.A., & DeGangi, G.A. (1983)
Western Psychological Services
1203 Wilshire Boulevard
Los Angeles, CA 90025
(310) 478-2061

### Denver Developmental Screening Test (Revised)

Frankenburg, W., Dodds, J., Archer, P., Bresnick, B.,
    Maschka, P., Edelman, N., & Shapiro, H. (1990)
Ladoca Publishing Foundation
University of Colorado
Denver, CO 80216

### Developmental Test of Visual Perception, 2nd ed.

(previously called the Marianne Frostig Developmental Test
    of Visual Perception)
Hammill, D.D., Pearson, N.A., & Voress, J.K. (1993)
Pro Ed
8700 Shoal Creek Boulevard
Austin, TX 78757-6897
(512) 451-3246

### Developmental Programming for Infants and Young Children

Schafer, D.S. & Moersch, M.S. (1981)
The University of Michigan Press
Ann Arbor, MI 48106
(313) 764-4392

### Early Coping Inventory

Zeitlin, S., Williamson, G.G., & Szczepanski, M. (1988)
Scholastic Testing Service
Bensenville, IL 60106-8056

**Early Intervention Developmental Profile**

Rogers, S.J., Donavane, C.M., D'Eugenio, D.B., Brown, S.L., Lynch, E.W., Moersch, M.S., & Schafer, D.S. (1981)
University of Michigan Press
Ann Arbor, MI 48106
(313) 764-4392

**Erhardt Developmental Prehension Assessment**

Erhardt, R.P. (1982)
Therapy Skill Builders
3830 E. Bellevue
P.O. Box 42050-TS4
Tucson, AZ 85733
(602) 323-7500

**Erhardt Developmental Vision Assessment**

Erhardt, R.P. (1988)
Therapy Skill Builders
3830 E. Bellevue
P.O. Box 42050-TS4
Tucson, AZ 85733
(602) 323-7500

**The First STEP**

Miller, L.J. (1993)
The Psychological Corporation
555 Academic Court
San Antonio, TX 78204
(210) 299-1061

**Gesell Preschool Test**

Ames, L.B., Gillespie, C., Haines, J., & Ilg, F.L. (1980)
Programs for Education, Inc.
P.O. Box 167
Rosemont, NJ 08556
(609) 397-2214

**Gross Motor Function Measure (GMFM)**

Russell, D., Rosenbaum, P., Cadman, D., Gowland, C., Hardy, S., & Jarvis, S. (1989)
Gross Motor Measures Group
c/o Dianne Russell
Building 74, Room 29
Station 9
Hamilton, ON
Canada L8N 3Z5

**Hawaii Early Learning Profile (HELP)**

Furuno, S., O'Reilly, K.A., Hosaka, C.M., Inatsuka, T.T., Allman, T.A., & Zeisloft, B. (1984)
Vort Corporation
P.O. Box 60123
Palo Alto, CA 94306
(415) 322-8282

**Home Observation and Measurement of the Environment (HOME)**

Caldwell, B. (1984)
Center for Early Development and Education
University of Arkansas
Little Rock, AR 77204

**In-Hand Manipulation Test**

Exner, C.E. (research edition only)
Occupational Therapy Department
Towson State University
Towson, MD 21204

**Miller Assessment for Preschoolers (MAP)**

Miller, L.J. (1982)
The Psychological Corporation
555 Academic Court
San Antonio, TX 78204
(210) 299-1061

**Motor-Free Visual Perception Test (MVPT)**

Colarusso, R.P., & Hammill, D.D. (1983)
Academic Therapy Publications
20 Commercial Boulevard
Novato, CA 94947-6191
(800) 422-7249

**Movement Assessment of Infants (MAI)**

Chandler, L.S., Andrews, M.S., & Swanson, M.W. (1980)
Movement Assessment of Infants
P.O. Box 4631
Rolling Bay, WA 98061

**Peabody Developmental Motor Scales**

Folio, R., & Fewell, R. (1983)
Riverside Publishing
8420 West Bryn Mawr Avenue
Chicago, IL 60631
(800) 767-8378
(800) 323-9540

## Pediatric Evaluation of Disability Inventory (PEDI)

Haley S.M., Coster W.J., Ludlow, L.H., Haltiwanger, J. T., & Andrellos, P.J. (1992)
PEDI Research Group
Department of Rehabilitation Medicine
New England Medical Center Hospital, #75K/R
750 Washington Street
Boston, MA 02111-1901
(617) 956-5031

## Pediatric Extended Examination at Three

Blackman, J.A., Levine, M.D., & Markowitz, M.
Educators Publishing Service, Inc.
75 Moulton Street
Cambridge, MA 02238-9101

## Pediatric Examination of Educational Readiness

Levine, M.D., & Schneider, E.A.
Educators Publishing Service, Inc.
75 Moulton Street
Cambridge, MA 02238-9101

## Quick Neurological Screening Test (QNST)

Mutti, M., Sterling, H.M., & Spalding, N.V. (1978)
Academic Therapy Publications
20 Commercial Boulevard
Novato, CA 94949
(415) 883-3314

## Sensory Integration and Praxis Tests (SIPT)

Ayres, A.J., & staff (1989)
Western Psychological Services
1203 Wilshire Boulevard
Los Angeles, CA 90025-1251
(310) 478-2061

## Test of Visual-Perceptual Skills (non-motor) (TVPS)

Gardner, M.F. (1982)
Psychological and Educational Publications, Inc.
1477 Rollins Road
Burlingame, CA 94010-2316
(800) 523-5775

## Test of Visual-Motor Skills (TVMS)

Gardner, M.F. (1986)
Psychological and Educational Publications, Inc.
1477 Rollins Road
Burlingame, CA 94010-2316
(800) 523-5775

## Test of Infant Motor Performance (TIMP)

Cambell, S.K., Osten, E.T., Kolobe, T.H.A., & Fisher, A.G. (1993)
Development of the Test of Infant Motor Performance
In Granger, C.V., & Gresham, G.E. (Eds.), New Developments in Functional Assessment
W.B. Saunders Company
Philadelphia, PA 19106

## Test of Sensory Functions in Infants (TSFI)

DeGangi, G.A., & Greenspan, S.I. (1989)
Western Psychological Services
1203 Wilshire Boulevard
Los Angeles, CA 90025-1251
(310) 478-2061

## Toddler and Infant Motor Evaluation (TIME)

Miller, L.J., & Roid, G.H. (1994)
Therapy Skill Builders
3830 E. Bellevue
P.O. Box 42050
Tucson, AZ 85733
(602) 323-7500

## Transdisciplinary Play-Based Assessment

Linder, T.W. (1993)
Paul H. Brookes Publishing Co.
P.O. Box 10624
Baltimore, MD 21285-0624
(800) 638-3775

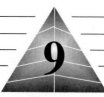

CHAPTER

# 9

# Use of Standardized Tests in Pediatric Practice

PAMELA K. RICHARDSON

## KEY TERMS

▲ Standardized Test
▲ Reliability
▲ Norm-Referenced Test
▲ Criterion-Referenced Test
▲ Normative Sample
▲ Measures of Central Tendency
▲ Measures of Variability
▲ Standard Score
▲ Correlation Coefficient
▲ Validity
▲ Ethics in Testing

## CHAPTER OBJECTIVES

1. Be aware of characteristics of commonly used standardized pediatric tests.
2. Describe the differences between norm-referenced and criterion-referenced tests, and the purpose for each type of test.
3. Understand the descriptive statistics used in standardized pediatric tests.
4. Understand the types of standard scores used in standardized pediatric tests.
5. Discuss the concept of reliability.
6. Discuss the importance of test validity.
7. Describe the procedures necessary to become a competent user of standardized tests.
8. Understand the ethical considerations when using standardized tests.
9. Apply knowledge of standardized test applications in a case study.

What is a standardized test, and why is it important to occupational therapists? A test that has been standardized has *uniform procedures* for administration and scoring (Anastasi, 1988). This means that examiners must use the same instructions, materials, and procedures each time they administer the test and must score it using criteria specified in the test manual. A number of standardized tests are in common use. Most schoolchildren have taken standardized achievement tests that assess how well the required grade-level material has been learned. College students are familiar with the Scholastic Aptitude Test (SAT), the results of which are used by many colleges and universities to make decisions about who should be admitted. Intelligence tests, interest tests, and aptitude tests are other examples of standardized tests that are used frequently with the general public. Pediatric occupational therapists are increasingly making use of standardized tests to determine eligibility of children for therapy services, to monitor progress in therapy, and to make decisions about what type of treatment intervention is most appropriate and effective. Standardized tests offer precise measurements of children's performance in a specific area and describe the child's performance as a standard score, which can be used and understood by other occupational therapists and child development professionals who are familiar with standardized testing procedures.

The initial concept of standardized assessments of human performance was developed by Galton and Cattell late in the nineteenth century, who attempted to use anthropometric measurements and psychophysical testing to measure intelligence. The first widespread use of human performance testing was initiated in 1904, when the minister of public education in Paris formed a commission to create tests that would help to identify "mentally defective children," with the goal of providing them an appropriate education. Binet and Simon developed the first intelligence test for this purpose. Terman and Merrill (1937) incorporated many of Binet and Simon's ideas in constructing the Stanford-Binet Intelligence Scale that remains widely used today (Sternberg, 1990).

Although intelligence was the first human attribute to be tested in a standardized manner, tests have been developed in the past 30 years that assess children's developmental status, cognition, gross and fine motor skills, language and communication skills, school readiness, school achievement, visual-motor skills, visual-perceptual skills, social skills, and other behavioral domains. Interestingly, although the number and types of tests have changed radically since the time of Simon and Binet, the basic reason for using standardized tests remains the same: to identify children whose performance in a given area is outside the "norm," or average, for their particular age and who may be in need of special intervention or programming.

The use of standardized tests requires a high level of responsibility on the part of the tester. The occupational therapist who uses a standardized test must be knowledgeable about scoring and interpreting the test, must be aware for whom the test is and is not appropriate, and must understand how to report and discuss a child's scores on the test. The tester must also be aware of the limitations of standardized tests in providing information about a child's performance deficits. This in turn requires a working knowledge of standardized testing concepts and procedures, familiarity with the factors that can affect performance on standardized tests, and awareness of the ethics and responsibilities of testers when using standardized tests. With this in mind, the purpose of this chapter is to provide an introduction to pediatric standardized testing for occupational therapists. Purposes and characteristics of standardized tests are discussed, technical information about standardized tests is presented, practical tips are given for becoming competent users of standardized assessments, and ethical considerations are discussed. The chapter concludes with a summary of the advantages and disadvantages of standardized tests, and a case study incorporates the concepts presented in the chapter into a "real-life" testing scenario. Throughout the chapter, several standardized assessments that are commonly used by pediatric occupational therapists are highlighted to illustrate the concepts of test administration, scoring, and interpretation.

## PURPOSES

Standardized tests are used for several reasons. First, a standardized test may be a screening tool. The purpose of a screening tool is to quickly and briefly assess large numbers of children to identify those who may have delays and are in need of more in-depth testing. Some examples of screening tests frequently used by occupational therapists include the Miller Assessment for Preschoolers (MAP) (Miller, 1982), the Denver Developmental Screening Test, revised (Denver-II) (Frankenburg, Fandal, Sciarillo, & Bur-

gess, 1981), Developmental Indicators for Assessment of Learning, revised (Mardell-Czudnoswki & Goldberg, 1983), and the First STEP (Miller, 1990). Screening tests typically assess several developmental domains, with each domain represented by a small number of items. Table 9-1 illustrates the domains assessed by the screening tools listed.

Screening tests generally take 20 to 30 minutes to administer and can be administered by professionals or by paraprofessionals such as classroom aides, volunteers, or parents. Although occupational therapists most frequently administer more in-depth assessment tools after a child has been referred to them with specific developmental concerns, therapists who work in settings that primarily serve typically developing children, such as public school systems or Head Start programs, may become involved in developmental screening activities. It is important for therapists who administer screening tests, or who receive referrals based on the results of screening tests, to be aware of the strengths and weaknesses of specific tests used in their settings. Although the screening tools mentioned are not discussed in greater depth, the concepts of developing, administering, scoring, and interpreting standardized tests (discussed later in this chapter) also should be considered when using screening tools.

Occupational therapists most frequently use standardized tests as in-depth assessments of various developmental or functional domains. Standardized tests are used for several purposes. The first purpose is for diagnosis. Specific areas

▲ Table 9-1  Developmental Domains Assessed in Four Screening Tools

| Screening Tool | Age Range | Domains Assessed |
| --- | --- | --- |
| Denver Developmental Screening Test, revised | 1 month to 6 years | Personal-social, fine motor-adaptive, language, gross motor |
| Developmental Indicators for Assessment of Learning, revised | 2½ to 6 years | Motor, language, concepts |
| First STEP: Screening Test for Evaluating Preschoolers | 2 years 9 months to 6 years 2 months | Cognition, communication, physical, social and emotional, adaptive functioning |
| Miller Assessment for Preschoolers | 2 years 7 months to 5 years 8 months | Foundations, coordination, verbal, nonverbal, complex tasks |

of strength and weakness can be identified, and performance can be compared with that of an age-matched sample of children. Standardized tests are frequently used to determine if a child has developmental delays or functional deficits that are significant enough to qualify for remedial services such as occupational therapy. Many funding agencies, early intervention programs, and public school programs use the results of standardized testing as a primary criterion for making the decision about whether a child will receive special education services or therapy intervention. Funding approval for special services is generally dependent on documentation of a predetermined amount of delay in one or more developmental domains, and standardized test results are an important component of this documentation. The results of standardized testing performed by occupational therapists, used in conjunction with testing done by other professionals, may also assist physicians or psychologists in arriving at a medical or educational diagnosis.

A second purpose for standardized testing is to document a child's current status. Many funding agencies and service agencies require periodic reassessment to provide a record of a child's progress and to determine if the child continues to qualify for services. Standardized tests are often a preferred way of documenting progress because the results from the most current assessment can be compared with the results of earlier assessments. Periodic formal reassessment can also provide valuable information to the treating therapist. Careful scrutiny of a child's test results can help identify areas of greatest and least progress. This can assist the therapist in prioritizing treatment goals. Many parents are also interested in seeing the results of their child's periodic assessments. However, care must be taken to put standardized test scores in perspective because gains in functional skills such as feeding, dressing, and toileting, for instance, may not be reflected in the child's scores on a comprehensive developmental or motor assessment. It is good practice to accompany the discussion of test performance with a discussion of the child's progress in other areas that may not be measured by standardized testing. Informal observations of the child's play and self-care behavior and interviews with the caretaker about the child's home routine, as well as review of pertinent medical or educational records, are equally important components of the assessment process. (See Chapter 8 for more information about the assessment process.)

A third purpose for standardized testing is for program planning. Standardized tests provide information about a child's level of function so that therapists can determine the appropriate starting point for therapy intervention. Most commonly, criterion-referenced standardized tests are used as the basis for developing goals and objectives for individual children and for measuring progress and change over time. Criterion-referenced tests are used extensively in educational settings and include such tools as the Hawaii Early

Learning Profile (HELP) (Furuno, O'Reilly, Hosaka, Inatsuka, Allman, & Zeisloft, 1979), the Assessment, Evaluation, and Programming System for Infants and Children (Bricker, 1993), and the Learning Accomplishment Profile, revised edition (Sanford & Zelman, 1981). Criterion-referenced tests are described in more detail in the following section.

## CHARACTERISTICS

Recall that, by definition, standardized tests have uniform procedures for administration and scoring. The characteristics of standardized tests, then, ensure that standard or uniform procedures are employed whenever the test is given. These standard procedures are what permit the results of a child's testing to be compared with either the child's performance on a previous administration of the test or with the test norms developed by administering the test to a large number of children.

First, standardized tests have a test manual that describes the purpose of the test, that is, what the test is intended to measure. The manual should also describe the intended population for the test. Generally for pediatric assessments, this refers to the age range of children for whom the test was intended. Test manuals also contain technical information about the test, such as a description of the test development and standardization process, characteristics of the normative sample, and studies done during the test development process to establish reliability and validity data. Finally, test manuals contain detailed information about administration, scoring, and interpretation of the test scores.

A second characteristic of standardized tests is that they are composed of a fixed number of items. Items may not be added or subtracted without affecting the standard procedure for test administration. Most tests have specific rules regarding how many items should be administered to have a standardized test administration. These may differ significantly from test to test. For instance, the Bruininks-Oseretsky Test of Motor Proficiency (BOTMP) (Bruininks, 1978) specifies that the entire item set be administered regardless of the age of the child. In contrast, the Bayley Scales of Infant Development, revised (BSID-II) (Bayley, 1993) has a number of item sets corresponding to age bands (e.g., 22 to 24 months). Testers are instructed to begin testing at the age band corresponding to the child's chronologic age (or corrected age, if the child was born prematurely) and to move either to higher or lower age bands if necessary, depending on the child's performance. The decision to move on to a different age band is made according to the number of items passed and failed at the initial age band. The decision rules are stated in the test manual.

The third characteristic of standardized tests is a fixed protocol for administration. A fixed protocol for administration refers to how each item is administered as well as how many items are administered. Generally the protocol for administration specifies what verbal instruction or demonstration is provided, how many times the instructions can be repeated, and how many attempts the child is allowed at the item. For some tests, instructions for each item are printed in the manual and the tester is expected to read the instructions verbatim to the child without deviating from the text.

The fourth characteristic of standardized tests is that there are fixed guidelines for scoring. Scoring guidelines usually accompany the administration guidelines and specify what the child's performance must look like to receive a passing score on the item. Depending on the nature of the item, there may be a description of the passing performance or a picture or diagram of the passing performance. Figures 9-1 and

---

Touching Thumb to Fingertips — Eyes Closed

With eyes closed, the subject touches the thumb of the preferred hand to each of the fingertips on the preferred hand, moving from the little finger to the index finger and then from the index finger to the little finger, as shown below. The subject is given 90 seconds to complete the task once. The score is recorded as a pass or a fail.

Trials: 1

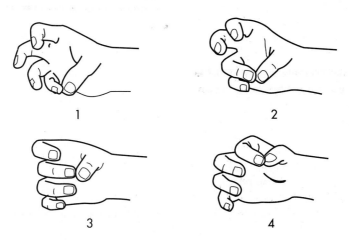

1  2

3  4

Administering and Recording

Have the subject sit beside you at a table. Have the subject extend the preferred arm. Then say, **You are to touch your thumb to each of the fingertips on this hand. Start with your little finger and touch each fingertip in order. Then start with your first finger and touch each fingertip again as you move your thumb back to your little finger** (demonstrate). **Do this with your eyes closed until I tell you to stop. Ready, begin.**

Begin timing. If necessary provide additional instruction. During the trial correct the subject and have the subject start over if he or she:
 a. fails to maintain continuous movements
 b. touches any finger except the index finger more than once in succession
 c. touches two fingers at the same time
 d. fails to touch fingers above the first finger joint
 e. opens eyes.

Allow no more than 90 seconds, including time needed for additional instruction, for the subject to complete the task once. After 90 seconds, tell the subject to stop.

On the Individual Record Form, record pass or fail.

---

**Figure 9-1** Administration and scoring protocol for Bruininks-Oseretsky Test of Motor Proficiency subtest 5, item 8. (From Bruininks, R.H. [1978]. *Bruininks-Oseretsky Test of Motor Proficiency.* Circle Pines, MN: American Guidance Service.)

9-2 illustrate the administration and scoring guidelines for two test items. Figure 9-1 is an item from the BOTMP. In this example the instructions to be given to the child are printed in bold type. Also included are the criteria for a passing score on the item, examples of incorrect responses, and the number of trials and time allowed to complete the item. Figure 9-2 is an item from the Motor Scale of the BSID-II. This example describes how to present the item and what constitutes a passing score, as well as a diagram of what a passing performance looks like. The BSID-II also provides scoring notes to provide cues to examiners when scoring a series of related items.

## TYPES OF STANDARDIZED TESTS

There are two main types of standardized tests: *norm-referenced* and *criterion-referenced*. Many pediatric occupational therapists use both norm-referenced and criterion-referenced tests in their practices. Each type of test has a specific purpose, and it is important for testers to be aware of the purpose for the test they are using.

A norm-referenced test has been developed by giving the test in question to a large number of children, usually several hundred or more. This group is called the *normative sample*, and the "norms," or average scores derived from this sample, provide the basis for comparison for the standard scores. When a norm-referenced test is administered, the performance of the child being tested is compared with this normative sample. The purpose of norm-referenced testing, then, is to determine how a child performs in relation to the average performance of the normative sample. Test developers generally attempt to include children from a variety of geographic locations, ethnic and racial backgrounds, and socioeconomic levels so that the normative sample is representative of the population of the United States, based on the most recent U.S. Census data. Generally the normative sample is composed of children who have no developmental delays or handicapping conditions, although some tests include smaller subsamples of clinical populations as a way to determine whether the test discriminates between children whose development is proceeding normally and children who have known developmental delays.

Norm-referenced tests tend to be rather general in content and cover a wide variety of skills. Some of the items may not have functional significance but give an indication of the child's ability level in a particular domain. For example, the BOTMP contains a subtest entitled *Bilateral Co-*

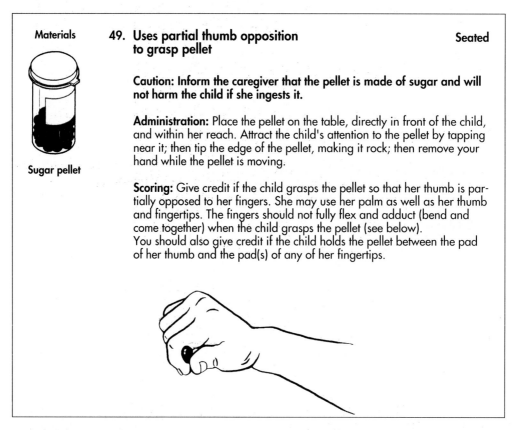

| Materials | 49. **Uses partial thumb opposition to grasp pellet** | Seated |

**Caution:** Inform the caregiver that the pellet is made of sugar and will not harm the child if she ingests it.

**Administration:** Place the pellet on the table, directly in front of the child, and within her reach. Attract the child's attention to the pellet by tapping near it; then tip the edge of the pellet, making it rock; then remove your hand while the pellet is moving.

**Scoring:** Give credit if the child grasps the pellet so that her thumb is partially opposed to her fingers. She may use her palm as well as her thumb and fingertips. The fingers should not fully flex and adduct (bend and come together) when the child grasps the pellet (see below).
You should also give credit if the child holds the pellet between the pad of her thumb and the pad(s) of any of her fingertips.

Sugar pellet

**Figure 9-2** Administration and scoring protocol for Bayley Scales of Infant Development—II motor scale item 49. (From Bayley, N. [1993]. *Bayley Scales of Infant Development* [2nd ed.]. San Antonio: The Psychological Corporation.)

*ordination.* Items in this subtest involve tapping fingers and feet simultaneously, jumping up and touching the feet, and performing running patterns with arms and legs. Although none of these activities is particularly functional in and of themselves, the standard score obtained from this subtest can tell the therapist whether a child is having difficulties with bilateral coordination. The therapist can then select related functional activities to address the child's performance deficits.

Norm-referenced tests have standardized protocols for administration and scoring. The tester must adhere to these protocols so that each test administration is as similar as possible to that of the normative sample. This is necessary to fairly compare any child's performance with that of the normative sample. Sometimes the examiner must deviate from the standard protocol because of special needs of the child being tested. For instance, a child with visual impairments may need manual guidance to cut with scissors, or a child with cerebral palsy may need assistance in stabilizing the shoulder and upper arm to reach and grasp a crayon. If changes are made in the standardized procedures, the examiner must indicate this in the summary of assessment, and standard scores cannot be used to describe that child's performance in comparison with that of the normative sample. Descriptive scores, such as age-equivalent scores, can be used on tests such as the Peabody Developmental Motor Scales (PDMS) (Folio & Fewell, 1983) and the BSID-II when the standardized protocol has been altered. In this way the examiner can obtain an approximate measurement of the child's developmental level. Age-equivalent scores are discussed in more detail in the section on standard scores.

Norm-referenced tests have specific psychometric properties. They have been analyzed by statisticians to obtain score distributions, mean or average scores, and standard scores. This is done to achieve the primary objective of norm-referenced tests, comparability of scores with the normative sample. The process of test development is also scrutinized statistically. A test under development initially has a much larger number of items than what ends up on the final version of the test. Through pilot testing, items are chosen or rejected based partially on how well they statistically discriminate between children of different ages and abilities. Items are not primarily chosen for their relevance to functional skills or developmental milestones. Consequently, norm-referenced tests are generally not intended to link test performance with specific objectives or goals for intervention.

Criterion-referenced tests, by contrast, are designed to provide information on how children perform on specific tasks. The term *criterion-referenced* refers to the fact that a child's performance is compared with a particular criterion, or level of performance of a particular skill. The goal of a criterion-referenced test is to determine which skills a child can and cannot accomplish, providing a focus for intervention. In general, the content of a criterion-referenced test is detailed and in some cases may relate to specific behavioral or functional objectives. Many developmental checklists have been field tested and then published as criterion-referenced tests. The HELP is a good example of a developmental checklist designed to be used with children from the ages of birth to 3 years. It contains a large number of items in each of the domains of gross motor, fine motor, language, cognitive, social-emotional, and self-help skills. Each item is correlated to specific intervention objectives. For instance, if a child is not able to pass Fine Motor item 4.81, *Snips with Scissors,* a list of intervention ideas are presented in the HELP activity guide (Furuno et. al., 1985) The activity guide is meant to accompany the test and is designed to help the therapist or educator by providing ideas for developmentally appropriate activities to address areas of weakness identified in the criterion-based assessment. The administration protocol for this item and the associated intervention activities are pictured in Figure 9-3. The intent of a criterion-referenced test is to measure a child's performance on specific tasks, rather than to compare the child's performance with that of his or her peers.

Administration and scoring procedures may or may not be standardized on a criterion-referenced test. The HELP has standard procedures for administering and scoring each item. There are also many other criterion-referenced tests that take the form of checklists in which the specific performance needed to receive credit on an item is not specified. Many therapist-designed tests for use in a particular facility or setting are nonstandardized criterion-referenced tests.

Criterion-referenced tests are not subjected to the statistical analyses that are performed on norm-referenced tests. No mean score or normal distribution is calculated; a child may pass all items or fail all items on a particular test without adversely affecting the validity of the test results. The purpose of the test is to learn exactly what a child can accomplish, not to compare the performance of the child with that of the peer group. This goal is reflected in the test development process for criterion-referenced tests, also. Items are chosen based on a process of task analysis or identification of important developmental milestones rather than for their statistical validity. Therefore the specific items on a criterion-referenced test have a direct relationship with functional skills and can be used as a starting point for generating appropriate goals and objectives for therapy intervention. The characteristics of norm-referenced and criterion-referenced tests are compared in Table 9-2. As the table indicates, some tests are both norm-referenced and criterion-referenced. This means that although the items have been analyzed for their ability to perform statistically, they also reflect functional or developmental skills that are appropriate for intervention. These tests permit the therapist to compare a child's performance with that of peers in the normative sample while providing information about specific skills that may be appropriate for remediation. The

**A**

**4.81** Snips with scissors    (23-25 months)

**Definition**: The child cuts a paper edge randomly one snip at a time, rather than using a continuous cutting motion.

**Example observation opportunities**: <u>Incidental</u>—may observe while child is preparing for a tea party with stuffed animals or dolls. Demonstrate making fringe on paper placemats and invite the child to help. <u>Structured</u>—using a half-piece of sturdy paper and blunt scissors, make three snips in separate places along the edge of the paper while the child is watching. Exaggerate the opening and closing motions of your hand. Offer the child the scissors and invite him or her to make a cut. Let the child explore the scissors (if interested), helping him or her position the scissors in his or her hand, as needed.

**Credit**: (see also Credit Notes in this strand's preface) + snips paper in one place, holding the paper in one hand and scissors in the other.

**B**

The child cuts with the scissors, taking one snip at a time rather than doing continuous cutting.

1. Let the child use small kitchen tongs to pick up objects and to practice opening and closing motions.
2. Let the child use child-sized scissors with rounded tips.
3. Demonstrate by placing your finger and thumb through the handles.
4. Position the scissors with the finger holes one above the other. Position the child's forearm in midsupination, that is, thumb up. Let the child place his or her thumb through the top hole and the middle finger through the bottom hole. If the child's fingers are small, place the index and middle fingers in the bottom hole. The child will adjust his or her fingers as experience is gained.
5. Let the child open and close the scissors. Assist as necessary by placing your hand over the child's hand.
6. Let the child snip narrow strips of paper and use it for fringe in art work.
7. The different types of scissors that are available for children are a scissors with reinforced rubber coating on the handle grips, a scissors with double handle grips for your hand as well as the child's hand, a left handed scissors, a scissors for a prosthetic hook. Use these different types of child's scissors appropriately as required.

**Figure 9-3**    **A,** Administration and scoring protocol for Hawaii Early Learning Profile item 4.81 and, **B,** item 4.81 activity guide suggestions. (**A** From Parks, S. [1992]. *Inside HELP: administration and reference manual for the Hawaii Early Learning Profile [HELP]*. Palo Alto, CA: Vort. **B** From Furuno, S., O'Reilly, K.A., Hosaka, C.M., Zeisloft, B., & Allman, T. [1985]. *HELP activity guide*. Palo Alto, CA: Vort.)

▲ **Table 9-2**    Comparison of Norm-Referenced and Criterion-Referenced Tests

| Characteristic | Norm-Referenced Test | Criterion-Referenced Test |
|---|---|---|
| Purpose | Comparison of child's performance with normative sample | Comparison of child's performance with a defined list of skills |
| Content | General; usually covers a wide variety of skills | Detailed; may cover specific objectives or developmental milestones |
| Administration and scoring | Always standardized | May be standardized or nonstandardized |
| Psychometric properties | Normal distribution of scores; means, standard deviations, and standard scores computed | No score distribution needed; a child may pass or fail all items |
| Test development | Items chosen for statistical performance; may not relate to functional skills or therapy objectives | Items chosen for functional and developmental importance; provides necessary information for developing therapy objectives |
| Examples | Bayley Scales of Infant Development revised, Peabody Developmental Motor Scales (PDMS), Bruininks-Oseretsky Test of Motor Proficiency, Pediatric Evaluation of Disability Inventory (PEDI) | PDMS, PEDI, Early Intervention Developmental Profile, Gross Motor Function Measure |

PDMS is one example of both a norm-referenced and a criterion-referenced test. Although the PDMS has been subjected to the statistical analyses used in norm-referenced tests, many individual items on the PDMS also represent developmental milestones that are frequent areas of focus for intervention. The PDMS test kit includes activity cards that correspond to each individual item, with specific suggestions for remediation activities. This permits examiners to generate specific intervention strategies based on how a child performed on the test items.

# TECHNICAL ASPECTS

The following discussion of technical aspects of standardized tests focuses on the statistics and test development procedures used for norm-referenced tests. It includes information on how standard scores are obtained and reported and how the reliability and validity of a test are determined. Although relevance of this material to new examiners may be questioned, it is important that all examiners be able to understand and make use of this information for three reasons: (1) occupational therapists need to be able to analyze and select standardized tests appropriately, according to the child's age, functional level, and the purpose of testing; (2) therapists need to be able to accurately interpret and report scores from standardized tests; and (3) therapists need to be able to explain test results to caregivers and other professionals working with the child in a clear and understandable manner. To do this, therapists need to be able to assess the strengths and weaknesses of a test relative to the intended use of the test. To do so, a basic understanding of test statistics and test development principles is necessary. Statistics that are commonly used in pediatric standardized tests are discussed first; then these statistics are applied in a discussion of the concepts of reliability and validity.

## Descriptive Statistics

*Descriptive statistics* inform us about the characteristics of a particular group. Many human characteristics such as height, weight, head size, and intelligence are represented by a distribution called the *normal curve* or bell-shaped curve (Figure 9-4). The pattern of performance on most norm-referenced tests also follows this curve. The largest number of people receive a score in the middle part of the distribution, with progressively smaller numbers of people receiving scores at either the high or the low end of the distribution. Descriptive statistics provide information about where members of a group are located on the normal curve. The two types of descriptive statistics are *measures of central tendency* and *measures of variability*.

Measures of central tendency indicate where the middle point of the distribution is for a particular group, or sample, of children. The most frequently used measure of central tendency is the *mean*. The mean is the sum of all the scores for a particular sample divided by the number of scores. It is computed mathematically through a simple formula:

$$M = \frac{\Sigma X}{n}$$

where $\Sigma$ means to sum up, $X$ = each individual score, and $n$ = the number of scores in the sample. The mean is also often called the average score.

A second measure of central tendency is the *median*. The median is simply the middle score of a distribution. Half the scores lie below the median and half the scores lie above the median. The median is the preferred measure of central tendency when there are outlying or extreme scores in the distribution. For instance, look at the following distribution of scores:

$$2 \quad 3 \quad 13 \quad 14 \quad 17 \quad 17 \quad 18$$

The mean score is $(2 + 3 + 13 + 14 + 17 + 17 + 18) \div 7 = 12$. The median, or middle score, is 14. In this case the score of 14 is a more accurate representation of the middle point of these scores than is the score of 12. This is because the two low scores, or outliers, in the distribution pulled down the value of the mean.

A second type of descriptive statistic is a *measure of variability* in a sample. These statistics determine how much the performance of the group as a whole deviates from the measure of central tendency (the mean or median). It is these measures of variability that are used to compute the standard scores used in standardized tests. As with the measures of central tendency, the measures of variability are derived from the normal curve. The two measures of variability discussed are the *variance*, and the *standard deviation (SD)*.

The variance is defined as the average of the squared deviations of the scores from the mean. In other words, it is a measure of how far the score of an average individual in a sample deviates from the group mean. The variance is computed using the following formula:

$$S^2 = \frac{\Sigma(X - \overline{X})^2}{n}$$

where $S^2$ is the variance, $\Sigma(X - \overline{X})^2$ is the sum of each individual score minus the mean score, and $n$ is the total number of scores in the group. The standard deviation is simply the square root of the variance. To illustrate, calculations are provided for the mean, the variance, and the standard deviation for the following set of scores from a hypothetical test:

$$17 \quad 19 \quad 21 \quad 25 \quad 28$$

To calculate the mean, the following equation is used:

$$\frac{(17 + 19 + 21 + 25 + 28)}{5} = 22$$

To calculate the variance, the mean must be subtracted from each score and then that value must be squared:

$$17 - 22 = (-5)^2 = 25$$
$$19 - 22 = (-3)^2 = 9$$
$$21 - 22 = (-1)^2 = 1$$
$$25 - 22 = (3)^2 = 9$$
$$28 - 22 = (6)^2 = 36$$

The squared values are then summed and then divided by the total number of scores:

$$25 + 9 + 1 + 9 + 36 = 80$$

$$\frac{80}{5} = 16$$

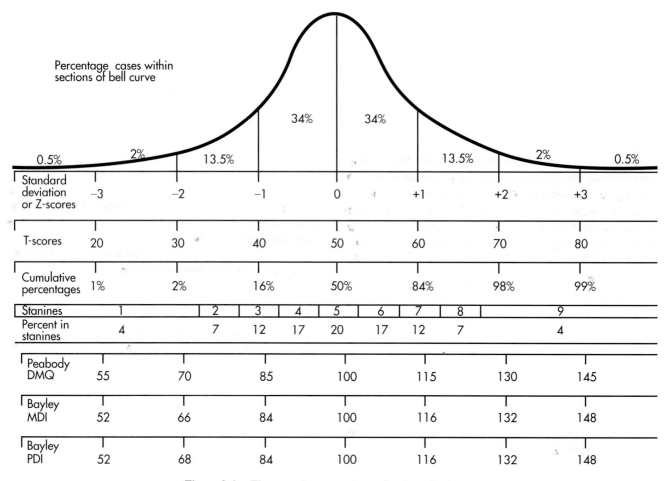

**Figure 9-4**   The normal curve and associated standard scores

The variance of this score distribution is 16. The standard deviation is simply the square root of the variance, or 4.

The standard deviation is an important number because it is the basis for computing many standard scores. In a normal distribution (Figure 9-4), 68% of the people in the distribution score within 1 SD of the mean (±1 SD), 95% score within 2 SD of the mean (±2 SD), and 99.7% score within 3 SD of the mean (±3 SD). In the score distribution with a mean of 22 and a standard deviation of 4, three of the five scores were within 1 SD of the mean (22 ± 4; a score range of 18 to 26), and all five scores were within 2 SD of the mean (22 ± 8; a score range of 14 to 30). The standard deviation, then, determines the placement of scores on the normal curve. By telling us the amount of variability in the sample, the standard deviation tells us how far the scores can be expected to range from the mean or median value.

## Standard Scores

Two standard scores that are computed using the standard deviation score are the *Z-score* and the *T-score*. The Z-score is computed by subtracting the mean for the test from the individual's score and dividing it by the standard deviation, using the following equation:

$$Z = \frac{X - \overline{X}}{SD}$$

Using the score distribution above, the person receiving the score of 17 would have a Z-score of 17 − 22 ÷ 4 = −1.25. The person receiving the score of 28 would have a Z-score of 28 − 22 ÷ 4 = 1.5. Note that the first score has a negative value. This indicates that the Z-score value is below the mean for the test. The second score has a positive value, indicating that the Z-score value is above the mean. Generally, a Z-score value of −1.5 or less is considered to be indicative of delay or deficit in the area being measured, although this can vary depending on the particular test.

The T-score is derived from the Z score. In a T-score distribution, the mean is 50 and the standard deviation is 10. The T-score is computed using the following equation:

$$T = 10(Z) + 50$$

So, for the two Z-scores computed above the T-score values are as follows: for the first Z-score of −1.25, the T score is $10(-1.25) + 50 = 39.75$. For the second Z-score of 1.5, the T-score is $10(1.5) + 50 = 65$. Note that all T-scores have positive values, but because the mean of a T-score distribution is 50, any number below 50 indicates a score below the mean. Because the standard deviation of the T distribution is 10, the first score of 39.75 is slightly more than 1 SD below the mean. The second score of 65 is 15 points, or 1.5 SD above the mean. Look at Figure 9-4 to determine where these Z- and T-scores are located on the normal curve.

Two other standard scores that are frequently seen in standardized tests include the *Deviation IQ Score* and *Developmental Index Score*. Deviation IQ scores have a mean of 100 and a standard deviation of either 15 or 16. These are the intelligence quotient (IQ) scores obtained from such tests as the Stanford-Binet (1972) or the Wechsler Intelligence Scale for Children (WISC) (Wechsler, 1974). On these tests, individuals who have IQ scores that are 2 SD below the mean (IQs of 70 and 68, respectively) are considered to be mentally retarded. Individuals who have IQ scores that are 2 SD above the mean (IQs of 130 and 132, respectively) are considered gifted.

Two other types of scores are frequently used in standardized tests. These are not standard scores in the strictest sense because they are computed directly from raw scores rather than through the statistically derived measures of central tendency and variability. However, they give an indication of a child's performance relative to that of the normative sample. The first of these scores is the *percentile score*. A percentile score is the percentage of people in a standardization sample whose score is at or below a particular raw score. A percentile score of 60, for instance, indicates that 60% of the people in the standardization sample received a score that was at or below the raw score corresponding to the 60th percentile. Tests that use percentile scores generally include a table in the manual by which raw scores can be converted to percentile scores. These tables generally also indicate at what percentile rank performance is considered deficient. Raw scores can be converted to percentile rank (PR) scores by a simple formula:

$$PR = \frac{(\text{Number of people below score} + \frac{1}{2} \text{ of people at score})}{\text{Total number of scores}} \times 100$$

Now convert the lowest and the highest scores from the distribution above to percentile ranks. The raw score of 17 is the lowest score in the distribution and is the only score of 17. Consequently, the equation is as follows:

$$\frac{(0 + \frac{1}{2})}{5} \times 100 = \frac{0.5}{5} \times 100 = 10$$

The highest score in the distribution is 28. Consequently, four people have lower scores and one person received a score of 28. The equation is as follows:

$$\frac{(4 + \frac{1}{2})}{5} \times 100 = \frac{4.5}{5} \times 100 = 90$$

In this distribution, then, the lowest score is at the 10th percentile and the highest score is at the 90th percentile.

Although percentile rank scores can be easily calculated and understood, they have one significant disadvantage. The percentile ranks are not equal in size across the score distribution. Distances between percentile ranks are much smaller in the middle of the distribution than at the ends of the distribution, so that improving a score from the 50th to the 55th percentile entails much less effort than improving a score from the 5th to the 10th percentile (Figure 9-4). Therefore an improvement in performance by a child who is functioning at the lower end of the score range may not be reflected in the percentile rank score the child achieves. Other standard scores are more sensitive in measuring changes in the performance of children who fall at the extreme ends of the score distribution.

Another score that is derived directly from the raw score is the *age-equivalent score*. The age-equivalent score is the age at which the raw score is at the 50th percentile. The age-equivalent score is generally expressed in years and months, for example, 4-3 (4 years 3 months). It is a score that is easily understood by parents and caregivers who may not be familiar with testing concepts or terminology, and for this reason it is used frequently. However, age-equivalent scores have some disadvantages. Although they may provide a general idea of a child's overall developmental level, for instance, saying that a 4-year-old child is functioning at the 2½-year level may be misleading. The age equivalent score may be more or less an average of several developmental domains, some of which may be at the 4½-year level and some of which may be at the 1½-year level. Therefore the child's performance may be highly variable and may not reflect that of a typical 2½-year-old child. Additionally, because the age-equivalent score only represents what a child of a particular age who is performing at the 50th percentile would receive, a child who is performing within normal limits for his or her age but whose score is below the 50th percentile would receive an age-equivalent score below his or her chronologic age. This can cause parents or caregivers to incorrectly conclude that their child has delays. Age equivalents, then, can be a useful way to describe a child's performance but should be used with caution.

## Correlation Coefficients

Another type of statistic that is important in the development of standardized tests is the *correlation coefficient*. A correlation coefficient tells the degree or strength of the relationship between two scores or variables. Although the standard scores are used to compute individual scores, correlation coefficients are used to determine the relationship between scores on one measurement and scores on another. Correlation coefficients range from −1.00 to +1.00. A correlation coefficient of 0.00 indicates that there is no relationship between the two variables being measured. Any relationship that occurs is strictly by chance. The closer the correlation coefficient is to either −1.00 or +1.00, the stronger the relationship is between the two variables. A negative correlation means that a high score on one variable is accompanied by a low score on the other variable. A positive correlation means that a high score on one variable is accompanied by a high score on the other variable and that a low score on one variable is accompanied by a low score on the other variable.

An example of two variables that generally have a fairly high positive correlation are height and weight. Individuals who are taller are also generally heavier than shorter individuals. However, this is not always true. There are tall individuals who are light and short individuals who are heavy. Consequently, the correlation between height and weight for a given population is a positive value but is not a perfect 1.00. An example of two variables that are unrelated are eye color and height. The correlation coefficient for these two variables for any population is close to zero because you cannot predict what a person's eye color is by knowing their height. An example of two variables that have a negative correlation might be hours spent studying and hours spent watching television. A student who spends many hours studying probably watches fewer hours of television, and a student who watches many hours of television probably spends fewer hours studying. Hence there is a negative relationship between these two variables. As one variable increases, the other decreases. Several different correlation coefficients may be calculated, depending on the type of data used. Some correlation coefficients commonly used in test manuals include the Pearson product-moment correlation coefficient, or Pearson $r$; the Spearman rank-order correlation coefficient, and the intraclass correlation coefficient (ICC). What is the importance of correlation coefficients? As the following sections on reliability and validity illustrate, correlation coefficients are important tools for evaluating the properties of a test. Knowledge of test characteristics helps testers know how best to use a test and be aware of the strengths and limitations of individual tests.

## Reliability

The *reliability* of a test describes the consistency or stability of scores obtained by one individual when tested on two different occasions with different sets of items or under other variable examining conditions (Anastasi, 1988). For instance, if a child is given a test and receives a score of 50 and 2 days later is given the same test and receives a score of 75, the reliability of the test is questionable. The difference between the two scores is called the *error variance* of the test, which is a result of random fluctuations in performance between the two testing sessions. It is expected that there is always some amount of random error variance in any test situation because of variations in such things as the child's mood, fatigue, or motivation or because of environmental characteristics such as light, temperature, or noise. However, it is important that error variance caused by the variations in the examiner or by the characteristics of the test itself be minimal. To have confidence in the scores obtained on a test, the test must be demonstrated to have adequate reliability over a number of administrations and less susceptibility to error variance. How is this done? There are a number of ways to calculate reliability. Most standardized tests evaluate two or three forms of reliability. The three forms of reliability most commonly used in pediatric standardized tests are *test-retest reliability, interrater reliability,* and *standard error of measurement (SEM)*.

Test-retest reliability is a measurement of the stability of the test over time. It is obtained by giving the test to the same individual on two different occasions. When evaluating test-retest reliability for a pediatric test, the time span between test administrations must be short to minimize the possibility of developmental changes occurring between the two test sessions but not so short that the child may recall items administered during the first test session and thereby improve his or her performance on the second test session. (This is called the learning or practice effect.) Generally the time span between testings is no more than 1 week for infants and toddlers and no more than 2 weeks for older children. During the process of test development, test-retest reliability is evaluated on a subgroup of the normative sample. The size and composition of the subgroup should be specified in the manual. The correlation coefficient between the scores of the two test sessions is calculated. This coefficient is the measure of the test-retest reliability of the test. A test that has a high test-retest reliability coefficient is more likely to yield relatively stable scores over time. That is, it is affected less by random error variance than a test that has a low test-retest reliability coefficient. The problem with a test that has a low test-retest reliability coefficient is that one has less confidence that the score obtained from testing a child is a true reflection of that child's abilities. If the child were tested at a different time of day or in a different setting entirely, different results might be obtained.

Test-retest reliability on the BSID was assessed by evaluating a sample of 175 infants twice within 2 weeks (about 4 days apart). Correlation coefficients were high but not perfect (0.83 for the Mental Scale and 0.77 for the Motor Scale). Scores increased slightly on the second testing, probably because of the rapid development of young infants and the practice effect. The test-retest reliability for the PDMS was high (0.95 for Gross Motor and 0.80 for Fine Motor) when 38 children were tested within a week's time. To evaluate test-retest reliability of the Developmental Test of Visual Perception (DTVP) (Hammill, Pearson, & Voress, 1993), 88 students were tested twice within 2 weeks. The correlation coefficients for the test's subsections ranged from 0.80 to 0.93. The reliability for the total test scores was 0.95. These three examples of good to excellent test-retest reliability are typical examples of pediatric sensorimotor tests. The rapid and variable development of young children and the practice effect are two factors that negatively influence the tests' stability over time. This test characteristic is critical to using the results as a measure of progress or intervention efficacy.

A second form of reliability is interrater reliability. This refers to the ability of two independent raters to obtain the same scores when scoring the same child simultaneously. The type of error variance being measured here is examiner variance, which is the differences between examiners in how they rate or score the test items. Interrater reliability is generally also measured on a subset of the normative sample during the test development process. This is often accomplished by having one rater administer and score the test while another rater observes and scores at the same time. The correlation coefficient calculated from the two raters' scores is the interrater reliability coefficient of the test. It is especially important to measure interrater reliability on tests where the scoring may require some judgment on the part of the examiner. Although the scoring criteria for many test items are specific on most tests, there is still some room for individual judgment, and this is a place where scoring differences can arise between different examiners. A test that has a low interrater reliability coefficient is especially sensitive to differences in scoring by different raters. This may mean that the administration and scoring criteria are not stated explicitly enough, requiring examiners to make judgment calls on a number of items. Alternatively, it can mean that the items on the test call for responses that are too broad or vague to permit precise scoring.

Examiners can exert some control over the interrater reliability of tests that they use frequently. It is good practice to check interrater reliability with more experienced colleagues when learning a new standardized test before beginning to administer the test to children in the clinical setting. Additionally, it is good practice to periodically check interrater reliability with colleagues who are administering the same standardized tests. There are some simple methods for assessing interrater reliability in the clinic. These are discussed in more depth on pp. 214 to 217.

What is an acceptable coefficient for test-retest and interrater reliability? There is no universal agreement regarding the minimum acceptable coefficient. The context of the reliability measurement, the type of test, and the distribution of scores are some of the variables that can be taken into account when determining an acceptable reliability coefficient. One standard suggested by Anastasi (1988) and used by a number of examiners is 0.80. The examples reported meet this criterion. Not all tests have test-retest or interrater reliability coefficients that reach the 0.80 level.

For example, the BSID-II Motor Scale has an interrater reliability of 0.75. This coefficient may indicate variability in scores by different raters. When examiners use a test that has a reliability coefficient below 0.80, scores must be interpreted with great caution. For example, if one subtest of a test of motor development has test-retest reliability of 0.60, care must exercised when using it to measure change over time, recognizing that a portion of the apparent change between the first and second test administration is a result of error variance of the test.

Interrater reliability was assessed for the BSID-II using 51 children of ages 2 to 30 months. Items were administered and scored by one examiner and were simultaneously scored by an observer. Interrater reliability coefficients were 0.96 for the Mental Scale and 0.75 for the Motor Scale. The correlation coefficient for the Motor Scale seemed to be lower because these items involved manipulation of the infant to score, placing the observer at a disadvantage (Bayley, 1993). Interrater reliability for the PDMS was evaluated using the same method; one tester administering and one observing the items. The resulting correlation coefficients were 0.97 for Gross Motor and 0.94 for Fine Motor, giving the tester strong confidence in the reliability of the scores across raters (Folio & Fewell, 1983). In a test such as the DTVP where scores are based on a written record of the child's response, interrater reliability is excellent. When two individuals scored 88 completed DTVP protocols, the interscorer reliability was 0.98 (Hammill, Pearson, & Voress, 1993).

When individual subtests of a comprehensive test have a low reliability coefficient, it is generally not recommended that the standard scores from the subtests be reported. Often the reliability coefficient of the entire test is much higher than that of the individual subtests. One reason for this is that reliability increases with the number of items on a test. Because subtests have fewer items than the entire test, they are more sensitive to fluctuations in the performance or scoring of individual items. When this occurs, it is best to describe subtest performance qualitatively but not to report standard scores. Standard scores can be reported for the total or comprehensive test score. Examiners should consult the reliability information in the test manual before deciding how to report test scores for individual subtests and for the test as a whole.

A third form of reliability is the SEM. This statistic is used to calculate the expected range of error for the test score of an individual. It is based on the range of scores that an individual might obtain if the same test were administered a number of times simultaneously with no practice or fatigue effects. Obviously this is impossible, so the SEM is a theoretic construct. It is, however, an indication of the possible error variance in individual scores. The SEM creates a normal curve for the individual's test scores, with the obtained score in the middle of the distribution. The child has a higher probability of receiving scores in the middle of the distribution than scores at the extreme ends of the distribution. The SEM is based on the standard deviation of the test, as well as the test's reliability (usually test-retest reliability). The SEM can be calculated using the following formula:

$$SEM = SD\sqrt{1 - r}$$

Once the SEM is calculated for a test, the value is added to and subtracted from the child's obtained score. This gives the range of expected scores for that child. This range is known as the *confidence interval*. The SEM corresponds to the standard deviation for the normal curve. Remember that 68% of the scores in a normal distribution fell within 1 SD on either side of the mean, 95% of the scores fell within 2 SD on either side of the mean, and 99.7% of the scores fell within 3 SD on either side of the mean. Similarly, a child receives a score within 1 SEM on either side of his or her obtained score 68% of the time, a score within 2 SEM of the obtained score 95% of the time, and a score within 3 SEM of the obtained score 99.7% of the time. Generally, test manuals report the 95% confidence interval. As you can see by the equation, when the standard deviation of the test is high or the reliability is low, the SEM increases. A larger SEM value means that there is potentially a much larger range of possible scores for an individual child (i.e., a larger confidence interval) and consequently a greater amount of possible error variance for the child's score. This means that an examiner can have less confidence that any score obtained for a child on that test represents the child's true score. An example here may help illustrate this point. Now consider two tests, both consisting of 50 items and both testing the same skill area. One test has a standard deviation of 1.0 and test-retest reliability coefficient of 0.90. The SEM for that test is calculated as follows:

$$SEM = 1\sqrt{1 - 0.90}$$
$$SEM = 0.32$$

The second test has a standard deviation of 5.0 and a test-retest reliability coefficient of .75. The SEM for that test would be calculated as follows:

$$SEM = 5\sqrt{1 - 0.75}$$
$$SEM = 2.5$$

Using the SEM, a 95% confidence interval can be calculated for each test. A 95% confidence interval is 2 SEM, so Test 1 has a confidence interval of ±0.64 points from the obtained score, or a total of 1.28 points. Test 2 has a confidence interval of ±5 points, or a total of 10 points. If both Tests 1 and 2 were available for a particular client, an examiner could use Test 1 with much more confidence that the obtained score is truly representative of that individual's abilities and is not caused by random error variance of the test. Occupational therapists who use standardized tests should be aware of how much measurement error a test contains so that the potential range of performance can be estimated for each individual.

Currently, the trend is to report standardized test results as confidence intervals rather than as individual scores (Deitz, 1989). The score tables for the BSID-II include confidence intervals for each index score. "The reporting of confidence intervals also serves as a reminder that the observed score contains some amount of measurement error" (Bayley, 1993, p. 192). The SEM is especially important to consider when evaluating the differences between two scores as when evaluating the progress a child has made over time with therapy (Anastasi, 1988). If the confidence intervals of the two test scores overlap, it may be incorrect to conclude that any change has been made. For instance, a child is tested in September and receives a raw score of 60. The child is tested again in June with the same test and receives a raw score of 75. From looking at the two raw scores, it appears that the child has made substantial progress. However, let us consider the scores in light of an SEM of 5.0. Using a 95% confidence interval (remember that the 95% confidence interval is 2 SEM on either side of the obtained score), the confidence interval for the first score is from 50 to 70, and the confidence interval of the second score is from 65 to 85. It cannot be conclusively stated that the child has made progress, based on the two test scores, because the confidence intervals overlap. It is conceivable that a substantial amount of the difference between the first and second scores is a result of an error variance of the test rather than of actual change in the child's abilities. See Cunningham Amundson and Crowe (1993) for a more in-depth discussion of the use of SEM in pediatric assessment, particularly the effect of SEM on interpretation of test scores and qualifying children for remedial services.

## Validity

*Validity* is the extent to which a test measures what it says it measures (Anastasi, 1988). It is important for testers to know that a test of fine motor development, for instance, actually measures fine motor skills and not gross motor or perceptual skills. The validity of a test must be established with reference to the particular use for which the test is being considered (Anastasi, 1988). For instance, the test of fine motor development is probably highly valid as a measure of fine motor skills. It is less valid as a measure of visual-motor skills, and has low validity as a measure of gross motor skills. Test manuals should report information about test validity that has been obtained during the test development process. Additionally, once a test is available commercially, clinicians and researchers continue to evaluate validity and publish the results of their validation studies. This information about test validity can help examiners make decisions about appropriate uses of standardized tests.

There are three categories of validity: *construct-related validity, content-related validity,* and *criterion-related validity.* Each is described in the following section.

Construct-related validity refers to the extent to which a tests measures a particular theoretic construct. Some constructs frequently measured by pediatric occupational therapists include fine motor skills, visual-perceptual skills, self-care skills, gross motor skills, and sensory integration. Construct validity must be obtained from a variety of sources, and it is a way of validating the theory underlying the domains being tested.

One way of establishing construct validity is by investigating how well a test discriminates between different groups of individuals. For instance, in a developmental test such as the BSID-II, the PDMS, and the BOTMP, it is expected that the test differentiates between the performance of older and younger children. Older children should receive higher scores than younger children, providing clear evidence of developmental progression with increasing age. Because these tests are also intended to discriminate normally developing children from children with developmental delays, children in specific diagnostic categories should receive lower scores than children who have no documented deficits. For example, during the development process of the BSID-II the performance of children in the following clinical groups was evaluated: premature birth, HIV-positive, prenatal drug exposure, perinatal asphyxia, Down syndrome, autism, developmental delay secondary to medical complications, and chronic otitis media. Performance of children in each of these groups was significantly lower than that of the standardization sample. Therefore the BSID-II was found to discriminate between children in the clinical groups and in the standardization sample, indicating that the BSID-II is able to differentiate the performance of children who have differing ability levels.

A second method of establishing construct validity is by the use of *factor analysis.* Factor analysis is a statistical procedure for determining relationships between test items. In a test of motor skills that includes gross motor items and fine motor items, factor analysis is expected to identify two factors where items showed the strongest correlation: one composed mostly of gross motor items, and one composed mostly of fine motor items. The factor analysis of the Sensory Integration and Praxis Tests (SIPT) resulted in identification of four primary factors. The constructs that emerged from the analysis demonstrated that the test primarily measures praxis (motor planning). One construct measures visual perceptual skills (related to praxis); one somatosensory-praxis skills; one, bilateral integration and sequencing of movements; and finally, praxis on verbal command (Ayres & Marr, 1991). The factor analysis helped establish what functions are measured by the SIPT and can be used to interpret the results of testing individual children.

A third way to establish construct-related validity is by repeated administration of a test before and after a period of intervention. For example, a group of children is given a test of visual-perceptual skills and then receives intervention focused on improving their visual-perceptual skills. They are then retested using the same test to determine if test scores improve. An increase in test scores supports the assertion that the test measured visual perceptual skills and provides evidence for construct-related validity.

*Content-related validity* is the extent to which the items on a test accurately sample a particular behavior domain. For instance, to test self-care skills, it is impractical to ask a child to perform every conceivable self-care activity. A sample of self-care activities must be chosen to be included on the test, and conclusions then can be drawn about the child's abilities on the basis of the selected items. Examiners must have confidence that self-care skills are adequately represented so that the conclusions drawn on the basis of the test can be considered to be an accurate representation of self-care skills.

Test manuals should show evidence that the authors have systematically analyzed the domain that is being tested. Content validity is established by review of the test content by experts in the field who reach some agreement that the content is in fact representative of the behavioral domain to be measured.

Criterion-related validity refers to the ability of a test to predict how an individual performs on other measurements or activities. To establish criterion-related validity, the test score is checked against a criterion, an independent measure of what the test is designed to predict. The two forms of criterion-related validity are *concurrent validity* and *predictive validity.*

Concurrent validity describes how well test scores predict present performance, and predictive validity describes how well test scores predict future performance. The degree of the relationship between the two measures is described with a correlation coefficient. Most validity correlation coefficients range from 0.40 to 0.80; a coefficient of 0.70 or above is considered to be desirable when comparing the performance of an individual on two different measures.

How is concurrent validity assessed? Concurrent validity is examined in the test development process to determine the relationship between a new test and existing tests that test a similar construct. For instance, during the development of the PDMS, children were tested with both the PDMS and the BSID (Bayley, 1969). The scores on the two tests were compared. A portion of the concurrent validity data are reproduced in Table 9-3.

As Table 9-3 shows, there are some areas of high correlation and one area of low correlation between the two tests. The BSID Mental Scale, which assesses a broad range of mental functions that include receptive and expressive language, problem-solving, and attention, also includes a number of items involving fine motor skills, visual-perceptual skills, and visual-motor skills. Not surprisingly, it has al-

▲ Table 9-3    Correlation Coefficients Between the
                Peabody Developmental Motor Scales and
                the Bayley Scales of Infant Development

|  | Bayley Mental Scale | Bayley Psychomotor Scale |
|---|---|---|
| Peabody Gross Motor Scale | −0.03 | 0.37 |
| Peabody Fine Motor Scale | 0.78 | 0.36 |

Modified from Folio, M.R. & Fewell, R.R. (1983). *Peabody Developmental Motor Scales and activity cards* (p. 118). Chicago: Riverside Publishers.

most no relationship with the PDMS Gross Motor Scale, which assesses an entirely different developmental area. However, the BSID Mental Scale correlates highly with the PDMS Fine Motor Scale, which is composed of fine motor items. The BSID Psychomotor Scale, which is composed of both gross motor and fine motor items, has moderate correlations with both the PDMS Gross Motor and Fine Motor Scales. This pattern of correlation coefficients is an expected finding when comparing the two tests and supports the concurrent validity of the PDMS as a measure of gross motor and fine motor skills.

In contrast to concurrent validity, predictive validity identifies the relationship between a test given in the present and some measure of performance in the future. Establishing predictive validity is a much lengthier process than other forms of validity because several years must often elapse between the first and second testing sessions. Often, the predictive validity of a test is not fully documented until it has been in use for several years.

An area of interest to many pediatric occupational therapists working in early intervention has been the ability of developmental tests to predict which infants and toddlers, who are identified as "high-risk" because of premature birth or perinatal medical complications, will have cerebral palsy or other developmental disabilities as they become older. Predicting outcomes necessitates testing the children as infants and then testing their developmental, physical, or cognitive status several months or years later. The second testing can use the same test if the child is still within the intended age range of that test, or another test that presumably tests the same construct as the first test and that is appropriate for the child's current age may be used. Palisano (1986) investigated the predictive validity of the PDMS and the BSID for full-term and premature infants who were given both tests at 12, 15, and 18 months. He found that scores obtained for either test at 12 months did not predict 18-month scores (i.e., the correlations between scores were low). Palisano concluded that the BSID and PDMS can be used only to describe current developmental status and should not be used for predictive purposes. Therefore an infant who achieves a low score on either of

these tests will not necessarily go on to have developmental delays. In contrast, BSID scores obtained at 12 months of age for children with biologic risk factors correlated with verbal and motor performance at 4½ years of age (Crowe, Deitz, & Bennett, 1987), and 6-month BSID Mental Scale scores for infants at risk because of environmental deprivation predicted Stanford-Binet IQ at 24 and 48 months for children who did not receive intervention (Farran & Harber, 1989). Thus the question of predictive validity of early developmental assessments for children at biologic or environmental risk remains unresolved. Therapists should conduct repeated testings when the child is at risk for developmental delays.

One final point about criterion-related validity: The meaningfulness of the comparison between a test and its criterion measure depends on both the quality of the test and the quality of the criterion. In the example of concurrent validity previously cited, the comparison of the PDMS and the BSID rests on the assumption that the BSID is an adequate measure of the criteria of gross and fine motor development. If the BSID was found to measure these criteria inaccurately, the validity of the PDMS would also be in question. Because no measure of criterion-related validity provides conclusive evidence of the test's validity, multiple investigations should be undertaken. Important developmental assessments such as the BSID undergo extensive evaluation of validity after publication. The resulting information helps the test user decide when and with whom the test results are most valid.

In summary, validity is an important but sometimes elusive concept that rests on a number of judgments by test authors, experts in the field, and by the users of the tests. It is important to remember that validity is not an absolute and that a test that is valid in one setting or with one group of children may not be valid for other uses. Test users must not assume that because a test has been developed and published for commercial distribution, it is universally useful and appropriate. An examiner must apply his or her knowledge of normal and abnormal development, clinical knowledge and experience, and understanding of an individual child's situation in deciding whether a test is a valid measure of the child's abilities.

## BECOMING A COMPETENT USER

The amount of technical information presented here might make the prospect of learning to administer a standardized test seem daunting. However, a number of specific steps that potential examiners can take ensure that they will be able to administer and reliably score a test and to interpret the results so as to give a valid representation of each child's abilities. This section discusses what is necessary to learn to administer and interpret any standardized test, whether it is a screening tool or a comprehensive assessment.

▲ Table 9-4    A Summary of Selected General Pediatric Standardized Tests

| Test Name | Age Range | Domains Tested | Standard Scores Used | Time to Administer |
|---|---|---|---|---|
| Bayley Scales of Infant Development—II | 1 to 42 months | Mental scale: cognitive, language and personal-social<br>Psychomotor scale: gross motor skills, fine motor skills, quality of movement, sensory integration, perceptual-motor integration<br>Behavior rating scale: Social interactions, orientation toward environment and objects, interests, activity level, and need for stimulation | Developmental index scores<br>Percentile rank scores<br>Developmental age-equivalent scores | 25 to 60 minutes, depending on child's age |
| Peabody Developmental Motor Scales | 1 to 84 months | Gross motor scale: reflexes, balance, locomotor, nonlocomotor, receipt, and propulsion<br>Fine motor scale: grasping, hand use, eye-hand coordination, manual dexterity | Percentile rank scores<br>Z-scores<br>T-scores<br>Age-equivalent scores<br>Developmental motor quotient scores<br>Scaled scores | 45 to 60 minutes for total test; 20 to 30 minutes for each scale |
| Bruininks-Oseretsky Test of Motor Proficiency | 4½ to 14½ years | Gross motor subtest: running speed and agility, balance, bilateral coordination, strength, and upper limb coordination<br>Fine motor subtest: response speed, visual-motor control, upper limb speed, and dexterity | Subtest and total test<br>Standard score<br>Percentile rank score<br>Stanine score<br>Age-equivalent scores | 45 to 60 minutes for long form; 15 to 20 minutes for short form |
| Pediatric Evaluation of Disability Inventory | 6 months to 7 years | Social function, self-care, mobility. Each domain is scored in each of the following areas: functional skills, caregiver assistance, and modifications | Normative standard score<br>Scaled score | 45 to 60 minutes when scoring by parent report |

The first step is to decide which tests to learn. A number of standardized tests used by pediatric occupational therapists address a wide age span and a number of different performance components and performance areas. A potential examiner must decide which tests will most likely meet the assessment needs for his or her particular caseload. For instance, an occupational therapist working in an early intervention setting might use the BSID-II. A therapist working with preschool-aged children might use the MAP (Miller,

1982) or the PDMS. A therapist working in a school-based setting might use the BOTMP. Table 9-4 summarizes selected pediatric standardized assessments. Additionally, a number of other standardized tests are available that assess more specialized areas of function, such as the SIPT (Ayres, 1989), the Developmental Test of Visual-Motor Integration (Beery, 1989), or the DTVP (Hammill, Pearson, & Voress, 1993). Potential examiners should consult with other therapists working in their practice settings to determine which tests are most commonly used. In addition, they should examine the characteristics of the children referred to them for assessment to determine which tests are most appropriate.

Once a decision is made about which test to learn, the therapist should thoroughly read the test manual. In addition to becoming familiar with administration and scoring techniques, the technical attributes of the test should be studied. Particular attention should be paid to the size and composition of the normative sample, the reliability coefficients, the validation data, and the intended population for the test. What are the standardized administration procedures, and can they be altered for children with special needs? How should the scores be reported and interpreted if the standardized procedure is changed? It may also be appropriate to consult other sources for information about a test. *The Eighth Mental Measurements Yearbook* (Buros, 1978), the *Ninth Mental Measurements Yearbook* (Mitchell, 1985), or *Tests in Print III* (Mitchell, 1983) publish descriptions and critical reviews of commercially available standardized tests written by testing experts. Published studies of validity or reliability of tests relevant to pediatric occupational therapists appear throughout the occupational therapy literature.

The next step in learning a test is to observe an experienced examiner administering the test, and, if possible, to discuss administration, scoring, and interpretation of the test results. One observation may suffice; however, it may be helpful to see several administrations of the test given to children of different ages and abilities. Observation provides an excellent way to see how other examiners manage the practical aspects of testing, such as arrangement of test materials, sequencing of test items, handling unexpected occurrences, and managing behavior. A discussion with the examiner regarding how a child's performance is interpreted can also be extremely helpful in understanding how observed behaviors are translated into conclusions and recommendations.

Once these preparatory activities are completed, the learner should practice administering the test. Neighborhood children, friends, or relatives can be recruited to be "pilot subjects." It is a good idea to test several children who are of similar ages to those with whom the test will be used. This more closely approximates the mechanical, behavioral, and management issues that will be faced with a clinical population. When possible, an experienced examiner should observe the testing and simultaneously score the items as a check of interrater reliability. A simple way to assess interrater agreement is by the use of *point-by-point agreement* (Kazdin, 1982). Using this technique, one examiner administers and scores the test while the other observes and scores. The two examiners then compare their scores on each item. The number of items on which the examiners agreed on the score are summed. The interrater agreement is then computed using the following formula:

$$\text{Point-by-point agreement} = \frac{A}{A + D} \times 100$$

A equals the number of items where there was agreement, and D equals the number of items where there was disagreement. Look at the following example of point-by-point agreement. A test of 10 items is scored by two examiners. The child receives either a pass (+) or fail (−) for each item. Scores for each examiner are shown in Table 9-5.

According to Table 9-5, the raters agreed on 7 of the 10 items. They disagreed on items 2, 7, and 9. Therefore their point-by-point agreement would be calculated as follows:

$$\frac{7}{(7 + 3)} = 0.70 \times 100 = 70\% \text{ point-by-point agreement.}$$

This means that they agreed on the scores for 70% of the items. To benefit from this exercise, the two examiners discuss the items where they disagreed on scores and their reasons for giving the scores that they did. A new examiner may not understand the scoring criteria and may be making scoring errors as a result. The experienced examiner can help clarify scoring criteria. This procedure helps bring the new examiner's administration and scoring techniques in line with the standardized procedures. The point-by-point agreement technique can also be used for periodic reliability checks by experienced examiners, and it is particularly important if the examiners may be testing the same children at different times. What is a minimum acceptable level for point-by-point agreement? No universally agreed-on standard exists; however, 80% is probably a good guideline for the minimum acceptable agreement. At the 80% level examiners disagree on one out of five items, which can potentially result in significant score differences over an entire test. Examiners would be well advised to aim for agreement in the range of 90% if possible.

Once adequate agreement has been established, the new examiner is ready to begin testing children from the clinical population. Some organizational tips make the testing proceed more smoothly and increase compliance with stan-

▲ **Table 9-5**   Rater's Scores for Point-by-Point Agreement

| Item | Rater 1 | Rater 2 |
|------|---------|---------|
| 1 | + | + |
| 2 | + | − |
| 3 | + | + |
| 4 | − | − |
| 5 | − | − |
| 6 | + | + |
| 7 | − | + |
| 8 | − | − |
| 9 | − | + |
| 10 | + | + |

dardized procedures. First, the testing environment should meet the specifications stated in the test manual. Generally, the manual specifies a well-lighted room free of visual or auditory distractions. If a separate room is not available, a screen or room divider can be used to partition off a corner of the clinic. Testing should be scheduled at a time when the child is able to perform optimally. For young children, caregivers should be consulted about the best time of day for testing so that the test session does not interfere with naps or feedings. Older children's school or other activities should be considered when scheduling assessments. For instance, a child who has just come from recess or a vigorous physical education session may have decreased endurance for gross motor activities.

The test environment should be ready before the child arrives. Furniture should be appropriately sized so children sitting at a table can rest their feet flat on the floor and can comfortably access items on the table. If a child uses a wheelchair or other adaptive seating, he or she should be allowed to sit in the equipment during testing. Infants or toddlers are generally best seated on the caregiver's lap, unless particular items on the test specify otherwise. The examiner should place the test kit where he or she can easily access the items but not where the child can see it or get into it. Often a low chair placed next to the examiner's chair is a good place to locate a test kit.

Each examiner should consider what adaptations are necessary to administer the test efficiently. In many cases a test manual is too large and unwieldy to have at hand during testing, and the score sheet does not provide enough information about administration and scoring criteria. Examiners have developed many ways to accommodate this need. One common method is a cue card, on which the examiner records specific criteria for administration and scoring, including the instructions to be read to the child. This can be accomplished by making a series of note cards, putting color codes on a score sheet or developing a score sheet with administration information. Reproduced below is a portion of a score sheet developed for the PDMS by the author and colleagues at the University of Washington (Figure 9-5). See also Hinderer, Richardson, and Atwater (1989).

Most importantly, the examiner has to be familiar enough with the test that attention can be focused on the child's behavior, not on the mechanics of administering the test. This is a critical part of preparation because much valuable information can be lost if the examiner is not able to carefully observe the quality of the child's responses and must instead devote energy to finding test materials or looking through the test manual. Additionally, young children's attention spans can be short, and the examiner must be able to take full advantage of the limited time that the child is able to attend to the activities. Familiarity with the test also allows the examiner to change the pace of activities if necessary or give the child a brief break to play, have a snack, or use the bathroom while interviewing the caregiver or jotting down notes. Most standardized tests have some flexibility about the order or arrangement of item sets, and an examiner who knows the test can use this to his or her advantage. Sometimes because of the child's fatigue, behavior, or time constraints, it is impossible to completely administer a test in one session. Most tests provide guidelines about how the test administration can be broken up, and examiners should be familiar with these guidelines before starting to test.

The final area of preparation is to evaluate the clinical usefulness of the test. Discuss the test with colleagues: What are its strengths and weaknesses? What important information does it give? What information needs to be collected through other techniques? For which children does it seem to work especially well or especially poorly? Can it be adapted for children with special needs? Does it measure what it says it measures? Are there other tests that do a better job of measuring the same behavioral domain? Is it helpful for program planning or program evaluation? An ongoing dialogue is an important way to ensure that the process of standardized testing meets the needs of the children, families, therapists, and service agencies who make use of the tests. The steps to becoming a competent user of standardized tests are summarized in the box below.

## ETHICAL CONSIDERATIONS IN TESTING

All pediatric occupational therapists who use standardized tests in their practice must be aware of the responsibilities they have to the children they test and their families. Following the framework outlined by Anastasi (1988), there are several ethical issues relevant to standardized testing.

The first ethical issue is that of examiner competency. This has been discussed in detail in the previous section, but it is important to reemphasize here that examiners need to achieve a minimal level of competency with a test before using it in practice. Along with knowing how to administer and score a test, a competent examiner should know who the test should be used with and for what pur-

---

### Steps to Becoming a Competent Test User

1. Study the test manual.
2. Observe experienced examiners; discuss observations.
3. Practice using the test.
4. Check interrater agreement with experienced examiner.
5. Prepare administration and scoring cue sheets.
6. Prepare the testing environment.
7. Consult with experienced examiners about test interpretation.
8. Periodically recheck interrater agreement.

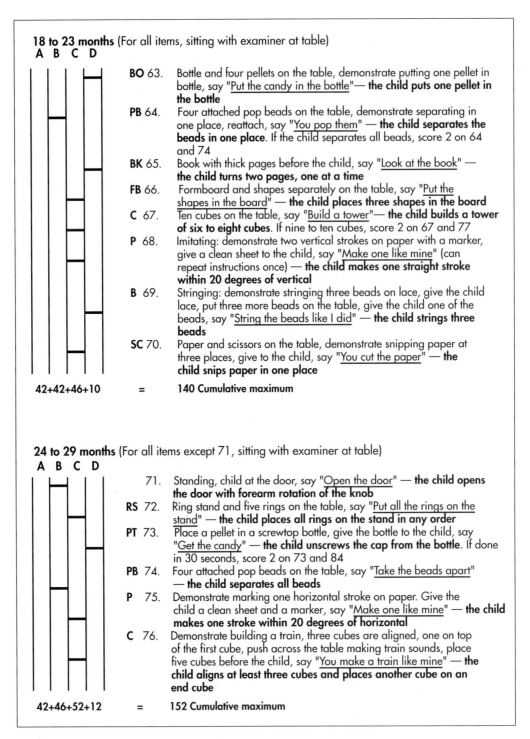

**18 to 23 months** (For all items, sitting with examiner at table)

A  B  C  D

**BO** 63. Bottle and four pellets on the table, demonstrate putting one pellet in bottle, say "Put the candy in the bottle"— **the child puts one pellet in the bottle**

**PB** 64. Four attached pop beads on the table, demonstrate separating in one place, reattach, say "You pop them" — **the child separates the beads in one place.** If the child separates all beads, score 2 on 64 and 74

**BK** 65. Book with thick pages before the child, say "Look at the book" — **the child turns two pages, one at a time**

**FB** 66. Formboard and shapes separately on the table, say "Put the shapes in the board" — **the child places three shapes in the board**

**C** 67. Ten cubes on the table, say "Build a tower"— **the child builds a tower of six to eight cubes.** If nine to ten cubes, score 2 on 67 and 77

**P** 68. Imitating: demonstrate two vertical strokes on paper with a marker, give a clean sheet to the child, say "Make one like mine" (can repeat instructions once) — **the child makes one straight stroke within 20 degrees of vertical**

**B** 69. Stringing: demonstrate stringing three beads on lace, give the child lace, put three more beads on the table, give the child one of the beads, say "String the beads like I did" — **the child strings three beads**

**SC** 70. Paper and scissors on the table, demonstrate snipping paper at three places, give to the child, say "You cut the paper" — **the child snips paper in one place**

42+42+46+10  =  **140 Cumulative maximum**


**24 to 29 months** (For all items except 71, sitting with examiner at table)

A  B  C  D

71. Standing, child at the door, say "Open the door" — **the child opens the door with forearm rotation of the knob**

**RS** 72. Ring stand and five rings on the table, say "Put all the rings on the stand" — **the child places all rings on the stand in any order**

**PT** 73. Place a pellet in a screwtop bottle, give the bottle to the child, say "Get the candy" — **the child unscrews the cap from the bottle.** If done in 30 seconds, score 2 on 73 and 84

**PB** 74. Four attached pop beads on the table, say "Take the beads apart" — **the child separates all beads**

**P** 75. Demonstrate marking one horizontal stroke on paper. Give the child a clean sheet and a marker, say "Make one like mine" — **the child makes one stroke within 20 degrees of horizontal**

**C** 76. Demonstrate building a train, three cubes are aligned, one on top of the first cube, push across the table making train sounds, place five cubes before the child, say "You make a train like mine" — **the child aligns at least three cubes and places another cube on an end cube**

42+46+52+12  =  **152 Cumulative maximum**

**Figure 9-5** Peabody Development Motor Scales cue sheet. (From OT/PT staff. (unpublished). *An adaptation of Peabody Developmental Motor Scales* by the OT/PT staff. Seattle Child Development and Mental Retardation Center, University of Washington.)

pose. This also means knowing when it is *not* appropriate to use a particular standardized instrument. The examiner should be able to evaluate the technical merits of the test and know how these characteristics may affect the administration and interpretation of the test. The examiner should be aware of the many things that can affect a child's performance on a test, including factors such as hunger, fatigue, illness, or distractions, as well as sources of test or examiner error. Finally, the competent examiner draws conclusions about a child's performance on a standardized test only after considering all available information about the child. This can include nonstandardized testing, informal observation, caregiver interview, and review of documentation from other professionals. It is extremely important to put a child's observed performance on standardized testing within the context of all sources of information about the child. This provides a more accurate and meaningful interpretation of standard scores.

The second ethical issue is the protection of privacy or confidentiality. Informed consent must be obtained from the child's legal guardian before testing is initiated. Agencies have different guidelines regarding how consent is obtained, and examiners should be aware of the guidelines for their particular institution. Informed consent is generally obtained in writing and consists of an explanation of the reasons for testing, the types of tests that will be used, the intended use of the test and its consequences (generally this refers to program placement or qualification for remedial services), and what testing information will be released and to whom it will be released. Caregivers should be given a copy of the summary report and should be informed about who will receive the additional copies.

Verbal conversations about the child should be limited. Although it is often necessary to discuss a case with a colleague for the purposes of information sharing and consultation, it is not acceptable to have a casual conversation about a particular child in the elevator, lunchroom, or hallway. If others overhear the conversation, this could result in a violation of confidentiality.

The third ethical issue is that of communicating test results. Reports should be written in a manner that is understandable to a nonprofessional, with a minimum of jargon. The report should be objective in tone, and the conclusions and recommendations should be clearly stated. When discussing the results of testing, the characteristics of the recipient should be taken into account. Different communication techniques are needed for speaking to other professionals than for speaking to family members. When sharing assessment results with family members, the examiner should be aware of the general level of education, and in the case of bilingual families, the level of proficiency with English. Even when family members have some fluency with the English language, it may be a good idea to have an interpreter available. Often the family members who are most skilled in English will act as an interpreter. This may not be an optimal arrangement for sessions where test results are being discussed because of the technical nature of some of the information. An ideal interpreter is one who is familiar with the agency and the kinds of testing and services it offers and who can help the examiner offer information in an understandable and culturally meaningful way.

Examiners must also consider the anticipated emotional response when presenting information. A parent who hears that his young child has developmental delays may be emotionally devastated, therefore the information should be sensitively communicated. Every child has strengths and attributes that can be highlighted when discussing overall performance. The examiner should also avoid any appearance of placing blame on the parent for the child's difficulties because many parents are quick to blame themselves for their child's problems. The tone of any discussion should be objective yet positive, with the emphasis placed on sharing information and joint decision making about a plan of action.

The final ethical issue relates to testing of children from diverse cultural groups. In recent years there has been a great deal of criticism about cultural bias in standardized tests. These criticisms raise many important points about the validity of tests developed primarily on a white, middle-class population when they are used with children from different cultural backgrounds. It is important for examiners to be aware of the factors that may influence how children from diverse cultures perform on standardized tests. First, children who do not have experience with testing may not understand the unspoken rules about test taking. They may not understand the importance of doing a task within a time limit or following the examiner's instructions. They may not be motivated to perform well on tasks because the task itself has no intrinsic meaning to them. The materials or activities may be seen as irrelevant, or, having had no experience with the kinds of materials used in the tests, they may not know how to interact with the materials. Establishing rapport may be difficult either because of language barriers or because there is a cultural mismatch between the social interaction patterns of the child and the examiner.

If the examiner is aware of these potential problems, some steps can be taken to minimize possible difficulties. The caregiver or an interpreter can be present to help the child feel more at ease. The caregiver can be questioned regarding the child's familiarity with the various test materials. This can give the examiner some information about whether the child's failure to perform individual items is caused by unfamiliarity with the materials or by inability to complete the task. The caregiver can also be shown how to administer some items, particularly those involving physical contact or close proximity to the child. This may make the situation less threatening for the child. Note, however, that if these adjustments are made, standard procedure has been violated and it may be inappropriate to compute a standard score. Even so, the test can provide a wealth of descriptive information about the child's abilities.

Clearly, occupational therapists must possess a number of skills beyond the ability to simply administer test items when using standardized tests. Professional communication skills are essential when administering tests and reporting information. Awareness of family and cultural values helps put the child's performance within a contextual framework. An understanding of the professional and ethical responsibilities involved in dealing with sensitive and confidential information is also extremely important. A competent examiner brings all of these skills into play when administering, scoring, interpreting, and reporting the results of standardized tests.

# PROS AND CONS

Standardized tests have permitted occupational therapists and other child development professionals to develop a more scientific approach to assessment. The use of tests that give statistically valid numeric scores has helped give more credibility to the assessment process. However, standardized tests are not without their drawbacks. The following section discusses the pros and cons of using standardized tests, along with suggestions regarding how to make testing results more accurate and meaningful.

## Advantages

Standardized tests possess several characteristics that provide a unique contribution to the assessment inventory of pediatric occupational therapists. First, they are tests that are, in general, fairly widely known and available commercially so that a child's scores on a particular test can be interpreted and understood by therapists in other practice settings or geographic locations. Standard scores generated by standardized tests allow testers from a variety of professional disciplines to "speak the same language" when it comes to discussing test scores. For instance, a child is tested by an occupational therapist for fine motor skills, a physical therapist for gross motor skills, and a speech pathologist for language skills. Each of the three tests expresses scores as T-scores. An average T-score is 50. The child receives a fine motor T-score of 30, a gross motor T-score of 25, and a language T-score of 60. It is apparent that although this child is below average in both gross and fine motor skills, language skills are an area of strength; and in fact, they are above average. These scores can be compared and discussed by the assessment team and used to identify areas requiring intervention and areas in which the child has particular strengths.

Standardized tests can be used to monitor developmental progress. Because they are norm-referenced according to age, the progress of a child with developmental delays can be measured against expected developmental progress as compared with the normative sample. In this way occupational therapists can determine if children receiving therapy are accelerating their rate of development as a result of intervention. Similarly, children who are being monitored after being discharged from therapy can be assessed periodically to determine if they are maintaining the expected rate of developmental progress or if they are beginning to fall behind their peers without the assistance of intervention.

## Disadvantages

Standardized tests are increasingly being criticized for giving therapists a false sense of accountability and security (Royeen, 1992). Much of the criticism centers around using standardized tests as a substitute for functional performance assessments. Because most standardized tests assess performance components such as balance, bilateral coordination, and visual-motor skills, rather than occupational performance areas such as play, activities of daily living, and educational or prevocational activities, the intervention goals that are generated as a result of standardized assessment frequently address these performance components rather than functional performance within the child's environmental context. As a result, occupational therapy intervention may not adequately address a child's occupational performance in a meaningful way. Stewart (Chapter 8) discusses the importance of placing standardized testing within the child's performance context. A standardized test cannot stand alone as a measure of a child's abilities. Clinical judgment, informal or unstructured observation, caregiver interview, and data gathering from other informants are all essential parts of the assessment process. These less structured evaluation procedures are needed to provide meaning and interpretation to the numeric scores obtained by standardized testing.

There are several other considerations that testers must take into account when using standardized tests. First, a test session provides only a brief "snapshot" of a child's behavior and abilities. The performance that a therapist sees in a 1-hour assessment in a clinic setting may be different from that seen on a daily basis at home or at school. Illness, fatigue, anxiety, or lack of familiarity with the test materials, the room, or the tester can adversely affect a child's performance. The tester must be sensitive to the possible impact of these factors on the child's performance. A competent tester can do a great deal to alleviate a child's anxiety about testing and to ensure that the experience is not an unpleasant one. However, it is important to remember that any test situation is artificial and usually does not provide an accurate indication of how the child performs on a daily basis. It is important to speak to the child's parent, caregiver, or teacher at the time of testing to determine if the observed behavior is truly representative of the child's typical performance. The representativeness of the behavior must then be taken into account in interpreting and reporting the child's test scores.

Another concern about standardized tests is the rigidity of the testing procedures themselves. Standardized tests specify both particular ways of administering test items and, in many cases, exactly what instructions the tester must give. Children with problems as diverse as hearing impairment, attention deficit, muscle weakness, or incoordination may not have an opportunity to perform optimally given these administration requirements. Many therapists believe that the standard score obtained by a standardized test administration is strongly affected by the child's particular deficits and does not accurately reflect the child's true abilities. Although this issue is not addressed by all standardized tests, some tests provide guidelines to use when attempting to administer the test under nonstandard conditions. For example, the PDMS provides case illustrations of how the test can be adapted for testing children with vision impairment and cerebral palsy. This provides testers with some guidance in the use of the test when special accommodations may need to be made. The BSID-II provides normative data for several clinical groups. It is important to reiterate that although it is permissible to alter the administration procedures of most tests to accommodate children's individual needs, the child's performance cannot be expressed as a standard score. Rather, the purpose of the testing is to provide a structured format for describing the child's performance. The test manual should always be consulted for guidelines related to alterations in test procedures.

Two standardized tests are available that have been developed specifically for use with children who have physical disabilities: the Pediatric Evaluation of Disability Inventory (PEDI) (Haley, Coster, Ludlow, Haitiwanger, & Andrellos, 1992) and the Gross Motor Function Measure (GMFM) (Russell et al., 1990). A unique characteristic of the PEDI is that it measures the amount of caregiver assistance and environmental modifications required for children to perform specific tasks. This provides a way to assess the level of independence and the quality of performance for children whose disabilities may prevent them from ever executing a particular task normally. The GMFM is a criterion-referenced test that measures the components of a gross motor activity that a child with cerebral palsy can accomplish. It is meant to provide information necessary for designing therapy programs and measuring small increments of change. These tests are among a new wave of tests designed by and for occupational and physical therapists, and they show promise in addressing the unique assessment and program planning needs of pediatric therapists.

### Referral Information

Caitlin is a 5-½-year-old kindergarten student referred for occupational therapy assessment by her teacher, Mrs. Clark. Mrs. Clark notes that Caitlin appears to be having a great deal of difficulty in learning to write; she holds her pencil awkwardly and either exerts too much or not enough pressure on the paper. She complains of fatigue during writing and coloring activities. On the playground and in physical education (PE) classes she has difficulty keeping up with the rest of the class. She falls frequently, appears uncoordinated, and has difficulty learning new motor skills. On several occasions she has complained of minor ailments; Mrs. Clark believes that she does this to avoid participating in PE. Mrs. Clark would like to know whether there are any underlying problems that may be causing Caitlin's school difficulties and if any special help is needed.

### Additional Information

Debra receives the occupational therapy referral. She speaks to Caitlin's parents before initiating her assessment and obtains additional information. She finds out that Caitlin received physical therapy briefly as an infant because of low muscle tone and slow achievement of developmental milestones. Although she appeared to make good progress in therapy, she has continued to lag be-

hind her peers somewhat. Her parents are particularly worried about how Caitlin will cope with the increased written requirements of first grade and how she will be accepted by other children if she continues to struggle in school. They do not have a great deal of free time but are willing to consider some home activities to help Caitlin along. They decline Debra's offer for them to be present at the testing session, citing concerns about Caitlin's behavior when they are present, but ask to meet with Debra after Caitlin's evaluation.

### Testing Information

Debra considers Caitlin's age (5½years) and the areas of concern expressed by Mrs. Clark and Caitlin's parents (gross and fine motor skills and social adjustment) in choosing which standardized test to use. She decides to administer the PDMS, along with clinical observations of Caitlin's posture, muscle tone, strength, balance, motor planning, hand use and hand preference, attention, problem-solving skills, and visual skills. Caitlin came enthusiastically to the testing session, which was scheduled at a midmorning time to avoid possible effects of fatigue or hunger. She attended well, although she needed encouragement for the more challenging items. By the end of the session she complained of fatigue, but Debra believed she was able to get a representative sample of Caitlin's motor skills and that the scores obtained were reliable.

### Test Results

Caitlin received a total gross motor raw score of 313, placing her in the 13th percentile for her age. Her total fine motor raw score was 205, placing her at the 5th percentile. These scores translate into Z-scores of $-1.13$ for gross motor and $-1.64$ for fine motor. In the gross motor area, ball skills were an area of relative strength but she had a great deal of difficulty with balance activities and activities involving hopping, skipping, and jumping. In the fine motor area, Caitlin used a static tripod grasp on the pencil, frequently shifting into a fisted grasp if the writing task was challenging. Based on the small number of visual-motor items on this test, visual-perceptual skills appeared to be an area of strength, whereas tasks involving speed and dexterity were particularly difficult. Debra found that Caitlin had low muscle tone overall, particularly in the shoulder girdle and hands, and strength was somewhat decreased overall. Caitlin's endurance was poor; for many tasks she performed well initially, but performance deteriorated as she continued. Motor planning difficulties were evident in the way she handled test materials and moved about the environment. She had difficulty devising alternate ways to accomplish tasks that were challenging for her and required Debra's manual guidance to complete some tasks. She became frustrated to the point of tears on two occasions, and needed a great deal of encouragement to continue when this occurred.

### Conclusions and Recommendations

According to her scores on the PDMS, Caitlin has mild delays in her gross motor skills and mild to moderate delays in her fine motor skills. Although Debra believed that the PDMS gave a good indication of what Caitlin could do under optimal circumstances (i.e., a nondistracting environment, individual attention and encouragement, and structuring of tasks to maximize success and minimize frustration), she also thought it did not represent the level of performance that would be seen over the course of a typical

## STUDY QUESTIONS

1. For what testing purposes is a criterion-referenced test preferred? A norm-referenced test?

2. You are testing 2-year-old Brandon using a standardized test. He refuses to attempt several items, throws test materials, and repeatedly tries to leave the test area. Brandon's mother states that this behavior is not typical, and that she knows that he is able to do many of the tasks that were presented to him. What statement can you make about the reliability of the test results? What strategies might you use to maximize the quantity and quality of information obtained during the test session?

3. Carmen, who is nine years old, is scheduled for her periodic formal school reassessment. Previous testing was done at age 6 using the PDMS. Now that Carmen is beyond the age range of the PDMS, what tests can be used and how can the score from this testing be compared with her previous test scores?

4. Jared, who is seven years old, is referred to you for assessment. You administer a standardized test, and he receives a raw score of 83. You then provide therapy services to Jared for 6 months. On reevaluation he receives a score of 98 on the same standardized test. The SEM of the test is 4.0. Using the 95% confidence interval, what is the potential range of scores for Jared for each testing? What can you conclude about the effect of your treatment?

5. You have just purchased a newly published test of visual-motor skills. You are interested in how a child's performance on this test relates to handwriting skills. What information would you look for in the test manual to answer this question?

6. You are learning to administer a standardized test. You check your interrater agreement on the test with another therapist in your department who frequently uses the test. Your point-by-point agreement on the test is 65%. What strategies can you use to improve interrater agreement, and what level of agreement should you aim to achieve?

7. A child is referred to you for assessment. When the child and her mother arrive, you discover that their English skills are extremely limited. Knowing that the test you plan to use requires you to give the child verbal instructions, how should you proceed in your testing and how should you discuss the results?

8. You are reviewing a new test that your department has purchased. The test manual reports concurrent validity of 0.85 with another well-known and well-regarded test that is used frequently by your department and other agencies in your area. What additional information should you look for to make a decision about which of these two tests to administer?

9. A 3-year-old child is referred to you with possible developmental delays. No other information is available on the referral note, but you know that he was recently screened in his preschool program. What information can you obtain that would help you decide what areas to test and the approximate developmental level to begin testing?

10. Given the following referral information, state what standardized tests and nonstandardized evaluation techniques you would use to assess this child.

Child's name: Natalie

Child's chronologic age: 3 years 3 months

Pertinent history and referral information: Natalie was born at 35 weeks' gestation to a mother who used cocaine and marijuana throughout her pregnancy. She had mild respiratory distress in the first few days of life. Natalie has had chronic middle ear infections and currently has ear tubes. She had early difficulties with sucking and is a picky eater. Her mother entered a drug treatment program during a subsequent pregnancy and has been clean and sober for 1½ years. Natalie lives with her mother and two siblings in a small apartment. Her mother states that Natalie is "different" than her other children and that she has difficulty controlling Natalie's behavior. Natalie seems to be bright but is active and easily frustrated with fine motor activities. She has frequent temper tantrums, refuses to nap, and wakes several times during the night. A public health nurse has been involved with the family since Natalie's birth, and she and Natalie's mother agree that some additional intervention may be necessary. Natalie is scheduled to enter a Head Start preschool program, and they would like recommendations for both home and school.

day. She spent a morning observing in Caitlin's classroom and discovered that Caitlin avoided fine motor and gross motor activities whenever possible and completed writing and drawing activities rapidly, resulting in poor quality of the end product. She was near tears on two occasions, after experiencing frustration with her attempts at an art activity. Her performance was clearly below that of her classmates, and it appeared that without intervention she would almost certainly fail in the first grade. In Caitlin's school district a child did not qualify for special education or related services unless scores in two or more developmental domains were below a Z-score of 1.5. In Caitlin's case only one Z-score (fine motor) was below this level. Because both Debra and Mrs. Clark felt strongly that Caitlin would not be successful without intervention, they met with the school psychologist, the school principal, and Caitlin's parents to determine a plan of action. It was determined that Debra would provide recommendations to Mrs. Clark about classroom modifications and activities that would increase Caitlin's success and build her motor skills. Debra provided a pencil gripper and a chair that fit Caitlin better and provided better positioning for writing. She provided Mrs. Clark with ideas for appropriate activities and ways of teaching Caitlin new motor skills. Debra provided Caitlin's parents with suggestions for family-oriented activities that would improve general strength and endurance (bicycle riding and swimming) and provided specific ideas for ways they could build Caitlin's fine motor skills at home. She also agreed to be available to Mrs. Clark for periodic informal consultation. It was agreed that a reassessment would be scheduled at the end of the school year so that the team could make a decision about further intervention and program planning for next school year.

## Conclusion

Standardized testing, specifically the PDMS, provided a helpful framework for Debra's assessment of Caitlin and gave specific information about areas of strength and difficulty. In this case Caitlin was unable to qualify for occupational therapy intervention because her standard scores did not satisfy the school's eligibility criteria. Debra made use of her clinical observations and information gathering from other sources to make a decision about what type of intervention was both necessary and feasible, given the constraints of the school district regulations. Clearly, if she had simply relied on standardized test scores, she would not have developed the breadth of knowledge that led to her decision-making process about intervention options. This example illustrates the important roles of both standardized testing and of other methods of data collection in arriving at meaningful and realistic conclusions about children's intervention needs and modes of service delivery.

## REFERENCES

Anastasi, A. (1988). *Psychological testing* (6th ed.). New York: Macmillan.

American Occupational Therapy Association. (1994). Occupational therapy code of ethics. *American Occupational Therapy Association, 48*(11), 1037-1038.

Ayres, A.J. & Marr, D. (1991). Sensory integration and praxis tests. In A. Fisher, E. Murray, & A. Bundy (Eds.). *Sensory integration: theory and practice* (pp 201-233). Philadelphia: F.A. Davis.

Bayley, N. (1969). *Bayley Scales of Infant Development*. New York: The Psychological Corporation.

Bayley, N. (1993). *Bayley Scales of Infant Development* (2nd ed.). San Antonio, TX: The Psychological Corporation.

Beery, K.E. (1989). *Developmental Test of Visual-Motor Integration: administration, scoring, and teaching manual—3rd revision.* Los Angeles: Western Psychological Services.

Bricker, D. (Ed.). (1993). *AEPS measurement for birth to three years.* Baltimore: Brookes.

Bruininks, R.H. (1978). *Bruininks-Oseretsky Test of Motor Proficiency.* Circle Pines, MN: American Guidance Service.

Buros, O.K. (Ed.). (1978). *The eighth mental measurements yearbook.* Lincoln, NE: Buros Institute of Mental Measurements.

Crowe, T.K., Deitz, J.C., & Bennett, F.C. (1987). The relationship between the Bayley Scales of Infant Development and preschool gross motor and cognitive performance. *The American Journal of Occupational Therapy, 41,* 374-378.

Cunningham Amundson, S.J. & Crowe, T.K. (1993). Clinical applications of the standard error of measurement for occupational and physical therapists. *Physical and Occupational Therapy in Pediatrics, 12*(4), 57-71.

Deitz, J.C. (1989). Reliability. *Physical and Occupational Therapy in Pediatrics, 9*(1), 125-147.

Farran, D.C. & Harber, L.A. (1989). Responses to a learning task at 6 months and IQ test performance during the preschool years. *International Journal of Behavioral Development, 12,* 101-114.

Folio, M.R. & Fewell, R.R. (1983). *Peabody Developmental Motor Scales and Activity Cards.* Chicago: Riverside Publishers.

Frankenburg, W.K., Dodds, J.B., Fandal, A.W., Kazuk, E., & Cohrs, M. (1975). *Denver Developmental Screening Test.* Denver: DDM.

Furuno, S., O'Reilly, K.A., Hosaka, C.M., Inatsuka, T.T., Allman, T.L., & Zeisloft, B. (1979). *The Hawaii Early Learning Profile.* Palo Alto, CA: Vort.

Furuno, S., O'Reilly, K.A., Hosaka, C.M., Inatsuka, T.T., Allman, T.L., & Zeisloft, B. (1985). *Hawaii Early Learning Profile Activity Guide.* Palo Alto, CA: Vort.

Gardner, M.F. (1982). *Test of Visual-Perceptual Skills (non-motor).* San Francisco: Children's Hospital of San Francisco.

Haley, S.M., Coster, W.J., Ludlow, L.H., Haltiwanger, J.T., & Andrellos, P.J. (1992). *Pediatric Evaluation of Disability Inventory: development, standardization and administration manual.* Boston: New England Medical Center Hospitals and PEDI Research Group.

Hammill, D.D., Pearson, N.A., & Voress, J.K. (1993). *Developmental Test of Visual Perception* (2nd ed.). Austin, TX: Pro Ed.

Hinderer, K.A., Richardson, P.K., & Atwater, S.W. (1989). Clinical implications of the Peabody Developmental Motor Scale: a constructive review. *Physical and Occupational Therapy in Pediatrics, 9*(2), 81-106.

Kazdin, A.E. (1982). *Single-case research designs.* New York: Oxford University Press.

Mardell-Czudnowski, C. & Goldenberg, D. (1983). *Developmental indicators for assessment of learning—revised.* Edison, NJ: Childcraft Educational Corporation.

McGavin, H., Cadman, D., & Jarvis, S. (1990). *Gross Motor Function measure.* Hamilton, Ontario: Gross Motor Measures Group.

Miller, L.J. (1990). *First STEP screening tool.* San Antonio, TX: The Psychological Corporation.

Miller, L.J. (1982). *Miller Assessment for Preschoolers.* San Antonio, TX: The Psychological Corporation.

Mitchell, J.V. (Ed.). (1983). *Tests in print III.* Lincoln, NE: Buros Institute of Mental Measurements.

Mitchell, J.V. (Ed.). (1985). *The ninth mental measurements yearbook.* Lincoln, NE: Buros Institute of Mental Measurements.

Palisano, R. (1986). Concurrent and predictive validities of the Bayley Motor Scale and the Peabody Developmental Motor Scales. *Physical Therapy, 66,*1714-1719.

Royeen, C.B. (1992). Measuring and documenting all services. In C.B. Royeen (Ed.). *AOTA self study series: school-based practice for related services.* Rockville, MD: American Occupational Therapy Association.

Sanford, A.R. & Zelman, J.G. (1981). *Learning Accomplishment Profile—revised.* Winston-Salem, NC: Kaplan.

Sternberg, R.J. (1990). *Metaphors of mind: conceptions of the nature of intelligence.* Cambridge, England: Cambridge University Press.

Terman, L.M. & Merrill, M.A. (1937). *Measuring intelligence.* Boston, MA: Houghton Mifflin.

Wechsler, D. (1974). *Wechsler Intelligence Scale for Children—revised.* San Antonio, TX: The Psychological Corporation.

## SUGGESTED READINGS

Anastasi, A. (1988). *Psychological testing.* New York: Macmillan.

Bailey, D.B. & Wolery, M. (1989). *Assessing infants and preschoolers with handicaps.* Columbus, OH: Merrill.

Campbell, S.K. (1990). Using standardized tests in clinical practice. In S. Campbell & R.E. Carter (coordinators). *Topics in pediatrics.* Alexandria, VA: American Physical Therapy Association.

Mitchell, J.V. (Ed.). (1983). *Tests in print III.* Lincoln, NE: Buros Institute of Mental Measurements.

Task force on standards for measurement in physical therapy. (1991). Standards for tests and measurements in physical therapy practice. *Physical Therapy, 71,* 589-622.

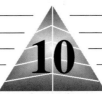

# Planning and Implementing Services

JANE CASE-SMITH

## KEY TERMS

▲ Intervention Goals and Objectives
▲ Documentation
▲ Best Practice Models
    Zone of Proximal Development
    Child-Centered Activity
    Motor Learning
    Clinical Reasoning
    Coping Model
▲ Team Interaction

## CHAPTER OBJECTIVES

1. Write functional, observable, and measurable objectives.
2. Write objectives that match team goals and environmental context.
3. Define activities within the child's zone of proximal development.
4. Describe and exemplify child-centered activity.
5. Describe principles of motor learning theory.
6. Explain the process of clinical reasoning when planning and implementing therapy with children and their families.
7. Explain the components and dynamics of the coping model, and apply this model to early childhood intervention.
8. Describe models of team intervention and the dynamics of team problem solving, negotiation, and decision making.

The process of linking evaluation to intervention is a challenging and essential part of occupational therapy. Through this process, occupational therapists interpret evaluation findings and use this information to derive meaningful goals and appropriate plans for their clients. This chapter explains the steps that link evaluation and intervention, that is, intervention planning with children. First, documentation of the occupational therapy plan is described and models of clinical decision making used by occupational therapists are explained. Then service delivery models, frames of reference, and team models used to plan comprehensive services are explained.

As described in Chapter 8, evaluation involves examination of performance components, performance areas, and performance context. Appendix 8-A lists the domains of concern of occupational therapy in the American Occupational Therapy Association's (AOTA's) *Uniform Terminology for Occupational Therapy,* 3rd ed (AOTA, 1994a). Performance areas, components, and context relate and interact. Performance components are addressed in intervention as they relate to performance areas (i.e., work, play, and daily living). Performance contexts are considered when evaluating function and dysfunction across performance areas and components (AOTA, 1994b).

To plan intervention, the occupational therapist gathers together all of the evaluation information, interprets its meaning, formulates goals and objectives, and then develops specific strategies and activities. Most often this process occurs within the context of a team. Therefore rather than one individual therapist making singular decisions about goals, objectives, strategies, and activities, a team of professionals that includes the consumer develops the plan (see Chapter 2). Accordingly, intervention planning is a process of decision making that involves negotiation and consensus building. Building team consensus about the goals for the child results in a cohesive plan. The plan should reflect team and family priorities and should define a long-range vision for the child.

The occupational therapist contributes to a written plan for the child. This written plan serves as a guideline or blueprint for intervention. It may be a legal contract such as an Individualized Education Program (IEP) that defines services and goals for the entire school year. Or the plan may be a highly flexible and easily modified guideline for intervention. With a written plan in place, the professionals are accountable for certain goals and objectives that the child is to achieve. The plan helps keep therapy activities on track with the priority goals for the child. It helps direct the team's efforts, including those of the child and family, toward important outcomes (Mager, 1975). It also defines specific behaviors that can be used to evaluate the child's progress and the effectiveness of intervention. The plan is a dynamic, vital document that not only guides the intervention process and provides a means for evaluating progress, but also helps team members work together toward common goals.

## DOCUMENTING THE INTERVENTION PLAN

The box at right lists the four components of an intervention plan as defined by the Standards of Practice for Occupational Therapy (AOTA, 1994b).

The Standards state that written goals are to be clear, measurable, behavioral, functional, and appropriate to the individual's needs. *Clear* means that the goals should be understandable and straightforward. For an objective to be useful, it must be meaningful to others. Technical terms are often misunderstood and are confusing rather than helpful to the parent or teacher.

*Measurable* goals allow for evaluation of goals. An objective that cannot be measured cannot be evaluated. Mager (1975) recommended that measurable objectives have three components:

1. Performance—What the student is expected to do (e.g., drink from a cup or draw a circle).
2. Conditions—The important conditions under which the performance is to occur or what the student uses to perform the activity (e.g., independence in word processing using a head pointer to access the keyboard or independence in lower extremity dressing using pants with Velcro closures).
3. Criterion—The quality or level of performance that is acceptable (e.g., exhibited accurate object placement at midline four of five times or demonstrated lip closure during chewing 50% of the meal).

Objectives that describe expected performance, including conditions and criteria, allow for specific measurement of objective achievement.

Performance-based objectives are also *behavioral;* they describe a child's behavior rather than a characteristic that may be reflected by that behavior. Therefore objectives that state that "the child will be more social" or "the child will demonstrate improved self-esteem" are not adequate because they do not describe measurable behaviors.

Examples of behavioral objectives for the goals stated above are "The child will verbalize positive comments about himself and his work four of five times when com-

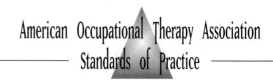

## American Occupational Therapy Association Standards of Practice

**STANDARD V: INTERVENTION PLAN**

1. An occupational therapist shall develop and document an intervention plan based on analysis of the occupational therapy assessment data and the individual's expected outcome after the intervention. A certified occupational therapist assistant may contribute to the intervention plan under the supervision of the therapist.
2. The intervention plan is stated in goals that are clear, measurable, behavioral, functional, and appropriate to the individual's needs, personal goal, and expected outcome after intervention.
3. The plan shall reflect the philosophic base of occupational therapy and be consistent with its established principles and concepts of therapy and practice. The intervention plan shall include the following:
   a. formulating a list of strength and weaknesses
   b. estimating rehabilitation potential
   c. identifying measurable short-term and long-term goals
   d. collaborating with the individual, family members, other caregivers, professionals, and community resources
   e. selecting the media, methods, environment, and personnel needed to accomplish the intervention goals
   f. determining the frequency and duration of occupational therapy services
   g. identifying a plan for reevaluation
   h. planning discharge
4. An occupational therapist shall prepare and document the intervention plan within the time frames and according to the standards established by the employing practice settings, government agencies, accreditation programs, and third-party payers.

From the American Occupational Therapy Association. (1994). Standards of Practice. *American Journal of Occupational Therapy, 48,* 1039-1043.

ments are solicited by the teacher," or "When praised by the therapist or teacher, the child will acknowledge and agree with the positive appraisal of his behaviors 90% of the time." By using behavioral terms, the team has a specific outcome in mind, which can be clearly communicated and measured.

*Functional* goals are those that clearly relate to the child's ability to function in his or her unique environments. They refer to important behaviors that enable the child to participate in the physical and social environment. *Functional goals* are important to the life roles that the child has in his or her everyday environments, for example, at home, in school, or in a child care center. The child's developmental level and age, in addition to the context of the behavior and the expectations of the educational curriculum, are considered.

The goals and objectives must also be appropriate to the child's individual needs, the family's or personal priorities, and hoped-for outcomes. Appropriate objectives are unique to each individual child; they specifically address needs that were identified through the assessment process. The objectives also carefully consider the expected outcome for the child as defined by the team. A team, including family members, develops a vision of the child in the near future, for example, at the end of 3 months, 6 months, or a year. This vision reflects the child's past developmental rate, the environmental supports and resources available, and information about the disability. The vision also considers the general expectations of the child's educational level. If the child is in the first grade, do the objectives meet the outcomes expected of all first graders? If the adolescent is ready to graduate from high school, does he or she have the skills required to enter an independent living situation? The expected outcome is therefore grounded in knowledge about the child's developmental course, the intervention services available, the school's curriculum, and the educational outcomes established for all children within a certain class or grade level. In medical settings, intervention outcomes consider the child's current medical status and prognosis in addition to context of his or her performance.

The written goals of the intervention plan are generally categorized as long-term goals and short-term objectives. The actual length of time to achieve the goals is determined by the nature of the environment (e.g., short-term hospital stay versus school setting), the age and type of disability of the child, and legal restrictions, state guidelines, or agency policies regarding documentation standards. During a hospital or rehabilitation stay, short-term objectives may be written for performance expected within 2 weeks. In early intervention programs, short-term objectives are often established for a 45-day period and long-term goals are established for a 6-month period. In school programs, long-term goals typically refer to performance at the end of an academic year. Annual goals may be broad and general, primarily serving as organizing end goals. Short-term objectives refer to performance at the end of 90 days. In general, short-term objectives describe the steps necessary to achieve the long-term goal. The objectives should be specific and well defined, including performance, conditions, and criteria. They state measurable behaviors to be observed as markers of intervention effectiveness and the child's progress. The following is an example of documentation using short-term objectives and long-term goals.

## Case Example
### History

Lindsey is a 12-month-old child who was diagnosed at birth with cytomegalovirus (CMV). Her early development was trau-

matic; she had seizures, feeding difficulties and poor weight gain, sensory defensiveness, and motor delays. In the first 4 months she was hypersensitive to all movement and touch, and as a result, she spent significant time in a quiet, darkened room to allow her periods of calm and rest.

### Assessment

By 12 months, her sensory defensiveness had resolved to the point that she could participate in most family activities and regularly attend an early intervention program. She remained fussy and would often fall asleep in the middle of a particularly stimulating activity or event. As a 1-year-old, Lindsey exhibited severe delays in motor skills. Her only form of mobility was spontaneous rolling from her stomach to back. She was unable to make transitions from one position to another, primarily because extensor postural tone dominated her movement. She lacked balanced activation of proximal flexor and extensor muscles to move reciprocally and segmentally. Axial rotation patterns were absent. She maintained static positions with minimal assistance from an adult, and therefore Lindsey sat by propping herself with her arms and with some support at the pelvis. She maintained a prone-on-elbows position with use of a roll under her chest and between her arms and trunk. In a supine position she demonstrated reciprocal kicking, and her hands were beginning to come to midline. Play skills were limited to basic sensory motor exploration of toys. In supported sidelying, she easily brought her hands together for play with objects; therefore this position was frequently used for play activities. Sitting in her corner chair with a tray in place offered another well-supported play position. She was beginning to transfer objects from hand to hand, to hold toys using a radial palmer grasp, and to wave and bang toys to produce a sound. Functional use of toys had not emerged. She demonstrated imitation and consistently repeated movements that were reinforced with social praise.

### Goals and Objectives
#### *Long-term goal*
I. Lindsey will exhibit trunk rotation and reciprocal extremity movement sufficient to move from a prone into a sitting position.

#### *Short-term objectives*
1. She will exhibit segmental rolling from a supine to prone position four of five times with the encouragement of her mother's verbal cuing.
2. She will demonstrate a sequence of two rolls toward an interesting toy three times within a therapy session.
3. When independently sitting on the mat, she will demonstrate an equilibrium response of lateral trunk flexion and reciprocal trunk elongation when tilted to the side, four of five times.

#### *Long-term goal*
II. Lindsey will demonstrate midline bilateral hand skills in play with toys.

#### *Short-term objectives*
1. While in supported sitting, she will transfer a toy from the right to left hand and left to right hand, three times each session.

2. Given a cube-shaped object, she will demonstrate a radial digital grasp three of four times.
3. Given a small, multiple-part toy, she will turn and rotate it using forearm rotation and isolated wrist extension, three of four times.

### Long-term goal
III. Lindsey will demonstrate tolerance to at least five new tactile and movement experiences.

### Short-term objectives
1. Given different textures placed on her tray (e.g., whipped cream, rice, sand, beans, cereal), she will actively explore the textures using a variety of hand and finger movements for a 5-minute period.
2. She will accept food consistencies of lumpy, soft (e.g., cottage cheese and eggs) and coarse, pureed (e.g., chunky apple sauce) twice each day.
3. She will tolerate fast movement experiences (e.g., bouncing on knee) without subsequent fussiness twice each day.

The short-term objectives provide specific descriptions of the steps involved in reaching the long-term goals. They also provide ways that achievement of the objectives can be measured through naturalistic observation, for example, in the therapy session. Three to four long-term goals is an appropriate number for the occupational therapist and parents to address at any one time. The selected goals reflect the therapist's and parents' *priorities* rather than an exhaustive list of possible objectives. The plan should be dynamic and allow for changes in priorities because changes are inevitable with young children and families.

## Team Objectives

When goals are written by a team, often the persons responsible for each goal or objective are listed. Generally, all the team members work on the agreed-on goals; however, the listed team member takes a leadership role in monitoring and evaluating that objective. This professional communicates with the family and other team members when an objective has been accomplished or needs to be changed. In the IEP or the Individualized Family Services Plan (IFSP), objectives often include the team members responsible and the measurement criterion to be used to evaluate achievement of each objective (see box at right).

Rainforth, York, and MacDonald (1992) provided examples of goals and objectives. They recommended that specific examples of context be embedded in the written objectives as a method to help the team develop strategies for addressing goals in the child's everyday environments. The following example demonstrates how short-term objectives can be used to provide contextual information about where the skill will be exhibited:

### Long-term goal
Kristen will exhibit a lateral pinch and thumb-to-finger tip grasp.

### Short-term objectives
1. Following verbal cuing Kristen will use a lateral pinch for finger foods at snack time for 3 consecutive days, four of five bites.
2. When seated at the table for art activities and handed a crayon in a vertical orientation, Kristen will grasp the crayon using a thumb-to-fingertip grasp four of five times. (The vertical orientation cues her to supinate and use her thumb actively in the grasp.)

The short-term objectives give the team a natural context for practice of the skills and for evaluation of accomplishment.

The process for developing goals and objectives is discussed in Chapters 8 and 9. These chapters define a process of identifying the child's strengths and limitations and the areas of concern and then developing an intervention program that targets the performance components and areas of concerns, considering the different contexts in which the child functions. It is suggested that therapists use different and often combined frames of reference to guide their decision making throughout this process.

### Examples of Team Objectives

**TEAM GOAL**

1. Jeremy will accurately select words using the switch-activated scanning system of his Liberator (Augmentative Communication Device by Prenke Romish Company, Wooster, Ohio).

**Short-Term Objectives**

a. Jeremy will consistently track the light scanning mechanism of his device 90% of the time.
   *Person responsible for evaluation:* Occupational therapist
   *Criterion:* Jeremy will exhibit smooth eye tracking of the Liberator's scanning mechanism set at a rate appropriate for conversation.
b. When positioned in good postural alignment with his Liberator, Jeremy will demonstrate sufficient eye-hand coordination to activate the switch with accurate word selection 90% of the time.
   *Person responsible for evaluation:* Occupational therapist
   *Criterion:* Using a plate switch to make word selections with device scanning, Jeremy selects the correct word 9 of 10 times.
c. Jeremy will successfully produce a sentence of four words within 30 seconds with 100% accuracy.
   *Person responsible for evaluation:* Teacher
   *Criterion:* When asked a question in class, Jeremy produces a four-word response within 30 seconds using his Liberator 100% of the time.

# INTERVENTION PLANNING PROCESS

Several comprehensive approaches are used by occupational therapists to develop intervention plans for children. These concepts provide therapists with general principles, rather than specific techniques, for designing intervention. They are approaches that are appropriate for many, if not most, children who are referred for occupational therapy services. One theme that transcends all of these concepts is that the client (that is, the child and family) is the center of occupational therapy practice. Law and Baum (1994) stated the following:

Client-centered practice is an approach to providing occupational therapy, which embraces a philosophy of respect for and partnership with people receiving our services. It recognizes the autonomy of individuals, the strengths clients bring to a therapy encounter, the need for client choice, and the benefits of client-therapist provider collaboration (p. 3).

Each of the following approaches illustrates this philosophy of practice and explains how the occupational therapist, in partnership with family and team members, makes decisions about intervention goals, objectives, and specific activities. The approaches include (1) the zone of proximal development, (2) child-centered activity, (3) motor learning theory, (4) clinical reasoning, and (5) the coping model.

## Zone of Proximal Development

In evaluating the child, the occupational therapist determines the child's current level of function. Based on an in-depth understanding of developmental principles, the therapist also assesses the child's potential for change or progress in performance areas. By estimating the child's potential for change, the therapist can plan outcomes for the child that are based on realistic expectations. The occupational therapist estimates the child's potential for improved performance by evaluating his or her response to intervention. The child's responses to supportive handling, specific sensory input, or adaptations to the environment that are designed to enhance performance give the therapist important information as to the potential effectiveness of those strategies. Initial trials of therapeutic strategies provide a basis for selecting therapy activities and for predicting how rapidly and to what degree improved performance will result.

Vygotsky (1978) defined the concept of the *zone of proximal development* to indicate the emerging skills that the child can not yet perform independently but that he or she can demonstrate with the help of the parent or therapist. For example, within the zone are the skills that the child can successfully perform with physical assistance or visual and verbal cuing. This "help" that a child needs to perform a skill is based on an understanding of what specifically is limiting performance and assessment of his or her performance with a variety of therapeutic inputs.

By defining the child's zone of proximal development, the therapist identifies the emerging skills that become the focus of intervention and defines the intervening methods that seem most helpful to the acquisition of new skills (Lyons, 1984). Published tests that explore the child's emerging skills and define a zone of proximal development include items that allow visual and verbal cues to be given that promote the child's performance. In some tests the materials or activities can be adapted to match the child's particular problem or limitation (e.g., Hawaii Early Learning Profile [Furuno et al., 1985] and Carolina Curriculum for Handicapped Infants and Infants at Risk [Johnson-Martin, Jens, & Attermeier, 1986]). Fewell's Play Assessment Scale (Fewell & Glick, 1993) records the child's performance with visual and verbal cuing. With an understanding of the zone of proximal development, the therapist can select activities that are "just right" for the child, that are challenging, and that can be successfully accomplished with specific therapeutic input. Working within this zone challenges the child to achieve higher-level developmental skills without frustrating him or her in tasks that are too difficult for possible success.

## Child-Centered Activity

Critical to any intervention plan is selection of activities that motivate the child and sustain his or her attention. An optimal level of arousal, alertness, attentiveness, and motivation is essential to learning any new task. Umphred and Appley (1990) explained the important role of the limbic system (as the neurologic center for controlling emotions and motivation) in learning new motor tasks. Most actions are influenced by the child's emotional state and feeling of well-being. The child attempts a new task when he or she is motivated and interested in that activity. Goal-directed and purposeful activities that match the child's developmental level and interests seem to motivate the child into active participation. A line of research to determine the importance of using activities that have meaning and purpose to elicit optimal performance has been pursued (Nelson, 1988; Nelson & Peterson, 1991). Campbell, McInerney, and Cooper (1984) suggested that the child's motivation and attention are increased in social situations. By including the child's peers in therapy activities, the activities become more motivating and reinforcing. The therapist can also promote the child's motivation by making an activity fun (playful) and by developing a relationship of trust with the child. Developing trust is critical to increasing the child's investment in the activity. Trust is enhanced when the therapist is playful, appears to enjoy the interaction, and is sensitive to the child's needs. DeGangi, Craft, and Castellan (1991) suggested a method for increasing the child's trust and positive feelings during the therapy session.

Child-centered activity is a model adapted from infant psychotherapy to children with sensorimotor and sensory processing problems (DeGangi, 1991). Its applications

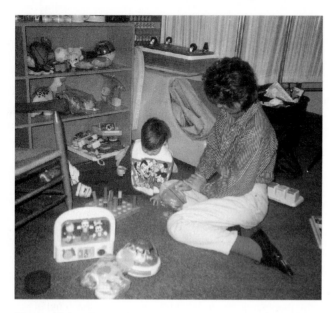

**Figure 10-1**  Occupational therapist watches a child in his selected play activity.

range from young children with emotional problems to those whose developmental delays appear to be related to sensory processing dysfunction. It is most appropriate for children with mild and moderate delays, rather than those with severe disabilities (e.g., spastic quadriparesis cerebral palsy). However, parts of this approach seem to have application to all children and their families.

Child-centered activity is based on the premise that play is the child's natural context for gaining new skills. The child seems to perform at the highest possible level in playful interaction with an adult who is trusted. The intervention approach is in contrast to more traditional and more structured approaches in which the therapist employs specific handling techniques, exercises, and skills-focused training. These approaches that involve direct instruction and skill training may not produce learning that can be generalized across environments.

The elements of child-centered activity include a flexible sequence of activity and involve the child's exploration of the environment and his or her own creative play. The child initiates play activities in an open space (e.g., on a mat) with interesting and developmentally appropriate toys available. The therapist selects toys with multiple uses, and an assortment of sensory qualities is desirable. Once the occupational therapist and the parents have structured the environment, their role is that of interested observers and facilitators (Figure 10-1). The child is encouraged to select activities that he or she enjoys. The child initiates the activity and interaction and experiences the parents' or the therapist's encouragement, which enhances feelings of competence and control (DeGangi, 1991). When the parent and therapist follow the child's

lead, the child gains a sense of effectiveness that can be generalized to other situations with peers and other adults.

DeGangi, Wietlisbach, Goodin, and Scheiner (1993) compared a child-centered activity program with a structured approach that used a predetermined sequence, repetitive drill, and adult direction that focused on teaching specific skills. Each sample was composed of 12 preschool children with a range of developmental, motor, emotional-behavioral, and sensory integrative disorders who received 8 weeks of each intervention type. Results of the study indicated that fine motor skills improved more as a result of the child-centered activities. In contrast, the structured sensorimotor therapy resulted in greater improvement in gross motor and functional skills. Repetition and practice of skills seemed to account for the improved performance. The authors concluded that different therapeutic strategies are needed to promote fine and gross motor skills. Gross motor skills are associated with the child's motivation to move about the environment. Fine motor skills depend on the child's motivation to seek and explore objects in the environment. The process of object exploration through creative play may be a critical aspect of gaining hand function. Specific handling techniques may be helpful in refining hand skills, but first the child must be interested and motivated to engage in manipulative play.

DeGangi (1991) described an example of child-centered activity with a boy who demonstrated hypersensitivity to touch and movement, postural instability, and low muscle tone. The child did not yet demonstrate symbolic play, and his manipulation of toys was highly stereotypic and immature for his age.

During the child-centered activity, Tommy spent considerable time lifting heavy push carts and pounding and pushing them on the floor, thus providing himself with heavy proprioceptive input. . . . Mother discovered that when she playfully imitated him, his pleasure and length of playing time increased. . . . mother was encouraged to allow Tommy to play in a large bin of styrofoam chips and to explore textured object (e.g., Slinky; rough hairbrushes) tactile activities that Tommy soon began to crave (p. 52-53).

Table 10-1 gives the primary goals of child-centered activity and examples of activities in which these goals can be accomplished.

Child-centered activity is most appropriate for achieving greater competence in fine motor play and social interaction. Therapy sessions should become more structured when the therapist and family are invested in specific skill development or when gross motor and postural skills, rather than fine motor and hand skills, are the focus of intervention.

Motor learning theorists have developed approaches and strategies that promote the child's acquisition of specific motor skills.

▲ Table 10-1   The Role of the Parent and Occupational Therapist in Child-Centered Activity

| General Goals of Child-Centered Activity | Activities of Parent and Therapist |
|---|---|
| Provide the child with focused, nonjudgmental attention from the parent | Watch the child, be relaxed, give accepting smiles, and imitate some of the child's actions |
| Facilitate initiative and problem-solving by the child | Offer simple cues (e.g., point where to place the object, position toys so that the child can better handle them) and wait for the child's response after each cue |
| Develop intentionality, motivation, curiosity, and exploration | Show interest, curiosity, and encouragement of exploration and play |
| Promote sustained and focused attention | Describe features of toys or objects to sustain attention (e.g., "Teddy's eyes are shiny today; do you think he is happy?") |
| Refine the child's signal-giving ability and performance | Repeat the child's verbalization to check intent; ask him or her to combine verbal and nonverbal communication by repeating his or her words; encourage a broad range of emotions in the child |
| Enhance mastering of sensorimotor developmental challenges within the context of play | Introduce play and playfulness into parent-child interaction, which may previously have been focused on caregiving and support; present the child with new challenges in play activities |

Modified from DeGangi, G.(1991). In S.S. Poisson & G. DeGangi (Eds.). *Emotional and sensory processing problems: assessment and treatment approaches for young children and their families.* (p. 50). Rockville, MD: Reginald Lourie Center for Infants and Young Children.

## Motor Learning Theory

What are the variables that promote skill acquisition? What principles guide the selection of activities that help the child learn new skills and generalize those skills to a variety of contexts? What factors need to be considered to develop an intervention plan? Recent research has demonstrated that the variables that influence skill acquisition involve interrelated systems (Brookes, 1986; Scholtz, 1990). Changes in motor performance are thought to be attributable to maturation of different subsystems, of which motor function is only one aspect. Somatosensory, musculoskeletal, affective organization, and cognition are important contributors to the child's performance (Bradley, 1994). The complexity of variables that influence the child's performance and learning suggests use of an ecologic approach that includes consideration of the influence of the child's everyday environment on his or her performance in designing intervention (Dunn, Brown, & McGuigan, 1994).

In motor learning theory the child's active participation in purposeful activity is the key to improving developmental and functional skills (Gliner, 1985). Evidence suggests that the individual who practices movements within the context of an activity that has a self-defined goal learns the movements more quickly and retains them longer than an individual who repeats meaningless movements (Kaplan, 1994; Nelson, 1988). When the child selects the activity and believes that he or she has control over how the activity is performed (e.g., when it begins and when it ends), learning from that activity is much more likely. The role of the therapist is to clarify for the child what is happening during the activity and to give reinforcing feedback. The feedback is specific and descriptive rather than general and globally positive. Theories about motor learning have helped therapists develop effective strategies for enhancing learning through use of *practice* and *feedback*.

### Practice

The most beneficial practice for learning a new skill occurs in the environment in which that skill must be performed. This is particularly true when the child first learns a new skill. Because the therapist cannot possibly be present for all of the opportunities that a child has during the day to practice a new skill, for example, cutting with scissors, pulling up his or her pants, or drinking from a cup, it is critical that the therapist teach the parents and child care providers methods used to assist the child in learning the skill. For example, if the child can don his or her coat given a simple series of physical and verbal cues, the therapist should instruct the child's teachers and parents in the cues needed to assist him or her in donning his or her coat. Involving other adults in teaching the skill to a child promotes learning and generalization of that skill. This concept reinforces the benefit of teaching others ways to handle and interact with the child and the importance of monitoring how well the child is performing the targeted skill with other adults in other environments.

Another principle that has been demonstrated in motor learning studies is that random practice is more effective in learning a novel task than repeated or blocked practice. Therefore the occupational therapist presents the same task at different times during the session and in different contexts as the ideal way to reinforce learning of that skill. If the targeted skill is tracing a circle, the child may trace a circle template on construction paper, trace a circle outlined by a string glued to the paper, and draw a circle around a small Frisbee to mark where it landed on the floor in a throwing game.

In addition, practice of a targeted skill within a natural whole task is beneficial in learning the skill. This is particularly true when skills need to be sequenced in a specific order with specific timing. When learning to feed with a spoon, working on the component of "scooping" by pretending to spoon-feed dried beans to a Teddy Bear does not necessarily generalize into independent self-feeding. The scooping action should be practiced in the context of self-feeding, which includes spoon entry into the child's mouth.

Skills learned in isolation in an intervention session are of little value unless they can be generalized to everyday function. Although this generalization often occurs naturally because the child becomes excited about a new skill and wants to practice it at every occasion, generalization does not always automatically occur. The child who demonstrates scissors skill by cutting a straight line across a narrow piece of paper will not automatically begin to cut out a circle, which requires higher-level bilateral skills to turn and position the paper. Once a child has achieved a skill, the therapist should provide examples of how the skill might be generalized and ways to promote its use in the child's everyday environments.

### Feedback

Another important variable in learning a new skill is the feedback that the child receives during and after skill performance. In the initial stages of learning a new skill, clear sensory feedback is important to refine how the skill is successfully performed. Intrinsic feedback refers to sensory information from the joint receptors, tendons, muscles, and skin. Visual and auditory feedback can also be intrinsic because it occurs naturally within the activity. Intrinsic feedback can be reinforced by the therapist's handling the child using touch, joint compression, and deep pressure. Two types of extrinsic feedback are useful to learning a new task: (1) knowledge of results and (2) knowledge of performance.

*Knowledge of results* refers to the child's awareness of what happened as a result of his or her movement. Did the ball reach the target? Did the circle he drew look like the circle printed on the paper? This type of feedback occurs naturally in the context of most activities. What appears to be most important is that the child receives accurate feedback. Therefore the child learns to recognize his or her errors as well as successes. Learning to discriminate how well a task is performed is important to learning to perform it better. By receiving immediate and accurate knowledge of results, the child can associate that knowledge with the intrinsic sensory feedback, thus reinforcing learning.

*Knowledge of performance* gives the child additional descriptive information about his or her performance. Important aspects of the child's performance can be reinforced verbally. The therapist can use gestures to reinforce movement or make comments about how the child's movement is forceful or gentle to reinforce those aspects of movement.

Kaplan (1994) summarized aspects of motor learning theory that fit with occupational therapy philosophy. These premises are basic to principles of practice:

1. Therapy activities that engage the child in purposeful activity, in a functional context, enhance skill learning.
2. A match between the learner and the environment is critical to increasing function and can be achieved by improving the child's skills or decreasing the demands of the environment. (This principle is discussed further in the following section on the coping model on p. 233.)
3. Sensory input is basic to learning motor skills. Sensory input can be enhanced by emphasizing important performance components, guiding the movement, and helping the child gain a clear understanding of the outcome.

### Clinical Reasoning

How does the occupational therapist apply the zone of proximal development, child-centered activity, or motor learning theory? The approach used by the therapist is uniquely applied to each child through a process of clinical reasoning. The therapist employs clinical reasoning to analyze important aspects of the child's behavior and the environment and to use this analysis to make decisions about intervention.

In a qualitative study of clinical reasoning, Mattingly and Fleming (1994) described four strategies used by occupational therapists to make intervention decisions. The strategies are used concurrently as the therapist contemplates the needs of the whole child. *Procedural and interactive reasoning* are employed to make the decisions that result in recommendations for an intervention plan. Given an understanding of the child's limitations and needs, *procedural reasoning* is used to identify specific methods designed to improve function. The therapist matches his or her understanding of the child's problem to the range of intervention approaches that appropriately address that problem. Procedural reasoning defines the process the therapist employs to identify the problems and then logically develops a goal and plan. This analysis is similar to the medical problem solving model in which a problem is identified, different solutions are tested, and intervention is defined.

Therapists also employed *interactive reasoning* to gain understanding of the child and family as individuals. This reasoning is used to understand the perspectives and experiences of the family from their point of view. Fleming (1994) listed a number of purposes for using interactive reasoning, some of which are listed below:

1. To engage the child in the treatment session
2. To know the child and family as individuals
3. To understand the disability from the family's point of view

4. To finely match the treatment goals and strategies to the particular child, with his or her disability and experience

5. To communicate a sense of acceptance, trust, and hope

Positive and meaningful interactions are essential to intervention. Therapists use interactive reasoning to assimilate the whole individual, including values and beliefs. The therapist then employs this understanding to guide decision making about intervention. In this form of reasoning the therapist responds to subtle cues of the child to select specific intervention activities and then adapts those activities to maintain the child's interest and attention. The result of interactive reasoning is that intervention activities are individualized to the child.

The therapist's thorough understanding of the child and the child's preferences and interests guides the selection of toys and activities that will engage the child in play and that will meet identified intervention goals. This process is intuitive rather than analytic. Although the therapist's *intuitive reasoning* often defies definition, the therapist's interpretation of the complex, subtle interactive cues is core to the effectiveness of intervention. When the occupational therapist accurately "reads" the child's mood, interests, and intentions, he or she can match these by offering appropriate activity choices that gain the interest and participation of the child. This intuitive activity selection is as important to the success of intervention as the analytic, procedural reasoning that matched activity selection directly to established goals. Once engaged in an activity with the child, the therapist continues to use his or her knowledge of intervention procedures and techniques to remediate the problem and his or her interactive abilities to individualize the activities to motivate and capture the child's attention.

A fourth type of reasoning appears to be used by many therapists to develop intervention plans. In *conditional reasoning,* the therapist thinks about the child's condition in three ways:

1. The therapist views the whole, that is, the child and his or her disability, the family, and the environment.
2. The therapist contemplates how the condition might change. He or she envisions a different child who can perform a skill at a higher level.
3. The therapist thinks about ways to ensure the child's participation. The therapist creatively develops activities that will interest and motivate the child with the realization that the success of intervention is based on the child's participation.

In conditional reasoning the therapist selects appropriate intervention activities based on the child's problem and his or her vision for the child in the future. This vision guides the therapist's decision to continue an emphasis on promoting developmental skills or to explore possible adapted methods for the child to compensate for functional limitations. The family's and the child's visions of the future also determine whether therapy should emphasize compensatory, functional strategies in lieu of developmental goals. Intervention is at high risk for failure when the therapist and family hold different visions for the future and therefore believe that different strategies should be employed.

For example, the parents of a 2-year-old with severe neuromotor delays envisioned that their child, Justin, would walk within a year. The occupational therapist believed that Justin would not achieve this goal but was a good candidate for a battery-powered wheelchair. The family preferred that therapy sessions focus on standing and walking activities; the occupational therapist preferred to focus on the eye-hand coordination needed to use a joystick to control a wheelchair. If each pursued their vision, it is likely that neither goal would be achieved. The therapist must develop an understanding of the family's vision and consider their perspectives of the child's problems. The therapist also needs to convey his or her vision and the rationale for such a vision. By sharing their individual goals for Justin, Justin's parents and the therapist can negotiate an intervention plan that clearly addresses the family's priorities and values and engages their participation in intervention. The occupational therapist and the parents reached consensus on the goal of improved trunk stability as a prerequisite skill for independent standing and for upright sitting in a wheelchair. By setting a common goal that both parties believed to be a priority, a basis for communication about the child's progress was established that helped the parents and the occupational therapist develop additional appropriate goals.

### Summary

Clinical reasoning describes the scientific and intuitive process that the occupational therapist employs to make decisions about intervention goals, strategies, and recommendations for children and their families. It involves logical, procedural reasoning from evaluation results to intervention methods; it also involves intuitive, tacit understanding of the child and family, which enables the therapist to engage the family as active participants in intervention. Important to this process is envisioning a future child, understanding the meaning of the disability to the child and family, and identifying variables that seem critical to developing positive relationships and trust.

## Coping Model

The *coping model* (Williamson, Szczepanski, & Zeitlin, 1993; Zeitlin & Williamson, 1988; Zeitlin & Williamson, 1994) is a comprehensive approach for designing an intervention program based on the child's and family's internal and external resources. The basic premise of the coping model is that the ability of the child to effectively function in his or her environment is primarily determined by the coping resources that are available to him or her.

### Internal Supports

*Beliefs and values* are internal resources and describe what the child holds as true about the self and the world.

Mastery of skills and performance is influenced by the child's sense of personal control, personal effectiveness, and self-esteem. The child's values reflect his or her desires or preferences. Families who value education may become more involved in intervention. Families who value physical prowess and strength may find raising a child with cerebral palsy particularly challenging and difficult. When family members and professionals have different beliefs, barriers are created that often interfere with communication (Zeitlin & Williamson, 1994).

*Physical and affect states* are other internal coping resources. Physical state includes one's general health and current physiologic condition (e.g., level of hunger or fatigue). The parents' health can affect their caregiving ability. Similarly, the child's health can affect his or her energy level, developmental progress, and ability to participate.

Affective state refers to the child's emotions and mood. Positive affect holds great benefits in promoting interaction; negative affect is stressful for caregivers and inhibits relationships with peers.

*Knowledge and skills* enable the child to interact in his or her environment with increasing confidence and independence. The goal of occupational therapy is to increase the knowledge and skills of both the child and the parents.

### External Supports

Two types of external supports are important coping resources. These are broadly categorized as human supports and material and environmental supports.

*Human support* is obtained from interpersonal relationships. Human support comes from informal sources (generally the family) and formal sources (e.g., occupational therapists or social workers). Interpersonal relationships are important to obtaining specific information and emotional support, as well as direct assistance (e.g., child care). Human supports and interpersonal relationships may change when the family has a child with a disability.

*Material and environmental supports* include aspects of the environment that help the child cope with stress. Material supports such as a new wheelchair or piece of adaptive equipment can be critical to the child's ability to interact with others and to explore and master his or her surroundings. Environmental supports that promote the safety and comfort of the child allow him or her to engage in play and social interactions.

### Goodness-of-Fit Model

Every individual has his or her own unique *coping style,* which defines the behaviors used to cope with stressful or challenging events. Coping style is based on temperament, competence, and prior experience. Children with effective coping styles often have positive self-concepts and take initiative in achieving their own goals.

The child exhibits the coping efforts that are required by environmental demands. When the child is introduced to a new activity or enters a new environment, he or she may

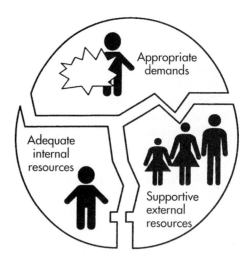

**Figure 10-2**    Coping Model: Goodness-of-Fit. (From Zeitlin, S. & Williamson, G. [1994]. *Coping in young children* [p. 21]. Baltimore: Brookes.)

withdraw or act out (less effective coping response) or may actively explore and investigate the new environment (more effective coping response). When the child has adequate internal resources and external supports to cope with the environmental demands, a "good fit" is achieved and the child successfully copes in that situation. Goodness-of-fit is a concept that helps therapists examine the whole picture of the child and evaluate the child's success or failure in light of the supports available in the environment and the appropriateness of the tasks demands. Goodness-of-fit, as defined by Zeitlin and Williamson (1994), has three components:

1. Demands are appropriate in that they are congruent with the individual's capability to meet them.
2. The individual has the personal resources (both internal and external) to make an effective coping effort.
3. The environment provides appropriate supportive and evaluative feedback.

These components that contribute to goodness-of-fit are illustrated in Figure 10-2.

The goodness-of-fit model gives the therapist a structure for designing intervention. To learn a new skill, the child must attempt new activities and accept new challenges. The child successfully copes with new challenges when (1) he or she has underlying skills that can be generalized to the new situation (i.e., the skill is within his or her zone of proximal development), (2) human supports are provided to facilitate his or her performance (e.g., the occupational therapist models the play activity and gives cues to direct reach [Figure 10-3]), and (3) environment supports are provided (e.g., the child is positioned well in a chair with firm back support and arm rests with feet supported to increase postural stability [Figure 10-4]).

In the goodness-of-fit model the occupational therapist continually evaluates whether the child's skills (internal resources) and environment supports (external resources) are

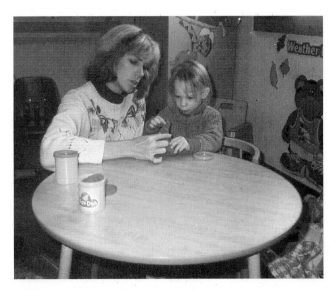

**Figure 10-3** Occupational therapist models an activity to promote the use of specific hand and finger movements.

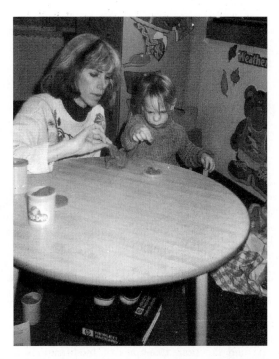

**Figure 10-4** Child sits in an adapted chair with firm back support and arm rests. Feet are also supported.

adequate to meet the demands of the activity. When the child begins to exhibit ineffective coping strategies, the therapist adjusts the task demands and provides more human or environmental support to enable the child to succeed in his or her coping effort. Unsuccessful coping can harm self-esteem and the belief that one can master the environment; however, failure in individual tasks does not need to be avoided. The child learns from the feedback that his or her movement was inadequate or that his or her efforts were insufficient. In giving constructive feedback the occupational therapist describes the task demands and the child's performance in a way that gives the child additional information about his or her effort. Feedback that helps the child evaluate his or her coping efforts, both successful and unsuccessful, helps the child develop effective action schemes that can be generalized to other situations.

Williamson, Szczepanski, and Zeitlin (1993) explained how the coping frame of reference can be employed in practice. Based on the components that contribute to goodness-of-fit, three principles guide how intervention activities are selected and adapted.

First, goodness-of-fit can be achieved by modifying the demands of the environment. For example, the environment can be adapted by reorganizing materials to reduce the amount of sensory stimulation the child receives and to help the child sequence a task; materials can be positioned within the reach of the child who does not yet have mobility skills. Positioning devices that provide external support can help the child focus on the fine motor skills required in a drawing activity or the oral motor skill required for feeding.

Second, intervention can enhance the child's internal resources to improve his or her ability to cope with environmental demands. Occupational therapists often focus on acquisition of developmental and physical skills. With higher-level skills the child can more successfully master expected roles, that is, independently perform self-care functions and demonstrate a greater repertoire of play skills. Williamson et al. (1993) recommended that priority be placed on the developmental skills the child needs to successfully cope in his or her everyday environment. Therefore in the exploratory phase of development the child can better cope if he or she has some form of mobility. Fine motor skills are critical to the child's ability to cope in the classroom (see Chapters 12 and 24). Developmental skills also seem to directly relate to the child's beliefs and values. Once the child gains the skills to master a task and become independent in an activity, self-esteem and sense of self-efficacy increase. Tailoring the environmental demands to enable success can also improve the child's belief in his or her ability to master and control the environment.

External supports are essential to the child's ability to cope. For the young child, a supportive, responsive family strengthens the child's ability to adapt to novel situations and take on new challenges. Positive family relationships are highly related to the child's acquisition of skills and ability to cope. Peer relationships become increasingly important to the older child. The social support of peers also enhances both the child's ability to cope and motivation to achieve and function independently. Social interaction in structured activities (e.g., in group therapy sessions) and unstructured activities (e.g., on the playground) enhances the child's emerging sense of self and ability to cope.

The occupational therapist also recommends adaptation to the physical environment to improve the child's ability

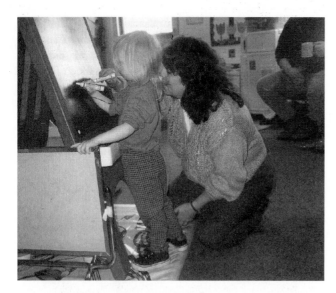

**Figure 10-5** Therapist follows the child's lead in drawing on an easel chalkboard.

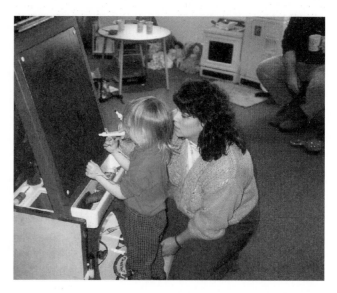

**Figure 10-6** Therapist makes descriptive remarks about the child's drawings.

to cope and function. Examples of modifications to the classroom include adapted seating so that visual perceptual tasks are less stressful and demanding or adapted writing and cutting utensils that are easily handled. The occupational therapist also makes recommendations regarding the home environment, for example, to help the parents provide sensory input that matches the child sensory processing abilities. Toy and play activities are often recommended.

The occupational therapist works with other team members to enhance the child's internal and external resources as these relate to the ability to cope and function in the child's natural environment. The emphasis of intervention depends on which resources, internal or external, seem to have the greatest relationship to the child's ability to cope and are most amenable to change. The therapist considers which developmental skills area seem most important to the child and family and which seem to relate to the coping style.

The third postulate proposed by Williamson et al. (1993) is that the child's coping effectiveness is enhanced when appropriate, contingent responses are given to the child's coping efforts:

> When feedback is timely, positive, clear, and accurate in response to productive coping efforts, the child experiences a sense of mastery that contributes over time to a belief system that addresses person worth and autonomy. Meaningful social feedback is not just verbal but can be expressed through smiles, frowns, and looks of admiration or consternation (Williamson et al., 1993, p. 426).

In this model, child-initiated activity is supported. The therapist and parents give responsive attention to the child's actions (Figure 10-5). Rather than providing continuous positive remarks, the adult describes the child's actions and the activity in ways that are helpful and show genuine in-

terest (Figure 10-6). This supportive interactional approach of waiting, watching, and then responding is in contrast to the typical adult-directed interaction that has been observed with children who have disabilities (Mahoney, Finger, & Powell, 1985).

## Example of the Coping Model

At 5 years of age, Phillip H. had 4 years of occupational therapy and by his mother's report "has made tremendous gains." Phillip first began occupational therapy when he was 18 months old. His motor skills were delayed; for example, he was not yet walking and had limited bilateral manipulation. He often used wave and bang strategies to play with objects. He had poor postural stability, with low muscle tone throughout, and poor cocontraction of shoulder muscles. He had never crept but had learned to roll from place to place and to crawl on his belly using a bilateral pull. Sensory processing was problematic; he exhibited tactile defensiveness that was extreme inside his hands and mouth. A sensory integration approach had been used by the occupational therapist and seemed to have been effective in improving postural stability, crossing the midline skills, and tactile integration.

At 5 years, his family moved to a new city and immediately sought occupational therapy services. Ms. H. found an occupational therapist in a private practice who was trained in the Sensory Integration and Praxis Test (SIPT) (Ayres, 1989). Phillip had never been tested using the SIPT, and the new occupational therapist thought that it would be helpful in planning services. Phillip's profile of SIPT results best aligned with generalized sensory integration dysfunction. He had low scores on the praxis tests and the bilateral integration and sequencing tests. The tactile perception tests were well below the norm. Testing using the Developmental Test of Visual Perception—2 (Hammill, Pearson, & Voress, 1993) indicated that his visual motor skills were delayed 1 year, and his visual perceptual skills were age appropriate. His tactile defensiveness seemed to have resolved, which his mother verified in description of his behavior at home. Phillip was hesitant to respond throughout the testing and continually looked to his mother for guidance and reassurance. His mother responded by instructing him to listen and attend to the therapist.

The occupational therapist and Ms. H agreed that activities based on the sensory integration approach should continue to be used. These strategies would help improve equilibrium, bilateral integration, and motor planning. However, the occupational therapist thought that other performance components and therefore frames of reference should be considered at this time to prepare Phillip for entry into school in the autumn. Using the coping frame of reference, the therapist identified the following issues:

*Beliefs and values:* Phillip's self-esteem was low, and he lacked confidence to try new activities. He relied on his mother to direct his actions.

*Physical skills:* He had made nice gains in gross motor skills and postural stability; however, motor planning was delayed, particularly when bilateral integration and sequencing were required. Visual motor skills were a year delayed.

*Affect:* Phillip was extremely shy and hesitant to respond. He generally clung to his mother for the first 5 minutes of the therapy session and looked to her for reassurance when a new activity was presented.

*Developmental skills:* Phillip demonstrated developmental skills of a 3- to 4-year-old child. In addition to delays in visual-motor and fine motor skills, he needed assistance in dressing (managing fasteners) and in bathing. He could not yet print any letters. Play skills were delayed, particularly with drawing and coloring, construction toys, and bicycle riding.

*Human support:* Ms. H. was supportive and a strong advocate of her son, seeking and investing resources into the services she believed he needed. Although she had always followed home program recommendations, she had recently discontinued implementing the specific activities the last occupational therapist had recommended. Ms. H. explained, "The therapy activities frustrate him and then he gets angry at me. I am tired of being the bad guy; I prefer to be just his mom." During the occupational therapy sessions her interactions with Phillip consisted of a string of directives closely followed with general praise of his efforts. She recognized his over-reliance on her and his low self-esteem but seemed unaware that her interactional style increased his dependence on her.

*Environmental support:* The H. home was comfortable and full of toys. Despite the toys available, Phillip played almost exclusively with his small cars and trucks, driving them on a large colorful plastic sheet that simulated town streets and buildings. He had recently learned to ride a three-wheel "tractor," which he seemed to thoroughly enjoy. His mother was thrilled that he had learned to use pedals. The family lived in a neighborhood full of children, but Phillip did not have any friends and almost always played alone. He occasionally played with this 3-year-old sister, Caitlyn, whose skills were comparable to his.

*Interpretation:* The occupational therapist was most concerned about Phillip's coping skills for entry into school. Given the high expectations in the areas of fine motor and visual motor skills, she thought that he would have difficulties in the classroom activities and assignments. She worried about his low self-esteem and lack of self-initiative. His performance seemed tightly tied to his mother's direction and reinforcement; the therapist could not imagine him spending an entire school day without his mother by his side.

*Recommendations and intervention:* The occupational therapist recommended goals that focused on developing the copying and drawing skills that are prerequisite to printing. She also recommended a focus on bilateral manipulation to prepare him to efficiently use scissors, writing utensils, paper, the computer, and other classroom materials.

Although the therapist employed some of the vestibular-based activities that he enjoyed, she spent most of the therapy session in art and play activities designed to improve visual-motor and bilateral hand skills. She also believed that peer interaction could be a helpful way to reduce Phillip's reliance on his mother's reinforcement. Although his mother seemed disappointed when the occupational therapist asked if she could schedule another boy of Phillip's age at the same time, she agreed to try a therapy program that included another child. Tommy, whose problems were similar to Phillip's, joined him in the next occupational therapy session. At first both boys were shy and reticent to engage in activities together. Initially the therapist selected fun activities in which both boys were assured of success. She designed cooperative activities that required efforts from both to accomplish, for example, pushing the barrel with the therapist inside, building an obstacle course with heavy equipment, blowing a ping pong ball down the length of the table with Phillip and Tommy on either side. Soon the two boys were great friends. Once an activity was introduced, they quickly took over directing it and creatively added new steps and different strategies. Their absorption in the activities allowed the occupational therapist to spend time with Ms. H. in quiet discussion about school and ways to promote Phillip's independence. Together they problem solved ways to encourage Phillip to play more often with neighborhood children. Ms. H. began to see that he could achieve and succeed without her direction. Throughout the session the occupational therapist had allowed him to choose the activities and had encouraged his self-direction. His self-direction increased exponentially as he plotted and planned activities with his new friend. The occupational therapist pointed out to Ms. H. how much his self-esteem seemed to improve when he was allowed to direct the activity.

Because the boys struggled most with bilateral manipulation and motor planning, they seldom selected fine motor tasks. Therefore the occupational therapist provided these when it was her turn to select the activity. She introduced art activities with neon-colored paints, stickers, and glitter because these materials resulted in interesting pictures with minimal skills required. The boys selected the themes for art each week, and the occupational therapist gradually introduced media that required developmentally higher visual motor skill. Often the boys made one large mural that was hung in the clinic room. Other fine motor activities included games with small pieces and cards, fishing for magnetic letters, mazes, and origami (paper folding).

Ms. H. reported that Phillip often initiated these activities at home once they had been introduced in the clinic. He demonstrated genuine pride in his artwork and began to show his new neighborhood friends how to make the origami figures. The summer before school began, Phillip told his mother that he could not wait until he went to school. Both the occupational therapist and Phillip's mother believed that this new eagerness, self-confidence, and change in self-esteem would assure his success in coping with his first school year.

## WHICH SERVICE DELIVERY MODEL?

The theoretical models described in the first part of this chapter help guide the occupational therapist in writing goals and objectives and in planning intervention activities and strategies. In addition to deciding on *what* services will meet the child's and family's needs and priorities, the team must decide on *how* the services should be delivered, for example, which service delivery model will effectively accomplish the intervention goals. Occupational therapists use a number of different service delivery models in association with different settings and arenas of practice (e.g., preschools, schools, hospitals, and home) and with different intervention purposes (e.g., a focus on psychosocial, play, fine motor, and self-care functions). The choice of service delivery model may also be influenced by the frame of reference (e.g., neurodevelopmental or occupational behavior) guiding intervention. The model of service delivery has implications for how the professionals of the interdisciplinary team interact, where and how frequently services are provided, and the nature of those services.

Three primary models of service delivery for children have been identified (AOTA, 1987). Most often the models are used in combination with each other. They can be used sequentially or together with a wide variety of options as to how they can be combined.

One model, *direct services,* focuses on the child and involves direction interaction with the child and family. *Monitoring and consultation* primarily involve interactions with others, either teaching or consulting, with the child being the focus of the adult interaction.

### Direct Services

In direct services the therapist works in one-on-one interaction with the child or leads a small group of children in intervention activities. Therapists select direct service models when specialized occupational therapy approaches and techniques are needed that are individualized to the child and require specific skills to administer. Direct services are appropriate when the intervention techniques cannot be safely administered by others or when the success of the technique relies on continually adjusting and adapting the input according to the child's unique responses. For example, the therapy approaches that require constant and ongoing monitoring of the child's autonomic nervous system and postural responses need to be implemented directly by the occupational therapist (Dunn & Campbell, 1991). Most often direct hands-on therapy involves use of neurodevelopmental, sensory integration, or play therapy, which are individually based techniques that require close monitoring of the child's responses and frequent adaptation of the

method (Dunn & DeGangi, 1992). Each action of the occupational therapist is closely tied to the child's responses and reactions. In addition to critical observation skills, the occupational therapist uses clinical reasoning to adapt or modify an activity or piece of equipment to ensure its therapeutic benefit. Activities are adapted so that a "just right" challenge is presented, so that the child effectively copes with that challenge, and so that the activity is intrinsically rewarding. Direct therapy is the best model when specific physical or behavioral handling is required and when a combination of verbal, visual, and physical cues are needed to assist in the child's performance.

Direct services are frequently provided in the child's natural environments (e.g., at home or in the classroom). Although services in the child's everyday environment promote generalizing of the skills learned, an isolated environment (e.g., the therapy clinic) is sometimes useful when the full attention of the child is needed, when a more intimate interaction is desirable, or when certain types of equipment are to be used. Direct services may be provided with intense frequency for a short period, then later with less frequency and with greater reliance on family members, teachers, and assistants to carry out the program.

### Monitoring

When the occupational therapist monitors the intervention program, he or she evaluates the child, develops a program, and then teaches others in the child's environment to implement the program. The therapist remains responsible for the outcome of the plan and oversees implementation to assure that the procedures are implemented on a consistent basis. Although the therapist may not directly interact with the child on an ongoing basis, he or she remains in regular contact with the persons who carry out the program, evaluates their verbal feedback about the child's progress, and suggests modifications of the program if needed.

Dunn and Campbell (1991) recommended that monitoring is an appropriate model of service delivery when three criteria are met: (1) the health and safety of the child are protected when the plan and procedures are carried out by the trained individual, (2) the implementor correctly demonstrates the implementor procedure, and (3) the implementor demonstrates knowledge of child cues that indicate that the procedure needs to be discontinued or modified.

To effectively use monitoring, the occupational therapist must demonstrate the ability to teach other adults and to share his or her knowledge in ways that enable the performance of others. Because the therapist remains responsible for the child's program, although he or she is not the daily implementor, monitoring involves trust in other team members, the ability to clearly articulate intent and specific activities, and skill in motivating, encouraging, and coaching other adults (Rainforth, York, & MacDonald, 1992).

## Consultation

Consultative services are designed to enable others to meet their expressed goals (Dunn, 1991, Dunn & Campbell, 1991). In consultation the therapist uses his or her knowledge to enable another person to successfully interact with the child or group of children in a way that promotes functional skills. Often the therapist provides consultation when a student or child problem arises that suggests that the expertise of the occupational therapist would be helpful. On request for consultation the therapist typically confers with the teacher to gain his or her perspective, observes the student or evaluates the student, and then makes recommendations. Consultation is an effective choice when skills need to be generalized to the natural environment or when the environment can be adapted to support improved functional skills. The therapist uses consultation with the teacher or other members of the team to establish therapeutic routines or to adapt specific tasks and activities expected of the child.

Dunn (1991) listed two goals in consultation: (1) to create solutions that remediate the immediate problems that the child is experiencing, and (2) to increase the consultee's skills so that he or she can respond more effectively to similar problems that arise in the future.

Commitment to the second goal implies that the occupational therapist help the consultee learn and generalize new skills and that this model of service delivery holds benefits beyond the specific child's problem that was the original reason for requesting occupational therapy consultation.

### Collaborative Consultation

Most of the work in developing consultative models has been done in the fields of education, psychology, and social work. Idol, Paolucci-Whitcomb, and Nevin (1987) described a model of collaborative consultation that meets the goals listed above; that is, this model helps remediate the student's problems and enables the consultee to manage future situations that involve similar problems.

In collaborative consultation, teams of professionals meet to solve problems and develop solutions. The therapist and consultee work together to identify the problem and solution, to formulate a plan, and to evaluate the recommendation. It is characterized by a trusting relationship in which each partner appreciates and respects the skills and ideas of the other. Each is committed to the plan, taking responsibility for portions of the plan. As a result of the collaboration, new strategies are tried, responses are evaluated, and adaptations to the strategies are made. To provide effective consultation, the occupational therapist directly interacts with the child. Opportunities to observe (and handle, when appropriate) the child help the therapist develop an understanding of strengths and limita-

tions that then guide his or her decision making (clinical reasoning). Once the occupational therapist and consultee have formulated a plan and the recommendations are implemented, the occupational therapy consultant regularly observes and interacts with the child to evaluate the effectiveness of the recommendations and to monitor changes in the child. Extensive follow-up and evaluation are important for effective results. An ongoing collaborative relationship between the occupational therapist and the consultee helps ensure that the plan is implemented, and, when needed, revised, and that the consultee gains new skills in working with the child and solving similar problems that may arise.

## COMPREHENSIVE MODEL FOR PLANNING AND IMPLEMENTING SERVICES

Occupational therapy services are almost always delivered in the context of interdisciplinary teams. The intervention program is planned and implemented by a group of professionals and the family, who have come to some consensus on the goals and priorities for the child. How the team members interact to develop the plan depends on a myriad of factors, for example, their opportunities to communicate, whether and how often they meet as a team, the sequence of events that preceded the written plan, and the role of the family. Teams with high levels of communication can provide well-integrated services; teams with few opportunities to communicate may provide less integrated services. Those teams with limited opportunity or ability to communicate are more at risk for providing fragmented or duplicative services. New teams need higher levels of communication, and well-established teams can provide integrated services with less communication. Because each child is unique and the environment is ever changing, intervention planning and review should involve a face-to-face meeting of team members. Teams that function effectively communicate at multiple levels. Written communication is a norm, and all team members should have access to important written communication about the child. Oral communication includes both informal (e.g., a problem-solving discussion regarding a child's behavior before a joint treatment session) and formal (e.g., an IEP meeting with the parents) interactions. Confidentiality is critical whenever information about the child and family is shared.

The goal in team communication is that the professionals and family members develop shared meaning about the child and their concerns and priorities for the child (Case-Smith & Wavrek, 1992). Because the language used by professionals is often technical and can be misunderstood by the general public, team members need to make specific efforts to develop shared meanings with family members. This goal is accomplished when professionals use clear, descriptive, everyday language and when they validate that the information given is understood by the recipient. Even when professionals use simple and direct language, how much of the message that is understood cannot be assumed. Parents are often preoccupied with their home and work situations, making listening with understanding difficult. The family's ability to assimilate information may also be limited in times of stress, for example, when the child is in the hospital.

Parents and professionals develop different understandings of a situation because they speak different languages. Common understanding is particularly difficult when the parent participates in a team meeting to develop plans for the child. In such a meeting, professionals typically communicate at two different levels, one technical and one nontechnical (McClelland, 1992). The use of specific medical terminology, although helpful to the physician and other professionals, can be baffling to the parent. Clear translation of technical terms for the parents should be offered without intimidating them and without losing the specific communication intent.

Parents are most likely to reinforce intervention goals when team members explain recommendations in sufficient depth, reinforce each other's suggestions, welcome parents' feedback, and incorporate the parents' ideas into a suggested activity. Such collaboration requires time and willingness to negotiate to develop a shared meaning of what is best for the child.

In teams who have developed effective communication systems, collaboration and integrated service delivery become possible. Teams use three methods for reaching decisions: (1) problem solving, (2) decision making by consensus, and (3) conflict resolution. All of these methods are based on open lines of communication, willingness and initiative in sharing information, and a commitment to team collaboration.

## Team Problem Solving

The advantages of team problem solving include the following: (1) more diverse knowledge and perspectives are brought to bear on the problem, (2) greater interest is stimulated in the problem as a result of attention by numerous individuals, (3) the resulting solution is greater than the sum of individual contributions, and (4) inappropriate solutions are rejected. Johnson and Johnson (1987) described problem solving as part of the team process (see the box on p. 241).

## Decision by Consensus

To produce an innovative and effective plan that the team and family can commit to implementing, all members should reach consensus on the plan. When all members agree about the intervention plan, the participation of all members increases and the plan is more likely to be successful. To reach team consensus all members must actively participate, with the voice of each member equally important. Decisions by consensus take more time than other decision-making models but are important to team cohesiveness around the needs of the child.

In team planning meetings that include parents (e.g., an IEP meeting), the parent's voice is the deciding one. To assume the role of decision maker, the parents need information about how the team operates, how they can participate in the process, and how an intervention plan is developed. Given clear and specific information about the team's assessment and planning process and the type of intervention the program offers, the parent can take a leadership role in building consensus for their important concerns about the child. Bailey (1989) described a strategy for organizing a team meeting that encourages the parent's full participation and leadership:

Another procedure for increasing the potential for parental involvement is to organize the meeting according to (the child's) skill areas and discuss first areas of high importance to families, such as self-help or motor skills. In each area, the parents are asked to describe how they perceive their child's skills and needs in the area being considered, such as toileting or feeding. . . . Once parents have provided detailed information about the skills being discussed, professionals supplement that information from their own assessments. Any discrepancies in perception of ability are discussed, and then parents are asked to identify priorities for intervention within that skill domain. Professionals attend to and reinforce those priorities whenever possible by establishing goals related to each. If additional goals are deemed important by professionals, they are then mentioned and discussed. This process sends a clear message to parents that they are important members of the decision-making team and that their perspectives and priorities for their children are valued by professionals seeking to provide the most appropriate early intervention services possible (p. 12).

Consensus on goals for the child and intervention strategies results when professionals communicate openly and clearly and when they consider child and family needs above their professional identities and personal interests. Additional discussion of communication strategies for consensus building may be found in Chapter 5. Team interaction is discussed in several chapters in Section IV of this book.

## Conflict Resolution

When disagreement arises regarding the intervention plan or service implementation, *negotiation* strategies should be employed to resolve the conflict in a positive and constructive way. Negotiation is a process by which people who want to come to an agreement, but disagree about the nature of the agreement, establish an plan accepted by all. Negotiation requires clear communication of all of the options and possible solutions. Team members should present clear rationales for the goals or solutions that they propose. The goals proposed should relate directly to the entire team's concerns and priorities, especially those of the family.

## Steps in Team Problem Solving

### STEP 1: DEFINE THE PROBLEM

Team members need to reach consensus about the definition of the problem. A clear definition of the problem enables the team members to agree on what the problem is. Therefore the first problem-solving step is to get valid, reliable, and correct information about the child and the environmental issues affecting the child's performance. Commitment to solving the problem rests with agreement as to the existence of the discrepancy between current and desired circumstances and an understanding of its importance.

### STEP 2: DIAGNOSE THE PROBLEM

The second step is to diagnose the dimension and causes of the problem. What variables are causing the problem? What barriers need to be overcome? What forces and factors are in place that might help solve the problem?

### STEP 3: FORMULATE ALTERNATIVE STRATEGIES

The third step is to formulate strategies and alternative ways to solve the problem. Creativeness, divergent thinking, opposition among ideas, and inventiveness are essential for this phase. Alternative solutions should address strengthening of the child's current skills, improving his or her functional level, and removing barriers of the environment that interfere with his or her functional performance. In specifying alternative strategies for change, the team members should think of as many ways as possible to solve the problem and promote the child's function. Outside consultation may be beneficial at this stage to increase the range of possible solutions. This step essentially involves brainstorming, and divergent thinking should be encouraged, with no right or wrong answers at this time.

### STEP 4: DECIDE ON AND IMPLEMENT A STRATEGY

Once all of the possible strategies have been identified and formulated in specific terms, the team selects a solution. First the team members engage in decision making by discussing the benefits for each alternative strategy, identifying resources needed to implement each alternative, and evaluating the probability of success if the alternative is implemented. Once a decision has been made, a plan is developed for implementing the solution. This may involve assigning specific team members to carry out parts of the plan and developing a timeline for complete implementation. A detailed plan is desirable for accountability. The plan should be evaluated for its fit with the overall intervention plan for the child. Adjustments may need to be made to the intervention plan or the newly formulated solution.

### STEP 5: EVALUATE THE SUCCESS OF THE STRATEGY

The decision is evaluated by determining (1) whether the strategies were successfully implemented and (2) what the effects of the strategies were. To effectively evaluate the strategy, criteria are needed.

---

Modified from Johnson, D. & Johnson, F. (1987). *Joining together: group therapy and group skills.* Englewood Cliffs, NJ: Prentice-Hall.

---

The first step in negotiation among team members is to identify the overall goal. When the team members disagree on specific objectives or activities, a global goal (such as promoting the child's optimal health and development) on which all members agree becomes the starting point for compromise. Common interest related to the general goal can be established by first reconfirming the common purpose. With an overall goal in mind, compatible intervention strategies can be identified. Conflicting interests need to be made explicit (Brandt, 1993).

Successful negotiation and problem resolution are more likely to be attained when (1) members are separated from the problem, (2) mutual interests and gains are accentuated, and (3) objective criteria are used to evaluate the solutions generated (Fisher & Ury, 1981). Therefore first the problem needs to be depersonalized or viewed as separate from the individuals involved and their interpersonal interactions. All common interests and concerns should be identified. These relate to the child but also might relate to concerns of family members. The solutions generated should be specific and concrete. They may need to be prioritized so that the team has an initial emphasis. Finally criteria must be established to evaluate progress toward resolution of the conflict. Short-term objectives with explicit criteria allow the family and team to measure immediate progress and make adjustments to the plan to avoid further negative feelings and conflict. These problem-solving strategies help the team reach agreement

## STUDY QUESTIONS

1. Use the example of Lindsey (pp. 227-228) to design an activity that would incorporate the principles of motor learning theory. Based on the listed objectives, describe a system of practice and feedback that would help her achieve those objectives.
2. Compare and contrast the tenets of motor learning theory and child-centered activity. In what ways are these two approaches similar? How do they differ?
3. Read the case study of Kevin in Chapter 8. Using the Coping Model, describe Kevin's (1) values and beliefs, (2) knowledge and skills, and (3) human and material supports. As his occupational therapist, explain how you would address each area of coping resources in your intervention. List one 6-month objective for each area. The identified objectives should be consistent with the goals listed on pp. 182-183.
4. Using the example of Phillip H. (pp. 236-238), describe two ways that consultative services might be provided as he begins the school year. Define the objectives for his transition into school.

about intervention goals and support each other and the family in reaching these goals.

## SUMMARY

Intervention planning requires careful interpretation of assessment information, clear communication of concerns about the child, and willingness to consider creative options for helping the child. The key to the process is the therapist's and team's ability to develop consensus around a plan that meets the child's needs, builds on current child and family strengths, addresses family priorities, and clearly reaches toward a future vision for the child. A written intervention plan provides the basis for communicating the occupational therapy goals, helps make the team accountable for services provided, and becomes a basis for measuring the effectiveness of intervention services.

## REFERENCES

Adelstein, L.A. & Nelson, D.L. (1985). Effects of sharing versus non-sharing on affective meaning in collage activities. *Occupational Therapy in Mental Health, 5,* 29-45.

American Occupational Therapy Association (1987). *Guidelines for school based practice.* Rockville, MD: American Occupational Therapy Association.

American Occupational Therapy Association (1994a). Uniform terminology—Third Revision. *American Journal of Occupational Therapy, 48,* 1047-1054.

American Occupational Therapy Association. (1994b). Standards of practice. *American Journal of Occupational Therapy, 48,* 1037-1038.

Ayres, J. (1989). *Sensory Integration and Praxis Tests.* Los Angeles: Western Psychological Services.

Bailey, D.B. (1989). Assessment and its importance in early intervention. In D. Bailey & M. Wolery (Eds.). *Assessing infants and preschoolers with handicaps* (pp. 1-21). Columbus, OH: Merrill.

Bradley, N.S. (1994). Motor control: developmental aspects of motor control in skill acquisition (pp. 39-78). In S. Campbell (Ed.). *Physical therapy for children.* Philadelphia: W.B. Saunders.

Brandt, P. (1993). Negotiation and problem-solving strategies: collaboration between families and professionals. *Infants and Young Children, 5*(4), 78-84.

Brooks, V.B. (1986). *The neural basis of motor control.* New York: Oxford University Press.

Bundy, A. (1991). Writing function goals for evaluation. In C. Royeen (Ed.). *AOTA self study series: school based practice for related services.* Rockville, MD: American Occupational Therapy Association.

Campbell, P.H., McInerney, W.F., & Cooper, M.A. (1984). Therapeutic programming for students with severe handicaps. *American Journal of Occupational Therapy, 38*(9), 594-600.

Case-Smith, J. & Wavrek, B.B. (1992). Models of service delivery and team interaction. In J. Case-Smith (Ed.). *Pediatric occupational therapy and early intervention.* Stoneham, MA: Andover Medical Publishers.

DeGangi, G.A. (1991). The fussy baby program: assessment and treatment of sensory, emotional and attentional problems. In S.S. Poisson & G.A. DeGangi (Eds.). *Emotional and sensory processing problems: assessment and treatment approaches for young children and their family* (pp. 41-58). Rockville, MD: Reginald Lourie Center for Infants and Young Children.

DeGangi, G.A., Craft, P., & Castellan, J. (1991). Treatment of sensory, emotional, and attentional problems in regulatory disordered infants. *Infants and Young Children, 3*(3), 9-19.

DeGangi, G.A., Wietlisbach, S., Goodin, M., & Scheiner, N. (1993). A comparison of structured sensorimotor therapy and child-centered activity in the treatment of preschool children with sensorimotor problems. *American Journal of Occupational Therapy, 47*(9), 777-786.

Dunn, W. (1991). Consultation as a process: how, when, and why? In C. Royeen (Ed.). *AOTA self study series: school-based practice for related services.* Rockville, MD: American Occupational Therapy Association.

Dunn, W., Brown, C., & McGuigan, A. (1994). The ecology of human performance: a framework for considering the effect of context. *American Journal of Occupational Therapy, 48*(7), 595-607.

Dunn, W. & Campbell, P. (1991). Designing pediatric service provision. In W. Dunn (Ed.). *Pediatric occupational therapy.* Thorofare, NJ: Slack.

Dunn W., & DeGangi, G. (1992). Sensory integration and neurodevelopmental treatment for educational programming. In C. Royeen (Ed.). *AOTA self study series: Classroom applications for school based practice.* Rockville, MD: American Occupational Therapy Association.

Exner, C.E. (1990). The zone of proximal development in in-hand manipulation skills of nondysfunction 3- and 4-year-old children. *American Journal of Occupational Therapy, 44*(10), 884-891.

Fewell, R. & Glick, M. (1993). Observing play: an appropriate process for training and assessment. *Infants and Young Children, 5*(4), 35-43.

Fisher, R. & Ury, W. (1981). *Getting to yes: negotiating agreement without giving in.* New York: Viking.

Fleming, M.H. (1994). The therapist with the three-track mind. In C. Mattingly & M.H. Fleming (Eds.). *Clinical reasoning: forms of inquiry in a therapeutic practice.* Philadelphia: F.A. Davis.

Furuno, S., O'Reilly, K.A., Hosaka, C.M., Inatsuka T.T., Allman, T.A., & Zeistoft, B. (1985). *Hawaii early learning profile.* Palo Alto, CA: Vort.

Gliner, J.A. (1985). Purposeful activity in motor learning theory: an event approach to motor skill acquisition. *American Journal of Occupational Therapy, 39,* 28-34.

Hammill, D.D., Pearson, N.A., & Voress, J.K. (1994). *Developmental test of visual perception—2.* Austin, TX: Pro Ed.

Idol, L., Paolucci-Whitcomb, P., & Nevin, A. (1987). *Collaborative consultation.* Austin, TX: Pro Ed.

Johnson, D.W. & Johnson, F.P. (1987). *Joining together: group theory and group skills.* Englewood Cliffs, NJ: Prentice-Hall.

Johnson-Martin, N., Jens, K., & Attermeier, S. (1986). *The Carolina curriculum for handicapped infant and infants at risk.* Baltimore: Brookes.

Kaplan, M.A. (1994). Motor learning: implications for occupational therapy and neurodevelopmental treatment. *Developmental Disabilities Special Interest Section Newsletter, 17*(3), 1-4.

Law, M. & Baum, C.M. (1994). *Creating the future: a joint effort.* Can Am Conference. Boston: American Occupational Therapy Association.

Lyons, B.G. (1984). Defining a child's zone of proximal development: evaluation process for treatment planning. *American Journal of Occupational Therapy. 38*(7), 446-451.

McClelland, M. (1992). *The discourse of interdisciplinary health care assessment: toward a biosocial model.* Dissertation at The Ohio State University, Columbus, OH.

McHale, K. & Cermak, S.A. (1992). Fine motor activities in elementary school: preliminary findings and provisional implications for children with fine motor problems. *American Journal of Occupational Therapy, 46,* 898-903.

Mager, R.F. (1975). *Preparing instructional objectives,* Belmont, CA: Pearson.

Mahoney, G., Finger, J., & Powell, A. (1985). The relationship of maternal behavior style to the developmental status of mentally retarded infants. *American Journal of Mental Deficiency, 90,* 296-302.

Mattingly, C. & Fleming, M.H. (1994). *Clinical reasoning: forms of inquiry in a therapeutic practice.* Philadelphia: F.A. Davis.

Nelson, D.L. (1988). Occupation: form and performance. *American Journal of Occupational Therapy, 42,* 633-641.

Nelson, D.L. & Peterson, C.Q. (1991). The effects of competitive versus cooperative structure on subsequent productivity in boys with psychosocial disorders. *The Occupational Therapy Journal of Research, 11* (2), 93-105.

Rainforth, B., York, J., & MacDonald, C. (1992). *Collaborative teams for students with service disabilities.* Baltimore: Brookes.

Scholtz, J.P. (1990). Dynamic pattern theory: some implications for therapeutics. *Physical Therapy, 70,* 827-843.

Umphred, D.A. & Appley, M.B. (1990). Limbic system: influence over motor control and learning, In D.A. Umphred (Ed.). *Neurological rehabilitation* (pp. 53-78). St. Louis: Mosby.

Vygotsky, L.S. (1978). *Mind in society: the development of higher psychological processes.* Cambridge, MA: Harvard University Press.

Williamson, G.G., Szczepanski, M., & Zeitlin, S. (1993). Coping frame of reference. In P. Kramer & J. Hinojosa (Eds.). *Frames of reference in pediatric occupational therapy* (pp. 395-436). Baltimore: Williams & Wilkins.

Williamson, G.G., Zeitlin, S., & Szczepanski, M. (1989). Coping behavior: implications for disabled infants and toddlers. *Infant Mental Health Journal, 10,* 3-13.

Zeitlin, S. & Williamson, G.G. (1988). Developing family resources for adaptive coping. *Journal of the Division for Early Childhood, 12,* 137-146.

Zeitlin, S. & Williamson, G.G. (1994). *Coping in young children: early intervention practices to enhance adaptive behavior and resilience.* Baltimore: Brookes.

# SECTION

# III

# Occupational Therapy Intervention:
# Performance Areas

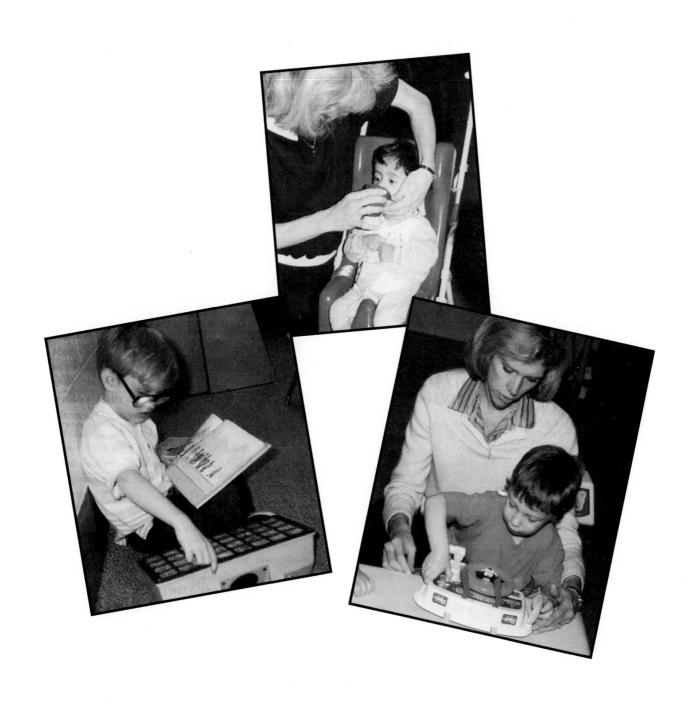

# CHAPTER

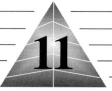

# The Development of Postural Control

DEBORAH S. NICHOLS

## KEY TERMS

▲ Neuromotor Control
▲ Postural Development
▲ Postural Control
▲ Righting Reactions
▲ Protective Reactions
▲ Equilibrium/Balance
▲ Reactive Postural Control
▲ Anticipatory Postural Control

## CHAPTER OBJECTIVES

1. Describe the development of postural control systems and the influence of that development on gross and fine motor development.
2. Discuss atypical development of postural control and its impact on the development of gross and fine motor skills.
3. Identify appropriate assessment tools available for the evaluation of postural control.
4. Identify appropriate treatment techniques for facilitating reactive and anticipatory postural control.
5. Apply the knowledge gained in this chapter to specific case situations of children with postural control deficits.

Early in life a child develops the ability to maintain body alignment while upright in space. Within the first year the child gains trunk stability sufficient for movement against gravity in a variety of upright positions, including stance. Postural control requires the development both of muscle strength that allows for antigravity movements and of proximal-axial muscle control, which results in dynamic patterns of cocontraction and mature equilibrium responses. In the past therapists have conceptualized postural devel-

opment as a hierarchy in which high-level brain structures (i.e., the cortex) controlled and mediated the functions of lower-level brain structures (i.e., the brainstem). Under the hierarchic model of neuromotor control, postural development was thought to be determined by maturation of the nervous system, resulting in the emergence of increasingly advanced reflex patterns and eventually voluntary movement (Woollacott, Shumway-Cook, & Williams, 1989). In addition, postural control was considered to mirror motor development and proceeded in a cephalocaudal manner (Bly, 1983; Connor, Williamson, & Siepp, 1978). However, this view of postural development is overly simplistic and, in some respects, incorrect. Recently system theories of neuromotor control have influenced the way therapists view postural development. System theories recognize that postural development results from more than maturation of a reflex hierarchy. These theories have acknowledged the importance of muscle strength, body mass, sensory system function, and environmental constraints on neuromotor and postural development.

This chapter uses recently developed theories to explain assessment and intervention for postural function in children. It includes descriptions of the development of antigravity movement, postural reactions and control, sensory processing associated with postural control, postural sway, and anticipatory postural control. Evaluations of all of these components of posture are described, and intervention strategies for improving postural control are provided.

## Development of Antigravity Movement

An important aspect of postural control is the development of antigravity movement. Margaret Rood proposed a four-stage sequence in the development of movement: (1) mobility, (2) stability, (3) mobility superimposed on stability, and (4) skill (Stockmeyer, 1967) (Figure 11-1). The stage of mobility was characterized by the development of antigravity movement. This stage was followed by the devel-

**PROGRESSION OF MOTOR DEVELOPMENT**

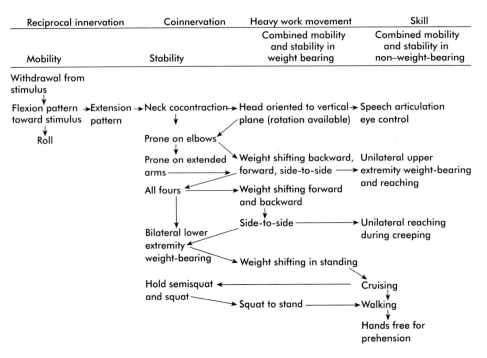

**Figure 11-1**    Rood's developmental progression.

opment of muscle cocontraction at the proximal joints, producing stability sufficient for the maintenance of weight-bearing postures. Once stability is achieved, the child superimposes movement on this stability, characterized by Rood as proximal movement on a fixed distal limb component. A perfect example of this behavior is the young child who assumes quadruped position and then begins to rock back and forth (proximal movement on a fixed distal limb component, the hands and knees). The last stage is characterized by skill or the ability to combine stability and mobility in non–weight-bearing postures (e.g., reach, grasp, and manipulation) (Stockmeyer, 1967).

As Rood's progression suggests, an important component of the development of both mobility and stability is the development of antigravity movement. Pountney, Mulcahy, and Green (1990) identified six levels in the development of antigravity movement, which were associated with more mature movement patterns, in both the prone and supine positions. The levels and their descriptions are shown in Figures 11-2 and 11-3. Using this sequence, the child develops an increased ability to move against gravity with all body parts, demonstrated by a shift from lateral movements to midline movements as antigravity muscle strength is achieved. The newborn infant is asymmetric, with the head turned to the side and arm and leg movements occurring in the lateral plane. The progression involves movement of the center of gravity from the upper body toward the pelvis; this is associated with increased freedom of movement of

the head and extremities, allowing head control and extremity weight-bearing to develop. Also, this progression includes a dissociation of the body segments so that the infant can roll segmentally, lift one leg, and reach across midline with one hand. Accordingly, the progression from one level to the next involves changes in head control, trunk control, and extremity movement and therefore does not follow a strict cephalocaudal progression. In addition, the change from one level to the next coincides with the integration of the preceding level in both prone and supine positions.

Similar changes in neck and trunk extension, including increased scapular stabilization, occur in the acquisition of independent sitting. The posture of a young infant when placed in a sitting position is one of total trunk flexion. This stage is followed by one in which the child exhibits increasing trunk extensor strength but has difficulty grading the activation of the back extensor muscles. When placed in a sitting position, the child frequently activates the back extensors without sufficient coactivation of the trunk flexors and, as a result, falls backward. At this time the child uses upper extremity weight-bearing (propping) to maintain the sitting position. Finally, the child develops sufficient strength of the trunk muscles to allow upright sitting. These changes in the development of antigravity trunk extension with reciprocal trunk flexion and the emergence of sitting stability are depicted in Figure 11-4.

The development of postural control is tightly linked to the acquisition of motor milestones. To review, the center

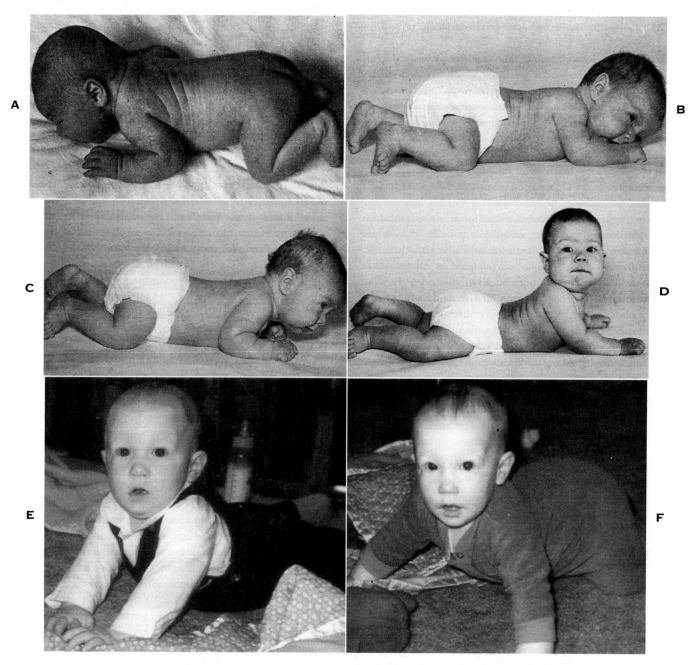

**Figure 11-2**    Prone development of antigravity movement. **A,** Level 1: "Top heavy." Weight-bearing is through chest, shoulders, and face. Pelvis is posteriorly tilted, hips and knees are flexed, and shoulder girdle is retracted. Chest turns flexed and adducted. Posture is asymmetric and head is to one side. **B,** Level 2: Child settles when placed. More generalized weight-bearing than level 1. Weight-bearing is through chest and upper abdomen. Pelvis is posteriorly tilted, shoulder girdle is retracted, shoulders are flexed and adducted, head is to one side, and child is beginning to lift it from floor with "flat back" profile but not sustaining. Posture is asymmetric and bottom is moving laterally as head turns side-to-side. **C,** Level 3: Child maintains prone position with neutral pelvis, and shoulder girdle is beginning to protract. Symmetric weight-bearing is through abdomen, lower chest, knees, and thighs. Child maintains head lift from floor with total trunk curvature—head is in line with spine. Child rocks anteroposteriorly. Child has no lateral weight shift and therefore often topples into supine position when lifting head and chest. **D,** Level 4: Pelvis is anteriorly tilted but not "anchoring." Shoulder girdle is protracted and child bears weight through abdomen and thighs, varying between forearm and hand propping with shoulders elevated. Head and upper trunk movement is dissociated from lower trunk, allowing lateral trunk flexion with lateral weight shift—a beginning of pivoting. Angular lateral profile of upper chest and bottom. Unilateral leg is kicking and hand and foot play is midline. **E,** Level 5: Pelvis is anteriorly tilted, shoulder girdle is protracted with hand propping, extended elbows, and lumbar spine extension. Weight-bearing is through iliac crest, thighs, and lower abdomen. Pelvic anchoring and upper body movement (extension and rotation) on it. Deft pivoting with lateral trunk flexion and moving backward on floor. Child rolls purposefully from prone to supine position. **F,** Level 6: Free movement of pelvis and shoulder girdle. Child begins to bear weight on all fours/anteroposterior, rocking on all fours.

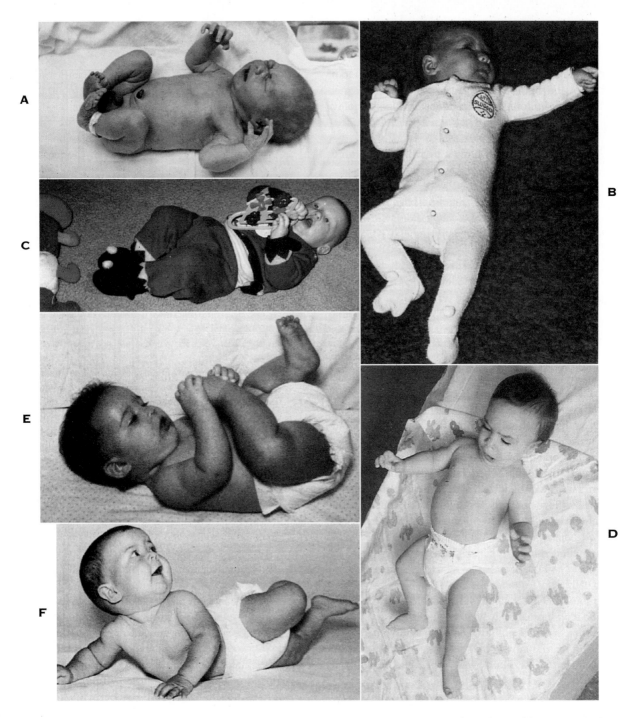

**Figure 11-3** Supine development of antigravity movement. **A,** Level 1: Child is unable to maintain supine position when placed, except momentarily, and then position is asymmetric. Child rolls into and maintains side-lying position—body follows head, turning in a total body movement. Weight-bearing is through lateral aspect of head, trunk, and thigh. Neck is extended with chin poke. **B,** Level 2: Child settles when placed on back ("top heavy"). Weight-bearing is through upper trunk and head. Pelvis is posteriorly tilted and shoulder girdle is retracted. Posture is asymmetric—head is to one side, and child has difficulty turning it side-to-side. Bottom moves laterally as the head is turned, resulting in a "corkscrew" appearance. **C,** Level 3: Child maintains supine position with neutral pelvic tilt, hip abduction, and shoulder girdle in neutral position. Posture is symmetric but "top heavy." Chin is tucked (not retracted) and head is in midline and able to move freely from side-to-side without lateral movement of bottom. Child is able to track objects visually and make eye contact. Weight-bearing is through pelvis and shoulder girdle, giving general curvature to trunk with "pot belly" lateral profile. Child begins unilateral grasp to side of body and takes fist and objects to mouth. Child may roll into prone position because of lack of lateral weight shift. **D,** Level 4: Symmetry of posture and movement is first seen at level 4. Pelvis is anteriorly tilted and shoulder girdle is protracted. Shoulders are flexing and adducting, allowing midline play above chest with hands and feet together. Posture is symmetric and weight-bearing is through upper trunk and pelvis. There is a definite lordotic curve and chin is retracted. "Free" pelvic movement is beginning, allowing child to touch knees with flexed hips (but not toes). Child can alternatively extend hips and knees; rests in crook-lying position. Child begins to be able to shift weight laterally and raise leg unilaterally, indicating independence of limbs from trunk. Adept finger movements toward end of this stage. **E,** Level 5: Free movement of shoulder girdle and pelvis on trunk. Pelvis has full range of movement, allowing child to play with toes with legs extended and to roll into side-lying position. Child is functional in side-lying position and can return to supine position. Weight-bearing is either on shoulder girdle and pelvis or on central trunk only. Child plays between these postures. Efficient limb movement—hand play and prehensile feet—crossing midline. **F,** Level 6: Pelvic and shoulder girdle move freely. Child is able to roll into prone position by achieving side-lying position (level 5) and then anteriorly tilting pelvis on trunk and extending hips.

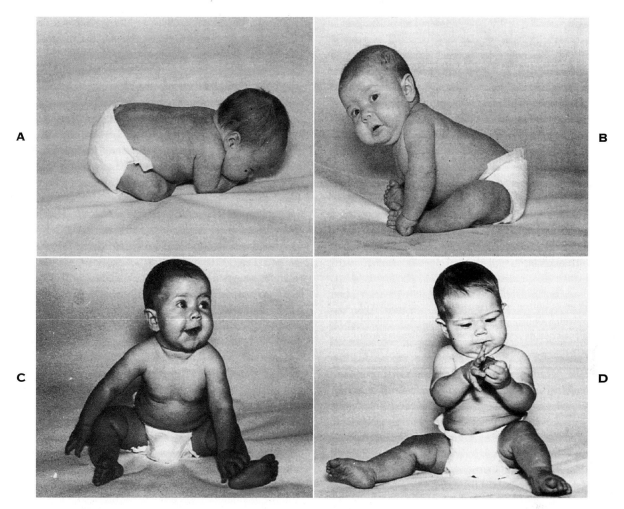

**Figure 11-4**   Development of antigravity movement in sitting. **A,** Total flexion posture of infant. **B,** Bursts of back extensor activity results in falling backward. **C,** Increased upper extremity strength allows stability in sitting with upper extremity weight-bearing. **D,** Mature sitting posture associated with antigravity trunk and neck extensor strength.

of gravity is initially located toward the head and then moves toward the pelvis. This shift frees the upper body from providing static stability to demonstrating dynamic mobility as the child moves in and out of upper extremity weight-bearing positions. As the center of gravity moves to the pelvis, the child demonstrates increased independence in extremity movement and dissociation of body parts, including rotation through the trunk and pelvis. When the child first attempts new postures against gravity, he or she tends to stiffen the trunk to achieve the stability needed. For example, when the child begins to sit and stand, he or she shows minimal rotation. With practice and experience the child uses rotation in each new posture. This rotation increases movement opportunities for the child and enables him or her to make transitions from one posture to another (e.g., sitting to quadruped) (Connor et al., 1978). The approximate ages of motor milestone acquisition are depicted in Table 11-1.

The development of antigravity control has also been found to coincide with the development of higher-level bal-

ance skills. In a study of children ages 4 to 5½, the ability to maintain the antigravity postures of prone extension and supine flexion was highly correlated with both static balance (e.g., single limb stance) and dynamic balance capabilities (e.g., balance beam activities) (Sellers, 1988). Therefore the development of antigravity movement is strongly associated with the development of higher levels of postural control or balance.

## Emergence of Postural Reactions

The development of the postural reactions (i.e., righting, protective, and equilibrium) has been reported to occur in a predictable sequence with reactions first appearing in prone, followed by supine, sitting, quadruped, and standing. It has been suggested that success in the development of these reactions in earlier positions is a prerequisite for their development in later positions (Connor et al., 1978).

A series of righting reactions develop in the first year of life that serve to maintain head alignment with the body as

▲ Table 11-1  Ages of Motor Milestone Acquisition

| Motor Milestone | Age (months) |
|---|---|
| **HEAD CONTROL** | |
| Prone | |
| Lifts head to 45 degrees | 2 |
| Lifts head to 90 degrees | 4 |
| Supine | |
| Maintains in midline | 2 |
| Lifts | 6 |
| **ROLLING** | |
| Prone to supine | |
| Without rotation | 4-6 |
| With rotation | 6-9 |
| Supine to prone | |
| Without rotation | 5-7 |
| With rotation | 6-9 |
| **SITTING** | |
| Unsustained with arm support | 4-5 |
| Sustained with arm support | 5-6 |
| Unsustained without arm support | 6-7 |
| Sustained without arm support | 7-9 |
| **MOBILITY** | |
| Crawling | 7-9 |
| Creeping | 9-11 |
| Cruising | 9-13 |
| Walking | 12-14 |

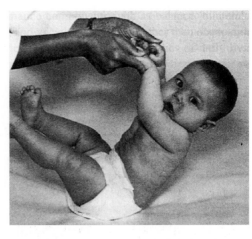

**Figure 11-5** Flexion response. The development of antigravity neck strength is first associated with the ability to maintain the head aligned with the body when pulled to a sitting position.

well as to maintain upper-body alignment with the lower body. When rotation is imposed on the body, these reactions serve to realign the segments of the body; these reactions also serve to maintain body alignment during forward flexion of the trunk or prone suspension (Barnes & Crutchfield, 1990). The neck on body righting reaction is observed in two forms. In the immature infant, turning of the head to the side results in a log roll to the sidelying position; in its mature form, turning of the head produces a segmental roll. The body on body righting reaction is similar; rotation of the infant's hips stimulates a log roll of the upper body in the immature form and a segmental roll of the upper body in the mature form to realign the body segments. A third reflex, the body on head righting reaction, serves to influence head position in response to a part of the body touching a support surface (i.e., in prone, the tactile input from the stomach touching the support surface stimulates head lifting). Two other reactions give the infant experiences of full body extension and full body flexion. The Landau reaction results in maintenance of body alignment during prone suspension, produced by neck, trunk, and leg extension. When the child is pulled to a sitting position, the development of antigravity neck flexion is associated with the child's ability to maintain head and trunk alignment against

the pull of gravity; this is sometimes referred to as the flexion righting reaction and is demonstrated in Figure 11-5. Table 11-2 should be consulted for approximate ages at which these reactions are seen.

Orientation of the body in space involves the maintenance of an upright posture under both static and dynamic conditions; this ability is more often called balance. The earliest form of body orientation is observed in two vertical righting reflexes: the optical righting reflex and the labyrinthine righting reflex. These two reflexes serve to realign the head in relation to vertical when the body is displaced and are mediated, respectively, by the visual and vestibular systems. The maintenance of balance also involves the child's ability to respond adequately to external disturbances (e.g., a push or trip) or internally generated movements (e.g., reaching).

Responses to external disturbances are reactive or compensatory and can be classified into equilibrium or protective reactions. These reactions emerge in lower-level positions (supine and prone) when the infant is aged 4 to 6 months. They continue to develop in more upright positions throughout the first 5 years. Equilibrium reactions, often called tilting reactions because of the way they are tested, serve to return the child's body to a vertical position after displacement. When the child is supine on a tiltboard, a lateral tilt to the right elicits trunk incurvation to the left, righting of the head, and abduction of the left arm and leg. These same movements are associated with equilibrium reactions in prone, sitting, quadruped, and standing to lateral tilt. Figure 11-6 demonstrates equilibrium reactions in sitting. In addition, when the child is in upright postures (i.e., sitting or kneeling), tilting anteriorly or posteriorly results in a corrective movement in the opposite direction to the tilt, returning the body to an upright position. Protective reactions differ from equilibrium reactions in that they protect the infant from a fall rather than correct a displacement. There-

▲ Table 11-2   Age of Postural Reactions Acquisition

| Balance Reactions | Age (months) |
| --- | --- |
| **RIGHTING REACTIONS** | |
| Neck on body | |
|   Immature | Birth |
| Neck on body | |
|   Mature | 4-5 |
| Body on body | |
|   Immature | Birth |
| Body on body | |
|   Mature | 4-5 |
| Body on head | |
|   Prone: | |
|     Partial | 1-2 |
|     Mature | 4-5 |
|   Supine | 5-6 |
| Landau | |
|   Immature | 3 |
|   Mature | 6-10 |
| Flexion | |
|   Partial (head in line) | 3-4 |
|   Mature (head forward) | 6-7 |
| Vertical | |
|   Partial (head in line) | 2 |
|   Mature (head to vertical) | 6 |
| **PROTECTIVE REACTIONS** | |
| Forward | 6-7 |
| Lateral | 6-11 |
| Backward | 9-12 |
| **EQUILIBRIUM REACTIONS** | |
| Prone | 5-6 |
| Supine | 7-8 |
| Sitting | 7-10 |
| Quadruped | 9-12 |
| Standing | 12-21 |

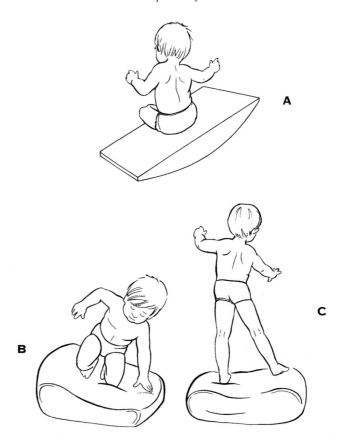

**Figure 11-6**   Equilibrium reactions in sitting, **(A)**, quadruped, **(B)**, and standing, **(C)**.

fore these reactions are characterized by extension of the extremities to "catch" the child as he or she falls, and they occur in the direction of the fall.

Haley (1986) assessed the emergence of a series of righting, protective, and equilibrium reactions in infants from 2 to 10 months of age. He reported that righting reactions emerged first in all positions, at least in their immature forms, before the development of any protective or equilibrium reactions in these postures. However, the development of protective and equilibrium reactions was overlapping within a given posture as well as between postures. For example, protective reactions in sitting developed at the same time as the equilibrium reactions. Also equilibrium reactions began to develop in higher-level positions (e.g., quadruped), and they continued to be refined in lower-level positions (e.g., supine) (Haley, 1986).

The amount of experience a child has in a given posture also relates to development of mature postural reactions as evidenced by patterns of muscle activation. Woollacott, Debu, and Mowatt (1988) found that infants younger than 5 months of age demonstrated inadequate or absent neck and trunk muscle activation patterns to linear translations in supported sitting. However, infants 6 to 8 months of age, who had experience in independent sitting, demonstrated appropriate activation patterns of the neck and trunk muscles. Similar differences in standing were identified between infants who had not yet developed independent stance and those who had. In addition, young children tend to demonstrate a larger amplitude of muscle activation as well as greater variability in the activation patterns (Shumway-Cook & Woollacott, 1985a; Williams, Fisher, & Tritschler, 1983). Therefore it appears that reactive postural reactions are dependent on experience in a given position as well as to neuronal maturation.

## Sensory Systems Associated with Postural Control

Three sensory systems contribute to the child's awareness of orientation in space: the visual system, the vestibular system, and the somatosensory system. The visual system provides a representation of the vertical plane that is dependent on the objects in the visual field. The child's somatosensory system provides input from proprioceptors, mechanoreceptors, and cutaneous receptors, which supply information about limb position and support surface characteristics. The vestibular system provides a constant gravitational reference for postural orientation, with which the child compares visual and somatosensory input. When the three sensory systems provide disparate information, a feeling of disequilibrium results. Discrepancies between the visual and somatosensory cues are decided in favor of the vestibular system (Horak & Nashner, 1986; Nashner, 1990).

## Changes in the Influence of Sensory Systems

As the infant matures, the relative influence of the sensory systems on postural control changes. Newborns demonstrate the ability to orient to a visual stimulus and are capable of tracking a moving object by turning their head if their head is supported (Bullinger, 1981). Initially young infants appear to rely more on visual than somatosensory information for use in postural control. Eventually, and with experience in each new posture, this reliance on vision is transferred to reliance on somatosensory cues (Woollacott, 1988; Woollacott et al., 1989). Studies have documented that the vestibular system is able to accurately detect postural disturbances at an early age (Jouen, 1984). Infants as young as 4 months make appropriate postural responses when they are tilted with their vision occluded. This early maturation of the vestibular system seems to be critical to the development of postural control. However, despite the integrity of the vestibular system early in life, when visual inputs are available, infants and young children tend to rely on them. This dominance of visual input is seen in each transitional state as the child acquires motor milestones. Thus the child first uses visual information to make postural adjustments in sitting. He or she later relies on vestibular and somatosensory input. Similar changes occur in quadruped and standing positions (Woollacott, 1988). The time course of this transition in standing is long; it is not until between the ages of 6 and 7 years that children appear to switch from a reliance on visual inputs to a reliance on somatosensory inputs similar to that of adults (Shumway-Cook & Woollacott, 1985a).

## Emergence of Anticipatory Postural Control

In addition to the automatic reactions described in the preceding paragraphs, postural control also involves the programming of postural muscle activation in association with voluntary movement. This activation occurs in a feedforward manner. *Feedforward* refers to the anticipatory strategies that are observed in the postural adjustments that the individual makes before voluntary movements. These postural adjustments can be observed before the onset of arm and hand movements or whole-body movements. This type of anticipatory control is dependent on the child's experience with the task and the environment in which the task takes place. It is also dependent on adequate postural muscle strength. The effect of the anticipatory muscle activation is the creation of a stable base on which the movement can take place (Bouisset & Zattara, 1981; Forrsberg & Nashner, 1982).

Infants as young as 10 months have been found to demonstrate anticipatory responses to an arm reach in sitting; yet these responses are inconsistent until the infant is independent in sitting and has had considerable experience with reaching in this position (von Hofsten, 1986). Investigations of reaching have identified the emergence of anticipatory postural activation in standing by 12 to 15 months of age (Forrsberg & Nashner, 1982). By age 4 children demonstrated a pattern similar to that found in adults (Hayes & Riach, 1989).

## Developmental Changes in Postural Sway and Muscle Activation

Postural sway can be defined as the natural movement of the child's center of gravity within a base of support. When standing, the child is not perfectly still but demonstrates a normal oscillatory movement from side to side and forward and back. With recent advances in technology, this postural sway has been evaluated and quantified by using several different techniques. Several studies have examined postural sway in children and have identified a developmental progression. Young children demonstrate significantly more postural sway than older children, with more variability between children and with less influence from closing the eyes (Forssberg & Nashner, 1982; Foudriat, DiFabio, & Anderson, 1993; Riach & Hayes, 1987). In studies that used the Pediatric Clinical Test of Sensory Integration for Balance (P-CTSIB) (Crowe, Deitz, Richardson, & Atwater, 1990; Deitz, Richardson, Atwater, Crowe, & Odiorne, 1991; Richardson, Atwater, Crowe, & Deitz, 1992), it was found that mature levels of postural sway in static standing seem to emerge somewhere around the age of 13. Children between the ages of 5 and 7 seemed to demonstrate greater sway than younger children (Dietz et al., 1991; Riach and Hayes, 1987); this may be attributable to the transition that occurs at this age between dominance of the visual system to dominance of the somatosensory system for the control of balance in standing (Deitz et al., 1991; Shumway-Cook & Woollacott, 1985a).

Not only does the amount of postural sway vary with age in children, but also the muscle activity elicited varies. In young children significantly greater amplitudes of muscle activity are used to maintain a posture than are demonstrated by older children (Berger, Quintern, & Dietz, 1985; Haas, Diener, Bacher, & Dichgans, 1986). Thus young children tend to use more muscles than do older children to maintain balance, and they require a greater degree of muscle contraction than do older children. Then, with experience in a given posture, there is a natural refinement in the muscle activity needed to maintain the posture (Shumway-Cook & Woollacott, 1985a; Williams et al., 1983; Woollacott & Sveistrup, 1992).

## ASSESSMENT OF POSTURAL CONTROL

The assessment of postural control takes different forms, depending on the age of the child and the nature of the postural control dysfunction. In young children postural assessment is linked to motor milestones and the development of antigravity movement and appropriate postural reactions. In children who have acquired ambulation, postural assessment has typically focused on balance capabilities such as single-limb stance and balance beam activities. More recently, evaluations of standing balance have begun to examine the functioning of sensory systems associated with balance function, the development of appropriate muscle synergies in response to perturbations, and the development of stability under various testing conditions.

### Assessment of Righting, Equilibrium, and Protective Reactions
#### Righting Reactions

The righting reactions, (neck on body, body on body, body on head, Landau, flexion, and vertical) are assessed through handling of the infant. The relative ages of emergence of these reflexes in their mature form are depicted in Table 11-2. To elicit the *neck on body reaction,* the child's head is manually turned to the side and the rolling response is observed. As stated earlier, the immature response is a log roll to realign the body, and the mature response is a segmental roll. The *body on body reaction* is evaluated in a similar fashion; the child's hips are rotated to the side and the upper body is observed. The immature response is, again, a log roll, and the mature response is a segmental roll. The *body on head reaction* is observed as the child is placed prone on a support surface. In the partial response the child lifts his or her head to 45 degrees vertical, and in the full response the child raises the head in midline to face vertical (90 degrees) and is able to maintain this upright position. The *Landau reaction* is observed in prone suspension; the examiner supports the child under the abdomen and looks for extension of both the neck and lower extremities. An immature response may be noted for the Landau; young infants may keep the head in line with the body before being able to demonstrate the mature response of head, trunk, and lower extremity extension. The *flexion response*

is assessed by pulling the child to sitting from supine and is considered present if the child can maintain the head in alignment with the body without any initial head lag. The *vertical reactions (optical and labyrinthine)* are typically evaluated by supporting the infant under the arms while the child is suspended vertically. Then the infant is laterally tilted about 45 degrees; the reaction is considered present if the infant rights his or her head to vertical. The *labyrinthine reaction* is tested either with a blindfold covering the eyes or in a dark room. Testing with the eyes open is considered to evaluate *optical righting* because vision dominates vestibular input in young infants (see previous section on sensory development). A partial response to vertical righting is often observed, characterized by the maintenance of the head in line with the body; this is considered an immature response (Barnes & Crutchfield, 1990).

Recently therapists and researchers have begun to question the relative importance of evaluating righting reactions. What does the presence or absence of righting reactions indicate? Although the emergence of mature responses is associated with a normally developing nervous system, delays in developing these reactions provide little insight into the cause. Delayed or deficient reactions can be secondary to neuromotor dysfunction, musculoskeletal abnormalities, or sensory system dysfunction.

### Equilibrium Reaction

Testing equilibrium and protective reactions has typically taken the form of placing the child on a tiltboard or other unstable surface (e.g., ball or bolster). The child's responses to displacement are observed in lateral, anterior, posterior, and diagonal directions. All appropriate developmental positions are used (i.e., prone, supine, sitting, quadruped, kneeling, and standing). An alternate form of testing involves observation of the child's response to manual displacement from a stationary support surface (i.e., the child is pushed in a given direction). A typical equilibrium reaction is characterized by movements of the trunk and extremities that oppose the imposed displacement and bring the center of gravity back within the base of support. For example, when the child is sitting, a posterior displacement results in contraction of the abdominals and neck flexors as well as the hip flexors and hamstrings to produce a forward movement of the body. Conversely, an anterior push or tilt is associated with neck, trunk, and hip extension; again, there may be hamstring activity to maintain the seated position. Similarly, lateral displacements are associated with trunk incurvation toward the elevated side if tilted or toward the pushed side if pushed. The child should rotate the upper body toward the elevated (pushed) side and often will extend the extremities on the elevated or pushed side (Figure 11-6). These responses to lateral tilting are consistent with those seen in all positions. Tilting in a diagonal direction is associated with increased trunk and neck rotation to oppose the movement. These rotary movements combine with trunk flexion when the child is tilted backward and trunk extension when he or she is tilted forward.

### Protective Reactions

Protective reactions, sometimes called parachute reactions, are also elicited by displacement on a tilting surface or manual displacement on a stable surface. These reactions differ from equilibrium reactions in that they are designed to protect the infant from a fall rather than to correct the displacement. Therefore these reactions are characterized by extension of the extremities to "catch" the child as he or she falls and occur in the direction of the fall. Forward protective reactions can be tested by suspending the child and then moving him or her forward toward a support surface. A positive response includes upper extremity extension and abduction sufficient to stop the forward movement. Testing in sitting also involves displacement in any direction sufficient to elicit upper extremity extension to stop the movement. The amount of displacement needed to elicit a protective reaction must be greater in degree than that used to elicit an equilibrium reaction (Figure 11-7).

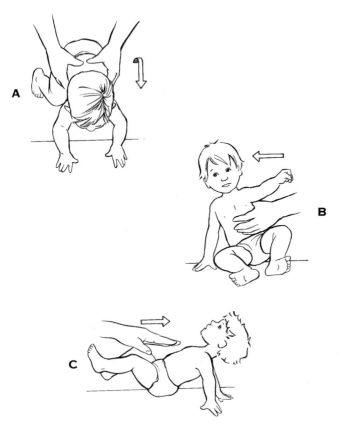

**Figure 11-7** Protective reactions forward, **(A)**, lateral, **(B)**, and backward, **(C)**.

### Neuromotor Assessment

Neuromotor assessments have been designed to evaluate the emergence and progression of postural reactions. The Milani-Comparetti Motor Development Screening Test tracks the emergence of these reactions as well as the emergence of antigravity movement and the integration of primitive reflexes (Milani-Comparetti & Gidoni, 1967). The Movement Assessment of Infants (MAI) (Chandler, Andrews, & Swanson, 1980) also examines postural reactions, or automatic reactions as they are referred to in the assessment, with an emphasis on examining asymmetries as well as the emergence of the reactions. Other neuromotor assessments include some, but not all, of the postural reactions in their assessment of motor milestones. Examples include the Infant Neurological International Battery (INFANIB) (Ellison, 1994), Alberta Infant Motor Scale (AIMS) (Piper & Darrah, 1994), and the Postural and Fine Motor Assessment (Case-Smith & Bigsby, 1993).

### Assessment of Antigravity Movement

The emergence of antigravity movement is assessed in most developmental tests through the appearance of motor milestones such as prone and supine head control and reaching. The six levels of prone and supine postural development described by Pountney et al. (1990) can be used to plot an infant's progression. In addition, the Milani-Comparetti Motor Development Screening Test (Milani-Comparetti & Gidoni, 1967), AIMS (Piper & Darrah, 1994), and MAI (Chandler et al., 1980) each have sections that address antigravity movement and the emergence of antigravity postures.

### Assessment of Sensory Organization

The initial evaluation of the child should include testing of sensory systems to determine function. The testing of optical and labyrinthine righting in young infants begins to explore the integrity of these systems for use in the control of balance. As described previously, these reactions are typically tested with the infant vertically suspended; this position is believed to eliminate somatosensory input. However, with the eyes open the vestibular system is also operating and can provide the needed input for balance control. Therefore the testing procedure for optical righting does not effectively evaluate the infant's ability to use visual information to provide spatial orientation.

Several tests have been designed for evaluation of sensory integrative function, including sensory organization, balance, and coordination. These tests are the DeGangi Berk Test of Sensory Integration (Berk & DeGangi, 1983) and the Sensory Integration and Praxis Tests (Ayres, 1989), which are described in Chapter 13. Further evaluation of each sensory system's role in postural control in young infants is difficult, requiring complex testing equipment. However, a new evaluation tool is available for use with older children that measures sensory organization in the control of balance: the Pediatric Clinical Test of Sensory Interaction for Balance (Crowe et al., 1991).

### Pediatric Clinical Test of Sensory Interaction for Balance

The Pediatric Clinical Test of Sensory Integration for Balance (P-CTSIB) is based on an adult version (CTSIB) developed by Shumway-Cook and Horak (1986). The P-CTSIB uses six testing conditions: three visual (eyes open, eyes closed, and conflict dome) and two somatosensory conditions (hard and flat surface and compliant foam surface) to evaluate the integrity of these systems (Figure 11-8). During two of the testing conditions a conflict dome is placed on the child's head. When the child is wearing the dome, his or her central and peripheral vision is blocked. However, the vertical lines of the dome provide a visual orientation for the child that is inconsistent with a true vertical orientation because the dome moves as the child sways.

Standing on the foam surface creates ambiguous somatosensory cues because the feet sink into the foam surface, making detection of sway difficult. Testing with the P-CTSIB is typically done with the feet together (malleoli touching) and with the feet in tandem (dominant foot behind the nondominant foot and the toes touching the heel). The duration that the child can maintain standing under each condition (maximum 30 seconds) and the amount of postural sway are recorded for each condition. Figure 11-9 depicts this measurement system. This test is one means of evaluating the child's ability to integrate sensory information and the relative reliance of the child on one sensory system or another. Although the P-CTSIB was designed to evaluate balance in standing, it would probably be effective to use the visual conflict dome or foam padding to evaluate balance responses in other postures (e.g., sitting or quadruped) and determine the child's ability to use visual or somatosensory cues in maintaining equilibrium.

### Posturography

The P-CTSIB is based on a sophisticated testing program, often referred to as *posturography*. Posturography typically

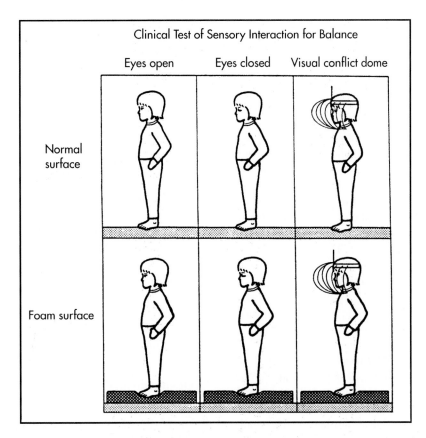

**Figure 11-8**  Six sensory conditions of the Pediatric Clinical Test of Sensory Interaction for Balance. (From Deitz, J., Richardson, P., Atwater, S., Crowe, T., & Odiome, M. [1991]. Performance of normal children on the Pediatric Clinical Test of Sensory Integration for Balance. *The Occupational Therapy Journal of Research, 7*[6], 343, 345.)

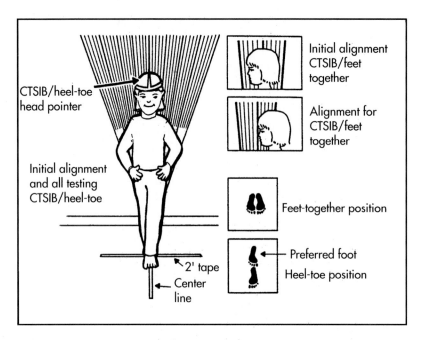

**Figure 11-9**   Measurement system and positioning for the Clinical Test of Sensory Interaction for Balance (CTSIB). (From Deitz, J., Richardson, P., Atwater, S., Crowe, T., & Odiome, M. [1991]. Performance of normal children on the Pediatric Clinical Test of Sensory Integration for Balance. *The Occupational Therapy Journal of Research, 7*[6], 343, 345.)

involves testing under six conditions, also involving sensory deprivation and conflict, using a computerized force platform system. The platform can be stable or sway referenced (moves as child sways such that the ankle joint remains in the same position); a curtainlike structure surrounds the child's entire visual field and can also be sway-referenced (sways with child). The six testing conditions are (1) eyes open, stable platform; (2) eyes closed, stable platform; (3) sway-referenced visual surround, stable platform; (4) eyes open, sway-referenced platform; (5) eyes closed, sway-referenced platform; (6) sway-referenced visual surround and platform (Nashner, 1990). This type of evaluation requires expensive equipment, but it is often used to assess vestibular dysfunction in adults and has been used with children (Forrsberg & Nashner, 1982; Horak, Shumway-Cook, Crow, & Black, 1988; Nashner, Shumway-Cook, & Marnin, 1983; Shumway-Cook, Horak, & Black, 1987).

Interpretation of both the P-CTSIB and posturography involves the examination of sway and the duration of time that the child can maintain each position. Individuals that have difficulty with a given condition demonstrate increased sway or lose their balance. Difficulty with condition 2 reflects an overreliance on the visual system. Although children and adults demonstrate a slight increase in sway in this condition, children as young as 4 have had no difficulty in maintaining stance for 30 seconds. Condition

3 examines the child's ability to remain standing in the presence of inaccurate visual cues but with accurate somatosensory and vestibular cues. Conditions 4 through 6 require stance in the presence of inaccurate somatosensory cues and varying visual input (present, absent, or conflicting). Individuals with sensory organization problems have difficulty with all conditions in which conflicting sensory cues are present (conditions 3 through 6). However, the last two conditions require the individual to rely on vestibular information only; therefore difficulties with only conditions 5 and 6 are typical of individuals with vestibular disorders. In testing with young children, a developmental progression occurs with an increase in stability between the ages of 3 and 6; 6-year-old children responded similarly to adults (Foudriat et al., 1993). However, even 3- and 4-year-old children were able to disregard misleading sensory inputs to maintain stance but with increased sway (Foudriat et al., 1993; Richardson et al., 1992).

## Assessment of Higher Level Balance Skills

More advanced balance skills are typically evaluated through parts of gross motor tests. Typical test items include single-limb stance (standing on one foot), balance beam activities, involving stance and ambulation, and other walking balance activities (walking heel-to-toe or walking in a straight line). For the most part, assessment of these skills involves timed tests of static stance capabilities (how long the child can stand on one foot) or frequency counts (how many consecutive heel-to-toe steps the child can take). The Bruininks-Oseretsky Test of Motor Proficiency can be used to examine these areas in children 4½ to 14½ years old (Bruininks, 1978). The Gross Motor Scale of the Peabody Development Motor Scale (PDMS) (Folio & Fewell, 1983) includes a number of items at ages 4 through 6 years that rate balance reactions in higher-level positions (e.g., on the balance beam, in one-foot stance, hopping).

## Assessment of Anticipatory Postural Control

Assessment of anticipatory postural control is accomplished through the observational skills of the therapist. Children who have delays in anticipatory postural control likely exhibit general delays in motor control. Children with limited anticipatory control have difficulty reaching, catching, or throwing in any posture. These activities involve sequential displacements of the child's center of gravity and require that postural tone remain activated (preset) for the child to be successful. An overreliance on protective and equilibrium reactions is another indication that anticipatory control is ineffective or limited. For example, a child who loses his or her balance when he or she attempts a reach may be demonstrating poor feedforward control.

## ATYPICAL POSTURAL DEVELOPMENT

Postural development is associated with maturational and experiential changes in the sensorimotor, musculoskeletal, and cognitive systems; therefore abnormal functioning of any of these systems can result in atypical postural development.

## Persistence of Primitive Reflexes

Primitive reflexes are those reflexes that are present at or soon after birth that disappear during the first year of life. The traditional hierarchic model proposed that these reflexes were controlled at lower levels of the central nervous system and that reflex integration was associated with maturation of patterns mediated by higher centers; that is, the higher centers inhibited the expression of these reflexes by the lower centers (Bobath & Bobath, 1954; Taylor, 1931; VanSant, 1993). The reemergence of these reflex patterns after brain injury in children and adults lent support to this concept. Indeed, the movement patterns of many children with cerebral palsy and children who have incurred traumatic brain injury are influenced by primitive reflex activity, including the asymmetric tonic neck, symmetric tonic neck, and tonic labyrinthine reflexes. The persistence of these reflexes or their reemergence after brain injury has been associated with delayed postural reflex development

(e.g., righting, protective, and equilibrium reactions) (Bobath & Bobath, 1954; Shumway-Cook, 1989).

## Abnormal Muscle Tone

The adequate development of postural reactions has also been linked to the presence of normal muscle tone (Bobath, 1966). Conversely, the presence of abnormal muscle tone in the form of hypertonia, hypotonia, athetosis, or rigidity (e.g., in cerebral palsy) has been associated with deficits in postural control mechanisms, including postural reactions, antigravity movement, proximal muscle cocontraction, and stability in upright postures (Bly, 1983; Bobath, 1966; Perin, 1989).

According to Bly (1983), the inability to develop antigravity movement and stability combined with the need to move result in fixing (or locking) of various body segments; this fixing provides some stability but also blocks more mature movement patterns, such as head control, extremity mobility, and dynamic weight-bearing. Blocks can occur at the neck, shoulder, and pelvis, depending on the positioning of the child, the underlying muscle tone, and the movements attempted.

Two types of *neck blocks* are described. The first type is characterized by neck hyperextension with compensatory shoulder elevation for stabilization of the head; this limits head mobility and midline activities. The second type is characterized by neck asymmetry associated with an asymmetric tonic neck reflex and poor development of bilateral antigravity neck flexion; this also limits head mobility and midline activities. The *shoulder block* is associated with poor development of scapular stability. This interferes with the child's ability to bear weight on the upper extremities in prone position, resulting in overuse of scapular adduction and spinal extension. This compensatory pattern blocks the emergence of midline activity in supine position. Two *pelvic blocks* are also described: an anterior pelvic block and a posterior pelvic block. Children with an anterior pelvic block assume a frog-legged position in association with failure to develop antigravity hip flexion and poor abdominal strength (most commonly in children with athetosis or hypotonia). The anterior pelvic block prevents rolling and lateral weight shift. The posterior pelvic tilt is most commonly found in children with a predominance of extensor tone, resulting in limited hip flexion with compensatory rounding of the back and increased knee flexion in supported sitting.

In addition to the delay or inability to develop antigravity movement and stability, many children with abnormal tone associated with cerebral palsy demonstrate hyperreflexia, which is characterized by exaggerated monosynaptic reflexes (e.g., deep tendon reflexes such as the patellar tendon reflex). Not only are these reflexes hyperexcitable, but also they have been found to be associated with activation of both the agonist and antagonist muscles. So in response to tapping of the patellar tendon, both the quadriceps muscle and hamstrings would be activated. As a result the child is unable to make a selective, graded movement. Also, in many children with cerebral palsy, muscle groups adjacent to those stimulated are activated as well; this response is termed *overflow*. Overflow is often seen in young, typically developing children, and it decreases after the first year of life. Normal overflow is not as widespread and does not involve as many muscles as the atypical overflow observed in children with cerebral palsy (Leonard, Hirschfeld, & Forrsberg, 1988). Because stretching of a spastic muscle activates this same monosynaptic reflex, this overflow pattern can be expected to occur in such activities as extending the arm quickly to protect from a fall. In the child with cerebral palsy the reflex activates the biceps, shoulder, and wrist muscles and results in failure to effectively stop the fall. In children with spasticity, then, the development of effective protective reactions is typically delayed and often absent (Bobath & Bobath, 1954).

### Musculoskeletal Abnormalities

Delays in the development of postural control have been described in conjunction with ligamentous laxity and decreased muscle strength in children with Down syndrome (Fetters, 1991). Musculoskeletal abnormalities are also associated with cerebral palsy and other developmental disabilities (e.g., arthrogryposis and muscular dystrophy). Contractures secondary to spasticity or soft tissue abnormalities can restrict movement and thereby disrupt the efficacy of postural reactions; thus changes in musculoskeletal alignment and joint biomechanics can reduce the child's ability to exhibit adequate protective reactions. Adequate muscle strength is also necessary to produce joint stability and adequate equilibrium reactions; therefore conditions that result in diminished muscle strength (e.g., muscular dystrophy and cerebral palsy) may be associated with deficits in postural control.

Not only are the development of equilibrium reactions affected by the presence of musculoskeletal abnormalities, but also the need for these reactions is altered. In any position there are limits to how far the child can lean before a fall occurs; these limits have been referred to as "the limits of stability" (Nashner, 1990). In children or adults with musculoskeletal limitations, these limits of stability are decreased; therefore it takes a smaller movement to elicit a loss of balance. A movement such as lifting the arm to reach for a toy may be sufficient to displace the child's center of gravity outside of the limits of stability and thereby elicit a fall. If the musculoskeletal change is asymmetric (e.g., in the child with hemiplegia), the decrease in the limits of stability occurs only on the side of the musculoskeletal abnormality (Nashner, 1990). Thus in a child with unilateral weakness the limits of stability on the involved side are decreased. To compensate for this, the child moves his or her

center of gravity toward the sound side to minimize the chance of falling, resulting in asymmetric postures.

### Altered Sensory Function or Integration

Postural control, according to Horak and Shumway-Cook (1990), "relies on 1) intact peripheral sensory pathways, and 2) the ability of the CNS to extract appropriate sensory information relevant to gravity, the surface, and visual environments" (p. 110). Postural control requires not only intact perception of visual, vestibular, and somatosensory stimulation but also the ability to determine the best source of information under the existing environmental conditions, especially if there are conflicting sensory inputs (e.g., unstable support surface resulting in inaccurate somatosensory inputs). When children with impairments in visual, somatosensory, or vestibular processing are required to resolve conflicting sensory input, they demonstrate deficits in postural control. Children with visual impairments typically demonstrate deficits in both static and dynamic balance skills when compared with sighted children (Johnson-Kramer, Sherwood, Frech, & Canabal, 1992; Ribaldi, Rider, & Toole, 1987). Similarly, about 60% of children with hearing impairments also demonstrate abnormal vestibular function and deficits in balance activities that rely on vestibular integrity (Horak et al., 1988) However, children with loss of only one sensory system are able to compensate in most conditions by use of the two remaining systems (Horak et al., 1988).

Shumway-Cook (1989) reported that children with impaired hearing and hypothesized vestibular dysfunction demonstrated normal postural reactions under conditions in which the sensory inputs were consistent but had difficulty in situations in which the sensory inputs were conflicting (e.g., on a moving platform with visual input that remained unchanged despite postural sway). This inability to interpret conflicting inputs and organize an appropriate response appears to be secondary to abnormalities within the central processes at the level of the cerebellum, brainstem, or cortex (Shumway-Cook, 1989). Children with a variety of other diagnoses, including cerebral palsy and learning disabilities, have been reported to have deficits in the selection of appropriate sensory inputs for postural control (Horak et al., 1988; Nashner et al., 1983; Shumway-Cook, Horak, & Black, 1987). Children with ataxic or diplegic cerebral palsy have demonstrated similar deficits in sensory organization under conditions of conflicting sensory cues (Nashner et al., 1983).

### Organization of the Motor Response

The child's motor response to tilt on an unstable surface or displacement of his or her center of gravity results in activation of the appropriate muscle groups to compensate for the loss of balance. An effective response to this displacement requires muscle activation that is accurately timed and of sufficient amplitude to reestablish the child's center of gravity. Abnormalities in the motor response result in inaccurate patterns of muscle activation and errors in the timing or amplitude, limiting the child's ability to maintain an upright posture.

A delay in the onset of muscle activity has been reported for children with Down syndrome (Shumway-Cook & Woollacott, 1985b) and children with cerebral palsy (both hemiplegic and ataxic)(Nashner et al., 1983; Shumway-Cook, 1989). This delay could result in use of an ineffective movement strategy when the child's center of gravity is displaced. In addition to a delay in the onset of muscle activity, children with cerebral palsy demonstrate patterns of muscle activation that are ineffective for maintaining postural control. The child may activate distal rather than proximal muscles, resulting in a stiffening of extremities instead of dynamic axial cocontraction. Also, overflow contractions that do not effectively contribute to the equilibrium response are observed (Leonard et al., 1988; Nashner et al., 1983).

## INTERVENTION

This chapter describes intervention as it relates to basic posture and movement. Subsequent chapters address the integration of postural control as a foundation of skilled activity performance. Specific occupational therapy approaches to intervention with children who have neurodevelopmental or musculoskeletal problems are presented elsewhere in this text.

Two frames of reference are widely used to facilitate the child's development of postural control: *neurodevelopmental treatment (NDT)* and *motor learning* theories. These frames of reference are often integrated in practice. Both are defined and illustrated in this section. The Bobaths (Bobath & Bobath, 1964) identified three principles as the basis of NDT: 1) The inhibition of abnormal postural reflex activity to reduce hypertonus in the spastic and athetoid patients; 2) The facilitation of potential normal postural and movement patterns on the basis of a more normal muscle tone, in order to maintain and secure normal tonus qualities obtained by inhibition; 3) The increase of postural reflex tone and the regulation of reciprocal muscle function (p. 3) Therefore the original purposes of NDT focused on the reflexive nature of postural control and described methods for inhibiting tone in children with hypertonus and for facilitating righting and equilibrium reactions.

An NDT approach involves *dynamic handling* in which the therapist helps the child grade transitional movements by facilitating the child's postural responses at key points, usually the neck, shoulders, and pelvis. Through facilitation of active weight shifts, mature righting and equilibrium reactions are promoted (Carrasco, 1989). Dynamic handling incorporates vestibular, proprioceptive, and tactile stimula-

tion to facilitate coactivation of muscle groups. Often therapists apply NDT techniques while the child is engaged in developmentally appropriate activities using toys and selected equipment such as therapy balls or benches.

Recently the focus of NDT includes methods to facilitate anticipatory postural reactions as well as compensatory postural reactions. Activities continue to emphasize the integration of visual, vestibular, and somatosensory information in the development of postural control.

Although NDT has been widely used by therapists to enhance postural control in children, motor learning theories are becoming more recognized and are providing therapists with a broader understanding of the development of posture and movement. Motor learning theories acknowledge that motor skills do not simply develop as a course of maturation and are more than the result of subcortical sensory experiences. A motor pattern is the result of learning and practice, with a permanent change in skill. Therapists who use motor learning theories stress the important role of motivation and volition in learning new skills (VanSant, 1994).

An individual learns a new motor skill from the intrinsic and extrinsic feedback received in association with the movement (Adams, 1971). Intrinsic feedback refers to the sensory information generated from the action or the perceptual experience. External feedback refers to the response of the environment produced as a result of the action. The therapist's response to the child's accomplishment or achievement reinforces the learner's "knowledge of results." The child's knowledge of the effects and results of his or her own movements is critical to learning and generalizing motor skills.

Although feedback appears important to learning new movements, not all movement is based on somatosensory feedback. Some is generated and carried out without feedback, (e.g., rapid movements such as throwing a ball). In a more recently developed learning theory, Schmidt (1988) hypothesized that recall and recognition schema are the basis for learning new motor skills. The schema are a set of rules learned about movement that are applied and generalized to new situations. The learner recognizes the relationships between the environment conditions, task requirements, and previously learned movements. The outcome of performance and the sensory consequences help the learner establish new motor skills based on an understanding of these relationships.

Motor learning theories emphasize the importance of practice and sensory feedback combined with knowledge of results. Implications of these theories on practice have been postulated and are currently topics of research. One implication is that random practice reinforces learning more than blocked practice. Blocked practice involves extended periods of repetitious movements with consistent reinforcement provided throughout the practice session. In random practice, an activity is practiced under constantly changing conditions (e.g., therapist changes direction and distance in practice of reach). Performance is reinforced on an intermittent or random schedule. Feedback during practice is also important to learning. High levels of feedback appear to be detrimental rather than helpful when learning a new motor task. Giving intermittent feedback and reducing feedback as the skill is achieved appear to be ideal ways to reinforce learning.

Another concept of motor learning is that practice of parts of skills should be followed by practice of the entire skill. Learning of skill parts might best occur within the context of the whole skill. It cannot be assumed that learning the parts of a skill necessarily means that the whole skill is achieved. These principles regarding learning and the system theories that relate postural development to the function of neurophysiologic and biomechanical variables in the child are the basis for the intervention activities described in the following section.

## Treatment of Musculoskeletal Abnormalities

To prepare the child to work on postural control, limitations in joint range of motion and problems in postural alignment need to be addressed (Effgen, 1993). Contractures or joint limitations secondary to spasticity or soft tissue changes often result in poor postural alignment (e.g., anterior or posterior pelvic tilt that blocks trunk rotation). Decreased range of motion limits mobility and decreases the base of support. As a result, adequate equilibrium or protective reactions do not develop and the child is limited in everyday play, self-care, and school activities.

A variety of inhibition techniques can be used to reduce muscle tone and improve range of motion. Most techniques focus on improving the child's range of motion and flexibility of the spine with the expected result of improved postural alignment and increased postural flexibility. Therapeutic techniques to increase muscle elongation are also used to help the child achieve extension of the extremities. Adequate arm and leg extension is needed for the development of protective extension responses. In particular, full knee and hip extension is required as a base for effective equilibrium responses in stance.

## Facilitation of Antigravity Movement

As previously described, normal postural control requires antigravity control in prone, supine, and upright postures. With the development of antigravity trunk flexion and extension the child achieves upright positions that allow for the development of skilled movements. When a child has not developed sufficient strength in the neck and trunk musculature to move against gravity, he or she is limited in activities such as prone extension and coming to sitting. These movements can be modified to diminish the pull of gravity so that the child can successfully practice the positions and

movements to increase neck and trunk strength. Use of a therapeutic ball or a wedge provides some assistance against gravity and reduces the range in which the child must move against gravity. A pull-to-sit activity can then be done from the incline or a ball (Figure 11-10). With the child's head and trunk inclined, less neck and trunk flexion is required to accomplish pull-to-sit activity. The degree of incline is gradually decreased as the child gains neck flexor strength. An alternative method for eliciting neck flexion is to help the child move from sitting toward the supine position. The therapist gradually lowers the child backward from the sitting position until the child starts to lose head control. The therapist then assists the child in returning to a sitting position. This activity requires neck flexor control in both directions (lowering from and returning to the sitting position). If the child does not have sufficient strength to perform either of these activities, neck and trunk flexion can be initiated in the sidelying position where gravity is eliminated and then progressed to the coming to sitting activities. Moving the child in lateral weight shifts while sitting also increases neck strength in a gravity-reduced plane. The therapist's support at the shoulders, trunk, and pelvis is necessary to allow isolation of the neck and trunk flexors. As the child's strength increases, the therapist introduces diagonal weight shifts that produce rotation. Diagonal or angular movements activate the transverse neck and trunk muscles (for example, the oblique abdominal muscles) that are required in mature equilibrium responses.

Similarly, neck and trunk extension can be elicited by working with the child in a variety of activities in the prone position over a ball, bolster, or wedge. When the child is positioned in a prone position on an inclined surface, the pull of gravity is reduced, allowing for more effective use of neck and trunk extension. Toys or the parent's voice is

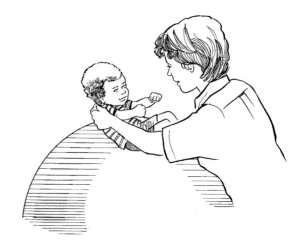

**Figure 11-10**   Facilitation of head righting from therapeutic ball. Other inclined surface could be used. Therapist supports child's shoulders, scapula, and trunk to encourage isolated activation of neck muscles.

used to motivate the child to raise the head while the therapist moves him or her in small ranges of anterior and posterior weight shift to stimulate a righting response. As the child's control of head and trunk extension improves, the degree of incline is gradually decreased. Engaging the child in reaching activities with one or both hands can facilitate antigravity trunk extension in the prone position (Figure 11-11). The therapist's handling should again provide stability so that specific extensor muscle activity is elicited and overflow contractions are inhibited (Bobath & Bobath, 1964; Perin, 1989; Sternat, 1993).

In addition to the traditional activities described previously, biofeedback devices are increasingly used with children who have muscular and neuromuscular disorders. Biofeedback can provide the needed feedback to the child about successful and unsuccessful muscle activation or positioning. In addition, it can provide the motivation for the child to attempt the activity. One example of biofeedback is a mercury switch strapped to the child's head and activated with upright head movement. Using this switch, the child can turn on the radio, tape recorder, or other battery-powered toy using simple head movements. Kramer, Ashton, and Brander (1992) found the mercury head switch to be effective in improving head control in prone and sitting over an 8-week period. Thus for some children, biofeedback can be used during therapy sessions or on a home-based program as a tool to increase the child's motivation and improve antigravity movement.

## Facilitation of Postural Reactions

The therapist can facilitate postural reactions using activities that displace the center of gravity and require corrective or protective responses. The speed, range, and direction of displacement determine whether righting or equilibrium responses are elicited. As previously mentioned, rapid movements in greater ranges elicit protective extension responses. These activities can also be performed on therapeutic balls, bolsters, equilibrium boards, or any other unstable surface (Figure 11-12). Reaching activities with the child positioned on an unstable surface can facilitate the development of these reactions because the child will displace his or her center of gravity during the reach, requiring a compensatory response. Initially, the therapist provides pelvic stability (e.g., with his or her hands) as a base from which the child can begin to produce the desired response. As postural reactions improve, this support is reduced and finally eliminated. Then the child practices skills unsupported on a stable surface, using first a wide base of support (most of his or her legs and buttocks are in contact with the supporting surface) and later a smaller base of support (only the buttocks are in contact with the surface). Postural reactions are refined by placing the child in a sitting position on an unstable surface. During advanced practice of these activities, the therapist moves the surface using a variety of speeds, ranges (degrees of tilt), and rhythms. Safety and protection of the child's fall become increasingly important as greater challenges to balance are imposed on the child. In addition to activities on an unstable surface, reaching activities that require the child to shift weight facilitate the development of equilibrium and righting reactions (Bobath & Bobath, 1964; Effgen, 1993; Perin, 1989).

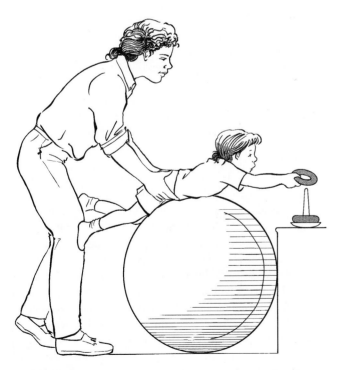

**Figure 11-11**   Facilitation of prone extension over therapeutic ball. Key point of control is at pelvis.

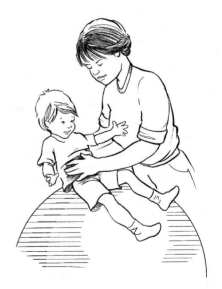

**Figure 11-12**   Facilitation of protective and equilibrium reaction to displacement on therapeutic ball.

Mature postural control and the motor patterns associated with these abilities develop through experience with the conditions in which they are required. Therefore the therapist provides the child with a variety of experiences that demand the use of postural reactions (VanSant, 1991). The therapist's role is to provide handling that is sufficient for these motor patterns to be expressed, motivate the child such that the activity is fun and meaningful, and provide feedback to the child about the appropriateness of the motor response. As skills develop, the child is encouraged to evaluate his or her own responses (Effgen, 1993). As described in the section on facilitating antigravity movement, biofeedback can be used as a method for reinforcing postural responses by providing additional feedback to the child. Research has demonstrated its successful use to increase head righting and control in prone and supine positions (Kramer et al., 1992) and to improve weight shift and ankle motion during walking (Conrad & Bleck, 1980; Seeger & Caudrey, 1983).

## Facilitation of Sensory Organization

As discussed previously, many children with developmental disorders demonstrate deficits in the organization of sensory inputs for use in balance. When sensory organization seems to be the basis for difficulty in postural control, it also becomes the focus of intervention. The therapist creates experiences with altered surfaces or visual contexts that match the identified needs of the child (Barnes and Crutchfield, 1990; Shumway-Cook et al., 1987). For example, children who demonstrate immature equilibrium responses when relying only on the somatosensory system benefit from activities that challenge this system, such as ball, bolster, or tilt board activities in a darkened room or with vision occluded (e.g., with the use of a blindfold). These activities should be designed so that the child does not feel threatened by the disruption of his or her vision and by the progress from easier positions to more complex positions (e.g., sitting to standing). Conversely, children with difficulty balancing when relying on visual information in the presence of conflicting somatosensory cues should benefit from practice of activities on unstable surfaces that challenge the somatosensory system. Movement on a surface padded with foam or covered with sand challenges balance with ambiguous information to the proprioceptive system. Combining the conflicting visual and somatosensory cues should require reliance on the vestibular system and would be appropriate to facilitate vestibular function in children with deficits in this area.

## Facilitation of Anticipatory Postural Control

Facilitation of anticipatory postural control requires that the child experience the need for this control. Reaching, catching, and throwing activities can be used to identify deficits

**CASE STUDY #1**

Marcy is a 2½-year-old child with a diagnosis of spastic diplegic cerebral palsy. She was born at 32 weeks' gestation, weighing 2 pounds 11 ounces. Her hospital stay was complicated by respiratory distress syndrome and a grade 2 intraventricular hemorrhage.

### Assessment

Marcy presents with spasticity in all four extremities, greater in the legs than in the arms. She demonstrates hypotonicity in the trunk. Her head control is good in all positions, but she continues to demonstrate an immature neck flexion response when pulled to sit. In sitting, she demonstrates a posterior pelvic tilt with weight-bearing primarily on her sacrum and her trunk flexed forward; she is able to free one hand for play but requires one hand support to maintain sitting. She lacks antigravity back extension sufficient for sitting without arm support. Forward protective reactions are present, and lateral protective reactions are developing but are inconsistent. Protective and equilibrium reactions backward are absent. Marcy is motivated to move about her environment and does so using a commando crawl-type movement of the arms with her legs tightly scissored. She is unable to assume or maintain quadruped.

### Interpretation

Marcy demonstrates gross motor skills at the 6- to 7-month age level. She also demonstrates delayed development of antigravity head and trunk control as well as delayed development of protective and equilibrium reactions. Her movement patterns are influenced by spasticity with overflow into synergistic and antagonistic muscles.

### Treatment

Treatment focuses on developing antigravity neck and trunk strength, facilitating protective and equilibrium reactions, and developing independent sitting without arm support. Antigravity neck flexion is facilitated by lowering from a sitting to a supine position and practicing small lateral weight shifts in sitting. Antigravity neck and trunk extension are promoted through activities that involved moving from a sidelying to a prone position on a large therapy ball. The movement of the ball is used to facilitate postural extension. Reaching activities in sitting on a ball or bolster are used to facilitate trunk strength as well as the development of trunk righting and equilibrium and protective reactions.

## CASE STUDY #2

John is a 5-year-old boy with Down syndrome. He is enrolled in a preschool program, and his teacher reports that he frequently falls and has difficulty keeping up with the other ambulatory children in the class. He tends to avoid situations that require walking on unstable surfaces such as gravel or stepping over obstacles. Prior testing has found vision and vestibular function to be within normal limits.

### Assessment

John presents with a mild degree of hypotonia, ligamentous laxity, and joint hypermobility at all peripheral joints. He walks with a stiff-legged, flat-foot gait characterized by minimal hip and knee flexion, knee recurvatum during stance, and an absent heel-strike. He is unable to achieve either a prone extension or supine flexion posture. On the Gross Motor Scale of the PDMS, John scored at the 30-month age level. Testing with the P-CTSIB showed that John had difficulty with balance when conflicting sensory input is given and seemed to overrely on vision to maintain his balance.

### Interpretation

John presents with generalized hypotonia and immature movement patterns in standing, associated with decreased antigravity muscle strength. John demonstrates a gross motor delay with function limited in activities of jumping and single-limb stance such as hopping, skipping, and alternating feet on walking up or down steps (These are the activities that John failed on the PDMS). The results of the P-CTSIB also suggest that John has difficulty with the organization of sensory cues for use in balance, resulting in difficulty under conditions of conflicting sensory cues from either the visual or somatosensory system.

### Treatment

Treatment focuses on developing antigravity muscle strength and facilitating the organization of sensory cues. Intervention to increase antigravity extension includes (1) reaching while prone on a ball or bolster; (2) activities in prone on a scooter board, such as pushing away from a wall or holding onto rubber tubing while being pulled around the room; and (3) reaching and throwing while lying prone in a hammock swing. Activities to increase supine flexion include (1) moving from supine position to sitting on an inclined surface; and (2) reaching while sitting on the therapy ball.

Activities that challenge the sensory organization system are helpful in facilitating the ability to deal with conflicting sensory cues, including walking on foam, sand, grass, or thick carpet in various visual conditions—eyes closed, dim lighting, conflicting conditions (e.g., conflict dome). In addition, standing activities that challenge the postural system facilitate more mature balance reactions. These activites include walking up and down stairs with an alternating step pattern, stepping over obstacles of various heights and widths, or kicking a ball.

---

in anticipatory control as well as to facilitate its use. The therapist uses handling and verbal instruction to stimulate anticipatory activity. Practice with weight-shifting may be necessary before practice of the displacing activity. Initially this may be enhanced by handling, but eventually the handling must be diminished and then curtailed so that the child experiences success or failure in the performance of the task; errors in task performance are important to the learning of the task (Schmidt, 1988). Experiences in reaching with and without handling allow the child to evaluate and learn from the sensory input during anticipatory weight-shift (i.e., to recognize errors in anticipatory postural control). Varying the direction, speed, and magnitude of the displacing activity is also important so that the child is required to reassess the intended movement and impose the appropriate anticipatory response (Barnes & Crutchfield, 1990).

## STUDY QUESTIONS

1. What are the roles of the visual, vestibular, and somatosensory systems in balance control? How do these roles change in the developing child?
2. What is the difference between compensatory postural reactions and anticipatory postural control? How can each of these be evaluated?
3. How is postural control affected by abnormalities of the musculoskeletal system, alterations in muscle tone, and abnormal motor pattern selection? How can treatment address these limitations?

## REFERENCES

Adams, J. A. (1971). A closed loop theory of motor learning. *Journal of Motor Behavior, 3,* 110-150.

Ayres, A. (1963). Occupational therapy directed toward neuromuscular integration. In H.S. Willard & C.S. Spackman (Eds.). *Occupational therapy* (pp. 358-466). Philadelphia: J.B. Lippincott.

Ayres, A. (1989). *Sensory Integration and Praxis Tests.* Los Angeles: Western Psychological Services.

Barnes, M. & Crutchfield, C. (1990). *Reflex and vestibular aspects of motor control, motor development and motor learning.* Atlanta: Stokesville.

Berger, W., Quintern, J., & Dietz, V. (1985). Stance and gait perturbation in children: developmental aspects of compensatory mechanisms. *Electroencephalographic Clinical Neurophysiology, 61,* 385-395.

Berk, R. & DeGangi, G. (1983). *DeGangi-Berk Test of Motor Proficiency examiner's manual.* Circle Pines, MN: American Guidance Service.

Bly, L. (1983). *The components of normal movement during the first year of life and abnormal development.* Oak Park, IL: Neurodevelopmental Treatment Association.

Bobath, B. & Bobath, K. (1954). A study of abnormal postural reflex activity in patients with lesions of the central nervous system. *Physiotherapy, 40,* 1-30.

Bobath, K. (1966). The motor deficit in patients with cerebral palsy. *Clinics in Developmental Medicine, 23,* 1-54.

Bobath, K. & Bobath, B.(1964). The facilitation of normal postural reactions and movements in the treatment of cerebral palsy. *Physiotherapy, 21,* 3-19.

Bouisset S. & Zattara, M. (1981). A sequence of postural movements precedes voluntary movement. *Neuroscience Letters, 22,* 263-270.

Bruininks, R. (1978). *Bruininks-Oseretsky Test of Motor Proficiency.* Examiners Manual, Circle Pines, MN: American Guidance System.

Bullinger, A. (1981). Cognitive elaboration of sensorimotor behavior. In G. Buttorworth, (Ed.). *Infancy and epistemology: an evaluation of Piaget's theory.* London: Harvester Press.

Carrasco, R.C. (1989). Children with cerebral palsy. In P.N. Pratt & A.S. Allen (Eds.). *Occupational therapy for children.* (2nd ed.). St. Louis: Mosby.

Case-Smith, J. & Bigsby, R. (1993). *Posture and Fine Motor Assessment of Infants: parts I and II.* Unpublished document, Columbus: Ohio State University.

Chandler, L., Andrews, M., & Swanson, M. (1980). *Movement assessment of infants manual.* Rolling Bay, WA.

Connor, F., Williamson, G., & Siepp, J. (1978). *Program guide for infants and toddlers with neuromotor and other developmental disabilities.* New York: Teachers College Press.

Conrad, L. & Bleck, E. (1980). Augmented auditory feedback in the treatment of equinus in children. *Developmental Medicine and Child Neurology, 22,* 713-718.

Crowe, T., Deitz, J., Richardson, P., & Atwater, S. (1990). Interrater reliability of the pediatric clinical test of sensory interaction for balance. *Physical and Occupational Therapy in Pediatrics, 10*(4), 1-27.

Dietz, J., Richardson, P., Atwater, S., Crowe, T., & Odiorne, M. (1991). Performance of normal children on the Pediatric Clinical Test of Sensory Interaction for Balance. *Occupational Therapy Journal of Research, 11*(6), 336-356.

Effgen, S. (1993). Developing postural control. In B. Connolly & P. Montgomery (Eds.). *Therapeutic exercise in developmental disabilities.* Hixson, TN: Chattanooga Group.

Ellison, P. (1994). *The INFANIB: a reliable method for the neuromotor assessment of infants.* Tucson: Therapy Skill Builders.

Fetters, L. (1991). Cerebral palsy: comtemporary treatment concepts. In M. Lister (Ed.). *Contemporary management of motor control problems proceedings of the II step conference.* Alexandria, VA: Foundation for Physical Therapy.

Folio, M. & Fewell, R. (1983) *Peabody developmental motor scales manual.* Chicago: Riverside Publishers.

Forssberg, H. & Nashner, L. (1982) Ontogenetic development of postural control in man: adaptation to altered support and visual conditions during stance. *Journal of Neuroscience 2*(5), 545-552.

Foudriat, B., DiFabio, R., & Anderson, J. (1993). Sensory organization of balance responses in children 3-6 years of age: a normative study with diagnostic implications. *International Journal of Pediatric Otorhinolaryngology, 27,* 255-271.

Haas, G., Diener, H., Bacher, M., & Dichgans, J. (1986). Development of postural control in children: short-, medium-, and long-latency EMG responses of leg muscles after perturbation of stance. *Experimental Brain Research, 64,* 127-132.

Haley, S. (1986). Sequential analyses of postural reactions in nonhandicapped infants. *Physical Therapy, 66*(4), 531-536.

Hayes, K. & Riach, C. (1989). Preparatory postural adjustment and postural sway in young children. In M. Woollacott & A. Shumway-Cook (Eds.). *Development of posture and gait across the life span.* Columbia: University of South Carolina Press.

Horak, F. & Nashner, L. (1986). Central programming of posture control: adaptation to altered support-surface configurations. *Journal of neurophysiology, 55,* 1368-1381.

Horak, F. & Shumway-Cook, A. (1990). Clinical implications of posture control research. In P. Duncan (Ed.). *Balance proceedings of the APTA forum.* Alexandria, VA: American Physical Therapy Association.

Horak, F., Shumway-Cook, A., Crow, T., & Black, F. (1988). Vestibular function and motor proficiency in children with hearing impairments and in learning disabled children with motor impairments. *Developmental Medicine and Child Neurology, 30,* 64-79.

Johnson-Kramer, C., Sherwood, D., Frech, R., & Canabal, M. (1992). Performance and learning of a dynamic balance task by visually impaired children. *Clinical Kinesiology, 1,* 3-6.

Jouen, F. (1984). Visual-vestibular interactions in infancy. *Infant Behavior and Development, 7,* 135-145.

Kramer, J., Ashton, B., & Brander, R. (1992). Training of head control in the sitting and semi-prone position. *Child Care, Health, and Development, 18,* 365-376.

Leonard, C., Hirschfeld, A., & Forrsberg, H. (1988). Gait acquisition and reflex abnormalities in normal children and children with cerebral palsy. In B. Amblard, A. Berthoz, F. Clarae, (Eds.). *Posture and gait development, adaptation, and modulation.* New York: Elsevier Science.

Milani-Comparetti, A. & Gidoni, E. (1967). Routine developmental examination in normal and retarded children. *Developmental Medicine and Child Neurology, 9,* 631-638.

Nashner, L. (1990). Sensory, neuromuscular, and biomechanical contributions to human balance. In P. Duncan (Ed.). *Balance proceedings of the APTA forum.* Alexandria, VA: American Physical Therapy Association.

Nashner, L., Shumway-Cook, A., & Marin, O. (1983). Stance posture control in selected groups of children with cerebral palsy: deficits in sensory organization and muscular coordination. *Experimental Brain Research, 49,* 393-409.

Perin, B. (1989). Physical therapy for the child with cerebral palsy. In J. Techlin (Ed.). *Pediatric physical therapy.* Philadelphia: J.B. Lippincott.

Piper, M. & Darrah, J. (1994). *Motor assessment of the developing infant.* Philadelphia: W.B. Saunders.

Pountney, T., Mulcahy, C., & Green, E. (1990). Early development of postural control. *Physiotherapy, 76*(12), 799-802.

Riach, C. & Hayes, K. (1987). Maturation of postural sway in young children, *Developmental Medicine and Child Neurology, 29,* 650-658.

Ribaldi, H., Rider, R., & Toole, T. (1987). A comparison of static and dynamic balance in congenitally blind, sighted, and sighted blindfolded adolescents. *Adapted Physical Activity Quarterly, 4,* 220-225.

Richardson, P., Atwater, S., Crowe, T., & Deitz, J. (1992). Performance of preschoolers on the pediatric clinical test of sensory interaction for balance. *American Journal of Occupational Therapy, 46*(9), 793-800.

Schmidt, R. (1988). *Motor control and learning* (2nd ed.). Champaign, IL: Human Kinetics.

Seeger, B. & Caudrey, D. (1983). Biofeedback therapy to achieve symmetrical gait in children with hemiplegic cerebral palsy: long term efficacy. *Archives of Physical Medicine and Rehabilitation, 64,* 160-162.

Sellers, J. (1988). Relationship between antigravity control and postural control in young children. *Physical Therapy, 68*(4), 486-430.

Shumway-Cook, A. (1989). Equilibrium deficits in children. In M. Woollacott & A. Shumway-Cook, A. (Eds.). *Development of posture and gait across the life span.* Columbia: University of South Carolina Press.

Shumway-Cook, A. & Horak, F. (1986). Assessing the influence of sensory interaction on balance. *Physical Therapy, 66,* 1548-1550.

Shumway-Cook, A., Horak, F., & Black, F. (1987). A critical examination of vestibular function in motor impaired learning disabled children. *International Journal of Otorhinolaryngology, 14,* 21-30.

Shumway-Cook, A. & Woollacott, M. (1985a). The growth of stability: postural control from a developmental perspective. *Journal of Motor Behavior, 17*(2), 131-147.

Shumway-Cook, A. & Woollacott, M. (1985b). Dynamics of postural control in the child with Down syndrome. *Physical Therapy, 9,* 1315-1322.

Sternat, J. (1993). Developing head and trunk control. In B. Connolly & P. Montgomery (Eds.). *Therapeutic exercise in developmental disabilities.* Hixson, TN: Chattanooga Group.

Stockmeyer, S. (1967). An interpretation of the approach of Rood to the treatment of neuromuscular dysfunction. *American Journal of Physical Medicine, 46,* 900-956.

Taylor, J. (1931). *Selected writings of John Hughlings Jackson,* Vol. II, London: Holder & Stoughton.

VanSant, A. (1991). Neurodevelopmental treatment and pediatric physical therapy: a commentary. *Physical Therapy, 3*(3), 137-140.

VanSant, A. (1993). Concepts of neural organization and movement. In B. Connolly & P. Montgomery (Eds.). *Therapeutic exercise in developmental disabilities.* Hixson, TN: Chattanooga Group.

VanSant, A. (1994). Motor control and motor learning. In D. Cech & S. Martin (Eds.). *Functional movement development across the life span.* Philadelphia: W.B. Saunders.

Von Hofsten, C. (1986). The emergence of manual skills. In M. Wade & A. Whiting, (Eds.). *Motor development in children: aspects of coordination and control.* Boston: Martinus Nijhoff.

Williams, H., Fisher, J., & Tritschler, K. (1983). Descriptive analysis of static postural control in 4, 6, and 8 year old normal and motorically awkward children. *American Journal of Physical Medicine, 62*(1), 12-26.

Woollacott, M. (1988). Posture and gait from newborn to elderly. In B. Amblard, A. Berthoz, & F. Clarae (Ed.). *Posture and gait development, adaptation, and modulation.* New York: Elsevier Science.

Woollacott, M., Debu, B., & Mowatt, M. (1988). Neuromuscular control of posture in the infant and child: is vision dominant? *Journal of Motor Behavior, 19*(2), 167-186.

Woollacott, M., Shumway-Cook, A., & Williams, H. (1989). The development of posture and balance control in children. In M. Woollacott & A. Shumway-Cook (Eds.). *Development of posture and gait across the lifespan.* Columbia: University of South Carolina Press.

Woollacott, M. & Sveistrup, H. (1992). Changes in the sequencing and timing of muscle response coordination associated with developmental transitions in balance abilities. *Human Movement Science, 11,* 23-36.

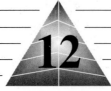

# Development of Hand Skills

CHARLOTTE E. EXNER

## CHAPTER OBJECTIVES

1. Describe typical development of hand skills in children.
2. Identify factors that contribute to typical or atypical development of hand skills.
3. Explain the implications of hand skill problems for play, self-care, and school performance.
4. Describe typical problems with children's development of hand skills.
5. Describe frames of reference and theories that may be used in structuring intervention plans for children who have problems with hand skills.
6. Identify evaluation tools and methods useful in assessing hand skills in children.
7. Describe treatment strategies for assisting children in improving or compensating for problems with hand skills.
8. Illustrate principles of evaluation and intervention with case examples of children.

Hand skills are critical to interaction with the environment. Hands allow us to act on our world through contact with our own and others' bodies and through contact with objects. Hands are the "tools" most often used to accomplish work, to play, and to perform self-maintenance tasks. The child who has a disability affecting hand skills has less opportunity to take in sensory information from the environment and to experience the effect of his or her actions on the world.

## COMPONENTS OF HAND SKILLS

Effective use of the hands to engage in daily occupational activities is dependent on a complex interaction of hand skills, postural mechanisms, cognition, and visual perception. The term *visual-motor integration* is used to refer to the interaction of visual skills, visual perceptual skills, and motor skills. The term *hand skills* may be used interchangeably with the term *fine motor coordination* or *fine motor skills*. Because this chapter refers to only those skills accomplished with hands to attain and manipulate objects, the more specific term *hand skills* is used here.

Although it is assumed that the development of hand skills is dependent on adequate somatosensory and postural functions and sufficient visual perceptual and cognitive development, these areas are not discussed in detail in this chapter. Hand skills are those patterns that normally rely on both tactile-proprioceptive and visual information for accuracy. However, these skills may be accomplished without visual feedback if somatosensory functions provide adequate information. The patterns include basic reach, grasp, carry, release, and the more complex skills of in-hand manipulation and bilateral hand use. Brief definitions of these patterns follow:

> *Reach:* Movement and stabilization of the arm and hand for the purpose of contacting an object with the hand
> *Grasp:* Attainment of an object with the hand
> *Carry:* The movement of the arm in space for the purpose of transporting a hand-held object from one place to another
> *Release:* The intentional letting go of a hand-held object at a specific time and place

*In-hand manipulation:* The adjustment of an object within the hand after grasp

*Bilateral hand use:* The effective use of two hands together to accomplish an activity

In this discussion, *hand-arm* refers to the interactive movement and stabilization of different parts of the hand and arm to accomplish a fine motor task.

*Visual skills* are the use of extraocular muscles to direct eye movements. These include the ability to visually fix on a stationary object and the smooth, accurate tracking of a moving target.

*Visual perceptual skills* are the recognition, discrimination, and processing of sensory information through the eyes and related central nervous system structures. Visual perceptual skills include the identification of shapes, colors, and other qualities, the orientation of objects or shapes in space, and the relationship of objects or shapes to one another and to the environment (see Chapter 14).

## CONTRIBUTIONS OF OTHER PERFORMANCE COMPONENTS TO HAND SKILLS

As children mature, they begin to effectively coordinate visual skills with hand skills, and later they combine eye-hand coordination with visual perceptual skills (Ayres, 1958). These skills in conjunction with cognitive and social development allow the child to engage in increasingly complex activities. Although motor issues are usually given the most attention, many other dimensions of development significantly impact effective hand use. These include the child's visual skills, somatosensory functions, sensory integration, visual perception, cognition, social factors, and culture.

### Visual Skills

Erhardt (1992) stresses the importance of visual skills and their major role in the development of hand function. Visuomotor development is expected to be mature by approximately 6 months of age in the normally developing infant. Erhardt outlined a theoretical framework for eye-hand function and developed tables to organize information about the relationship between visual development and hand skill development. This information is useful to the occupational therapist in assessing and planning intervention for any child who has difficulty in using visual control to effectively guide the hands.

### Somatosensory Functions

Pehoski (1992) used research from several disciplines to illustrate the important role of somatosensory information and feedback in the development of children's hand skills, particularly those that involved isolated movements of the fingers and thumb. Children who have poor tactile discrimination receive less feedback about how their fingers move together and independently of one another. Children with cerebral palsy and those with sensory integration problems are likely to have tactile discrimination problems or tactile defensiveness. However, despite the strong theoretical link between tactile perception and hand skills and reports between the 1950s and 1970s of tactile dysfunction in children with cerebral palsy (Kenney, 1963; Monfraix, Tardieu, & Tardieu, 1961; Tachdjian & Minear, 1958; Twitchell, 1965), recent research with this population of children has been minimal.

In a more recent study, Lenti, Radice, Cerioli, and Musetti (1991) discussed the results of a tactile extinction study in children, adolescents, and young adults with hemiplegia. Approximately 60% of the individuals in this study were unable to identify two textures presented simultaneously.

Case-Smith (1991) studied the relationship between both tactile defensiveness and tactile discrimination and in-hand manipulation skills in 50 children between the ages of 4 and 6 years. In this sample, which included 80% nondysfunctional children, those having problems with either tactile defensiveness or decreased tactile discrimination showed no significant problems with performing the in-hand manipulation tasks presented. However, those who had both tactile discrimination problems and tactile defensiveness did have difficulty with performance of the in-hand manipulation tasks that were timed. Their performances were significantly slower than the children in the other groups. Further investigation of the relationship between tactile functioning and various hand skills is needed.

### Sensory Integration

The types of sensory integration problems (see Chapter 13) that are most likely to influence hand use are tactile defensiveness, poor bilateral integration, and dyspraxia. The child with tactile defensiveness is likely to avoid contact with certain materials, thus limiting exposure to various objects. Bilateral integration dysfunction limits development of in-hand manipulation and bilateral hand use. Motor planning deficits may be associated with poor body scheme (particularly poor awareness of the fingers as individual units) and poor tactile discrimination (Ayres, 1979). In many cases children have difficulty motor planning and with motor control.

### Visual Perception and Cognition

Perceptual and cognitive development can be difficult to isolate from one another, particularly as they relate to object-handling skills in children; therefore these areas are addressed together in this section. Visual perceptual, tactile perceptual, and cognitive development interact with development of hand skills. Development in hand skills allows for more complex interaction with objects, and perceptual and cognitive development allow the child to know the possibilities available for object use and interactions.

The child's perception of object characteristics, movement speed required, and power needed affect his or her ability to effectively control objects (Elliott & Connolly, 1984). Certain aspects of knowledge about objects are typically acquired through object manipulation.

During an infant's first 6 months, visual and tactile stimuli are used to guide fine motor development as the infant begins to develop an awareness of object placement in space (Corbetta & Mounoud, 1990). In the second half of the first year, the infant adjusts actions of the hand in response to object characteristics such as size, shape, and surface qualities (Corbetta & Mounoud, 1990). Ruff, McCarton, Kurtzber, and Vaughan (1984) emphasized the importance of object manipulation between 6 and 12 months of age for learning of object characteristics because this learning was believed to be important for concept and language development. Infants reflect their perceptual and cognitive skills in preparation for object contact. Corbetta and Mounoud (1990) noted that, by 9 to 10 months of age, infants adapt their arm positions to horizontal versus vertical object presentations and shape their hands appropriately for convex and concave objects.

During the second year infants learn to relate objects to one another with more accuracy and purpose. Before 18 months of age infants modify their movement approach to the anticipated weight of the object (Corbetta & Mounoud, 1990).

Exner and Henderson (1995) discussed the interaction of cognition and hand skill development. Like perceptual development, cognitive development seems to influence and be supported by development of hand skills. For example, changes in attentional control and development of problem-solving strategies are seen in the gradual improvement in infants' ability to handle two objects. Without this development in cognition, bilateral skills would not be possible because the infant must be able to attend to two objects simultaneously to be able to bang objects together, to stabilize an object with one hand while manipulating with the other, and to manipulate two or more objects simultaneously (e.g., in buttoning or tying). Corbetta and Mounoud (1990) noted that attention and planning demands were much greater for two-handed activities than for one-handed activities; thus bilateral skill development tends to lag behind unilateral skill development.

## Social Factors

Social factors that may affect the development of hand skills include socioeconomic status, gender, and role expectations. Like culture, these factors are less likely to affect development of more basic hand skills but may have a greater impact on skills needed for the complex manipulation of objects and tool use. For example, children in conditions of poverty may not have exposure to writing utensils, scissors, and other materials common to children from middle class environments.

## Cultural Factors

Object manipulation is done with objects that are important in a particular culture. The tools important in one culture may not be available in another culture; therefore children may not have the opportunity to develop some tool-specific skills. For example, eating utensils may vary from chopsticks to forks and spoons. Scissor use may be important for school performance in some cultures but not addressed in others.

In addition, the age at which children are expected to achieve skill in object manipulation may vary. Safety concerns may influence parents in some cultural groups to delay the introduction of a knife to their child, whereas other parents may encourage independence in knife use. The use of writing materials may be introduced by some cultures to children younger than age 1 year; yet in other groups children would not be given these materials until they could be consistently expected to adhere to requirements such as only using them on paper (vs. on the wall or on clothing).

Another factor that is influenced by culture is children's need for manipulative materials. Linked to this is the cultural group's view of the importance of play. Play materials that provide opportunities for development of manipulative skills (such as building sets, beads, puzzles, and table games) are highly valued in some cultural groups, whereas in other groups, play with gross motor objects such as balls and riding toys or play with animals may be more valued. In some cultural groups, children's play may not be viewed as highly important; thus few play materials of any type are available.

Apparently, although types of activities encouraged may promote the development of specific skills, acquisition of basic hand skills of reach, grasp, release, and manipulation does not rely on the availability of any particular materials. However, it does rely on reasonable exposure to a variety of materials with the opportunity to handle them.

## MOTOR AND PHYSICAL FACTORS
### Integrity of the Hand

The integrity of the hand is an important consideration in hand function. Children with congenital hand anomalies may be missing one or more digits, thus significantly affecting the variety of possible prehension patterns. Refined finger movements and in-hand manipulation skills may also be limited or absent. Severe congenital anomalies can affect bilateral hand use. Involvement of the thumb has a more significant effect on hand function development than impairment of any other digit.

## Range of Joint Motion

Range of joint motion has a significant effect on positioning the arm for hand use and reaching and carrying skills. Effective hand function is also dependent on adequate mobilization of distal muscle groups that control palmar arches. Limitations in range may occur as a result of abnormal joint structure, muscle weakness, and joint inflammation. Any of the problems that decrease range of motion are likely to affect the child's ability to grasp larger objects or to flatten the hand for use in stabilizing materials.

## Strength

Sufficient strength is necessary to initiate all types of grasp patterns and to maintain these patterns during carrying. Children with poor strength may be unable to initiate the finger extension or the thumb opposition pattern necessary before grasp. They also may not have the flexor control to hold a grasp pattern. Many children with decreased strength are unable to use patterns that rely on the intrinsic muscles for control and are therefore unable to use thumb opposition or metacarpophalangeal (MCP) joint flexion with interphalangeal (IP) joint extension. Children with fair strength may be able to initiate a grasp pattern but may be unable to lift an object against gravity while maintaining the grasp. Endurance during an activity can be a problem for children with mildly decreased strength, particularly in situations in which they must use a sustained grasp pattern or use the object as it is held against resistance.

## Tone

Tone within muscle groups affects the stability of parts of the upper extremities during activities as well as the types of movements possible. Tone abnormalities, caused by damage to the central nervous system, can affect range of joint motion and, in general, decrease speed of movement. Increased tone tends to result in loss of range; decreased tone results in exaggerated joint range and decreased stability. Children with fluctuating tone typically have full range, but they can maintain joint stability only at the extreme end of a joint position (full flexion or full extension). In addition, movements are less controlled and often appear to be random or unrelated to the task.

## GENERAL DEVELOPMENTAL CONSIDERATIONS

The following are several key principles that have been used to describe the development of motor skills:

▲ Mass to specific
▲ Gross to fine
▲ Proximal to distal

The mass to specific principle indicates that less differentiated movement patterns precede discrete, highly specialized skills. For example, all fingers are used in early grasping; later only the specific number of fingers needed for object contact are used.

The gross to fine principle suggests that gross motor patterns emerge before fine motor patterns. This principle is questioned on the basis of the extensive data that demonstrate infants' early development of visuomotor skills and their ability to use basic forms of reach and grasp before 6 months of age. Both gross and fine motor skills develop substantially during the infant's first year. Refinement in these basic skills and acquisition of complex gross and fine motor skills continue through the preschool and early school years. Gradually more integration of gross and fine motor skills occurs, as is seen in the child's ability to sustain and adjust postural control while engaged in complex fine motor tasks such as typing, writing, and shoe tying.

The proximal to distal principle of development has been used to suggest that development initially occurs proximally (in the head and trunk) and then gradually progresses toward the distal parts of the body (hands and feet). This principle has been used by therapists in planning and explaining intervention for children who have difficulty with hand skills. Therapists have often considered that it was necessary for a child to develop improved proximal skills before it was appropriate to address distal skills in treatment. Sometimes the inference has been that when a child's proximal skills improved, distal skills would automatically improve as well. However, this principle has been called into question by several clinical research studies (Case-Smith, Fisher, & Bauer, 1989; Wilson & Trombly, 1984) and by Pehoski (1992) in her chapter addressing central nervous system control of precision movements of the hand. The clinical studies have yielded correlations between postural or proximal control and hand function of approximately 0.20 to 0.35. Only in the Case-Smith et al. (1989) study was the obtained correlation ($r = 0.35$) statistically significant. However, even this correlation is low and indicates that the relationship between proximal and distal control is not a strong one. Case-Smith et al. (1989) stated that "the correlations between the proximal and distal motor functions would be markedly higher if proximal motor control were necessary for the development of distal motor skill" (p. 661). The relationship between proximal and distal control is a functional one or a biomechanical one in which postural control is necessary for placement of the hand in space and support of the hand during its execution of skills. Case-Smith et al. (1989) emphasized that "therapists should not assume that proximal control is a necessary precursor to fine motor skill; they should, however, assume that treating proximal weakness may affect distal function" (p. 661).

Pehoski (1992) used work by Lawrence and Kuypers (1968) to explain why distal control is not directly linked to proximal control. She described two motor systems used in upper extremity control. One system is responsible for postural control and proximal control, including integrated body-limb and body-head movements. This system comprises the medial and lateral brainstem pathways; synapses are primarily with interneurons for trunk and proximal muscles (Pehoski, 1992). In contrast, the corticospinal track system has its origin in the primary motor cortex, and its fibers directly synapse with the motoneurons for hand muscles. The latter system allows for isolated finger movements, which are needed for a precise pincer grasp and fine manipulation that is quick and precise (Pehoski, 1992). Thus development of upper extremity skills and hand skills may be described as occurring because of proximal *and* distal control mechanisms, rather than one proximal *to* distal mechanism.

Refined movements are also dependent on the ability to effectively combine *patterns of stability and mobility* (Bobath, 1978). The child must develop the ability to stabilize the trunk effectively and maintain it in an upright position without relying on frequent use of one or both arms to maintain balance. Also, the child sequentially develops patterns of stability and mobility in the scapulohumeral, elbow, and wrist joints. This permits arm use that is independent from, but effectively used with, trunk movement. Eventually the ability to use stability and mobility in the hand emerges.

For normal functioning, joints must be able to stabilize at any point within the normal range of movement and to move within small, medium, or large segments of range. At times during upper extremity fine motor activities, the proximal joints are more stable. Grasp is an example because the arm is stable while the fingers move. However, in carrying, the distal joints are more stable. In mature handwriting, the elbow, forearm, and wrist joints are stable and the shoulder and finger joints are mobile.

An important sequence in the development of motor control is the use of straight movement patterns before the emergence of controlled rotation patterns. For example, the baby first develops controlled stability and mobility in basic flexion and extension of the shoulder, elbow, and wrist. This is followed by control of internal and external rotation of the shoulder and pronation and supination of the forearm. In normal development the infant progresses from gross asymmetric patterns to generalized symmetries and then to mature, voluntarily controlled asymmetric patterns. This sequence is dependent on the child's maturing ability to dissociate movements from one another for specialized purposes. The baby uses the upper extremities initially in patterns that are not coordinated. Movements of one arm often elicit reflexive, nonpurposeful reactions in the other arm. Gradually, the baby develops the ability to move the two arms together in the same pattern. As skilled use of symmetric hand and arm patterns is refined, the baby begins to use the two arms discriminatively for different parts of an activity. For example, an object is stabilized with one hand while the other hand is used to manipulate it. Overflow and associated movements gradually decrease to allow separate but coordinated action of the two hands together.

## DEVELOPMENT OF HAND SKILLS

As in all areas of occupational therapy, academic study of hand skill development and treatment must be supplemented with clinical awareness. Directed observation in practice settings is highly recommended. In addition, it is helpful to imitate each of the normal and abnormal movements and patterns described in the text, both as isolated actions and within the context of activity performance.

### Reach

The random arm movements of the newborn are asymmetric. Soon, however, the baby shows increasing visual regard of the hands and objects close to him or her. This visual awareness is followed by swiping or batting objects, with the arm abducted at the shoulder. Objects are rarely grasped, and then only by accident, because the baby is not yet able to sustain an open hand while stabilizing the arm away from the body.

Gradually a midline orientation of the hands develops. Initially the hands are held close to the body, but, with an increased desire for visual regard and greater control of postural extension, the child holds the hands further away to view them. This pattern precedes the onset of symmetric bilateral reaching, usually first in supine and then in sitting. Reach is initiated with humeral abduction, partial shoulder internal rotation, forearm pronation, and full finger extension.

As the baby shows increasing dissociation of the two body sides during movement, unilateral reaching begins. Abduction and internal rotation of the shoulder are less prominent, but the hand is usually more open than necessary for the size of the object. As scapular control and trunk stability mature, the baby begins to use shoulder flexion, slight external rotation, full elbow extension, forearm supination, and slight wrist extension during reaching. It should be noted that active supination of the forearm is not seen until some external rotation is used to stabilize the humerus. Mature reach is usually seen in conjunction with sustained trunk extension and a slight rotation of the trunk toward the object of interest. Over the next few years the child refines this unilateral reaching pattern, increasing accuracy of arm placement and grading of finger extension as appropriate to a specific object (Figure 12-1).

### Hand Reflexes: Influence on Arm and Hand Use

Twitchell (1965) described a series of hand reflexes occurring in the young infant. These reflexes influence the normal infant's hand use and may predominate when the child with central nervous system damage is unable to inhibit the reflexive movements. Although strong influence usually diminishes within the first year, Twitchell found that elements of the hand reflexes may be seen through the preschool years.

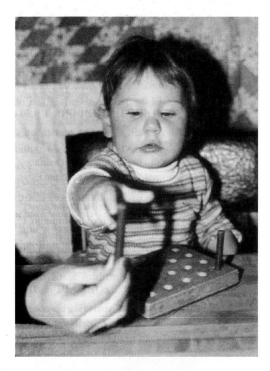

**Figure 12-1** This normal child demonstrates reach with trunk rotation, full elbow extension, slight forearm rotation, and wrist stability, yet some degree of excess finger extension before grasp. (Photograph by Ed Exner.)

The earliest occurring hand reflex is the *traction response* (Twitchell, 1965). This is a pattern of strong flexion throughout the upper extremity when the shoulder is passively abducted. This response is present in newborns and gradually diminishes in strength over the next 5 months.

The *grasp reflex* (Twitchell, 1965) may be a full reaction or a less complete response, called fractionation of the grasp reflex. When the baby is about 4 weeks old, tactile stimulation to the radial portion of the palm and web space of the thumb elicits a response of thumb and index finger adduction. Over the following weeks, broader contact with the palm and proximal surface of the finger is needed to elicit the reflex, but the response is also one of more complete finger flexion and adduction.

By 3 to 4 months, stimulation of the grasp reflex must include proprioceptive and tactile qualities. Contact must originate in the radial part of the palm and move toward the distal part of the hand. The baby responds with rapid, mass finger flexion. If resistance is given to the baby's finger movement, flexion is sustained. This reflex is usually no longer evident at 4 to 5 months of age, at which time more isolated hand use is established.

As the full grasp reflex diminishes, the fractionated pattern occurs. Ammon and Etzel (1977) identified the stimulus for this reaction as proprioceptive input to one finger on its palmar surface. Presence of the fractionated reflex is evidenced by flexion of an isolated finger.

The *avoiding reaction* (Twitchell, 1965) appears in the neonatal period and persists throughout infancy. However, it is not fully integrated until the child is 6 to 7 years old. This reaction occurs in response to stimuli that is applied to the back of the hand and fingers, the ulnar border of the hand, or the palmar surface of the fingertips. The reflex reaction acts to move the hand away from the stimulation by pronating or supinating differentially in response to radial or ulnar hand contact.

The *instinctive grasp reaction* (Twitchell, 1965) helps the baby develop an appropriate orientation of the hand to the object being grasped. The stimulus may be either stationary or moving light touch along either the radial or ulnar side of the hand. At 4 to 5 months, radial contact elicits a slight supination of the forearm, but by 7 to 8 months the hand gropes to find an object presented at either side. By 8 to 10 months the baby follows a moving stimulus with his or her hand.

## Grasp

### Classifications of Grasp Patterns

Napier (1956) proposed two basic terms to describe hand movements: prehensile and nonprehensile. *Nonprehensile movements* involve pushing or lifting the object with the fingers or the entire hand. In contrast, *prehensile movements* involve grasp of an object and may be further divided according to purpose of the grasp: precision or power. *Precision grasps* are characterized by opposition of the thumb to fingertips to hold an object. *Power grasps* involve the entire hand and are used to resist forces on the object being held. The thumb may be held flexed or abducted to other fingers according to control requirements.

The grasp pattern used is usually determined by the intended activity and characteristics of the object. Small objects are generally held in a precision grasp primarily because of the large amount of sensory feedback that is available through the fingertips and the control that can be used to move them. Medium objects may be held with either pattern, and large objects are held with a power grasp. Napier (1956) noted a frequent interplay between precision and power handling of different objects according to the activity.

A slightly different method of classification, described by Weiss and Flatt (1971), also uses thumb position as a determinant. Grasps with no thumb opposition include hook and power grasps and lateral pinch. The patterns that use thumb opposition include tip and palmar pinches. The palmar pinch category is further divided into standard, spherical, cylindrical, and disc grasps.

The *hook grasp* is used when strength of grasp must be maintained to carry objects. The transverse metacarpal arch is essentially flat, fingers are adducted with flexion at the IP joints, and flexion or extension occurs at the MCP joints (Weiss & Flatt, 1971) (Figure 12-2).

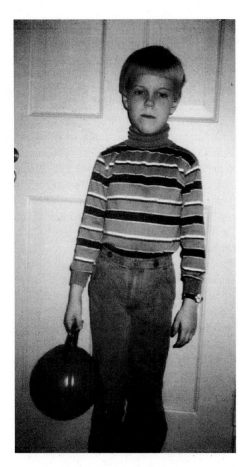

**Figure 12-2**    Hook grasp.

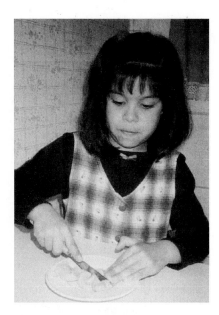

**Figure 12-3**    Power grasp with the right hand.

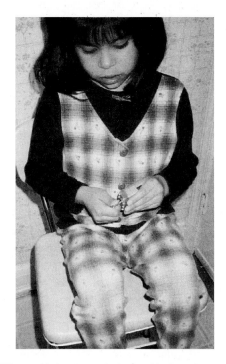

**Figure 12-4**    Lateral pinch with the left hand.

In contrast, the *power grasp* is often used to control tools or other objects. Maximum power is obtained with horizontal placement of the object in the palm and full thumb and finger flexion (Weiss & Flatt, 1971). Precision handling with this grasp, for hairbrushing as an example, is facilitated by oblique placement in the hand, more finger extension on the radial side of the hand, and thumb extension and adduction. Thus the object is stabilized with the ulnar side of the hand and controlled for position and use by the radial side of the hand (Weiss & Flatt, 1971) (Figure 12-3).

*Lateral pinch* is used to exert power on or with a small object. This pattern is characterized by partial thumb adduction, MCP extension, and IP flexion. The index finger is held in a slightly flexed position. The pad of the thumb is placed against the radial side of the index finger at or near the distal interphalangeal (DIP) joint (Figure 12-4).

There are two types of *standard* palmar pinches. When the thumb is opposed to the index finger pad only, this pattern may be referred to as pad to pad (Smith & Benge, 1985), standard palmar pinch (Weiss & Flatt, 1971), two-point pinch (Smith & Benge, 1985), or pincer grasp (Figure 12-5) (Gesell & Amatruda, 1947). Opposition of the thumb simultaneously to index and middle finger pads, which provides increased stability of prehension, has been

called three-point pinch (Smith & Benge, 1985), three-jaw chuck (Erhardt, 1982), and radial digital grasp (Gesell & Amatruda, 1947) (Figure 12-6).

*Tip pinch* is characterized by opposition of the thumb and index fingertip so that a circle is formed (Figure 12-7). All joints of the finger and thumb are partially flexed. This pinch pattern is used to obtain small objects.

Differences in hand posture characterize the other palmar grasps. *Spherical grasp* is marked by significant wrist

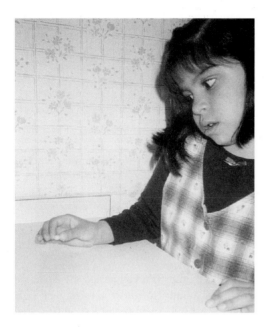

**Figure 12-5**    Pincer grasp.

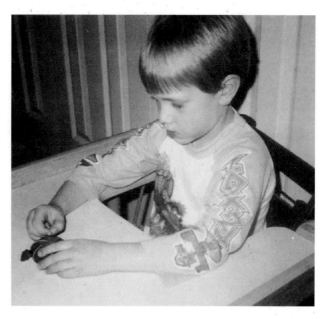

**Figure 12-7**    Tip pinch. Normal radial grasps, such as tip pinch, are accompanied by slight forearm supination.

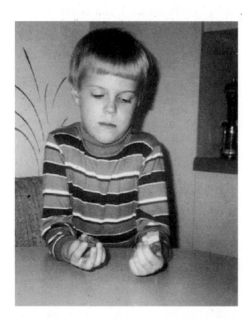

**Figure 12-6**    This child is using a three-jaw chuck grasp with his left hand and a variation of this grasp pattern with the right.

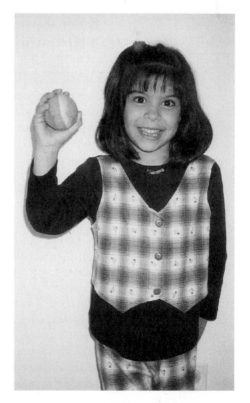

**Figure 12-8**    Spherical grasp.

extension, finger abduction, and even flexion at the MCP and IP joints (Figure 12-8). Stability of the longitudinal arch is necessary to use this pattern to grasp large objects. The hypothenar eminence lifts to assist the cupping of the hand for control of the object (Weiss & Flatt, 1971).

In the *cylindrical grasp* the transverse arch is flattened to allow the fingers to hold against the object. The fingers are only slightly abducted, and IP and MCP joint flexion is graded according to the size of the object. When additional force is required, more of the palmar surface of the hand contacts the object (Weiss & Flatt, 1971) (Figure 12-9).

*Disc grasp* (Weiss & Flatt, 1971) is characterized by finger abduction that is graded according to the size of the object held, hyperextension of the MCP joints, and flexion of the IP joints (Figure 12-9). This wrist is more flexed when objects are larger, and only the pads of the fingers contact

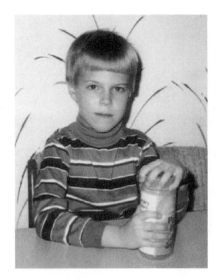

**Figure 12-9**   The child uses a cylindrical grasp with his right hand and a disc grasp with his left.

the object. The amount of thumb extension also increases with object size. The transverse metacarpal arch is flattened in this prehension pattern.

### Sequential Development of Grasp Patterns

Several developmental trends affect the particular type of grasp pattern that an infant is able to use at any time. The following sequences interact and overlap (see box).

These motor sequences are influenced by the baby's growing interest in objects, desire to attain them, and desire to explore them and how they can relate to other objects. Visual perceptual development contributes to the baby's ability to shape the hand appropriately for the object and to approach the object with optimal orientation of the arm and hand.

Other aspects of motor development that contribute to the baby's use of increasingly mature and greater variety of patterns is the ability to use thumb opposition, internal stability throughout the upper extremity, and forearm supination. Thumb activity and control are necessary to allow for patterns other than palmar grasp. Hirschel, Pehoski, and Coryell (1990) discussed the impact of increasing arm stability on the baby's use of a mature pincer grasp. The ability to stabilize the wrist in a slightly extended position is important for grasp patterns that use distal (fingertip) control. Slight forearm supination is important because it positions the hand so that the thumb and radial fingers are free for active object exploration and it allows the baby to view his or her fingers and thumb during grasp.

The following sequence is typical during the infant's first 6 months. Initially the infant appears to have no voluntary hand use. The hands alternately open and close in response to various sensory stimuli. Gradually, the traction response and grasp reflex decrease and a voluntary ulnar grasp be-

## Sequential Development of Grasp

▲ Ulnar grasp → palmar grasp → radial grasp
▲ Palmar contact → finger surface contact → finger pad contact (Hohlstein, 1982)
▲ Use of long finger flexors → use of intrinsic muscles with extrinsic muscles (long flexors and extensors)

gins to emerge. Within the next few months the baby progresses to being able to use a palmar grasp (by approximately 6 months).

The second 6 months is a key period for development of hand skills. The ability to grasp a variety of objects increases significantly between 6 and 9 months of age. During this time grasp patterns with active thumb use emerge. Crude raking of a tiny object is present by about 7 months of age, and by 9 months the infant is able to attain a tiny object on the finger surface and with the thumb. However, on larger objects, the infant's grasp appears much more mature. By 8 to 9 months of age a radial digital grasp pattern (thumb opposed to two or more fingers) is present and can be readily varied to the shape of the object. However, intrinsic muscle control does not appear to be present because the infant does not use grasp with MCP flexion and IP extension. Between 9 and 12 months refinement occurs in the ability to use thumb and finger pad control for tiny and small objects. This refinement also is characterized by more precise preparation of the fingers before initiating grasp, more inhibition of the ulnar fingers, and slight wrist extension and forearm supination.

After 1 year of age, further refinement occurs in grasp patterns that were seen earlier and more sophisticated patterns emerge. Between 12 and 15 months of age increasing control of the intrinsic muscles may be seen in the baby's ability to hold crackers, cookies, and other flat objects. Although studies are limited in terms of grasp development for patterns other than the pincer grasp, it appears that between 18 months and 3 years of age most children with typical development acquire the ability to use a power grasp, a disc grasp, a cylindrical grasp, and a spherical grasp with control. The pattern for a lateral pinch may be present by 3 years of age, but children may not be able to functionally use this pattern until later in the preschool years.

### In-Hand Manipulation Skills
#### Classifications

Three basic patterns of in-hand manipulation have been identified: translation, shift, and rotation. More recently, in-hand manipulation was described as including five basic types of patterns: finger-to-palm translation, palm-to-finger translation, shift, simple rotation, and complex rotation (Exner, 1992). Long, Conrad, Hall, and Furler (1970) described translation as a linear movement of the object from the palm to the fingers or the fingers to the palm: the object stays in constant contact with the thumb and fingers during this pattern—the fingers and thumb maintain grasp but then move into and out of MCP and IP flexion and extension. In contrast, in Exner's descriptions of the pattern of finger-to-palm translation, the object is grasped at the pads of the fingers and thumb but then is moved into the palm (Exner, 1992). The finger pad grasp is released so that the object rests in the palm of the open hand or is held in a palmer grasp at the conclusion of the pattern. The object moves in a linear direction within the hand, and the fingers move from a more extended position to a more flexed position during the translation. An example of this skill is picking up a coin with the fingers and thumb and moving it into the palm of the hand.

Palm-to-finger translation is the reverse of the finger-to-palm translation pattern. However, palm-to-finger translation requires isolated control of the thumb and use of a pattern beginning with finger flexion and moving to finger extension. This pattern is linear but is more difficult for the child to execute than is finger-to-palm translation. An example of this skill is moving a coin from the palm of the hand to the finger pads before placing the coin in a vending machine.

Shift involves a linear movement of the object on the finger surface (Exner, 1992) to allow for repositioning of the object relative to the pads of the fingers. In this pattern the fingers move just slightly at the MCP and IP joints, and the thumb typically remains opposed or adducted with MCP and IP extension throughout the shift. The object usually is held solely on the radial side of the hand. Examples of this skill include separating two pieces of paper when they seem slightly stuck together, moving a coin from a position against the volar aspect of the DIP joints to a position closer to the fingertips (e.g., so that the coin can be placed easily into the slot on the vending machine), and adjusting a pen or pencil after grasp so the fingers are positioned close to the writing end of the tool. This skill seems to be used frequently in dressing tasks such as buttoning, fastening snaps, putting laces through the holes on shoes, and putting a belt through beltloops.

Two patterns of rotation have been identified: simple and complex. Simple rotation involves the turning or rolling of an object held at the finger pads approximately 90 degrees or less (Exner, 1992). The fingers act as a unit (little or no differentiation of action is shown among them), and the thumb is in an opposed position. Unscrewing a small bottle cap and picking up a small peg from a surface and rotating it from a horizontal to a vertical position for placement into a pegboard are examples of simple rotation. Another example is reorienting a puzzle piece within the hand by turning it slightly before placing it into the puzzle.

Complex rotation involves the rotation of an object 180 to 360 degrees once or repetitively (Exner, 1992). During complex rotation the fingers and thumb alternate in producing the movement, and the fingers typically move independently of one another. An object may be moved end over end, such as in turning a coin or a peg over or in turning a pencil over to use the eraser.

## In-Hand Manipulation Skills Without and With Stabilization

Exner (1990a, 1992) has described all in-hand manipulation skills as being used when one object is held in the hand and when several objects are held in the hand and manipulation of one object occurs while simultaneously stabilizing the others. For example, a child typically unscrews a bottle lid with no other objects in his or her hand; this illustrates the skill of simple rotation. However, a child may have two or more pieces of cereal in his or her hand but only bring one piece out to the finger pads before placement in the mouth; this illustrates the use of palm-to-finger translation with stabilization. Thus the term *with stabilization* refers to the use of an in-hand manipulation skill while other objects are being stabilized in the hand. Any of the in-hand manipulation skills done with stabilization is more difficult than the same skill done without the simultaneous stabilization of objects in the hand.

## Developmental Considerations

Motor skill prerequisites for in-hand manipulation include the following:

▲ Movement into and stability in various degrees of supination
▲ Wrist stability
▲ An opposed grasp with thumb opposition and object contact with the finger surface (not in the palm)
▲ Isolated thumb and radial finger movement
▲ Control of the transverse metacarpal arch
▲ Disassociation of the radial and ulnar sides of the hand

Children who are unable to use in-hand manipulation skills are likely to substitute other patterns. These patterns appear to be part of the normal developmental process for acquisition of in-hand manipulation skills, so their use does not necessarily represent abnormal fine motor control. Typical patterns used when the child has no evidence of in-hand manipulation are a change of hands—to put the object in the other hand for use—and transferring from hand to hand—to move the object from one hand to the other and back to the hand that held it first. These patterns are used after the initial grasp when the child realizes that the object within his or her hand needs to be repositioned to use it, but the child cannot readily adjust the object within that hand. To adjust the position the child moves the object to the other hand (and perhaps back to the first hand). A typical example is for a child to pick up a crayon or marker with one hand but not be able to shift it so that the fingers are near the writing end so he or she grasps the object with the other hand with the fingers appropriately positioned. Some children seem to preplan for this by picking up the crayon with the nonpreferred hand then changing it to the preferred hand.

Several skills may be observed in children who are beginning to use in-hand manipulation skills or are preparing for the use of these skills. The substitutions or precursors involve supporting the object while the hand is changing position on it. The type of support used may depend on the type of in-hand manipulation skill being used. Infants typically engage in bilateral manipulation of objects by moving an object between the two hands. As the object is moved between the hands it is turned and repositioned within the hands. Children may use this strategy, called a *hand assist,* when faced with the need to rotate an object, or they may use palm-to-finger translation. In this case the object does not leave the hand that grasped it initially, but the other hand helps with repositioning of the object. There is clear use of the fingers to assist with the repositioning of the object; the fingers participate in the object manipulation.

Other common types of assists for beginning manipulation include the body assist and the surface assist. In the body assist, the object is supported on a part of the body (typically the chest or the face) while the fingers change position on the object. For the surface assist, the object is supported on a surface (such as a table) while the fingers change position on the object. All of the assist strategies seem to be most commonly used for shift and complex rotation.

Ongoing research by Exner (1990a, 1993) is directed toward determining a sequence for in-hand manipulation skill development and an instrument useful for clinical and research purposes for these skills. The following developmental sequence has been identified. By approximately 12 to 15 months of age, toddlers seem to use finger-to-palm translation to pick up and "hide" small pieces of food in their hands. By 2 to 2½ years of age, toddlers use palm-to-finger translation and simple rotation with some objects, although these skills may not be seen with stabilization of other objects in the hand simultaneously. By 3 to 3½ years of age, children begin to use shift and complex rotation with easy-to-handle objects. Between 3½ and 5½ years of age children develop skills in rotating a marker (regardless of its initial orientation) and shifting it into an optimal position for coloring and writing. Combinations of in-hand manipulation skills that must be used within an activity, such as palm-to-finger translation with stabilization followed by complex rotation with stabilization, become more consis-

tently used between the ages of 6 and 7. Ongoing research suggests that in-hand manipulation skills continue to be refined through at least 8 years of age.

However, the presence of a skill with one type of object is not always associated with the child being able to use the skill with another size or shape of an object. For example, the child may be able to use simple rotation to turn a small peg but may not use simple rotation to orient a crayon for coloring. In general, it appears that small objects (e.g., the smaller-diameter crayons) are easier for children to manipulate than are slightly larger objects (e.g., the larger-diameter crayons) or tiny objects. Tiny objects require precise fingertip control, whereas medium and larger objects require control with more fingers than do small objects.

Skills with stabilization always emerge after the child has developed some competency with the skill while holding only the one object to be manipulated. The easiest skill with stabilization is finger-to-palm translation with stabilization. The most difficult skills are shift with stabilization and complex rotation with stabilization.

In addition to object characteristics and the need for using an in-hand manipulation skill with or without stabilization, other factors may contribute to the child's use of these skills with any particular materials. These factors include the cognitive-perceptual demands of the activity, the child's interest in the manipulative materials or the activity, and the child's motor planning skills. Problems in any of these areas or in processing tactile-proprioceptive information or in visual acuity could affect development of in-hand manipulation skills.

## Carry

Carrying involves a smooth combination of body movements while stabilizing an object in the hand. Small ranges of movements are used and adjusted in accordance with the demands of the tasks. Cocontraction often occurs in the more distal joints of the wrist and hand. The forearm must be able to be held stable while in any position. Frequently the forearm position and the wrist position must be able to be modified during the carry so that the object remains in an optimal position. Similarly, the child must be able to use shoulder rotation patterns simultaneously with shoulder flexion and abduction.

## Voluntary Release

Voluntary release, like grasp, depends on control of arm movements. To place an object for release, the arm needs to move into position accurately and then stabilize as the fingers and thumb extend. Ayres (1954) stated that the development of smooth, accurate release of small objects normally takes several years. Initially, the baby does not voluntarily release an object, and often objects either must be forcibly removed from the baby's hand in the presence of a strong grasp reflex or they drop involuntarily from the hand.

As the baby's nondiscriminative responses to tactile and proprioceptive stimuli decrease and visual control and cognitive development increase, more volitional control of release occurs. As mouthing of objects increases and the baby becomes more proficient in bringing both hands to midline and playing with them there, the transfer of objects from one hand to another emerges. Initially the object is stabilized in the mouth during transfers or is pulled out of one hand by the other. Soon the baby begins to freely transfer the object from one hand to another. The object is stabilized by the receiving hand, and the releasing hand is fully opened.

By 9 months of age the baby begins to release objects without stabilizing with the other hand. The arm is fully extended during release (Connor, Williamson, & Siepp, 1978). Shoulder control appears to develop in conjunction with voluntary release as the baby freely drops objects. The next step is development of elbow stability in various positions, and the baby begins to release with the elbow in more flexion. The arm or hand may be stabilized on the surface during release. At about 1 year, objects are released with shoulder, elbow, and wrist stability, but the MCP joints remain unstable during this pattern so that the child continues to show excess finger extension (Figure 12-10). Gradually the child develops the ability to release objects into smaller containers (Figure 12-11) and to stack blocks (Figure 12-12). The release pattern is refined over the next few years until the child can release small objects with graded

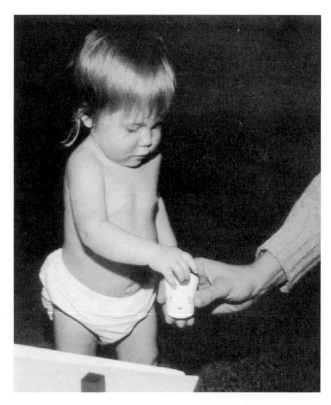

**Figure 12-11** Shoulder, elbow, and wrist are stable and less finger extension occurs with release. The child can release objects into a small container. (Courtesy Kennedy Kreiger Institute, Baltimore, MD.)

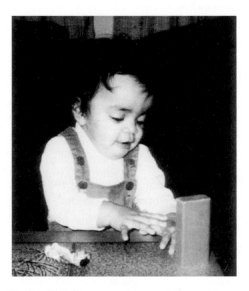

**Figure 12-10** Full finger extension and some wrist movement occur with voluntary release.

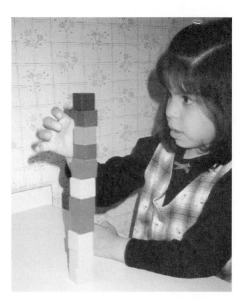

**Figure 12-12** Shoulder, elbow, forearm, wrist, and finger stability combines with perceptual development to promote accurate placement of objects off a surface.

extension of the fingers, indicating control over the intrinsic muscle groups of the hand.

## Bilateral Hand Use

As discussed earlier, the normal baby progresses from asymmetry to symmetry to differentiated asymmetric movements in bilateral hand use. Asymmetric movements occur up to about 3 months. Symmetric patterns predominate between 3 and 10 months, when bilateral reach, grasp, and mouthing of the hands and objects occur. These movements are controlled primarily at the shoulder, with the hands engaged at midline. By 9 to 10 months the baby can hold one object in each hand and bang them together. More complex bilateral symmetric skills, such as catching or bouncing a large ball, develop later in childhood.

The ability to use differentiated movements begins at about 8 to 10 months. Initially, arm movements are reciprocal or alternating. However, by 12 to 18 months materials are stabilized with and without grasp, (Connor et al., 1978). For these skills to emerge, the baby must be able to dissociate the two sides of the body and begin to use the two hands simultaneously for different functions. Effective stabilization of materials, of course, also depends on adequate shoulder, elbow, and wrist stability.

Between 18 and 24 months the child begins to develop skills that are precursors to simultaneous manipulation. Bilateral skill refinement is heavily dependent on continuing development of reach, grasp, release, and in-hand manipulation skills. Visual-perceptual, cognitive, and motor skills development become more integrated, leading to the child's effective use of motor planning for task performance. Simultaneous manipulation is demonstrated at 2 to 3 years (Connor et al., 1978). The mature stage of bilateral hand use, which is the ability to use opposing hand and arm movements for highly differentiated activities such as cutting with scissors, begins to emerge at about 2½ years. Patterns from each stage of bilateral hand use are applied and refined through different activities throughout the child's development.

## Ball-Throwing Skills

Ball-throwing skills may be viewed as reflecting the child's ability to use voluntary release skills. In throwing a small ball the child must sequence and time movements throughout the entire upper extremity. The child must bring the arm into a starting position, then prepare for projection of the ball into space by moving first the trunk with the scapulohumeral joint, then stabilize the shoulder while beginning to extend the elbow, then stabilize the elbow while moving the wrist from extension to a neutral position and simultaneously forcefully extending the fingers and thumb.

Children move through a progression of levels of skill before they can smoothly sequence these movements and project the ball to the desired location. By 2 years the child is expected to be able to throw a ball forward and to maintain balance so that his or her body also does not move forward (Sheridan, 1975); Folio and Fewell (1983) described the child as using extensor movements to fling the ball but not being able to sustain shoulder flexion during the toss. These descriptions illustrate the child's ability to disassociate trunk and arm movement by stabilizing the trunk while the arm is moving but not the ability to disassociate humeral and forearm movements. By 2½ to 3 years of age the child is able to aim the ball toward a target and project the ball approximately 3 feet forward (Folio & Fewell, 1983). This ability to control the direction of the ball to some degree implies that the child can control the humerus so that the elbow is in front of the shoulder when the ball is released. Thus the humerus is now able to be moved into a position and be stabilized there while the elbow and fingers move. By 3½ years of age the child is able to throw the ball 5 to 7 feet toward a target with little deviation from a straight line (Folio & Fewell, 1983). For this to occur the elbow must be positioned in front of the shoulder before the ball is released. Further refinement of ball throwing skills occurs over the next few years in distance and accuracy of the throw; such changes demonstrate the greater scapulohumeral control, the ability to sustain the humerus above the shoulder at least briefly, and the ability to control the timing of elbow, wrist, and finger extension. Thus at approximately 5 years of age a child is able to use an overhand throw to fairly consistently hit a target 5 feet away (Folio & Fewell, 1983). Six- to seven-year-olds are able to hit a target 12 feet away by using an overhand throw (Folio & Fewell, 1983). Underhand throws to contact a target are also possible in children who are 5 years old and older. This skill requires the ability to move the humerus into flexion while sustaining full external rotation.

## Tool Use

Connolly and Dalgleish (1989) defined a tool as being "a device for working on something . . . tools serve as extensions of the limbs and enhance the efficiency with which skills are performed" (p. 895). They defined *tool use* as "a purposeful, goal-directed form of complex object manipulation that involves the manipulation of the tool to change the position, condition or action of another object" (p. 895). A child's development of skill in using tools is critical for accomplishment of a wide variety of self-care, play and leisure, and school and work tasks. Skills in tool use for eating and play typically begin to emerge during the second year, after the child has mastered the basic skills of reach, grasp, and release. The skills seem to emerge concurrently with in-hand manipulation skills. In-hand manipulation skills are necessary for progression of tool use skills beyond grasp and release of the tool and relatively crude tool use because they allow for the tool to be adjusted in the hand after it is grasped. Tool use skills take several years to develop (Connolly & Elliott, 1972; Gilfoyle, Grady, & Moore, 1990).

A key factor in acquisition of skills with tool use skills is the reliance of these skills on cognitive development. Connolly and Dalgleish (1989) emphasized that an individual needs to know both what he or she wants to do (the intentional aspect of the task) and how he or she can accomplish the task (the operational aspect of the task). Both of these elements require development of the child's cognitive skills, with the latter relying on the child's motor skills as well.

Tool use skills in children seem to develop in a manner similar to grasp skills and in-hand manipulation skills in that initially the skills are not present, then they are accomplished with varying strategies (a child may show multiple strategies for the same task), and gradually the strategies are limited so that the focus is on efficiency in the skill and accomplishment of the goal. At this latter point elements of the entire process may be varied, but the basic motor pattern used is fairly consistent unless demands are significantly changed. Inconsistency is seen both within a child during the skill acquisition stage on different trials even within the same session, and across children of the same age, in whom multiple strategies are likely to be recorded for children who are beginning to use a particular skill. Thus inconsistency in the strategy used for performing a skill should be considered to be an important stage in the skill acquisition process.

Practice is important for any skill to be able to move from being performed with a high level of attention to a more automatic level. With such practice, performance becomes faster, more accurate, and smoother. Practice is typically necessary for a skill to become truly functional for execution in daily life tasks.

Acquisition of children's skills in using three tools have received some degree of study. The area receiving the most study has been in the drawing and writing tool use. For a description of this type of tool use see Chapter 19.

Schneck and Bataglia (1992) provide a description of the development of scissors skills in young children. This skill emerges when the child first learns to place his or her fingers in the holes and open and close the scissors. Initial cutting is actually snipping, a process of simply closing the scissors on the paper, but with no movement of the paper and with no ability to repetitively open and close the scissors while flexing the shoulder and extending the elbow to move across the paper. Snipping may be done while the child's forearm is pronated. Three-year-old children may use a pronated forearm position or a forearm-in-midposition placement (Schneck & Battaglia, 1992), or they may alter-

nate between the two forearm positions. By 4 years of age children typically hold both forearms in midposition for the cutting activity.

According to the Peabody Developmental Motor Scales (Folio & Fewell, 1983), by 2 years of age children can snip with scissors, by 2½ years of age most children can cut across a 6-inch piece of paper, by 3 to 3½ years they can cut on a line that is 6-inches long, by 3½ to 4 years they can cut a circle, and by 4½ to 5 years they can cut a square. More complex cutting skills develop between 6 and 7 years of age. Other factors that need to be considered in assessing the child's skill in cutting include the width of the line to cut on, the size of the paper, the size of the design to be cut, and the complexity of the design.

The child's grasp on the scissors can be expected to change over time. The thumb position in one hole tends to remain fairly consistent, but the finger positions change (Schneck & Battaglia, 1992). In a mature grasp, which may not be achieved until after the age of 6 years, the child has the middle finger in the lower hole of the handle, the ulnar two fingers flexed, and the index finger positioned to stabilize the lower part of the scissors (Myers, 1992; Schneck & Battaglia, 1992).

The general ages at which a child learns to use various utensils in eating has been described as spoon use by 18 months of age, fork use by 2½ years, and knife use by 6 years of age (Erhardt, 1992). However, documentation regarding how these skills are acquired and how various components of movement interact to produce skill has been limited. To address this issue, Connolly and Dalgleish (1989) conducted a longitudinal study of babies between 11 and 23 months of age to document their acquisition of spoon use skills. They analyzed videotapes of the infants' grasp patterns on the spoon; the placement of the spoon within the hand; movements used in filling the spoon, bringing it to the mouth, clearing the spoon, and taking it out of the mouth; and visual monitoring of the pattern, timing, and use of the nonpreferred hand in the eating process. They found that the mean number of grasp patterns decreased during the ages of 11 and 17 months and that the majority of 17-month-old and older infants showed a clear hand preference for eating. Ten different grasp patterns were used by the infants, but none used an adult pattern. The most commonly used pattern was a transverse palmar grasp with all four fingers flexed around the handle of the spoon. The next two most commonly used patterns were ones in which the fingers were flexed but the handle was on the finger surface rather than in the palm. In the 17- to 23-month-old infants this pattern was accompanied by some degree of index finger extension, which is a precursor to manipulation of the spoon's orientation within the hand. The infants became increasingly efficient in spoon use during this period and improved their visual monitoring of the process.

Another component to be considered in viewing the development of tool use in children is the role of the assisting hand. In handwriting and coloring, the assisting hand plays an important role in stabilizing the paper. In using scissors and eating, however, the role of the assisting hand is likely to be much more active. In cutting, this hand must hold the paper and orient it through rotation by moving in the same or opposite direction as the hand with the scissors. In eating, the child's assisting hand may be involved in a variety of activities, depending on the child's age and the utensils used. Connolly and Dalgleish (1989) found that infants between 18 and 23 months of age showed significantly more involvement of the assisting hand in stabilizing a dish during spoon feeding than did infants between 12 and 17 months of age. Learning to use a knife entails learning to stabilize food with one hand or with another tool while the preferred hand is used with the knife for spreading or cutting.

## RELATIONSHIP OF HAND SKILLS TO FUNCTIONAL PERFORMANCE OF DAILY LIFE SKILLS

Hand skills are vital to the child's interaction with the environment. Functional performance of daily life skills requires object handling; except in rare individuals who must compensate for lack of hand use with foot or mouth use, this object handling must be accomplished with the hands. Usually greater impairment of hand use results in the need for increased adaptations if the child is to function independently in daily life skills.

### Play

Although young infants engage with people and objects through their visual and auditory senses, these are distant senses and do not readily bring the infant the salient information that can only be gained through touch. Ruff (1980) described the importance of object handling in conjunction with visual exploration as a key vehicle for an infant learning object properties. It appears that the visual-haptic (touching) interaction serves to enhance the infant's ability to integrate sensory information and to learn that objects remain the same regardless of visual orientation. Typically this object handling in infants is called *play* because it is purposeful and done with pleasure. With increasing age, until at least the early school years, a great deal of play is dependent on competence in fine motor skills. These skills are reflected in the child's interest in activities such as cutting with scissors, dressing and undressing dolls, putting puzzles together, constructing with various types of building materials and model sets, participating in sand play, completing craft projects, and playing with jacks. Video games and computer use also require fine motor control but may not demand isolated finger control for game playing.

Some children may pursue play and leisure activities through organized groups such as Girl or Boy Scouts and 4-H, which tend to use projects that require manual skills as a key component of their programs.

### Self Care

Self-care skills also depend on the child's ability to use all types of fine motor skills. In the area of dressing, complex grasp patterns and in-hand manipulation skills are most evident in the use of fasteners, but the ability to use all types of bilateral skills and a wide variety of grasp patterns is useful for putting on and removing shirts, shoes, socks, and pants. The ability to handle jewelry relies on the ability to use delicate grasp patterns and in-hand manipulation.

Hygiene skills depend on the child's increasing ability to use fine motor skills with objects that are often slippery (e.g., the soap). In addition, these skills are likely to be done in a standing position, such as when brushing teeth, shaving, and applying makeup. A high level of skill in tool use is needed for complex hygiene activities such as shaving, makeup application, tweezer use, nail cutting, and hair styling (using barrettes, rubber bands, curling iron, brush, and hair dryer).

Eating skills rely on refinement of the ability to use forearm control with a variety of grasp patterns and tools. The ability to use both hands together effectively is necessary for spreading and cutting with a knife, opening all types of containers, pouring liquids, and preparing food. In-hand manipulation skills are used to adjust eating utensils and finger foods in one's hand, handle a napkin, and manipulate small packages of condiments and seasonings.

### School

Functioning within the school environment also requires the presence of effective fine motor skills. The preschool classroom presents children with a wide variety of manipulative activities, including use of crayons, scissors, small building materials, and puzzles and simple cooking and art projects. In kindergarten and the early elementary school years, children are expected to use fine motor skills most of the school day. In fact, McHale and Cermak (1992) found that 30% to 60% of the day for the first- and third-grade children in their study was spent in fine motor activities, and the primary fine motor activity was paper-pencil tasks. Any writing activity includes preparing one's paper, using an eraser, and getting writing tools in and out of a box. Other typical fine motor activities in childrens' classrooms include cutting with scissors, folding paper, using paste and tape, carrying out simple science projects, assuming responsibility for managing one's own snack and lunch items, and organizing and maintaining one's desk. Computer skills are also needed in most elementary classrooms.

For older children and adolescents, fine motor skills are needed for science projects, vocational courses (e.g., woodworking, metal shop, and home economics), art classes, music classes (other than vocal music), managing a high volume of written work and notebooks, and maintaining one's locker. Adolescents with learning disabilities and fine motor limitations have problems in these areas.

## GENERAL MOTOR PROBLEMS AFFECTING HAND SKILLS

Impairment of basic hand function (reach, grasp, carry, and release) in early childhood necessarily precludes emergence of more advanced hand skill and bilateral hand use. One of the more common problems is *inadequate isolation of movements.* Children who demonstrate this problem tend to use total patterns of flexion or extension throughout the upper extremities; they are unable to combine wrist extension with finger flexion or elbow flexion with finger extension. Similarly, the child is unable to perform differentiated motions with each arm and hand. Inadequate isolation of movements is handicapping even in early infancy because of the impact on the most basic reach and grasp skills.

Another common problem is *poorly graded movements.* Usually the extent of a movement is too great for the task, thus impairing accuracy of performance. This problem occurs when joint stability in the hand or proximal to the hand is not effective. For example, the child may be unable to hold the elbow in approximately 90 degrees of flexion and the wrist in neutral position during a grasp activity. Thus when initiating the grasp the child may overflex the fingers in an attempt to obtain the object before the arm posture is lost. Children with poorly graded movements lack the ability to effectively use the middle ranges of movement; instead they use too much flexion, extension, or any other movement. To compensate, some children learn to hold one or more joints in a locked position during attempts at hand use (Figure 12-13). Typical patterns used to increase stability include internal rotation of the shoulder, elbow extension, and hyperextension of the MCP joints. Problems with grading of movement are typically associated with abnormal tone, muscle weakness, or sensory integrative dysfunction. In the latter situation the child has difficulty perceiving and evaluating sensory feedback and so cannot accurately plan the extent of movements needed for a task. Disorders that cause poorly graded movements in infancy particularly affect the development of effective reach and release, as well as in-hand manipulation and bilateral hand use.

*Poor timing of movements* may also be a problem. Inadequate timing of muscle contractions leads to the use of movements that are too fast or too slow for the intended purpose. Movements that are too fast also tend to be poorly graded. Disorders of tone or muscle weakness are often the underlying factors in movement that is too slow. Instability

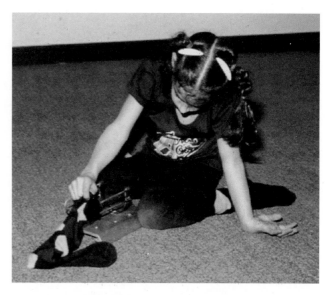

**Figure 12-13**   This child, who has involuntary movement, demonstrates the attempt to find stability by locking the elbows in extension and by elevating her right shoulder during hand use. She also has difficulty isolating upper extremity movements and using both hands together at midline. (Courtesy Kennedy Kreiger Institute, Baltimore, MD.)

at joints tends to cause disordered sequences of hand and arm movements. For example, wrist extensions may not be combined with the reach for an object but instead may occur after the grasp.

A fourth problem that affects hand function is a *disorder in bilateral integration of movements.* This affects both the normal symmetric and asymmetric movements needed to develop and use hand functions. Some children are unable to effectively bring both hands to midline or to maintain use of both hands at midline long enough to accomplish a task. Other children can hold objects symmetrically at midline but are unable to dissociate movements of the two upper extremities. Therefore they have difficulty with activities that require refined forms of bilateral hand use.

Many children have difficulty with hand use because of *limitations in trunk movement and control.* Central nervous system dysfunction or generalized muscle weakness may impair development or effective use of equilibrium reactions. Therefore the child may use one or both arms for support in maintaining sitting or standing positions. This significantly limits bilateral hand use and may limit the development of fine motor skills in the hand that the child most often uses for support.

Children with trunk instability or abnormal posture tend to have difficulty with smooth and accurate placement of the hand and arm that is being used for a fine motor task. When the trunk is postured in flexion, functional range of motion in the arm is limited (Figure 12-14). Conversely, hy-

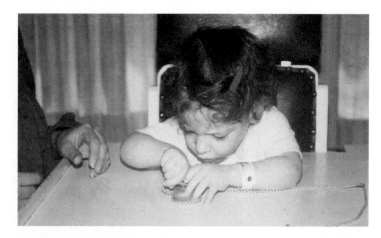

**Figure 12-14**   Poor trunk stability affects the upper extremity range of motion this child can use. Note her forearm pronation and wrist flexion on the right. She is unable to effectively use a three-jaw chuck or a pincer grasp on the materials. (Courtesy Kennedy Kreiger Institute, Baltimore, MD.)

perextension of the trunk tends to be accompanied by hyperextension of the humerus. The latter pattern typically causes one of three patterns of shoulder and elbow positioning: external rotation with elbow flexion, neutral rotation with elbow flexion, or internal rotation with elbow extension. Frequent posturing in any of these arm patterns affects the development of hand skills. Similarly, lateral trunk flexion causes the child to lean to one side and thus affects the child's ability to use the arm on the flexed side.

Any of these problems can contribute to the child's use of *compensatory patterns of movement.* In an effort to increase function the child seeks another pattern to substitute for movements impaired by the primary problem. For example, the child with weakness or instability may learn to use lateral trunk flexion to increase the height of the arm during reach. Or a child with increased tone may compensate for limited finger extension by using a wrist tenodesis action. Although these patterns may be effective initially, and in some cases may provide all of the independent function that is available to a child, development of higher level skills may be hindered by continued use of compensatory movements.

## ANALYSIS OF A HAND SKILL PROBLEM

A sample analysis of a functional problem that is at least partially caused by hand skill difficulties is presented in the box on p. 285. In this example the therapist has identified two main components of this functional problem: the lack of in-hand manipulation skills and the breakage of materials be-ing handled. The therapist then attempts to determine the motor and other factors that are elements of these problems; these are referred to in the example as subcomponents. They include factors that are usually identified in the

evaluation process and may include problems with wrist and MCP joint stability, midrange movement control, lack of isolated finger movement, and excessive use of flexion. Based on evaluation findings and the therapist's frames of reference, potential causes for these difficulties are identified. The causes may include sensory disorders, problems with tone or strength in particular muscle groups, associated reactions, sensory integrative dysfunction, or cognitive-perceptual factors.

## THEORIES AND FRAMES OF REFERENCE USED IN ASSESSING AND INTERVENING FOR HAND SKILL PROBLEMS IN CHILDREN

Once the therapist has described the child's functioning, he or she needs to determine the probable underlying causes of the child's difficulties. Although description of the child's performance is affected by the theory or frame of reference the therapist is using, delineation of the probable causes of the performance problems and decisions about how intervention should be structured are clearly influenced directly by this theory or frame of reference. Chapter 3 presents descriptions of theoretical foundations for pediatric occupational therapy. Therefore this section refers to the most commonly used theories or frames of reference in assessing children who have problems with hand skills and intervening for those problems.

### Biomechanical Frame of Reference

The biomechanical frame of reference is used primarily in assessing and treating children with limitations in range of

## Problem: Unable to Effectively Engage in Constructive Manipulative Play

**COMPONENTS, SUBCOMPONENTS, AND CAUSES**

1. No in-hand manipulative skills
   a. Wrist not stable in neutral position or extension, uses wrist flexion—possible causes:
      (1) Decreased tone in wrist extensors
      (2) Increased tone in wrist flexors
   b. Metacarpophalangeal (MCP) joints not stable—possible causes:
      (1) Poor cocontraction in finger joints
      (2) Increased pull of extensor digitorum
   c. Unable to indentify finger being touched, resulting from decreased tactile discrimination
   d. Lacks midrange movements of finger joints—possible causes:
      (1) Decreased proprioception
      (2) Poor cocontraction in MCP and interphalangeal flexors and extensors
      (3) Increased tone in intrinsics and long finger flexors
2. Breaks materials often as a result of dropping and crushing them
   a. Unable to sustain finger pad grasp—possible causes:
      (1) Poor tactile or poor proprioceptive awareness
      (2) Poor cocontraction of muscle groups
   b. Shows excessive finger flexion in grasp—possible causes:
      (1) Poor proprioceptive awareness of size, and weight of object
      (2) Increased finger flexor tone
      (3) Associated reactions
      (4) Inactivity in intrinsics
   c. Bilateral handling is ineffective—possible causes:
      (1) Poor spatial relations
      (2) Grasp unstable as a result of poor wrist extension caused by increased flexor tone
      (3) Overflow in one upper extremity
      (4) Unilateral disregard

motion, strength, or endurance that affect their hand skills. It has been used to explain difficulties in arm use for reach caused by problems in postural alignment or impaired ability to use the arms against gravity (Colangelo, 1993). Biomechanics helps the therapist understand the principles involved in tenodesis grasping patterns and the relationship of intrinsic and extrinsic muscle control in grasp and in-hand manipulation patterns. Activities are designed based on these principles of hand function. Splinting for hand problems most often relies on the biomechanical frame of reference.

## Developmental Frame of Reference

The developmental frame of reference focuses on describing the sequences of skills as they are observed in typically developing children. For example, this frame of reference has been used to describe children's progression from an ulnar grasp pattern to a pincer grasp. This frame of reference is used in developmental curricula that present tasks in a sequential order and are grouped under age levels. In planning intervention for hand skill problems, occupational therapists often rely on an understanding of the developmental sequences of skills that children typically follow; these sequences are either used as a basis for sequencing goals and treatment, or the therapist makes a decision not to use the typical sequence of skill acquisition. This frame of reference also helps the therapist understand how hand skills relate to other developmental skills.

## Neurodevelopmental Treatment Frame of Reference

The neurodevelopmental treatment frame of reference focuses on understanding the child's difficulties with postural tone, postural control, and stability and mobility and presents interventions to address these areas of difficulty (Schoen & Anderson, 1993). Although this frame of reference has been used most to address the development of equilibrium and controlled movement against gravity, it also includes methods to improve arm and hand motor control (Boehme, 1988; Danella & Vogtle, 1992). Some splinting techniques that use the neurodevelopmental treatment principles have been developed.

## Sensory Integration Frame of Reference

The sensory integration frame of reference addresses the importance of sensory functioning and the integration of sensory functions to allow for adaptive responses. Occupational therapists may use this frame of reference to describe hand skill problems that seem to be caused by problems with integrating tactile or proprioceptive information. These problems may be seen in children who appear to be unaware of having five digits on each hand; these children function as if they were wearing mittens and thus lack adaptive hand use. This frame of reference may be used in assessing and treating children who the therapist believes have fine motor dyspraxia. Bilateral integration problems also may be viewed from this frame of reference.

## Motor Learning Theory

Motor learning theories are within the category of acquisitional theories. Use of motor learning theories is increasing in occupational therapy practice. When using this theory, therapists focus on the child's actual acquisition of specific new motor skills and how the learning of these motor skills occurs. Children are assisted in acquiring these skills through structure and feedback and are provided with structured practice to refine the skills. The type of practice that is used and the feedback that the child is given while practicing are considered important. Motor learning theories may be used by the therapist in assisting the child with developing a particular grasp pattern or in-hand manipulation skill or with developing speed in a motor skill, such as buttoning.

## Behavioral Theory

The behavioral frame of reference focuses on reinforcing children's performances through specific feedback. In contrast to motor learning theory, this acquisitional theory usually focuses on tasks or functional activities that involve more than motor components. Therapists often structure activities by using backward shaping in which the child first performs the last step of the desired skill, then other elements of the skills are added in a backward order so that the first step of the process is learned last. For example, in teaching shoe tying the therapist may first have the child pull the loops of the bow tight. Eventually each step of the process is added to the sequence until the last step is beginning to form the bow. In addition, therapists typically use positive verbal feedback to the child to indicate success with performance of the task or a component of it. Therapists often have the child choose an activity that he or she will complete after doing a nonpreferred activity.

## EVALUATION OF HAND SKILLS IN CHILDREN
### Rationale

An evaluation of a child's hand skills is done when the occupational therapist has sufficient evidence to suggest that problems with performance of one or more daily life skills is at least partially attributable to the child's problems with hand skills. A fine motor evaluation should not be done simply because one of the occupational therapist's roles is to assess these skills and to provide this information to the team. The occupational therapist must first have evidence to suggest that the child has at least one problem with daily life skills. Parents, teachers, and the child are often the best sources of information about difficulties with daily life skills.

## Screening for Hand Skill Problems

When a functional problem with a daily life skill is identified, the therapist needs to continue the data-gathering process to determine if it is reasonable to carry out a full evaluation of fine motor performance. This information needs to include data about the child's age, gross and fine motor functioning, cognitive and perceptual skills, sensory pro-

cessing, social situation and skills, and emotional development. Screening information of this type may be obtained from parents, teachers, the child, other professionals or reports of other professionals, and a screening conducted by the occupational therapist.

The hand skills part of the screening may include the observations in Table 12-1. This list of observations of fine motor skills was structured to include reach, grasp, release, in-hand manipulation, and bilateral skills. It is not meant to be a standardized test or to replace standardized testing of a child. However, because few standardized tests include assessment of specific hand skills, this form may be used to make observations about the child's quality of hand skills. The sections of this chapter on normal development of the various hand skills may be used as a basis for determining if the child has difficulty with a particular skill.

Information gathered in this screening can be useful in determining if further observation of the child's hand skills is necessary or if a standardized test should be administered. In addition, parents or teachers and the child may find that these tasks are useful to them in delineating the areas that are difficult for the child versus those with which the child may be more successful. Discussing the observations during or after the screening often serves as a basis for collaborative treatment planning to address the areas of difficulty.

In addition to providing the therapist with information about hand skills and tool use, observations of the child during performance of hand skills may yield information useful about the child in the following areas:

▲ Psychosocial functioning, particularly interest in objects and activities, social conduct and interpersonal skills, and self-control
▲ Cognitive skills particularly in regard to level of arousal, attention span and ability to shift attention, direction following, and to some extent, sequencing
▲ Sensory skills, particularly visual and tactile awareness and processing
▲ Perceptual skills, particularly kinesthesia, form constancy, position in space, figure-ground, and depth perception
▲ General neuromuscular functioning, particularly muscle tone, strength, and postural control
▲ Praxis abilities

Information about these areas is critical to planning intervention and may suggest the need for observation or testing to delineate problems in areas other than in hand skills.

## Activities for Fine Motor Screening

The activities listed in Table 12-1 are appropriate for use in screening a child's fine motor abilities. Because some skills are inappropriate for younger children, an "X" has been used to designate the age-group for which any activity may be used. When a skill may emerge within a particular age-group, ages have been used rather than an "X." For block

▲ Table 12-1  Hand Skills Screening Activities

| Activities | Age-Groups | | | |
| --- | --- | --- | --- | --- |
| | 6-12 mos | 1-2 yrs | 3-5 yrs | 6 yrs + |
| **REACH** | | | | |
| Move *both* arms full ROM | X | X | X | X |
| Reach to midline, extended elbow | X | X | X | X |
| Reach across midline | | X | X | X |
| **GRASP** | | | | |
| Use full palmar grasp | X | X | X | X |
| Use radial-digital grasp | 9 mo | X | X | X |
| Use standard pincer grasp | 10 mo | X | X | X |
| Use spherical grasp | | X | X | X |
| Use intrinsic-plus grasp | | X | X | X |
| Use power grasp on tool | | | X | X |
| **RELEASE** | | | | |
| Release object freely | X | X | X | X |
| Release 1-inch object into container | | X | X | X |
| Stack 1-inch blocks* | | 2-6 | 9-10 | 10 |
| Release tiny object into small hole | | X | X | X |
| Throw small ball at least 3 feet | | | X | X |
| **IN-HAND MANIPULATION** | | | | |
| Manipulate object between two hands | X | X | X | X |
| Use finger-to-palm translation, small object† | | X | X | X |
| Use palm-to-finger translation | | | | |
| One object† | | 2 yrs | X | X |
| Two to three objects† | | 2 yrs | X | X |
| With coin | | | X | X |
| Unscrew bottle top | | 2 yrs | X | X |
| Use shift to separate magazine pages or cards | | | X | X |
| Roll piece of clay into a ball‡ | | | X | X |
| Pick up marker or crayon using rotation | | | 4 yrs | X |
| Shift on marker or pencil | | | 5 yrs | X |
| Rotate pencil to use eraser and back | | | | X |
| **BILATERAL SKILLS** | | | | |
| Hold or carry large ball with 2 hands | X | X | X | X |
| Stabilize paper during coloring or writing | | | X | X |
| Hold paper during scissors use | | | X | X |
| Manipulate paper during scissors use | | | | X |
| **TOOL USE** | | | | |
| Use scissors to cut | | | | |
| Line | | | 3 yrs | X |
| Simple shapes | | | 4 yrs | X |
| Complex shapes | | | | X |
| Scribble with marker | | X | | |
| Copy appropriate forms | | | X | X |
| Handwriting appropriate for grade | | | | X |

*Block stacking allows for assessment of arm stability in space, spatial orientation of the objects, and controlled finger extension. Voluntary release of objects other than blocks may be used. Screening should include placement of objects when arm is not supported and placement that requires precision.
†An object that is not flat should be used. Examples include small pieces of cereal (appropriate for children under 3 years or those who still mouth objects), small beads, or small pegs.
‡A piece of clay that is approximately ¼-inch thick and 1-inch in diameter is placed in the palm of the child's hand. The child is asked to form the clay into a ball without using the other hand or the table surface. Palm-to-finger translation, finger-to-palm translation, simple rotation, and sometimes complex rotation may be observed.
*ROM,* Range of motion.

stacking, the number represents the number of blocks that a child within that age-group may be expected to stack. The therapist may vary materials used for some of the items so that many of these skills can be assessed during a mealtime, dressing, hygiene, or play activity. For all categories except *Bilateral Skills* and *Tool Use,* both hands should be presented with the activities.

## Evaluation Content

A child with functional problems who shows difficulties on screening for hand skills should be evaluated further to carefully delineate the characteristics of the problem and the optimal situations for the child's performance. For example, the therapist may need to determine if the child is able to use any type of functional grasp, if wrist extension is possible in any grasp patterns, the situations under which voluntary release is most feasible for the child, the types of objects that are easiest for the child to handle when using the in-hand manipulation skill of simple rotation, and whether the child is able to stabilize materials better when the materials are closer or further from his or her body.

In the process of determining the child's performance in the area of hand skills and potential reasons for any problems, the occupational therapist often uses a variety of standardized and nonstandardized assessments. All children should receive an assessment of hand skills in functional activities such as dressing, eating, hygiene skills, school activities, and play activities. Other standard testing may be done if this testing meets one or more of the following purposes:

It is likely to yield information that will be

1. Valuable for documenting the child's current status to later determine if the child has shown progress in hand skills, has remained the same, or has lost skills
2. Helpful in determining if the child qualifies for occupational therapy services by clarifying the degree of the child's disability
3. Useful in determining the causes of the child's hand skill problems
4. Helpful in determining the child's potential for improvement in hand skills and in selecting specific treatment goals
5. Helpful in planning treatment strategies

References and description for the tests listed below are found in Chapters 8 and 9.

### For children with strength or range of motion problems:

1. Measurement of active and passive range of motion
2. Evaluation of strength
   a. Muscle testing
   b. Grip and pinch strength testing

(See Ager, Olivett, & Johnson [1984]; Latch, Freeling, & Powell [1993]; and Mathiowetz, Weimer, & Federman [1986])

### For children with moderate to severe impairment due to abnormal tone:

1. Assessment of range of motion, with documentation of contractures
2. Assessment of tactile and proprioceptive functioning using standard method (without norms)
3. Administration of the Erhardt Developmental Prehension Assessment (EDPA, 1982)

### For children with mild to moderate impairment caused by abnormal tone and sensory or sensory integration problems:

1. Assessment of range of motion, with documentation of contractures
2. Assessment of tactile and proprioceptive functioning, using one of the following:
   a. Standard method (without norms)
   b. Sensory Integration and Praxis Tests (see Chapter 13)
3. Administration of a standardized developmental test that includes a fine motor section (see Appendix 8-A)
   a. Learning Accomplishment Profile (LAP)
   b. Hawaii Early Learning Profile (HELP)
   c. Bayley Scales of Infant Development-Revised
   d. Early Intervention Development Profile (EIDP)
   e. Brigance
4. Administration of a developmental motor test
   a. The Toddler and Infant Motor Evaluation (TIME)
   b. Peabody Fine Motor Scale
   c. Bruininks-Oseretsky Test of Motor Performance
5. Administration of the In-Hand Manipulation Test (IMT)

The IMT is being developed by Exner (1993) to assess the quality and speed of in-hand manipulation skills in children between the ages of 3 and 8 years. The test uses age-appropriate materials presented in the context of play. Children are not cued as to how to perform the skills. Those who demonstrate the ability to use a variety of in-hand manipulation skills are timed when performing additional items. The test is expected to take approximately 30 minutes to administer. It is designed to yield information useful in clinical practice, such as comparing a child's performance with that of age-peers, treatment planning, and documenting progress. It also is designed for research use to assess the relationship between in-hand manipulation skills and other aspects of functioning.

The IMT has been assessed for content validity, which was reported to be good (Exner, 1993). Results of preliminary studies also indicate high interrater and test-retest reliability. Preliminary validity studies will be conducted before the test is available for clinical use.

6. Administration of a visual-motor integration test
   a. Test of Visual Motor Skills (TVMS)
   b. Developmental Test of Visual Motor Integration (VMI)

*The adolescent with hand skill problems:*
1. Assessment of range of motion, with documentation of any contractures
2. Assessment of hand skills in prevocational or work tasks
3. Administration of a standardized motor test
   a. The Purdue Pegboard Test (Mathiowetz, Rogers, Dowe-Keval, Donohoe, & Rennells, 1986)
   b. The Bruininks-Oseretsky Test of Motor Performance

# GUIDELINES FOR INTERVENTION
## Setting Goals

The child's functional problems and number and types of problems in the hand skill area, the therapist's frame of reference, and the setting in which services are to be provided influence the types of goals that are developed in the area of hand skill, as well as other areas of the child's functioning. In general, developmental sequences of skills affect the selection of goals, but with the child with a motor disability, other factors should affect the goals established and the strategies selected for intervention. These factors include the types of functional skills the child needs, the complexity of the child's problems, and the human and nonhuman resources available to support the intervention program.

Goals for hand skill problems are addressed in each of the sections that follows. The therapist must be realistic in the number and types of goals that can be established relative to any other goals for the child. In addition, the therapist needs to consider hand skill goals that are feasible for the child to accomplish and within the child's behavioral repertoire. Such goals may be limited for children with severe disabilities. In all cases, hand skill goals should be linked to the child's ability to more effectively engage in daily life skills.

## Sequencing Treatment Sessions

When direct treatment is provided to improve hand and arm function, it is usually carried out in the following sequence:
Preparation:
1. Positioning of the child
2. Inhibition or facilitation of tone
3. Activities to improve postural control (i.e., pelvic, shoulder, and head control)
Hand skill development:
4. Activities that emphasize isolated arm and hand movements, such as external rotation, supination, and wrist extension
5. Reach, grasp, carry, and release activities
6. Isolated finger movement activities
7. In-hand manipulation activities
8. Bilateral hand use activities
Generalizing skills:
9. Integration of hand skills into functional activities

Not all children need all of the steps of this sequence. In addition, intervention for all areas is rarely done in one treatment session.

## Preparation for Hand Skill Development

Many children require preparation of the total body in each treatment session before intervention for specific hand skill problems are addressed. In addition to intervention to improve motor function, specific attention should be given to the child's sensory functioning. Tactile and proprioceptive input to the arms and hands may be provided to enhance sensory awareness and discrimination. Stimuli may be provided by lotion, toys, the child's own clothing, or, preferably, active movements of the child's hands, with or without assistance. Normal children, as well as those with developmental dyspraxia, have greater tactile sensitivity when performing an activity that involves active touching rather than being touched (Haron & Henderson, 1985). Visual awareness of the hands in conjunction with tactile and proprioceptive input should also be encouraged.

### Positioning Considerations

In selecting positioning of the therapist and the child for fine motor intervention, the therapist must consider the position that is the most optimal for eliciting the particular skills desired in that child and the position in which the child will use the skills. When these positions are different, the therapist needs to consider whether to use only one position at this time and to introduce the other position later or whether to use both positions at this time. For example, the child may be able to bring both hands to midline and to reach with the greatest elbow extension in sidelying. However, for functional use the child may need to be able to contact a switch on a surface while in an adapted sitting position. In a treatment session with this child the therapist may initially work with the child in sidelying, then move to supported sitting to help the child generalize the skills to a functional position. The therapist may choose to address reaching skills only in sidelying for a few sessions before combining both positions. Eventually the therapist may work with the child primarily in a supported sitting position. In any case the therapist almost always needs to specifically address carryover of skills across positions with the child. Often this carryover can be done through activities developed collaboratively with the parents or the teacher.

Certain body positions can be used more effectively in treatment of some hand skills than others. Supine is an effective position for working with young children on arm movements and visual regard of the hands during movement. Prone on forearms is an appropriate position for addressing shoulder stability and cocontraction in 90 degrees of elbow flexion, dissociation of the two sides of the body during weight bearing on one arm while manipulating with the other, gross bilateral manipulation of objects, and visual regard of the hands. Sidelying can be an effective position for encouraging unilateral arm movement to bat at an object and for hand-to-hand play. Visual regard of the hands and of objects is difficult to address in sidelying.

Sitting at a table is often the position in which children are most likely to use fine motor skills. For optimal hand use children need a stable chair with adequate foot support. Usually a child who is not yet independent in sitting should not be expected to work on sitting stability while working on hand skills. Such children need adaptations for sitting, for example, lateral supports and chest straps. A tray or table surface should be a working surface rather than a supporting surface in intervention to improve fine motor skills. The table or tray should be only slightly above elbow height. A lower table promotes use of body flexion, and a higher surface promotes use of abduction and internal rotation of the arms. The therapist also may treat the child in sitting on the floor or sitting in a chair with no table, particularly when working on reaching skills or gross bilateral skills.

For children with mild to moderate motor involvement, standing may be an appropriate position for treatment of hand skills. Many daily living skills that rely on hand skills are most commonly done while standing, such as brushing teeth, zipping and buttoning clothing, shaving and applying makeup, and cooking. For children who have substantial difficulties with standing or performing hand skills, standing should be used only after the child has mastered the skills in a sitting position.

### Managing Tone and Improving Postural Control

The child with increased tone throughout the body may need overall inhibition of tone before participation in hand skill activities. Finnie (1975) suggested several helpful techniques, including the use of slow rotary movements at the shoulder and forearm. These movements may be performed within a small range of motion between internal and external rotation of the shoulder and between forearm pronation and supination. Boehme (1988) and Danella and Vogtle (1992) discussed other handling techniques to address problems with tone in the child's arms and hands.

Upper extremity weight bearing is particularly useful as a treatment technique for improving postural control and improving stability in the scapulohumeral area. It also can be used to encourage the child to maintain elbow cocontraction and some degree of wrist extension while engaging in slight weight shifting. Proprioceptive input is provided during weight bearing. The primary focus should be on helping the child increase overall stability rather than concentrating on achieving full elbow, wrist, or finger extension. Weight-bearing activities can be carried out with the child in prone position on forearms, prone position on extended arms, side-sitting, or long-sitting, depending on the child's skill level.

Effectively controlling the child who has significant wrist flexion in an upper extremity weight-bearing position is often difficult. The most appropriate positions for these chil-

dren to use include prone on forearms and sidelying. The therapist can help the child position wrists in neutral position, but may not expect extension beyond neutral.

Mildly and moderately involved children often can work toward maintaining full finger extension during weight bearing. However, this may not be feasible for children with moderate or severe involvement. Finger flexion may be permitted during weight bearing as long as the thumb is not in an abnormal position. If the child's thumb is tightly adducted and flexed, the therapist should use handling techniques before weight bearing. The therapist can use his or her own hand to provide firm pressure over the first metacarpal and relax the child's hand through slow, small rotary and flexion-extension movements.

Using multiple baseline single subject design, Barnes (1986, 1989a, 1989b) found that subjects with cerebral palsy demonstrated increased use of wrist extension and finger extension after upper weight bearing. Grasp and voluntary release quality and skill were not affected by the weight bearing other than through increased wrist extension. Chakarian and Larson's study (1993) of weight bearing with 10 children with cerebral palsy also found improvements in wrist and finger extension.

Activities that inhibit and facilitate changes in muscle tone often simultaneously address postural control. The development of postural control is described at length in Chapter 11.

## HAND SKILL DEVELOPMENT
### Isolated Movement Control

The therapist may choose to address specific movements in the upper extremity in isolation of specific hand skills. For example, the therapist may assist the child in using elbow flexion-extension or supination-pronation or wrist flexion-extension movements before integrating these movements into reaching, grasping, or releasing patterns. Using this strategy is an example of the use of motor learning theory. Such an approach appears to be most successful with children who are able to follow verbal instructions and participate actively in working on specific hand skills. Games or songs may be used in conjunction with practicing use of these movements. Emphasis on specific movements needs to be followed immediately in the treatment session with use of these movements within a functional context.

Supination control seems to be one of the greatest areas of difficulty for children with disabilities, particularly for those with tone problems. Difficulties with initiating or sustaining forearm supination are often compensated for with abnormal posturing at the trunk, shoulder, elbow, or wrist.

Supination is easiest to use when the elbow is fully flexed and most difficult to use with full elbow extension. Therefore activities that position the elbow in more than 90 degrees of flexion can be used to facilitate supination. If the child can initiate supination but has poor control of this pattern, he or she can benefit from activities with the elbow held in 90 degrees, with the forearm stabilized on a surface and an object presented vertically (Figure 12-15). Gradually materials are moved to encourage the child to use more elbow extension while maintaining the supinated position. Children with more severe involvement may only be able to achieve about 30 degrees of supination—the minimum amount needed to effectively handle materials on a table. Children with less motor impairment should be encouraged to obtain at least 90 degrees of supination to accomplish functional activities such as drinking, eating with utensils, or turning a doorknob. It is also helpful to facilitate supination in the nonpreferred arm so that the hand can more effectively stabilize materials.

## Reach
### Problems

Children with neuromotor disabilities exhibit typical problems in reach that limit the range and control. Examples of problems in reach include the following:

1. Use of abduction and internal rotation to initiate reach
2. Use of shoulder elevation and lateral trunk flexion to increase the height of the arm for reaching
3. Inability to coordinate the hand position with the timing of the reach
4. Difficulty maintaining an upright body posture when reaching forward or across midline

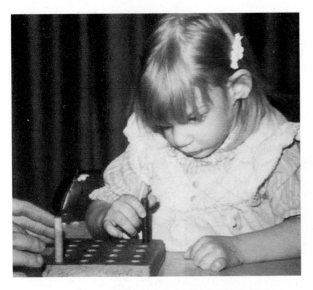

**Figure 12-15** Arm support on the surface, elbow flexion, and vertical orientation of materials encourage this child's use of forearm supination. Note this child's lack of spontaneous stabilization of the pegboard with her right hand. (Courtesy of Kennedy Kreiger Institute, Baltimore, MD.)

### Goals

The following are examples of goals that may be used for children with a variety of levels of disabilities. The goals are in approximate order of difficulty, although difficulty in using any one pattern may vary with individual children. The child will do the following:

1. Maintain visual regard of the object while contacting the object with the hand
2. Contact objects in various planes
3. Sustain some degree of finger extension while reaching for objects in various planes
4. Reach with both hands together for an object presented at midline
5. Orient the forearm appropriately for object contact during bilateral reaching
6. Reach with 45 degrees of shoulder flexion, using neutral rotation of the humerus and elbow extension
7. Reach with 90 degrees of shoulder flexion, using slight external rotation of the humerus, elbow extension, and forearm supination to midposition
8. Use appropriate hand positioning for grasp in conjunction with a mature reaching pattern
9. Reach across midline with an erect trunk posture and humeral external rotation, elbow extension, and forearm supination to midposition
10. Reach above the head with control

### Intervention Strategies

When the child initiates little movement or is unable to open the hand during arm movement the primary focus of intervention is on controlled initiation of arm movements. This includes using various types of arm movements and being able to place and hold the arm to allow for contact with objects. This type of reaching goal is a priority for children with extremely limited movement control or strength and those whose degenerative disease process results in skill regression. These movements are important for contact with others and can be used to activate switches for toys and electronic adapted equipment.

To facilitate arm movements and contact with objects, the therapist must identify the best position to promote postural stability and visual regard. The most commonly used position is sitting, with attention given to head and trunk control, visual regard, and visual tracking. However, supine and sidelying positions can be used effectively as well.

Children with severe motor involvement need toys and materials that are easy to activate and have no "failure" elements. Such toys include play foam, beans, rice, musical toys that are activated by light touch, and soap bubbles. Best results are usually obtained through proximal handling at the shoulders and upper arms, as the therapist assists the child with movements of either or both arms. Initial emphasis is on general arm movement, then on hand and arm placement, and finally on finger extension during arm movement as a precursor for reach with grasp.

When children are able to contact objects with some control, the therapist should introduce structured activities to assist the child with using elements of a more mature reaching pattern. Gradually these elements are combined for a smooth direct reach. The therapist needs to determine the placement of objects in relation to the child's body that allows the child to use the best reaching pattern he or she can. From that position the therapist can begin to vary object placement and orientation. For example, because presentation of objects at shoulder height often results in reaching with internal rotation and elbow flexion, initial presentation of objects at a level below the child's shoulder may facilitate the use of shoulder flexion and neutral rotation. Gradually objects can be raised higher as the child develops more control. Lateral reaching may be used to promote shoulder abduction and slight external rotation during reach. The child should also be encouraged to reach behind his or her body, combining humeral hyperextension with controlled internal rotation and various elbow positions. Many children have difficulty with this posterior reaching pattern, which is required in dressing and other daily living skills.

Some children are able to use neutral to slight external shoulder rotation in combination with humeral flexion if provided with a minimal amount of handling at the humerus or elbow (Figure 12-16). However, if such handling techniques are required for a child to use a mature reaching pattern, ipsilateral reaching activities are recommended. The child is probably not yet ready to practice reaching across the midline for an object, especially if elbow extension is required.

To encourage reaching that incorporates neutral to slight external rotation of the shoulder and forearm supination, objects need to be oriented vertically. Horizontal orientation of an object and large objects tend to encourage use of forearm pronation. Children with muscle weaknesss are better able to reach objects when they are provided with a table or tray surface that is at or slightly above elbow height. Mobile arm suspension systems can be used for support and to assist with movements of the child with muscle grades of fair-minus or lower.

Children with attentional problems or visual impairment should be presented with objects that have high color contrasts or bright solid colors. In the presence of severe visual impairment, objects may combine both auditory stimuli and varied textures. If the child has not developed the ability to search for objects, materials should be presented within a confined space or tied to strings so that they can be easily retrieved after dropping (Fraiburg, Smith, & Adelson, 1969).

## Grasp
### Problems

The child who has difficulty opening the hand for grasp may have significantly increased tone, muscle weakness, or joint limitations. The following problems have been observed in development of effective grasp:

1. Fisting or finger flexion that prevents hand opening
2. Wrist flexion (often with ulnar deviation) in combination with finger extension

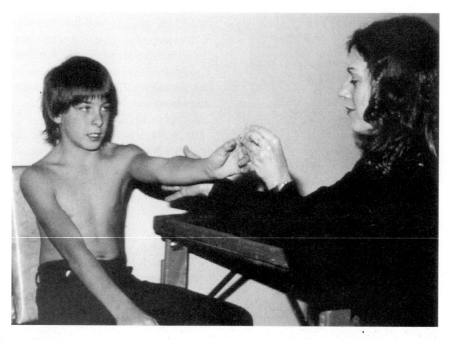

**Figure 12-16**   Facilitation is provided to prompt use of slight humeral external rotation and forearm supination. The object is held vertically to assist this reaching pattern. (Courtesy Kennedy Kreiger Institute, Baltimore, MD.)

3. Sustained forearm pronation, which interferes with use of radial finger grasp patterns
4. Thumb adduction, often with MCP or IP flexion; the lack of ability to use thumb abduction and adduction with MCP and IP extension
5. The lack of ability to initate or sustain thumb opposition
6. Inability to use grasp patterns that involve control of the intrinsic finger muscles
7. Inability to vary grasp in accordance with object characteristics

## Goals

The following are examples of goals that may be used for children with a variety of levels of disabilities. The goals are in approximate order of difficulty, although difficulty in using any one pattern may vary with individual children. The child will do the following:

1. Use a sustained palmar grasp with the arm in a variety of positions
2. Use a finger surface grasp on a variety of objects (rather than using a palmar grasp)
3. Use a finger pad grasp with thumb opposition and one, two, or three fingers on objects that are small or have a small diameter
4. Vary the type of opposed grasp pattern used in accordance with object shapes and characteristics
5. Use an effective lateral pinch grasp pattern
6. Use a grasp with MCP flexion and IP extension to hold thin, flat objects
7. Use a power grasp on a variety of tools in daily living tasks

## Intervention Strategies

For children with delays and functional difficulties in grasp, the therapist needs to match preparation techniques such as positioning, handling, or strengthening to the child's problem.

Some children make fists with their hands or refuse to grasp objects because of tactile defensiveness. If this problem appears to be present, treatment should follow principles appropriate for the child with tactile defensiveness (see Chapter 13). In addition, weight bearing with the hand closed and graded tactile input are useful. Usually firm objects with smooth surfaces and contours are tolerated best initially. Maintenance of grasp may also be influenced by tactile defensiveness.

Children with tactile discrimination problems also may have problems with grasp. These difficulties include problems with accurate use of grasp patterns and with regulation of pressure in grasp as seen in either dropping of objects or inappropriate squeezing of objects. Regardless of the cause of a somatosensory deficit, most children seem to benefit from graded sensory input and increasing attention to sensory discrimination as part of the intervention for

grasp skills. Having the child actively explore the sizes, shapes, and textures of objects can precede emphasis on grasp in a treatment session.

In planning intervention that addresses grasp problems, objects should be selected with consideration of the child's interests, sensory needs, and motor skills. Properties to consider include the size, shape, color, weight, and texture of objects.

***Children with severe disabilities.*** Children with severe disabilities need to develop an effective palmar grasp and, if possible, grasp using the finger surface. If possible, independent initiation of grasp should be stressed as well as the ability to sustain grasp with the arm in a variety of positions. If the child is unable to open the hand readily for grasp, the therapist may explore other body positions. Sidelying may decrease stress on overall body posture and make it possible for the child to open the hand more easily. In supported sitting the child may find opening the hand easier if objects are placed below the seat of the chair and lateral to the child's body. Other handling techniques described by Boehme (1988) may be needed to assist the child with hand opening.

For the child who can independently open the hand but who shows wrist flexion with grasp, the therapist may emphasize development of on a palmar grasp. The therapist may find activities that promote squeezing of clay or dowel-shaped objects with the child's wrist in extension to be helpful. Once the child can sustain this pattern, he or she can be assisted or encouraged to move the arm while grasping an object. Activities that may be effective include using a small stick to hit a suspended balloon or to break soap bubbles blown by the therapist, touching pictures on a wall or mirror with a stick, or holding onto clothing items while they are pulled up or down. Children who are able to begin working on grasp with the finger surface benefit from the use of techniques discussed in the next section.

The child with a severe disability may wear a splint or other orthotic device during treatment as well as at other times of the day. Splinting techniques that may be useful in supporting hand function during treatment are described later in this chapter. For many of these children, adaptations to materials are needed to support their performance of activities at home, school, and play. Built-up handles (that accommodate a palmar grasp pattern) and larger objects, such as game pieces and blocks, may be used instead of smaller ones. Use of standard tools such as pencils and scissors may not be possible. If the child is able to participate in classroom and play activities that use these tools, adaptive devices or strategies are needed.

***Children with moderate disabilities.*** Children with moderate disabilities typically have difficulties with forearm control, wrist extension, thumb opposition, and control of the MCP and IP joints. They can initiate grasp, although this initiation may be with wrist flexion. Grasp goals for these children usually are designed to address use of opposed grasp patterns and use of grasp patterns in which the hand effectively accommodates to objects.

Development of opposed grasp patterns and those grasps in which the fingers and thumb accommodate to the size and shape of the object begin with emphasis on grasp alone, rather than on grasp combined with reach. Selection of objects for use in developing these grasp patterns is critical. Objects must to be able to be used within the context of an activity that is interesting and meaningful to the child. Games and imaginary play materials can provide opportunities for repetitive presentation of objects to the child. Opposed grasp patterns are used with medium- and small-sized objects as well as tiny ones. In treatment, children often can demonstrate better thumb and finger control with small- or medium-sized objects that have well-defined edges. Tiny objects require too much precision, such that the child often resorts to a more primitive grasping pattern. In fact, skill in using a pincer grasp usually is less critical for the child's functional performance of daily life tasks than skill in using and varying a three-point opposed grasp pattern. Once the child begins to acquire an opposed grasp pattern, objects can be varied in size, shape, texture, and weight. To begin developing an opposed grasp pattern, the therapist needs to ensure that the child's arm is well stabilized when objects are presented. Having the wrist in a neutral or slightly extended position is critical; if appropriate, the volar surface of the child's forearm can be stabilized on his or her leg while the therapist gives support over the dorsum of the forearm (Figure 12-17). Objects are presented in line with the shoulder and not at midline, because midline positioning has a tendency to encourage the use of pronation. With positioning in line with the shoulder, at least neutral rotation of the humerus is encouraged and slight forearm supination is likely to occur. The therapist holds the object with his or her fingers and presents the object directly to the child's fingers (Figure 12-17). After grasp, the child carries the object to a nearby container or surface. The therapist repeats this strategy for grasp, carry, and release of several more objects. Once the child is able to use this pattern well, the therapist can move to the next skill level.

At this level the therapist places the object in his or her cupped hand so that the object is stable and asks the child to grasp the object. The object is positioned in line with the child's shoulder. When this strategy is used, the child needs to use more internal stability of the arm and some degree of prepositioning before grasp.

As the child develops skill in grasping from the therapist's hand, the therapist can begin to place an object on the table surface. As at the prior two levels, the object is in line with the child's shoulder; it is not at midline. The therapist may need to stabilize the object or place it on a nonskid surface for the child who does not yet have sufficient arm stability to grasp without unintentionally moving the object.

After the child is able to grasp from the table surface with the object in line with the shoulder, the therapist can begin

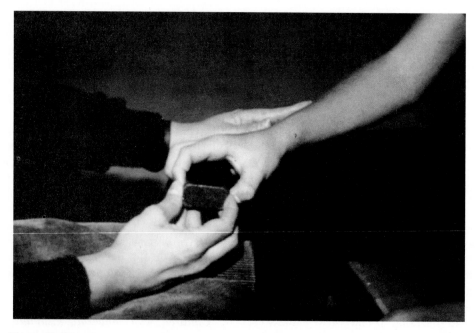

**Figure 12-17** The child is assisted with using grasp with thumb opposition and finger pad contact by stabilization of his forearm and presentation of the object directly to his fingers. (Courtesy Kennedy Institute, Baltimore, MD.)

to move the object further away on the table surface and closer to midline. Eventually the therapist can begin to structure activities to combine reach with grasp. This requires the child to stabilize the arm in space while controlling finger movements. The therapist may need to consider using a variety of these object placements in a therapy session to elicit the child's best skills. Different object placements may be needed with various sizes and shapes of objects.

***Children with mild disabilities.*** Children with mild disabilities typically have difficulties with small ranges of movements in supination and wrist extension. Sustained control with the intrinsic muscles of the hand may be difficult for these children to achieve. Fingertip control in grasp is often poor, as is the ability to control the palmar arches and to achieve radial-ulnar dissociation of movements within the hand.

Goals for grasp skills for these children usually are focused on use of an effective lateral pinch grasp pattern, use of a grasp with MCP flexion and IP extension to hold thin, flat objects, or use of a power grasp on a variety of tools in daily living tasks. Both the lateral pinch pattern and the grasp for thin, flat objects require wrist stability and use of the intrinsics. Verbal cuing and structuring of activities to elicit intrinsic muscle activity may be used with children who are appropriate for these skills. Activities can include holding all fingers in adduction and extension while rolling out clay, using finger abduction to stretch rubber bands placed around two or more fingers, playing finger games that require isolation and small ranges of finger movements, holding or hiding objects in a cupped hand, and squeezing clay or other objects between the pad of the thumb and the pads of one or more fingers.

Emphasis on radial-ulnar disassociation in the hand and on grasp with MCP flexion and IP extension can be helpful as precursors to the precision grasp pattern. To address radial-ulnar disassociation, the therapist can have the child hold two objects in one hand and release one at a time, hold an object in the ulnar side of the hand with the ring and little fingers while grasping and releasing with the radial fingers and thumb, and engage in activities that develop finger-to-palm translation with stabilization skills. Myers (1992) presented additional activities for developing higher-level grasp skills. Schneck and Battaglia (1992) discussed specific strategies for assisting children with mild disabilities in the development of scissors skills.

In addressing the power grasp within functional activities, the therapist carefully selects the type of tool the child handles. Tools that have a narrow surface for index finger contact are particularly difficult for children to control. Verbal cues, stickers, or other dots on the handles of the tools may be used to encourage appropriate finger placement. Built-up handles may be needed to facilitate the child's performance initially.

## Carrying

The child must maintain grasp of an object during the carry phase. Therefore the therapist needs to attend to the child's ability to vary all joint positions in the arm while sustaining grasp. Wrist extension with sustained finger flexion usually needs to be emphasized. The therapist should be especially attentive to the child's use of compensatory trunk movements. If these are present, the child may need intervention to improve sustained trunk control in midline and trunk rotation in conjunction with arm movements. The use of adapted equipment to support the trunk in a symmetric, erect posture is helpful for many children. Stabilization of the shoulder to prevent scapular elevation also may be necessary.

Facilitation of arm movements in a manner similar to that described for reaching may be used to encourage carry patterns of shoulder rotation, graded elbow movements, and forearm supination. Most children with increased tone or stability problems have more difficulty carrying small or thin objects. Use of objects that are larger in diameter, such as those adapted with built-up handles, can promote wrist extension and management of carrying.

## Voluntary Release
### Problems

Treatment for problems with voluntary release is commonly combined with intervention for grasp. Children with difficulty in releasing objects may exhibit the following:

1. Fisting and tight finger flexion
2. Difficulty with sustained arm position during object placement and release
3. Difficulty combining wrist extension with finger extension
4. Inability to use slight forearm supination to allow for release in small areas or near other objects and with visual monitoring of the placement
5. Overextension of the fingers in release, limiting control of specific object placement

### Goals

The following are examples of goals that may be used for children with a variety of levels of disabilities. These goals specifically define the size of area in which the object can be released (i.e., into a container with a 4-inch opening) or the height of surface on which the object can be released (i.e., stack six cubes). The following goals incorporate these commonly used strategies and are in an approximate order of difficulty, although difficulty in using any one pattern may vary with individual children. The child will do the following:

1. Release objects into a container with the container placed on the floor
2. Release objects into a container placed on a table surface with the container at arms' length from the child's

body (to encourage wrist extension with finger extension)

3. Release objects into a container at midline while using wrist extension
4. Stack three (or more, up to 10 to 12) 1-inch cubes
5. Release tiny objects into a container with a small opening
6. Place objects within 1 inch of other objects without making other objects move or fall
7. Release unstable, lightweight objects while keeping them in an upright position

## Intervention Strategies

Intervention focuses on one or more of the following areas, depending on the child's problems: hand opening for object release, arm placement and stability for release, or accuracy of object placement. The therapist should attend carefully to the child's grasp pattern because the quality of voluntary release can be no better than the quality of the grasp. A child who uses a palmar grasp uses full-finger extension to release the object. A child who uses a pincer grasp has the opportunity to use voluntary release with good control of the intrinsic muscles as balanced with the extrinsics. To initiate hand opening, some children who have high tone and fisting or muscle weakness use tenodesis. When the child shows excessive finger flexion (fisting), initial treatment for voluntary hand opening focuses on the child's ability to move the arm while maintaining some finger extension. Splinting may be helpful in supporting the child's wrist or facilitating increased wrist and finger extension. When fisting is a problem, asking the

child to place the object in a container tends to increase the child's fisting. Therefore an effective strategy can be to place a large object in the child's hand, then encourage the child to move the elbow into extension and let the object fall to the floor. Some children have more success releasing to the side of their body because movement toward midline tends to increase the pronation-flexion posturing. If the child is able to accomplish this level of voluntary release, release of medium- and large-sized objects into a container with a large opening that is placed on the floor may be attempted next. For some children, transfer of objects from hand to hand is a reasonable strategy for encouraging release with object stabilization, but for many children with fisting, using elbow flexion tends to increase the fisting.

Children who are able to voluntarily open their hands but who use tenodesis patterns may benefit from intervention to increase voluntary finger extension while sustaining the wrist in neutral. For some children structured activities and handling are effective, but many children appear to benefit from wearing a dorsal wrist splint (see Figure 12-19). A therapist may have the child wear a splint during part of the therapy session and encourage finger extension through a variety of activities, including voluntary release. Similar activities can be used after splint removal.

Children who use wrist flexion with voluntary release may benefit from structured activities in which a container for objects is placed slightly laterally from the child's midline and at a sufficient distance from the child's body that elbow extension is needed (Figure 12-18). This level of control is similar to that of a baby who releases objects with

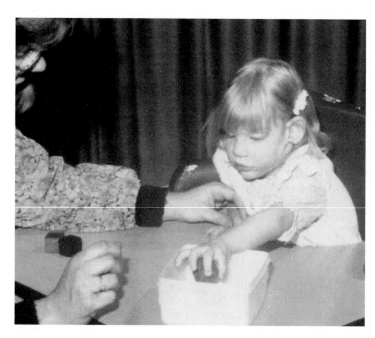

**Figure 12-18** Positioning materials to elicit elbow extension during release encourages this child's use of wrist extension. (Courtesy Kennedy Institute, Baltimore, MD.)

the arm held in a total extension pattern. Over time, target containers for release of objects can be brought closer to the body, requiring gradually increasing elbow flexion with wrist extension. Sometimes this pattern can be facilitated if containers are set at an angle. Once the child can release medium-sized objects into a container at midline while maintaining wrist extension to at least neutral, the size of the container opening can be decreased.

Children with overextension of the fingers during voluntary release may benefit from activities previously described that address development of intrinsic muscle control. They also may need intervention to improve somatosensory awareness of their hands. Activities for these children often incorporate the use of lightweight materials and objects that vary in size and stability. Verbal cuing of the child to attend to object and hand placement and graded activities to facilitate increasing accuracy and visual monitoring of materials is often helpful.

## In-Hand Manipulation
### Problems

Children who have difficulty with in-hand manipulation skills tend to drop objects, use surfaces for support during manipulation, or be slow in the execution of skills (Exner, 1990a). Case-Smith (1993) found empirical support for these problems in her study of children with and without fine motor delays. These problems may be associated with tactile problems (Case-Smith, 1991). Motor control problems, particularly of the intrinsic and praxis problems, also may be major causes of limited in-hand manipulation skill development. Attentional and cognitive problems contribute to these problems in some children. Problems that limit in-hand manipulation include the following:

1. Limited finger isolation and control
2. Inability to effectively cup the hand to hold objects in the palm
3. Inability to hold more than one object in the hand at the same time
4. Insufficient stability to control object movement at the finger pads, thus objects are dropped frequently

### Goals

The following are examples of goals that may be used for children with a variety of levels of in-hand manipulation skill. The goals are in approximate order of difficulty, although difficulty in using any one pattern may vary with individual children. The child will do the following:

1. Use the skill of finger-to-palm translation to hold a coin in the palm of the hand
2. Use finger-to-palm translation with stabilization skills to hold several coins in one hand
3. Use shift skills to adjust a coin for placement into a slot in a bank
4. Use simple rotation skills in adjusting utensils during eating or brushing teeth

5. Use palm-to-finger translation (and palm-to-finger translation with stabilization) while eating small finger foods
6. Use simple rotation with stabilization in playing a board game with markers in the shape of little people
7. Use complex rotation skills to erase with the eraser end of the pencil

### Intervention Strategies

Intervention goals and strategies are influenced by the therapist's assessment of the causes of the child's problems and the therapist's determination of the child's potential for acquiring specific in-hand manipulation skills. Many children with moderate and severe disabilities who lack the necessary prerequisite skills will not be able to develop these skills. Children with mild disabilities usually can develop at least the lower-level in-hand manipulation skills.

Specific activity suggestions are given in the box on p. 298. The following sections provide suggestions of strategies to use with children who differ in their level of skills. See Exner (1995) for additional information on treatment of in-hand manipulation skills.

***Children with no in-hand manipulation skills.*** With children who show no in-hand manipulation skills or who have only finger-to-palm translation, the therapist may encourage the child to use bilateral manipulation of objects and use of support surfaces to assist in the manipulation. Use of these strategies can be helpful in allowing the child to begin to move the fingers actively over object surfaces. Objects such as cubes that have pictures on all sides, kaleidoscopes, and textured toys can be used. When the child can effectively move the fingers over this type of object, the therapist can introduce finger-to-palm translation activities in the context of "hiding object games" using various objects. Finger isolation games can be useful; the thumb should be incorporated into these activities too. The child should be assisted in developing and functionally using a wide variety of grasp patterns, including those that combine flexion at the MCP joints with extension at the IP joints. Tactile discrimination and proprioception activities can be used to enhance awareness of the various fingers and areas of the palm of the hand.

***Children with beginning in-hand manipulation skills.*** Children who have the ability to use finger-to-palm translation and beginning simple rotation, or shift, or palm-to-finger translation skills can work on refinement of these skills, expanding their repertoire of skills used without stabilization and beginning their ability to stabilize objects in the ulnar side of the hand while manipulating with the radial fingers.

Object selection for in-hand manipulation skills is important. Objects that do not roll and that are small are often the easiest for the child to handle. Examples include dice-

## PREPARATION ACTIVITIES
### General Tactile Awareness Activities

1. Using crazy foam
2. Using shaving cream
3. Applying hand lotion
4. Finger painting

### Activities Involving Proprioceptive Input

1. Weight bearing—wheelbarrow, activities on a small ball
2. Pushing heavy objects (boxes, chairs, benches, etc.)
3. Pulling (tug-of-war)
4. Pressing different parts of the hand into clay
5. Pushing fingers into clay or therapy putty
6. Pushing shapes out of perforated cardboard
7. Tearing packages or boxes open
8. Playing clapping games

### Activities Involving Regulation of Pressure

1. Tearing edges off of computer paper
2. Rolling clay into a ball
3. Squeezing water out of a sponge or washcloth
4. Pushing snaps together

### Activities Involving Tactile Discrimination

1. Doing finger games and songs
2. Playing finger identification games
3. Discriminating objects with the object stabilized
4. Discriminating shapes with the shape stabilized
5. Writing on the body and identifying the shape, letter, or object drawn
6. Discriminating textures

## SPECIFIC IN-HAND MANIPULATION ACTIVITIES
### Translation—Fingers to Palm

1. Getting a coin out of a change purse
2. Hiding a penny in the hand (magic trick)
3. Crumpling paper
4. Picking up and bringing small piece of food into the palm

### Translation—Fingers to Palm With Stabilization

1. Getting two or more coins out of a change purse, one at a time
2. Taking two or more chips off a magnetic wand, one at a time
3. Picking up pegs or paper clips one at a time to hold two or more in the hand at one time
4. Picking up several utensils one at a time to hold two or more in the hand at one time

### Translation—Palm to Fingers

1. Moving a penny from the palm to the fingers
2. Moving a chip to the fingers to put on a magnetic wand
3. Moving an object to put it into a container
4. Moving a food item to put it in the mouth

### Translation—Palm to Fingers With Stabilization

1. Holding several chips to put on a wand, one at a time
2. Handling money to put it into a bank or soda machine
3. Putting one utensil down when holding several
4. Holding several game pieces (chips, pegs, or markers)

### Shift

1. Turning pages in a book
2. Picking up sheets of paper, tissue paper, or dollar bills
3. Separating playing cards
4. Stringing beads (shifting string and bead as string goes through the bead)
5. Shifting a crayon, pencil, or pen for coloring or writing
6. Shifting paper in the nonpreferred hand while cutting
7. Playing with tinkertoys (the long, thin pieces)
8. Moving a cookie while eating
9. Adjusting a spoon, fork, or knife for appropriate use
10. Rubbing paint, dirt, or tape off the pad of a finger

### Shift With Stabilization

1. Holding a pen and pushing the cap off with the same hand
2. Holding chips while flipping one out of the fingers
3. Holding fabric in the hand while attempting to button or snap
4. Holding a key ring with the keys in hand, shifting one for placement in a lock

### Simple or Complex Rotation (Depending on Object Orientation)

1. Removing or putting on a small jar lid
2. Putting on or removing bolts from nuts
3. Rotation of a crayon or pencil—tip oriented ulnarly (simple rotation)
4. Rotation of crayon or pencil—tip oriented radially (complex rotation)
5. Removing a crayon from the box and preparing it for coloring
6. Rotating a pen or marker to put the top on
7. Rotating toy people to put them in chairs, a bus, or a boat
8. Rotating a puzzle piece for placement in the board
9. Feeling objects or shapes to identify them
10. Handling construction toy pieces
11. Turning cubes that have pictures on all six sides.
12. Constructing twisted shapes with pipe cleaners
13. Rotating a toothbrush or eating utensils during use

### Simple or Complex Rotation With Stabilization

1. Handling parts of a small-shape container while rotating the shape to put it into the container
2. Holding a key ring with keys, rotating the correct one for placement in the lock

sized cubes, nickels, game pieces, and other small toys. Larger objects require the child to involve all fingers in the manipulation, so these are more difficult for the child to handle. Tiny objects require excellent tactile discrimination and fingertip control, so they are also more difficult to handle.

The therapist structures the presentation of objects to assist the child in using a particular in-hand manipulation skill and often cues the child in the use of the skill. For example, in addressing palm-to-finger translation, the therapist first places the object on the middle phalanx of the child's index finger. When the child is able to move the object from this position out to the pads of the fingers, the therapist places the object on the volar surface of the proximal phalanx of the index finger. Later the therapist may be able to place the object in the palm of the child's hand. At this point a great deal of thumb isolation and control are needed to move the object.

Simple rotation skills can be structured by placing the object in the child's hand (in a radial grasp pattern) and asking the child to turn it upright. Pegs and peglike objects, such as candles and objects that look like little people, can be helpful in developing these skills. Verbal cuing to make the child stand up are used to support the child's performance.

Finger-to-palm translation with stabilization is the one skill with stabilization that is likely to be feasible for these children. This skill often can be facilitated during finger-feeding activities and in play with coins. The therapist first encourages the child to hold one object in the hand while picking up and hiding another. After the child is able to manage two objects, the therapist can progress to using three; progression to handling four or more objects may be feasible in time.

***Children with basic in-hand manipulation skills.*** For children with basic in-hand manipulation skills, emphasis is placed on developing complex rotation skills and the use of stabilization with the other skills. Small- and medium-sized objects are introduced, and emphasis is placed on use of the skills in a variety of functional activities such as dressing, hygiene, and school tasks. Combinations of skills such as finger-to-palm translation, then palm-to-finger translation, and then simple rotation are practiced. Speed of skill use also may be stressed by using timing of skills and reporting the speed to the child. Children who are working at this level of skill typically respond well to verbal cuing for strategies to use in performing skills and to feedback about the effectiveness and speed of their skills.

## Bilateral Hand Use
### Problems

Difficulties with bilateral hand use tend to result from a combination of problems, of which motor factors may be

only one component. Some children with significant cognitive delays cannot attend to two objects simultaneously, thus alternating hand use or stabilization with one hand combined with manipulation with the other hand is not possible. Deficits in integration of the two body sides may be present (see Chapter 13). Impaired sensation may contribute to a lack of attention to one body side. Finally, lack of bilateral motor experience, as in children with hemiplegia or brachial plexus injuries, can cause children to approach all tasks in a one-handed manner. Other problems include the following:

1. The child cannot effectively sustain both hands at midline
2. The child has difficulty using supination during bilateral activities
3. The child has overflow movement and associated reactions in one upper extremity when using the other

### Goals

The following are examples of goals that may be used for children with a variety of levels of disabilities. These goals are written to fit the categories of gross symmetric bilateral skills, stabilizing or manipulating with one hand and bilateral simultaneous manipulation with the other hand. The following goals show increasing levels of difficulty that are consistent with a developmental perspective. This progression in skills may not be appropriate for children with a particular weakness or paresis of one body side. The child will do the following:

1. Bring both hands to midline for grasp of a medium- or large-sized object
2. Use both hands together to push large objects
3. Use both hands together to lift and carry large objects
4. Stabilize materials on a table surface with one open hand while the other hand manipulates materials (e.g., coloring, writing, or holding a puzzle board while putting pieces in it)
5. Stabilize materials using a palmar grasp while the other hand manipulates materials (e.g., holding the handle of a small pan while pretending to cook)
6. Stabilize materials using a variety of grasp patterns while the other hand manipulates materials (e.g., holding a cup while pouring liquid into it or holding a slice of bread while spreading butter on it)

The focus of treatment goals varies, depending on the severity of the child's disability and the level of skills the child is anticipated to be able to use eventually. The therapist must consider the child's need and potential for developing gross symmetric hand use, stabilizing with one hand while manipulating with the other, and bilateral simultaneous manipulation. Following a developmental sequence for intervention may be inappropriate.

## Intervention Strategies

***Children with severe disabilities.*** Treatment of the child with significantly increased tone or marked asymmetry focuses on promoting ability to stabilize materials with the more involved upper extremity while manipulating with the more proficient hand or arm. Activities that require stabilization with grasp (rather than stabilization without grasp) are often easier for these children. However, stabilization without grasp may be accomplished as long as the child can use his or her hand in a fisted position with the wrist in neutral to slight extension. Symmetric bilateral hand use may receive some attention. Simultaneous bilateral manipulation skills usually are inappropriate for these children unless adaptations can be used.

Special handling techniques can promote the child's ability to stabilize objects while manipulating them or use gross bilateral skills. The therapist can sit behind the child and stabilize both shoulders to help the child bring and keep both hands at midline. Trunk rotation should also be encouraged so that the child can cross midline more effectively.

Toys and materials selected for program activities must require bilateral hand use, particularly in the early phases of treatment. Initially the child may be more successful with gross bilateral skills if he or she can sustain grasp and keep the forearms pronated, such as in holding a stick horizontally to hit a balloon. For the child who is working on stabilizing with one hand while manipulating with the other, if objects are presented on a slippery surface the child will have more incentive to stabilize them than if a nonskid surface is used. Objects that have handles are useful when working on stabilization with grasp. Stabilizing without grasp is initially addressed with activities that are simple for the manipulating hand so the child can focus on the role of the stabilizing hand.

Usually materials are placed at midline. However, the therapist and the child should explore other positions if midline positioning does not appear optimal.

When a child cannot successfully stabilize materials and does not show potential for this skill in the near future, adaptations should be considered. Nonskid surfaces and other devices can assist in stabilization with table activities. Various commercial adaptations are available to aid accomplishment of other types of daily living activities with one hand (see Chapter 17).

***Children with moderate disabilities.*** Intervention for children with low tone or some degree of involuntary movement may be able to approximate the normal sequence of bilateral hand skill development. Therapy may initially focus on improving symmetry and stability and proceed through stabilizing with and without grasp. These children may benefit from working on a slightly unstable surface, because this environmental change may prompt more spontaneous stabilization of materials during manipulation. Adaptations may be needed for certain activities in which one hand needs to be an effective stabilizer, such as in handwriting. In general, simultaneous bilateral manipulation is not feasible for these children.

***Children with mild disabilities.*** Activities for children with mild disabilities may require gross symmetric bilateral skills and stabilizing with one hand while manipulating with the other. These children may also be able to develop or improve their simultaneous bilateral manipulation skills. To enhance development of simultaneous bilateral manipulation, activities that elicit these skills are carefully selected, graded, and structured. Functional activities of daily living may also be used in treatment of these skills.

***Children with muscle weakness.*** Children with muscle weakness can often manage simultaneous manipulation activities well because little hand strength and movement of the arms against gravity is required. These children often need assistance or adaptations to develop the ability to stabilize materials with one hand because this demands more strength in the stabilizing arm. Gross symmetric bilateral skills may be able to be accomplished only on table surfaces that provide arm support.

## GENERALIZATION OF SKILL INTO FUNCTIONAL ACTIVITIES

Most children do not readily generalize skills from isolated activities presented in therapy to their everyday life activities without assistance. Therefore activities for children with hand or arm function problems should be presented to the child in a meaningful context. For example, reaching program activities can be carried out during dressing and hygiene training or while playing with a toy that has many different parts. Grasp activities can be incorporated into independent eating and vocational readiness tasks. In-hand manipulation can be facilitated by having the child use materials from his or her pencil or crayon box or through building with construction toys. Voluntary release can be structured into a game that uses moveable pieces. Bilateral hand use can be developed through meal preparation activities, play, and schoolwork. Many other combinations are possible to help the child develop mature function of hand or arm skills in conjunction with increasing competence in daily life activities.

## SPLINTING FOR CHILDREN

Splinting is often a component of occupational therapy intervention for children with hand function problems. Children who have one or more of the following problems may benefit most:

1. Deformities
2. Sustained abnormal posturing

3. Increased tone
4. Limited movement of the hand
5. Limitations in functional skills secondary to problems with hand functions

Any one or a combination of these problems may make splinting for a child with severe motor disability as a result of central nervous system damage an appropriate type of intervention. Children with moderate motor impairment are less likely to require splinting to prevent or correct a deformity, but they may benefit from splints to reduce tone or improve mobility and functional skills. The child with minimal involvement secondary to central nervous system damage may have more difficulty with thumb use than wrist or finger control. Therefore this child needs a thumb splint to decrease tone or provide stability so that function is enhanced. Children who do not have central nervous system damage may require splinting for any of the previously mentioned problems, except increased tone.

## Precautions and Indications for Splint Use

Precautions for splint use are always in order, particularly for young and nonverbal children who may have poor sensation. These factors make them vulnerable to skin irritations and pressure problems. Children may be unable to report sensory problems during or after splint application; therefore the therapist must carefully instruct the child's parents regarding the wearing schedule, possible problems, and postural changes to note.

Static splints generally are worn for shorter periods than splints that allow hand movement. Initially, children may only tolerate 5- to 10-minute splint-wearing periods. Usually these periods can be gradually increased. If the child has increased tone, maximum wearing time for a static splint is usually 6 to 8 hours per day. However, if splints allow some hand movement and are used to aid accomplishment of functional activities, additional hours may be tolerated. Night splints are generally worn all night. At least a portion of each 24-hour period should be spent without splints.

Not all children with increased tone need night resting splints. In many cases their hands are more relaxed during sleep, and arms and hands can be positioned in neutral by parents. Children who have neutral positioning at night generally are at less risk for development of contractures. The child who shows abnormal hand posturing during the day but not at night may, however, require daytime splint application to increase function.

Boehme (1985) noted that some children have learned to use abnormal patterns of wrist flexion and ulnar deviation or thumb adduction to accomplish their daily activities. If this pattern is inhibited by a splint, the child may compensate by using another abnormal position of the hand or arm. Therefore before a splint is applied, the therapist must determine whether functional skill patterns that the child has

been using will be lost. Frequently an increased level of treatment, not a decreased level, needs to be provided to children who are wearing splints so that they can develop better quality patterns of hand use.

The use of splinting has rarely been questioned for children who have muscle weakness, traumatic injury of the hand or arm, or joint inflammation. However, splinting has been more controversial in its abnormal tone. Most of the related literature addresses problems of adults with abnormal tone; fewer studies (Exner & Bonder, 1983; MacKinnon, Sanderson, & Buchanan, 1975; McPherson, 1981) report the use of splints with children. This topic is explored further in conjunction with splint descriptions.

## Types of Splints Used With Children

Splints may be categorized into those that allow hand movement and those that do not. *Static* splints include resting pan splints, other volar and dorsal full hand and wrist splints, spasticity reduction splints, and thumb positioning splints. *Dynamic splints* assist the child with a particular wrist, finger, or thumb movement. A third type of *neurophysiologically based* splint may provide stimulation to the hand or arm or assist with stabilization of one or more joints during hand or arm activities.

Doubilet and Polkow (1977) and Snook (1979) reported case studies suggesting that *spasticity reduction splints* help decrease tone in adults. McPherson (1981) used an empirical design to study the effectiveness of Snook's spasticity reduction splint for five adolescents with severe disabilities. Splint-wearing time was gradually increased from 15 minutes the first day to 2 hours daily by the fourth week. The outcome measure was passive muscle tone at the wrist, which was documented on a daily basis through use of a scale that measured pounds of force when the individual assumed wrist flexion. During the 4 weeks of splint application, the subjects' wrist tone decreased significantly. When they did not wear the splints for a week, their tone increased again. In contrast, Mathiowitz, Bolding, and Trombly (1983) found that four adult subjects showed no reduction in tone during or immediately after use of finger spreaders and hard cone splints.

A concern with many spasticity reduction splints is that they control the thumb over the first and second phalanges but not over the metacarpal. Phelps and Weeks (1976) noted that control of the first metacarpal is essential when a thumb-index finger web space contracture is present. Distal force on the thumb can result in ". . . stretch or even rupture of the ulnar collateral ligament of the MCP joint of the thumb . . . " (Phelps et al., 1976, p. 545) as well as subluxation of the MCP joint. Because children with spasticity usually demonstrate marked thumb adduction, distal control of the thumb moves the MCP and IP joints into hyperextension but does not abduct or extend the first metacarpal. Thus if a splint does not control the carpometacarpal (CMC) joint of the thumb, joint damage can occur, further impairing thumb and hand use.

*Resting pan splints* may provide more support to and control of the thumb than some of the spasticity reduction devices. However, splints should be planned and monitored carefully for reactions at the wrist and fingers. The classic position for a resting hand splint in which the wrist is in 20 to 30 degrees of extension and fingers are in slight flexion may not be appropriate or tolerated by children with increased tone. The child with moderately increased tone may have more tolerance for a resting splint that holds the wrist in neutral position and the fingers in slight flexion. However, if flexor spasticity is severe, the child often pull out of such splints. In this instance, splinting that begins with the wrist in marked flexion and emphasizes slightly increased finger extension (out of full fisting) may be most effective. Initially, wrist position should be stabilized in just slightly more extension than the child normally achieves, but still less than neutral (Boehme, 1985). Splints are then adjusted or reconstructed to position at the wrist, thumb, and fingers. In general, extension is increased at only the wrist or fingers at one time to prevent the occurrence of flexion or extension deformities in the fingers.

Other *volar splints,* such as the wrist cock-up splint, may be used with children who respond to control of wrist flexion but who do not need or cannot tolerate positioning of the fingers or thumb simultaneously. The cock-up splint also allows the child to use the hand to perform functional activities. Volar cock-up splints may also require serial refitting to promote progression in controlled finger use of finger extension during activities. Ulnar deviation should be controlled by the wrist cock-up splint as well.

Controversy regarding the use of dorsal versus volar static splints is long-standing and has yet to be resolved. From a functional perspective it appears that dorsal splints are most effective with children who have muscle weakness and those with mild to moderately increased tone. The dorsal splint shown in Figure 12-19 has been used on children with high tone and those with low tone to hold their wrists in a neutral position. The splint is designed to provide support to the palmar arch. Although the child cannot use extreme wrist flexion, a small degree of wrist flexion

may be used in functional activities. Because of the small amount of contact with the volar surface of the hand and forearm, this splint interferes less with controlled arm use on a surface than a volar splint would; children have responded favorably to this splint. However, use of dorsal static splints to control abnormal finger position in children with central nervous system deficit is sometimes difficult.

Thumb splints are indicated when a child has difficulty with thumb control but can adequately coordinate movements in other parts of the wrist and hand or when the thumb seems to be the greatest problem. Exner and Bonder (1983) reported a study of short opponens thumb splint use with 12 children who had cerebral palsy with spastic hemiplegia. These splints controlled the thumb over the first metacarpal and extended onto the distal phalanx (Figure 12-20). Splints were used 8 hours daily for 6 weeks. When tested with the splints off, two children showed improvement in bilateral hand use and three children showed improved grasp. Some children in the study found that wearing the splints on the nonpreferred hand interfered with stabilization of materials that could not be grasped. In clinical use the splint has been beneficial in improving children's abilities to use their hands functionally.

The Neoprene or Neoplush soft-splint for the thumb is made of two straight pieces of the material, which is about ¼-inch thick and has a slight stretch. This design appears best suited for control of only mildly increased tone. Use of an opponens splint pattern using the design for the splint described above is more suitable when higher tone is present (Figure 12-21). Hill (1988) described other splinting techniques for thumb adduction problems.

Several therapists have explored the effectiveness of other orthotic devices to provide specific types of sensory stimulation and thereby inhibit or facilitate tone. The hard cone, dowel, and orthokinetic cuff are examples. Farber and Huss (1973) stated that the purpose of the cone was to activate golgi tendon organs and inhibits muscle contraction through pressure on the finger flexor tendons. Hard cones should be fabricated to the shape of the hand, with a narrower diameter on the radial side and larger area on the ulnar side. However, hard cones do not seem to effectively

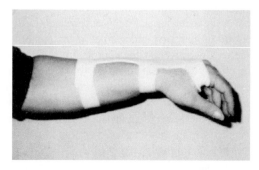

**Figure 12-19**   Dorsal splint to support the wrist in extension.

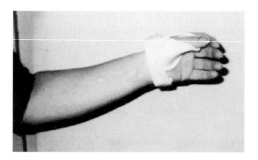

**Figure 12-20**   Short opponens thumb splint.

control the first metacarpal. Therefore they should be used with caution if the child shows a thumb adduction pattern.

MacKinnon, Sanderson, and Buchanan (1975) introduced the *MacKinnon splint,* a device that uses a dowel in the child's hand to provide pressure against the metacarpal heads. A piece of rubberized tubing is attached to each end of the dowel and connects to a small band that fastens around the child's wrist. Contact of the dowel with the metacarpal heads is believed to stretch and facilitate the intrinsic muscles of the hand and inhibit the long finger flexors. MacKinnon et al. (1975) reported that children with spastic cerebral palsy improved in hand awareness and bilateral hand use and showed a decrease in fisting.

Exner and Bonder (1983) modified the MacKinnon splint. The forearm piece was enlarged, and two straps were used to provide better stabilization (Figure 12-22). They found that stabilization of the dowel against the metacarpal heads did not occur, but the dowel did remain in contact with the palm of the child's hand. The orthotic was fitted with the child's hand in its most typical wrist position (in flexion, if necessary) so that firm dowel contact with the palm could be maintained. Wrist positioning is not a function of this splint. Children in their study wore the modified MacKinnon splints 8 hours daily for 6 weeks. Seven of the 12 children showed improvement secondary to use of this splint. Three children improved in both grasp and bilateral hand skills, two improved in both grasp only, and two improved in bilateral hand skills alone. The children with improved skills all had moderate to severe upper extremity motor involvement. All children tolerated the splint well and found that weight bearing could be accomplished comfortably during application periods.

Several precautions regarding use of the MacKinnon splint should be noted. The splint is usually constructed by attaching aquarium tubing to the dowel with small nails. Even though these nails are covered with moleskin, the splint should not be used if the child is likely to put objects in his or her mouth. An alternative is to roll thermoplastic material around the tubing in place of using a dowel. This alternative is not as readily adjustable, however.

Hill (1988) noted that some children may experience instability of the upper extremity in conjunction with decreased tone secondary to MacKinnon splint use. Therefore careful monitoring, particularly in number of weeks for use, is recommended.

*Orthokinetic devices* are applied to facilitate tone in one muscle group and inhibit tone in the opposing muscles. These cuffs are made of elastic and nonelastic segments. Blashy and Fuchs (1959) postulated that the elastic portion activates afferent fibers of skin exteroceptors and possibly the proprioceptors and thus affects the motor neurons that innervate the muscles underlying the stimulated skin area. It is unclear whether the effectiveness of the device is attributable to its inhibitory or facilitory functions or a combination of both. However, the authors noted that orthokinetic cuffs were more effective when tone imbalance between the muscle groups was pronounced.

The Exner and Bonder (1983) study of splint use with 12 children with cerebral palsy also tested application of orthokinetic cuffs. Evaluation of effects was tested over a 6-week period, with 8 hours of daily use. Cuffs were placed on the forearm, with the elastic (facilitory) portion over the muscle bellies of the finger and wrist extensors. Four children demonstrated improvement in both functions. The study indicated that the device helped encourage wrist or finger extension when the child was able to use some active contraction of the muscles being facilitated.

Orthokinetic cuffs are made from three layers of elastic bandage material, with nonstretch fabric sewn into the areas that are to be inhibitory. The cuff should be carefully

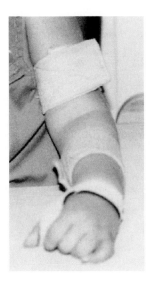

**Figure 12-21** A neoplush thumb splint is worn with orthokinetic cuffs on the forearm and arm. Both orthokinetic cuffs are designed to promote extension and inhibit flexion.

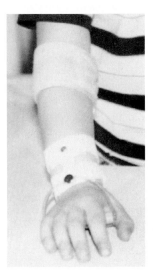

**Figure 12-22** MacKinnon splint and forearm orthokinetic cuff.

fitted before final sewing so that it is snug and the elastic portion does not extend onto the muscles to be inhibited. For facilitation of elbow extension, the active (elastic) area of the cuff is placed over the triceps and the inactive area over the biceps. Orthokinetic cuffs can easily be used with other hand splints. They can also be worn during treatment activities.

Other orthotic devices have been developed for children with increased tone or contractures. Positioning children who have had head injuries to prevent loss of range is particularly important during extensive comatose, semicoma-

tose, and recovery periods. Inflatable air (pneumatic) splints (Hill, 1988) are used to decrease tone, maintain and increase joint range, and stimulate somatosensory function. Casting is used with increasing frequency with children who exhibit spasticity and soft contractures secondary to cerebral palsy or head injury (Yasukawa & Hill, 1988). Tona and Schneck (1993) conducted a single-subject study using upper-extremity casting. Their findings were positive regarding the effectiveness for that child.

## SUMMARY

A description of the components of hand and arm function that are instrumental in the performance of play, self-maintenance, schoolwork, and vocational readiness activities have been presented in this chapter. Factors that influence the development of hand function, as well as generic types of problems in hand and arm use, were discussed. The normal sequences of development for basic skills of reach, grasp, release, and carry, as well as advanced functions of in-hand manipulation and bilateral hand use, were presented. Treatment strategies for development of hand skills were described, as well as the appropriate uses of splinting with children. Assessment and treatment of hand and arm function problems should be seen within the context of the child's daily life tasks.

---

## STUDY QUESTIONS

1. What are the major considerations for intervention with an adolescent who has spastic hemiplegia, demonstrates elbow flexion, forearm pronation, and fisting in the nonpreferred hand; and is having difficulty completing manual dexterity tasks in his or her vocational readiness program?

2. A 5-year-old girl with marked involuntary movements in the upper extremities and poor postural stability would like to feed herself. What aspects of arm and hand function would you assess to determine if she can do this with or without adaptive equipment? What treatment strategies could be used to promote the most effective grasp of the spoon and cup and achievement of the plate-to-mouth pattern? What types of splinting could be considered?

3. An 8-year-old boy has sloppy handwriting. How may problems with bilateral hand use and in-hand manipulation skills interact with short attention span and somatosensory problems to contribute to his handwriting difficulties?

4. What aspects of reach, grasp, release, and bilateral hand use should be addressed with a 15-month-old Down syndrome baby who shows low tone, low hand function, and cognitive skills at the 8- to 10-month level?

5. A 10-year-old girl sustained a head injury 2 months ago. Before the accident she was left hand dominant. She is now alert but has some memory deficits and motor planning problems. She has a left elbow contracture and shows moderately increased tone in wrist flexion, thumb adduction, and finger flexion. What types of splinting or casting could be considered? How could you determine if the splinting or casting devices are effective treatment?

## REFERENCES

Ager, C.L., Olivett, B.L., & Johnson, C.L. (1984). Grasp and pinch strength in children 5 to 12 years old. *The American Journal of Occupational Therapy, 38,* 107-113.

Ammon, J.E. & Etzel, M.E. (1977). Sensorimotor organization in reach and prehension. *Physical Therapy, 57,* 7-14.

Ayres, A.J. (1954). Ontogenetic principles in the development of arm and hand function. *The American Journal of Occupational Therapy, 8,* 95-99.

Ayres, A.J. (1958). The visual-motor function. *The American Journal of Occupational Therapy, 12,* 130-138.

Ayres, A.J. (1979). *Sensory integration and the child.* Los Angeles: Western Psychological Services.

Barnes, K.J. (1986). Improving prehension skills of children with cerebral palsy: a clinical study. *Occupational Therapy Journal of Research, 6*(4), 227-239.

Barnes, K.J. (1989a). Relationship of upper extremity weight bearing to hand skills of boys with cerebral palsy. *Occupational Therapy Journal of Research, 9,* 143-154.

Barnes, K.J. (1989b). Direct replication: relationship of upper extremity weight bearing to hand skills of boys with cerebral palsy. *Occupational Therapy Journal of Research, 9,* 235-242.

Blashy, M.R.M. & Fuchs, R.L. (1959). Orthokinetics: a new receptor facilitation method. *The American Journal of Occupational Therapy, 13,* 226-234.

Bobath, B. (1978). *Adult hemiplegia: evaluation and treatment* (2nd ed.). London: Heinemann Educational Books.

Boehme, R.H. (1985). *NDT advanced course for treatment of the upper extremities.* August. Denver.

Boehme, R.H. (1988). *Improving upper body control: an approach to assessment and treatment of tonal dysfunction.* Tucson: Therapy Skill Builders.

Case-Smith, J. (1991). The effects of tactile defensiveness and tactile discrimination on in-hand manipulation. *The American Journal of Occupational Therapy, 45,* 811-818.

Case-Smith, J. (1993). Comparison of in-hand manipulation skills in children with and without fine motor delays. *Occupational Therapy Journal of Research, 13,* 87-100.

Case-Smith, J., Fisher, A.G., & Bauer, D. (1989). An analysis of the relationship between proximal and distal motor control. *The American Journal of Occupational Therapy, 43,* 657-662.

Chakarian, D.L. & Larson, M. (1991, September). The effects of upper extremity weight bearing on hand function in children with cerebral palsy. *NDTA Newsletter,* pp. 4-5.

Colangelo, C.A. (1993). Biomechanical frame of reference. In P. Kramer & J. Hinojosa (Eds.). *Frames of reference for pediatric occupational therapy* (pp. 233-305). Baltimore: Williams & Wilkins.

Conner, F.P., Williamson, G.G., & Siepp, J.M. (1978). Movement. In *Program guide for infants and toddlers.* New York: College Press.

Connolly, K. & Dalgleish, M. (1989). The emergence of a tool-using skill in infancy. *Developmental Psychology, 25,* 894-912.

Connolly, K. & Elliott, J. (1972). The evolution and ontogeny of hand function. In B. Jones (Ed.). *Ethological studies of child behaviour* (pp. 329-383). London: Cambridge University.

Corbetta, D. & Mounoud, P. (1990). Early development of grasping and manipulation. In C. Bard, M. Fleury, & L. Hay (Eds.). *Development of eye-hand coordination across the life span* (pp. 188-213). Columbia: University of South Carolina.

Danella, E. & Vogtle, L. (1992). Neurodevelopmental treatment for the young child with cerebral palsy. In J. Case-Smith & C. Pehoski (Eds.). *Development of hand skills in the child* (pp. 91-110). Rockville, MD: AOTA.

Doubilet, L. & Polkow, L.S. (1977). A classification of manipulative hand movements. *Developmental Medicine and Child Neurology, 26,* 283-296.

Elliott, J.M. & Connolly, K.J. (1984). A classification of manipulative hand movements. *Developmental Medicine and Child Neurology, 26,* 283-296.

Embry, D.G. (1993). Efficacy studies in children with cerebral palsy: focus on upper extremity function. *Physical and Occupational Therapy in Pediatrics, 12* (4), 89-95.

Erhardt, R.P. (1982). *Erhardt developmental prehension assessment.* Tucson: Therapy Skill Builders.

Erhardt, R.P. (1992). Eye-hand coordination. In J. Case-Smith & C. Pehoski (Eds.). *Development of hand skills in the child* (pp. 13-33). Rockville, MD: AOTA.

Exner, C.E. (1990a). In-hand manipulation skills in normal young children: a pilot study. *Occupational Therapy Practice, 1* (4), 63-72.

Exner, C.E. (1990b). The zone of proximal development in in-hand manipulation skills of non-dysfunctional 3- and 4-year-old children. *The American Journal of Occupational Therapy, 44,* 884-891.

Exner, C.E. (1992). In-hand manipulation skills. In J. Case-Smith & C. Pehoski (Eds.). *Development of hand skills in the child* (pp. 35-45). Rockville, MD: AOTA.

Exner, C.E. (1993). Content validity on the in-hand manipulation test. *The American Journal of Occupational Therapy, 47,* 505-513.

Exner, C.E. (1995). Remediation of hand skill problems in children. In A. Henderson & C. Pehoski (Eds.). *Hand function in the child: foundations for remediation* (pp. 197-222). St. Louis: Mosby.

Exner, C.E. & Bonder, B.R. (1983). Comparative effects of three hand splints on the bilateral hand use, grasp, and arm-hand posture in hemiplegic children: a pilot study. *Occupational Therapy Journal of Research, 3,* 75-92.

Exner, C.E. & Henderson, A. (1995). Cognition and motor skill. In A. Henderson & C. Pehoski (Eds.). *Hand function in the child* (pp. 93-110). St. Louis: Mosby.

Farber, S.D. & Huss, J. (1973). *Sensory motor evaluation and treatment procedures for allied health personnel.* Indianapolis: Indiana University—Purdue University at Indianapolis.

Finnie, N.R. (1975). *Handling the young cerebral palsied child at home* (2nd ed.). New York: E.P. Dutton.

Folio, R.M. & Fewell, R. (1983). *Peabody developmental motor scales.* Chicago: Riverside.

Fraiberg, S.A., Smith M., & Adelson, E. (1969). An educational program for blind infants. *Journal of Special Education, 3,* 121-139.

Gesell, A. & Amatruda, C.S. (1947). *Developmental diagnosis.* New York: Harper & Row.

Gilfoyle, E.M., Grady, A.P., & Moore, J.C. (1990). *Children adapt* (2nd ed.). Thorofare, NJ: Slack.

Haron, M. & Henderson, A. (1985). Active and passive touch in developmentally dyspraxic and normal boys. *Occupational Therapy Journal of Research, 5,* 101-112.

Hill, J. (1994). The effects of casting on upper extremity motor disorders after brain injury. *The American Journal of Occupational Therapy, 48,* 219-224.

Hill, S.G. (1988). Current trends in upper-extremity splinting. In R. Boehme (Ed.). *Improving upper body control* (pp. 131-164).Tucson: Therapy Skill Builders.

Hirschel, A., Pehoski, C., & Coryell, J. (1990). Environmental support and the development of grasp in infants. *The American Journal of Occupational Therapy, 44,* 721-727.

Hohlstein, R.R. (1982). The development of prehension in normal infants. *The American Journal of Occupational Therapy, 36,* 170-176.

Kenney, W.E. (1963). Certain sensory defects in cerebral palsy. *Clinical Orthopedics, 27,* 193-195.

Latch, C.M., Freeling, M.C., & Powell, N.J. (1993). A comparison of the grip strength of children with myelomeningocele to that of children without disability. *The American Journal of Occupational Therapy, 47,* 498-503.

Lawrence, D.G. & Kuypers, H.G. (1986). The functional organization of the motor system in monkey. Parts I & II. *Brain, 91,* 1-36.

Lenti, C., Radice, L., Cerioli, M.I., & Musetti, L. (1991). Tactile extinction in childhood hemiplegia. *Developmental Medicine and Child Neurology, 33,* 789-794.

Long, C., Conrad, P.W., Hall, E.A., & Furler, S.L. (1970). Intrinsic-extrinsic muscle control of the hand in power grip and precision handling. *Journal of Bone and Joint Surgery, 52A,* 853-913.

MacKinnon, J., Sanderson, E., & Buchanan, J. (1975). The MacKinnon splint: a functional hand splint. *Canadian Journal of Occupational Therapy, 42,* 157-158.

Mathiowitz, V., Bolding, P.J., & Trombly, C.A. (1983). Immediate effects of positioning devices on the normal and spastic hand measured by electromyography. *The American Journal of Occupational Therapy, 37,* 247-254.

Mathiowitz, V., Rogers, S.L., Dowe-Keval, M., Donohoe, L., & Rennells, C. (1986). The Purdue Pegboard: Norms for 14- 19-year olds. *The American Journal of Occupational Therapy, 40,* 174-179.

Mathiowitz, V., Weimer, D.M., & Federman, S.M. (1986). Grip and pinch strength: norms for 6- to 19-year olds. *The American Journal of Occupational Therapy, 40,* 705-711.

McHale, K. & Cermak, S.A. (1992). Fine motor activities in elementary school: preliminary findings and provisional implications for children with fine mot or problems. *The American Journal of Occupational Therapy, 46,* 898-903.

McPherson, J.J. (1981). Objective evaluation of a splint designed to reduce hypertonicity. *The American Journal of Occupational Therapy, 35,* 189-194.

Monfraix, C., Tardieu, G., & Tardieu, C. (1961). Disturbances of manual perception in children with cerebral palsy. *Developmental Medicine and Child Neurology, 22,* 454-464.

Myers, C.A. (1992). Therapeutic fine-motor activities for preschoolers. In J. Case-Smith & C. Pehoski (Eds.). *Development of hand skills in the child* (pp. 47-59). Rockville, MD: AOTA.

Napier, J.R. (1956). The prehensile movements of the human hand. *Journal of Bone Joint Surgery, 38B,* 902-913.

Pehoski, C. (1992). Central nervous system control of precision movements of the hand. In J. Case-Smith & C. Pehoski (Eds.). *Development of hand skills in the child* (pp. 1-11). Rockville, MD: AOTA.

Phelps, R.E. & Weeks, P.M. (1976). Management of thumb-in-palm web space contracture. *The American Journal of Occupational Therapy, 30,* 543-556.

Ruff, H.A. (1980). The development of the perception and recognition of objects. *Child Development, 51,* 981-992.

Ruff, H.A., McCarton, C., Kurtzber, D., & Vaughan, Jr., H. G. (1984). Preterm infants' manipulative exploration of objects. *Child Development, 55,* 1166-1173.

Schneck, C. & Battaglia, C. (1992). Developing scissors skills in young children. In J. Case-Smith & C. Pehoski (Eds.). *Development of hand skills in the child* (pp. 79-89). Rockville, MD: AOTA.

Schoen, S. & Anderson, J. (1993). Neurodevelopmental treatment frame of reference. In P. Kramer & J. Hinojosa (Eds.). *Frames of reference for pediatric occupational therapy* (pp. 49-86). Baltimore: Williams & Wilkins.

Sheridan, M.D. (1975). *From birth to five years: children's developmental progress.* Atlantic Highlands, NJ: Humanities Press.

Smith, R.O. & Benge, M.W. (1985). Pinch and grasp strength: standardization of terminology and protocol. *The American Journal of Occupational Therapy, 39,* 531-535.

Snook, J.H. (1979). Spasticity reduction splint. *The American Journal of Occupational Therapy, 33,* 648-651.

Tachdjian, M.O. & Minear, W.I. (1958). Sensory disturbances in the hands of children with hemiplegia. *Journal of the American Medical Association, 155,* 628-632.

Tona, J.L. & Schneck, C.M. (1993). The efficacy of upper extremity inhibitive casting: a single-subject pilot study. *The American Journal of Occupational Therapy, 47,* 901-910.

Twitchell, T.E. (1965). The automatic grasping responses of infants. *Neuropsychologics, 3,* 247-259.

Weiss, M.W. & Flatt, A.E. (1971). Functional evaluation of the congenitally anomalous hand. Part II. *The American Journal of Occupational Therapy, 25,* 139-143.

Wilson, B. & Trombly, C.A. (1984). Proximal and distal function in children with and without sensory integrative dysfunction: an EMG study. *Canadian Journal of Occupational Therapy, 51,* 11-17.

Yasukawa, A. (1992). Upper-extremity casting: adjunct treatment for the child with cerebral palsy. In J. Case-Smith & C. Pehoski (Eds.). *Development of hand skills in the child* (pp. 111-123). Rockville, MD: AOTA.

Yasukawa, A. & Hill, J. (1988). Casting to improve upper extremity function. In R. Boehme (Ed.). *Improving upper body control* (pp. 165-188). Tucson: Therapy Skill Builders.

## SUGGESTED READINGS

Duff, S.V. (1995). Prehension. In D. Cech & S. Martin (Eds.). *Functional movement development across the life span* (pp. 313-353). Philadelphia: W.B. Saunders.

Eliasson, A.C., Gordon, A.M., & Forsaberg, H. (1991). Basic co-ordination of manipulative forces of children with cerebral palsy. *Developmental Medicine and Child Neurology, 33,* 661-670.

Henderson, A. & Pehoski, C. (1995). *Hand function in the child.* St. Louis: Mosby.

Jensen, G.D. & Alderman, M.E. (1963). The prehensile grasp of spastic diplegia. *Pediatrics, 31,* 470-477.

Kopp, C.B. (1974). Fine motor abilities of infants. *Developmental Medicine and Child Neurology, 16,* 629-636.

Ruff, H.A. (1982). Role of manipulation in infants' responses to invariant properties of objects. *Developmental Psychology, 18,* 682-691.

Sugden, D.A. & Keogh, J.F. (1990). *Problems in movement skill development.* Columbia: University of South Carolina.

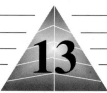

# Sensory Integration

L. DIANE PARHAM ▲ ZOE MAILLOUX

## KEY TERMS

- ▲ Sensory Nourishment
- ▲ Adaptive Responses
- ▲ Neural Plasticity
- ▲ Ontogeny of Sensory Integration
- ▲ Sensory Modulation
- ▲ Sensory Defensiveness
- ▲ Sensory Discrimination
- ▲ Vestibular Processing Disorders
- ▲ Dyspraxia
- ▲ Classical Sensory Integration Treatment
- ▲ Compensatory Skill Development
- ▲ Group Therapy Program
- ▲ Expected Outcomes of Sensory Integration Treatment
- ▲ Efficacy Research

## CHAPTER OBJECTIVES

1. Explain the neurobiologic concepts that are basic to an individual's sensory integrative function.
2. Explain the link between sensory input from the environment and the child's adaptive response.
3. Describe the development of sensory integration from prenatal life through childhood.
4. Explain the clinical picture and hypothesized basis for problems in sensory modulation, defensiveness, and discrimination.
5. Describe vestibular processing disorders and the types of behaviors that characterize children with vestibular processing problems.
6. Define developmental dyspraxia, and identify examples of behaviors that might be observed in a young child with dyspraxia.
7. Identify and describe tests, interviews, and instruments used in evaluation of sensory integration.

8. Define and explain classical sensory integrative treatment, and discuss limitations and benefits of using such an intervention approach.
9. Explain when individual therapy should focus on compensatory skill development.
10. Describe group therapy programs and consultative models, and explain the benefits of using these models in combination with classical treatment.
11. Identify the expected outcomes of occupational therapy using a sensory integrative approach.
12. Discuss the published research on the effectiveness of sensory integration.

The term *sensory integration* holds special meaning for occupational therapists. In some contexts it is used to refer to a particular way of viewing the neural organization of sensory information for functional behavior. In other situations this term refers to a clinical frame of reference for the assessment and treatment of persons who have functional disorders in sensory processing. Both of these meanings originated in the work of A. Jean Ayres, an occupational therapist and educational psychologist whose brilliant clinical insights and original research revolutionized occupational therapy practice with children.

Ayres' ideas ushered in a whole new way of looking at children and understanding many of the developmental, learning, and emotional problems that arise during childhood. Her innovative practice and groundbreaking research met a tremendous amount of resistance within the profession when introduced in the late 1960s and 1970s. Today the treatment methods that she pioneered continue to be questioned and investigated; yet there is little doubt that her perspective has had a profound influence on occupational therapy practice. The presence of sensory integration concepts in nearly all of the chapters of this book attests to the extent to which these ideas have affected the thinking of pediatric occupational therapists. Furthermore, the research base of the sensory integration frame of reference is extensive. Indeed, more research has been conducted in the area of sensory integration than in any other area of occupational therapy.

This chapter provides an in-depth orientation to this fascinating aspect of occupational therapy practice. The reader will gain a general sense of how sensory integration as a brain function is related to everyday occupations. Following is a description of how sensory integration is manifested in typically developing children and then in relation to the daily-life problems of children who experience difficulty with sensory integration. The history of research on sensory integrative dysfunction is reviewed to give the reader a perspective on how this field came into being, what the major constructs are, and how they have changed—and continue to change—over time. Sensory integration, as a clinical frame of reference, is described by identifying types of sensory integrative dysfunction, reviewing approaches to clinical assessment, and outlining the characteristics of both direct and indirect modes of intervention. The issue of effectiveness research is addressed. Finally, case examples of children who have been helped by occupational therapists using sensory integrative principles are presented.

## SENSORY INTEGRATION IN CHILD DEVELOPMENT

One of the most distinctive contributions that Ayres made to understanding child development was her focus on sensory processing, particularly with respect to the proximal senses: vestibular, tactile, and proprioceptive. In the sensory integration viewpoint, these senses are emphasized because they are primitive and primary: they dominate the child's interactions with the world early in life. Certainly, the distal senses of vision and hearing are critical and become increasingly more dominant as the child matures. Ayres believed, however, that the body-centered senses are a foundation on which complex occupations are scaffolded. Furthermore, when Ayres began her work, the vestibular, tactile, and proprioceptive senses were virtually ignored by scholars and clinicians who were interested in child development. She devoted her career to studying the roles that these forgotten senses play in development and in the genesis of developmental problems of children.

A basic assumption made by Ayres (1972b) was that brain function is a critical factor in human behavior. She reasoned, therefore, that knowledge of brain function and dysfunction would give her insight into child development and would help her understand the developmental problems of children. However, Ayres also had a pragmatic orientation that sprang from her professional background as an occupational therapist. Consequently, her work represents a fusion of neurobiologic insights with the practical, everyday concerns of human beings, particularly children and their families.

As Ayres developed her ideas about sensory integration, she used terms such as *sensory integration, adaptive response,* and *praxis* in ways that reflected her orientation. A glossary of terms that are commonly used within the framework of sensory integration theory is presented in Appendix 13-A. It may be helpful to the reader to refer to these definitions frequently while reading this chapter. Some of the terms in Appendix 13-A were coined by Ayres, whereas others were drawn from the literature of other fields. When Ayres borrowed a term from another field, however, she imparted a particular meaning to it. Consider, for example, *sensory integration.* Ayres did not use this term to refer solely to intricate synaptic connections within the brain, as neuroscientists typically do. Rather, she applied it to neural processes as they relate to functional behavior. Hence, her definition of sensory integration is the "organization of sensation for use" (Ayres, 1979, p. 5). It is the inclusion of the final clause "for use" that is a hallmark of Ayres because it ties sensory processing to the person's occupation.

Not only did Ayres introduce a new vocabulary of sensory integration theory, but she also synthesized important concepts from the neurobiologic literature to organize her views of child development and dysfunction. Many of these ideas were first published in her classic book, *Sensory Integration and Learning Disorders* (Ayres, 1972b). Later she wrote a book for parents, *Sensory Integration and the Child* (Ayres, 1979) outlining the behavioral changes that can be observed in a child as sensory integration develops. Major points made in these books regarding, first, neurobiologic concepts in relationship to development, and second, the ontogeny of sensory integration, are presented in the following sections.

## NEUROBIOLOGICALLY BASED CONCEPTS
### Sensory Nourishment

Sensory input is necessary for optimal brain function. The brain is designed to constantly take in sensory information, and it malfunctions if deprived of it. Sensory deprivation experiments conducted in the 1950s and 1960s make it clear that without an adequate inflow of sensation, the brain generates its own input in the form of hallucinations and subsequently distorts incoming sensory stimuli (Solomon et al., 1961). Developmentally, it is known that if adequate sensory stimulation is not available at critical periods in development, brain abnormalities and resulting behavioral disorders result (Hubel & Wiesel, 1963; Kolb & Whishaw, 1985).

Ayres (1979) considered sensory input to be nourishment for the brain, just as food is nourishment for the body. Wilbarger (1984), a colleague of Ayres, built on this concept with her notion of the *sensory diet* designed specially for the child with sensory integrative dysfunction. The therapeutic sensory diet provides the optimal combination of sensations at the appropriate intensities for an individual child.

For most typically developing children, the sensory diet does not require conscious monitoring by caregivers. The environment continuously "feeds" the child a variety of nourishing sensations in the flow of everyday life.

As critical as input is to the developing brain, the mere provision of sensory stimulation is limited in value. In fact, too much stimulation can generate stress that is detrimental to development. To have an optimal effect, the child must actively *use* sensory input to act on the environment.

## Adaptive Response

A child is not a passive sponge for whatever sensations come along. Rather, the child actively selects those sensations that are most useful at the time and organizes them in a fashion that facilitates accomplishing goals. This is the process of *sensory integration*. When this process is going well, the child organizes a successful, goal-directed action on the environment. This is what we call an *adaptive response*. When a child makes an adaptive response, he or she successfully meets some challenge presented in the environment. The adaptive response is possible because the brain has been able to efficiently organize incoming sensory information, which then provides a basis for action (Figure 13-1).

Adaptive responses are powerful forces that drive development forward. When a child makes an adaptive response that is more complex than any previously accomplished response, the brain attains a more organized state and its capacity for sensory integration is enhanced. Thus sensory integration leads to adaptive responses, which, in turn, results in more efficient sensory integration.

Ayres (1979) provided the example of learning to ride a bicycle to illustrate this process. The child must integrate sensations, particularly from the vestibular and proprioceptive systems, to learn how to balance on the bicycle. The senses must accurately and quickly detect when the child begins to fall. Eventually, perhaps after many trials of falling, the child integrates sensory information efficiently enough to make the appropriate weight shifts over the bicycle to maintain balance. This is an adaptive response, and once made, the child is able to balance more effectively on the next attempt to ride the bike. The child's nervous system has changed and now is more adept at the business of bicycle riding.

In making adaptive responses the child is an active doer, not a passive recipient. Adaptive responses come from within the child. No one can force a child to respond adaptively, although a situation may be set up that is likely to elicit adaptive responses from the child. For typically developing children and for most children with disabilities, there is an innate drive to develop sensory integration through adaptive responses. Ayres (1979) called this *inner drive* and speculated that it is generated primarily by the limbic system of the brain, a structure known to be critical

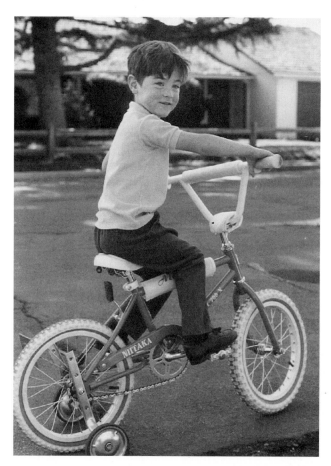

**Figure 13-1** Adaptive responses help the child acquire skills such as riding a bicycle. Although training wheels reduce the challenge for this boy, his nervous system must integrate vestibular, proprioceptive, and visual information adequately to successfully steer the bicycle while it is moving. (Courtesy of Shay McAtee.)

in both motivation and memory. Ayres designed therapeutic activities and environments to engage the child's inner drive, elicit adaptive responses, and in so doing, advance sensory integrative development.

## Neural Plasticity

It is thought that when a child makes an adaptive response, change occurs at a neuronal synaptic level. This change is a function of the brain's plasticity. Plasticity is the ability of a structure and concomitant function to be changed gradually by its own ongoing activity (Ayres, 1972b). It is well established in the neuroscientific literature that when organisms are permitted to explore interesting environments, significant increases in dendritic branching, synaptic connections, synaptic efficiency, and even size of brain tissue result (Rosenzweig, Bennett, & Diamond, 1972). These changes are most dramatic in a young animal and probably represent a major mechanism of brain development, although it is clear that such manifestations of plasticity are characteristic of optimal brain functioning throughout the lifespan (Bach-Y-Rita, 1981). Studies of the effects of enriched environments on animals indicate that the essential ingredient for positive brain changes is that the organism actively interacts with a challenging environment (Bennett, Diamond, Krech, & Rosenzweig, 1964). Passive exposure to sensory stimulation does not produce these same positive changes (Dru, Walker, & Walker, 1975). It can be hypothesized from these findings that adaptive responses activate the brain's neuroplastic capabilities. Furthermore, the brain's plasticity makes it possible for an adaptive response to increase the efficiency of sensory integration at a neuronal level.

Schaaf (1994) used the activity of learning to ride a bicycle to illustrate how neuroplasticity may operate in development. She pointed out that a child first practices the basic skill of maintaining balance on the bicycle, but then once this is mastered, the child uses it repeatedly in riding up and down the sidewalk for hours. After this is mastered, the child looks for greater challenges, such as riding up and down hills or jumping curbs. Schaaf (1994) interpreted these behaviors using concepts of developmental plasticity. First the child solidifies the necessary neural pathways for bike riding and then later enhances or modifies these pathways by creating challenging environments. Schaaf (1994) further drew a parallel between this process and the opportunities that are afforded a child during sensory integrative treatment.

## Central Nervous System Organization

Ayres (1972b) looked to the organization of the central nervous system (CNS) for clues as to how children organize and use sensory information and how sensory integration develops over time. At the time she was developing her theory, *hierarchic* models of the CNS-dominated thinking in the neurosciences.

Hierarchic models view the nervous system in terms of vertically arranged levels, with the spinal cord at the bottom, the cerebral hemispheres at the top, and the brainstem sandwiched in between. These levels are interdependent yet reflect a trend of ascending control and specialization. Thus the cerebral cortex at the top of the hierarchy is highly specialized and analyzes precise details of sensory information. Ordinarily the cortex assumes a directive role over lower levels of the hierarchy. For example, the cortex may command lower centers to "ignore" certain stimuli deemed unimportant. This process is called *descending inhibition* and is critical in enabling higher brain functions to work efficiently (Ayres, 1972b). The lower levels of the CNS, however, have functions that are more diffuse, primitive, less specialized, and yet potentially more pervasive in influence compared with those of the higher levels. One of the important responsibilities of the lower levels is to filter and refine sensory information before relaying organized sensory messages upward to the cerebral cortex. Thus cortical centers are dependent on lower centers for the receipt of essential, well-organized sensory information to analyze in preparation for the planning of action. According to hierarchic views, the higher levels of the CNS superimpose more sophisticated functions on the lower levels, but these do not replace the important lower-level functions (Ayres, 1972b).

Ayres (1972b) believed that critical aspects of sensory integration are seated in the lower levels of the CNS, particularly the brainstem and thalamus. Most of the CNS processing of vestibular information occurs in the brainstem, and much somatosensory processing takes place there and in the thalamus. One of the basic tenets of Ayres' theory is that because of the dependence of higher CNS structures on lower structures, increased efficiency at the levels of the brainstem and thalamus enhance higher-order functioning (Ayres, 1972b). This view is in sharp contrast to mainstream neuropsychology and education, which tend to emphasize the direct study and remediation of high-level, cortically directed skills such as reading and writing.

In adopting a hierarchic view of the CNS, Ayres (1972b) also assumed that the CNS develops hierarchically from bottom to top, with spinal and brainstem structures maturing before higher-level centers. At the time that Ayres was developing her theory, this was somewhat speculative although generally accepted by neuroscientists. In more recent years the use of positron electron tomography (PET) scans in research on infants has provided direct support for the notion that brain development proceeds in a bottom-to-top direction (Chugani & Phelps, 1986).

The hierarchic approach to CNS functioning and development led Ayres to emphasize the more primitive vestibular and somatosensory systems in her work with young children. These systems mature early and are seated in the lower CNS centers. Using the logic of hierarchy, Ayres reasoned that the refinement of primitive functions such as postural control, balance, and tactile perception provides a sensorimotor foundation for higher-order functions such as academic ability, behavioral self-regulation, and complex motor skills such as those required in sports. Thus she viewed the developmental process as one in which primitive body-centered functions serve as building blocks on which complex cognitive and social skills can be scaffolded. This view undergirds a basic premise of the therapy approach that she developed: that by enhancing lower-level functions related to the proximal senses, one might have a positive influence on higher-level functions.

On some points Ayres (1972b) departed from a strictly hierarchic view of the CNS. For example, she noted that each level of the nervous system can function as a self-contained sensory integration system. Therefore the brainstem has the capacity to independently direct some sensorimotor patterns without being directed by the higher-level cortex. Furthermore, the sensory integrative process involves the brain working as a whole, not simply as a series of hierarchically controlled messages, as rigid hierarchic models might suggest. These ideas are more consistent with the view of some contemporary biologists that the brain is a *heterarchic* system. A heterarchy is a system in which different parts may assume the controlling role in different situations; control does not always flow in a top-down direction (Salthe, 1985). Ayres was ahead of her time in suggesting that the brain does not operate exclusively as a hierarchy but has holistic characteristics. These heterarchic notions strengthened her view that functions considered to be primitive were worthy of serious consideration in therapy.

## ONTOGENY OF SENSORY INTEGRATION

Ayres (1979) believed that sensory integration develops primarily in the first 7 years of life. She drew this conclusion not only from her many years of observing children, but also from research in which she gathered normative data on tests of sensory integration (Ayres, 1972b). By the time most children reach 7 or 8 years of age, their sensory integrative capabilities are almost as mature as an adult's.

Development, from a sensory integrative standpoint, occurs as the CNS organizes sensory information and adaptive responses with increasing degrees of complexity. Sensory integration, of course, enables adaptive responses to occur, which in turn promote the development of sensory integration. As this process unfolds in infancy, the developing child begins to attach meaning to the stream of sensations experienced. The child becomes increasingly adept at shifting attention to what he or she perceives as meaningful, tuning out that which is irrelevant to current needs and interests. As a result the child can organize play behavior for increasing lengths of time and gains control in the regulation of emotions. Inner drive leads the child to search for opportunities in the environment that are "just right challenges." These are challenges that are not so complex that they overwhelm or induce failure, nor so simple that they are routine or disinteresting. The just right challenge is one that requires effort but is accomplishable for the child. Because there is an element of challenge, a successful adaptive response engenders feelings of mastery and a sense of self as a competent being.

It is fascinating to watch this process unfold in typically developing children. They require no adult guidance or teaching to acquire basic developmental skills such as manipulating objects, sitting, walking, and climbing. Little if any step-by-step instruction is needed to learn daily occupations such as playing on playground equipment, dressing and feeding oneself, drawing and painting, and constructing with blocks. These achievements seem to just happen. They are the product of an active nervous system busily organizing sensory information and searching for challenges that bring forth more and more complex behaviors.

In the following sections, developmental hallmarks of sensory integration are identified. The proximal senses dominate early infancy and continue to exert their influence in critical ways as the visual and auditory systems gain ascendancy. Also, because development is highly canalized (genetically programmed) in infancy, there is limited variation across children in the sequence in which developmental achievements unfold during the first year of life. Developmental variability becomes increasingly apparent after this first year. By kindergarten age, skills vary tremendously among children because of differences in environmental opportunities, familial and cultural influences, and personal experiences, as well as genetic endowment.

### Prenatal Period

The first known responses to sensory stimuli occur early in life, at approximately 5.5 weeks after conception (Humphrey, 1969; Short-DeGraff, 1988). These first responses are to tactile stimuli. Specifically, they involve reflexive avoidance reactions to a perioral stimulus: the embryo bends its head and upper trunk away from a light touch stimulus around the mouth. This is a primitive protective reaction. It is not until about 9 weeks gestational age that an approach response, a moving of the head toward the chest, occurs (Humphrey, 1969), probably as a function of proprioception. The first known responses to vestibular input in the form of the Moro reflex also appear at about 9 weeks postconception. The fetus continues to develop a repertoire of reflexes such as rooting, sucking, Babkin, grasp, flexor withdrawal, Galant, neck righting, Moro, and positive supporting in utero that are fairly well established by the time of birth. Thus when the time comes to leave the uterine home and enter the outside world, the newborn is well equipped with responses that enable a strong connection with a caregiver to be made, as well as protection of the newborn's own physical integrity primarily through the tactile, proprioceptive, and vestibular senses. These innate reactions require rudimentary aspects of sensory integration that are built into the nervous system.

### Neonatal Period

Touch, smell, and movement sensations are particularly important to the newborn infant, who uses these to maintain contact with a caregiver. Tactile sensations, especially, are critical in establishing a mother-infant bond and thus play a key role in fostering feelings of security in the infant.This is just the beginning of the important role that the tactile system plays in a person's emotional life because it is directly involved in making physical contact with others (Figure 13-2). Proprioception is also critical in the mother-infant relationship, enabling the infant to mold to the adult caregiver's body in a cuddly manner. The phasic movements of the infant's limbs generate additional proprioceptive inputs. Together, all of these proprioceptive inputs set the stage for the eventual development of body scheme (the brain's map of the body and how its parts interrelate).

The vestibular system is fully functional at birth, although refinement of its sensory integrative functions, particularly its integration with visual and proprioceptive systems, continues through childhood. Of all the sensory systems, the vestibular system is the first to mature (Maurer & Maurer, 1988). The influence of vestibular stimuli on the infant's arousal level is appreciated instinctively by most caregivers, who use rocking and carrying to soothe and calm the infant. Ayres (1979) pointed out that sensations such as these, which make a child contented and organized, tend to be integrating for the child's nervous system. Vestibular stimuli have other integrating effects on the infant as well. Being lifted into an upright position against the caregiver's shoulder is known to increase alertness and visual pursuit (Gregg, Hafner, & Korner, 1976). While being held in such a position, the young infant's vestibular system detects the pull of gravity and begins to stimulate the neck muscles to raise the head off the caregiver's shoulder. This adaptive response reaches full maturation within 6 months. In the first month of life, head righting may be minimal and intermittent with much wobbling, but it will gradually stabilize and become firmly established as the baby assumes dif-

ferent positions, first when the baby lies in a prone position, and later in supine.

The visual and auditory systems of the newborn are immature. The neonate orients to some visual and auditory inputs and is particularly interested in human faces and voices, although meaning is not yet attached to these sensations (Short-DeGraff, 1988). Visually the infant is attracted to high-contrast stimuli, such as black and white designs, and the range of visual acuity for most stimuli is limited to approximately 10 inches. The infant's visual acuity and responsiveness to visual patterns expand dramatically over the first few months of life (Maurer & Maurer, 1988).

## First Six Months

By 4 to 6 months of age a shift occurs in the infant's behavioral organization. The sensory systems have matured to the extent that the baby has much greater awareness and interest in the world, and developing vestibular-proprioceptive-visual connections provide the beginnings of postural control. During the first half of the first year the infant begins to show a strong inner drive to rise up against gravity (Figure 13-3). Body positions during the first 6 months characteristically involve the prone position with gradually increasing extension from the neck down through the trunk, and arms gradually bear more weight to help push the chest off the floor. By 6 months of age, many infants spend a great deal of time in a prone position with full active trunk extension, and most are able to sit independently, at least if propped with their own hands. These milestones are reflective of the maturing lateral vestibulospinal tract. Head control is well established by now and provides a stable base for control of eye muscles. This, of course, reflects the growing integration of vestibular, proprioceptive,

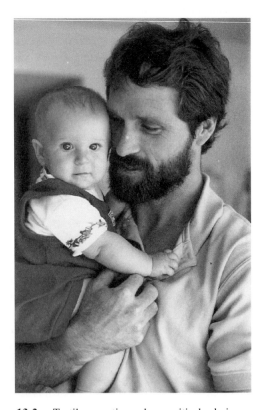

**Figure 13-2**   Tactile sensations play a critical role in generating feelings of security and comfort in the infant and are influential in emotional development and social relationships throughout the life span. (Courtesy of Shay McAtee.)

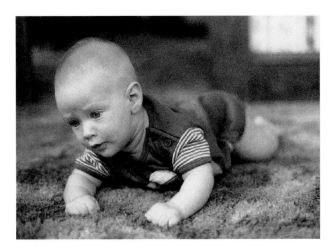

**Figure 13-3**   Strong inner drive to master gravity is evident in this infant's efforts to lift his head and shoulders off the floor. This is an early form of the prone extension posture. (Courtesy of Shay McAtee.)

and visual systems, which become increasingly important in providing a stable visual field as the baby becomes mobile.

Somatosensory achievements at this time are particularly evident in the infant's hands. The infant uses tactile and proprioceptive sensations to grasp objects, albeit with primitive grasps. Touch and visual information are integrated as the baby begins to reach for and wave or bang objects. The infant has a strong inner drive to play with the hands by bringing them to midline while watching and touching them. Connections between the tactile and visual systems are being made that pave the way for later eye-hand coordination skills. In addition, midline hand play is a significant milestone in the integration of sensations from the two sides of the body.

By now neonatal reflexes no longer dominate behavior; the baby is beginning to exercise voluntary control over movements. The earliest episodes of motor planning occur as the infant works to produce novel actions. This becomes evident as the infant handles objects and begins to initiate transitions from one body position to another, as in rolling from prone position to supine. Although reflexes may play a role in such actions (such as grasp and neck righting reflexes), the infant's actions have a goal-directed, volitional quality and are not stereotypically reflex bound but are responsive to changing characteristics of the environment.

## Second Six Months

Another major transition occurs during the latter half of the first year: infants become mobile in their environments, and by the first birthday they can willfully move from one place to another, many walking while others creep or crawl. These locomotor skills, of course, are the product of the many adaptive responses that have gone before, resulting in increasingly more sophisticated integration of somatosensory, vestibular, and visual inputs.

As the infant explores the environment, greater opportunities are generated for integrating a variety of complex sensations, particularly those responsible for developing body scheme and spatial perception. The child is learning about environmental space and about the body's relationship to external space through sensorimotor experiences.

During the second 6 months of life, tactile perception becomes further refined and plays a critical role in the child's developing hand skills. The infant relies on precise tactile feedback in developing a fine pincer grasp, which is used to pick up small objects. Proprioceptive information is also an important influence in developing manipulative skills, and now the baby experiments with objects using a wide variety of actions. These somatosensory-based adaptive responses contribute to development of motor planning ability. Further development of midline skills is also apparent as the baby easily transfers objects from one hand to the other, and the infant may even occasionally cross the midline while holding an object.

All through the first year, auditory processing has played a significant role in the infant's awareness of environment, especially the social environment. Auditory information is integrated with tactile and proprioceptive sensations in and around the mouth as the infant vocalizes. The fruits of this process begin to blossom in the latter half of this first year, when the infant begins to experiment with creating the sounds of the language used by caregivers. Vocalizations such as consonant-vowel repetitions ("baba" and "mamama") are common. Parents often attach meaning to these infant vocalizations and strongly encourage them, thus leading the infant also to begin to attach meaning to these sounds. By their first birthday many infants have a small vocabulary of words or wordlike sounds that they use meaningfully to communicate desires to caregivers.

Another major landmark toward the end of the first year is beginning independence in an occupation that is universal to the human race: feeding oneself. This complex achievement requires refined somatosensory processing of information from the lips, the jaw, and inside the mouth to guide oral movements in the chewing and swallowing of food. Taste and smell sensations are also integral to this process. But self-feeding involves more than the mouth. All of the acquired sensory integrative milestones involving eye-hand coordination are important to self-feeding. The infant at this period of life uses the fingers directly to feed himself or herself and to explore the textures of foods. At this stage, use of a utensil such as a spoon is not very functional and is messy business because motor planning skills have not progressed to the point that the child can manipulate it successfully. However, many infants begin to demonstrate a drive to use the spoon in self-feeding by the end of the first year. It is noteworthy that for many contemporary American infants, use of a spoon is the first real experience in using a tool (Figure 13-4).

The occupation of dining, then, begins to emerge in infancy as sensory integrative abilities mature, allowing the child to engage in self-feeding. As an occupation, however, dining in its fullest sense goes far beyond the physical, sensorimotor act. It usually takes place within a social context, whether a family dinner at home or a date in a formal restaurant, so social standards for acceptable behavior and etiquette become increasingly important as the child develops. Furthermore, partaking in a meal gradually comes to take on personal symbolic meanings that tend to be powerful. The sensory integrative underpinnings of the dining experience influence how mealtimes are experienced by the child and how others view the child as a dining partner, thus playing a role in shaping the social and symbolic aspects of this vitally important occupation.

## Second Year

As the child moves into the second year of life, the basic vestibular-proprioceptive-visual connections that were laid

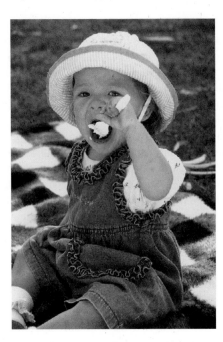

**Figure 13-4**   Because somatosensory processing and visual-motor coordination strongly influence self-feeding skills, sensory integration is an important contributor to development of dining, a fundamental occupation. (Courtesy of Shay McAtee.)

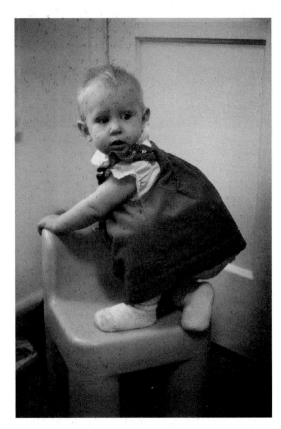

**Figure 13-5**   As motor planning develops during the second year of life, the infant experiments with a variety of body movements and learns how to transition easily from one position to another. These experiences are thought to reflect development of body scheme. (Courtesy of Shay McAtee.)

down earlier continue to refine, resulting in growing finesse in balance and fluidity of dynamic postural control. Discrimination and localization of tactile sensations also become much more precise, allowing for further refinement of fine motor skills.

Increasingly complex somatosensory processing furthermore contributes to the continuing development of body scheme. Ayres (1972b) hypothesized that as body scheme becomes more sophisticated, so does motor planning ability. This is because the child draws on knowledge of how the body works to program novel actions (Figure 13-5). Throughout the second year the typically developing toddler experiments with many variations in body movements. Imitation of the actions of others contributes further to the child's movement repertoire. In experiencing new actions, the child generates new sensory experiences, thus building an elaborate base of information from which to plan future actions.

While motor planning ability becomes increasingly more complex in the second year, another aspect of praxis, ideation, begins to emerge. Ideation is the ability to conceptualize what to do in a given situation. Ideation is made possible by the cognitive ability to use symbols, first expressed gesturally and then vocally during the second year of life (Bretherton et al., 1981). Symbolic functioning enables the child to engage in pretend actions and to imagine doing actions, even actions that the child has never before done. By the end of the second year the toddler can join together several pretend actions in a play sequence (McCune-Nicolich, 1981). Furthermore, the 2-year old child demonstrates that

he or she has a plan before performing an action sequence, either through a verbal announcement or through a search for a needed object (McCune-Nicolich, 1981). Thus a surge in practic development occurs in the second year as the child generates many new ideas for actions and begins to plan actions in a systematic sequence.

The burgeoning of praxis abilities plays an important role in the development of self-concept. Infant psychiatrist Daniel Stern (1985) has suggested that the sense of an integrated core self begins in infancy as an outcome of the volition and the proprioceptive feedback involved in motor planning. The consequences of the child's voluntary, planned actions add to the developing sense of self as an active agent in the world. As praxis takes giant leaps during the second year, so does this sense of self as an agent of power. The child feels in command of his or her own life when sensory integration allows the child to move freely and effectively through the world (Ayres, 1979).

## Third Through Seventh Years

The child's competencies in the sensorimotor realm mature in the third through seventh years of life, which Ayres (1979) considered to be a crucial period for sensory inte-

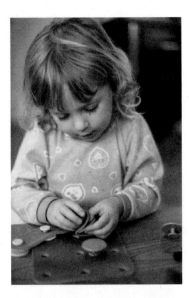

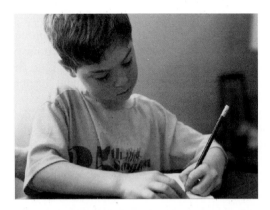

**Figure 13-7** By the time a child reaches school age, sensory integrative capacities are almost mature. The child now can devote full attention to demands of academic tasks because basic sensorimotor functions, such as maintaining an upright posture and guiding hand movements while holding a tool, have become automatic. (Courtesy of Shay McAtee.)

**Figure 13-6** Adaptive responses involved in this activity require precise tactile feedback and sophisticated praxis. During activities such as this one, the preschooler becomes adept at handling tools and objects that are encountered in daily occupations throughout life. (Courtesy of Shay McAtee.)

gration because of the brain's receptiveness to sensations and its capacity for organizing them at this time. This is the period when sensorimotor functions become entrenched as a foundation for higher intellectual abilities. Although further sensory integrative development can and usually does occur beyond the eighth birthday, the changes that take place are likely to be far more limited than those that occurred earlier.

In the third through seventh years, children have strong inner drives to produce adaptive responses that not only meet complicated sensorimotor demands but also sometimes require interfacing with peers. The challenges posed by children's games and play activities attest to this complexity. In the visual-motor realm, sophistication develops through involvement in crafts, drawing and painting, constructional play with blocks and other building toys, and video games (Figure 13-6). Children are driven to explore playground equipment by swinging, sliding, climbing, jumping, riding, pushing, pulling, and pumping. Toward the end of this period they enthusiastically grapple with the motor planning challenges posed by games such as jump rope, jacks, marbles, and hopscotch. Many children begin to participate in occupations that present sensorimotor challenges for years to come, such as soccer, softball, karate, gymnastics, playing a musical instrument, and ballet. It is also during this period that children become expert with household tools such as scissors, pencils, zippers, buttons, forks and knives, pails, shovels, brooms, and rakes (Figure 13-7).

As children participate in these occupations, their bodies are challenged to maintain balance through dynamic changes in body position. They must frequently anticipate how to move in relation to changing environmental events

by accurately timing and sequencing their actions (Fisher, Murray, & Bundy, 1991). This is particularly challenging in sports when peers, with their often unpredictable moves, are involved. In fine motor tasks, children must efficiently coordinate visual with somatosensory information to guide eye and hand movements with accuracy and precision while maintaining a stable postural base.

Children meet these challenges with varying degrees of success. Some are more talented than others with respect to sensory integrative abilities, but most children eventually achieve a degree of competency that allows them to fully participate in the daily occupations they are expected to do and wish to do at home, in school, and in the community. Furthermore, most children experience feelings of satisfaction and self-esteem as they master those occupations that are heavily dependent on sensory integration.

## WHEN PROBLEMS IN SENSORY INTEGRATION OCCUR

Unfortunately, not every child experiences competency in sensory integration. When some aspect of sensory integration does not function efficiently, the child may experience stress in the course of everyday occupations because processes that should be automatic or accurate are not. It may be stressful, for example, to simply maintain balance when sitting in a chair, to get dressed in the morning before school, to attempt to play jump rope, or to eat lunch in a socially acceptable manner. The child is aware of these difficulties and becomes frustrated by frequent failure when confronted with ordinary tasks that come easily for other children. Many children with sensory integrative problems develop a tendency to avoid or reject simple sensory or motor challenges, responding with refusals or tantrums when pushed to perform. If this becomes a long-term pattern of behavior, the child may miss important experiences, such as playing games with peers, that are critical in building feelings of competency, mastering a wide repertoire of useful skills, and developing flexible social strategies. Thus the capacity to participate fully in the occupations that the child wants to do and needs to do is compromised.

Often behavioral, social, or motor coordination concerns are cited when a child with a sensory integrative dysfunction is referred to occupational therapy. The occupational therapist needs to evaluate whether a sensory processing problem may underlie these concerns. The therapist then must decide on a course of action to help the child move toward the goal of greater success and satisfaction in doing meaningful occupations. These challenges to the therapist—to identify a problem that may be hidden and to figure out how to best help the child—were the challenges to which Ayres devoted most of her career.

Earlier we discussed how Ayres turned to the neurobiologic literature to give her insight into understanding children's learning and behavior problems. Ayres also took on the responsibility of conducting research to develop her theory of sensory integration. In doing so she produced a diagnostic system for clinical evaluation of children through the use of standardized tests. She also conducted research that was designed to evaluate the effectiveness of her treatment methods. After each study, Ayres always returned to her theory to revise and refine it in light of research findings. While she was doing this, she maintained a private practice; thus she had many years of firsthand, clinically based experience on which to ground her theoretic work.

The following sections examine the research that Ayres conducted to identify different types of sensory integrative dysfunction in children. The general categories of sensory integrative dysfunction that concern clinicians today, based on research findings and clinical experience are discussed. The field of sensory integration continues to be a dynamic field that changes as future research generates new findings and as future experiences of clinicians generate new ways of interpreting those findings.

## RESEARCH BASE FOR SENSORY INTEGRATIVE DYSFUNCTION

Throughout her entire professional career, Ayres was guided by her keen observation skills and her search to reach a deeper understanding of the clinical problems she encountered in practice. To begin answering the questions that arose as she worked with children, Ayres initiated the process of developing standardized tests of sensory integration during the 1960s. Interestingly, she originally developed these tests solely as research tools to aid in theory development. At the time, she was working with children with learning disabilities, many of whom she suspected had covert difficulties processing sensory information, and she sought to uncover the nature of whatever sensory integrative difficulties might exist. It was after her initial efforts at research using her tests that other therapists asked to have access to the tests, instigating their publication by Western Psychological Services.

The first group of tests created by Ayres were published as the Southern California Sensory Integration Tests (SC-SIT) (Ayres, 1972c). These were later revised and renamed as the Sensory Integration and Praxis Tests (SIPT) (Ayres, 1989). Normative data were collected on a regional scale for the SCSIT and on a national scale for the SIPT. The tests were designed to measure aspects of visual, tactile, kinesthetic, and vestibular sensory processing as well as motor planning abilities.

Using first the SCSIT and later the SIPT with samples of children, Ayres used a statistic procedure called factor analysis to develop a typology of sensory integrative function and dysfunction. Tables 13-1 and 13-2 summarize results of her factor analytic studies. In factor analysis, sets of test scores are grouped according to their associations with each other. The resulting groups of associated test scores are called factors. Ayres interpreted the factors that emerged from her studies as representative of neural substrates underlying learning and behavior in children. For example, in her 1965 study, Ayres found that the tactile tests correlated highly with the motor planning tests, forming a factor. She hypothesized that there is an ability called *motor planning* that is dependent on somatosensory processing and influences one's interactions with the physical world. *Apraxia* was the term she used to identify a disorder in this ability. In her later work she subsumed the notion of motor planning under the construct of praxis and replaced the term *apraxia* with *dyspraxia* when referring to children.

In her last set of analyses with the SIPT, just before her death in 1988, Ayres used both factor analysis and another statistical technique called cluster analysis, which groups together children with similar SIPT profiles (Table 13-1). This approach was used to further carve out diagnostic groupings of children that might prove to be useful clinically. Today, consideration of cluster groupings, along with factor analysis results, is a critical component in the interpretation of a child's SIPT scores.

Through the years as Ayres conducted her studies with different groups of children, she continually revisited her theory, bringing along new hypotheses based on new research results. Of particular interest were the patterns that recurred despite being generated from different samples of children. Among the most consistent findings was that children who had been identified as having learning or developmental problems often displayed difficulties in more than one sensory system. Ayres (1972b) interpreted this finding in light of the neurobiologic literature on intersensory integration, which indicates that the sensory systems tend to function synergistically with each other rather than in isolation. Thus the idea of intersensory integration as critical to human function became one of the major tenets of sensory integration theory.

Another finding that emerged in early studies, as well as in later SIPT studies, was that some patterns of scores were seen only in groups of children who had been identified as having disorders. In other words, some factors were not evident in typically developing children at any age. This led to the proposal that the sensory integrative disorders associated with these particular patterns were representative of neural dysfunction rather than developmental lag.

Yet another recurrent pattern was a relationship between tactile perception and praxis scores. This association appeared again and again in her studies and led Ayres to theorize that the tactile system contributes importantly to the development of efficient practic functions. The robustness of this finding across many studies influenced Ayres to emphasize the relationship between the tactile system and praxis, a relationship that became a cornerstone of sensory integration theory.

Throughout her research, several patterns emerged that Ayres suspected were related to a discrete involvement of cortical rather than brainstem or intersensory dysfunction. Ayres came to view these types of problems as different than those classified as sensory integrative disorders and less likely to be responsive to the treatment techniques she was developing. An example is the association of low Praxis on Verbal Command scores with high Postrotary Nystagmus scores. Praxis on Verbal Command is the only item on the SIPT with a strong language comprehension component. Postrotary Nystagmus is a test that may reflect cortical dysfunction if scores are extremely high. In this example it is hypothesized that an underlying cortical dysfunction, possibly involving the left hemisphere (where language centers are located), is responsible for the pattern of scores. Ayres did not view this particular pattern as a sensory integrative dysfunction, although it could be detected by her tests.

As Fisher and Murray (1991) have pointed out, Ayres' factor analytic studies are limited by some design flaws. Specifically, sample sizes were small in relation to the number of tests studied, and she repeated exploratory techniques with different groups of tests in her studies, rather than using confirmatory factor analysis to replicate results using the same group of tests. The presence of these flaws makes results vulnerable to instability because of associations that may occur by chance. It is important to note, however, that similar factors did recur across her studies, despite these limitations (Tables 13-1 and 13-2). The resilience of some of these factors in the face of design limitations actually strengthens the hypothesis that they do indeed reflect underlying patterns of function.

Ayres conducted her factor and cluster analyses to shed light on the types of sensory integrative dysfunctions that children experience, yet she did not view the resulting typologies as specific diagnostic labels to pin on individual children. Rather, the typologies were seen as general patterns exhibited time after time by groups of children who were struggling in school or with some other aspect of behavior or development. They provide the therapist with relevant information to consider when conducting clinical assessments. They do not provide prefabricated slots in which to fit children. Ultimately, the important job of interpreting an individual child's pattern of scores in relation to his or her unique life situation lies in the purview of the therapist's judgment.

## SENSORY INTEGRATIVE DISORDERS

The results of research, combined with the experiences of clinicians and the work of scholars in the field, have generated many different ways of conceptualizing sensory integrative disorders over the past 30 years. The complexity of this domain can be initially confusing to the novice therapist, but it is also one of the most intriguing aspects of the field. The term *sensory integrative disorder* does not refer to one particular type of problem but to a heterogeneous group of disorders that are thought to reflect subtle, primarily subcortical, neural dysfunction involving multisensory systems. These disorders affect human behavior in ways that are often difficult to interpret unless seen through the eyes of someone with special training in sensory integration.

Most discussions of sensory integrative problems assume normal sensory receptor function. In other words, sensory integrative disorders involve central, rather than peripheral, sensory functions. For instance, when sensory integrative disorders involving the vestibular system are discussed, these problems are generally thought to be based within brainstem structures and pathways (namely, the vestibular nuclei and its connections) rather than the vestibular receptor (i.e., the semicircular canals, utricle, or saccule). This has been a point of confusion in some studies. Polatajko (1985), for example, used measures of peripheral vestibular functioning to evaluate Ayres' hypothesis that some learning-disabled children have vestibular dysfunction. Because Polatajko failed to measure the kind of vestibular function that was of concern to Ayres, it is no surprise that she found no differences in vestibular functioning between children with and without learning disabilities. Wiss (1989) has provided an excellent discussion of this issue in relation to vestibular processing. The same point could apply to other sensory systems as well. In this chapter, the discussions of sensory integrative problems assume that peripheral function is normal.

As noted above, different conceptualizations of sensory integrative disorders have been generated over the years. Recent categorical systems of sensory integrative dysfunction include, for example, those of Clark, Mailloux, and Parham (1989); Fisher et al. (1991); Kimball (1993); and the theory and treatment course syllabi of Sensory Integration International. Although perfect consensus on how to catego-

*Text continued on p. 324.*

▲ **Table 13-1**   Purpose, Hypotheses, Design, Results, and Contributions of Ayres' Studies of Dysfunctional Patterns

| Year | Purpose | Hypothesis | Instruments | Design | Subjects | Results | Contribution to Theory |
|------|---------|------------|-------------|--------|----------|---------|------------------------|
| 1965 | Identify relationships among sensory perception, motor performance, laterality in normal and children with perceptual problems<br><br>Establish construct and discriminant validity | Test results would identify factors for children with and without dysfunction<br><br>Normal and dysfunctional children will demonstrate different factors | Early versions of the Southern California Sensory Integration Tests (SCSIT), additional perceptual-motor and laterality tests, also freedom from hyperactivity and tactile defensiveness | Thirty-three tests<br><br>Two behavioral parameters<br><br>Analysis of difference between group means<br><br>Q- and R-technique factor analysis | n = 100 dysfunctional<br><br>n = 50 normal<br><br>Dysfunctional children had learning or behavioral disorders | Tests discriminated between normal and dysfunctional groups<br><br>Five patterns detected:<br>Apraxia<br>Dysfunction form and space perception<br>Deficit bilateral integration<br>Visual figure-ground perception<br>Tactile defensiveness | Established discriminant validity of early versions<br><br>Most children demonstrated more than one factor, therefore factors related<br><br>Sensory integration-clusters were not by sensory systems<br><br>Praxis and tactile functions linked<br><br>Tactile defensiveness, hyperactivity, distractibility linked<br><br>Cognitive aspects deemphasized<br><br>Eye-hand agreement not discriminative<br><br>Empirical support for syndromes |
| 1966a | Explore perceptual-motor relationships in a normal sample and compare with prior studies<br><br>Establish construct validity | That factors would emerge | Frostig tests, early versions of the SCSIT<br><br>Also freedom from hyperactivity and tactile defensiveness | Seventeen tests<br><br>R-technique factor analysis (simplified matrix) | n = 92<br><br>Formed normal distribution, 10% abnormal, three with mild cerebral palsy | Praxis accounted for most variance<br><br>Motor planning, Kinesthesia, tactile functions, Motor Accuracy, Bilateral Coordination<br><br>Visual perception factor: Ayres Space Test, Frostig | More support for praxis syndrome<br><br>Visual component without motor element<br><br>Perceptual-motor functions correlate as a whole in normative sample<br><br>Kinesthesia closer to tactile than visual perception as in prior study |

*Continued.*

| | | | | | | | |
|---|---|---|---|---|---|---|---|
| 1966b | Provide an understanding of whether syndromes represent dysfunction or developmental lag Establish construct validity | Nearly the same as 1966a | That variation in perceptual-motor abilities would be small in a group of typical children | Sixteen tests Two behavioral parameters R-technique factor analysis | n = 64 Adopted, all normal on Gesell | Visual motor ability accounted for most variation Praxis and tactile perception were least variable Hyperactivity, distractibility, tactile defensiveness factor Factors weak because of lack of variance in performance of normal children | Suggested that low scores in praxis and tactile perception represent developmental deviation, not delay Little systematic variation when tests given to normal children Tactile defensiveness-hyperactivity may have a maturational component |
| 1969 | To provide an in-depth analysis of dysfunctional patterns in children with learning handicaps Establish construct validity | Sixty-four tests and observations: SCSIT, psycholinguistic, intelligence, auditory, postural-ocular reactions, academic achievement | Brain functions involve several levels and will cluster accordingly | Q-technique factor analysis | n = 36 Educationally handicapped children | Five factors identified: Auditory language, sequencing Postural and bilateral integration Right hemisphere dysfunction Apraxia Tactile defensiveness | Hints to left hemisphere dysfunction |
| 1971 | To identify predictors of severity of sensory integrative syndromes | Forty-eight tests and observations: SCSIT, psycholinguistic, intelligence, eye-hand usage, postural responses | That predictive equations would emerge | Ten-step regression equations for each syndrome calculated | n = 140 Educationally handicapped children | Presence of more than one type of disorder was the norm Prone extension best predictor of postural-bilateral integration Imitation of postures best predictor of praxis | Somatosensory and praxis linked again Elucidated best predictors of syndromes As many children may have apraxia as have postural and bilateral coordination problems |

Modified from Ayres, A.J. (1964). Tactile functions: their relation to hyperactive and perceptual motor behavior. *American Journal of Occupational Therapy, 18*(1), 6-11; Ayres, A.J. (1965). Patterns of perceptual-motor dysfunction in children: a factor analytic study. *Perceptual and Motor Skills, 20,* 335-368; Ayres, A.J. (1966a). Interrelationships among perceptual-motor functions in children. *American Journal of Occupational Therapy, 20*(2), 68-71; Ayres, A.J. (1966b). Interrelations among perceptual-motor abilities in a group of normal children. *American Journal of Occupational Therapy, 20*(6), 288-292; Ayres, A.J. (1969). Deficits in sensory integration in educationally handicapped children. *Journal of Learning Disabilities, 2*(3), 44-52; Ayres, A.J. (1971). Characteristics of types of sensory integrative dysfunction. *American Journal of Occupational Therapy, 26*(1), 13-18; Ayres, A.J. (1972a). Cluster analyses of measures of sensory integration. *American Journal of Occupational Therapy, 25*(7), 329-334; Ayres, A.J. (1972d). Types of sensory integrative dysfunction among disabled learners. *American Journal of Occupational Therapy, 31*(6), 362-366; Ayres, A.J., Mailloux, Z., & Wendler, C.L.W. (1987). Development apraxia: is it a unitary function? *Occupational Therapy Research, 7*(2), 93-110; Ayres, A.J. (1989). *Sensory Integration and Praxis Tests manual.* Los Angeles: Western Psychological Services; and Ayres, A.J. & Marr, D. (1991). Sensory Integration and Praxis Tests. In A.G. Fisher, E.A. Murray, & A.C. Bundy (Eds.), *Sensory integration: theory and practice* (pp. 203-250). Philadelphia: F.A. Davis.

▲ **Table 13-1**  Purpose, Hypotheses, Design, Results, and Contributions of Ayres' Studies of Dysfunctional Patterns—cont'd

| Year | Purpose | Hypothesis | Instruments | Design | Subjects | Results | Contribution to Theory |
|---|---|---|---|---|---|---|---|
| 1972 | To further analyze and refine factors. Establish construct validity | That similar factors as previously would emerge | Same as above | R-technique factor analysis | n = 148 Educationally handicapped children | Six factors identified: Form and space perception, Auditory language, Postural ocular, Motor planning, Reading-spelling and IQ, Hyperactivity, tactile perception | Further confirmed left hemisphere dysfunction. Reconfirmed syndromes found in other samples of learning-disabled children |
| 1977 | To further analyze interrelationships (add Southern California Postrotary Nystagmus Test [SCPNT]) so that differential diagnosis can be further refined | That clusters would continue to be refined | SCSIT, SCPNT, postural-ocular and lateralization measures, dichotic listening, Illinois Test of Psycholinguistic Abilities (ITPA), intelligence, academic achievement, Flowers-Costello (auditory) | Series of R-technique factor analyses (not all measures entered each time) | n = 128 Learning disabled children | Five major domains identified: Somatosensory-motor planning, Auditory-language, Postural-ocular, Eye-hand coordination, Postrotary nystagmus | Further elucidated nature of interhemispheric integration. Role of vestibular system clarified |
| 1987 | To continue to attempt to differentiate types of sensory integration dysfunction. New praxis tests as well as many of the tests that had been used in past studies | Is praxis a unitary function? Would computer-generated clusters match those that had been identified clinically and through factor analysis? | SCSIT, SCPNT, selected ITPA test, sentence repetition. Clinical observation of prone extension, supine flexion, ocular pursuits. Preliminary versions of newly designed praxis tests: Sequencing Praxis, Praxis on Verbal Command, Oral Praxis, Block Building Test | Screen plot factor analyses, correlation coefficients. Comparison of test profiles of children with diagnoses. Use of computer-generated clusters | n = 182 Learning or behavior disorders | Praxis tests were related with one another. Visual tests correlated with tactile tests. Somatovisual-practic factor identified. Tactile scores and praxis related; short duration postrotary nystagmus; statistical association with praxis | Suggestion of a general somatopractic function. Further verified close association of tactile score and praxis. Computer-generated clusters were not meaningful |

| Year | Purpose | Test | Hypothesis | Type of Analysis | Sample | Results | Implications |
|---|---|---|---|---|---|---|---|
| 1989 | Factor analyses: to clarify the nature of the constructs measured by the Sensory Integration and Praxis Tests (SIPT) | SIPT (17 tests) | That factors related to those of the SCSIT would emerge | Principal components analysis | Three analyses: n = 1750 Normative sample n = 125 Learning or sensory integrative disorders n = 293 Combined sample of learning or sensory integrative disorders and matched children from normative sample | Visuopraxis and somato-praxis factors emerged in all three analyses. Bilateral integration and sequencing factor and praxis on verbal command factor seen only in dysfunctional sample Other factors related to vestibular and somatosensory processing identified | Expanded understanding of vestibular-bilateral disorders to include sequencing element Somatopraxis factor reinforced previous findings linking tactile perception and praxis Visuopraxis factor provided support for previous visual-motor linkages |
| 1989 | Cluster analyses: to assist in identifying children in need of different types of remediation or services | SIPT (17 tests) | That meaningful diagnostic groupings would emerge | Agglomerative cluster analysis, Ward method | n = 293 Same sample as above, combined dysfunctional and normative | Six cluster groups identified: Low average bilateral integration and sequencing Generalized sensory integrative dysfunction Visuo- and somato-dyspraxia Low average sensory integration and praxis Dyspraxia on verbal command High average sensory integration and praxis | Children with and without dysfunction can be differentiated on the basis of SIPT profiles Identified specific SIPT profile that may be characteristic of left hemisphere dysfunction |

▲ **Table 13-2**    Factors and Clusters Identified in Studies by Ayres (1965-1977)

| Date of Study | Dyspraxia | Deficit in Visual Perception and Visual-Motor Functions | Deficit in Vestibular, Postural, and Bilateral Integration | Deficit in Auditory and Language Functions | Tactile Defensiveness | Miscellaneous |
|---|---|---|---|---|---|---|
| 1965: 100 dysfunctional, 50 normal | Tactile tests Motor planning (Imitation of Posture, Motor Accuracy, Grommet) Eye pursuits | Frostig tests Kinesthesia Manual Form Perception Ayres' Space Test | Right-left discrimination Avoidance crossing midline Rhythmic activities | Not tested | Poor tactile perception Hyperactive-distractible behavior Tactile defensiveness | Figure-ground a separate factor Eye-hand agreement not related to perceptual-motor dysfunction |
| 1966a: Normal distribution of Gesell developmental quotients | Accounted for most variance Motor planning Tactile and kinesthesia Motor accuracy Figure-ground Frostig tests | Figure-ground Frostig spatial relations Ayres' Space Test | | Not tested | Low association of tactile defensiveness with praxis factor | Identified two main factors in normal sample: General perceptual-motor (somatosensory and motor) Visual perception |
| 1966b: Only normal children | | Frostig tests Ayres' Space Test Motor Accuracy Figure-ground | Integration two sides of body and tactile perception | Not tested | Tactile defensiveness and hyperactivity—may be a maturational factor involved | Visual-motor ability accounted for most variation in normal children Poor motor planning—tactile perception not seen in normal children |
| 1969: Educationally handicapped children | Tactile Motor Planning | Most Southern California Sensory Integration Tests (SCSIT); visual tests not included in analysis Possible right hemisphere dysfunction: eye movement deficits, better right- than left-sided function | Bilateral integration Postural reactions Reading and language problems | Possible left hemisphere dysfunction: Auditory-language Reading achievement Auditory and visual-motor sequencing | Tactile defensiveness and hyperactivity—loaded together but not a separate factor | |

| | | | | | | |
|---|---|---|---|---|---|---|
| 1972: Educationally handicapped children | Motor planning; Hyperactivity; Tactile defensiveness (more emphasis on motor than tactile) | Position in Space; Illinois Test of Psycholinguistic Abilities (ITPA) visual closure; Space Visualization; Design Copying; Tactile tests | Poor ocular control; Excessive residual primitive postural responses; Relatively good left-hand coordination; Bilateral integration symptom did not load | Auditory language; Intelligence | Hyperactivity-distractibility; Tactile perception | Reading-spelling load together; Motor accuracy highly associated with all parameters |
| 1977: Learning disabled children | *Analysis 5:* Imitation of Postures; Composite tactile; Kinesthesia | *Analysis 3:* Four SCSIT visual tests; Manual Form Perception | *Analysis 5:* Prone extension; Composite postural; Flexion posture; Composite tactile; Kinesthesia; Bilateral integration symptom did not load | *Analysis 5:* Composite language (ITPA); Dichotic listening; Flowers-Costello (auditory) | Not measured | Visual tests have strong cognitive component (loaded with IQ on Analysis 2); Space Visualization Contralateral Use (SVCU) score associated with lateralization indices; Motor accuracy loaded separately on all |
| 1989: Children with learning disorders and sensory integrative deficits and children from normative sample of Sensory Integration and Praxis Tests (SIPT) | Somatopraxis (Oral Praxis, Postural Praxis, Graphesthesia; Visuo- and somatodyspraxia cluster | Visuopraxis (Constructional Praxis, Design Copying, Space Visualization, Figure-Ground) | Bilateral integration and sequencing (Sequencing Praxis, Bilateral Motor Coordination, Standing and Walking Balance); Low average bilateral integration and sequencing cluster | Praxis on Verbal Command; Dyspraxia on verbal command cluster (high Postrotary Hystagmus with low Praxis on Verbal Command) | Not measured | High functioning group identified within normative sample; Generalized dysfunction group identified within group with learning disorders and sensory integrative dysfunction |

Modified from Ayres, A.J. (1964). Tactile functions: their relation to hyperactive and perceptual motor behavior. *American Journal of Occupational Therapy, 18*(1), 6-11; Ayres, A.J. (1965). Patterns of perceptual-motor dysfunction in children: a factor analytic study. *Perceptual and Motor Skills, 20,* 335-368; Ayres, A.J. (1966a). Interrelationships among perceptual-motor functions in children. *American Journal of Occupational Therapy, 20*(2), 68-71; Ayres, A.J. (1966b). Interrelations among perceptual-motor abilities in a group of normal children. *American Journal of Occupational Therapy, 20*(6), 288-292; Ayres, A.J. (1969). Deficits in sensory integration in educationally handicapped children. *Journal of Learning Disabilities, 2*(3), 44-52; Ayres, A.J. (1972d). Types of sensory integrative dysfunction among disabled learners. *American Journal of Occupational Therapy, 26*(1), 13-18; Ayres, A.J. (1977a). Cluster analyses of measures of sensory integration. *American Journal of Occupational Therapy, 31*(6), 362-366; Ayres, A.J. (1989). *Sensory Integration and Praxis Tests manual.* Los Angeles: Western Psychological Services; Ayres, A.J. & Marr, D. (1991). Sensory Integration and Praxis Tests. In A.G. Fisher, E.A. Murray, & A.C. Bundy (Eds.). *Sensory integration: theory and practice* (pp. 203-250). Phildaelphia: F.A. Davis.

rize sensory integrative dysfunctions does not exist, clearly there are recurring themes across all authors. For the purposes of this chapter the following categories are used: problems with sensory modulation, problems with sensory discrimination and perception, vestibular processing disorders, and dyspraxia. The first two of these categories involve direct expressions of sensory processing; the latter two expressions involve indirect, motoric outcomes of sensory integration.

## Sensory Modulation Problems

*Modulation* refers to the central nervous system's regulation of its own activity (Ayres, 1979). With respect to sensory systems, this term is used to refer to the tendency to generate responses that are appropriately graded in relation to incoming sensory stimuli, rather than underreacting or overreacting to them. Cermak (1988) and Royeen (1989) have hypothesized that there is a continuum of sensory responsivity, with hyporesponsivity at one end and hyperresponsivity at the other. An optimal level of arousal and orientation lies in the center of the continuum (Figure 13-8).

Royeen and Lane (1991) point out that, ordinarily, individuals experience fluctuations across this continuum in the course of a day, with most activity falling in the midrange. Dysfunction is indicated when the fluctuations within an individual are extreme or when an individual tends to function primarily at one extreme end of the continuum or the other.

An individual who tends to function at the extremely underresponsive end of the continuum may be said to have diminished sensory registration. This is the person who fails to notice sensory stimuli that elicits the attention of most people. At the other extreme of the continuum is the individual with sensory defensiveness. This is the person who is overwhelmed and overstressed by ordinary sensory stimuli. Because these problems tend to manifest themselves differently and are handled differently in treatment, they are discussed separately.

Originally, Ayres (1979) thought of sensory registration problems as different in nature from sensory modulation problems such as tactile defensiveness. Soon after she introduced the concept of sensory registration, however, other experts in the field of sensory integration suggested that sensory registration and tactile defensiveness were indeed related and that both are mediated by limbic system functions. Dunn and Fisher (1983) first posited this important idea, which eventually led to the creation of the sensory modulation continuum model described here, wherein sensory registration problems and defensiveness are seen as two ends of the same continuum of function.

## Sensory Registration Problems

As we noted earlier in this chapter, sensory integration is the "organization of sensory input for use" (Ayres, 1979, p. 184). However, before sensory information can be used functionally, it must be registered within the CNS. When the CNS is working well, it knows when to "pay attention" to a stimulus and when to "ignore it." Most of the time this process occurs automatically and efficiently. For example, a student may not be aware of the noise of traffic outside the window of a classroom while listening to a lecture, instead focusing his or her attention on the sound of the lecturer's words. In this situation the student registers the auditory stimuli generated by the lecturer but not the stimuli generated by the traffic. The process of sensory registration is critical in enabling efficient function so that persons pay attention to those stimuli that enable them to accomplish desired goals. Simultaneously, if the process is working well, energy is not wasted attending to irrelevant sensory information.

Traditionally, occupational therapists, beginning with Ayres (1979), have used the term *sensory registration problem* to refer to the difficulties of the person who frequently fails to attend to (or register) relevant environmental stimuli. This kind of problem is often seen in individuals with autism, but it may also be seen in other individuals with developmental problems. When a sensory registration problem is present, the child often seems oblivious to touch, pain, movement, taste, smells, sights, or sounds. Usually more than one sensory system is involved, but for some children one system may be particularly affected. Sometimes the same child who does not register relevant stimuli may be overfocused on irrelevant stimuli; this is commonly seen in children with autism. It is also common for children with severe developmental problems, such as autism, to lack sensory registration in some situations but react with extreme sensory defensiveness in other situations.

Safety concerns are frequently an important issue among children with sensory registration problems. The child who does not register pain sensations, for example, has not learned that certain actions naturally lead to negative consequences, such as pain, and therefore may not withdraw adequately from dangerous situations. Instead of avoiding situations likely to result in pain, the child may repeatedly engage in activities that actually may be injurious, such as jumping from a dangerous height onto a hard surface or

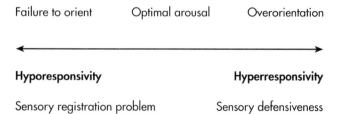

| Failure to orient | Optimal arousal | Overorientation |
|---|---|---|
| **Hyporesponsivity** | | **Hyperresponsivity** |
| Sensory registration problem | | Sensory defensiveness |

**Figure 13-8**   Continuum of sensory responsivity and orientation. (Modified from Royeen, C.B. & Lane, S.J. [1991] In A.G. Fisher, E.A. Murray, & A.C. Bundy (Eds.). *Sensory integration: theory and practice.* Philadelphia: F.A. Davis.)

touching a hot object. Other children may not register noxious tastes and smells that warn of hazards. Similarly, sights and sounds su~~ch as~~ sirens, flashing lights, firm voice commands, and ⌐          ¬nt to warn of perils go          an be life endangerin~~g~~          child steps in front of

A se          vith the child's abili~~ty~~          uation. Consequ          nner drive that          hildhood occu-          unmotivated to          . The long-term          re, can be pro-          n children with          rs them among          g a sensory inte-          nefit from indi-          y be slow to un-          l experience and          can be enhanced          ation, particularly          nput, particularly          traction (Ayres,          Green, & Ayres,          ss          t are underrespon-          these children have          but others seem to          ory modality that is          vestibular stimuli          imulation when in-          clinic setting. This          sensations and usu-          sensations, but the

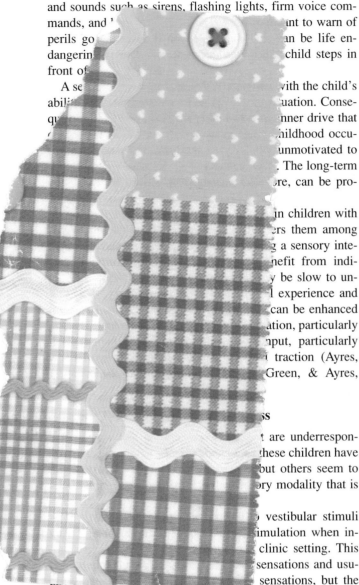

input does not impact the nervous system to the extent that it does for most other children. The underresponsive child may not become dizzy or show any autonomic responses in response to intense stimulation that is be overwhelming for most peers. This is called hyporesponsivity because it refers to the underlying mode of sensory processing rather than to observable motor behavior. Although the child may appear to be active motorically, the child is not reacting to intense vestibular stimuli to the degree that most children do. In everyday settings these children often appear to be restless, motorically driven, and thrill seeking.

Some children seem to seek greater than average amounts of proprioceptive input. These children may be underresponsive to proprioceptive input. Typically these children often seek a great deal of active resistance to muscles, deep touch pressure stimulation, or joint compression and trac-

tion, for example, by stomping instead of walking, intentionally falling or bumping into objects (including other people), or pushing against large objects. They may tend to use strong ballistic movements such as throwing objects forcefully. Some of these children may not seem to register the positions of body parts unless intense proprioceptive stimulation is present.

The behaviors generated by underresponsive children may be disruptive or inappropriate in social situations. Safety issues frequently are of paramount concern, and often these children are labeled as having social or behavioral problems. A challenge for the occupational therapist working with these children may be to identify strategies by which they can receive the high levels of stimulation they seek without being socially disruptive, inappropriate, or dangerous to self or others.

### Sensory Defensiveness

At the opposite end of the sensory modulation continuum are problems associated with hyperresponsivity or sensory defensiveness. The child who has sensory defensiveness is overwhelmed by ordinary sensory input and reacts defensively to it, often with strong negative emotion and activation of the sympathetic nervous system. This condition may occur as a general response to all types of sensory input or it may be specific to one or a few sensory systems.

The term *sensory defensiveness* was first used by Knickerbocker (1980) and later by Wilbarger and Wilbarger (1991) to describe sensory modulation disorders involving multisensory systems. The Wilbargers suggest that more than one sensory system is typically involved when signs of hyperresponsivity are present. These include overreactions to touch, movement, sounds, odors, and tastes, any of which may create discomfort, avoidance, distractibility, and anxiety. Most of our knowledge regarding hyperresponsivity is related to the two systems that occupational therapists have focused their research and clinical efforts on, the tactile and vestibular systems. We shall now examine the characteristics of hyperresponsivity in these two systems.

*Tactile defensiveness.* Tactile defensiveness involves a tendency to overreact to ordinary touch sensations (Ayres, 1964; 1972b; 1979). It is one of the most commonly observed sensory integrative disorders involving sensory modulation. Individuals with tactile defensiveness experience irritation and discomfort from sensations that most people do not find bothersome. Light touch sensations are especially likely to be disturbing. Common irritants include certain textures of clothing, grass or sand against bare skin, glue or paint on the skin, the light brush of another person passing by, the sensations generated when having one's hair or teeth brushed, and certain textures of food. Common responses to such irritants include anxiety, distractibility, restlessness, anger, throwing a tantrum, aggression, fear, and emotional distress.

Common self-care activities such as dressing, bathing, grooming, and eating are often affected by tactile defensiveness. Classroom activities such as fingerpainting, sand and water play, and crafts may be avoided. Social situations involving close proximity to others, such as playing near other children or standing in line, tend to be uncomfortable and may be disturbing enough to lead to emotional outbursts; thus ordinary daily routines can become traumatic for children with tactile defensiveness and for their parents. Teachers and friends are likely to misinterpret the child with tactile defensiveness as being rejecting, aggressive, or simply negative.

It is difficult for individuals with tactile defensiveness to cope with the fact that their discomfort is not shared by others and that situations they find so upsetting actually may be enjoyed by others. For a child with this disorder, who may not be able to verbalize or even recognize the problem, the accompanying feelings of anxiety and frustration can be overwhelming and the impact on functional behavior is likely to be significant.

An occupational therapist working with a child who is tactually defensive must become aware of the specific kinds of tactile input that are aversive and the kinds that are tolerated well by that particular child. Usually light touch stimuli are aversive, especially when they occur in the most sensitive body areas such as the face, abdomen, and palmar surfaces of upper and lower extremities. Generally, tactile stimuli that are actively self-applied by the child are tolerated much better than stimuli that are passively received, as when being touched by another person. Tactile stimuli may be especially threatening if the child cannot see the source of the touch. Most individuals with tactile defensiveness feel comfortable with deep touch stimuli, and may experience relief from irritating stimuli when deep pressure is applied over the involved skin areas. Knowledge of these characteristics of tactile defensiveness helps the occupational therapist identify strategies that help the child and others who interact with the child to cope with this condition. For example, the occupational therapist may recommend to the teacher that if the child needs to be touched, it should be done with firm pressure in the child's view, rather than with a light touch from behind the child.

***Gravitational insecurity.*** Gravitational insecurity is a form of hyperresponsivity to vestibular sensations, particularly sensations from the otolith organs, which detect linear movement through space as well as the pull of gravity (Ayres, 1979). Children with this problem have an insecure relationship to gravity characterized by excessive fear during ordinary movement activities. The gravitationally insecure child is overwhelmed by changes in head position and movement, especially when moving backward or upward through space. Fear of heights, even those involving only slight distances from the ground, is a common problem associated with this condition.

Children who display gravitational insecurity often show signs of inordinate fear, anxiety, or avoidance in relation to stairs, escalators or elevators, moving or high pieces of playground equipment, and uneven or unpredictable surfaces. Some children are so insecure that only a small change from one surface to another, as when stepping off the curb or from the sidewalk to the grass, is enough to send them into a state of high anxiety or panic.

Common reactions of these children include extreme fearfulness during low-intensity movement or when anticipating movement and avoidance of tilting the head in different planes (especially backward). They tend to move slowly and carefully, and they may refuse to participate in many gross motor activities. When they do engage in movement activities such as swinging, many of these children refuse to lift their feet off the ground. When threatened by simple motor activities, they may try to gain as much contact with the ground as possible or they may tightly clutch a nearby adult for security. These children often have signs of poor proprioception in addition to the vestibular hyperresponsivity.

Playground and park activities are often difficult for children with gravitational insecurity, as are other common childhood activities such as bicycle riding, iceskating, rollerskating, skateboarding, skiing, and hiking. Ability to play with peers and to explore the environment is therefore significantly impacted. Functioning in the community may also be affected when the child needs to use escalators, stairs, and elevators.

A distinction can be made between gravitational insecurity and a similar condition called *postural insecurity.* Postural insecurity was the term originally used by Ayres to refer to all children with fears related to movement. Over the years, however, it became clear that some children moved slowly and displayed fears of movement not because of a hyperresponsivity to vestibular input but because they lacked adequate motor control to perform many activities without falling. The fears of these children, then, seemed to be based on a realistic appraisal of their motor limitations. The term *posturally insecure* is used to refer to these children. Often it is difficult to discern whether a child's anxiety is based on sensory hyperresponsivity or limited motor control because these two conditions can, and often do, coexist in the same child. Sometimes, however, the distinction is clear. Children with mild spastic diplegia, for example, commonly have postural but not gravitational insecurity. These children typically (and appropriately) react with anxiety when faced with a minimal climbing task; however, they may show pleasure at receiving vestibular stimulation, including having the head radically tilted in different planes as long as they are securely held and do not have to rely on their own motor skills to maintain a safe position.

***Defensiveness in other sensory modalities.*** Although little is known about hyperresponsivities in sensory systems other than tactile and vestibular, there is no doubt that they exist and can make a significant impact on people's lives. Some of the types of heightened responsivity that often create problems for children include overreactions to sounds, odors, and tastes. These types of problems, like hyperresponsivity to touch and movement, may create discomfort, avoidance, distractibility, and anxiety. The raucous sounds found at birthday parties, parades, playgrounds, and carnivals are interpreted by most people as happy sounds, but they can be overwhelming to a child with auditory defensiveness. A visually busy and unfamiliar environment may evoke an unusual degree of anxiety in a child with visual defensiveness. Similarly, the variety of tastes and odors encountered in some environments may be disturbing to a child with hyperresponsivity in these systems.

## Sensory Discrimination and Perception Problems

Sensory discrimination and perception allow for refined organization and interpretation of sensory stimuli. Some types of sensory integrative disorders involve inefficient or inaccurate organization of sensory information, for instance, difficulty differentiating one stimulus from another or difficulty perceiving the spatial or temporal relationships among stimuli. A classic example involving the visual system is the older child with a learning disability who persists in confusing a *b* with a *d*. A child with an auditory discrimination problem may be unable to distinguish between the sounds of the words *doll* and *tall*. A child with a tactile perception problem may not be able to distinguish between a square block and a hexagonal block using touch only, without visual cues.

Some children with perceptual problems have no difficulty whatsoever with sensory modulation. However, modulation problems often do coexist with perceptual problems. It makes sense that these two types of problems would be associated. A child who often does not register stimuli probably has deficit perceptual skills because of a lack of experience interacting with sensory information. Conversely, the child who has sensory defensiveness may exert a lot of energy trying to avoid certain sensory experiences. Defensive reactions may make it difficult to attend to the detailed features of a stimulus and thereby may impede perception.

Discrimination or perception problems can occur in any sensory system. They are best detected by standardized tests, except in the case of proprioception, which is difficult to measure in a standardized manner. Professionals in many different fields, such as clinical psychology, special education, and speech pathology, are trained to evaluate perceptual problems, and their focus usually is on the visual and auditory systems. In contrast, occupational therapists are somewhat unique in their emphasis on somatosensory perception.

### Tactile Discrimination and Perception Problems

Poor tactile perception is one of the most commonly found sensory integrative disorders. Children with this disorder have difficulty interpreting tactile stimuli in a precise and efficient manner. They may have difficulty, for example, localizing precisely where an object has brushed against them or using stereognosis to manipulate an object that is out of sight. Fine motor skills are likely to suffer when a tactile perception problem is present, especially if tactile defensiveness is also present (Case-Smith, 1991).

As discussed earlier in this chapter, the tactile system is a critical modality for learning during infancy and early childhood. Tactile exploration using the hands and mouth is particularly important. If tactile perception is vague or inaccurate, the child is at a disadvantage in learning about the different properties of objects and substances. It may be difficult for a child with such problems to develop the manipulative skills needed to efficiently perform tasks such as connecting pieces of constructional toys, fastening buttons or snaps, braiding hair, or playing marbles. Inadequate tactile perception also interferes with the feedback that is normally used to precisely guide motor tasks such as writing with a pencil, manipulating a spoon, or holding a piece of paper with one hand while cutting with the other.

Tactile perception is associated with visual perception (Ayres, Mailloux, & Wendler, 1987), thus it is fairly common to see children with problems in both of these sensory systems. Not surprisingly, these children tend to have concomitant problems with eye-hand coordination.

One of the most striking findings in Ayres' factor analytic studies was the link between tactile perception and motor planning, which recurred in different studies (Ayres, 1965, 1966a, 1966b, 1971, 1972a, 1977a; Ayres, et al., 1987). These findings led Ayres to hypothesize that tactile perception is an important contributor to the ability to plan actions. She speculated that the tactile system is responsible for the development of body scheme, which then becomes an important foundation for praxis.

Ordinarily, tactile perception operates at such an automatic level that, when it is impaired, compensation strategies take a great deal of energy. Consider, for example, the child who cannot make the subtle manipulations needed to fasten a button without looking at it. Because this child needs to use compensatory visual guidance, the task of buttoning, which is usually performed rapidly and automatically, becomes a tedious, tiring, and frustrating task. The necessity of using such compensatory strategies throughout the day tends to interrupt the child's ability to focus on the more complex conceptual and social elements of tasks and situations.

### Proprioception Problems

Another type of perceptual problem involves proprioception, which arises from the muscles and joints to inform the brain about position of body parts. This is a difficult area to research, because direct measures of proprioception are not available. However, the experience of many master clinicians indicates that a number of children have serious difficulties interpreting proprioceptive information.

Children who do not receive reliable information about body position often appear clumsy, distracted, and awkward. As with poor tactile perception, these children must often rely on visual cues or other cognitive strategies (for example, use of verbalizations) to perform simple aspects of tasks, such as staying in a chair or using a fork correctly. Other common attributes of children with poor proprioception include using too much or too little force in activities such as writing, clapping, marching, or typing. Breaking toys, bumping into others, and misjudging personal space are other ramifications of poor proprioception, which have strong social implications.

Many children with this condition seek firm pressure to their skin, or joint compression and traction. These sensation-seeking behaviors may be an attempt to gain additional feedback about body position, or they may reflect a concomitant hyporesponsiveness to proprioceptive sensations. In any case, if these behaviors are done in socially inappropriate ways or at inopportune times, such as leaning on another child during circle time or hanging from a doorway at school, the child's behavior may be misinterpreted as being willfully disruptive.

### Visual Perceptual Problems

Visual perception is an important factor in the competent performance of many constructional play activities and fine motor tasks. Tests are available to measure figure-ground perception, spatial orientation, depth perception, and visual closure, to name just a few of the many aspects of visual perception that have been of concern to professionals in many disciplines.

Problems with visual perception are commonly seen in children with sensory integrative disorders, particularly when poor tactile perception or dyspraxia is present (Ayres, et al., 1987; Ayres, 1989). However, some children have only a specific visual perception problem without any other sign of a sensory integrative dysfunction. Generally, therapists do not consider that these children have a sensory integrative disorder. A classic sensory integrative treatment approach, as described later in this chapter, is inappropriate for these children, although an occupational therapist might choose to work with the child using another treatment approach, such as visual perception training (Todd, 1993), use of compensatory strategies, or skill training in specific occupations.

### Other Perceptual Problems

Many other dimensions of perception and sensory discrimination exist. For example, perception of movement through space involves the integration of vestibular, proprioceptive, and visual integration and may be affected in children with vestibular-proprioceptive problems. Auditory perception is an important function that may be involved in some children with sensory integrative disorders. However, it often exists as a discrete problem in children with language disorders. A discrete auditory perception problem, therefore, usually would not be considered a sensory integrative dysfunction but probably would be addressed by the speech pathologist. Many areas of perception are not well understood and warrant further research.

### Vestibular Processing Disorders

Over the years the research of Ayres identified a class of disorders termed *vestibular processing disorders*. These disorders are thought to reflect a problem in central vestibular processing. The clinical signs related to this type of disorder involve the motor functions that are outcomes of vestibular processing, such as poor equilibrium reactions and low muscle tone, particularly of the extensor muscles, which are strongly influenced by the vestibular system. Signs of vestibular processing dysfunction can be observed informally, but these disorders are best assessed using formal clinical observations and standardized test scores.

Different names have been applied to vestibular processing disorders at different points in time because of the changing patterns of research findings. In her early factor analytic studies, Ayres identified a linkage between postural-ocular mechanisms and integration of the two sides of the body. Clinically, she called the related dysfunction a disorder in "postural and bilateral integration," and she noted that it often occurred in children with learning disabilities, especially those with reading disorders (Ayres, 1972b). Additional problems commonly seen in this disorder included low muscle tone, immature righting and equilibrium reactions, poor right-left discrimination, and lack of clearly defined hand dominance.

Later in the 1970s Ayres included the Southern California Postrotary Nystagmus Test (SCPNT) (Ayres, 1975), in her research as a more specific measure of vestibular processing. This test continues to be used and is part of the SIPT. Ayres (1978) found that this measure seemed to be related to the clinical pictures of children who responded well to her therapy, and she began to emphasize what appeared to be a vestibular processing component to the postural and bilateral integration (PBI) disorder that she had identified earlier. At this point she replaced the old PBI concept with the term *vestibular-bilateral integration* (VBI) disorder. One of the main characteristics of this problem was depressed postrotary nystagmus scores, suggesting inefficient central processing of vestibular input. Also characteristic were other signs of vestibular-related dysfunction such as low muscle tone, postural-ocular deficits, and diminished balance and equilibrium reactions. In addition, poor bilateral coordination was implicated in VBI.

With the advent of the SIPT, new factor and cluster analyses led to further evolution of the concept of vestibular processing disorders. The SIPT studies identified a *bilateral integration and sequencing (BIS)* problem characterized by poor bilateral coordination and difficulty sequencing actions (Ayres, 1989). Ayres suggested that vestibular functioning was an important component of this set of dysfunctions, but she was only able to make preliminary conjectures about this before her death in 1988. Building on Ayres' ideas, Fisher (1991) also suggested that a vestibular-proprioceptive disorder is the basis for a bilateral and sequencing deficit, but she recommended that continued research is needed to investigate this putative relationship.

Fisher (1991) introduced an interesting new concept in relation to bilateral integration and sequencing, that is, the notion of *projected action sequences*. A projected action sequence involves anticipating how to move as one's relationship to the environment changes, as when moving to kick a ball or catching a moving ball. Fisher suggested that difficulty with projected action sequences is related to poor vestibular-proprioceptive processing, and further, that such deficits are a form of motor planning disorder. Thus Fisher has proposed a formal link between vestibular processing and praxis through the production of bilateral and sequenced movements.

Despite the variety of ways that have been used to describe vestibular processing disorders, there are classic clinical signs that are common to all, such as poor equilibrium reactions. In general, many children with vestibular processing disorders do not appear to have the level of dysfunction associated with other types of sensory integrative disorders; thus the problem is easy to overlook. Lower than average muscle tone, particularly in extensor muscles, may lead to poor endurance, a tendency toward slouching, or difficulty in keeping the head upright. Impaired balance and equilibrium reactions are likely to affect function in activities such as bicycle riding, rollerskating, skiing, and playing games such as hopscotch. Poor bilateral integration interferes with these activities as well. In addition, poor bilateral integration makes activities such as cutting with scissors, buttoning a shirt, or doing jumping jacks especially challenging. Vestibular processing problems that involve the vestibular-ocular pathways may adversely affect function when directing eye movements while moving, as when watching a rolling soccer ball while running to kick it. Neurologic connections between the reticular activating system and the limbic system also put children with vestibular processing disorders at risk for problems with attention, organization of behavior, communication, and modulation of arousal.

## Dyspraxia

Praxis is the ability to conceptualize, plan, and execute a nonhabitual motor act (Ayres, 1979). Dyspraxia refers to a condition characterized by difficulty with praxis that cannot be explained by a medical diagnosis or developmental disability and that occurs despite ordinary environmental opportunities for motor experiences. When Ayres originally wrote about this condition, she used the term *developmental apraxia* (Ayres, 1972b). Because the term *apraxia* is often associated with brain damage in adults, however, she later replaced this term with *developmental dyspraxia* (Ayres, 1979, 1985). The prefix *developmental* implies that the condition emerges in early childhood development and is not the result of traumatic injury.

As noted earlier, Ayres was struck with the relationship between tactile perception and praxis that emerged in study after study. She hypothesized that good tactile perception contributes to development of an accurate and precise body scheme, which serves as a reservoir of knowledge to be drawn on when planning new actions. Her interest in praxis appeared to grow over time, as is evident in the number of praxis tests included in the SIPT as opposed to the older SCSIT. When Ayres (1989) discussed praxis in relation to her SIPT studies, she introduced the idea that praxis problems may be manifested in different forms, not all of which are sensory integrative in nature. She coined the term *somatopraxis* to refer to the aspect of praxis that is sensory integrative in origin and grounded in somatosensory processing. At the same time she introduced the term *somatodyspraxia* to refer to a sensory integrative deficit that involves poor praxis as well as impaired tactile and proprioceptive processing. By definition, then, somatodyspraxia involves a disorder in tactile discrimination and perception. Cermak (1991) noted that not all children with developmental dyspraxia demonstrate poor tactile perception; the term *somatodyspraxia* applies only to those who do.

The child with somatodyspraxia appears clumsy and awkward. Novel motor activities are performed with great difficulty and often result in failure. Transitioning from one body position to another may pose a great challenge, as well as sequencing and timing the actions involved in a motor task. These children typically have difficulty relating their bodies to physical objects in environmental space. They often have difficulty accurately imitating actions of others. Directionality of movement may be disturbed, resulting in toys being broken unintentionally when the child forcefully pushes an object that should be pulled. Many of these children have difficulties with oral praxis, which may affect eating skills or speech articulation.

Some children with dyspraxia have problems with ideation; that is, they have difficulty generating ideas of what to do in a novel situation. When asked to simply play, without being given specific directions, these children may not initiate any activity or they may initiate activity that is habitual and limited or seems to lack a goal. Typical responses, for example, are to wander aimlessly, to perform simple repetitive actions such as patting or pushing objects around, to randomly pile up objects with no apparent plan, or, for the more sophisticated child, to wait to observe others doing an activity and then imitate them rather than initiating an activity independently.

For children with dyspraxia, skills that most children attain rather easily can be excessively challenging, for example, donning a sweater, feeding self with utensils, writing the alphabet, jumping rope, and making a pop-up toy work. These skills can be mastered only with high motivation on the part of the child, coupled with a great deal of practice, far more than most children require. Participation in sports is often embarrassing and frustrating, and organization of schoolwork may be a problem of particular concern. Children who have somatodyspraxia and are aware of their deficits often avoid difficult motor challenges and may attempt to gain control over such situations by assuming a directing or controlling role over others.

Praxis is best evaluated using the SIPT, which is sensitive to difficulties in this area. However, parent interview and informal observations provide critical pieces in the assessment process. In fact, these are essential in evaluating ideation because standardized tests are extremely limited in their measurement of this aspect of praxis.

## Secondary Problems Related to Sensory Integrative Dysfunction

In addition to the primary characteristics of sensory integrative dysfunctions, secondary problems may arise in the child's functioning at home, in school, and in the community. Following is an explanation of these indirect, but significant, influences on the child and family.

First, sensory integrative dysfunction is an "invisible" disability (that is, not directly and easily seen by the casual observer) that is easily misinterpreted. Sensory integrative disorders can fluctuate in severity from one time to another within the same child. Moreover, the severity of dysfunction and the ways dysfunction is expressed vary tremendously from one individual to another. This makes it difficult to predict which situations cause problems for a particular child, how much discomfort results, and when distress is likely to occur. Parents and teachers of children with these disorders often find the unpredictability of the child's behavior to be frustrating and difficult to understand. As a result, sensory integrative problems are frequently misinterpreted as purely behavioral or psychological issues.

A second indirect effect of sensory integrative dysfunction on the child's life is its negative impact on skill development secondary to limited participation in childhood occupations. The child who avoids fingerpainting because of tactile defensiveness or rarely attempts climbing on the jungle gym because of dyspraxia, misses more than these singular experiences. The child also misses experiences that hone underlying functions such as tactile discrimination, hand strength and dexterity, shoulder stability, balance and equilibrium, eye-hand coordination, bilateral coordination, ideation, and motor planning. In addition to interference with the development of sensorimotor functions, interactions important to the development of communication and social skills do not occur. Thus some children with sensory integrative disorders may lack the ability to play successfully with peers partially because they have not been able to participate fully in the play occupations in which sensory, motor, cognitive, and social skills emerge and develop. The fear, anxiety, or discomfort that accompany many everyday situations are also likely to work against the expression of the child's inner drive toward growth-inducing experiences. Therefore lack of experience, as well as diminished drive to participate, compound the direct effects of a sensory integrative disorder. Consequently, the development of competence in many domains of development may be seriously compromised.

Finally, a third indirect effect of sensory integrative dysfunction is the undermining of self-esteem and self-confidence over time. Children with sensory integrative dysfunction are often aware of their struggles with commonplace tasks, so it is natural for them to react with frustration. Frustration is likely to mount as the child observes peers mastering these same tasks effortlessly. Chronic frustration can negatively affect and detract from the child's feelings of self-efficacy. Instead the child may develop feelings of helplessness. This, of course, leads to further limitations in the child's experiences because the child becomes less likely to attempt challenging activities.

## ASSESSMENT OF SENSORY INTEGRATIVE FUNCTIONS

Assessment of sensory integration, like all other areas addressed in occupational therapy, requires a multifaceted approach because of the need to understand presenting problems not only in relation to the individual who is being assessed, but also with respect to the family and environments in which that individual lives. A variety of tools are needed to help the therapist identify whether a sensory integrative disorder is a factor in the child's life and, if so, what the nature of the problem is and whether any intervention should be recommended. Assessment tools employed by occupational therapists using a sensory integration perspective include interviews and questionnaires, informal and formal observations, standardized tests, and consideration of services and resources available to the family.

### Interviews and Questionnaires

The potential need for an occupational therapy assessment of sensory integration usually arises with a referral from someone who knows the child and something about the problems the child is experiencing. The time of referral, therefore, is often ideal for initiating the assessment process. The referral source, family members, and others who work with the child may all be valuable sources of information through interview or questionnaire (Figure 13-9). This initial phase of evaluation serves to identify the presenting problems, or main concerns, about the child and begins the process of determining whether a sensory integra-

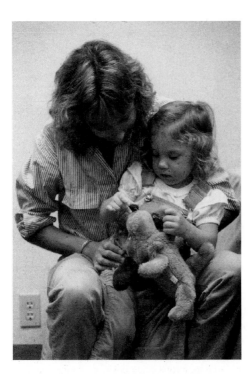

**Figure 13-9** Because parents know their child better than anyone else, they are invaluable sources of information to the therapist, especially in beginning phases of the assessment process. (Courtesy of Shay McAtee.)

tive dysfunction is a significant influence on the child's ability to function.

During the initial interview, as the parent, teacher, psychologist, physician, or other referral source describes the child's difficulties, the therapist may gather important information by probing to uncover hidden signs of sensory integrative dysfunction that may be present. For example, the teacher may report that the child is always fighting while standing in line and cannot seem to stay seated during reading circle time. Further questioning by the therapist may disclose signs of possible tactile defensiveness that might explain the child's behavior but were not considered important by the teacher who is unfamiliar with this condition. A parent may be able to provide critical information about the child's development, which may be helpful in identifying early signs of sensory integrative dysfunction. For instance, parents may have noticed that it always took the child longer than others to learn new tasks such as cutting with scissors or riding a tricycle, possible signs of dyspraxia. Another important role of the interview is to uncover alternative explanations of the child's difficulties that may rule out sensory integrative dysfunction such as when a recent emotional crisis, such as a divorce or death, coincides with the onset of problems.

Questionnaires, checklists, and histories given by caregivers and other adults who know the child well are other means for gathering information that aid in identifying presenting problems, estimating how long they have been a

concern, and clarifying the priorities of the family. One such instrument is a sensory history or similar questionnaire. Originally developed as an unpublished questionnaire by Ayres, this instrument asks parents specific questions regarding child behaviors indicative of sensory integrative dysfunction. Many therapists over the years have modified this instrument, so many versions of it exist. Researchers are currently working to evaluate reliability and validity of these kinds of questionnaires to increase their clinical value (Carrasco, 1990; Dunn, 1994; LaCroix, 1993; Spyropulos, 1991).

Behavior checklists and other questionnaires that address classroom performance are often a convenient way to elicit information from teachers (Carrasco & Lee, 1993). An additional way to gather information in the initial phases of assessment is through clinical records, including reading previous reports from other professionals and reviewing medical histories.

Finally, it may be useful to talk with the child directly when this is possible. Royeen and Fortune (1990) developed a child questionnaire for the assessment of tactile defensiveness, called the *Touch Inventory for Elementary School-Aged Children (TIE)*. Children with enough verbal skills to discuss their own abilities, perceptions, and difficulties can sometimes provide invaluable insight into their condition through such a questionnaire-based interview. One 5-year-old girl, when asked, "Do fuzzy shirts bother you?" (an item on the TIE), responded with a 10-minute discussion regarding the types of clothes she could and could not wear. Even at this young age, she had developed a clear awareness of her own tactile preferences and aversions.

The information garnered through the initial interview process is used to decide whether further assessment is warranted, and if so, which evaluation procedures are most appropriate. This information is also critical in interpreting the final pool of information gathered through assessment and in prioritizing goals for the child in light of the main concerns of the family.

## Informal and Formal Observations of the Child

Direct observation of the child is essential to the evaluation of sensory integration. Both informal, unstructured observations and structured, testlike observations are commonly used.

### Informal Observations

Informal observation of the child in natural settings, such as a classroom, playground, or home, is informative and should be done whenever feasible. Not only will this influence the conclusion as to whether a sensory integrative disorder is present, but it will, perhaps more importantly, indicate how the child's difficulties are interfering with daily occupations. For example, an experienced therapist can often detect signs of poor body awareness by observing the child at school. Such signs might include exerting too much pressure on a pencil, standing too close to classmates in line, misstepping when climbing on a jungle gym, and sitting in an ineffective position in a chair while doing class assignments. Teachers may not necessarily report these behaviors to the therapist if they perceive them as typical signs of inattentiveness or clumsiness.

Informal observation of the child in the clinical setting can also be useful in that it shows how the child responds to situations that are novel or unpredictable. A child with dyspraxia may have a great deal of difficulty figuring out how to mount an unfamiliar climbing structure in the clinic, even though performance is adequate on similar tasks at home or at school where the child has practiced them. The novelty of the clinical therapy room elicits responses from children that may be diagnostically relevant. For children with good ideation and sensory processing abilities, the endless opportunities afforded by sensory integration equipment in the clinic can be exhilarating. For the child with a disorder like dyspraxia, the same environment may be confusing, puzzling, or frustrating. A child with gravitational insecurity may be terrified by the prospect of equipment that moves, whereas a child with autism may be distressed by the clinic environment because of its unpredictability and discrepancy from familiar settings. Parham (1987) has provided some guidelines for organizing informal observations in the clinic, with special attention to issues related to praxis. Although her suggestions are focused on the assessment of preschoolers, they can also be applied to older children and may be particularly helpful in evaluating older children who are unable to cooperate with standardized testing.

### Clinical Observations

Formal observations that are highly structured and somewhat testlike are often used in an occupational therapy assessment of sensory integration. Usually referred to as *clinical observations*, these typically involve a set of specific tasks, reflexes, and signs of nervous system integrity that are associated with sensory integrative functioning. Ayres (1965, 1966a, 1966b, 1969, 1971, 1972d, 1977a, 1987) included measures of such formal observations in her factor analytic studies, along with standardized tests. She also developed a set of clinical observations that she used in clinical practice. These unpublished, nonstandardized evaluation tools were intended to supplement standardized test scores and subsequently were revised and expanded upon by many other therapists over the years. Examples of some of the most commonly used clinical observations are described in the box at right.

One of the difficulties in using clinical observations as an assessment tool is that administration and scoring criteria have not been standardized. This means that they are administered using different procedures from one clinician

## Examples of Commonly Used Clinical Observations

*Crossing body midline:* The ability to cross the body midline with one or both hands to manipulate objects in contralateral space. Deficits in this area may be associated with inadequate bilateral integration or poor trunk rotation and may also be indicative of deficits in the development of hand preference.

*Equilibrium reactions:* Compensatory movements of body parts that serve to maintain the center of gravity over the base of support when either the center of gravity or support surface is displaced.

*Hypotonicity:* Exaggerated mobility at the joints (i.e., joint laxity or hyperextensibility) or "soft" muscle bellies on palpation may be indications of hypotonicity.

*Prone extension:* The ability to simultaneously lift the head, flexed arms, upper trunk, and extended legs up against gravity from the prone-lying position. Poor prone extension often is associated with inadequate processing of vestibular-proprioceptive inputs.

*Supine flexion:* Simultaneous flexion against gravity of the knees, hips, trunk, and neck from a supine-lying position; the top of the head should approximate the knees. The ability to assume this position has been related to somatosensory function and praxis.

Excerpted from material prepared by Susanne Roley and Anne Fisher for Sensory Integration International. Reprinted by permission from Sensory Integration International, 1602 Cabrillo Avenue, P.O. Box 9013, Torrance, CA 90508.

to another. Furthermore, most of them lack any normative data to aid in interpretation of any scores that might be obtained. Only a few clinical observations have any research behind them to inform interpretation (e.g., Dunn, 1981; Gregory-Flock & Yerxa, 1984; Magalhaes, Koomar, & Cermak, 1989; Wilson, Pollock, Kaplan, & Law, 1994). Occupational therapists must rely on the information from these studies, as well as their personal expertise and judgment, to interpret the results of clinical observations. Without the requisite data in hand, occupational therapists are cautioned to avoid overinterpretation of clinical observations in light of the lack of standardized procedures and inadequate information regarding expected performance across age, gender, and other demographically related groups. Perhaps most problematic is that most clinical observations primarily address motor functions that may be strongly affected by conditions other than sensory integrative dysfunction. Advanced knowledge of sensory integration theory, therefore, must be mastered by the therapist before meaningful interpretations of these observations can be made.

## Standardized Testing

Standardized tests are frequently used by occupational therapists in the evaluation of sensory integration. Although most relevant tests are not labeled as tests of sensory integration per se, they do include items or subtests from which inferences regarding sensory integration may be drawn. For example, the Miller Assessment for Preschoolers (Miller, 1988) includes tests of stereognosis, tactile perception, and some vestibular functions. Many tests, such as the Bruininks-Oseretsky Test of Motor Proficiency (Bruininks, 1978), measure aspects of fine and gross motor skills (such as bilateral coordination) that are related to sensory integrative functions. Other tests, such as the Developmental Test of Visual Motor Integration (Beery, 1989), provide specific information related to visual-perceptual and perceptual-motor skills.

Whereas a number of tests are available that contribute incidental information regarding sensory integrative functions, the SIPT are the only set of standardized tests designed specifically for in-depth evaluation of sensory integration. The SIPT evolved from a series of tests that Ayres developed in the 1960s (Ayres, 1963, 1964, 1966a, 1966b, 1969) and later published as the SCSIT (Ayres, 1972c) and the SCPNT (Ayres, 1975). The standardization process used in the development of the SIPT was rigorous, involving normative data on approximately 2000 children in North America and extensive reliability and validity studies (Ayres, 1989). Its 17 tests measure tactile, vestibular, and proprioceptive sensory processing; form and space perception and visuomotor coordination; bilateral integration and sequencing abilities; and praxis (Ayres & Marr, 1991). A list of the 17 tests and the functions measured by each is presented in Table 13-3.

The SIPT require about 2 hours to administer and another 30 to 45 minutes to score. Test score sheets may be sent to the publisher, Western Psychological Services (WPS), for computerized scoring or may be scored by the therapist, using a software scoring program available from the publisher. After test scores are obtained, they are critically examined by the therapist to detect whether any known patterns of sensory integrative dysfunction are evident. Not only are patterns of test scores scrutinized, but also the observations that the therapist has made of child behavior during testing are considered in interpreting test scores. Finally, test scores and test behaviors are integrated with all other sources of information from the assessment in reaching a conclusion regarding the status of sensory integrative functioning.

Because it is a standardized test, the SIPT must be administered with great care to adhere strictly to standardized procedures (Figure 13-10). Specialized training is required to administer and interpret the SIPT. It is a complex set of

▲ Table 13-3   Functions Measured by the Sensory Integration and Praxis Tests

| Function | Description |
|---|---|
| Space Visualization | Motor-free visual space perception; mental manipulation of objects |
| Figure-Ground Perception | Motor-free visual perception of figures on a rival background |
| Manual Form Perception | Identification of block held in hand with visual counterpart or with block held in other hand |
| Kinesthesia | Somatic perception of hand and arm position and movement |
| Finger Identification | Tactile perception of individual fingers |
| Graphesthesia | Tactile perception and practic replication of designs |
| Localization of Tactile Stimuli | Tactile perception of specific stimulus applied to arm or hand |
| Praxis on Verbal Command | Ability to motor-plan body postures on the basis of verbal directions without visual cures |
| Design Copying | Visuopractic ability to copy simple and complex two-dimensional designs, and the manner or approach one uses to copy designs |
| Constructional Praxis | Ability to relate objects to each other in three-dimensional space |
| Postural Praxis | Ability to plan and execute body movements and positions |
| Oral Praxis | Ability to plan and execute lip, tongue, and jaw movements |
| Sequencing Praxis | Ability to repeat a series of hand and finger movements |
| Bilateral Motor Coordination | Ability to move both hands and both feet in a smooth and integrated pattern |
| Standing and Walking Balance | Static and dynamic balance on one or both feet with eyes open and closed |
| Motor Accuracy | Eye-hand coordination and control of movement |
| Postrotary Nystagmus | Central nervous system processing of vestibular input assessed through observation of the duration and integrity of a vestibuloocular reflex |

Reprinted from Mailloux, Z. (1990). An overview of the Sensory Integration and Praxis Tests. *American Journal of Occupational Therapy, 44,* 589-594.

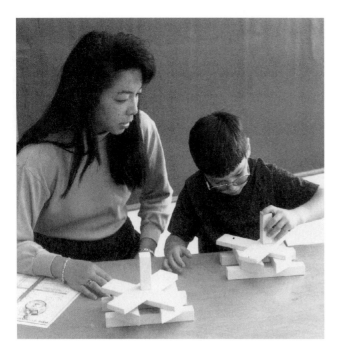

**Figure 13-10**   Constructional Praxis Test is one of 17 tests of the Sensory Integration and Praxis Tests (SIPT). The SIPT must be administered individually with strict adherence to standardized procedures. (Courtesy of Shay McAtee.)

tests and, unlike most published tests, cannot be self-taught by simply reading the manual. A certification process in SIPT administration and interpretation is offered through Sensory Integration International. To become certified, a therapist must take prerequisite coursework in statistics and sensory integration theory, followed by courses in SIPT administration and interpretation, an observation of test administration skills, and passage of a competency examination. (Appendix 13-B.) In addition to formal training for the SIPT, it is strongly recommended that therapists practice administration of the tests with children who do not have any known problems, as well as with children who have recognized difficulties. With this experience and training, the therapist can administer the tests in a manner that produces reliable scores while also allowing for observation of behaviors that provide additional information about the child's sensory integration and praxis abilities.

## Consideration of Available Services and Resources

In addition to the information that is gathered about the child, an occupational therapy assessment of sensory integration should take into consideration the services and resources that are available to the child. Information regarding the type of services the child is currently receiving, how he or she is responding to these services, and what services, programs, and resources are available to the child need careful consideration in light of the purpose and findings of the

evaluation before recommendations can be formulated. For example, an occupational therapist may be asked to provide a reevaluation of a child who has been receiving occupational therapy for several years. If the child continues to demonstrate significant sensory integrative dysfunction and has shown a diminishing response to treatment using a classical sensory integration approach, the recommendations would be different than if the child no longer showed evidence of a significant sensory integrative dysfunction. Similarly, a child who lives in an area in which there are no therapists qualified to provide occupational therapy using a classical sensory integration approach needs a different program recommendation than a child who has easy access to this type of service. Understanding family resources in terms of funding, transportation, time, and available caregivers is also critical in identifying what kinds of services are most helpful to the child and family. These issues are just as important to the assessment process as the within-child factors that are addressed in a sensory integration evaluation.

## Interpretation of Assessment Findings

Once all of the information from interviews, questionnaires, informal and formal observations, standardized tests, and consideration of available services and resources has been collected, the occupational therapist must integrate and interpret these data to reach meaningful conclusions and appropriate recommendations for the individual child under consideration. One of the first steps in this process is to evaluate whether a sensory integrative dysfunction is a contributor to the presenting problems of the child. To do this, data are classified into categories that either support or refute the presence of particular types of sensory integrative dysfunction. Following a detailed analysis of the constellation of assessment findings, a hypothesis is generated as to whether a sensory integrative dysfunction appears to be present. If a sensory integrative dysfunction is thought to be present, the type of disorder is tentatively identified.

Whether a sensory integrative dysfunction is evident, it is critical to relate the findings to the presenting problems and initial concerns of the family or referral source. For example, an assessment may uncover signs of tactile defensiveness in a child described by the parents as destructive and impulsive. The evaluating therapist must explain how tactile defensiveness may be related to the child's behavior problems. Because sensory integrative problems are not commonly recognized, the therapist usually includes an educational component in the evaluation report to link assessment findings to the daily life experiences of the child and family.

If an assessment leads to a recommendation for intervention, it generally includes an estimate of the duration of time the child should receive therapy, some indication of prognosis, and a statement regarding expected areas of change.

The anticipated gains can be further clarified through the establishment of specific goals and objectives. The format in which goals are specified is often a function of the setting in which therapy is delivered. For example, a school district may tend to include certain types of goals as part of an individualized education plan, whereas a hospital setting may lean toward more medically related outcomes. Whatever the case, goals should be established in a manner that is culturally relevant for the family and considers the needs and wishes of the individual child.

## SENSORY INTEGRATIVE DYSFUNCTION INTERVENTION

Planning an occupational therapy program for a child with a sensory integrative disorder requires the same careful analysis that is used when applying any theoretical framework in clinical practice. That is, the constellation of child and family characteristics is analyzed in relation to the occupations of the individuals involved. In a sensory integration approach to intervention, the unique ways in which sensory integrative problems affect the occupations of the particular child and his or her family provide the cornerstone on which decisions regarding treatment are made.

The assessment process aids the therapist in deciding whether any intervention is recommended and, if so, in what format: individual therapy, group sessions, collaborative problem solving with parents and teachers, or consultation. Regardless of the form in which intervention is delivered, theory-based concepts regarding the nature of sensory integration are applied whenever a sensory integrative approach is selected. Six guiding principles from the work of Ayres (1972b, 1979, 1981) are summarized in the box at right. The key ideas behind these principles were introduced earlier in this chapter in the sections on sensory integrative development and sensory integrative disorders.

Making decisions regarding the manner in which occupational therapy should be provided for children with sensory integrative disorders requires a great deal of expertise that is developed through advanced training and years of practice. The field of sensory integration is a complex, specialized area of occupational therapy practice that demands that the therapist synthesize information from many sources, and because it is a dynamically changing field of practice, it is important that the therapist stay abreast of new developments in sensory integration theory, practice, and research. These sources of information, in combination with the unique situation of the child and family being helped, all come to bear on the decision of whether to intervene and, if so, how. In the following section, three of the primary methods of service delivery are described: individual therapy, group sessions, and consultation. Most of the time, in clinical practice, these forms of intervention are used in combination, rather than as isolated treatments. They may also be used in conjunction with interventions based on

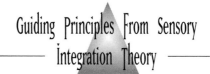

## Guiding Principles From Sensory Integration Theory

1. Controlled sensory input can be used to elicit an adaptive response.
2. Registration of meaningful sensory input is necessary before an adaptive response can be made.
3. An adaptive response contributes to the development of sensory integration.
4. Better organization of adaptive responses enhance the child's general behavioral organization.
5. More mature and complex patterns of behavior are composed of consolidations of more primitive behaviors.
6. The more inner-directed a child's activities are, the greater the potential of the activities for improving neural organization.

other frames of reference, such as neurodevelopmental treatment or training of in-hand manipulation, as long as the underlying assumptions of the interventions are mutually compatible.

### Individual Therapy

Individual occupational therapy for a sensory integrative disorder is the most intensive form of intervention. Individual therapy is usually recommended as the most effective way to initially help a child gain improved capabilities when sensory integrative problems are interfering with the child's occupations at home, in play, at school, or in the community. Individual occupational therapy for sensory integrative disorders can generally be classified into two categories: classical sensory integration treatment and compensatory skill development.

#### Classical Sensory Integrative Treatment

In this section the term *classical sensory integration treatment* refers to the kind of individual occupational therapy that Ayres developed specifically to remediate sensory integrative dysfunction in children. Although she originally designed this therapy for children with learning disabilities (Ayres, 1972b), she and many other expert clinicians have used this kind of intervention to help children with other kinds of problems as well, including autism and other developmental disabilities.

In designing this specialized form of occupational therapy, Ayres was influenced by the neurobiologic literature, which shows that nervous systems have plasticity or changeability. Plasticity is particularly characteristic of the developing young child. This led Ayres to hypothesize that the neural systems that impair function may be remediable, especially in the young child. Accordingly, she set out to design a therapy that capitalized on the plasticity of the nervous system to remediate sensory integrative dysfunction. This is *not* to say that sensory integrative treatment cures conditions such as learning disability, autism, or developmental delays. Rather, the intent is to improve the efficiency with which the nervous system interprets and uses sensory information for functional use. In a classical sensory integration approach, therefore, therapy is aimed at promoting underlying capabilities and minimizing abnormal function to the greatest degree possible.

Classical sensory integrative treatment has a number of defining characteristics. It is virtually always applied on an *individual* basis because the therapist must adjust therapeutic activities moment by moment in relation to the individual child's interest in the activity or response to a specific challenge or sensory experience (Clark et al., 1989; Kimball, 1993; Koomar & Bundy, 1991). This requires the therapist to continually focus attention on the child while being mindful of opportunities in the environment for eliciting adaptive responses. The therapist's decisions regarding how and when to intervene involve a delicate interplay between the therapist's judgment regarding the potential therapeutic value of an activity and the child's motivation to do the activity. The therapist does not use a "cookbook" approach in providing this therapy, for example, by entering the therapy situation with a predetermined schedule of activities that the child is required to follow. Rather, the therapist enters into a relationship with the child that fosters the child's inner drive to actively explore the environment and to master challenges posed by the environment.

Treatment involves a *balance between structure and freedom* (Ayres, 1972b, 1979), and its effectiveness is contingent on the proficiency of the therapist in making judgments regarding when to step in to provide structure and when to step back and allow the child to choose activities. The therapist's job is to create an environment that evokes increasingly complex adaptive responses from the child, and this is done by respecting the child's needs and interests while looking for opportunities to help the child successfully meet a challenge. For example, consider a child who needs to develop more efficient righting and equilibrium reactions and chooses to sit and swing on a platform swing. The therapist may allow the child to swing awhile to become accustomed to the vestibular sensations. Once the child seems comfortable, the therapist steps in to jiggle the swing to stimulate the desired responses. However, if the child responds to this challenge with signs of anxiety or fear, the therapist needs to intervene quickly to help the child feel safer. For example, the therapist might set an inner tube on the swing to provide a base to stabilize the lower part of the child's body and increase feelings of security while the child's upper body is free to make the required righting reactions. Therapeutic activities thus emerge from the interaction between therapist and child. Such individualized

treatment can be fully realized only when there is a one-to-one ratio between therapist and child (Figure 13-11).

The emphasis on the *inner drive* of the child is another key characteristic of classical sensory integration therapy (Ayres, 1972b, 1979; Clark et al., 1989; Koomar & Bundy, 1991). Self-direction on the part of the child is encouraged because therapeutic gains are maximized if the child is fully invested as an active participant. This is not to say that the child is permitted to engage in free play with no adult guidance, however. The optimal therapy situation is one in which a balance is struck between the structure provided by the therapist and some degree of freedom of choice on the part of the child (Ayres, 1972b, 1981). Drawing on the child's interests and imagination is often a key to encouraging a child to exert more effort on a difficult task or to stay with a challenging activity for a longer time. However, because children with sensory integrative problems do not always demonstrate inner drive toward growth-inducing activities, it is often necessary to modify activities and to find ways to entice a child toward interaction. A high degree of directiveness often is needed when working with children with autism or other children whose inner drive is limited. Occasionally a therapist may use a high degree of directiveness within the context of a particular activity to show

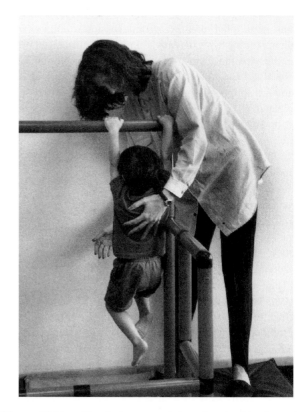

**Figure 13-11** Classical sensory integration treatment requires the therapist to attend closely to the child on a moment-by-moment basis to ensure that therapeutic activities are individually tailored to changing needs and interests of the child. (Courtesy of Shay McAtee.)

a child that the challenging activity is possible not only to achieve, but also to enjoy.

Related to inner drive is another key feature of sensory integration treatment, the valuing of *active participation,* rather than passive, on the part of the child. Because the brain responds differently and learns more effectively when an individual is actively involved in a task rather than merely receiving passive stimulation, it is considered optimal for a child to be an active participant to the greatest degree possible. For example, sensory integration theory posits that a child experiences a greater degree of integration from pumping a swing or pulling on a rope to make it go than from being swung passively. Generally speaking, maximal active involvement takes place when therapeutic activities are at just the right level of complexity, wherein the child not only feels comfortable and nonthreatened but also experiences some challenge that requires effort. The course of therapy usually begins with activities in which the child feels comfortable and competent and then moves toward increasing challenges. For children with gravitational insecurity, for example, therapy usually begins with activities close to the ground and with close physical support from the therapist to help the child feel secure. Gradually, over weeks of therapy, activities that require stepping up on different surfaces and moving away from the floor are introduced as the therapist subtly withdraws physical support. Introducing just the right level of challenge, while respecting the child's need to feel secure and in control, is a key to maximizing the child's active involvement in therapy (Figure 13-12).

However, there are situations in which passive stimulation is needed to help prepare a child for more complex or challenging activities. The child with autism, for example, may show improved sensory registration after receiving

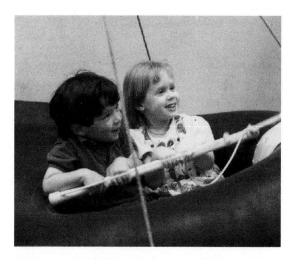

**Figure 13-12** Rather than passively imposing vestibular input on the child, classical sensory integration treatment emphasizes active participation and self-direction of the child. (Courtesy of Shay McAtee.)

passive linear vestibular stimulation (Slavik et al., 1984). The improved registration means that the child has greater awareness of the environment, and thus the passive stimulation is a stepping stone toward active involvement in an activity. Another example is the use of passive tactile stimulation as a means for reducing tactile defensiveness (Ayres, 1972b; Wilbarger & Wilbarger, 1991). This aspect of therapy, however, is seen as only a limited component of a sensory integrative treatment program and then only as a step toward facilitating more active participation.

Another key characteristic of sensory integrative treatment is the *setting* in which it takes place. The provision of a special therapeutic environment is an important aspect of this kind of intervention and has been described in detail by other authors (Slavik & Chew, 1990; Walker, 1991). Based on the research that shows that brain structure and function is enhanced when animals are permitted to actively explore an interesting environment (Rosenzweig et al., 1972), a sensory-enriched environment is designed to evoke active exploration on the part of the child. The clinic that is designed for classical sensory integrative treatment contains large activity areas with an array of specialized equipment. The availability of suspended equipment is a hallmark of this treatment approach (Clark et al., 1989; Koomar & Bundy, 1991). Suspended equipment provides rich opportunities for stimulating and challenging the vestibular system. In addition, equipment and materials are available that provide a variety of somatosensory stimuli, including tactile, vibratory, and proprioceptive. Mats and large pillows are used for safety. Overall, this special environment provides the child with a safe and interesting place in which to explore his or her capabilities. At the same time it provides the therapist with a tool kit for creating sensory experiences that are enticing and for gently guiding the child toward activities that challenge sensory modulation, perception, dynamic postural control, and motor planning (Figure 13-13).

Because of the prominence of vestibular stimulation in the classical sensory integration treatment environment, a few cautionary words are in order regarding this powerful tool. Vestibular stimulation, most often in the form of linear movement, is commonly introduced early in the course of treatment for many children because it is believed to have an organizing effect on other sensory systems (Ayres, 1972b, 1979, 1981). However, it can have a highly disturbing and disorganizing effect on the child if used carelessly. Vestibular stimulation may produce strong autonomic responses, such as blanching and nausea. It directly influences the arousal level, and if not regulated carefully, may produce hyperactive, distractible states or lethargic, drowsy states. Used in classical sensory integration treatment, vestibular stimulation is not passively imposed on the child. Rather, the child is allowed to initiate and actively control vestibular input as much as possible, with the therapist stepping in to help modulate it when indicated. For example, if a child is actively rotating while sitting in a tire swing and

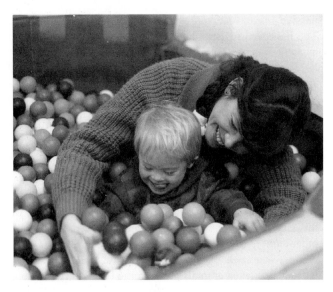

**Figure 13-13**   Setting in which classical sensory integration treatment takes place provides variety of sensory experiences. Immersion in a pool of balls presents challenges to sensory modulation. (Courtesy of Shay McAtee.)

begins to exhibit mild signs of autonomic activation, the therapist might intervene by having the child reduce the intensity of the swinging by guiding the child to shift to slow linear swinging or by offering the child a trapeze to pull to increase the amount of proprioceptive input. Proprioceptive input is believed to have an inhibiting effect on vestibular input, based on results of animal research (Fredrickson, Schwartz, & Kornhuber, 1966). Knowledge of the effects of vestibular stimulation and its interactions with other sensory systems, therefore, is critical in this treatment approach. Responsible use of vestibular stimulation as a treatment modality absolutely requires advanced training in sensory integration.

To summarize the key features of classical sensory integrative treatment, therapeutic activities are neither predetermined nor are they simply free play. The flow of the treatment session results from a collaboration between the therapist and child in which the therapist encourages and supports the child in a way that moves the child toward therapeutic goals. This all takes place within a special environment that is safe yet challenging. The use of special equipment and powerful sensory modalities requires that the therapist have special training well beyond the entry level of practice in occupational therapy.

Classical sensory integration treatment is an intensive, long-term intervention. Although treatment schedules vary, a typical schedule involves two sessions per week, each lasting 45 minutes to 1 hour. A typical course of therapy lasts for about 2 years. Most experts agree that at least 6 months of therapy are needed to detect results.

After Ayres (1972b, 1979) developed the classical sensory integrative treatment approach, her colleagues and stu-

dents continued to further develop and expand on her intervention concepts. Koomar and Bundy (1991) provided a particularly thorough description of the application of sensory integration procedures for specific types of sensory integrative disorders. Oetter, Richter, and Frick (1993) described a therapeutic program that incorporates specific techniques for oral motor function, respiration, and posture into classical sensory integration treatment. Others have imported classical sensory integration treatment concepts into the neonatal intensive care unit (Holloway, 1993), where the treatment principles are used to help children with the most plastic and vulnerable of developing nervous systems.

Use of the classical sensory integration treatment approach requires advanced study and training. Koomar and Bundy (1991) advocated a mentorship process as the best preparation for learning how to clinically apply sensory integration principles. Ayres also advocated this and established a 4-month course in which therapists receive experience treating children under close supervision. Ayres believed that this level of intensity was required to master the classical sensory integration approach. Several facilities across the United States provide formal mentoring experiences in sensory integration for occupational therapists. Some of these are listed in Appendix 13-C. Additionally, mentorship experiences may be independently set up by contacting therapists who have widely recognized expertise in this form of practice.

Sensory Integration International, a nonprofit organization that supports and promotes education, treatment, and research related to sensory integration, has published a Standards of Practice statement (Appendix 13-B) that provides guidelines for therapist qualifications in relation to the provision of sensory integrative treatment. Because of the highly specialized and complex nature of the classical sensory integration approach, it is important that occupational therapists follow the recommended guidelines for developing skills and experience in this area before independently engaging in this form of practice.

### Compensatory Skill Development

In contrast to the classical sensory integrative treatment approach, the compensatory skill development approach does not attempt to remediate an underlying sensory integrative disorder, but instead it aims to help the child and family develop specific skills or coping strategies in the face of a sensory integrative disorder. This approach may be used to supplement or to replace classical sensory integrative treatment.

The compensatory approach may be appropriate when a therapist trained in classical sensory integrative treatment is not available. It may also be selected as the treatment of choice for a child who urgently needs to accomplish specific tasks or skills and cannot wait for the longer-range but more widely generalizable outcomes of classical sensory integrative treatment. It may also be a desirable alternative for the child who has reached an age at which expected gains from the classical treatment are minimal. Finally, the compensatory approach may be introduced to a child who has been involved with classical sensory integrative treatment. Such cases include children who (1) have responded well to a classical sensory integrative treatment for some time but have reached a plateau in gains; (2) are approaching or have reached ages at which expected gains from the classical treatment are minimal; (3) do not appear motivated to participate or show waning interest in the classical approach; (4) do not demonstrate improvement in response to the classical sensory integrative approach after a reasonable amount of time (usually a 6-month trial) or (5) urgently need to accomplish specific tasks or skills that could be trained as a supplement or replacement for classical sensory integrative treatment.

When the compensatory skill approach is selected, therapy is aimed at training specific skills or using techniques that permit better performance on a given task. For example, a child with poor proprioceptive feedback may need to keep up with handwriting exercises assigned in his or her second grade class. The child is involved with classical sensory integrative treatment, which aims to help him or her develop better body awareness that eventually will help him or her not only with writing, but also with catching, throwing, cutting, buttoning, and many other proprioception-related difficulties. However, because of the everyday stress of the demands of handwriting, the child may not be able to afford to wait for these generalized capabilities to develop through sensory integrative treatment. For this child, specific handwriting training may be used to help him or her develop better handwriting skills, despite poor proprioceptive feedback. Adaptations may also be introduced to help the child compensate for the problem. For instance, a weighted pencil may provide augmented proprioceptive feedback regarding the position of the child's hand. Additionally, arrangements may be made with the child's teacher for the child to enter part of his or her schoolwork on a computer or to dictate it into a tape recorder to prevent poor writing skills from impeding other aspects of academic performance.

The therapist who chooses to use the compensatory skill development approach to individual therapy can do so while being mindful of the guiding principles of sensory integration theory presented in the box on p. 335. For example, it is optimal to involve self-direction and active participation as much as possible. This might be accomplished with our example child by having the child write his or her own stories related to his or her interests and experiences. Handwriting exercises that require active movement are expected to accomplish much more than any that are dependent on passive guidance of the child's hand. The therapist's ability to read the child's responses to writing activities helps ensure that the activities remain motivating and appropriately challenging. However, this approach generally tends to be much more therapist directed than the child-centered classical sensory integration approach.

Use of a compensatory skill approach for children with sensory integrative disorders requires that the therapist know enough about sensory integration to make sound judgments regarding when this approach is appropriate. Understanding the underlying sensory integrative disorder adequately is also essential so that the therapist does not misinterpret sensory-based problems as behavioral or neuromuscular in origin. Finally, continuing education courses in specific training methods are available, particularly in the area of fine motor skills, and should be actively pursued by therapists desiring to use this approach.

## Group Therapy Programs

Group rather than individual occupational therapy is sometimes recommended for children experiencing sensory integrative disorders. Sometimes group programs are used as a transition from individual therapy so that the child can apply newly developed skills in a social peer context with less intensive support from a therapist (Figure 13-14). The need to help a child learn to function in the context of school- and community-based groups, such as in classrooms or on sports teams, is another important reason to consider placing the child in a therapeutic group setting. Furthermore, sensory integrative disorders often create social problems for children, and treatment in groups can provide an opportunity to help the child develop important peer interaction skills.

Of course, the occupational therapist working with a group of children cannot provide the same level of vigilance to individual responses that takes place during individual therapy. Therefore some of the more intense applications of sensory stimulation or risk-taking behaviors that might be encouraged during classical sensory integrative treatment cannot be used within a group, nor can the therapist give the close guidance that is finely tuned to the individual child's needs every moment of the treatment session. Again, however, the principles of sensory integration theory outlined in the box on p. 335 are important concepts to incorporate into the group format as much as possible.

Working with children in a group affords the opportunity to observe some of the ways in which sensory integrative disorders interrupt functional behavior in a social context. Some problematic child behaviors emerge only in a group situation and may not be evident during individual therapy. For example, tactile defensiveness may not be apparent in the safe constraints of individual therapy but may become obvious as a child tries to participate within a group of people who are brushing by in an unpredictable manner. Observing how the group dynamic affects the child can help the therapist know what aspects of the classroom, playground, park, or after-school activities are likely to pose a threat or challenge.

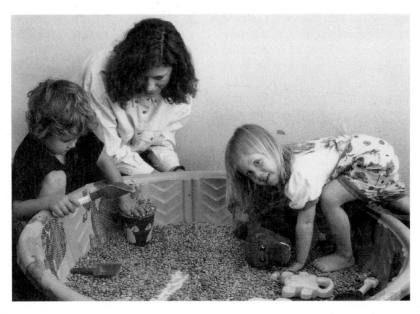

**Figure 13-14**    Group programs provide opportunities for children with sensory integrative disorders to develop coping skills that help them function in social context with peers. (Courtesy of Shay McAtee.)

In some situations, external variables such as funding limitations, availability of staff, or organizational policies create the need for children to receive therapy in a group setting. It is important that occupational therapists make recommendations based primarily on the needs of the children being served, taking into consideration such outside factors, rather than allowing the external factors to dictate the type of intervention that is provided. It is also important to differentiate what can be accomplished within a group versus individual therapy sessions. Because group programs do not permit the same degree of intensive therapy as the classical sensory integration approach, they are not expected to lead to the same outcomes. Moreover, group programs usually resemble the compensatory skill approach more closely than classical sensory integrative treatment in aim and process, although some do aim to facilitate and maintain sensory integrative functions.

A number of resources are available to the therapist interested in developing group programs based on sensory integration concepts. Sensory Integration International has published a *Sensory Motor Handbook* that includes group activities meant to be used in classroom settings (Bissell, Fisher, Owens, & Polcyn, 1988). Young (1988) produced a program of activities for preschool-aged children that are organized into categories of sensory and motor challenges. An especially innovative application of sensory integration concepts to groups is reflected in the work of Williams and Shellenberger (1994). Through a group format, their *Alert Program* helps children learn to recognize how alert they are feeling, to identify the sensorimotor experiences that they can use to change their level of alertness, and to monitor their arousal levels in a variety of settings.

To apply sensory integration principles to a group program, an occupational therapist should be familiar enough with sensory integration theory to understand precautions and general effects of various sensory and motor activities. Experience and training in working with groups, including how to maintain the attention of children in a group, how to address varying skill and interest levels, and how to deal with behavioral issues, are also recommended for occupational therapists applying sensory integration in group programs.

## Consultation

Sensory integrative disorders are complex and are often misinterpreted as behavioral, psychologic, or emotional in origin. Helping family members, teachers, and others who come into contact with the child to understand the nature of the problem can be a powerful means toward helping the child. The provision of information to those who are in ongoing contact with the child and the development of strategies through collaboration with them are important ways that the therapist can indirectly intervene to impact the child's life positively across a variety of settings. The term *consultation* broadly refers to this indirect form of intervention.

Although many of the concepts that make up sensory integration theory and practice are not usually familiar to family members, teachers, or other professionals, once they are explained in everyday terms, a newfound understanding of the child often ensues. Cermak (1991) aptly referred to this process as demystification. Parents commonly express relief at finally having a name for behaviors they have ob-

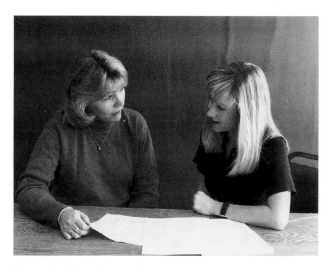

**Figure 13-15** Consultation in school involves joint problem solving between the occupational therapist and the teacher. (Courtesy of Shay McAtee.)

served, and they may experience release from feeling that they have caused these problems through a maladaptive parenting style. Teachers also may be appreciative of having an alternative way to view child behaviors, especially when this new perspective is coupled with the application of strategies that promote more productive responses from the child.

Helping those around the child understand their own sensory integrative processes is sometimes a good way to make these new concepts more meaningful. Williams and Shellenberger (1994) use this tactic when introducing their Alert Program to promote optimal arousal states. They encourage the adults who are involved with the program to develop awareness and insight into their own sensorimotor preferences. This first step of the consultation process, increasing an understanding of sensory integration, can be achieved through a number of avenues, including parent conferences, experiential sessions, lecture and discussion groups, professional in-services, and ongoing education programs. Whatever format is used, it is likely that the greater the understanding of the basic concepts of sensory integration, the greater is the openness and willingness to address these problems (Figure 13-15).

Perhaps the most important component of any consultation program is providing guidance for how to cope with the problems that stem from the sensory integrative dysfunction. Sometimes specific activities can be suggested that will help a child to prepare for a challenging task. For example, a child who has tactile defensiveness may be better able to tolerate activities such as fingerpainting or sand play if some desensitization techniques such as applying firm touch-pressure to the skin are used just before the activity. Promoting success in activities can also be accomplished by suggesting individualized ways to help a child through difficult tasks. For instance, some children with

dyspraxia are likely to be more successful in completing a novel task when they receive verbal directions, whereas others respond optimally to visual demonstrations, and still others need physical assistance with the motion. Determining which method or combination of methods is most likely to help the individual child can assist adults in facilitating success. Making adjustments in the environment can also be an important component of a consultation program for sensory integrative disorders. For example, children with autism often are highly affected by the sensory characteristics of their environments. Finding ways to manage sound, lighting, contact with other people, environmental odors, and visual distractions can make a great deal of difference in attention, behavior, and, ultimately, performance.

Consultation services may be provided before, in conjunction with, or after direct occupational therapy intervention, or they may be recommended as the intervention of choice instead of direct individual or group therapy. Whichever the case, the consultation should not be used to take the place of direct intervention if this would be most beneficial to the child. As previously mentioned external pressures should not be allowed to unduly influence the form of therapy provided to a child with sensory integrative disorders. Nor should procedures or techniques that require advanced training of an occupational therapist be recommended to parents and other professionals. For instance, an appropriate consultation program never attempts to train a parent or teacher to provide individual therapy using the classical sensory integration approach. Therapists should also be familiar enough with the child to be aware of any precautions that might apply before suggestions are made. For example, some children display delayed responses to vestibular stimulation and can become overstimulated or lethargic hours after such stimulation is received. Many aspects of sensory integrative techniques can lead to adverse reactions and must be used with care.

At its best, consultation as a form of intervention for sensory integrative disorders requires training and experience at the most advanced levels. However, therapists with lesser degrees of experience and training can use this approach successfully, albeit to a more limited extent, providing they do not overstep the bounds of their knowledge. The same background and training that is needed to provide individual therapy for sensory integrative dysfunction is desirable for this approach because the therapist needs to be able to predict what the child's likely responses will be to various activities and situations, given the characteristics of the child's sensory integrative disorder. In addition, the therapist should be well enough versed in sensory integration concepts to be able to explain them in simple yet meaningful terms. Finally, it is imperative that the therapist have excellent communication skills and respect for the various people and environments that are involved. Bundy (1991) provided an excellent description of the communication process involved in a good consultation program.

## Expected Outcomes of Occupational Therapy

As we pointed out earlier, occupational therapy is not expected to "cure" sensory integrative disorders. Rather, occupational therapy aims first to reduce the problem by providing a therapy program that helps to normalize function to the greatest possible extent, and second, to help minimize the effects of the disorder by providing strategies and compensatory models for coping with the dysfunction. The goals and objectives that are formulated as part of a child's treatment plan target the specific behavioral outcomes that are most critical to the individual child and his or her family. These goals and objectives can be conceptualized as falling into six general categories of expected outcomes. They are summarized in the box below.

### Increase in the Frequency or Duration of Adaptive Responses

As discussed in the introduction, adaptive responses occur when an individual responds to environmental challenges with success. Application of sensory integration principles helps the therapist envision how to create opportunities for the child to make adaptive responses. This may be accomplished through the use of controlled sensory input that promotes organization within the child's nervous system. Ensuring that the sensory inputs inherent in activities are organizing rather than disorganizing and integrating rather than overwhelming requires careful monitoring on the part of the therapist, who must be sensitive to the child's response to each aspect of an activity and to each type of sensory input involved. The classical sensory integrative treatment approach intensively focuses on the child's demonstration of higher-level adaptive responses. However, compensatory skill approaches, group programs, and consultation services may also boost the frequency and duration of adaptive responses by changing the child's everyday environments in ways that enable the child to make adaptive responses more easily.

Increasing the duration and frequency of adaptive re-

## Expected Outcomes of Occupational Therapy Using Sensory Integration Principles

1. Increase in the frequency or duration of adaptive responses.
2. Development of increasingly more complex adaptive responses.
3. Increase in self-confidence and self-esteem.
4. Improvement in gross and fine motor skills.
5. Improvement in daily living and personal-social skills.
6. Improvement in cognitive, language, and academic performance.

sponses is an important outcome of sensory integration because it is on simple adaptive responses that functional behavior and skills are developed. For example, a child who has difficulty staying with an activity for more than a few seconds tends to shift from one activity to another. A desirable outcome for that child might be to stay for a longer time with a simple activity, such as swinging, in a therapy environment. Achievement of this simple adaptive response may eventually contribute to the functional behavior of staying with the reading circle in the school classroom for the required amount of time, despite the many distractions and cognitive challenges imposed by this occupation.

### Development of Increasingly More Complex Adaptive Responses

Adaptive responses can vary in complexity, quality, and effectiveness (Ayres, 1981). A simple adaptive response might be simply holding onto a moving swing. A more complex adaptive response involving timing of action might be releasing grasp on a trapeze at just the right moment to land on a pillow. Effective intervention is expected to enable the child to make more complex adaptive responses over time. This outcome is based on the assumption that sensory integrative procedures promote more efficient brainstem organization of multisensory input. Better neural organization of primitive functions is expected to enhance more complex functions. Put into functional terms, the result is an improvement in the child's ability to make judgments about the environment, what can be done with objects, and what specific actions need to be taken to accomplish a goal (Ayres, 1981).

Although repetition of a familiar activity may be important while a child is assimilating a new skill and may be useful in helping a child get ready for another more challenging activity, development of increasingly more complex abilities occurs only when tasks become slightly more challenging than the child's prior accomplishments. This is one of the main tenets of classical sensory integrative treatment. Because of the high degree of personal attention continuously given to the child during this kind of therapy, a fine gradient of complexity can be built into therapeutic activities while simultaneously ensuring that the child experiences success and a growing sense of "I can do it!" Group program activities, compared with individual therapy, tend to place greater demands on children for several reasons, including limited opportunity for individualization of activities, the presence of other children with their unpredictable behaviors, and reduced opportunity for direct assistance from the therapist. Thus a limitation posed by group programs is that challenges imposed on the group may at times be too great for an individual child, leading to frustration and failure. The therapist who provides a group program needs to be alert to the potential for this undesirable effect and strive to avoid it as much as possible. Whatever format for intervention is used, the therapist uses activity analysis, assessment information, ongoing observations, and knowledge of child development to ensure that the program engages the child's inner drive as much as possible to draw forth increasingly more complex interactions within the clinical, home, or community environments.

## Increase in Self-Confidence and Self-Esteem

Ayres (1979) asserted that enhanced ability to make adaptive responses promotes self-actualization by allowing the child to experience the joy of accomplishing a task that previously could not be done. The final outcome of therapy that encourages successful, self-directed experiences is a child who perceives the self as a competent actor in the world. Individual and group programs and direct and indirect services all can be geared to helping the child master the activities that are personally meaningful and essential to success in the world of everyday occupations. Mastery of such activities is expected to result in feelings of personal control that, in turn, lead to increased willingness to take risks and to try new things (Ayres, 1979). For example, a child with gravitational insecurity may experience not only fear responses to climbing and movement activities, but also feelings of failure and frustration at not being able to participate in the play of peers. In such a case, an increase in self-confidence and comfort in one's physical body is often accompanied by a general boost in feelings of self-efficacy and worth.

## Improvement in Gross and Fine Motor Skills

The child who makes consistent and more complex adaptive responses shows evidence of improved sensory integration. Moreover, this child meets new challenges with greater self-confidence. A net result of these gains frequently is greater mastery in the motor domain. An example is the child with a vestibular processing disorder who exhibits greater competency and interest in playground activities and sports after classical sensory integrative treatment, even though these activities were not practiced during therapy. Motor skills may be among the earliest complex skills to show measurable change in response to a classical sensory integrative approach, probably because of the extent of the motor activity that is inherent in this treatment approach. Compensatory skill treatment, group intervention, or consultation for children with sensory integrative disorders should result in improvement of specific motor skills if these are targeted by the intervention. For example, if a compensatory approach to handwriting is used to help a child with poor somatosensory perception, specific gains in handwriting performance should follow if the intervention is successful.

## Improvement in Daily Living and Personal-Social Skills

Occupational therapy programs that address sensory integrative dysfunction encourage the child to organize his or her own activity, particularly in the classical sensory integration approach. As the child develops general sensory integrative capabilities and improved strategies for planning action, gains are expected in relation to ability to organize behavior, to cope with daily routines, and to master self-care tasks (Ayres, 1979). For example, treatment may help the child who is overly sensitive to touch or movement to deal with sensations in a more adaptive manner. As a result, the child is enabled to approach and engage in the challenges of everyday occupations such as dining, dressing, and bathing with greater security and confidence. Not only are daily living skills improved, but also relationships with others are likely to become more comfortable and less threatening. Group therapy programs are an ideal arena in which the increases in self-confidence made in individual therapy can be tried out in the more challenging context of a social setting. Gains in personal-social skills, as well as mastery of self-care tasks, are among the most significant of intervention outcomes.

## Improvement in Cognitive, Language, or Academic Performance

Although cognitive, language, and academic skills are not specific objectives of occupational therapy for sensory integrative disorders, improvement in these domains has been detected in some intervention studies involving the provision of classical sensory integration treatment (Ayres, 1972a, 1976, 1978; Ayres & Mailloux, 1981; Cabay, 1988; Magrun, Ottenbacher, McCue, & Keefe, 1981; Ray, King, & Grandin, 1988; White, 1979). Application of classical sensory integration procedures is thought to generate broad-based changes in these areas secondary to enhancement of sensory modulation, perception, postural control, or praxis (Ayres, 1979, 1981; Cabay & King, 1989). For example, a child with autism may be helped through a sensory integrative approach to respond in a more adaptive way to sights, sounds, touch, and movement experiences that initially were disturbing. This improvement in sensory modulation may lead to a better ability to attend to language and academic tasks; thus improvement in these areas may follow. A child who has a vestibular processing disorder may improve in postural control and equilibrium, freeing the child to more efficiently concentrate on academic material without the distraction of frequent loss of sitting balance or loss of place while copying from the blackboard. This child's vestibular-related improvements are also likely to have a positive effect on playground and sports activities because effects of classical sensory integration treatment are expected to generalize to a wide range of outcome areas.

Occupational therapy aimed at developing compensatory skills such as improved handwriting also may free the child to focus on the conceptual aspects of academic tasks, rather than the perceptual-motor details of how to write letters on a page or how to keep a sentence on a printed line. In such compensatory programs, effects on outcome skills tend to

CASE STUDY #1

## History

Drew was diagnosed with autism (high functioning) when he was 7 years old. His mother is Korean, and his father is American. All of Drew's early developmental milestones were attained within normal limits, except for language acquisition. He did not speak any words until 2 years of age, and by age 3 his family was concerned about his development because of delayed language skills. Drew attended an English language preschool at age 3, and then a Korean language preschool. (His family speaks both Korean and English at home.) He was asked to leave the second preschool because of aggressive behavior. At age 4 years Drew attended a private special education school where he received speech therapy and participated in a language-intensive playgroup. When Drew reached kindergarten age, he was enrolled in public special education programs where he attended specialized classrooms for speech and language disorders, autism, and multiple handicaps over the elementary school years.

## Reason for Referral

Drew initially was referred by the state regional center for developmental disabilities to an occupational therapy private practice for evaluation when he was nearly 8 years old. His regional center counselor thought that Drew had signs of a sensory integrative disorder, and he believed that Drew might benefit from occupational therapy. Drew's mother reported that her main concerns for Drew were related to his poor socialization skills, his limited ability to play with games and toys, and his tendency to become easily frustrated.

## Evaluation Procedure

Although the Sensory Integration and Praxis Tests (SIPT) were attempted during the initial occupational therapy assessment, Drew was unable to follow the directions or attend to the tests sufficiently to obtain reliable scores. His occupational therapy evaluation, therefore, consisted of a parent interview, including completion of a developmental and sensory history, and observation of Drew in a clinical therapy setting. At the time of assessment it was not possible to interview Drew's teacher. However, information about Drew's performance at school was obtained from his mother, who often observed him in the classroom.

## Evaluation Results

Drew demonstrated inefficiencies in sensory processing in a number of sensory systems. During the assessment, signs of inconsistent responses to tactile input were evident. For example, Drew demonstrated a complete lack of response to some stimuli such as a puff of air on the back of his neck or the light touch of a cotton ball applied to his feet when he was not visually attending. However, he withdrew in an agitated fashion when the therapist attempted to position him. His mother reported that he showed extreme dislike for certain textures of food and clothing and that he disliked being touched. She also stated that he seemed to become irritated by being near other children at school and sometimes pinched or pushed peers who came close to him. Drew also appeared easily overstimulated by extraneous visual and auditory stimuli. His mother stated that he often covered his ears at home when loud noises were present and that at school he sometimes seemed confused as to the direction of sounds. He was observed to pick up objects and look at them very closely, and he appeared to rely on his vision a great deal to complete tasks. In response to movement, he enjoyed swinging slowly but became fearful with an increase in velocity. His mother stated that he often became fearful at the park when climbing. Drew's balance was observed to be poor, and his equilibrium reactions were inconsistent. He also had trouble positioning himself on various pieces of equipment, showing poor body awareness. During the assessment he appeared to seek touch-pressure stimuli, including total body compression. He was reported to jump a great deal at home and at school. These types of proprioception-generating actions appeared to have a calming effect on Drew.

In the areas of praxis, Drew was able to imitate positions and follow verbal directions to complete motor actions, but he had a great deal of difficulty initiating activities on his own or attempting something that was unfamiliar to him. He also had difficulty timing and sequencing his actions. His mother reported that he tended not to participate in sports or in park activities and that he had trouble throwing, catching, and kicking balls. Drew was able to complete puzzles, string beads, and write his name; however, bilateral activities such as cutting and pasting were difficult for him.

Socially, Drew demonstrated poor eye contact and tended to use repetitive phrases he had heard in the past. His mother stated that he wanted to play with peers but found it hard to make friends. Drew was independent in all self-care skills, except for tying shoes and managing some fasteners.

Based on an interview and questionnaire with Drew's mother, as well as observation of Drew in a clinical therapy setting, it was determined that he displayed irregularities in sensory processing, including hypersensitivity to some aspects of touch, movement, visual, and auditory stimuli. He also demonstrated difficulty with position sense, balance, bilateral integration, and the ideation, timing, and sequencing aspects of praxis. These difficulties were thought to interfere with Drew's ability to play purposefully with toys and to participate in age-appropriate games and sports. These problems, in combination with his language delays, were interfering significantly with his social skills, ability to make friends, and tendency to become frustrated, which were the major concerns of his parents.

### Recommendation

Individual occupational therapy was recommended to address Drew's sensory integrative dysfunction, as well as the development of specific fine and gross motor skills. Because socialization issues were such a major concern for Drew's family and were interfering with his performance at school, the evaluating therapist also recommended that Drew participate in an after-school group occupational therapy program to facilitate the acquisition of social skills.

### Occupational Therapy Program

Drew received individual occupational therapy in a therapy clinic for 1 year after the evaluation. This individual therapy involved a combination of classical sensory integration and a compensatory skill development approach. During this time, Drew demonstrated significant gains in sensory processing with no further significant signs of tactile defensiveness or fear of movement activities. Motor planning of novel actions improved but continued to be of some concern for Drew. He did make notable gains in being able to catch and throw a ball and in writing and scissors skills. Through the group occupational therapy program, Drew became able to initiate and maintain interaction with peers, share objects, and play cooperatively with some assistance and structure from adults.

After this year of clinically based individual and group occupational therapy, it was recommended that individual therapy be continued at school. The focus of this occupational therapy program was to help Drew apply his improved sensorimotor and social skills in the natural context of school. Through a combination of direct service and consultation, a number of activities and adaptations were made to facilitate his performance at school. Because the initial year of intensive therapy using a classical sensory integrative approach had helped Drew tolerate and respond appropriately to sensory information and because he had developed many of the specific skills he needed in the classroom during individual therapy, he was much better able to focus on the demands expected of him at school at that time. By the end of the school year, Drew's occupational therapist recommended that occupational therapy be discontinued because she believed that his teacher would be able to continue to help him in the areas that had been addressed through the consultation program.

However, when the individual educational plan (IEP) team met to discuss Drew's transition to a new school, there was significant concern about the possibility of Drew regressing in a new setting where he would need to adjust to many different routines. The IEP team requested that occupational therapy continue to ensure a smooth transition for Drew and to put in place a plan that would continue to help him develop socially. When school resumed in the fall, the occupational therapist had arranged a "big buddy" program with a local high school. Two high school seniors worked with Drew as part of a social service assignment during recess for the fall semester. The occupational therapist trained the high school students to carry out a socialization program aimed at helping Drew feel comfortable with a new set of peers. Drew seemed to look up to the high school students and responded well to the "big buddy" program. By the end of the fall semester in the new school, Drew played cooperatively with peers, interacting independently and communicating appropriately. His occupational therapy program was formally discontinued at this time, although the occupational therapist continued to check in with Drew's teacher when at his school site to work with other children. No additional intervention has been needed, but the option for further consultation or direct intervention is available, should the need arise.

be limited to the specific task of concern. Similarly, consultation programs may enhance language, cognitive, or academic skills by providing strategies for reducing the effect of sensory integrative disorders on these functions. For instance, helping a teacher understand how best to seat a child in class (such as in a bean bag chair versus a firm wooden chair or in the front corner of the room near the teacher's desk) may assist in reducing the effects of a sensory integrative disorder by making it easier for the child to attend to instruction in the classroom.

## Research on Effectiveness of Intervention

There is little question that more effectiveness research exists in the area of sensory integration than in any other practice area of occupational therapy. Most of the research studies on effectiveness of intervention using sensory integration principles have been directed toward the classical sensory integration approach, although some studies have involved group treatment programs. Virtually no research has focused on compensatory skill training or consultation programs that are guided specifically by sensory integration principles. Therapists who wish to use a sensory integration approach in practice need to keep themselves up to date on the most recently published research literature. A helpful reference containing reviews of effectiveness studies was recently published by Sensory Integration International (Daems, 1994).

Most of the effectiveness studies indicate that classical sensory integration treatment produces gains in participants' motor, language, cognitive, or academic skills. Early studies were particularly encouraging in this regard (for example, Ayres, 1972a, 1976, 1978; Ayres & Mailloux, 1981; Cabay, 1988; Magrun et al., 1981; Ottenbacher, 1982; White, 1979). However, some of the more recent studies have found that, although children receiving sensory integration treatment make gains after intervention, they do not significantly outperform other children receiving an alter-

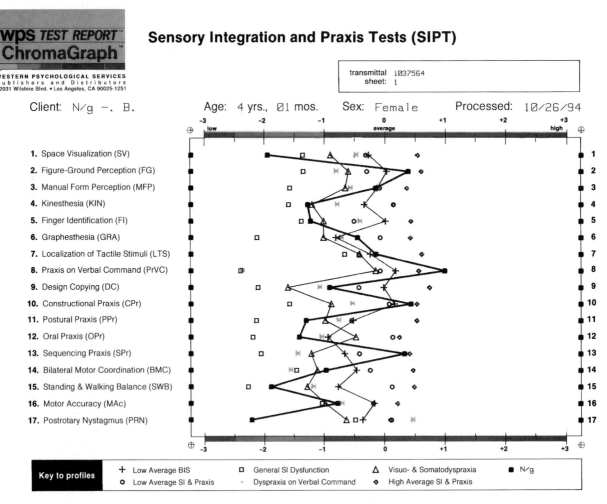

**Figure 13-16** Karen's Sensory Integration and Praxis Tests profile. (From Western Psychological Services [1988]. *Sensory Integration and Praxis Tests*. Los Angeles: Western Psychological Services.)

CASE STUDY #2

## History

Karen was born after a full-term pregnancy complicated by gestational diabetes. Labor, which was induced at 40 weeks, was long, and it was believed that Karen broke her right collar bone during delivery. Karen achieved her early motor and language milestones within average age ranges. However, she was described as an irritable baby who had difficulty breastfeeding, startled easily, and could only be calmed by swinging. Karen attended a parent cooperative child development program as a toddler, and at age 4 she was found eligible for a special education preschool program through her school district. She has not been given any specific medical or educational diagnosis.

## Reason for referral

Karen's mother expressed concern about Karen's fine and gross motor skills to a neurologist, who referred Karen for an occupational therapy assessment when she was 4 years old. When asked why she was seeking an evaluation for Karen, her mother wrote, "Up until recently I had been very patiently waiting for normal development to occur (for example, handedness, fine motor). The school psychologist feels this still may occur, but I am convinced something isn't right. Karen's increasing frustration and decreasing belief in herself prompted me to seek evaluations. While a part of me wishes to have a 'normal child,' the other part will be relieved to find that the child I have had so many doubts about since infancy does indeed have some behaviors and actions that are unusual."

## Evaluation Procedures

The Sensory Integration and Praxis Tests (SIPT) were administered in one testing session. Karen was also observed in a clinical therapy setting and at home. In addition, Karen's mother was interviewed, and she completed a developmental and sensory history on which she provided detailed accounts of Karen's early and current sensorimotor, language, cognitive, social, and self-care development.

## Evaluation Results

On the SIPT, Karen scored below average for age expectations on 7 of 17 tests. Her profile of SIPT scores is shown in Figure 13-16. This profile, called a ChromaGraph, was generated through computer scoring by the test publisher. The unit of measure represented by the scores is a statistic measure called a standard deviation, which represents how different the child's score is from that of an average child the same age. The closer a child's score is to 0 on the horizontal axis, the closer to average was the child's performance on that test. Karen's scores are plotted as solid squares that are connected by a dark line on the ChromaGraph. Scores falling below −1 on the horizontal axis are considered to be possibly indicative of dysfunction.

One of Karen's scores was low on a motor-free visual perception test (Space Visualization), and it was noted that she had difficulty fitting a geometric form into a puzzle board during this test. Her mother reported that she knew colors at 18 months of age but had trouble learning shapes. However, she was reported to have a strong visual memory for roads, signs, and faces. These findings suggested difficulty with spatial orientation of objects but relative strengths in visual memory.

Karen had several low scores and showed signs of difficulty performing on several of the tests of somatosensory and vestibular processing. A low score on Finger Identification suggested inefficient tactile feedback involving the hands. This was corroborated by observations of poor manipulative skills during activities such as buttoning and using utensils. She was also observed to have signs of tactile defensiveness, also corroborated by her mother's report. Her low score on Kinesthesia, as well as her difficulty in exerting the appropriate amount of pressure on pencil and in positioning her body for dressing, suggested problems with proprioceptive feedback. Karen's lowest score on the SIPT was on the Postrotary Nystagmus test (−2.2 standard deviations). This low score, as well as below average scores on Standing and Walking Balance, observations of poor functional balance in dressing and playground activities, a tendency not to cross her body midline, poor bilateral coordination in activities such as cutting, and reports that she never appeared to get dizzy all pointed to the probability of vestibular processing problems.

Karen showed above average performance on a praxis test on which she could rely on verbal directions. However, tests of motor planning that were more somatosensory dependent (Oral Praxis and Postural Praxis) were substantially more difficult for her. Karen was unable to ride a tricycle, pump a swing,

CASE STUDY #2–cont'd

or skip. She had extreme difficulty planning her movements to dress herself or even to let someone else dress her. She also had a great deal of difficulty using utensils during eating and often choked on food and drinks. Writing skills have been particularly difficult for Karen, and her lack of hand preference, immature grasp, and hesitancy to cross her midline have hampered her attempts at drawing or writing.

Karen was reported to be a social child who was liked by adults and younger peers. However, her mother worried that she did not seem able to "pick up on the hints and unwritten rules of her peers" and was "definitely starting to march to her own beat." She noticed increasing signs of frustration that she thought were beginning to impinge on Karen's willingness to participate with peers.

Overall, the evaluation results suggested deficits in sensory processing of some aspects of visual, tactile, proprioceptive, and vestibular sensory information. These difficulties were seen as related to somatodyspraxia, poor balance and bilateral integration, difficulties with specific gross and fine motor skills, and emerging concerns around socialization. Karen's strengths included age-appropriate cognitive and language skills, good ability to motor plan actions using verbal directions, and an exceptionally supportive and involved family.

### Recommendations

Based on the evaluation results and a meeting of Karen's individual educational plan (IEP) team, who met shortly after the assessment, it was recommended that Karen receive individual occupational therapy using a sensory integration approach to enhance foundational sensory and motor processes. This program was funded by the school district as part of her special education program, but because of her significant sensory integrative problems and need for a specialized approach, the therapy was recommended to initially occur in a therapy clinic equipped for classical sensory integrative treatment.

### Occupational Therapy Program

In the first 6 months of individual occupational therapy a classical sensory integration approach was used. In addition to the classical treatment, a brushing program (Wilbarger & Wilbarger, 1991) and a series of oral motor activities (Oetter et al., 1993) were initiated to attempt to reduce Karen's tactile defensiveness and her habit of frequently sucking in her cheeks. These aspects of her individual occupational therapy, although not part of the classical sensory integration treatment per se, used principles of sensory integration theory to help Karen overcome specific difficulties related to her sensory integration problems.

After 6 months of therapy Karen has shown decreasing tactile defensiveness, a reduced tendency to choke on food, acquisition of the ability to ride a tricycle, and an improved ability to plan new or unusual motor actions. Although these are significant gains for Karen, she continues to exhibit substantial difficulties with many aspects of sensory processing, general motor planning ability, and many age-appropriate fine and gross motor skills. If she continues to respond to occupational therapy using a classical sensory integration approach, it is expected that by the beginning of the next school year (in about 6 months) she will have improved in basic sensory and motor functions to the extent that some specific skill training will become more appropriate. It is likely that at that time some therapy will occur at school with the introduction of a consultation program for her teacher. Her parents have already begun a home program, and that also appears to be supporting the gains she is making through direct services. Karen's young age and initial positive response to therapy make her an optimal candidate for application of the sensory integration approach, and the outlook for her in the long term is excellent.

native treatment such as tutoring (Wilson, Kaplan, Fellowes, Gruchy, & Faris, 1992) or perceptual-motor training (Humphries, Wright, Snider, & McDougall, 1992; Polatajko, Law, Miller, Schaffer, & Macnab, 1991). Although these studies may be interpreted negatively, it should be pointed out that it is striking that classical sensory integrative treatment, which does not directly train specific motor or academic skills, results in improvements in motor and academic skills that are comparable to the gains made by interventions that do train these skills specifically.

Over the years researchers have become increasingly critical of studies examining effectiveness of treatment in large part because of the growing sophistication of researchers regarding the design and interpretation of this type of research. Virtually every study suffers from flaws in research design, some more serious than others. For example,

**STUDY QUESTIONS**

1. How did A. Jean Ayres use the term *sensory integration*?
2. Describe how sensory integration plays a role in normal development. Provide specific examples of behaviors seen in infancy and early childhood, and explain how they relate to the development of sensory integration.
3. Identify the four main types of sensory integrative dysfunction, and describe some of the ways that each can impact daily function.
4. Imagine that you are explaining sensory modulation to a teacher who has never heard of this concept before. How would you communicate to this person that sensory modulation disorders affect classroom functioning?
5. What types of analyses did Ayres conduct to develop sensory integrative theory? What were some of the main tenets of sensory integration theory that emanated from these research studies?
6. Discuss the different methods that can be used as part of an occupational therapy assessment using a sensory integration approach.
7. Describe the Sensory Integration and Praxis Tests and the general domains that they assess.
8. Contrast the application of the classical sensory integration treatment approach with the compensatory skill approach. What would be the rationale for using one versus the other?
9. Under what circumstances would a group occupational therapy program or a consultation program be the intervention of choice for a child with a sensory integrative disorder?
10. How might expected outcomes of treatment differ for classical sensory integrative treatment versus compensatory skill, group, or consultation approaches?

many studies use unclear or unsound methods to identify who is to receive sensory integration treatment; this creates the possibility that some children who do not have sensory integrative dysfunction are assigned to this treatment inappropriately. Another common flaw is that researchers attempt to use a standard treatment protocol to ensure that the sensory integration treatment is well defined and adheres to strict criteria. The problem associated with this is that the highly individualized, child-centered, fluid nature of classical sensory integration treatment is lost; therefore results of the study do not represent the effects of the classical treatment. A problem that is difficult to circumvent is

related to selection of outcome measures. Often children's responses to classical sensory integration treatment are as individualized as the methods used with them in intervention, making it difficult, perhaps impossible, for the researcher to select tests and other measurements that target the precise areas of gain for individual children. Moreover, it is likely that children with different types of sensory integrative dysfunction respond to this treatment with different kinds of gains. For example, children with tactile defensiveness are likely to show gains in different outcome domains than children with vestibular processing disorders; yet almost all of the research studies lump children together with sensory integrative dysfunction as if they should have similar responses to a standard treatment. This certainly was not Ayres's view, as she spent considerable effort attempting to identify subgroups of children with sensory integrative dysfunction who might differ from each other with respect to degree and type of responsiveness to intervention (Ayres, 1972a, 1978; Ayres & Tickle, 1980). Hopefully researchers who conduct future effectiveness studies will become more sensitive to this important issue.

Despite the methodologic problems that characterize effectiveness studies, the studies clearly indicate that children who participate in classical sensory integrative treatment are likely to benefit. However, it is not clear that the gains they make are superior to gains that might be made through other forms of treatment. A great deal of investigation remains to be done to explore questions regarding effectiveness of sensory integration treatment. It would be particularly beneficial to be able to better predict who will be the best responders to the classical sensory integration approach and who may be better served by other interventions. The effectiveness of combining classical sensory integration treatment with compensatory skill treatment, group programs, or consultation is another area in need of research, particularly because such intervention combinations are what is typically done in clinical practice. The kinds of outcomes likely to proceed from various treatment approaches and the timeframes in which those outcomes can be expected to emerge deserve close examination in effectiveness studies. Finally, studies need to explore which intervention outcomes are most meaningful to the families of children with sensory integrative dysfunction to ensure that intervention programs are responsive to the needs of the people served.

## REFERENCES

Ayres, A.J. (1963). The Eleanor Clark Slagle Lecture. The development of perceptual-motor abilities: a theoretical basis for treatment of dysfunction. *American Journal of Occupational Therapy, 17*(6), 221-225.

Ayres, A.J. (1964). Tactile functions: their relation to hyperactive and perceptual motor behavior. *American Journal of Occupational Therapy, 18*(1), 6-11.

Ayres, A.J. (1965). Patterns of perceptual-motor dysfunction in children: a factor analytic study. *Perceptual and Motor Skills, 20,* 335-368.

Ayres, A.J. (1966a). Interrelationships among perceptual-motor functions in children. *American Journal of Occupational Therapy, 20*(2), 68-71.

Ayres, A.J. (1966b). Interrelations among perceptual-motor abilities in a group of normal children. *American Journal of Occupational Therapy, 20*(6), 288-292.

Ayres, A.J. (1969). Deficits in sensory integration in educationally handicapped children. *Journal of Learning Disabilities, 2*(3), 44-52.

Ayres, A.J. (1971). Characteristics of types of sensory integrative dysfunction. *American Journal of Occupational Therapy, 25*(7), 329-334.

Ayres, A.J. (1972a). Improving academic scores through sensory integration. *Journal of Learning Disabilities, 5,* 338-343.

Ayres, A.J. (1972b). *Sensory integration and learning disorders.* Los Angeles: Western Psychological Services.

Ayres, A.J. (1972c). *Southern California Sensory Integration Tests.* Los Angeles: Western Psychological Services.

Ayres, A.J. (1972d). Types of sensory integrative dysfunction among disabled learners. *American Journal of Occupational Therapy, 26*(1), 13-18.

Ayres, A.J. (1975). *Southern California Postrotary Nystagmus Test.* Los Angeles: Western Psychological Services.

Ayres, A.J. (1976). *The effect of sensory integrative therapy on learning disabled children: the final report of a research project.* Los Angeles: Center for the Study of Sensory Integrative Dysfunction.

Ayres, A.J. (1977a). Cluster analyses of measures of sensory integration. *American Journal of Occupational Therapy, 31*(6), 362-266.

Ayres, A.J. (1977b). Dichotic listening performance in learning-disabled children. *American Journal of Occupational Therapy, 31*(7), 441-446.

Ayres, A.J. (1978). Learning disabilities and the vestibular system. *Journal of Learning Disabilities, 11*(1), 30-41.

Ayres, A.J. (1979). *Sensory integration and the child.* Los Angeles: Western Psychological Services.

Ayres, A.J. (1981). *Aspects of the somatomotor adaptive response and praxis.* (Audiotape). Pasadena, CA: Center for the Study of Sensory Integrative Dysfunction.

Ayres, A.J. (1985). *Developmental dyspraxia and adult-onset apraxia.* Torrance, CA: Sensory Integration International.

Ayres, A.J. (1986). *Sensory integrative dysfunction: test score constellations. Part II of a final project report.* Torrance, CA: Sensory Integration International.

Ayres, A.J. (1989). *Sensory Integration and Praxis Tests manual.* Los Angeles: Western Psychological Services.

Ayres, A.J. & Mailloux, Z. (1981). Influence of sensory integration procedures on language development. *American Journal of Occupational Therapy, 35*(6), 383.

Ayres, A.J., Mailloux, Z., & McAtee, S. (1985). An update of the Sensory Integration and Praxis Tests. *Sensory Integration Special Interest Section Newsletter,* p. 1.

Ayres, A.J., Mailloux, Z., & Wendler, C. L. W. (1987). Developmental apraxia: is it a unitary function? *Occupational Therapy Research, 7*(2), 93-110.

Ayres, A.J. & Marr, D. (1991). Sensory Integration and Praxis Tests. In A.G. Fisher, E.A. Murray, & A.C. Bundy (Eds.). *Sensory integration: theory and practice* (pp. 203-250). Philadelphia: F.A. Davis.

Ayres, A.J. & Tickle, L. (1980). Hyperresponsivity to touch and vestibular stimuli as a predictor of positive response to sensory integration procedures in autistic children. *American Journal of Occupational Therapy, 34,* 375-381.

Bach-Y-Rita, P. (1981). Brain plasticity. In J. Goodgold (Ed.). *Brain plasticity.* St. Louis: Mosby.

Beery, E. (1989). *The Developmental Test of Visual-Motor Integration* (3rd ed.). Cleveland: Modern Curriculum.

Bennett, E.L., Diamond, M.C., Krech, D., & Rosenzwieg, M.R. (1964). Chemical and anatomical plasticity of brain. *Science, 146,* 610-619.

Bissell, J., Fisher, J., Owen, C., & Polcyn, P. (1988). *Sensory motor handbook: a guide for implementing and modifying activities in the classroom.* Torrance, CA: Sensory Integration International.

Bretherton, I., Bates, E., McNew, S., Shore, C., Williamson, C., & Beeghly-Smith, M. (1981). Comprehension and production of symbols in infancy: an experimental study. *Developmental Psychology, 17,* 728-736.

Bruininks, R.H. (1978). *Bruininks-Oseretsky Test of Motor Proficiency examiner's manual.* Circle Pines, MN: American Guidance Service.

Bundy A.C. (1991). Consultation and sensory integration theory. In A.G. Fisher, E.A. Murray, & A.C. Bundy (Eds.). *Sensory integration: theory and practice* (pp. 318-332). Philadelphia: F.A. Davis.

Cabay, M. (1988). *The effect of sensory integration–based treatment on academic readiness of young, "at risk" school children.* Annual conference of the American Occupational Therapy Association, Phoenix, AZ.

Cabay, M. & King, L.J. (1989). Sensory integration and perception: the foundation for concept formation. *Occupational Therapy in Practice, 1,* 18-27.

Carrasco, R.C. (1990). Reliability of the Knickerbocker Sensorimotor History Questionnaire. *Occupational Therapy Journal of Research, 10,* 280-282.

Carrasco, R.C. & Lee, C.E. (1993). Development of a teacher questionnaire on sensorimotor behavior. *Sensory Integration Special Interest Section Newsletter, 16* (3), 5-6.

Case-Smith, J. (1991). The effects of tactile defensiveness and tactile discrimination on in-hand manipulation. *American Journal of Occupational Therapy, 45,* 811-818.

Cermak, S. (1988). The relationship between attention deficits and sensory integration disorders (Part I). *Sensory Integration Special Interest Section Newsletter, 11*(2), 1-4.

Cermak, S.A. (1991). Somatodyspraxia. In A.G. Fisher, E.A. Murray, & A.C. Bundy (Eds.). *Sensory integration: theory and practice* (pp. 137-170). Philadelphia: F.A. Davis.

Chugani, H.T. & Phelps, M.E. (1986). Maturational changes in cerebral function in infants determined by 18FDG positron emission tomography. *Science, 231,* 840-843.

Clark, F.A., Mailloux, Z., & Parham, D. (1989). Sensory integration and children with learning disorders. In P.N. Pratt & A.S. Allen (Eds.). *Occupational Therapy for Children* (2nd ed.) (pp. 457-509). St. Louis: Mosby.

Daems, J. (Ed.). (1994). *Reviews of research in sensory integration.* Torrance, CA: Sensory Integration International.

Dru, D., Walker, J.P., & Walker, J.B. (1975). Self-produced locomotion restores visual capacity after striate lesion. *Science, 187,* 265-266.

Dunn, W.W. (1981). *A guide to testing clinical observations in kindergartners.* Rockville, MD: American Occupational Therapy Association.

Dunn, W.W. (1994). *Performance of typical children on the sensory profile: An item analysis.* Paper presented at the annual conference of the American Occupational Therapy Association, Boston, MA.

Dunn, W. & Fisher, A.G. (1983). Sensory registration, autism, and tactile defensiveness. In J. Melvin (Ed.). *Occupational therapy in practice* (Vol. 1) (pp. 181-182). Rockville, MD: American Occupational Therapy Association.

Fisher, A.G. (1991). Vestibular-proprioceptive processing and bilateral integration and sequencing deficits. In A.G. Fisher, E.A. Murray, & A.C. Bundy (Eds.). *Sensory integration: theory and practice* (pp. 69-107). Philadelphia: F.A. Davis.

Fisher, A.G. & Murray, E.A. (1991). Introduction to sensory integration theory. In A.G. Fisher, E.A. Murray, & A.C. Bundy (Eds.). *Sensory integration: theory and practice* (pp. 3-26). Philadelphia: F.A. Davis.

Fisher, A.G. Murray, E.A., & Bundy, A.C. (Eds.). (1991). *Sensory integration: theory and practice.* Philadelphia: F.A. Davis.

Fredrickson, J.M., Schwartz, D.W., & Kornhuber, H.H. (1966). Convergence and interaction of vestibular and deep somatic afferents upon neurons in the vestibular nuclei of the cat. *Acta Otolaryngologica, 61,* 168-188.

Gregg, C.L., Hafner, M.E., & Korner, A. (1976). The relative efficacy of vestibular-proprioceptive stimulation and the upright position in enhancing visual pursuit in neonates. *Child Development, 47,* 309-314.

Gregory-Flock, J.L. & Yerxa, E.J. (1984). Standardization of the prone extension postural test on children ages 4 through 8. *American Journal of Occupational Therapy, 38,* 187-194.

Holloway, E. (1993). Early emotional development and sensory processing. In J. Case-Smith (Ed.). *Pediatric occupational therapy and early intervention* (pp. 163-197). Boston: Andover Medical Publishers.

Hubel, D.H. & Wiesel, T.N. (1963). Receptive fields of cells in striate cortex of very young, visually inexperienced kittens. *Journal of Neurophysiology, 26,* 994-1002.

Humphrey, T. (1969). Postnatal repetition of human prenatal activity sequences with some suggestions of their neuroanatomical basis. In R.J. Robinson (Ed.). *Brain and early behavior.* New York: Academic Press.

Humphries, T., Wright, M., Snider, L., & McDougall, B. (1992). A comparison of the effectiveness of sensory integrative therapy and perceptual-motor training in treating children with learning disabilities. *Journal of Developmental and Behavioral Pediatrics, 13,* 31-40.

Kimball, J.G. (1993). Sensory integrative frame of reference. In P. Kramer & J. Hinojosa (Eds.). *Frames of reference for pediatric occupational therapy* (pp. 87-167). Baltimore: Williams & Wilkins.

Knickerbocker, B.M. (1980). *A holistic approach to learning disabilities.* Thorofare, NJ: C.B. Slack.

Kolb, B. & Whishaw, I.Q. (1985). *Fundamentals of human neuropsychology* (2nd ed.). New York: W.H. Freeman.

Koomar, J.A. & Bundy, A.C. (1991). The art and science of creating direct intervention from theory. In A.G. Fisher, E.A. Murray, & A. C. Bundy (Eds.). *Sensory integration: theory and practice* (pp. 251-317). Philadelphia: F.A. Davis.

LaCroix, J.E. (1993). *A study of content validity of the Sensory History Questionnaire.* Unpublished master's thesis, University of Southern California, Los Angeles.

Magalhaes, L.C., Koomar, J., & Cermak, S.A. (1989). Bilateral motor coordination in 5- to 9-year old children. *American Journal of Occupational Therapy, 43,* 437-443.

Magrun, W.M., Ottenbacher, K., McCue, S., & Keefe, R. (1981). Effects of vestibular stimulation on spontaneous use of verbal language in developmentally delayed children. *American Journal of Occupational Therapy, 35,* 101-104.

Maurer, D. & Maurer, C. (1988). *The world of the newborn.* New York: Basic Books.

McCune-Nicolich, L. (1981). Toward symbolic functioning: structure of early pretend games and potential parallels with language. *Child Development, 52,* 785-797.

Miller, L.J. (1988). *Miller Assessment for Preschoolers manual* (rev. ed). San Antonio, TX: Psychological Corporation.

Oetter, P., Richter, E., & Frick, S. (1993). *MORE: integrating the mouth with sensory and postural functions.* Hugo, MN: PDP Press.

Ottenbacher, K. (1982). Sensory integration therapy: affect or effect. *American Journal of Occupational Therapy, 36,* 571-578.

Parham, L.D. (1987). Evaluation of praxis in preschoolers. *Occupational Therapy in Health Care, 4*(2), 23-36.

Polatajko, H.J. (1985). A critical look at vestibular dysfunction in learning-disabled children. *Developmental Medicine and Child Neurology, 27,* 283-291.

Polatajko, H.J., Law, M., Miller, J., Schaffer, R., & Macnab, J. (1991). The effect of a sensory integration program on academic achievement, motor performance, and self-esteem in children identified as learning disabled: results of a clinical trial. *Occupational Therapy Journal of Research, 11,* 155-176.

Ray, T., King, L.J., & Grandin, T. (1988). The effectiveness of self-initiated vestibular stimulation in producing speech sounds in an autistic child. *Occupational Therapy Journal of Research, 8,* 186-190.

Rosenzweig, M.R., Bennett, E.L., & Diamond, M.C. (1972). Brain changes in response to experience. *Scientific American, 226* (2), 22-29.

Royeen, C.B. (1989). Commentary on "Tactile functions in learning-disabled and normal children: reliability and validity considerations." *Occupational Therapy Journal of Research, 9,* 16-23.

Royeen, C.B. & Fortune, J.C. (1990). TIE: Touch Inventory for Elementary school-aged children. *American Journal of Occupational Therapy, 44,* 165-170.

Royeen, C.B. & Lane, S.J. (1991). Tactile processing and sensory defensiveness. In A.G. Fisher, E.A. Murray, & A.C. Bundy (Eds.). *Sensory integration: theory and practice* (pp. 108-136). Philadelphia: F.A. Davis.

Salthe, S.N. (1985). *Evolving hierarchical systems.* New York: Columbia University.

Schaaf, R. (1994). Neuroplasticity and sensory integration. Part 2. *Sensory Integration Quarterly, 22* (2), 1-7.

Short-DeGraff, M.A. (1988). *Human development for occupational and physical therapists.* Baltimore: Williams & Wilkins.

Slavik, B.A. & Chew, T. (1990). The design of a sensory integration treatment facility: the Ayres Clinic as a model. In S.C. Merrill (Ed.). *Environment: implications for occupational therapy practice* (pp. 85-101). Rockville, MD: American Occupational Therapy Association.

Slavik, B.A., Kitsuwa-Lowe, J., Danner, P.T., Green, J., & Ayres, A. J. (1984). Vestibular stimulation and eye contact in autistic children. *Neuropediatrics, 15,* 333-336.

Solomon, P., Kubzansky, P,E., Leiderman, P.H., Mendelson, J.H., Trumball, R., & Wexler, D. (Eds.). (1961). *Sensory deprivation.* Cambridge: Harvard University.

Spyropulos, P. (1991). *Sensory History Survey: the relationship between sensory responsiveness, sensory integration, and learning* handicaps. Unpublished master's thesis, University of Southern California, Los Angeles.

Stern, D.N. (1985). *The interpersonal world of the infant.* New York: Basic Books.

Todd, V.R. (1993). Visual perceptual frame of reference: An information processing approach. In P. Kramer & J. Hinojosa (Eds.). *Frames of reference for pediatric occupational therapy* (pp. 177-232). Baltimore: Williams & Wilkins.

Walker, K.F. (1991). Sensory integrative therapy in a limited space: an adaptation of the Ayres Clinic design. *Sensory Integration Special Interest Section Newsletter, 14* (3), 1, 2, 4.

White, M. (1979). A first-grade intervention program for children at risk for reading failure. *Journal of Learning Disabilities, 12,* 26-32.

Wilbarger, P. (1984). Planning an adequate "sensory diet": application of sensory processing theory during the first year of life. *Zero to Three*, pp. 7-12.

Wilbarger, P. & Wilbarger, J.L. (1991). *Sensory defensiveness in children aged 2-12.* Denver, CO: Avanti Educational Programs.

Williams, M.S. & Shellenberger, S. (1994). *"How does your engine run?" A leader's guide to the Alert Program for Self-regulation.* Albuquerque, NM: TherapyWorks.

Wilson, B.N., Kaplan, B.J., Fellowes, S., Gruchy, C., & Faris, P. (1992). The efficacy of sensory integration treatment compared to tutoring. *Physical and Occupational Therapy in Pediatrics, 12,* 1-36.

Wilson, B.N., Pollock, N., Kaplan, B.J., & Law, M. (1994). *Clinical Observations of Motor and Postural Skills (COMPS).* Tucson: Therapy Skill Builders.

Wiss, T. (1989). Vestibular dysfunction in learning disabilities: differences in definitions lead to different conclusions. *Journal of Learning Disabilities, 22,* 100-101.

Young, S.B. (1988). *Movement is fun: a preschool movement program.* Torrance, CA: Sensory Integration International.

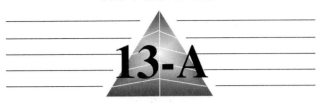

## Definitions of Terms

**Adaptive response:** a successful response to an environmental challenge (Ayres, 1979). The adaptive response is an important mechanism of sensory integrative development and is a central concept in classical sensory integration treatment.

**Bilateral coordination:** the ability of the two sides of the body to work together motorically.

**Bilateral integration:** the brain function that enables coordination of functions of the two sides of the body.

**Body scheme:** an internal representation of the body; the brain's "map" of body parts and how they interrelate.

**Dyspraxia:** a condition in which the individual has difficulty with praxis. In children, this term is usually used to refer to praxis problems that cannot be accounted for by a medical condition, developmental disability, or lack of environmental opportunity.

**Gravitational insecurity:** a condition in which there is a tendency to react negatively and fearfully to movement experiences, particularly those involving a change in head position and movement backward or upward through space.

**Hyperresponsivity:** a disorder of sensory modulation in which the individual is overwhelmed by ordinary sensory input and reacts defensively to it, often with strong negative emotion and activation of the sympathetic nervous system.

**Hyporesponsivity:** a disorder of sensory modulation in which the individual tends to ignore or be relatively unaffected by sensory stimuli to which most people respond.

**Ideation:** the ability to conceptualize a new action to be performed in a given situation (Ayres, 1981, 1985). This aspect of praxis involves generating an idea of what to do. It precedes motor planning, which addresses the plan for how to do the action.

**Motor planning:** the process of organizing a plan for action. This aspect of praxis is a cognitive process that precedes the performance of a new action.

**Perception:** the organization of sensory data into meaningful units. For example, stereognosis, a type of tactile perception, involves the organization of tactile details so that an object can be recognized by touch.

**Praxis:** the ability to conceptualize, organize, and execute nonhabitual motor tasks (Ayres, 1979, 1981).

**Sensory defensiveness:** a condition characterized by hyperresponsivity in multisensory systems (Wilbarger & Wilbarger, 1991).

**Sensory discrimination:** the ability to distinguish between different sensory stimuli. This term is usually used to refer to the ability to make fine distinctions between stimuli of one sensory modality, such as discriminating between two points of tactile contact, or differentiating between similar sounds.

**Sensory integration:** the organization of sensation for use (Ayres, 1979), a primary function of the central nervous system. This term is also used to refer to a frame of reference for treatment of children who have difficulty with this neural function.

**Sensory modulation:** the tendency to generate responses that are appropriately graded in relation to incoming sensations, neither underreacting nor overreacting to them.

**Sensory registration:** the process by which the central nervous system attends to stimuli; this usually involves an orienting response.

**Sequencing:** the ability to appropriately order a series of actions, an important element of motor planning. This term also is sometimes used to refer to the ability to replicate a series of sensory stimuli in the correct order.

**Somatopraxis:** an aspect of praxis that is heavily dependent on somatosensory processing (Ayres, 1989). An impairment of this aspect of praxis is termed *somatodyspraxia* (Cermak, 1991) and is characterized by poor tactile and proprioceptive processing as well as poor praxis.

**Somatosensory:** pertaining to the tactile and proprioceptive systems.

**Tactile defensiveness:** a condition in which there is a tendency to react negatively and emotionally to touch sensations (Ayres, 1979).

**Vestibular:** pertaining to the inner ear receptors, the semicircular canals and otolith organs, that detect head position and movement as well as gravity.

APPENDIX

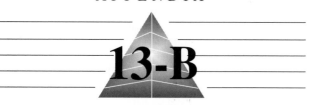

## Sensory Integration International Standards of Practice*

## EVALUATION AND TREATMENT OF SENSORY INTEGRATIVE DYSFUNCTION

This statement presents the official position of Sensory Integration International (SII) regarding the minimum guidelines for qualifications needed for the evaluation and treatment of sensory integrative dysfunction. This statement is intended to promote uniform standards of professional practice in the delivery of services for individuals with sensory integrative disorders for (1) the protection of consumers in need of such services, (2) provision of guidelines for qualified professionals in the delivery of these services, and (3) the promotion of the understanding and appropriate application of Sensory Integrative Theory.

### Background

Sensory integration, as a neurobiologic process, is the organization of sensory information for use in human function. *Sensory Integrative Theory* is a set of assumptions, principles, and techniques, first proposed by A. Jean Ayres, PhD, OTR, for the understanding and assessment of sensory integrative function and therapeutic intervention for sensory integrative dysfunction. Sensory integrative dysfunction is an irregularity or disorder in brain function that makes it difficult to organize sensory input and may result in varying degrees or problems in development, learning, and behavior. Sensory Integrative Theory has developed from the study of neurosciences, normal and abnormal development, and neuromuscular function and dysfunction as an occupational therapy frame of reference. Although many aspects of Sensory Integrative Theory, as developed by Ayres, are unique to the field of occupational therapy, there is the potential for diverse application of these concepts to other professions.

### Evaluation

Assessment of basic sensory integrative processes may be part of many occupational therapy and physical therapy evaluations. Clinical observation of the individual, medical and developmental histories, and performance on a variety

*From the Professional Standards & Practice Committee. Shay McAtee & Zoë Mailloux. November 5, 1994. Reprinted with permission from Sensory Integration International 1602 Cabrillo Avenue, P.O. Box 9013, Torrance, CA 90508.

of tests may be used to form impressions of sensory integrative functioning.

Standardized evaluation of sensory integrative functioning is available through the **Sensory Integration and Praxis Tests (SIPT),** which were formulated for assessing children aged 4 years to 8 years 11 months. The SIPT are a set of rigorously designed tests standardized on children from the United States and Canada; they replace the **Southern California Sensory Integration Tests (SCSIT).**

Knowledge of Sensory Integrative Theory and knowledge of tests and measurement are necessary to administer and interpret the SIPT. This background knowledge is part of standard curricula within most U.S. bachelor's and master's degree occupational therapy programs.

To assure that competently trained and responsible persons are administering and interpreting the SIPT, certification by SII was established.

SII has established the following criteria for certification in administration and interpretation of the **SIPT.** The criteria for admission to the certification process include the following:

1. Current registration as an occupational therapist, physical therapist, or neuropsychologist
2. Completion of an SII-approved theory course
3. Satisfactory completion of an accredited college-level statistics course

The criteria for completion of the SIPT certification process include the following:

1. Completion of an SII-approved SIPT Administration course
2. Completion of an SII-approved SIPT Interpretation course
3. Completion of a test administration observation
4. A passing score on the SIPT Competency Examination

### Treatment

SII recommends that treatment for the remediation of sensory integrative dysfunction be provided by registered occupational therapists who have had specialized training in sensory integration. The basic education for these professions provides a uniquely appropriate foundation of knowledge on which to build sensory integration treatment skills. This foundation includes the study of neurosciences, normal and abnormal development, neuromuscular function and dysfunction, psychosocial development, daily life tasks, activity analysis, and the treatment planning process.

SII also recognizes that the sensory integration concepts may contribute to intervention strategies used by a wide variety of professionals outside of occupational therapy. It is expected that any professional would interpret, integrate, and practice sensory integration–related information in accordance with the broader practices and established standards of their professions.

All professionals need specialized training for qualified application of sensory integration principles. Suggested credentials include the completion of the following:

1. An SII-approved theory course or university-sponsored theory course
2. Course that present application of sensory integration to practice settings
3. Advanced training in sensory integration within a university curriculum of advanced training using sensory integration intervention techniques for 3 months under the direct supervision of a professional who has had at least 3 years of experience in the application of sensory integration principles, including evaluation
4. Demonstration of participation in ongoing continuing education courses specifically addressing sensory integration intervention techniques and neurobiologic theories.

In addition, the knowledge gained in completing the **SIPT** certification process is advantageous to the competent provision of sensory integration treatment procedures.

APPENDIX

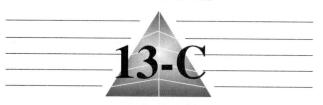

**13-C**

Resources for Mentorship Experiences in Sensory Integration

*Center for Neurodevelopmental Studies*
8434 N. 39th Avenue
Phoenix, AZ 85051
(602) 433-1400

*Cincinnati Occupational Therapy Institute*
4440 Carver Woods Drive
Cincinnati, OH 45242
(513) 791-5688

*Occupational Therapy Associates*
124 Watertown Street
Watertown, MA 02172
(617) 923-4410

*Research and Development in Pediatric Therapy*
Nancy Lawton-Shirley
Special Children's Center
1810 Crestview Drive
Hudson, WI 54016

*Sensory Integration International*
1602 Cabrillo Avenue
P.O. Box 9013
Torrance, CA 90508
(213) 533-8338

*USC Occupational Therapy Department*
1540 Alcazar Street—CHP 133
Los Angeles, CA 90033
(213) 342-2879

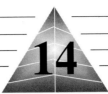

# Visual Perception

COLLEEN M. SCHNECK

## KEY TERMS

▲ Visual-Receptive Component
▲ Visual-Cognitive Component

## CHAPTER OBJECTIVES

1. Define visual perception.
2. Describe typical development of visual perceptual skills.
3. Identify factors that contribute to typical or atypical development of visual perception.
4. Explain the implications of visual perceptual problems for performance of play, self-care, and school performance.
5. Describe models and theories that may be used in structuring intervention plans for children who have problems with visual perceptual skills.
6. Identify evaluation tools and methods useful in assessing visual perceptual skills in children.
7. Describe treatment strategies for assisting children in improving or compensating for problems with visual perceptual skills.
8. Illustrate principles of evaluation and intervention with case examples of children.

Although one may question which of our senses is the most important for performance, some consider vision to be the most influential sense in humans (Bouska, Kauffman, & Marcus, 1990; Hellerstein & Fishman, 1987; Nolte, 1988). There is little argument that vision is the dominant sense in human perception of the external world; it helps us monitor what is happening in the environment outside our bodies. Because of the complexity of the visual system, it is difficult to imagine the impact of a visual perceptual deficit on daily living. Functional problems that may result from a visual perceptual deficit include difficulties with eating, dressing, reading, writing, locating objects, driving, and many more activities necessary for functional independence. Given that occupational therapists focus on functional independence in the performance of activities of daily living, work and productive activities, and play and leisure activities, the focus on the performance component of visual perception is critically important. Although visual perception is a major treatment emphasis of occupational therapists working with children, it is one of the least understood areas of evaluation and treatment (Warren, 1993a). The information presented in this chapter describes current information on visual perception that relates to evaluation and intervention with children. The information in this area of visual perception is evolving and will change as new research is presented.

## DEFINITIONS

*Visual perception* is defined as the total process responsible for the reception and cognition of visual stimuli (Zaba, 1984). The visual-receptive component is the process of extracting and organizing information from the environment (Solan & Ciner, 1986), and the visual cognitive component is the ability to interpret and use what is seen. These two components allow us to understand what we see, and they are both necessary for functional vision. Visual perceptual skills include the recognition and identification of shapes, objects, colors, and other qualities. Visual perception allows a person to make accurate judgments of the size, configuration, and spatial relationships of objects.

Kwatney and Bouska (1980) defined the following as functions of the mature visual system. These functions demonstrate the interaction of the visual-receptive and visual-cognitive components:

1. Respond and adjust to retinal stimuli (anatomic and physiologic integrity)
2. Move both the head and eyes to collect raw data (oculomotor and vestibuloocular control)

3. Effectively interpret visual information (visuoperceptual ability)
4. Respond to visual cues through efficient limb movements (visuomotor ability)
5. Accomplish integration of all these abilities

## PERFORMANCE COMPONENTS
### Visual-Receptive Components

Hearing and vision are the distant senses that allow us to understand what is happening in the environment outside our bodies or in extrapersonal space. These sense organs transmit information to the brain, whose primary function is to receive information from the world for processing and coding. The visual sensory stimuli are then integrated with other sensory input and associated with past experiences. The eye, oculomotor muscles and pathways, optic nerve, optic tract, occipital cortex, and associative areas of the cerebral cortex (parietal and temporal lobes) are all included in this process. As an occupational therapist, it is impera-

tive to understand the neurophysiologic interactions in the central nervous system to effectively evaluate and treat children with problems in the visual system. This discussion begins with the sensory receptor, the eye.

### Anatomy of the Eye

A basic understanding of the anatomy and physiology of the eye aids in understanding its impact on perception (Figure 14-1). The eye functions to transmit light to the retina. It focuses images of the environment onto the retina. The eye is shaped to refract the rays of light so that the most sensitive part of the retina receives rays at one convergent point. The cornea covers the front of the eye and is part of the outermost layer of the eyeball. It plays a large part in focusing or bending the rays of light entering the eye. Behind the cornea is the aqueous humor, which is a clear fluid. The pressure of this fluid helps maintain the shape of the cornea and helps in focusing the rays. The colored part of the eye, or iris, with its center hole, the pupil, is directly behind the cornea. The iris governs the amount of light en-

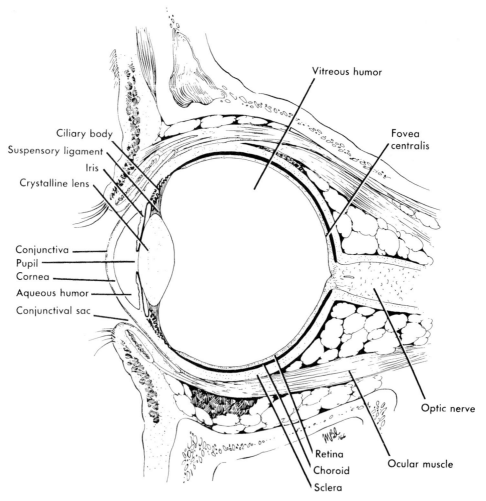

**Figure 14-1** Cross-section of the eye. (From Ingalls, A.J. & Salerno, M.C. [1983]. *Maternal and child health nursing* [5th ed.]. St. Louis: Mosby.)

tering the eye by increasing or decreasing the size of the pupil. The light then progresses through the crystalline lens, which does the fine focusing for near or far vision, and through the jellylike substance called the vitreous humor. The eye has three layers: the sclera is fibrous and elastic, helping to hold the rest of the eye structure in place; the choroid is primarily blood vessels that nourish the eye; and the retina is the innermost layer. The retinal layer is composed of receptor nerve cells that contain a chemical that is activated by light. The retina has three types of receptor cells:

1. *Cones*—Used for color perception and visual acuity
2. *Rods*—Used for night and peripheral vision
3. *Pupillary cells*—Controls opening (dilation) and closing (constriction) of the pupil

The fovea centralis (located in the retina) is the point of sharpest and clearest vision. It is most responsive to daylight and must receive a certain quantity of light before it transmits the signal to the optic nerve. The retina responds to spatial differences in intensity of light stimulation, especially at contrasting border areas, and it provides basic information about light and dark areas. Light stimulates the visual receptor cells in the retina, causing electrochemical changes that trigger an electrical impulse to flow to the optic nerve. The optic nerve (cranial nerve II) transmits the visual sensory messages to the brain for processing. This information travels to the brain in a special way. Fibers from the nasal half of each retina divide, and half of these fibers cross to the contralateral side of the brain. Fibers from the outer half of each retina do not divide and so carry visual information ipsilaterally. Therefore visual information from either the left or right visual field enters the opposite portion of each retina and then travels to the same hemisphere of the brain. This organization means that even with the loss of vision in one eye, information is transmitted to both hemispheres of the brain. This also means that damage in the region of the left or right occipital cortex can cause a loss of vision that is referred to as a *field cut* in the opposite visual field. The optic nerve leads from the back of the eye to the lateral geniculate nucleus in the optic thalamus. It is here that binocular information is received and integrated at a basic level, which may contribute to crude depth perception. Information then passes from the two lateral geniculate bodies of the thalamus to the visual cortex in the occipital lobe (area 17). From the occipital cortex the refined visual information is sent in two directions via visual areas 18 or 19 (Rafal & Posner, 1987; Ratcliff, 1987). Some impulses flow upward to the posterior parietal lobe where visual spatial processing occurs, focusing on the location of objects and their relationships to objects in space. Other impulses flow downward to the temporal lobe where visual object processing takes place. Information sent here is analyzed for the specific details of color, form, and size needed for accurate object identification; the focus is on pattern recognition and detail and remembering the qualities of objects.

## Oculomotor System

The oculomotor system makes possible the reception of visual stimuli (visual-receptive). The visual-receptive components include *fixation, pursuit and saccadic eye movements, acuity, accommodation, binocular vision and stereopsis,* and *convergence and divergence. Visual fixation* on a stationary object is a prerequisite skill for other ocularmotor responses such as shifting gaze between objects (scanning) or tracking. Each eye is moved by the coordinated actions of the six extraocular muscles. These are innervated by the third, fourth, and sixth cranial nerves: the oculomotor, the trochlear, and the abducens. The oculomotor nuclei are responsible for automatic conjugate eye movements: lateral, vertical, and convergence. They also help regulate the position of the eyes in relation to the position of the head. The nuclei receive most of their information from the superior colliculus. Two types of eye movements are used to gather information from the environment: pursuit eye movements, or tracking, and saccadic eye movements, or scanning. *Visual pursuit* or *tracking* involves the continued fixation on a moving object so that the image is maintained continuously on the fovea. The smooth pursuit system is characterized by slow, smooth movements. Tracking may occur with eyes and head together or with eyes moving independently from the head. *Saccadic eye movements* or *scanning* are defined as a rapid change of fixation from one point in the visual field to another. A saccade may be voluntary, as when localizing a quickly displaced stimulus or when reading, or it may be involuntary, as during the fast phases of vestibular nystagmus. A saccadic movement is precise, although the presence of a slight overshoot or undershoot is normal. In addition to voluntary control of eye movements, the vestibular-ocular pathways control conjugate eye movements reflexively in response to head movement and position in space. These pathways enable the eyes to remain fixed on a stationary object while the head and body move.

In addition to the tasks of visual fixation, pursuit movements, and saccadic movements, other visual-receptive components include the following:

▲ *Acuity*—The capacity to discriminate the fine details of objects in the visual field (20/20 means that a person can perceive as small an object as an average person can perceive at 20 feet).

▲ *Accommodation*—The ability of each eye to compensate for a blurred image. Accommodation refers to the process used to obtain clear vision, that is, to focus on an object at varying distances. This occurs when the internal ocular muscle (the ciliary muscle) contracts and causes a change in the crystalline lens of the eye to adjust for objects at different distances. Focusing must take place efficiently at all distances, and the eyes must be able to make the transition from focusing at nearpoint (a book or a paper) to farpoint (the teacher and the blackboard) and vice versa. It should take only a split second for this process of accommodation to occur.

▲ *Binocular fusion*—The ability to mentally combine the images from the two eyes into a single percept. There are two prerequisites for binocular fusion to occur. The first is that the two eyes must be aligned on the object of regard. This is termed *motor fusion;* it requires coordination of the six extraocular muscles on each eye and precision between the two eyes. *Sensory fusion* is the second aspect. This requires that the size and clarity of the two images be compatible. Only when these two aspects have occurred can the brain combine what the two eyes see into a single percept, and binocular fusion has taken place.

▲ *Stereopsis*—Binocular depth perception or three-dimensional vision.

▲ *Convergence and divergence*—The ability of both eyes to turn inward toward the medial plane and outward from the medial plane.

Skeffington (1963) recognized that vision was more than light coming from the physical environment, entering the eye, and then becoming transformed into an external phenomenon. He believed that vision cannot be separated from the total individual nor from any of the sensory systems because it is integrated into all human performance. He proposed a model that describes the visual process as the meshing of audition, proprioception, kinesthesia, and body sense with vision. This interaction is presented by four connecting circles, each denoting one important subsystem (Figure 14-2). The core, where each circle connects with the others, is vision. It should be clear from this model that visual perception is not obtained by vision alone. It comes from combining visual skills with all the other sensory modalities, including the proprioceptive and vestibular systems.

## Visual-Cognitive Components

Interpretation of the visual stimulus is a mental process involving cognition, which gives meaning to the visual stimulus (visual-cognitive). The visual-cognitive components include *visual attention, visual memory, discrimination,* and *integration of the visual stimulus* with other sense modalities.

### Visual Attention

Visual attention involves the selection of visual input. It also provides an appropriate time frame through which visual information is passed by the eye to the primary visual cortex of the brain, where visual perceptual processing can occur. Voluntary eye movements of localization, fixation, ocular pursuit, and gaze shift lay the foundation for optimal functioning of visual attention (Erhardt, 1989). The four components of visual attention are alertness, selective attention, vigilance, and shared attention. The first level, alertness, is reflective of the child's natural state of arousal. Alerting is the transition from an awake to an attentive and

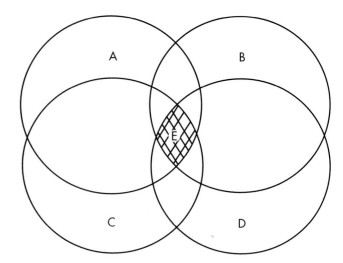

**Figure 14-2** *Skeffington model of vision. A,* Antigravity: coming to terms with gravity to move. *B,* Centering: ability to locate objects in space. *C,* Identification: ability to focus on information, to refine and discriminate detail, and to save that information in the brain. *D,* Speech audition: ability to communicate through speech and gesture and to use hearing. *E,* Vision: interweaving of all these modalities *(A through D)*. (From Optometric Extension Program, Inc. [1963]. *The Skeffington Papers.* Series 36, No.2, p. 11.)

ready state needed for active learning and adaptive behavior. Selective attention is the next level. This is the ability to choose relevant visual information while ignoring the less relevant information; it is conscious, focused attention. Visual vigilance, the third level, is the conscious mental effort to concentrate and persist at a visual task. This skill is exhibited when a child plays diligently with a toy or when writing a letter. Divided or shared attention is the ability to respond to two or more simultaneous tasks. This skill is exhibited when a child is engaged in one task that is automatic while visually monitoring another task.

### Visual Memory

Visual memory involves the integration of visual information with previous experiences. Long-term memory is the permanent storehouse, which has expansive capacity; in contrast, short-term memory can hold a limited number of unrelated bits of information for approximately 30 seconds.

### Visual Discrimination

Visual discrimination is the ability to detect features of stimuli for recognition, matching, and categorization. The specific visual discrimination abilities require the ability to note similarities and differences among forms and symbols with increasing complexity and then relate these back to information previously stored in long-term memory. These three abilities are described below:

1. *Recognition*—the ability to note key features of a stimulus and relate them to memory

2. *Matching*—the ability to note the similarities among visual stimuli
3. *Categorization*—the ability to mentally determine a quality or category on which similarities or differences can be noted

Visual perceptual abilities aid in the manipulation of a visual stimulus for visual discrimination (Todd, 1993). Resources on visual perception use different terms and categories to define the same visual perceptual skills. This contributes to much confusion because each discipline may define the same terms differently.

It is also important to note that a distinction exists between object (form) vision and spatial vision (Mishkin, Ungerleider, & Macko, 1983). Object vision is implicated in the visual identification of objects by color, texture, shape, and size: what things are. Spatial vision is concerned with the visual location of objects in space: where things are. These two classes of function are mediated by separate neural systems. The cortical tracts for both object vision and spatial vision are projected to the primary visual area, but the object vision pathway goes to the temporal lobe and the spatial vision pathway goes to the parietal lobe.

Based on studies after brain damage, these two functions have been shown to be independent (Necombe & Ratcliff, 1989). That is, disturbances of object recognition can occur without spatial disability, and spatial disability can occur with normal object perception. The following are definitions of the object (form) and spatial perceptual skills. Although they may not be separate entities, these groups of abilities or skills are labeled as follows:

1. Object (form) perception
   a. Form constancy: The recognition of forms and objects as the same in various environments, positions, and sizes. Form constancy helps a person develop stability and consistency in the visual world. It enables the person to recognize objects even when there are differences in orientation or detail. Form constancy enables a person to make assumptions regarding the size of an object even though visual stimuli may vary under different circumstances. The visual image of an object in the distance is much smaller than the image of the same object at close range, yet the person knows that the actual sizes are equivalent. An example of form constancy is that a school-aged child can identify the letter *A* whether it is typed, written in manuscript, written in cursive, written in upper- or lower-case letters, or written in italics.
   b. Visual closure: The identification of forms or objects from incomplete presentations. This enables the person to quickly recognize objects, shapes, and forms by mentally completing the image or by matching it to information previously stored in memory. This allows the person to make assumptions regarding what the object is without having

to see the complete presentation. For example, a child working at his or her desk is able to distinguish a pencil from a pen, even though both are partially hidden under some papers.
   c. Figure-ground: The differentiation between foreground and background forms and objects. It is the ability to separate essential important data from distracting surrounding information and the ability to attend to one aspect of a visual field while perceiving it in relation to the rest of the field. It is the ability to visually attend to what is important. For example, a child is able to visually find a favorite toy in a toy box filled with toys.
2. Spatial perception
   a. Position in space: The determination of the spatial relationship of figures and objects to oneself or other forms and objects. This provides the awareness of an object's position in relation to the observer or the perception of the direction in which it is turned. This perceptual ability is important in understanding directional language concepts such as in, out, up, down, in front of, behind, between, left, and right. In addition, position in space perception provides the ability to differentiate letters and sequences of letters in a word or in a sentence (Frostig, Lefever, & Whittlesey, 1966). For example, the child knows how to place letters equal spaces apart, touching the line; he or she is able to recognize letters that extend below the line, such as p, g, q, or y.
   b. Depth perception: The determination of the relative distance between objects, figures, or landmarks and the observer and changes in planes of surfaces. This provides an awareness of how far away something is. This perceptual ability also helps us move in space, for example, walk down the stairs.
   c. Topographical orientation: The determination of the location of objects and settings and the route to the location. *Wayfinding* is dependent on a cognitive map of the environment. These maps include information about the destination, spatial information, instructions for execution of travel plans, recognizing places, keeping track of where one is while moving about, and anticipating features. These are important means of monitoring one's movement from place to place (Garling, Book, & Lindberg, 1984). For example, the child is able to leave the classroom for a drink of water from the water fountain down the hall and then return to his or her desk.

## Visual Imagery

Another important component in visual cognition is visual imagery, or visualization, as it is often called. Visual imagery refers to the ability to "picture" people, ideas, and objects in the mind's eye, even when the objects are not physically present. Developmentally, the child is first able to picture objects that make certain sounds and those that are familiar by taste or smell. The ability to picture what words say is the next step. This level of visual-verbal matching provides the foundation for reading comprehension and spelling.

## Developmental Framework for Intervention

Warren (1993a) presented a developmental framework based on a bottom-up approach to evaluation and treatment. Using the work of Moore (Gilfoyle, Grady, & Moore, 1990), Warren suggested that with knowledge of where the deficit is located in the visual system, the therapist can design appropriate evaluation and treatment strategies to remediate basic problems and improve perceptual function. To apply this approach, it is necessary for the occupational therapist to have an understanding of the visual system, including both the visual-receptive and visual-cognitive components. Although Warren's model was presented as a developmental framework for evaluation and treatment of visual perceptual dysfunction in adults with acquired brain injuries, it is useful as a model for children with visual perceptual deficits. A hierarchy of visual perceptual skill development in the central nervous system is presented in Figure 14-3. The definitions of components of each level are provided below and are used in later descriptions of evaluation and treatment.

1. Three primary visual skills form the foundation for all visual functions.
   a. Oculomotor control—The efficient eye movements that ensure the scan path is accomplished.
   b. Visual fields—Register the complete visual scene.
   c. Visual acuity—Ensures that the visual information sent to the central nervous system is accurate.
2. Visual attention—The thoroughness of the scan path depends on visual attention.
3. Scanning—Pattern recognition is dependent on organized, thorough scanning of the visual environment. The retina must record all of the detail of the scene systematically through the use of a scan path.
4. Pattern recognition—The ability to store information in memory requires pattern detection and recognition. This is the identification of the salient features of an object.
   a. Configural aspects (shape, contour, and general features).
   b. The specific features of an object (details of color, shading, and texture).
5. Visual memory—The mental manipulation of visual information needed for visual cognition requires the ability to retain the information in memory for immediate recall or to store for later retrieval.
6. Visual cognition—The ability to mentally manipulate visual information and integrate it with other sensory information to solve problems, formulate plans, and make decisions.

## DEVELOPMENTAL SEQUENCE
### Visual-Receptive Components

Like other areas of development, the development of visual-receptive components takes place according to a prescribed timetable, which begins in the womb. By the 24th gestational week, gross anatomic structures are in place, and the visual pathway is complete. Between the 24th and 40th gestational weeks, the visual system, particularly the retina and visual cortex, undergo extensive maturation, differentiation, and remodeling (Glass, 1993). As early as the fifth gestational month, eye movements are produced by vestibular influences (DeQuiros & Schranger, 1979). At birth the infant has rudimentary visual fixation ability and brief reflexive tracking ability. The visual system at this age is relatively immature compared with other sensory systems, with considerable development occurring over the next 6 months (Glass, 1993). Toward the end of the second month, accommodation, convergence, and oculomotor subsystems are established (Bouska et al., 1990). Maximum accommodation is reached at 5 years, and the child should be able to sustain this skill effort for protracted periods of time at a fixed distance.

Controlled tracking skills progress in a developmental pattern from horizontal eye movements to eye movements in vertical, diagonal, and circular directions. By kindergarten a child should be able to move his or her eyes with smooth control and coordination in all directions. This can be demonstrated by asking the child to follow a moving ob-

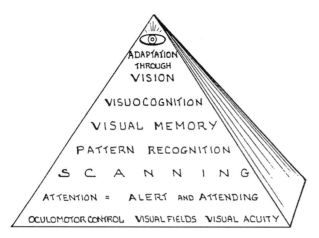

**Figure 14-3** Hierarchy of visual perceptual skill development. (From Warren, M. [1993]. A hierarchial model for evaluation and treatment of visual perceptual dysfunction in adult acquired brain injury. Part 1. *American Journal of Occupational Therapy, 47,* 42-54.)

ject at 8 to 12 inches. If the child moves his or her head along with the eyes, this skill is still developing. Visual acuity is best at age 18 and begins to decline until age 40.

## Visual-Cognitive Components

Some visual-cognitive capacities are present at birth, and other higher-level visual-cognitive tasks are not fully developed until adolescence. This development occurs through perceptual learning, the process of extracting information from the environment. This increases with experience and practice and through stimulation from the environment.

### Object (Form) Vision

Long before infants can manipulate objects or move around space, they have well-developed visual perceptual abilities, including pattern recognition, form constancy, and depth perception. Infants as young as 1 week show a differential response to patterns, with complex designs and human faces receiving more attention than simple circles and triangles. The infant learns to attend to relevant aspects of visual stimuli, to make discriminations, and to interpret available cues according to past experiences.

Visual perception develops as the child matures, with the bulk of it taking place by age 9. However, children vary in the rate at which they acquire perceptual abilities, in their effective use of these capacities, and in the versatility and comfort with which they apply these functions (Levine, 1987). In the developing child there is a systematic increase in the ability to perceptually analyze and discriminate objects. It is generally believed that visual perception develops in the following ways:

▲ General to specific
▲ Whole to parts
▲ Concrete to abstract
▲ Familiar to novel

However, these sequences have not been proven, and in certain instances the opposite may actually occur. For example, the development may follow specific to general. The child first learns to recognize an object based on its general appearance and not by spectific details. As the child learns to classify objects into categories and types, it becomes apparent that the child is able to extract the features that make the object part of that category (Mussen, Conger, & Kagan, 1979). For example, the child learns to categorize cars as certain types or classify animals according to their species. Further study is needed in this area. Williams (1983) suggested the developmental guidelines outlined in Table 14-1.

Bouska et al. (1990) described three areas in which a normally developing child demonstrates increasing ability to visually discriminate. These include the ability to (1) recognize and distinguish specific distinctive features (i.e., that *b* and *d* are different because of one feature), (2) observe invariant relationships in events that occur repeatedly over time (i.e., a favorite toy is the same even when distance

makes it appear smaller), and (3) find a hierarchy of pattern or structure allowing the processing of the largest unit possible for adaptive use during a particular task (i.e., a map is scanned globally for the shape of a country, but subordinate features are scanned for the route of a river) (Gibson & Levin, 1975).

The child's first perceptions of the world develop primarily from tactile, kinesthetic, and vestibular input. As these three basic senses become integrated with the higher-level senses, vision and audition gradually take over. Young children or beginning readers tend to prefer learning through their tactile and kinesthetic senses and have lower preferences for visual and auditory learning (Carbo, 1980, 1983). At the age of 6 or 7, most children appear to prefer kinesthetic, tactile, visual, and auditory learning, in that order. They learn easily through their sense of touch and whole-body movement and have difficulty learning through listening activities. Generally, boys are less auditory and verbal and remain kinesthetic longer than girls (Restak, 1979). Around third grade most children become highly visual, and not until fifth grade do many children learn well through their auditory sense.

In the young child, visual discrimination of forms precedes the visual motor ability of copying forms by years. Throughout elementary school, the child is able to handle more and more internal detail of figures and to understand, recall, and recreate such configurations (Levine, 1987). Children begin to use simultaneous and sequential data to develop strategies, and cognitive or learning styles begin to emerge. In addition, children learn best through their dominant sensory input channel. It is interesting to note that 40% of school-aged children remember visually presented information, whereas only 20% to 30% recall what is heard (Carbo, Dunn, & Dunn, 1986).

▲ **Table 14-1** Developmental Guidelines for Visual Perception

| Object (Form) Perception | Developmental Age |
|---|---|
| Figure-ground perception | Improves between the ages of 3 to 5 years, stabilized growth at 6 to 7 years of age |
| Form constancy | Dramatic improvement between the ages of 6 to 7 years, with less improvement from 8 to 9 years of age |

| Spatial perception | Developmental Age |
|---|---|
| Position in space | Development complete at 7 to 9 years of age |
| Spatial relationships | Improves to approximately 10 years of age |

Modified from Williams, H. (1983). *Perceptual and motor development.* Englewood Cliffs, NJ: Prentice Hall.

Information processing in the visual perceptual–motor domain has been identified as one of the major factors that can predict readiness for the first grade. There is evidence that the child who enters school with delayed perceptual development may not catch up with his or her peers in academic achievement (Morency & Wepman, 1973). Adequate perceptual discrimination is considered necessary for the development of reading and writing skills (Moore, 1979).

Children gradually develop the abilities to attend to, integrate, sort, and retrieve increasingly larger chunks of visual data. These stimuli from the environment usually arrive for processing either in a simultaneous array or in a specific serial order (Levine, 1987). Much of one's experience with simultaneous processing has *spatial overtones,* and we interpret much of this spatial information visually. As an example of simultaneous processing, consider observing and later trying to recall what someone wore. Sequential processing involves the integration of separate elements into groups whose essential nature is temporal where each element leads only to one another. It enables the child to perceive an ordered series of events (Kirby & Das, 1978). An example of sequential processing is the visual information given to assemble a plastic model or macrame a plant hanger. An effective learner in the classroom needs to be able to evaluate, retain, process, and produce both simultaneous and sequential packages of information or action. In addition, children must learn to analyze and synthesize material containing more detail at a faster rate.

In adolescence, perceptual skills are enhanced by their interrelationship with expanding cognitive skill. Thus the adolescent can imagine, create, and construct complex visual forms. The adolescent is able to mentally manipulate visual information to solve increasingly complex problems, formulate plans, and make decisions.

### Development of Spatial Vision

In the developmental process of organizing space the child first acquires a concept of vertical dimensions, followed by horizontal dimensions. Oblique and diagonal dimensions are more complex, and perception of these spatial coordinates matures later. The 3- to 4-year-old child can distinguish vertical lines from horizontal ones but is unable to discriminate vertical, horizontal, and oblique lines until about age 6 (Cratty, 1970). The ability to discriminate between mirror or reversed imaged numbers and letters, such as *b* and *d* and *p* and *q,* does not mature until around age 7 (Ilg & Ames, 1981).

The child develops an understanding of left and right from the internal awareness that his or her body has two sides (Suchoff, 1987). This understanding of left and right is called *laterality* and proceeds in stages, according to Cratty (1970). A child's awareness of his or her own body is generally established by the age of 6 or 7. Before age 7 a child is not yet ready to handle spatial concepts on a strictly visual basis. The child must relate them back to his or her own body.

Around the eighth year the child begins to project the laterality concepts outside himself or herself. The child then develops *directionality,* or the understanding of an external object's position in space in relationship to himself or herself. This allows the child to handle spatial phenomena almost exclusively in a visual manner. By sensing a difference between body sides, the child becomes aware that figures and objects also have a right and a left. The child "feels" this visually.

Directionality is thought to be important in the visual discrimination of letters and numbers for both reading and writing. First a child learns these concepts on himself or herself, and then transfers them to symbols and words.

## SPECIFIC VISUAL PERCEPTUAL PROBLEMS
### Visual-Receptive Components

The importance of good vision for classroom work cannot be emphasized enough. More than 50% of a student's time is spent working at near point visual tasks such as reading and writing. Another 20% is spent on tasks that require the student to shift focus from distance to near and near to distance, such as copying from the board. Thus for more than 70% of the day, tremendous stress is being put on the visual system (Ritty, Cool, & Solan, 1992). Many students with vision dysfunctions can have difficulty meeting the behavioral demands of sitting still, sustaining attention, and completing their work.

Figure 14-4 presents a sample list of behaviors noted in children with specific visual problems (Optometric Extension Program Foundation, 1985). In addition to these behaviors noted in the list, Seiderman (1984) suggested that individuals with functional vision problems may use any of the following compensatory techniques:

▲ Avoidance of reading work
▲ Asthenopic symptoms (visual fatigue)
▲ Adaptation through the development of a refractive error to perform near-centered visual task demands

Disruption of oculomotor control can occur through disruption of cranial nerve function or disruption of central neural control. The pattern of oculomotor dysfunction depends on the areas of the brain that have been injured and the nature of the injury (Leigh & Zee, 1983). Oculomotor problems can limit ability to control and direct gaze. In addition, when large amounts of energy must be used on the motor components of vision, little energy may be left for visual cognitive processing (Hyvarinen, 1988). See Warren (1993a) for a detailed description of oculomotor deficits and other deficits seen in visual-receptive components.

### Refractive Errors

The child who is nearsighted has blurred distant vision, but generally experiences clarity at near point. The child who is farsighted frequently has clear distant and near vision, but has to exert extra effort to maintain clear vision at

1. **Appearance of eyes**
   One eye turns in or out at any time _____
   Reddened eyes or lids _____
   Eyes tear excessively _____
   Encrusted eyelids _____
   Frequent styes on lids _____

2. **Complaints when using eyes at desk**
   Headaches in forehead or temples _____
   Burning or itching after reading or desk work _____
   Nausea or dizziness _____
   Print blurs after reading a short time _____

3. **Behavioral signs of visual problems**
   a. Eye movement abilities (ocular motility)
      Head turns as reads across page _____
      Loses place often during reading _____
      Needs finger or marker to keep place _____
      Displays short attention span in reading
        or copying _____
      Too frequently omits words _____
      Repeatedly omits "small" words _____
      Writes up or down hill on paper _____
      Rereads or skips lines unknowingly _____
      Orients drawings poorly on page _____

   b. Eye teaming abilities (binocularity)
      Complains of seeing double (diplopia) _____
      Repeats letters within words _____
      Omits letters, number, or phrases _____
      Misaligns digits in number columns _____
      Squints, closes, or covers one eye _____
      Tilts head extremely while working
        at desk _____
      Consistently shows gross postural
        deviations at all desk activities _____

   c. Eye-hand coordination abilities
      Must feel things to assist in any
        interpretation required _____
      Eyes not used to "steer" hand movements
        (extreme lack of orientation, placement
        of words or drawings on page) _____
      Writes crookedly, poorly spaced: cannot
        stay on ruled lines _____
      Misaligns both horizontal and vertical
        series of numbers _____
      Uses hand or fingers to keep place on
        the page _____
      Uses other hand as "spacer" to control
        spacing and alignment on page _____
      Repeatedly confuses left-right directions _____

   d. Visual-form perception (visual comparison,
      visual imagery, visualization)
      Mistakes words with same or similar
        beginnings _____
      Fails to recognize same word in next
        sentence _____
      Reverses letters and/or words in writing
        and copying _____
      Confuses likenesses and minor differences _____
      Confuses same word in same sentence _____
      Repeatedly confuses similar beginnings
        and endings of words _____
      Fails to visualize what is read either
        silently or orally _____
      Whispers to self for reinforcement
        while reading silently _____
      Returns to "drawing with fingers" to
        decide likes and differences _____

   e. Refractive status (e.g., nearsightedness,
      farsightedness, focus problems)
      Comprehension reduces as reading
        continued; loses interest too quickly _____
      Mispronounces similar words as continues
        reading _____
      Blinks excessively at desk tasks and/or
        reading; not elsewhere _____
      Holds book too closely; face too close
        to desk surface _____
      Avoids all possible near-centered tasks _____
      Complains of discomfort in tasks that
        demand visual interpretation _____
      Closes or covers one eye when reading
        or doing desk work _____
      Makes errors in copying from chalkboard
        to paper on desk _____
      Makes errors in copying from reference
        book to notebook _____
      Squints to see chalkboard, or requests
        to move nearer _____
      Rubs eyes during or after short periods
        of visual activity _____
      Fatigues easily; blinks to make chalkboard
        clear up after desk task _____

---

NOTE: Students found to have any of the visual or eye problems on the checklist should be referred to a behavioral optometrist. Referral lists of behavioral optometrists are available from Optometric Extension Program Foundation, 2912 S. Daimler, Santa Ana, CA 92705.

**Figure 14-4** Checklist of observable clues to classroom vision problems.

near. The child with astigmatism experiences blurred vision at distance and near, with the degree of loss of clarity depending on the amount of astigmatism. Measures of visual acuity alone do not predict how well children interpret visual information (Hyvarinen, 1988). Other determinants include the ability to see objects in low-contrast lighting conditions, the ability of the eye to adapt to different lighting conditions, visual field problems, accommodation, and other oculomotor functions (Hyvarinen, 1988).

If accommodation takes longer than previously described, words appear blurry and the child tends to lose his or her place, missing important information and understanding. When accommodation for near objects is poor, presbyopia exists; this individual is described as farsighted.

When the conditions of motor fusion and sensory fusion have not been met for binocular fusion to occur (this process was described earlier), single binocular vision is at best difficult, and at worst, impossible. If one eye overtly turns in, out, up, or down because of muscular imbalance, the condition is known as *strabismus,* sometimes referred to as a crossed or wandering eye. This can result in double vision or a mental suppression of one of the images. This, in turn, can have effects on the development of visual perception. Some children have surgery to correct an eye turn. Although this intervention can correct the eye cosmetically, it does not always result in binocular vision.

Another type of binocular dysfunction is termed *phoria.* Phoria refers to a tendency for one eye to go slightly in, out, up, or down but with the absence of overt misalignment of the two eyes. A phoria requires that the child expend additional mechanical effort to maintain motor fusion of the two eyes, whether focusing near or far. The extra effort frequently detracts from the child's ability to process and interpret the meaning of what he or she sees.

## Visual-Cognitive Components
### Attention

To review, visual attention is composed of alertness, selective attention, vigilance, and shared attention. If the child's state of alertness or arousal is impaired, the child may demonstrate behaviors of overattentiveness, underattentiveness, or poor sustained attention (Todd, 1993). Children who are overattentive may be compelled to respond to visual stimuli around them rather than attend to the task at hand, may be easily distracted by visual stimuli, and may demonstrate continual visual searching behaviors. Children who are underattentive may have difficulty orienting to visual stimuli, may habituate quickly to a visual stimulus, and may fatigue easily. At this level a child may refrain from attending to a familiar stimulus. A child with poor sustained attention may demonstrate a high activity level and be easily distracted.

Selective attention is the next level of visual attention, and a child with difficulty in this area demonstrates a reduced ability to focus on a visual target. The child may have

difficulty screening out unimportant or irrelevant information, focus on irrelevant stimuli, and be distracted by irrelevant stimuli. A child with difficulty in selective attention is easily confused. The child may focus on unnecessary tasks or information and therefore not obtain the specific information needed for the task.

A child with reduced vigilance skills shows reduced persistence on a visual task and poor or cursory examination of visual stimuli. The child cannot maintain visual attention. The more complex the visual structure of an object, the lengthier the process of visual analysis and the greater vigilance skills are needed. A child with deficits in shared attention can only focus well on one task at a time. He may be easily confused or distracted if required to share visual attention between two tasks.

Enns and Cameron (1987) suggested that visual inattention is the result of an inability to select the features that differentiate objects in a visual array. The child cannot see, recognize, or isolate the salient features and therefore does not know where to focus visual attention. Luria (1966) suggested that problems of visual recognition represent a breakdown of active feature-by-feature analysis necessary for interpreting a visual image.

### Memory

The child with visual memory deficits has poor or reduced ability to recognize or retrieve visual information and to store visual information in short- or long-term memory. The child may fail to adequately attend, to allow for storage of visual information, or may show a prolonged response time. The child may demonstrate the inability to recognize or match visual stimuli presented previously because he or she has not stored this information in memory or he or she may not be able to retrieve it from memory (Todd, 1993). The child may have good memory for life experiences but not for factual material and may fail to relate information to prior knowledge. The child may demonstrate inconsistent recall abilities, and the child may demonstrate poor ability to use mnemonic strategies for storage.

### Visual Discrimination

The child with poor discrimination abilities may demonstrate an inadequate ability to recognize, match, and categorize. Ulman (1986) proposed that a finite set of visual operations or "routines" are performed to extract shape properties and spatial relations. Object recognition is frequently determined by what is taken to be the top or the bottom of the object. A child with poor matching skills may demonstrate difficulty matching the same shape presented in a different spatial orientation or may confuse similar shapes. A child with poor matching skills may have difficulty in recognizing form within a complex field.

*Object (form) vision.* Children with form constancy problems may have difficulty recognizing forms and objects presented in different sizes, different orientations in space, or when there are differences in detail. This interferes with the child's ability to organize and classify perceptual experiences for meaningful cognitive operations (Piaget, 1964). This may result in difficulty recognizing letters or words in different styles of print or in making the transition from printed letters to cursive ones.

A child with a visual closure deficit may be unable to identify a form or object if an incomplete presentation is made. Therefore the child would always need to see the complete object to identify it. For example, a child completing work at his or her desk would not be able to differentiate between the pencil and the pen when they are partially covered by paper.

The child with figure-ground problems may not be able to pick out a specific toy from a shelf. The child may have difficulty with sorting and organizing personal belongings. The child may overattend to details and miss the big picture or may overlook details and miss the important information. Children with figure-ground problems may have difficulty attending to a word on a printed page because they cannot block out other words around it. The child with figure-ground difficulties may not have good visual search strategies. Marr (1982) suggested that control of the direction of gaze is a prerequisite for efficiency of visual search. Cohen (1981) described these visual search strategies:

1. The reviewer looks for specific visual information and makes crude distinctions between figure and ground by isolating one figure from another.
2. The viewer determines which figures are most meaningful (the process stops here when recognition is immediate).
3. When recognition is not immediate, the viewer makes a hypothesis about the visual information received and directs attention to selected items to test the hypothesis.

Rogow and Rathwill (1989) found that good readers more frequently proceeded from the left to the right and from the top down to find "hidden figures" than did poor readers. Good readers were also more flexible in their approach; they rotated the page as needed and were not content until they found as many hidden as possible. The good readers also were less distressed by ambiguity, and they understood that pictures could be viewed in different ways.

*Spatial vision.* A child with position-in-space difficulty has trouble discriminating among objects because of their placement in space. These children also have difficulty planning their actions in relation to objects around them. They may show letter reversals past the age of 8 and may show confusion regarding the sequence of letters or numbers in a word or math problem (e.g., was/saw). Writing and spacing letters and words on paper may be a problem. The children may show difficulty in understanding directional language such as in, out, on, under, next to, up, down, in front of.

Decreased depth perception can affect the child's ability to walk through spaces and to catch a ball. The child may

be unable to visually determine when the surface plane has changed and may have difficulty with steps and curbs. Transference of visual spatial notations across two visual planes can make copying from the blackboard difficult. Faulty interpretation of the spatial relationships can contribute to a problem with sorting and organizing personal belongings.

A child who has diminished topographic orientation may be easily lost and unable to find his or her way from one location to the next. The child may also demonstrate difficulty determining the location of objects and settings.

## Diagnoses With Problems in Visual Perception

When children with handicapping conditions have visual problems, the impact of the visual disabilities can be tremendous. Numerous studies have found a high frequency of vision problems among individuals with disabilities (Ciner, Macks, & Schanel-Klitsch, 1991; Duckman, 1979; Fanning, 1971; Scheiman, 1984). Severe refractive errors are common among children with developmental problems (Rogow, 1992). Impaired skills of visual attention are often exhibited through the functional behavior of these children. Often considered distractable, some children may be able to locate objects yet demonstrate an inability to sustain eye contact or recognize objects visually (Rogow, 1992).

Retinopathy of prematurity is the single most often cited cause of blindness in preterm infants. Cortical visual impairment also occurs in preterm infants and is generally associated with severe central nervous system damage such as periventricular leukomalacia. Other visual disorders common in preterm children include lenses that are too thick, poor visual acuity, astigmatism, extreme myopia, strabismus, amblyopia, and anisometropia (unequal refraction of the eyes) (Fledelius, 1976). These children also have difficulty processing visual information. Measures of visual attention, pattern discrimination, visual recognition, memory, and visual motor integration are lower than those for full-term infants (Caron & Caron, 1981; Rose, 1980; Sigman & Parmelee, 1974). Studies of older children suggest that these problems often persist (Siegel, 1983).

Children with cerebral palsy (CP) have frequently been identified as a group with visual perception deficits (Abercrombie, 1963; Breakey, Wilson, & Wilson, 1994). Children with CP often have a strabismus, ocular motor problems, convergence insufficiencies, or nystagmus. These problems may also limit ability to control and direct visual gaze (Rogow, 1992).

Early research indicated that the degree of perceptual impairment in persons with CP was related to the type and severity of the motor impairment (Birch, 1964). Children with athetosis have been found to have fewer visual perceptual disorders than children with spasticity (Abercrombie, 1963). Although the research findings differ as to the presence or absence of visual perceptual problems in children who have a right or left hemiplegia, Abercrombie

(1964) stated that both groups of children have visual perceptual problems. A recent study showed that 24 children with CP obtained significantly lower scores than did 24 normal children on a motor-free test of visual perception (Menken, Cermak, & Fisher, 1987). These findings supported earlier studies in that the group with spastic quadriplegic involvement scored lowest on six of the seven subtests on the Motor Free Test of Visual Perception. Further study is needed to determine differences among subgroups of children with CP.

In children with language delay, poorly developed visual perception may contribute to their language difficulties. For example, language moves from the general to the specific. Young children call every animal with four legs a dog. Eventually they are able to visually discriminate between dogs and lions, and the vocabulary follows the visual perceptual lead. Next, they can tell dalmatians from dachshunds, but they are unable to recognize that they are both dogs. Finally, the ability to categorize and generalize emerges somewhere between the ages of 7 and 9. In addition, the child who has visual spatial perception deficits may show difficulty in understanding directional language such as *in, on, under,* and *next to.*

Not all children with learning disabilities have visual perception problems (Hung, Fisher, & Cermak, 1987). However, visual perceptual problems are found more frequently in persons who show significantly higher verbal scores than performance scores on intelligence testing. Children with learning disabilities may have difficulty filtering out irrelevant environmental stimuli and therefore present with erratic visual attention skills. Children who have difficulty interpreting and using visual information effectively are described as having visual perceptual problems because they have not acquired adequate visual perceptual skills in spite of normal vision (Todd, 1993).

The incidence of visual perceptual and visual motor deficits in children with psychiatric disorders was studied by Daniels and Ryley (1991). In this study visual-motor skills deficits occurred far more frequently than visual perception skills deficits. When visual perception problems did occur, they were in conjunction with visual-motor skill problems. Some children with autism have demonstrated poor oculo-motor function (Rosenhall, Johansson, & Gilberg, 1988). Children with autism often do not appear to focus their vision directly on what they are doing (Wing, 1976). A possible explanation is that they are using peripheral vision to the exclusion of focal vision.

## Effects of Visual Perceptual Problems on Performance Areas

The effects of visual perceptual problems may be subtle in nature, with no obvious disabilities. However, when the child is asked to perform a visual perceptual task, he or she may be slow or unable to perform the task. Visual percep-

tion dysfunction affects the child's ability to use tools and relate materials to one another (Ayres, 1979); thus bilateral manipulative skills are affected to a greater degree than the child's basic prehension patterns indicate (see Chapter 12). The child with visual perceptual deficits may show problems with cutting, coloring, constructing with blocks or other construction toys, doing puzzles, using fasteners, and tying shoes. Visual perception deficits can influence children's self-care, work, and play and leisure performance.

Children with visual perception problems may demonstrate difficulty with activities of daily living tasks. In grooming, the child may have difficulty obtaining the necessary supplies and using a mirror to comb and style hair. Applying toothpaste to the brush may be difficult for the child. Fasteners; donning and doffing clothing, prostheses, and orthoses; tying shoes; and matching clothes may present problems. The skilled use of handwriting, telephones, typewriters, computers, and communication devices may all present difficulty for the child with visual-cognitive problems. Community mobility may be difficult because the child is unable to locate objects and find his or her way. In play, the child may demonstrate difficulty with playing games and sports, drawing and coloring, cutting with scissors, pasting, constructing, and doing puzzles.

Work and productive activities such as home management and classroom assignments may present problems for the child with visual perceptual problems. For example, the child may have trouble sorting and folding clothes as a home management task. Educational activities such as reading, spelling, writing, and math may be difficult for the child. The following section elaborates on the educational problems seen in the school-aged child.

### Problems in Reading

Gibson (1971) has delineated different characteristics of printed (written) information necessary for reading. These include a word's graphic configuration, orthography (order of letters), phonology (sounds represented), and semantics (meaning). The child benefits from these multiple simultaneous clues in reading. If the child has difficulty with one characteristic, he or she can use the clues from the other features.

In early reading, children first encounter the visual configuration (graphics) and orthographics in a printed word. The child then must break the written word into its component phonemes (phonology), hold them in active working memory, and then synthesize and blend the phonemes to form recognizable words (semantics). After practice, this step is accomplished and the word can then be dealt with as a gestalt and added to the child's growing sight vocabulary. Sight vocabulary consists of words that are instantly recognized as gestalts. As a child's reliance on sight vocabulary increases, decoding takes less time and the child develops automaticity, which allows the child to begin to concentrate on comprehension and retention.

Understanding sentences requires adding two more variables: context and syntax (word order and grammatic construction, respectively), to the skills previously discussed (Levine, 1987). To read paragraphs, chapters, and texts, it is assumed that decoding is well automatized. A hierarchy can be assumed here in that any developmental dysfunctions that impair decoding or sentence comprehension impede text reading.

The segmenting of written words in early reading calls for a variety of skills. First, children must be able to recognize individual letter symbols. This requires visual attention, visual memory, and visual discrimination. In the presence of severe dysfunction, recognition of words may be impaired (Levine, 1987) and thus interfere with the acquisition of sight vocabulary. Problems with visual perception might be suspected in a child who appears to be better at understanding what was read than at actually decoding the words. This child has good language abilities but some trouble processing written words.

Visual perceptual attributes are different from the capacity to assimilate visual detail. The child may be diagnosed as having visual perceptual problems when he or she is limited in attending to or extracting data presented simultaneously. In this instance the child does not have difficulty with the specific perceptual content but with the amount of information that must be simultaneously perceived to understand the whole.

Memory deficiencies also present reading problems (Levine, 1987). Children with visual memory problems may be unable to remember the visual shape of letters and words. Such children may also demonstrate the inability to associate these shapes with letters, sounds, and words (Greene, 1987). Children with weaknesses of visual-verbal associative memory have difficulty establishing easily retrievable or recognizable sound-symbol associations. They are unable to associate the sound, visual configuration, or meaning of the word with what is seen or heard.

Children with difficulty with active working memory cannot hold one aspect of the reading process in suspension while pursuing another component. It is closely related to perceptual span, or the ability to recall the beginning of the sentence while reading the end of it. The child must take a second look at the beginning of a sentence after reading the end of it.

Children with visual discrimination deficits may not be able to recognize symbols and therefore may be slow to master the alphabet and numbers. Their relatively weak grasp of constancy of forms may make visual discrimination an inefficient process. Some children, therefore, cannot readily discern the differences between visually similar symbols. Confusions over the letters *p, q,* and *g* and *a* and *o,* as well as letter reversals, may ensue such as the notorious differentiation between *b* and *d*. Visual discrimination abilities (form perception and spatial perception) are somewhat less important at advanced stages of the learning-to-read process than they are during the initial stages of reading acquisition (deHirsch, Jansky, & Langford, 1966; Jansky & deHirsh, 1972; Lyle, 1969).

Confusion over the directionality and other spatial characteristics of a word may result in weak registration in visual memory, again possibly creating significant delays in the consolidation of a sight vocabulary. Thus even frequently encountered words need to be analyzed anew each time they appear. A child with visual spatial deficits has difficulty with map reading and interpretation of instructional graphics such as charts and diagrams. Graphic representations require the child to integrate, extract the most salient elements from, condense, and organize the large amount of stimuli presented at once. Again, the child may not have difficulty with the perceptual content, but the amount of information to be simultaneously assimilated is more than the child can integrate and remember (Levine, 1987).

## Problems in Spelling

Children with impaired processing of simultaneous visual stimuli may have difficulty with spelling (Boder, 1973). Their inability to visualize words may result from indistinct or distorted initial visual registration. Such children who have a strong sense of sound-symbol association may make what Boder calls *dyseidetic errors*—spelling words phonetically (e.g., lite for light), yet incorrectly. They exhibit spelling inaccuracies that reflect good phonetic approximations but are inaccurate. Visual sequential memory is necessary for remembering the sequence of letters in a word. The child may exhibit poor spelling and be unaware of letters omitted.

## Problems in Handwriting

Pilot studies have begun to explore the relationship between visual-cognitive skills and handwriting (Chapman & Wedell, 1972; Yost & Lesiak, 1980; Ziviani, Hayes, & Chant, 1990). Tseng and Cermak (1993) suggested that the role of visual perception shows little relationship to handwriting, whereas kinesthesia, visual motor integration, and motor planning appear to be more closely related to handwriting. However, further research is necessary to provide information concerning the role of visual perception in handwriting.

Visual-cognitive abilities may affect writing in any one or any combination of the following. Children with problems in attention may have difficulty with the correct letter formation, spelling, mechanics of grammar, punctuation, and capitalization and the formulation of a sequential flow of ideas necessary for written communication. For the child to write spontaneously, he or she must be able to revisualize letters and words without visual cues. Therefore if the child has visual memory problems, he or she may have difficulty recalling the shape and formation of letters and numbers. Other problems seen in the child with poor visual memory would be the child mixing small and capital letters within a sentence, the same letter written many ways on the same page, and the inability to print the alphabet from memory. In addition, legibility may be poor, and the child may need a model to write.

Visual discrimination problems may affect the child's handwriting. The child with poor form constancy does not recognize errors in his or her own handwriting. The child may be unable to recognize letters or words in different prints and therefore have difficulty in copying from a different type of print to handwriting. The child may also show poor recognition of letters or numbers in different environments, positions, or sizes. If the child is unable to discriminate a letter, he or she may show poor letter formation. A child with visual-closure difficulty always needs to see the complete presentation of what he or she is to copy. If the child has figure-ground problems, he or she may have difficulty in copying because he or she is unable to determine what it is he or she should be writing. The child, therefore, may omit important segments.

Visual spatial problems can affect the child's handwriting in many ways. The child may show reversals of letters such as *m, w, b, d, s, c,* and *z* and of numbers *2, 3, 5, 6, 7,* and *9.* If the child is unable to discriminate left from right, he or she may have difficulty with the left to right progression of writing words and sentences. The child may demonstrate overspacing or underspacing and have trouble keeping within the margins. He or she may be unable to relate one part of the letter to another part of the letter and therefore show inconsistency in letter size. The child may have difficulty with the placement of letters on a line and the ability to adapt the letter sizes to the space provided on the paper or worksheet.

### Visual-Motor Integration

In handwriting, the ability to integrate the visual image of letters or shapes with the appropriate motor response is necessary. Visual-motor integration is not well understood because it is not a unitary process and consequently can be disrupted for a variety of reasons. Failure on visual-motor tests may be caused by underlying visual-cognitive deficits including visual discrimination, poor fine motor ability, inability to integrate visual-cognitive and motor processes, or a combination of these abilities. Therefore careful analysis is necessary to determine what is the underlying problem. Tseng and Murray (1994) examined the relationship of perceptual motor measures to legibility of handwriting in Chinese school-aged children, and visual-motor integration was found to be the best predictor of handwriting.

### Math

The child with visual perceptual problems has difficulty correctly aligning columns for calculation and therefore the answers are incorrect because of alignment and not because of calculation skills. Worksheets with many rows and columns of math problems may be disorganizing to children with figure-ground problems. Children with poor visual memory may have difficulty using a calculator. Visual memory may also present problems for students when addition and subtraction problems require multiple steps. Geometry, because of its spatial characteristics, present much difficulty for the child with visual spatial perception problems. Problem solving often involves recognizing, discriminating, and comparing object form and space as a foundation for higher-level mathematic skills. Visual imagery required to match and compare forms and shapes is difficult for students with visual perceptual problems and interferes with learning these underlying skills.

## EVALUATION METHODS

In evaluation of visual perceptual function, the therapist considers the entire process of vision and examines the relationship of visual function to behavior and performance (Seiderman, 1984). Visual-receptive and visual-cognitive components may represent different issues in a child's school performance. Problems can and do exist in either area, with differing effects on the learning process. However, visual-receptive components can influence the information obtained for visual-cognitive analysis. Because receptive and cognitive components are important in the visual processing of information, individual assessment of the child should be conducted within a multidisciplinary approach, realizing that the interplay between visual-receptive, visual-cognitive, and school success is different for each child (Flax, 1984). Thus the occupational therapist's findings can be integrated with those of the reading specialist, psychologist, speech-language pathologist, and classroom teacher as a part of the multidisciplinary team. By combining test results and analysis of the child's performance the team ascertains the nature of the interaction of the disability with the activity. A vision specialist, such as an opthalmologist or an optometrist, may be needed to assess visual-receptive dysfunction and to remediate the condition.

### Visual-Receptive Assessment

Evaluation should begin by focusing on the integrity of the visual-receptive components including visual fields, visual acuity, and oculomotor control (Warren, 1993b). If deficits occur in these foundation skills, then insufficient or inaccurate information regarding the location and features of objects is sent to the central nervous system. Therefore the quality of learning through the visual sense is severely affected. Warren (1990) suggested that what sometimes appear to be visual-cognitive deficits are actually visual receptive problems, which may include oculomotor disturbances; therefore visual-receptive and visual-cognitive deficits may be misdiagnosed. The occupational therapist should be familiar with visual screening because the assessment of vision and oculomotor skills assists in assessing and analyzing their influence on visual perception and functional performance (Todd, 1993).

Visual screening consists of basic tests administered to select those children who are at risk for inadequate visual functions (Bouska et al., 1990). The purpose of the screening is to determine those children who should be referred for a complete diagnostic visual evaluation. Therefore the purpose of the screening of the visual-receptive system is to determine how efficient the eyes are in acquiring visual information for further visual-cognitive interpretation. The observational checklist in Figure 14-4 assists in alerting the therapist to visual symptoms commonly found in those who demonstrate poor visual performance.

Perimetry, confrontation, and careful observation of the child as he or she performs daily activities gives useful information regarding field integrity in measuring visual fields (Warren, 1993a). Missing or misreading the beginning or ends of words or numbers may indicate the presence of a central field deficit.

The child's refractive status, which is the clinical measurement of the eye, should be measured. This is usually conducted by a school nurse or vision specialist. A student's refractive status determines whether there is nearsightedness (myopia), farsightedness (hyperopia), or astigmatism. There are several methods used to measure the child's refractive status. One method, the Snellen Test, is used to screen children at school or in the physicians office. However, this test measures only eyesight (visual acuity) at 20 feet. This figure, expressed commonly as x/20 has little predictive value for how well a child uses his or her vision. It is estimated that this measurement shows less than 5% of visual problems (Seiderman & Marcus, 1990). When a child passes this screening, he or she may be told that his existing vision is fine. However, it is only the eyesight at 20 feet that is fine.

Some schools and clinics use a Telebinocular or other similar instrument in vision screening. This provides information on clarity or visual acuity at both near and far distances, as well as information on depth perception and binocularity (two-eyed coordination). Warren (1993b) suggested that the Contrast Sensitivity Test is best for measuring acuity. A pediatric version is available (Vistech Consultants Inc., Dayton, OH).

The occupational therapist may observe oculomotor dysfunction in the child. The screening test should answer several questions: Do the eyes work together? How well? Where is visual control the most efficient? The least efficient? What types of eye movements are the most efficient? The least efficient? (Warren, 1993b). Screening tools that can be used by occupational therapists are presented in Table 14-2. In the presence of oculomotor impairment the child should be referred to an appropriate vision specialist, such as an optometrist, because of the complexity of oculomotor problems.

In addition, the child's ocular health should be ascertained. The presence of a disease or other pathologic condition such as glaucoma, cataracts, or a deterioration of the nerves or any part of the eye, for instance, must be ruled out. An interview with the family regarding significant visual history helps identify any conditions that may be associated with visual limitations. A record review can also help obtain this information, as can a consultation with other professionals involved in direct care of the child (e.g., teacher or physician).

When visual problems are detected in screening, the child may be referred to a vision specialist such as an optometrist. The specialist can help determine if the child has a visual problem that might be causing or contributing to school difficulties. The therapist will then be able to understand what effect those deficits have on function and the strategies needed for intervention. With this information the therapist can design and select appropriate activities that are within the visual capacity of the child (Bouska et al., 1990).

## Visual-Cognitive Assessment

Clinical evaluation and observation may be the occupational therapist's most useful assessment methods. The therapist should observe for difficulty in selecting, storing, retrieving, or classifying visual information. Observations could include visual search strategies used during visual perceptual tasks (e.g., outside borders to inside), how the child approaches the task, how the child processes and interprets visual information, the child's flexibility in analyzing visual information, methods used for storage and retrieval of visual information, and amount of stress associated with visual activities. The therapist should carefully analyze the tasks observed to determine what visual skills are needed and to identify where the child has difficulty.

Visual-cognitive evaluations that are typically administered by occupational therapists and those typically administered by other professionals are presented in Tables 14-3 to 14-6. Currently, the best evaluation method of visual attention in children is informal observation during occupational performance tasks. Further description of some the assessments as well as other assessments that may be used follow:

▲ Bruininks-Oseretsky Test of Motor Proficiency (Bruininks, 1978)
▲ The Reversals Frequency Test (Gardner, 1978)—A norm-referenced test for children between ages 5 and 15 years. This test measures reversals in a recognition and execution mode and includes a questionnaire for the teacher to complete that indicates the type and frequency of a child's reversals in both reading and writing.
▲ Test of Pictures, Forms, Letters, Numbers, Spatial Orientation, and Sequencing Skills (Gardner, 1992)—This test measures the ability to visually perceive forms, let-

▲ Table 14-2   Vision Screening Tests

| Test | Author (Date) | Description |
|---|---|---|
| Functional Visual Screening | Langley (1980) | Screening developed for the severely or profoundly handicapped, which consists of 12 items including pupillary reactions, blinking, peripheral orientation, fixation, gaze shift, tracking, and convergence |
| Visual Screening | Bouska, Kauffman, & Marcus (1990) | Comprehensive screening of distance and near vision, convergence near point, horizontal pursuits, distant and near fixations, and stereoscopic visual skills to select those children who should be referred to a qualified vision specialist for a complete diagnostic visual evaluation |
| Erhardt Developmental Vision Assessment | Erhardt (1989) | Assessment that measures motor components of vision from fetal and natal periods to 6 months of age; the 6-month age level is considered to be a significant stage of maturity, and this is appropriate for older children; the motor components of vision measured include both reflexive visual patterns and voluntary eye movements of localization, fixation, ocular pursuit, and gaze shift |
| Sensorimotor Performance Analysis | Richter & Montgomery (1991) | Assessment of visual tracking, visual avoidance, visual processing, and eye-hand coordination during gross and fine motor tasks |
| Crane-Wick Test | Crane & Wick (1987) | A norm-references test that can be administered individually or in a group, for children in kindergarten through grade 12; a sustained nearpoint visual skills test that is used to identify children with vision problems that interfere with learning and work activities; subtests included are accommodation, saccadic eye movement, near point of convergence, eye teaming, pursuit of movement, visual processing, and functional hearing |
| Visual Skills Appraisal | Richards & Oppenheim (1984) | An individually administered norm-referenced test for children ages 5 to 9 years; six subtests include pursuit, scanning, alignment, locating movements, eye-hand coordination, and fixation unity; resulting subtest scores are converted to a scale, and cutoff points are provided to indicate whether a student requires further examination by a specialist |
| OK Vision Kit | Williamson (1993) | A test that measures visual acuity using observable reflexive optokinetic nystagmus |
| Pediatric Clinical Vision Screening for Occupational Therapists | Schierman (1991) | A test that screens accommodation, binocular vision, and ocular motility |
| Clinical Observations of Infants | Ciner, Macks, & Schanel-Kiltsch (1991) | Description methods for testing vision in early intervention programs |
| Clinical Observation for Adults | Warren (1993b) | Detailed description of visual screening is outlined for adults, but many items may be applied to children |

▲ Table 14-3    Assessments of Visual Attention

| Description | Test | Author (Date) |
|---|---|---|
| **SCANNING** | | |
| Saccadic eye movements. Rapid change of fixation from one point in the visual field to another. | Line Bisection* Letter Cancellation* | Warren (1993a) |
| **VISUAL VIGILANCE** | | |
| Ability to handle substantial simultaneous detail. The task requires the child to sustain attention and emphasizes visual attention to detail by having the child find a particular rarely occurring design embedded in many others. | Matching Familiar Figures Test* Visual Vigilance task on the Pediatric Early Elementary Examination (PEEX) Visual Vigilance task on the Pediatric Examination of Educational Readiness at Middle Childhood (PEERAMID) | Cairns & Cammock (1978) Levine & Rapport (1983) Levine (1985) |
| **VISUAL SEQUENCING** | | |
| Registration and immediate recall of visual sequences. | Picture Arrangement subtest of Wechester Intelligence Scale for Children (WISC-III) Visual Sequential memory subtest of the Test of Visual Perception Skills (Nonmotor)* | Wechsler (1991) Gardner (1982) |

*Tests administered by occupational therapists.

▲ Table 14-4    Assessments of Visual Memory

| Description | Test | Author (Date) |
|---|---|---|
| **VISUAL RETRIEVAL MEMORY TESTS** | | |
| Visualization and recall of entire configurations. In these tests a child studies a geometric form and then is asked to reproduce it from memory. | Benton Visual Retention Test* Memory for Designs Test* Visual Memory Scale* Spatial Memory subtest from the Kaufman Assessment Battery for Children | Benton (1974) Graham & Kendall (1960) Carroll (1975) Kaufman & Kaufman (1983) |
| **VISUAL RECOGNITION MEMORY** | | |
| Short-term visual memory. The child is shown a design and later asked to select it from among similar sets of stimuli. | Visual recognition subtests of Pediatric Early Elementary Examination (PEEX) Visual recognition subtests of Pediatric Examination of Education Readiness at Middle Childhood (PEERAMID) Visual Memory subtest of the Test of Visual Perception Skills (Nonmotor)* | Levine & Rapport (1983) Levine (1985) Gardner (1982) |

*Tests administered by occupational therapists.

ters, and numbers in the correct direction and to visually perceive words with letters in the correct sequence. There are seven subtests in this norm-referenced test for children ages 5 to 9 years; it can be administered individually or in a group.

▲ Concepts of Left and Right Test (Laurendau & Pinard, 1970)—This instrument evaluates the child's understanding of left and right, from total lack of understanding to full internalization.

▲ The Birch-Belmont Auditory-Visual Integration Test (Suchoff, 1968)— This test involves an auditory-visual pattern-matching task. The child is asked to identify an array of dots corresponding to a series of taps that he or she hears.

▲ Test of Visual Perceptual Skills (TVPS) (Gardner, 1982)

▲ Test of Visual Analysis Skills—This is an individually administered criterion-referenced test for children ages 5 to 8 years. The child taking this untimed test is asked to copy simple to complex geometric patterns. The purpose of the assessment is to determine if the child is competent or in need of remediation in perceiving

▲ Table 14-5   Assessments of Visual Discrimination

| Description | Test | Author (Date) |
|---|---|---|
| **OBJECT (FORM) PERCEPTION** | | |
| Matching one design with another or finding a specific stimuli embedded within a complex background (usually administered as a motor-free assessment). | Motor Free Visual Perception Test* | Colarusso & Hammill (1972) |
| | Test of Pictures, Forms, Letters, Numbers, and Spatial Orientation* | Gardner (1992) |
| | Developmental Test of Visual Perception (2nd Ed)* | Hammill, Pearson, & Voress (1993) |
| | Subtests of the Test of Visual-Perception Skills (Nonmotor)* | Gardner (1982) |
| **SPATIAL PERCEPTION** | | |
| Match a design to one that has experienced some transformation but retains its identity (mirror image or rotation). | Position in Space subtest of the Frostig* | Frostig, Lefever, & Whittlesey (1966) |
| | Visual Form Constancy subtest of the Test of Visual-Perception Skills (Nonmotor)* | Gardner (1982) |
| | Matrix Analogies subtest of the Kaufman Assessment Battery of Children (ABC) | Kaufman & Kaufman (1983) |
| | Raven's Progressive Matrices* | |
| | The Reversals Frequency Test* | Gardner (1978) |
| | Jordon Left-Right Reversal Test—Revised* | Jordon (1980) |
| | Concepts of Left and Right Test* | Laurendau & Pinard (1970) |
| | Block Design and Object Assembly subtest of Wechsler Intelligence Scale for Children (WISC-III) | Wechsler (1991) |

*Tests administered by occupational therapists.

▲ Table 14-6   Assessment of Visual Motor Integration

| Description | Test | Author (Date) |
|---|---|---|
| Integration of spatial input with fine motor production. The child is shown a geometric form and asked to copy it. | Bender Visual Motor Gestalt* | Bender (1963) see Koppitz scoring, ages 5-10 years, Koppitz (1963) |
| | Benton Visual Retention Test | Benton (1974) |
| | Developmental Test of Visual Motor Integration (VMI)* | Beery & Buktenica (1989) |
| | Test of Visual Analysis Skills* | |
| | Memory for Design Test* | Graham & Kendall (1960) |

*Test administered by occupational therapists.

the visual relationships necessary for integrating letter and word shapes.

▲ Developmental Test of Visual Perception (DTVP) (2nd ed.) (Hammill, Pearson, & Voress, 1993)—This is the 1993 revision of Frostig's DTVP. This test is unbiased relative to race, gender, and handedness. It is a norm-referenced test for children ages 4 to 10 years. There are eight subtests, which include eye-hand coordination, copying, spatial relations, position in space, figure-ground, visual closure, visual-motor speed, and form constancy.

▲ Jordon Left-Right Reversal Test—Revised (Jordon, 1980)—This is a standardized test for children ages 5 to 12 years that can be administered individually or in a group. It is an untimed test that takes about 20 min-

utes to administer and score. The test is used to detect visual reversals of letters, numbers, and words. The manual includes remediation exercises for reversal problems.

These tests can be used to evaluate how the child is processing, organizing, and using visual-cognitive information. Care in interpreting and reporting test results should be taken because it is not always clear what visual perceptual tests are measuring. Because of the complexity of the tests, it is certain that they tap different kinds and levels of function, including language abilities. The effectiveness of any treatment method is largely determined by how the child is diagnosed; therefore careful analysis of test results and observations is important.

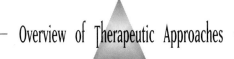

## Overview of Therapeutic Approaches

**Occupational Performance Skills**
↑
Adaptation and compensation
↑
Skill training
↑
Developmental stimulation
↑
**Occupational Performance Components**
↑
Behavioral approaches
↑
Biomechanical approaches
↑
Sensory integration therapy
↑
Neurophysiologic approaches (preparation for treatment)

From Cowan, M.K. (1993). Overview of therapeutic approaches. Lecture notes from OTS 352, *OT For Infants and Children.* Richmond, KY: Eastern Kentucky University.

## INTERVENTION

### Theoretic Approaches

The theoretical approaches that guide evaluation and treatment of visual perceptual skills can be categorized as *developmental* or *compensatory.* Warren's (1993a,b) developmental model, described in an earlier section, is based on the concept that higher-level skills evolve from integration of lower-level skills and are subsequently affected by disruption of lower-level skills. Skill levels within the hierarchy function as a single entity and provide a unified structure for visual perception. As pictured in Figure 14-1, oculomotor control, visual field, and acuity form the foundation skills, followed by visual attention, scanning, pattern recognition or detection, memory, and visual cognition. The identification and remediation of deficits in lower-level skills permit integration of higher-level skills. Occupational therapists who follow this model need to evaluate lower-level skills before proceeding to high-level skills to identify where the deficit is in the visual hierarchy and to design appropriate evaluation and intervention.

Cowan (1993) described a hierarchy of therapeutic approaches, as diagrammed in the box above, and provided a framework for discussing the occupational therapy treatment of children with visual perception problems. The *neurophysiologic* approaches aim to address the maturation of the human nervous system and the link to human behavior. These approaches help create a therapeutic environment, inhibit abnormal movement and sensory hypersensitivity, and facilitate normal patterns of movement and sensory reception. In addition, these approaches work on positioning for function. For example, postural stability is important for oculomotor efficiency. Sensory integration provides preparation for functional performance and is discussed in Chapter 13. The neurophysiologic approaches focus on improving occupational performance components necessary for visual-receptive and visual-cognitive functioning.

In *skill development* approaches an attempt is made to improve the child's ability to profit from standard instruction. Many remedial treatment programs teach the child visual analysis skills. The goal is to teach the child a systematic method for identifying the pertinent, concrete features of spatially organized patterns, thereby enabling the child to recognize how new information may link up with previously acquired knowledge on the basis of similar and different attributes. The child should be able to transfer across dissimilar tasks so that improvement in visual perceptual skills should lead to improvement in all functional activities requiring those skills. Perceptual training programs fall in the skill development category. These programs to remediate deficit or prerequisite skills have been implemented in the public schools over the past two decades (e.g., Frostig, Kephart). Occupational therapists have adapted many activities from these approaches.

In *compensatory approaches* classroom materials or instructional methods are modified to accommodate the child's limitations. The environment can also be altered or adapted. Adaptation and compensation techniques can include special techniques, adaptive equipment, and technology. For motor skills, adaptations can be made for decreased skill in posture, movement, and eye-hand skills. In daily living skills, adaptations to increase grooming, dressing, eating, and communication skills can be made. In play situations, toys can be made more accessible, and in work activities, adaptations to promote copying, writing, and organizational skills can be made. The box on p. 376 outlines compensatory instruction guidelines.

### Optometry

Optometry and occupational therapy have common goals related to the effects of vision on performance (Kalb & Warshowsky, 1991). Collaboration is frequent. When a visual dysfunction is identified, sometimes only environmental modifications, such as changes in lighting, desk height, or surface tilt, may alleviate the problem. In many cases glasses (lens therapy) are prescribed to reduce the stress of close work or to correct refractive errors. Other times optometric vision therapy may be prescribed by an optometrist. Through vision therapy, optometrists provide structured visual experiences to enhance basic skills and perception.

### Intervention Strategies

Treatment suggestions are given according to age-groups. However, activities should be analyzed and then selected

**376** *Occupational Therapy Intervention: Performance Areas*

## Compensatory Instruction Guidelines

1. Limit the amount of new material presented in any single lesson.
2. Present new information in a simple, organized way that highlights what is especially pertinent.
3. Be sure the child has factual knowledge.
4. Link up the new information with the information the child already knows.
5. Use all senses.
6. Provide repeated experiences to establish the information securely in long-term memory—practice until the child knows it and does not need to figure it out.
7. Group children with similar learning styles together.

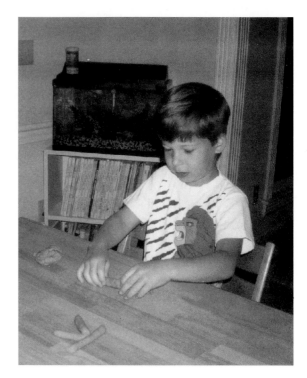

**Figure 14-5** Kyle making letters with clay.

according to the child's needs, rather than according to his or her age-group. These activities illustrate both the developmental and compensatory approaches. Often activities combine approaches. For example, when classroom materials are adapted so that the print is larger and less visual information is presented (compensatory approach), the child might be better able to use visual percetual skills with resulting improvement in those skills (developmental approach).

### Infants

Glass (1993) presented a protocol for working with preterm infants in a neonatal intensive care unit. Dim lighting allows the newborn to spontaneously open his or her eyes. Stimulating the more mature senses (i.e., tactile-vestibular) influences the development of the later maturing ones such as visual (Rose, 1980; Turkewitz & Kenny, 1985). Based on research of neonatal vision, Glass suggested ways to use the human face as the infant's first source of visual stimulation. The intensity, amplitude, and distance of the stimulus are dependent on whether the intent is to arouse or quiet the infant. Glass also recommended beginning with softer, simpler forms and three-dimensional objects and to vary the stimuli on the intent to soothe or arouse the infant. Mobiles hung over cribs should be placed approximately 2 feet above the infant and slightly to one side. This allows for selective attention by the infant. In addition, she suggested that black and white patterns be reserved for full-term infants who are visually impaired and unable to attend to a face or toy. Once a visual response is elicited with the high-contrast pattern, a shift to a pattern with less contrast should be made.

### Preschool and Kindergarten

Occupational therapists can help preschool and kindergarten teachers organize the classroom activities to help children develop the readiness skills needed for visual per-

ception. Teachers should understand the increased need for a multisensory approach with young children who are struggling with shape, letter, and number recognition. For example, the child might benefit from tactile input to help learn shapes, letters, and numbers. By using letters with textures the child has additional sensory experiences on which he or she can rely when visual skills are diminished. Children should be encouraged to feel shapes, letters, and words through their hands and bodies. Letters can be formed with clay, sandpaper, beads, or in chocolate pudding (Figure 14-5).

All preschool, kindergarten, and primary classes should include frequent activities that develop body-in-space concepts. Even with a wide range of levels of understanding among young students, group projects that reinforce body-in-space comprehension through rhyming, joint responses, and paired learning can reach all children.

In the occupational therapy literature a number of publications detail activities for both classroom teachers and therapists and are presented in Appendix 14-A.

### Grade School

Therapy should begin at the level of the visual hierarchy where the child is experiencing difficulty. If the child is experiencing difficulty with visual-receptive skills, the cooperative efforts between the occupational therapist and the optometrist may be necessary.

***Organizing the environment.*** Visual perception affects a child's view of the entire learning environment. Visually distracting and competing information can be problematic

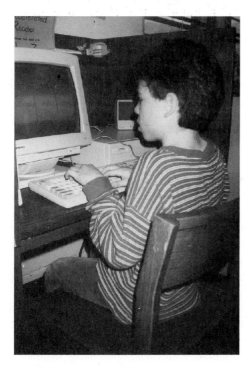

**Figure 14-6**    Todd in a study carrel.

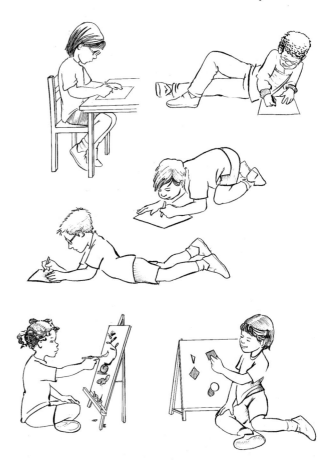

**Figure 14-7**    Alternate positions for visual perceptual activities.

to the child who has not yet fully developed his or her skills. The child may require that the classroom be less "busy" visually to be successful. Limiting a distractable child's peripheral vision by using a carrel is often helpful (Figure 14-6). In addition, levels of illumination and the control of glare needs to be monitored.

The child needs a stable postural base that allows his or her eyes to work. Children often sit at ill-fitting furniture, which can compound their problems. The occupational therapist can assist the teacher in properly positioning children. The therapist could add bolsters to seat backs, put blocks under a child's feet, or provide the child with a slantboard if any of these materials will help the child use vision better or be more productive. The therapist could also stress the importance of encouraging different positions for visual activity. Figure 14-7 illustrates such alternate positions as prone, TV sit position, and side-lying for visual perceptual activities such as reading. Each position should place the child in good alignment and should offer adequate postural support.

Children may benefit from color-coded worksheets to assist them in attending to what visually goes together. However, children with color vision problems have difficulty with educational materials that are color-coded, particularly when the colors are pastel or muddy. Therefore it is important to differentiate an actual visual color deficit from a problem with either color naming or color identification (Ciner et al., 1991).

Christenson and Rascho (1989) proposed strategies to assist the elderly in topographic orientation, which can also be adapted for children. These authors found that use of landmarks and signage can enhance way-finding skills and topographic orientation. They recommended the use of pictures or signs that are realistic, simple, and of high color contrast. For example, a simple, graphic depiction of a lunch tray with food could be used for the cafeteria door.

***Visual attention.*** Following a neurophysiologic frame of reference, general sensory stimulation or inhibition may be done during or before visually oriented activities to improve visual attending skills. If the child is overaroused, the therapist can apply sensory inhibition to calm him or her; if the child is underaroused the therapist selects stimulation activities to alert him or her.

For the child with impaired visual attention, the therapist addresses goals using varied activities and time segments that are achievable. The therapist identifies activities that are intrinsically motivating to the child because these will help maintain the child's attention. The therapist should plan activities together with the child and use as many novel activities as possible. Most challenging to the therapist is the ability to adapt or modify task activities while maintaining a playful learning environment for the child. Elimination of extraneous environmental stimuli is helpful at each level of visual attention.

Developmentally appropriate and visually and tactilely stimulating activities enhance visual attention skills. Manual activities of drawing or manipulating play dough or clay encourage the eyes to view the movements involved (Rogow, 1992). In addition, the hand helps educate the eye about object qualities such as weight, volume, and texture and helps direct the eye to the object (Rogow, 1987). Simultaneous hand and eye movements construct internal representations of objects and serve the function of object recognition.

Activities to compensate for limitations in attention include using a black mat that is larger than the worksheet placed under it to increase high contrast to assist in visual attention to the worksheet, drawing lines to group materials, and reorganizing worksheets (Todd, 1993). Visual stimuli on a worksheet or in a book can be reduced by covering all of the page except the activity on which the student is working or by using a mask that uncovers one line at a time (Figure 14-8). Reducing competing sensory input in both the auditory and visual modalities can be helpful for some students with poor visual attention. For example, headphones can be worn when working on a visual task. Good lighting and use of pastel-colored paper helps reduce the glare. Additionally, encouraging children to search for high-interest photographs or pictures can help increase visual attention skills (Rogow, 1992). *Where's Waldo* and other similar books are highly motivating and encourage children to develop search strategies and visual attention. Other suggestions include cuing the child to important visual information by using a finger to point, a marker to underline, or therapist verbalization to help the child maintain visual attention. Cooper (1975) found that subjects tended to look at a picture when it was named. The therapist can use large colorful pictures combined with rhyming chants to encourage attention to the pictures (Rogow, 1992). Vi-

sual work should be presented when the student's energy is highest and not when he or she is fatigued (Rogow, 1992).

***Visual memory.*** Children with visual memory problems need repeated consistent experiences; therefore the therapist should consult with the parents and teachers so that these activities can be done at home and in the classroom. Grouping information in ways that provide retrieval cues can help a child remember interrelated data. Several strategies may be helpful. "Chunking" is organizing information into smaller units or chunks. This can be done by cutting up worksheets and presenting one unit or task at a time. "Maintenance rehearsal" (repetition) helps the child hold information in his or her short-term memory but seems to have no effect on long-term storage. An example of this strategy would be repeating a phone number until the number is dialed. "Elaborative rehearsal" is a strategy in which new information is consciously related to knowledge already stored in long-term memory. By the time a child is 8 years old, he or she can rehearse more than one item at a time and can rehearse information together as a set to remember. Children can also relate ideas to more than one other idea. Mnemonic devices are memory-directed tactics that help transform or organize information to enhance its retrievability through use of language cues such as songs, rhymes, and acronyms. Gibson (1971) suggested that memory is composed primarily of distinctive features (what makes something different). Occupational therapists can help the child determine differences in visual stimuli to promote storage into memory. Games such as concentration, copying a sequence after viewing it for a few seconds, or remembering what was removed from a tray of several items can be enjoyable ways to increase visual memory. The therapist first provides the student with short, simple tasks that the child can complete quickly and with success; then gradually, as the student accomplishes tasks, the therapist increases the length and complexity of the tasks.

***Visual discrimination.*** The therapist must use task analysis to design an intervention program. By analyzing the continuum of a task, the therapist can grade the activity from simple to complex to allow success while challenging the child's visual abilities (Blanksby, 1992). Remediation therefore should follow an orderly design (Bouska et al., 1990) so that the child can make sense of each performance. Intervention strategies should aim to help children recognize and attend to the identifying features by teaching them to use their vision to locate objects and then to use object features as well as other cues to form identification hypotheses. Teaching children to visually scan or search pictures instructs the child on the value of looking and finding meaning. With high-interest materials the therapist can teach the child to look from top to bottom and left to right (Rogow, 1992). Using pictures from magazines, the therapist removes an important part of a picture and asks the student

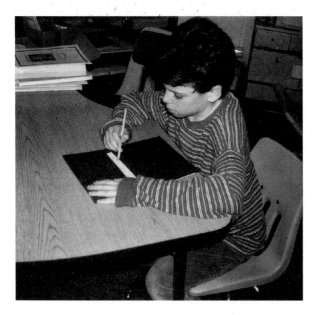

**Figure 14-8** Todd's mask uncovers one line at a time.

to identify what part is missing. Drawing, painting, and other art and craft activities encourage exploration and manipulation of visual forms. As the child moves from awareness to attention and then to selection, he or she becomes better able to discriminate between the important and unimportant features of the environment.

Occupational therapists can assist teachers in reorganizing the child's worksheets. Color coding different problems may assist the child in visually attending to the correct section. Worksheets can also be cut up and reorganized to match the child's visual needs. It is important to gradually fade out the restructuring of the worksheets so the child can eventually use the sheets as they are presented in the workbooks.

When a child has problems copying from the chalkboard, an occupational therapist might recommend that the chalkboard be regularly cleaned in an effort to provide high contrast for chalk marks. Notations on chalkboard, bulletin boards, or overhead transparencies should be color coded, well spaced, and uncluttered. These practices may reduce figure-ground problems. The therapist may also suggest that a teacher reduce use of the chalkboard by having the children copy from one paper to another with both papers in the same plane. A teacher may be encouraged to try bean bag games in which the targets are placed at approximately the same distance from the child's eyes as is the chalkboard so that a student can practice focusing and fixating eyes near and far in play.

Students with figure-ground difficulties are helped by reducing the amount of print on a page (less print, fewer math problems) and providing math problems on graph paper so that the numbers are in columns in the ones, tens, and hundreds places. Masking the part of the worksheet that is not being worked on can help the child focus on one problem at a time. Cooper (1985) proposed a theoretical model for the implementation of color contrast to enhance visual ability in the elderly. Principles of color contrast and the ways in which color contrast can be achieved by varying hue, brightness, or color saturation of an object in relation to its environment is the foundation of the method of intervention. This helps a child identify the relevant information, such as the classroom materials and supplies.

***Decoding problems in reading.*** Children with difficulty distinguishing between similar visual symbols may benefit from a multisensory approach. This includes tracing the shapes and letters, hearing them, saying them, and then feeling them. This permits a number of routes of processing to help supplement weak visual perceptual processing. Thus the child sees it, hears it, traces it, and writes it. Eating letters is an activity loved by children; alphabet cereal, gelatin jigglers, cookies, and french fries in the shape of letters can be served for snack. The children can trace the letters with frosting from tubes onto cookies and catsup from packets for french fries.

For children with word recognition difficulty, the initial emphasis should be on recognition rather than retrieval. The child can be given a choice of visually similar words to complete sentences that have single words missing. In addition, word recognition skills can be enhanced by using word families (ball, call, and tall) to increase sight vocabulary. Phonic approaches may also be the best reading instruction method for children with poor word recognition. Textbooks recorded on audiotape cassettes can be ordered from local and state libraries from the American Printing House for the Blind, Louisville, Kentucky. The student can then hear the textbook as well as read it.

If the child has strong verbal skills, verbal mediation (talking through) printed words should be stressed, and the child could be encouraged to describe what he or she sees to retain the information. A strategy that may assist a child who reverses letters in words is to follow along the printed lines with a finger. This technique helps stress reading the letters in the correct sequence. Reading material rich in pictorial content such as comic books, pictures with captions and cartoons, and computer software designed to enhance sight vocabulary can strengthen these associations.

***Visualization.*** The development of visualization techniques or visual imagery may be delayed. Like all skills, this proceeds from the concrete to the abstract. Therapists can start by helping students picture something they can touch or feel. Using a grab bag while the child has vision occluded is a good way to do this.

As material becomes less concrete, more visual skills are drawn into play. A student might be asked to visualize something he or she has done. The occupational therapist can facilitate the child's thinking by reminding him or her to consider various factors such as color, brightness, size, sounds, temperature, space, movement, smells, and tastes. Hopefully once the child practices orally, he or she will generalize the visualization process to reading. There are a number of good resources that detail the development of visualization (Bell, 1991; Vitale, 1982).

Children with poor visualization may have difficulty spelling and may need to learn spelling rules thoroughly. They may also demonstrate reading comprehension problems. In addition, they may have difficulty forming letters because they are unable to visualize them. In handwriting, the child may reverse letters and may have difficulty aligning numbers in columns for math.

***Learning styles.*** All students have a preferred learning style (Carbo, Dunn, & Dunn, 1986). When a student is taught through his or her preferred style, the child can learn with less effort and remember better. Figure 14-9 illustrates diagnostic learning styles. All students need to be taught through their strongest senses and then reinforced through their next strongest sense.

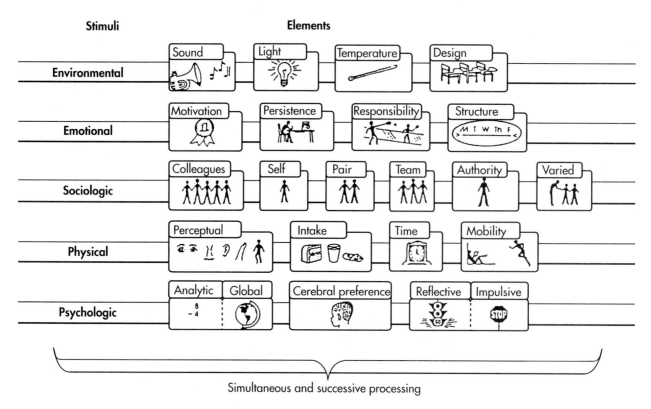

**Figure 14-9** Diagnostic learning styles. (From Rita Dunn, Ed.D. Director, Learning Styles Network, The Center for the Study of Learning and Teaching Styles, School of Education & Human Services, St. John's University, Jamaica, NY.)

Auditory learners are those who recall at least 75% of what is discussed or heard in a normal 40- to 45-minute period (Carbo, Dunn, & Dunn, 1986). Visual learners remember what they see and can retrieve details and events by concentrating on the things they have seen. Tactual and kinesthetic learners assimilate best by touching, manipulating, and handling objects. They remember more easily when they write, doodle, draw, or move their fingers. It is best to introduce material to them through art activities, baking, cooking, building, making, interviewing, and through acting experiences. If a child has weaknesses in visual processing, it is more difficult for him or her to learn through the visual sense. Therefore the occupational therapist can assist the teacher in identifying a child's perceptual strengths for learning. This child may learn more effectively through the kinesthetic and tactile senses. (See the box on p. 381 for suggestions for kinesthetic learning.)

Occupational therapists can greatly assist teachers by helping to determine a child's perceptual strengths and weaknesses so that an appropriate reading program can be matched to the child's preferred perceptual modality. Once the child is in first grade, it is important to determine what reading program the teacher is using. Table 14-7 matches reading methods to perceptual strengths and weaknesses and global and analytic styles. For example, the Orton-Gillingham method (Gillingham & Stillman, 1968; Orton, 1937) teaches decoding through a multisensory approach.

In addition to perceptual strengths, the therapist must also keep in mind the child's preferred manner of approaching new material. For instance, global learners require an overall comprehension first and then can attend to the details. Analytic learners piece details together to form an understanding.

**Visual-Motor Integration**

To review, the therapist should first focus on the underlying visual-receptive functions and then focus on the visual-cognitive functions. This should precede in the sequence of visual attention, visual memory, visual discrimination, and finally focusing on specific visual discrimination skills. A multisensory approach to handwriting may be helpful to a child with visual-cognitive problems. Working with eyes closed can be effective in reducing the influence of increased effort that vision can create as well as lessen the visual distractions. Keeping the eyes closed can also improve the awareness of the kinesthetic feedback from letter formation.

Use of a vibrating pen provides augmented tactile input to the child's hand during handwriting and can reinforce learning correct letter formation. The child whose preferred learning style is through the auditory system can be assisted in learning handwriting through use of a talking pen. The kinesthetic writing program described by Benbow, Hanft, and Marsh (1992) has many strategies for teaching hand-

▲ Table 14-7  Matching Reading Methods to Perceptual Strengths

| Reading Method | Description | Reading-Style Requirements |
|---|---|---|
| Phonics | Isolated letter sounds or letter clusters are taught sequentially and blended to form words. | Auditory and analytic strengths. |
| Linguistic | Patterns of letters are taught and combined to form words. | Auditory and analytic strengths. |
| Orton-Gillingham | Method consists of phonics and tactile stimulation in the form of writing and tracing activities. | Auditory and analytic strengths combined with visual weaknesses. |
| Whole-word | Before reading a story, new words are presented on flash cards and in sentences, with accompanying pictures. | Visual and global strengths. |
| Language-experience | Students read stories that they write. | Visual, tactile, and global strengths. |
| Fernald | Language-experience method and student traces over new words with index finger of writing hand. | Tactile and global strengths combined with visual weaknesses. |
| Choral reading | Groups read a text in unison. | Visual and global strengths. |
| Recorded book | Students listen two or three times to brief recordings of books, visually track the words, then read the selection aloud. | Visual and global strengths. |

From Carbo, M. (1987). Deprogramming reading failure: giving unequal learners an equal chance. *Phi Delta Kappan, Nov.,* p. 35.

# Suggestions for Tactile and Kinesthetic Learners

▲ At storytime give the child a prop that relates to the story—the child could act out something they just heard using the prop
▲ Provide letter cubes to make words
▲ The student can build models and projects following simple written and recorded directions (see and hear written directions simultaneously, which increases their understanding and retention) (Carbo, Dunn, & Dunn, 1986)
▲ Use games such as bingo, dominoes, or card games to teach or review reading skills—these activities allow movement as well as peer and adult interaction
▲ Use writing activity cards—paste colorful, high-interest pictures on index cards and add stimulating questions (Carbo, Dunn, & Dunn, 1986)
▲ Use a tape player and filmstrips
▲ Children could actively participate while they read—for example, children could write while they read, underline or circle key words, place an asterick in the margin next to an important section, and inscribe comments when appropriate
▲ Use glue letters
▲ Use blocks from Boggle game
▲ Play Scrabble

writing through kinesthesia. Handwriting programs that are easier for children with visual-cognitive problems include D'Nealian, Loops and Other Groups (Benbow, 1990), and Printing Power and Cursive Writing (Olsen, 1993a,b). Olsen described strategies to help children correct or avoid reversals. During handwriting lessons the child should proofread his or her own work and circle the best-formed letters. Chapter 19 has comprehensive information on developing handwriting skills.

Children with visual spatial problems often choose random starting points, which can confuse the writing task from the onset. Concrete cues must be used to teach abstract handwriting concepts. For example, colored lines on the paper or paper with raised lines can be helpful for the child who is having trouble knowing where to place the letters on the page. In addition, green lines drawn to symbolize *go* on the left side of the paper and red lines to symbolize *stop* on the right side may help a child know which direction to write his or her letters and words. Upright orientation of the writing surface may also lessen directional confusion of letter formation (up means up and down means down) versus at a desk on a horizontal surface, where up means away from oneself and down means toward oneself.

Directional cues can be paired with verbal cues for the child who commonly reverses letters and numbers. These cognitive cues rely on visual images for distinguishing letters and include the following:

1. With palms facing the chest and thumbs up, the student makes two fists. The left hand will form a *b* and the right hand will form a *d*.
2. Lower-case *b* is like *B*, only without the top loop.
3. To make a lower case *d,* remember *c* comes first, then add a line to make a *d*.

The therapist can develop cue cards for the student to keep at his or her desk with common reversals.

Children with visual-cognitive problems often overspace or underspace words. The correct space should be slightly more than the width of a single lower-case letter. When a child has handwriting spacing problems, the occupational therapist may recommend a decorated tongue depressor to

## CASE STUDY #1

Todd was a 9-year-old student in the third grade. The majority of his day was spent in the regular third-grade classroom, where he functioned at grade level in all areas of academics except in reading. Todd received daily resource room instruction in this area. His resource instruction consisted of copying, worksheet completion, and drill and repetition techniques and did not include opportunities for manipulative activities.

An occupational therapy evaluation indicated that Todd's perceptual skills were about 2 years delayed, with weaknesses noted in visual-spatial relations, figure-ground perception, and visual sequential memory. From interviewing the teacher the therapist learned that Todd was not moving from learning to read to reading to learn. His decoding was not automatic, and therefore he spent considerable time figuring out what the words were rather than comprehending what he was reading. He also reported that his eyes tired easily while reading. Good eye movements were now needed to sustain reading for longer periods. Because of poor spatial abilities, Todd had difficulty discerning differences in visually similar symbols and had difficulty with words that only differed by sequence (*three* and *there*) or spatial orientation (*dad* and *bad*). The third-grade reading books had more print per page and fewer illustrations to give cues. Too many words on the page made it difficult for Todd because of his poor figure-ground abilities. He demonstrated an inability to recall exact order of words, poor sight vocabulary, and poor spelling caused by poor visual sequential memory.

The therapist referred Todd for optometric evaluation because of his reported visual fatigue during reading tasks. Planning together with Todd, the therapist developed strategies to assist him in increasing his visual memory. Initially short visual memory tasks were used, and then gradually the length of tasks was increased. This was done using visual memory games and activities on the computer. In addition, visual discrimination tasks were started, beginning with simple forms and moving to more complex forms.

In consultation with the teacher, the therapist recommended decreasing the amount of print per page and masking what was not immediately needed, when this could not be done. Phonics approaches to word recognition were recommended (Table 14-7), as was using verbal mediation to decode words.

## STUDY QUESTIONS

1. Describe the relationship of the visual receptive and the visual cognitive components.
2. What are the differences between object (form) vision and spatial vision? Describe different forms of each.
3. What could an occupational therapist recommend to a second-grade teacher for a child with difficulties in visual attention?

use for spacing words, a pencil, or simply have the child use his finger as a guide. The child can also imagine a letter in the space to aid in judging the distance.

When students need additional help to stop at lines, templates with windows can be used in teaching handwriting. These templates can be made out of cardboard with three windows; one for one-line letters (*a, c, e, i, m,* and *n*), one for two-line letters (*b, d, k, l,* and *t*), and another window for three-line letters (*f, g, j, p, q, z,* and *y*). It is important to consider that visual memory is used to recognize the letters or words to be written, and motor memory starts the engram for producing the written product. Therefore it may be that motor memory, not visual memory, is the basis for the problem (see Chapter 19).

### Computers

Many wonderful educational computer programs for young children are already on the market that the occupational therapist could use. Computers with a CD-ROM have software programs available that are highly motivating for children of all ages. Living books on the computer reinforce the written word with the spoken word and assist in developing a sight word vocabulary.

The computer can be used as a motivational device to assist in increasing the child's attention to the task. The computer also provides a way to practice skills in an independent manner. Drill and practice software record data on accuracy and time taken to complete the drills, thus allowing the therapist to record the child's progress. The computer program can be adapted by the therapist by changing the background colors to those that enhance the child's visual perceptual skills. The therapist can also enlarge the written information so that there is less information on the screen.

## SUMMARY

Children with visual perceptual problems often receive the services of occupational therapists. This chapter described a developmental approach in which the underlying components of visual receptive and visual cognitive skills were identified. The relationship of these components to various performance areas was described. Using the developmental approach, the occupational therapist helps the child increase his visual perceptual skills by improving his or her underlying components of performance. By adapting classroom materials and instruction methods, the therapist also helps the child compensate for visual perception problems. Intervention often includes a combination of developmental and compensatory activities. This holistic approach enables the child with visual perceptual problems to achieve optimal function and learning.

## REFERENCES

Abercrombie, M.L.J. (1963). Eye movements, perception, learning. In *Visual disorders and cerebral palsy*. London: William Heinemann.

Ayres, A.J. (1979). *Sensory integration and the child*. Los Angeles: Western Psychological Services.

Beery, K.E. (1989). *Developmental Test of Visual-Motor Integration*. Cleveland: Modern Curriculum Press.

Bell, N. (1991). *Visualizing and verbalizing for language comprehension and thinking*. Paso Robles, CA: Academy of Reading Publishers.

Benbow, M. (1990). *Loops and other groups*. Tucson: Therapy Skill Builders.

Benbow, M., Hanft, B., & Marsh, D. (1992). Handwriting in the classroom: improving written communication. In C.B. Royeen (Ed.). *AOTA self study series: classroom applications for school-based practice*. Rockville, MD: AOTA.

Bender, C.L. (1963). *Bender Visual-Motor Gestalt Test*. Cleveland: The Psychological Corporation.

Benton, A.L. (1974). *Benton Visual Retention Test* Chicago: The Psychological Corporation.

Birch, H.G. (1964). *Brain damage in children: the biological and social aspects*. New York: Williams & Wilkins.

Blanksby, B.S. (1992). Visual therapy: a theoretically based intervention program. *Journal of Visual Impairment and Blindness, 86*, 291-294.

Bouska, M.J., Kauffman, N.A., & Marcus, S.E. (1990). Disorders of the visual perception system. In D. Umphred (Ed.). *Neurological rehabilitation* (2nd ed.). St. Louis: Mosby.

Boder, E. (1973). Developmental dyslexia: a diagnostic approach based on three atypical reading-spelling patterns. *Developmental Medicine and Child Neurology, 15*, 661.

Breakey, A.S., Wilson, J.J., & Wilson, B.C. (1994). Sensory and perceptual functions in the cerebral palsied. *Journal of Nervous and Mental Diseases, 158*, 70-77.

Bruininks, R.H. (1978). *Bruininks-Oseretsky Test of Motor Proficiency*, Circle Pines, MN: American Guidance Service.

Cairns, E. & Cammock, T. (1978). Development of a more reliable version of the matching familiar figures test. *Developmental Psychology, 14*,555.

Carbo, M. (1980). An analysis of the relationship between the modality preferences of kindergartners and selected reading treatments as they affect the learning of a basic sight-word vocabulary. Doctoral Dissertation, Jamaica, NY: St. John's University.

Carbo, M. (1983). Reading styles change from second to eighth grade. *Education Leadership, 40*, 56-59.

Carbo, M. (1987). Deprogramming reading failure: giving unequal learners an equal chance. *Phi Delta Kappan, Nov.*, p. 35.

Carbo, M., Dunn, R., & Dunn, K. (1986). *Teaching students to read through their individual learning styles*. Englewood Cliffs, NJ: Prentice-Hall.

Caron, A. & Caron, R. (1981). Processing of relational information as an index of infant risk. In S. Friedman & M. Sigman (Eds.). *Preterm birth and psychological development*. New York: Academic Press.

Carroll, J.L. (1975). *Visual memory scale*. Mt Pleasant, MI: Carroll Publications.

Chapman, L.J. & Wedell, K. (1972). Perceptual-motor abilities and reversal errors in children's handwriting. *Journal of Learning Disabilities, 5*, 321-325.

Christenson, M.A. & Rascho, B. (1989). Environmental cognition and age-related sensory change. *Occupational Therapy Practice, 1*, 28-35.

Ciner, E.B., Macks, B., & Schanel-Klitsch, E. (1991). A cooperative demonstration project for early intervention vision services. *Occupational Therapy Practice, 3*(1), 42-56.

Cohen, K.M. (1981). The development of strategies of visual search. In D.F. Fisher, R.A. Monty, & J.W. Senders (Eds.). *Eye movements: cognition and visual perception*. Hillsdale, NJ: Lawrence Erlbaum.

Colarusso, R.P.& Hammill, D.D. (1972). *Motor-Free Visual Perception Test*. Novato, CA: Academic Therapy Publications.

Cooper, B.A. (1985). A model for implementing color contrast in the environment of the elderly, *American Journal of Occupational Therapy, 39*, 253-258.

Cooper, L.A. (1975). Mental rotation of random tow-dimensional shapes. *Cognitive Psychology. 7*(2), 20-43.

Cowan, M.K. (1993). *Overview of therapeutic approaches*. Lecture notes from OTS 352, Occupational Therapy for Infants and Children. Richmond: Eastern Kentucky University.

Crane, A. & Wick, B. (1987). *Crane-Wick Test*. Houston: Rapid Research Corporation.

Cratty, B.J. (1970), *Perceptual and motor development in infants and children*, New York: Macmillan.

Daniels, L.E. & Ryley, C. (1991). Visual perceptual and visual motor performance in children with psychiatric disorders. *Canadian Journal of Occupational Therapy, 58*(30), 137-141.

deHirsch, K., Jansky, J., & Lanford, W. (1966). *Predicting reading failure*. New York: Harper & Row.

DeQuiros, J.B. & Schranger, O.L. (1979), *Neuropsychological fundamentals in learning disabilities*. Novato, CA: Academic Therapy Publications.

Duckman, R. (1979). The incidence of anomalies in a population of cerebral palsied children. *Journal of the American Optometric Association, 50*, 1013.

Enns, J.T. & Cameron, S. (1987). Selective attention in young children: the relation between visual search, filtering, and priming. *Journal of Experimental Child Psychology, 44*, 38-63.

Erhardt, R.P. (1989). *Erhardt Developmental Vision Assessment (EDVA)* (rev. ed.).Tucson: Therapy Skill Builders.

Fanning, G.S. (1971). Vision in children with Down's syndrome. *Australian Journal of Optometry, 54*, 74.

Flax, N. (1984). Visual perception versus visual function. *Journal of Learning Disabilities, 17*, 182-185.

Fledelius, T. (1976). Prematurity and the eye. *Acta Ophthalmology*, 128-134.

Frostig, M., Lefever, W., Whittlesey, J.R.B. (1966). *Administration and scoring manual for the Marianne Frostig Developmental Test of Visual Perception*. Palo Alto, CA: Consulting Psychologists Press.

Gardner, M.F. (1982). *Test of Visual-Perceptual Skills (TVPS)*. Seattle: Special Child Publications.

Gardner, M.F. (1992). *Test of Pictures-Forms-Letters-Numbers-Spatial Orientation & Sequencing Skills,* Burlington, CA: Psychological and Educational Publications.

Gardner, R.A. (1978). *Reversals frequency test.* Cresskill, NJ: Creative Therapeutics.

Garling, R., Book, A., & Lindberg, E. (1984). Cognitive mapping of large-scale environments: the interrelationship of action plans, acquisition and orientation. *Environment and Behavior, 16,* 3-34.

Gibson, E.J. (1971). Perceptual learning and the theory of word perception. *Cognitive Psychology, 2,* 351.

Gibson, E.J. & Levin, H. (1975). *The psychology of reading.* Cambridge, MA: The MIT Press.

Gilfoyle, E., Grady, A. & Moore, J. (1990). *Children adapt.* (2nd ed.). Thorofare, NJ: Slack.

Gillingham, A. & Stillman, B. (1968). *Remedial teaching for children with specific disability in reading, spelling and penmanship.* Cambridge, MA: Educator's Publishing Service.

Glass, P. (1993). Development of visual function in preterm infants: implications for early intervention. *Infants and Young Children, 6*(1), 11-20.

Graham, F.K. & Kendall, B.S. (1960). Memory for Designs Test-revised. *Perceptual Motor Skills (Monograph Supplement 2-VII), 11,* 147-188.

Greene, L.J. (1987). Learning disabled and your child: a survival handbook. New York: Ballantine Books.

Hammill, D.D., Pearson, N.A., & Voress J.K. (1993). *Developmental Test of Visual Perception* (2nd ed.). Austin, TX: Pro Ed.

Hellerstein, L. & Fishman, B. (1987). Vision therapy and occupational therapy: an integrated approach. *American Occupational Therapy Sensory Integration Special Interest Section Newsletter, 10*(3), 4-5.

Hung, S.S., Fisher, A.G., & Cermak, S.A. (1987). The performance of learning-disabled and normal young men on the test of visual-perceptual skills. *American Journal of Occupational Therapy, 41,* 790-797.

Hyvarinen, L. (1988). *Vision in children: normal and abnormal.* Medford, Ontario: Canadian Deaf, Blind and Rubella Association.

Ilg, F.L., & Ames, L.B. (1981). *School readiness.* New York: Harper & Row.

Jansky, J. & deHirsh, K. (1972). *Preventing reading failure: prediction, diagnosis, and intervention.* New York: Harper & Row.

Jordon, B.A. (1980). *Jordon Left - Right Reversal Test* (2nd ed.). Los Angeles: Western Psychological Services.

Kalb, L. & Warshowsky, J.H. (1991). Occupational therapy and optometry: principles of diagnosis and collaborative treatment of learning disabilities in children. *Occupational Therapy Practice, 3*(1), 77-87.

Kaufman, A.S. & Kaufman, N.L. (1983). *Kaufman Assessment Battery for Children.* Circle Pines, MN: American Guidance Service.

Kirby, J. & Das, J.P. (1978). Information processing and human abilities. *Journal of Educational Psychology, 70.*

Koppitz, E.M. (1963). *The Bender Visual-Motor Gestalt Test for Young Children.* New York: Grune & Stratton.

Kwatney, E. & Bouska, M.J. (1980). Visual system disorders and functional correlates: final report. Philadelphia: Temple University Rehabilitation and Training Center No. 8.

Langley, M.B. (1980). *Functional vision inventory for the severely/profoundly handicapped.* Chicago: Stoelting.

Laurendau, M. & Pinard, A. (1970). *Development of the concept of space in the child.* New York: International University Press.

Leigh, R.J. & Zee, D.S. (1983). *Neurology of eye movements.* Philadelphia: F.A. Davis.

Levine, M. (1985). *The ANSER system.* Cambridge, MA: Educator's Publishing Service.

Levine, M. (1987). *Developmental variation and learning disorders.* Cambridge, MA: Educators Publishing Service.

Levine, M. & Rapport, L. (1983). *The ANSER system.* Cambridge, MA: Educator's Publishing Service.

Luria, A. (1966). *Higher cortical functions in man.* New York: Basic Books.

Lyle, J.G. (1969). Reading retardation and reversal tendency: a factorial study. *Child Development, 40,* 833-843.

Marr, D. (1982). *Vision.* San Francisco: Freeman.

Menken, C., Cermak, S.A., & Fisher, A.G. (1987). Evaluating the visual-perceptual skills of children with cerebral palsy. *American Journal of Occupational Therapy, 41*(10), 646-651.

Mishkin, M., Ungerleider, L., & Macko, K. (1983). Object vision and spatial vision: two cortical pathways. *Trends in Neuroscience, 6,* 414-417.

Moore, R.S. (1979). *School can wait.* Provo, UT: Bigham Young University Press.

Morency, A. & Wepman, J. (1973). Early perceptual ability and later school achievement. *Elementary School Journal, 73,* 323.

Mussen, P.H., Conger, J.J., Kagan, J. (1979). *Child development and personality.* (5th ed.). New York: Harper & Row.

Necombe, F. & Ratcliff, G. (1989). Disorders of spatial analysis. In E. Boller & J. Grafman (Eds.). *Handbook of Neuropsychology. Vol. 2.* New York: Elsevier Science.

Nolte, J. (1988). *The human brain,* (2nd ed.). St. Louis: Mosby.

Olsen, J.Z. (1993). *Cursive handwriting.* Potomac, MD: Olsen.

Olsen, J.Z. (1993). *Printing power.* Potomac, MD: Olsen.

Optometric Extension Program Foundation. (1985). Santa Ana, CA: 92705.

Orton, S.T. (1937). *Reading, writing, and speech problems in children.* New York: W.W. Norton.

Piaget, J. (1964). *Development and learning.* Ithaca, NY: Cornell University Press.

Rafal, R.D. & Posner, M.I. (1987). Cognitive theories of attention and the rehabilitation of attentional deficits. In M. J. Meier, A. L. Benton, & L. Diller (Eds.). *Neuropsychological rehabilitation.* New York: Guilford.

Ratcliff, G. (1987). Perception and complex visual processes. In M. J. Meier, A.L. Benton, & L. Diller (Eds.). *Neuropsychological rehabilitation* (pp 182-201). New York: Guilford.

Restak, R. (1979). *The brain: the last frontier.* New York: Doubleday.

Richards, R.G. & Oppenheim, G.S. (1984). *Visual skills appraisal.* Novato, CA: Academic Therapy Publications

Richter, E. & Montgomery, P. (1991). *The sensorimotor performance analysis.* Hugo, MN: PDP Products.

Ritty, J.M., Solan, H., & Cool, S.J. (1993). Visual and sensory-motor functioning in the classroom: a preliminary report of ergonomic demands. *Journal of the American Optometric Association 64*(4), 238-244.

Rogow, S.M. (1987). The ways of the hand: hand function in blind, visually impaired, and visually impaired multiply handicapped children. *British Journal of Visual Impairment, 5*(2), 58-63.

Rogow, S.M. (1992). Visual perceptual problems of visually impaired children with developmental disabilities. *Review, 25*(2), 57-64.

Rogow, S.M. & Rathwill, D. (1989). Seeing and knowing: an investigation of visual perception among children with severe visual impairments. *Journal of Vision Rehabilitation, 3*(3), 55-66.

Rose, S.A. (1980). Enhancing visual recognition memory in preterm infants. *Developmental Psychology, 16,* 85.

Rosenhall, J., Johansson, E., & Gilberg, C. (1988). Oculomotor findings in autistic children. *Journal of Laryngeal Otology, 102,* 435-439.

Scheiman, M. (1984). Optometric findings in children with cerebral palsy. *American Journal of Optometric Physiology Opt., 61,* 321-323.

Scheirman, M. (1991). Pediatric clinical vision screening for occupational therapists. Pennsylvania College of Optometry.

Seiderman, A.S. (1984). Visual perception versus visual function. *Journal of Learning Disabilities, 17,* 182-185.

Seiderman, A.S. & Marcus, S.E. (1990). *20/20 is not enough: the new world of vision.* New York: Alfred B. Knopf.

Sigman, M. & Parmelee, A. (1974). Visual preferences of four month old premature and fullterm infants. *Child Development, 45,* 969-965.

Siegel, L. (1983). The prediction of possible learning disabilities in preterm and fullterm children. In T. Field & A. Sostek (Eds.). *Infants born at risk: physiological, perceptual, and cognitive processes.* New York: Grune & Stratton.

Skeffington, A.N. (1963), *The Skeffington Papers,* November, 1963, Series 36, #2 (p. 11). Santa Ana, CA: Optometric Extension Program.

Solan, H.A. & Ciner, E. B. (1986). *Visual perception and learning: issues and answers.* New York: SUNY College of Optometry.

Suchoff, I.B. (1968). *Birch-Belmont Auditory-Visual Integration Test (AVIT).* Santa Ana, CA: Optometric Extension Program.

Suchoff, I.B. (1987). *Visual-spatial development in the child.* 2nd Printing. New York: State University of New York, State College of Optometry.

Todd, V.R. (1993). Visual perceptual frame of reference: an information processing approach. In P. Kramer & J. Hinojosa (Eds.). *Frames of reference for pediatric occupational therapy* (pp.177-232). Baltimore: Williams & Wilkins.

Tseng, M.H. & Cermak, S.A. (1993). The influence of ergonomic factors and perceptual-motor abilities on handwriting performance. *The American Journal of Occupational Therapy, 47*(10), 919-926.

Tseng, M.H. & Murray, E.A. (1994). Differences in perceptual-motor measures in children with good and poor handwriting. *The Occupational Therapy Journal of Research, 14*(1), 19-36.

Turkewitz, G. & Kenny, P.A. (1985). The role of developmental limitations of sensory input on sensory/perceptual organization. *Developmental Behavioral Pediatrics, 6,* 302.

Ulman, S. (1986). Visual routines. In S. Pinker (Ed.). *Visual cognition.* Cambridge: MIT Press.

Vitale, B. (1982). *Unicorns are real.* Hill Estates, CA: Jalmar Press.

Warren, M. (1990). Identification of visual scanning deficits in adults after CVA. *American Journal of Occupational Therapy, 44,* 391-399.

Warren, M. (1993a). A hierarchical model for evaluation and treatment of visual perceptual dysfunction in adult acquired brain injury. Part 1. *American Journal of Occupational Therapy, 47*(1), 42-54.

Warren, M. (1993b). A hierarchical model for evaluation and treatment of visual perceptual dysfunction in adult acquired brain injury. Part 2. *American Journal of Occupation Therapy, 47*(1), 55-66.

Wechsler, D. (1991). *Wechsler Intelligence Scale for Children-III.* New York: Psychological Corporation.

Williams, H. (1983). *Perceptual and motor development.* Englewood Cliffs, NJ: Prentice-Hall.

Williamson, T. (1994). *OK Vision Test.* Farmersville, OH: Vision Lyceum.

Wing, L. (1976). *Early childhood autism* (2nd ed.). New York: Pergamon Press.

Yost, L. W. & Lesiak, J. (1980). The relationship between performance on the developmental test of visual perception and handwriting ability. *Education, 101,* 75-77.

Zaba, J. (1984). Visual perception versus visual function. *Journal of Learning Disabilities, 17,* 182-185.

Ziviani, J., Hayes, A., & Chant, D. (1990). Handwriting: a perceptual motor disturbance in children with myelomeningocele. *Occupational Therapy Journal of Research, 10,* 12-26.

# APPENDIX

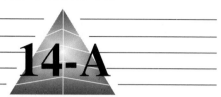

## 14-A

## Publications on Classroom Activities

1. *Sensory Motor Handbook* (Bissell et al., 1988). A wonderful guide for implementing and modifying activities in the classroom. Both visual perceptual and spatial concerns are addressed. Exercises are indexed according to the skill that they are designed to remediate.

2. *Little Kim's Left and Right Book* (McMonnies, 1992). A picture book for preschoolers that is very appealing.

3. *A Practical Guide for Remedial Approaches to Left/Right Confusion and Reversals,* (McMonnies, 1991).

4. *Overcoming Left/Right Confusion and Reversals: A Classroom Approach* (McMonnies, 1992). Includes group and individual remediation exercises for older children. These 18 remedial procedures outlined by McMonnies follow a developmental sequence, starting with body awareness in regard to oneself, which is used as a basis for acquiring an ability to project that internal awareness into space (directionality). The aim is to provide variety to activities that will establish an internal/automatic/reflex/somatesthetic awareness of right and left that does not depend on external cues such as identifying the writing hand, watch-wearing hand, or ring-wearing hand. Specific activities are used to help children overcome difficulty with left-to-right reading. All of McMonnies materials are being distributed in this country through the Optometric Extension Program (OEP), Santa Ana, CA.

5. *Reversal Errors: Theories and Therapy Procedures* (Lane, 1988), and *Developing Your Child for Success* (Lane, 1991). For use by the school-based practitioner, teachers, and parents.

6. *Classroom Visual Activities* (CVA) (Richards, 1988). More than two dozen exercises are provided to remediate underlying laterality, directionality, and midline problems, as well as activities focused on the underlying visual skills necessary to achieve efficient visual perception. They have categorized these exercises by the areas addressed, which include muscle movement, oculomotor skills, accommodation, and visualization.

7. *Songs for Sensory Integration, The Calming Tape, and The Vision Tape* (Hickman, 1992). Auditory tapes. The latter is narrated by optometrist Lynn Hellerstein. Included is a clear, simple explanation of vision and exercises that can be used to supplement optometric vision therapy.

8. For children who are having trouble remembering letters, and their sounds, Pavlak (1985) presents 41 letter- and letter-sound recognition activities and 52 consonant- and vowel-recognition activities.

## REFERENCES

Bissell, J., Fisher, J., Owens, C., & Polcyn, P. (1988). *Sensory motor handbook.* Torrance, CA: Sensory Integration International.

Hickman, L. (1992). *Songs for sensory integration. The calming tape, and* The vision tape. Boulder, CO: Belle Curve Records.

Lane, K.A. (1988). *Reversal errors theories and therapy procedures.* Santa Ana, CA: Vision Extension.

Lane, K.A. (1991). *Developing your child for success.* Santa Ana, CA: Vision Extension.

McMonnies, C.W. (1991). *A practical guide for remedial approaches to left/right confusion and reversals.* Sydney, Australia: Superior Educational Publication.

McMonnies, C.W. (1992). *Little Kim's left and right book.* Sydney, Australia: Superior Educational Publications.

McMonnies, C.W. (1992). *Overcoming left/right confusion and reversals: a classroom approach.* Sydney, Australia: Superior Educational Publications.

Pavlak, S.A. (1985). *Classroom activities for correcting specific reading problems.* West Nyack, NY: Parker Publishing.

Richards, R.G. (1988). *Classroom visual activities (CVA).* Novato, CA: Academic Therapy Publications.

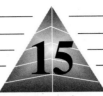

CHAPTER

# 15

# Psychosocial and Emotional Domains of Behavior

ANNE F. CRONIN

## KEY TERMS

- ▲ Temperament
- ▲ Temperament Types
- ▲ Goodness of Fit
- ▲ Social Competence
- ▲ Cultural Social Norms
- ▲ Social Referencing
- ▲ Mastery Motivation
- ▲ Self-Esteem
- ▲ Personal Causation
- ▲ Locus of Control
- ▲ Learned Helplessness
- ▲ Anxiety Disorders
- ▲ Disruptive Behavior Disorders
- ▲ Eating Disorders
- ▲ Mood Disorders
- ▲ Organic Mental Disorders
- ▲ Task Impersistence
- ▲ Cognitive Organizing Processes
- ▲ Child Abuse
- ▲ Pediatric Pain
- ▲ Sensory Integration
- ▲ Model of Human Occupation
- ▲ Model of Social Interaction
- ▲ Self-Management and Values Clarification
- ▲ Interest Groups
- ▲ Socratic Questioning
- ▲ Child-Centered Intervention
- ▲ Affirmation and Praise
- ▲ Performance Contingencies
- ▲ Reinforcement Menu
- ▲ Behavior Recording Systems
- ▲ Time-Out
- ▲ Performance Contracts
- ▲ Overcorrection
- ▲ Career Exploration and Planning

## CHAPTER OBJECTIVES

1. Understand the stages of psychosocial and emotional development.
2. Explain how temperament and social learning influence behavior.
3. Describe psychosocial and behavioral problems that can occur in childhood and adolescence.
4. Apply occupational therapy frames of reference to intervention for psychosocial problems.
5. Describe evaluation of psychosocial function through interviews, inventories, and observation.
6. Explain environmental factors that influence psychosocial development and issues of child abuse and family mental illness.
7. Describe secondary emotional and behavioral problems associated with physical disabilities, long-term health problems, or pain.
8. Discuss methods to enhance psychosocial development and to establish a positive therapy environment.
9. Describe behavioral management strategies.
10. Describe intervention strategies to enhance psychosocial development in the transition to adult life, career planning, and community living.

It is growing ever more apparent that babies are more complex than a bundle of reflexes. There is an increasing sensitivity to the distinctly individual behavior observed as early as the neonatal period. Research suggests that a large part of what is called *personality* is inborn. Studies of

387

social-cognitive development identify true social and emotional responses in young infants. Social and emotional development is a product of inborn characteristics, the child's human and nonhuman environment, and the child's sum of experience. Children with atypical development, including invisible problems like attention deficit disorder and visible problems like Down syndrome, are likely to have difficulties in psychosocial and emotional development.

Parents often have difficulty distinguishing between the normal emotional turmoil of childhood and problems requiring professional intervention (Turecki & Wernick, 1994). Occupational therapists in traditional pediatric settings often overlook the child's psychosocial problems and focus on their sensorimotor delays. In spite of the psychosocial emphasis in occupational therapy education, psychosocial intervention in pediatrics is often treated as an isolated specialty (Schultz, 1992). There are normal developmental transitions that stress all children, like starting school and puberty. These normal stresses may be enough to challenge some children's ability to adapt. Most children need social and emotional support at some point in their school years. This support is particularly needed when the child moves to new programs, environments, or situations. The sensitive therapist can ease these normal transitions as a part of meeting their client's developmental needs.

Occupational therapists who work with children in all types of practice settings need to recognize their social and emotional skills and whether these match the demands of the environment. Because the occupational therapy population consists largely of children at risk for psychosocial problems, it is crucial to understand and incorporate the psychosocial and emotional domains of behavior in interventions. The challenge to the therapist is to develop both the cultural and the ethnic sensitivities to support children and their families without being prescriptive about social values (Dillard et al., 1992). A positive and objective understanding of social behavior and emotional development is one goal of this chapter.

This chapter has been organized with three sections. The first section presents normal developmental issues in the psychosocial and emotional domains of behavior. Key to this section are the discussions of temperament and social learning as the building blocks of psychosocial and emotional behavior. This section offers the occupational therapist a neutral and objective basis for analyzing child behavior.

The second section includes occupational therapy interventions and an overview of psychosocial dysfunction in children and adolescents. Some important developmental issues in child psychopathology are included. Several common psychosocial diagnostic categories of children and adolescents are briefly discussed. Also discussed is the role of the environment in the development of social and emotional skills. The determination of childhood function or dysfunction is greatly influenced by the performance expectations in the child's everyday environments. Occupational therapy theory and frames of reference are discussed as they apply to pediatric psychosocial interventions. The remediation of psychosocial function and childhood performance and its effects on the areas of self-care, play, communication, and school performance described. Clinical examples offer insights into the environmental influences and cultural contexts of social and emotional behavior.

The third section focuses on the everyday clinical setting and the promotion of psychosocial development in all children. The focus of this section is establishing and maintaining a positive therapy environment. Behavior management strategies are reviewed for use in the clinical, home, and classroom settings. This section ends with a discussion of issues surrounding the transition to adult life that are common to persons at risk for psychosocial and emotional difficulties.

## ▲ Development of Emotional and Social Functions

Early research implied that there were predictable, orderly sequences of social and emotional development evolving from sensorimotor reflexes and neural responses (Freud, 1933; Piaget, 1952, 1954). Rather than modeling after the developmental sequence models of Piaget and others, recent studies have supported a more complex, integrated model of genetic predisposition and experience (Carpenter, 1975; Kaye, 1982). New theories, focusing on temperament and mastery, offer occupational therapy tools for more effective intervention in all pediatric clients. Temperament has been described as a continuum of normal patterns and of high-risk patterns. The occupational therapist working with children can effectively use the construct and elements of temperament to assess the child's social and emotional functioning.

### TEMPERAMENT AND PERSONALITY
#### Temperament Defined

Personality has long been considered a composite of nature and nurture. In this conception nature represents inborn characteristics, both genetic and congenital. Nurture consists of environmental influences such as social expectation, opportunity, and mastery experiences. Nature, or the child's inborn characteristics, is where this discussion begins.

For the past 20 years the pioneering work of Chess and Thomas (1983, 1984, 1987) has suggested that the role of nurture in social and emotional development is strongly influenced by the child's nature. It is now clear that there is a genetic predisposition in personality and behavioral style. Chess and Thomas (1987) describe this predisposition as temperament.

Wide variations in the rate of skill acquisition are reflected on all standardized pediatric tests. Children also vary in the development of interests, habits, talents, and social competence. Little attention was previously paid to the range of differences in social and emotional development. These differences in behavior were the focus of Chess and Thomas' research. They studied child behavior in terms of the individual's style of responding to various stimuli and experiences (Chess & Thomas, 1987). They considered information on caretakers' behavior and expectations as well as the child's specific environmental experience. Of particular interest to the occupational therapist, the research focused on "children's individual differences in carrying out the activities of their lives: sleeping and eating, exploring objects, and so on with the more and more complex activities of older children" (Chess & Thomas, 1987, p. 23). The outcome of this research was *temperament,* the style of a person's behavior in completing daily tasks.

Although this concept has been expanded by some authors, basic temperament research suggests nine characteristics of temperament. The nine categories with their definitions are given in the box at right. In reviewing these characteristics it is important to note that no behavior is inherently good or bad. Temperament characteristics are neutral. No child or parent is at fault for a child's activity level, intensity, or mood. Temperament is an individual's genetic predisposition to certain types of behavior in each category.

## Clinical Examples of Temperament

All of the characteristics listed in the box at right are important in describing a child's behavioral style. Many of these attributes are not obvious in a therapy setting. Typical examples of a high and low rating for each category are given in Figure 15-1. As noted before, there is no value of "good" or "bad" placed on high or low ratings. Children who are not at extremes in any direction may have the easiest time negotiating the social and emotional demands of childhood, but the determination of function or dysfunction has much to do with *goodness of fit.*

## Temperament Types

Chess and Thomas (1983) described three patterns of temperament that occurred commonly and resulted in patterns of behavior. These combinations were given the labels the easy child, the difficult child, and the slow-to-warm-up child (Figure 15-1).

The *easy* child is positive in mood and approach to new stimuli. This child is calm, expressive, malleable, and has a low to moderate activity level. Children characterized as easy may vary greatly. They may vary in activity level (high activity is generally considered difficult), distractibility, and attention span. The *difficult* child is at the opposite end of the temperament spectrum. Characteristics that make a child difficult are a negative mood and approach, slow adaptability, a high activity level, and emotional intensity. Extremes

### Categories of Temperament

1. **Activity level:** Motor activity and the proportion of active and inactive periods
2. **Rhythmicity:** The predictability or unpredictability of the timing of biologic functions, such as hunger, sleep-wake cycle, and bowel elimination
3. **Approach or withdrawal:** The nature of the initial response to a new situation or stimulus—a new food, toy, person, or place. Approaches are more positive and may be displayed by mood expression (smiling, speech, or facial expression) or motor activity (swallowing a new food or reaching for a new toy). Withdrawal reactions are negative and may be displayed by mood expression (crying, fussing, speech, or facial expression) or motor activity (moving away, spitting new food out, or pushing new toy away)
4. **Adaptability:** Long-term responses to new or altered situations. The concern is not the nature of the initial responses but the ease with which they are modified by the child in desired directions
5. **Sensory threshold:** The intensity level of stimulation necessary to evoke a discernible response, irrespective of the specific form the response may take
6. **Quality of mood:** The amount of pleasant, joyful, friendly mood expression as contrasted with the amount of crying, unfriendly behavior, and mood expression
7. **Intensity of reactions:** The energy level of response, positive or negative
8. **Distractibility:** The effectiveness of an outside stimulus in interfering with or changing the direction of the child's ongoing behavior
9. **Persistence and attention span:** Persistence refers to the continuation of an activity in the face of obstacles or difficulties. Attention span concerns the length of time an activity is pursued without interruption.

Modified from Chess, S. & Thomas, A. (1987). *Know your child.* (pp. 28-31). New York: Basic Books.

of sensory threshold often are found among children having a difficult temperament pattern. Finally, a *slow-to-warm-up* child demonstrates mild-intensity negative reactions to new stimuli in combination with slow adaptation. These children require several therapy sessions to become comfortable with the therapy environment and do not change therapists easily. Once a slow-to-warm-up child has established a routine, this child functions well. Transitions are problematic for children of this temperament type.

Turecki and Wernick (1994) elaborate on these temperament categories. For greater clarity the original nine categories are expanded to 18 categories. They also depart from Chess and Thomas' neutral *high* and *low* designations

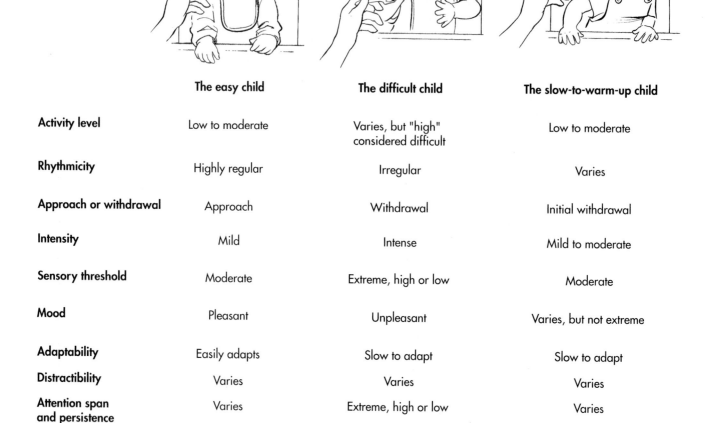

| | The easy child | The difficult child | The slow-to-warm-up child |
|---|---|---|---|
| **Activity level** | Low to moderate | Varies, but "high" considered difficult | Low to moderate |
| **Rhythmicity** | Highly regular | Irregular | Varies |
| **Approach or withdrawal** | Approach | Withdrawal | Initial withdrawal |
| **Intensity** | Mild | Intense | Mild to moderate |
| **Sensory threshold** | Moderate | Extreme, high or low | Moderate |
| **Mood** | Pleasant | Unpleasant | Varies, but not extreme |
| **Adaptability** | Easily adapts | Slow to adapt | Slow to adapt |
| **Distractibility** | Varies | Varies | Varies |
| **Attention span and persistence** | Varies | Extreme, high or low | Varies |

**Figure 15-1**   Temperament types.

to the terms *easy (potential asset)* and *difficult (potential liability)*. Children who do not fit all of the criteria of Chess and Thomas' difficult child may still have difficult aspects of their personality. Occupational therapists usually see children at risk for delays in social and emotional development secondary to disability or physical injury. With the added stress of disability and illness, the impact of difficult personality traits is exaggerated.

Temperament assessment provides a tool for the therapist to identify personality strengths and potential risk factors. It is useful in dealing with families because it can be interpreted neutrally without implying poor parenting and further stressing or alienating the family. Many instruments to assess temperament are listed later in this chapter.

Turecki and Wernick (1994) described behavior characteristics that place the child at risk for developing positive relationships with others. These categories apply when the described behaviors are persistent. Occasional gloominess or impulsive behavior is normal and not a risk. The temperament characteristics Turecki and Wernick identified as potential liabilities are shown in the box on p. 391.

## Social and Emotional Aspects

A child's temperament can actively influence his or her interaction with other children and adults. For example, a child with a generally gloomy mood may be viewed as unfriendly and uncooperative. Recognizing predominant mood as a personality characteristic may not change the therapy goal but will influence the therapist's approach to the goal. Helping the parents realize that their child's negative mood is not a reflection of their parenting may greatly improve the parent-child interactions. Children with difficult temperaments are at greater risk for child abuse and school difficulties (Guralnick & Groom, 1990; Kaplan & Sadock, 1988; Keogh & Burstein, 1988). The occupational therapist may pull away too quickly from a negative or moody child, not understanding the nature of temperament.

# Potential Liability Temperament Characteristics

Predominant mood: gloomy
Disposition: high-strung
Consistency of mood: changeable
Emotional sensitivity: high
Sociability: shy, timid
Expressiveness: reserved, taciturn
Initial response: withdrawal
Expression of anger: hot-tempered
Self-control: impulsive
Intensity: loud, forceful
Activity level: very high
Concentration: distractible
Regularity: irregular
Adaptability: poor; is upset by transitions
Sensory threshold: low
Preferences: particular, strong preferences
Negative persistence: stubborn, resistant
Positive persistence: gives up easily

Modified from Turecki, S. & Wernick, S. (1994). *The emotional problems of normal children.* (pp. 102-105). New York: Bantam Books

Temperament literature supports that although some behavior styles are innate, the child is not intentionally difficult. The therapist working with this child needs to look objectively at the child's interpersonal skills. Social skills training may help the difficult child function socially in challenging situations like the classroom.

Chess and Thomas (1987) were interested in learning about the influence of personality characteristics on the parent-child relationship and the child's development. They took the statistic concept, *goodness of fit,* and applied it to interpersonal relationships. In a nutshell, when the demands and expectations of persons important to the child are compatible with the child's temperament, there is a good fit. With this combination healthy development can be expected. Although Chess and Thomas focused on parent-child fit, other research has supported the findings in teacher and peer relationships (Keogh, 1986; Keogh & Burstein, 1988). Temperament and fit can be valuable teaching tools for therapists working to improve parent-child dynamics.

Most children have a combination of temperament strengths and liabilities. The liabilities, especially in the presence of other stresses, can be considered risk factors in social and emotional development. This does not mean that a liability in temperament alone limits the child; the whole picture matters. Temperament interacts with whatever stressor a child experiences. For example, children with lan-

guage delays are often mistakenly thought to be less intelligent than articulate children. The intelligent child with developmental aphasia may be frustrated and limited in social situations. This, in a child with a negative mood or a slow-to-warm-up child, could be a devastating combination.

Another example would be the verbally precocious 2-year-old child who, although her language makes her seem older, is developmentally unable to meet the behavioral expectations of an older child. If a child constantly fails to meet the expectations of others, he or she begins to believe something is wrong with him or her. When this lack of *fit* between abilities and demands exceeds the child's ability to adapt, intervention is warranted. Intervention, in this case, focuses on understanding of the child's temperament and adaptation of the social and physical environment to reduce the stress on that child.

## SOCIAL COMPETENCE

The child is not a passive recipient of social and environmental experiences. Even in infancy active social patterns can be observed. Active synchrony between infant movement and the structure of adult speech has been demonstrated (Condon & Sander, 1974). Young infants imitate simple adult facial expressions (Meltzoff & Moore, 1983). The infant is socially aware and socially active. The research on the social and cognitive behavior of neonates affirms that infants identify with other human beings and respond with some self-awareness (Field & Fox, 1985).

As a result of the complex influence of learning and social experience, there are not universally accepted milestones for either social or emotional development. Children develop skills for the environments in which they must function. Children in limiting environments may be as capable as children in enriched environments but possess different skills.

Social competence is the result of the diverse skills and behaviors that allow individuals to learn, to care for their daily needs, and to maintain satisfactory human relationships within their cultural context. Social competence provides the foundation from which an individual can successfully negotiate social and emotional challenges. Social competence in an infant includes sensory and perceptual skills, such as orienting to smiles and imitating facial expressions.

A socially competent 3-year-old child demonstrates a wide variety of complex skills. He or she reads the nonverbal cues of adults in the environment to learn about the desirable or dangerous aspects of unfamiliar situations. The 3-year-old child has mastered the nonverbal and gestural communication appropriate to his or her culture and imitates expected social behaviors well. Although the child may not understand the meaning or intent of certain learned behaviors, he or she understands that the performance of the behavior is expected. An example of this would be the 3-year-old child who folds his hands in prayer before meals.

The child is imitating the behavior but is unlikely to understand *prayer.*

Assessment of social competence should include the child's function in natural environments. If a specific social skill area is deficient, the therapist needs to analyze the behavior and the environment to determine what is causing the limitation. Intervention differs for developmental, cognitive, motor, or sensory problems.

Play is one of the earliest and most important arenas for learning social competence. Children who do not imitate or initiate play are likely to have difficulty in some area of childhood performance that limits their ability to respond. Competent play strengthens the child's motivation and encourages a positive sense of self. Parent-child interactions may help or hinder a child's ability to organize and then master developmental tasks.

Four-year-old Rex seldom attempted to interact with toys or persons in the play environment. He sat quietly, taking toys that were offered to him, but he did not reach for distant toys. Rather than attempting it himself, he handed his toys to adults and gestured for the adults to activate them. Although he liked to watch toys that were activated by others, he did not initiate interactions with toys. Rex's mother expressed frustration in encouraging the type of activity recommended in his home program. She tried leaving him in a room with toys around him, thinking that if no one entertained him with toys, he might play with them on his own, but he either sat quietly or cried.

The occupational therapist explained to Rex's mother that his motor-planning and problem-solving skills were limited. Unlike other children he could not watch a movement and then imitate it. To enhance his ability to play, the mother was taught to organize the task into small steps, including hand-over-hand physical prompts. These motor prompts were paired with playful social interactions that Rex understood. During the practice setting he began to actively hammer pegs. Within the month he had learned to play several other hammering and pounding games.

Social competence usually involves interpersonal communication. Communications may be simple and nonverbal, like the infant's expression of distress or pleasure. Communication becomes more complex as children develop language. As the child gains language skills, social behaviors are more easily assessed and interpreted. The communication skills of a 3-year-old child include an effective vocabulary that includes the understanding of the intangible meaning of words for emotions and thoughts. Although the child may not be able to define the words, words like *happy, angry, understand, scared, feel, sad,* and *sorry* are correctly used by a 3-year-old child (Bretherton & Beeghly, 1982; Wellman & Estes, 1987). By the age of 3, social competence has become dynamic and interactive.

Most 3-year-old children have formed selective attachments to certain adults in their world. This social attachment emotionally grounds the child and facilitates the child's ability to form new attachments. Children who do not have a stable home environment and do not form strong attachments early in life may still form loving attachments with adults. Children placed in healthy foster or adoptive homes usually rebound and are able to form loving relations with their new family. A lack of security in early social relationships does seem to influence peer relationships several years later. Children without secure adult relationships in early life often have difficulty making and sustaining friendships (Rutter, 1987).

Social competence requires communication, motor, cognitive, emotional, and sensory perceptual skills. Deficits in any of these performance areas places the development of social competence at risk.

Visual impairment is an example of a sensory processing impairment that influences social competence development. Vision helps the child identify distant features in their world. Distant features are important in interpersonal activity and in recognizing context specific behavior. Recognition of facial, gestural, and other behavioral cues that encourage a child to engage socially is limited in children with visual impairment. When visual or other sensory deficits limit the child, the occupational therapist can help provide an enriched environment and consistent social information to enhance the child's awareness and the development of compensatory behaviors to provide the needed social information.

One aspect of social competence is the ability to appropriately adjust social behavior according to location and audience. For example, most children play differently with peers than with adults. Social and emotional behaviors are greatly shaped by the child's cultural experience and environmental pressures. This is an important consideration when evaluating social competence. Social behavior is difficult to measure objectively in children who are not members of the predominant social group. For example, developmental assessments may have social items, but these items reflect cultural norms. Comparison with social-cultural norms is appropriate when the child tested has the same cultural background as the standardization sample. Such comparison can identify risk areas for children whose social skills developed in another cultural milieu but who must function in the mainstream. For example, a 5-year-old child raised in a Vietnamese community may fail to prepare cereal and play board or card games when given the Denver Developmental Screening Test—Revised (Frankenburg, Dodds, & Fandal, 1990). This should be considered as an indication that the child may have some social difficulties with middle-class suburban playmates in the United States. However, such test item failures should not be considered a delay in the absence of further indicators of social problems in the child's actual home, play, or school environments.

In another example of social learning, Ivan, an 11-year-old boy from Bulgaria, conversed at length about the difficulty of having friends come to his house because he did not own a video game system. When asked generally about his family in Bulgaria, he expounded on the lack of personal computers and video games. This is an example of good social learning. Ivan had learned that American children appreciate and sympathize with hardships like the absence of Nintendo.

Other aspects of Ivan's life in Bulgaria were unfamiliar to his American peers. After growing up sharing his living quarters with a large, extended family, Ivan felt lonely living only with his parents. The schools he was used to offered intensive science and math programs that far exceeded the programs available to him now. Ivan talked to adults about how frustrated he was with the slow pace of his math class but avoided the subject with peers. An 11-year-old boy complaining about a too-easy math class may be socially excluded from his peers.

## COMPONENTS OF SOCIAL COMPETENCE

Social competence requires an ability to imitate and learn social behaviors. In addition to social learning, children need some intrinsic motivation for social interaction. Intrinsic motivation develops from a sense of mastery and personal causation.

### Mastery Motivation

Children exhibit pleasure and confidence on mastering desired skills. When a child achieves a goal independently, it helps him or her open up to new challenges. Rex's mother announced that his personality changed during his first year in the Early Intervention Center program; "I never would have expected it, but suddenly I have a confident, independent little boy on my hands." Rex continued to have difficulty problem solving new tasks and needed encouragement to play in novel ways, but his sensorimotor skills grew with his sense of mastery.

Theories of mastery motivation emphasize the child's active role in his or her own learning. At around 9 months of age, children begin to engage in task-directed behavior. At this time the child can be observed repeating successful cause-and-effect tasks like operating a pop-up box or ringing a toy telephone. Gentle praise of the child's play, especially focusing on what he or she does independently, reinforces the child's pleasure in the achievement.

Critical to the growth of mastery motivation is the freedom to initiate activity (Linder, 1990). Parents or therapists who are too invested in the child's performance may not allow the child the freedom to experiment in play. It is especially hard to watch a child get frustrated when working toward a goal. Both occupational therapists and parents are often too quick to rescue the struggling child. While relieving the child's frustration, this "help" may also reduce the child's sense of competence.

Two-year-old Bronwyn declares her need for independence by pushing her mother away, announcing, "No Mommy! Me do it myself!" as she shoves both legs into the same leg of her pajamas. Bronwyn is an intense and persistent child. She has begun to understand the function of objects and to connect that new understanding with her own growing skills.

Achieving task competence requires the understanding of the function of any objects involved, the sensorimotor skill to act on that object in an effective manner, and the mastery motivation to accept the task challenge. Bronwyn should be allowed to persist at this task as long as she is interested. Her mother can participate and gently guide her explorations through social interactions like "You are working very hard at that. . . . Look at your silly feet in the same hole; can you think of a way to fix that?" When Bronwyn is ready for help, she will let her mother know.

An important part of task mastery is the challenge and practice with gradually increasing skills. Parents and therapists need to encourage independence without giving the child insurmountable tasks. Bronwyn's mother can help her daughter gain skill and a sense of mastery by selecting clothing items appropriate to her daughter's developmental level. Slightly oversized elastic waist shorts may make Bronwyn's explorations more positive than a pair of tights.

### Self-Esteem

Mastery motivation, and the degree to which it is nurtured, provides the basis for self-esteem, a sense of self as individual and vital. This sense of personal value, that one can accept challenges and potentially master them, is considered the core of self-esteem (Chess & Thomas, 1983). Average, or typical, children begin creating ideas about themselves and about their emotions between the ages of 18 months and 3 years (Greenspan & Greenspan, 1985). As young children begin to understand and remember the emotional aspects of their interactions, they begin to form ideas about their own value and the value of others. They play with language labels. "You are my very best friend" and "I love you" may be offered indiscriminantly to toys, family members, and strangers. Through the fourth year children sort out *me* and *you*, and the idea of social expectations and standards. The therapist can enhance this developmental process by providing an emotionally supportive environment and modeling appropriate means of expressing difficult emotions like anger, fear, and sadness.

In older children and in children with atypical development, the nurturing adult often has to contend with a social environment that frustrates the child's abilities and has to combat the social learning associated with failures. Tools to help the challenged child develop a sense of personal value include guidance in reality testing. Can the child separate reality from fantasy? Is he or she right in deciding all of the other children are better at cartwheels? Talking through these observations can help the child understand his or her own unique abilities and to distinguish feelings from perceived abilities. Research suggests that before the age of 7, children's self-assessments are not based on normative information (Butler, 1989; Ruble, 1983). Children are likely to vary their comparison standard with the expectations of children and adults in the immediate environment. Helping children, their families, and their teachers develop realistic expectations is an important step in enhancing a positive self-esteem.

Another useful strategy is to help the child develop a sense of personal time. Understanding the concepts of present, past, and future can help the child test reality. The child who has had orthopedic surgery or has just started medications to improve attention needs to learn that what used to be difficult or painful is now possible. The child should also learn to set realistic personal goals, such as to decide how he or she wants to be in the future and work with the therapist and family toward that goal.

## Personal Causation

Personal causation is the sense that one can influence the people and events within one's environment. It is an individual's perception of who (or what) is in control. Who is responsible for the bad (and the good) things that happen? Perception of control is fluid. A child may feel in control on the soccer field but not in the classroom. Likewise a child may have a healthy sense of personal control in familiar environments yet feel helpless when hospitalized.

One of the first clear developmental demonstrations of personal control is learning to use the toilet. Through successful toilet learning, Rex now learns that he can control an important part of his life. This is a step toward developing an internal perception (or locus) of control. The individual feels powerless when all control is externally provided. The hospitalized child often feels powerless and responds passively to people or things in the environment. Children's perception of themselves varies much more than that of adults. Changes in the environment can result in dramatic changes in self-concept. Commonly noted changes in a child's self-concept in response to illness include the following (Cherry, 1989; Frank, Huecker, Segal, Forwell, & Bagatell, 1991; Kielhofner, 1995):

1. Impaired sense of mastery motivation and personal causation
2. Change in, or lower-than-expected, academic performance
3. Social immaturity, isolation, unpopularity, or deviance
4. Instability or lack of persistence in activity
5. Dissatisfaction with all personal performances
6. Learned helplessness and low motivation and initiative

The Model of Human Occupation places personal causation central to occupational therapy interventions (Kielhofner, 1995). Perception of control is a dynamic state that is not easily measured by simple standard scales (Coster & Jaffe, 1991). This construct follows a developmental process encompassing discrete aspects.

[J]udgment of control is the end product of the integration of several other judgments. Among these are judgements of contingency and competence, which then involve assessment of task difficulty and of personal effort required and a comparison of self to a standard (Coster & Jaffe, 1991, p. 21).

As the child matures, perception of control becomes a multidimensional construct that includes a child's perceived competence, social experience, and internal motivation. Young children with atypical development may not be fully aware of their differences until about the age of 7 (Butler, 1989). At this time these children are likely to be more emotionally and socially vulnerable than the average child. Even typical school-aged children sometimes assume that they are responsible for major negative events in their lives like the death of a sibling or their parents' divorce (Rothbaum & Weisz, 1989).

Children who need a great deal of adult direction and support are less likely to demonstrate initiative in learning and play. Returning to the example of Bronwyn, if her independence is consistently squelched in the interest of efficiency, Bronwyn will begin to lose her motivation to initiate self-care independently. In therapy sessions, children with atypical aspects to their development are more likely to look externally for motivation and direction of their activity. The following are observations of personal causation as children react to the therapy environment.

When he entered the therapy room, Andre (6-½ years old) exploded with activity. He found the large balls irresistible. He rolled forward onto the mat, and made himself an obstacle course in the moments before the therapist began his intervention. He showed good internal motivation in his attempts to organize and stay with his undertaking. He quickly responded to verbal prompts and needed a minimum of adult reinforcement in exploratory play.

Michael (age 7) bounced into the therapy room and flitted from one piece of equipment to another. He pulled a large ball out of the box, then abandoned it to investigate the rope ladder. He spread toys all over the floor but did not stay with any undertaking. He had little internal motivation to persist. With suggestions offered by the therapist, Michael was a little more organized but continued to need verbal praise and extravagant gestures of encouragement to persist.

## Learned Helplessness

Learned helplessness is a concept from social psychology describing problems in learning to initiate social behaviors. Learned helplessness is that pattern of behavior that occurs when a child is exposed to unsolvable problems. In other words, learned helplessness is believed to be the behavioral result of a strongly externalized locus of control. Children who have learned that they fail in school no matter how hard they try soon quit trying. Learned helplessness is the actualization of the individual's perception of hopelessness. "Nothing that I do matters; why try?"

Kaplan and Sadock (1988) describe this concept as a type of depression that results in a person feeling "helpless, without options, and unable to control events" (p. 88). Kashani, Soltys, Dandoy, Vaidya, and Reid (1991) looked at patterns of hopelessness in children with psychiatric problems. These researchers noted that children with high hopelessness demonstrated lower cognitive performance, had difficult temperament characteristics, more anxiety, lower self-esteem, and were more psychopathologic than children with low hopelessness.

The occupational therapist often needs to motivate and direct skill development in children who have long experience with failure. This requires much active listening and environmental modification on the part of the therapist. The therapist must provide the child with assured and valued successes to offset their earlier experience. This is relatively easy with preschool children. Repetition of simple bean-bag or obstacle course games provides the child security while improving basic skills. Because school-aged children have a sense of normative reference (they know how they compare with classmates), providing successes often requires creativity.

Robert (age 9) was referred for work on his handwriting. He announced that his writing looked stupid and that people laughed at it. Robert balked at the introduction of activities centered on writing. Although he recognized his handwriting as a problem, he did not believe that doing "baby" stuff would improve it. Robert had no motivation and was not cooperative in therapy until the therapist used novelty to provide Robert with some success.

Robert loved comic books and was introduced to the *Drawing with Language* program (Lindamood, 1981) as a means of learning to copy cartoons. This approach teaches him language to describe the various parts of complex figures and a problem-solving approach to describe and copy these figures. As Robert gained skill in this area, copying cartoons was added to therapy.

The therapist's respect for Robert's pride and interests paid off in regaining his motivation. With his success in copying cartoons, Robert was able to tackle the disliked task of handwriting practice. He still did not want to work on handwriting in therapy and was allowed to take worksheets as homework. As long as Robert did his homework and made progress, he was allowed to work on cartoons and other skilled hand tasks in treatment sessions. Robert's handwriting became legible in a short time. He seemed surprised by this, describing it as "awesome." Robert returned to his classroom armed with the new problem-solving strategies and personal confidence.

Learned helplessness is combatted by an environment that allows a child to initiate activities and to be supported as they learn to persist at challenging tasks. Children who have experienced many failures lose the intrinsic motivation to master tasks. Notice if the child is performing an activity to please adults or solely for external reinforcement (praise or rewards). If a child is not strongly motivated internally, the therapist needs to build support and encouragement into all interventions and home programs. As the child

begins to succeed and a sense of mastery develops, the reinforcement should be discontinued.

## DEVELOPMENT OF INTERPERSONAL RELATIONSHIPS (IN CHILDREN AT RISK)

The child's first social relationship is with the immediate family or other caregivers. From the start the parent and the child are equal contributors to their social interactions. This is an important idea because difficulties with interpersonal relationships can occur when the parent and child have clashing temperament styles (Linder, 1990). Children who are atypical in their development may show less affect than other children, or they may show atypical affect. Parents may perceive that lack of affect reflects lack of attachment or desire to interact, thus negatively influencing the parents' early feelings of competence. The quality of their child's affect, its readability, and its predictability appear to be highly related to the parents' interactional style with the child (Linder, 1990).

Interpersonal reciprocity occurs naturally between most human infants and their mothers (Brazelton, Tronick, Adamson, Als, & Wise, 1975). This reciprocity relies on both parties reading and interpreting the other's nonverbal cues. The social interactions of the child with a disability or with atypical development also tend to be atypical. Low muscle tone results in minimal to absent facial expression (Goldberg, 1977). A difficulty in reading adult or infant cues can strain this crucial relationship.

Children with low muscle tone or multiple sensory impairments are also likely to be less active and less likely to initiate interaction than other children (Field, 1983; Linder, 1990). Unusual interactions persist well beyond infancy in many children. In time, families can learn to read and respond to their atypical children. However, communication with the world outside remains a problem. These children often become increasingly socially isolated at the developmental period when their age peers have mastered language and begin to expand their social horizons. Added to this, the unusual physical appearance and stigma associated with handicaps may further impede social development (Bracegirdle, 1990).

Children with less obvious developmental deviations may also have persistent difficulties with interpersonal relationships. Right-hemisphere deficit syndrome is common among children who have attention deficit disorder (Voeller, 1986). This syndrome results in a difficulty interpreting social cues and expressing feelings. In a study of social competence and peer rejection in a psychiatric inpatient setting,

. . . children with externalizing disorders (conduct or attention deficit disorders) and children with concurrent depressive and externalizing disorders were the most rejected, least liked, and least socially competent children (Asarnow, 1988, p. 151).

Clearly the growth of social competence has an important developmental influence on the child. Poor social skills may affect both self-esteem and personal causation in the preschool-aged and elementary school-aged child. Social awareness and sensitivity to the child's particular needs can reduce family stress and allow the family to focus on more positive interactions. In many cases it is the child's aberrant or immature social behavior, rather than specific cognitive or physical limitations that restricts the child's community contact. Especially in older children and adolescents, social difficulties exaggerate other difficulties that the child may have and may isolate them from normal friendships and opportunities for peer support.

Derrick (age 9) was seen by his family and teachers as a sensitive, gentle child. Derrick sometimes got overexcited in play, but he was not an aggressive child. Somehow, he was always in trouble on the playground. He was frequently suspended for hitting and fighting on the playground and was being considered for special placement as a "behavior disorder" because of these playground fights. When questioned, Derrick seemed confused by it all. He did not know why the other kids did not like him. He felt singled out and picked on by both his classmates and teachers.

After observing Derrick during social interactions, it became clear that some of the other children were taunting him. Derrick did not seem to be able to distinguish sarcasm or teasing from direct insults. He responded intensely and physically to these perceived insults, striking out and yelling. It was clear that some classmates had recognized and played with this weakness. With discussion and role playing Derrick was able to develop some other responses to his peers, and all of the adults in his world worked to help him sort out the subtle cues that distinguish playful teasing from true insult.

Derrick has attention deficit disorder hyperactivity type (ADDH). He also is an intense, emotional child with a low sensory threshold. His difficulty with perception of nonverbal social cues suggests some difficulty with right-hemisphere processing. Derrick needs special coaching, demonstration, and language cues to respond in a socially appropriate way. This may not be the only occupational therapy goal but should be addressed because of the impact it has on his ability to perform in normal childhood environments.

Language is an important asset to the development of interpersonal skills. Other types of communication were previously reviewed. Nonverbal gestures, referencing behaviors, and facial expression are all important social communication tools. Language is a specialized form of communication. "(L)anguage refers to a rule-governed system for representing concepts through symbols, which can be verbal or nonverbal" (Linder, 1990, p.151). Occupational therapists may not be directly involved in assessing or remediating language, but the role of language in development is so crucial that the pediatric therapist must understand some basics about language in the assessment of the whole child.

Although the occupational therapist may not be the primary team member planning language remediation, developmental issues involving language can affect the child's occupational performance. The pragmatics of language, the social rules governing the use of language, are especially important for the occupational therapist to understand because of their influence on interpersonal relationships.

Many interpersonal skills are based on language pragmatics. Pragmatics are context and audience specific. Pragmatics also involves active listening and respect for the communication of others. Highly verbal children may still have difficulty with pragmatics. For example:

Hello, my name is Clariece Parker. I live at 1114 Long Street, Lake City, Florida 66602. My subdivision is Pine Knoll, and I have a dog named Skip. This may seem an impressive greeting from a 4-year-old child, but when it is presented in its entirety every time Clariece faces a new person or a new situation, it is socially inappropriate.

In play with peers and in the therapy session Clariece would seldom respond to conversations around her. When she wanted to interact with another person, she would interject, into whatever conversation had been going on, a long discourse on one of her "topics." Clariece had monologues on listing the full addresses of everyone she knew, the eating habits and life cycle of hermit crabs, and her bedtime routine. Although this did impress some adults, it was generally alienating to peer interactions and significantly limited her social experience.

The following questions can serve as a guide to assess pragmatic language. First, what meaning is implied by the child's gestures, vocalizations, and verbalizations? For example, is the child seeking attention? requesting an object or action? requesting information? protesting? greeting?. Second, what functions does the child's communication fulfill? For example, does it satisfy needs? control the behavior of others? define the social interchange? express feelings? provide or obtain information?. Finally, what discourse skills does the child demonstrate? For example, attending to a speaker? initiating conversation? turn-taking? maintaining a topic? questioning? responding to requests for clarification? (Linder, 1990, pp. 179 to 180).

Clariece's speech was often attention seeking. She appropriately requested things and protested things. In these areas her meaning was appropriate. Other aspects of implied meaning, that her greetings were stereotypic, and not tailored to the environment and that Clariece often did not acknowledge the speech of others, caused social problems for her. In addition, Clariece had significant difficulties with discourse skills. She would only attend inconsistently to a speaker and then she would attend primarily to adults. She did not appropriately take turns, maintain a topic, or change the topic. Attempts to verbally direct her in therapy or in the classroom were frustrating. Clariece was disliked and avoided by peers in her preschool and church group.

These language skills could be easily and appropriately prompted and reinforced as a part of the occupational therapy intervention. In particular, Clariece's family needs to be educated about her social language difficulties. Family members often grow so familiar with their child and his or her behavior that they have difficulty seeing how it might interfere outside of the home. This was particularly true of Clariece because her performance was better with adults than with children. Adults notice her memory and vocabulary more than the inappropriate timing and poor conversational relevance of her speech. Peers, however, are put off by her interruptions and self-centered focus. Before the problem was identified and explained to them, Clariece's family had no idea why their articulate daughter had so much difficulty making friends.

## Goodness of Fit

Two children having identical temperament types adapt differently based on the parent's temperament and style of caregiving. The interaction of child and adult temperaments on a day-to-day basis is called *goodness of fit* (Chess & Thomas, 1987). With a healthy parent-child fit, "the demands and expectations of the parents and other people important to the child's life are compatible with the child temperament, abilities, and other characteristics" (Chess & Thomas, 1987, p. 56).

As discussed earlier, research suggests that there is a range of measurable individual differences in behavioral style. Temperament is easiest to study and identify in young children because it has not yet been mediated by experience. Teens and adults have their own characteristic temperaments, and goodness of fit relates to the compatibility of temperaments between individuals. A parent with a low activity level and a low sensory threshold may have difficulty with an intense, high-activity child. Teachers, therapists, and any other adult who has behavioral expectations for the child must balance their own expectations against that of the child.

Goodness of fit includes a child's social context, behavior expectations, and family and social values. Current research has focused on the social and emotional performance of the child at risk because of disability or chronic illness (Bracegirdle, 1990; Cherry, 1989; Kielhofner, 1995; Schultz, 1992). Figure 15-2 outlines the continuum from biologic impairment to behavioral outcome. *Social fit* is the heart of the interaction. It is the fit of the child's performance with social demands, both at home and in the community, that determines whether a child must deal with the stress and frustration of social failure. It is also the fit that the occupational therapist must consider in establishing therapy goals. Will intensive therapy for increasing tongue lateralization improve the occupational performance of a 15-year-old child with athetoid cerebral palsy? What are the concerns and interests of this child? What are his or her family, school, and community demands? Although tongue lateralization may be an appropriate intervention, such a focus is unlikely to address this child's difficulties with social fit.

The school-based occupational therapist working with

developmentally delayed preschoolers may have difficulty adjusting behavior expectations when assigned to a third grader with ADDH. The impulsive, disruptive, and labile behavior associated with ADDH is rude and offensive, but it is part of the disability. The therapist needs to look at the whole child, not just at his ability to tie his shoes. Many school-aged children are more academically limited by poor social competence than they are by motor incoordination.

The adults in a child's world have a large impact on a child's goodness of fit. For example, Rodney's working mother may consider her active, intense, low-sensory–threshold child as a problem. He has difficulty staying in his seat in the structured nursery school program that provides day care. He is easily distracted and often fights with the other children. The nursery school has asked Rodney to leave. It is the third day care placement his mother has tried in as many months. Because Rodney's mother must work and must have reliable care for Rodney, Rodney's behavior is unacceptable and causes stress in the parent-child relationship. This illustrates a poor fit between parent needs and child temperament. Sometimes helping a parent or teacher understand a child's temperament defuses the negative emotion and leads to creative solutions to the problem.

A child is at greater-than-average risk for social and emotional problems when the parent has a history of emotional and social problems (Kaplan & Sadock, 1988). In many therapy environments the therapist is expected to focus on

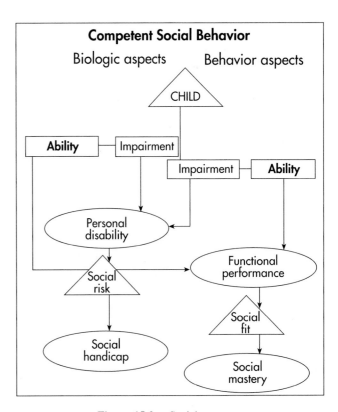

**Figure 15-2**   Social mastery.

the child's development. If a parent's social and emotional problems are contributing to the difficulties the child has, the mental health needs of the parent must be addressed by the intervention team.

Children who are perceived as socially competent are spoken to in a more affirming manner than are those children with low perceived social competence (Wichstrom, Holte, Husby, & Wynne, 1993). Parents' perceptions of their children influence the emotional and behavioral outcome in children. The most obvious case is child abuse. Abused children are often perceived by parents as different or difficult. Parents who abuse their children often have unmet dependency needs and seek emotional gratification through their children. This places inappropriate behavior expectations on the child. The resulting social conflict can lead to problems at home, at school, and throughout the child's life (Kaplan & Sadock, 1988).

## SUMMARY

This section focused on temperament and issues in the development of emotional and social functions that are consistent across children and across disability type. Assessment and remediation strategies for difficulties in development are discussed in the next section.

## ▲ Occupational Therapy Theory and Interventions for Children With Psychosocial and Emotional Dysfunctions

### PSYCHOSOCIAL DYSFUNCTION IN CHILDREN

Studies indicate that approximately 2% of children and adolescents receive intervention for psychosocial problems (Cohen, Cohen, & Brook, 1993; National Advisory Mental Health Council, 1990). Epidemiologic studies of the general population of children suggest that about 20% of children have psychosocial behavior that meets psychiatric diagnostic standards. Some of the 20% of children with psychosocial problems are expected to have transitory problems, and not all cases require intervention. Nonetheless, large number of children with psychosocial problems are not gaining access to formal intervention. With the probable incidence of about 20% of all children, the occupational therapist working with children is likely to see some children with psychosocial problems.

### Recognizing Psychosocial and Behavioral Disorders

In assessment and intervention the therapist needs to be sensitive to the social and emotional needs of their child clients. Most children occasionally behave in unusual ways.

For this reason it is sometimes difficult to discriminate ordinary behavior from dysfunctional behavior. Many emotional problems in children are a combination of problems in the child, the family, and the environment. Children's behavior patterns can be divided into four general categories:

1. Ordinary behavior: The child occasionally does unusual or destructive things, but the behavior is well within expectations for his or her developmental age and situation.
2. Problem behavior in response to extraordinary circumstances: This is the ordinary child facing a specific personal, health, or family crisis. When the child's crisis is resolved, the child functions adequately.
3. Problem behavior in response to home environment: This is the ordinary child facing chronic upheaval or dysfunction in the home environment. If the problems with the family or the physical environment are removed, the child functions normally.
4. Troubled behavior: This is the child that carries his or her own pathologic condition. The problems are persistent and impair the child's ability to function and learn.

The degree and persistence of the problem are critical considerations in identifying mental health problems in children. The first approach to the first three types of behavior is to provide emotional support and promote self-awareness, self-esteem, and interpersonal skills. When a child's problematic behavior persists and the behavior is unusual for the child's developmental level, a specialist should be consulted. Consider the following guidelines for determining whether to refer a child for psychosocial interventions: (1) Is the child self-destructive? This includes behaviors like substance abuse, physical harm to themselves, and suicidal talk or gestures. (2) Are the child's behaviors destructive to others? This includes starting fires and injuring animals. (3) Does a child (older than 3 years) know real from make-believe? (4) Is there a sudden change in personality? If so, is there a clearly identifiable cause for the change in a child's behavior such as a death or serious illness in the family?

When a positive relationship exists, family members may look to the occupational therapist as a resource when determining whether to seek help. The occupational therapist should be able to determine whether the problem can be handled simply at home, whether the family may benefit from support in occupational therapy, and when referral to a specialist is indicated. Because motivation plays such a key role in therapy success, ignoring social and emotional problems diminishes the effectiveness of all occupational therapy interventions.

### Major Classification of Psychosocial Dysfunction Used with Pediatric Populations

Before entering into a discussion of psychosocial classifications, it is critical to remember that only 2% of children actually carry these diagnostic labels. Labels can be useful and enhance understanding in a pediatric psychosocial intervention setting. However, psychosocial labels are also stigmatizing and sometimes seduce people into responding to the diagnosis rather than the child. The general trend has been to decrease the use of diagnostic labels.

Medical or psychosocial diagnosis is more subjective than it seems. In a child with multiple problems the diagnosis may be influenced by how the health care system allocates resources. For example, if state funding for mental retardation programs has been increased, dually diagnosed clients (those with mental illness and mental retardation) may have mental retardation listed as the primary disability.

A basic summary of common pediatric psychosocial classifications follows. It is not comprehensive, and the practitioner specializing in this area should review this topic in greater depth.

### Anxiety Disorders

*Separation anxiety and social phobia.* Separation anxiety and social phobia usually center on separation from a major attachment figure or place. The child with separation anxiety disorder experiences excessive anxiety, sometimes to the point of panic, when leaving a parent, the home, or some other secure fixture in the child's life. Degrees of separation anxiety are normal in the preschool years. This disorder reaches clinical proportions when the behavior extends beyond the expected developmental level (as in a middle-school child) or when it occurs to such a degree that it interferes with normal activities. Separation anxiety and social phobia are usually accompanied by morbid fears, preoccupations, and nightmares. The diagnosis of social phobia has been extended in the Diagnostic and Statistical Manual, 4th ed. (DSM-IV) (APA, 1994) to include what has been traditionally called school phobia (Frances, First, Pincus, Davis, & Vettorello, 1994).

*Overanxious disorder.* Overanxious disorder is believed to result from unusual pressure for performance. It is characterized by extreme self-consciousness, excessive and unrealistic worries, and anxiety about competence. Worrisome thoughts are intrusive and are out of proportion to the actual likelihood or impact of the feared event. These children may complain of stomachaches, headaches, and difficulty falling asleep. Rates are comparable for boys and girls in childhood. In adolescence (and throughout adulthood) the rate for this disorder is greater among girls and women (Cohen, et al., 1993). Overanxious disorder is also considered to be more common in urban areas than in rural areas (Kaplan & Sadock, 1988).

*Posttraumatic stress disorder.* Traditionally posttraumatic stress disorder (PTSD) has been reserved for adults. It is applied to persons who have experienced traumatic emotional or physical stress. Research now suggests that this diagnosis is appropriate for some victims of child abuse (APA, 1994; Famularo, Kinscherff, & Fenton, 1990; Rowan & Foy, 1993). The most notable effects of childhood PTSD are poor emotional bonding to children or adults, difficulty making friends, apathy, and depression. Children may demonstrate an acute form of PTSD with a relative increase in spontaneously acting as though the trauma were recurring, difficulty falling asleep, hypervigilance, nightmares, and generalized anxiety and agitation. A more chronic form of PTSD, and that most likely to be seen in occupational therapy, includes detachment, restricted range of affect, dissociative episodes, and sadness (Famularo et al., 1990).

### Disruptive Behavior Disorders

*Conduct disorder.* Conduct disorder is characterized by behaviors that are distressing to others. This child exhibits repetitive and persistent patterns of behavior that violate social expectations. Many children occasionally behave in ways that violate the rights of others or offend social sensibilities. This diagnosis is reserved for serious and persistent infractions of social rules. Types of behaviors included in this disorder are aggression toward people or animals, destruction of property, deceitfulness or theft, and serious violations of rules. Overall, conduct disorder is about twice as common in boys. Interestingly, the peak incidence in boys is around age 10, with a steady rate decline throughout adolescence. In girls the rate begins increasing at age 10 to age 16. At age 16 there is little gender difference in incidence. After age 16 the rate for girls abruptly decreases. This suggests that there are developmental periods during which a child is at risk for this type of problem. The most common explanation for these findings are the role transitions the child experiences (Cohen et al., 1993). The ages and the incidence of this disorder are likely to vary within cultural groups because the disorder is defined by cultural expectations.

*Oppositional defiant disorder.* Oppositional defiant disorder includes negative, hostile, and defiant behaviors often directed toward authority figures. Oppositional defiant disorder differs from conduct disorder primarily in that the disruptive behavior does not violate the rights of others. Behaviors common to this disorder include exhibiting temper tantrums, actively defying adult direction, and blaming others for their own actions. The individual is often angry and resentful (APA, 1994). This disorder shows similar prevalence and age patterns for boys and girls. The incidence rises to a high in the 13- to 16-year-old period and then becomes much less common (Cohen et al., 1993). Like conduct disorder, the incidence of this disorder is likely to vary within different ethnic groups, based on cultural expectations.

*Attention deficit/hyperactivity disorder.* ADHD is the most common behavioral disorder in childhood and occurs nearly twice as often in boys (Friedman & Doyal, 1992).

Unlike other disruptive behavior disorders, ADHD is believed to have a neurobiologic basis rather than a basis in social learning (Voeller, 1991; Zametkin et al., 1990). It includes a cluster of behavioral limitations that may include a short attention span, poor impulse control (including poor safety awareness), difficulty completing tasks, high levels of motor activity, emotional lability, and poor interpersonal awareness. This disorder is especially difficult to diagnose objectively because the clinical manifestations of the disorder are likely to be modified by the age and gender of the client. ADHD is also difficult to identify because children with this disorder may not exhibit attentional deficits and may behave relatively normally in situations that are highly motivating to them.

Children with ADHD have cognitive deficits that impair social learning and affect the child's innate ability to mediate behavior. Many children with ADHD have secondary psychosocial diagnoses. Secondary labels like conduct disorder or overanxious disorder may result as the child attempts to compensate for the hyperactivity and limited ability to attend (Friedman & Doyal, 1992).

### Eating Disorders

***Anorexia nervosa.*** Anorexia nervosa is an eating disorder that generally occurs in females between the ages of 10 and 30. It is characterized by secret, self-imposed dietary limitations that result in a body weight less than 85% of that expected for height and build (APA, 1994). Although its incidence is relatively small, this disorder is life threatening and usually results in hospitalization. Perons who are admitted to university hospitals for treatment have shown to have a mortality rate of 10%, usually caused by starvation, suicide, or electrolyte imbalance (APA, 1994). Individuals with anorexia are considered to have highly distorted body images and experience intense fear of gaining weight, despite being emaciated. Because teenage girls often have distorted body images, they are developmentally more vulnerable to this problem. The mean age of onset is 17 years. Atkins and Silber (1993) suggested that the development of anorexia nervosa in children relates to a complex combination of factors, including physical maturation, entry into junior high, loss of friendships, or some combination of these factors.

***Bulimia nervosa.*** Bulimia nervosa is like anorexia nervosa in that it seems to be a response to a distorted body image and occurs most frequently in young women. This disorder is less destructive and life threatening than anorexia and is less likely to require hospitalization. Bulimia involves recurrent episodes of binge eating followed by a self-induced purging. Although anorexia is often episodic, this disorder is more likely to be chronic over a period of many years. Mental disorders often seen with bulimia include depression, anxiety, and substance abuse of alcohol or stimulants (APA, 1994).

### Affective Disorders

***Major depressive disorder.*** The essential feature of major depressive disorder is a disturbance of mood. In children and adolescents the prevailing mood can be either depression or irritability. Depressed children may fail to gain weight as expected with normal growth. In most other aspects this disorder mirrors the adult condition. Children have little interest in daily activities and often fall behind in their schoolwork. Excessive fatigue and sleep disorders are common. All areas of development are likely to be impaired during a depressive episode and may be misdiagnosed as a learning disability (Kaplan and Sadock, 1988, p. 633). These disorders tend to be insidious, and in adolescents they often are associated with substance abuse. Other symptoms may include suicidal thoughts or actions or psychotic symptoms (APA, 1994). In childhood and late adolescence, rates for major depression are low, with no significant gender differences. Cohen et al. (1993) observed a sharp increase in the incidence of major depression in girls around the age of puberty. This finding suggests that the biologic changes of puberty predispose young women to this problem. Another hypothesis is that changing social expectations play a role. Depression is 1.5 to 3 times more common among children with a depressed parent than in the general population (APA, 1994).

### Neurologically Based Mental Disorders

This is a catch-all category for mental and behavioral impairment that is secondary to neurologic dysfunction. This includes mental retardation, closed head injury, problems after brain surgery, seizure disorder, and substance-induced dementias. There is no single set of symptoms in this classification because of the variability of organic problems involved. Common problems associated with neurologically based mental disorders include the following:

1. Memory impairment, specifically short-term recall
2. Impaired abstract thinking, generalization, logical reasoning, and conceptualization
3. Impaired ability to problem solve in social and play environments
4. Impaired ability to learn and perform novel tasks
5. Impulsivity in language and behavior
6. Impaired ability to attend to salient features of tasks or spoken directions
7. Decreased or absent safety awareness
8. Decreased sensitivity to and awareness of consequences
9. Impaired orientation to time and space
10. Distorted perception of one's body and environment

For more information on this category of psychosocial problems, the therapist should refer to texts specific to the diagnostic problem.

***Cognitive dysfunction.*** Many children seen in occupational therapy have cognitive difficulties. Cognitive dysfunction can impair a child's social function and often occurs in children with brain injury, ADHD, and other conditions related to neurologic dysfunction.

TASK IMPERSISTENCE. Task impersistence describes difficulty with orienting and attending to tasks. Children with this problem have difficulty completing tasks, particularly challenging ones, without being prompted. Task impersistence is critically limiting to the social and emotional development and the school performance of the child. Children with this problem have difficulty sustaining participation in games and often cooperate poorly. They have little sense of the overall task, or the "whole picture," in terms of organized games. These children are often avoided, or even ostracized, in middle childhood because of their flighty or disruptive influences into organized group activities.

COGNITIVE ORGANIZING PROCESSES. In addition to attending to and persisting at tasks, independent task completion requires mental analysis and organization of the task. A child with difficulties in cognitive organizing processes is likely to sit and stare at a task, even a familiar one, rather than initiate activity. Knowing where and how to start and then how to proceed with a task requires specific cognitive skills.

Cognitive organizing processes include analyzing, classifying, integrating, sequencing, identifying relevant features of objects and events, comparing for similarities or differences, and detecting errors. Organization is a cognitive product. For example, the child can be guided to organize his or her bureau drawers to make getting ready for school more efficient. Organization can also be an active process. Organization can be the process of taking in environmental information and organizing the information in a meaningful way to plan behavioral output. The following examples clarify the functional outcomes and potential degrees of impairment of these problems (Szejeres, Ylvisaker, & Holland, 1985).

A moderate to severe impairment would include weak or bizarre associations, disorganized sequencing of events, difficulty analyzing objects in terms of features, difficulty identifying the main idea in a task or activity, difficulty cognitively organizing information as "tools" to task.

A mild impairment would include subtler versions of the earlier problems, difficulty maintaining goal-directed thinking, difficulty discerning the main idea and integrating the main idea into a broader theme, may easily get lost in details.

## Pervasive Developmental Disorders

Children with pervasive development disorders (PDD) share severe and consistent abnormalities in their abilities to form reciprocal social relationships and to verbally and nonverbally communicate. They may also demonstrate repetitive movements, extremely limited interests or preoccupations, or ritualized patterns of behavior. Diagnoses that fall within the category of PDD include autistic disorder,

Rett's syndrome, childhood disintegrative disorder, and Asperger's disorder (see Chapter 7).

Children with PDD are often unable to participate in most family, community, and school activities without extensive support and accommodation. Their lack of comprehension of and motivation by social interaction often results in disruptive, uncooperative behavior. Mental retardation is commonly, although not always, concomitant with these disorders (APA, 1994). Most children with PDD receive special education services for cognitive and behavioral problems. Behavior modification approaches are often used to teach daily living skills and basic social interaction. Sensory integration approaches have also been found effective for some children with autistic disorder. The problems faced by these children and their families are lifelong and neccessitate planning for the child's entire course of development.

## Developmental Issues in Psychosocial Diagnosis

The frequency and persistence of childhood and adolescent emotional problems vary with the child's age and gender. Cohen et al. (1993) demonstrated developmental stage–associated risk factors. For example, major depression is seen most often in girls, specifically around the onset of puberty. The incidence of this disorder is low and similar in both genders before and after puberty (Cohen et al., 1993). ADHD and conduct disorders are identified twice as often in boys, and in both cases the incidence rate drops about 20% per year beginning around age 10.

Many children who have psychosocial problems have been given multiple diagnoses. This is most likely with children obtaining any disruptive diagnosis; nearly half of these children received more than one diagnosis (Cohen et al., 1993). ADHD is often the primary diagnosis in these cases. This supports the idea that ADHD creates greater than average social and emotional stress. Table 15-1 shows that boys have a steady decline in all disruptive behavior disorders throughout their teen-age years. Where incidence rates decline steadily, the gradual growth in skills, self-control, social maturity, and conformity to gender role expectations probably account for the improvement (Cohen et al., 1993). This suggests that developmental skill training in these areas may alleviate some problems in the younger child and help speed the resolution of the disorder.

As was previously noted, the pattern for disruptive behavior disorders in girls is initially low, peaks in the 14- to 16-year-old age-group, and then quickly diminishes. Cohen et al. (1993) speculated that the physiologic changes of puberty trigger the peak incidence. Again, occupational therapists can provide support and specific social skill training to help provide the young teenager with positive behavior to help her weather this biologically stressful time.

In contrast to the behavioral disorders only 20% of children with mood disorders received more than one diagnosis (Cohen et al., 1993). With the exception of major depression, there is a steady decline in incidence of all these

▲ Table 15-1  Disruptive Behavior Disorders (Prevalence in Percent)

| Age (Years) | Attention Deficit Disorder | | Conduct Disorder | | Oppositional Disorder | |
|---|---|---|---|---|---|---|
| | Girls | Boys | Girls | Boys | Girls | Boys |
| To 13 | 8.5 | 17.1 | 3.8 | 16.0 | 10.4 | 14.2 |
| 14-16 | 6.5 | 11.4 | 9.2 | 15.8 | 15.6 | 15.4 |
| 17-20 | 6.2 | 5.8 | 7.1 | 9.5 | 12.5 | 12.2 |

Modified from Cohen et al. (1993). An epidemiological study of disorders in late childhood and adolescence: I. Age- and gender-specific prevalence. *Journal of Child Psychology and Psychiatry, 34*(6), 858.

▲ Table 15-2  Common Mood Disturbances (Prevalence in Percent)

| Age (Years) | Overanxious Disorder | | Separation Anxiety | | Major Depression | |
|---|---|---|---|---|---|---|
| | Girls | Boys | Girls | Boys | Girls | Boys |
| to 13 | 15.4 | 12.8 | 13.1 | 11.4 | 2.3 | 1.8 |
| 14-16 | 14.1 | 5.3 | 4.6 | 1.2 | 7.6 | 1.6 |
| 17-20 | 13.8 | 5.4 | 1.8 | 2.7 | 2.7 | 2.7 |

Modified from Cohen et al. (1993). An epidemiological study of disorders in late childhood and adolescence: I. Age- and gender-specific prevalence. *Journal of Child Psychology and Psychiatry, 34*(6), 855.

disorders throughout the teen-age years. The rates for boys drop off much more abruptly than those for girls (Table 15-2). The gender differences in incidence may be caused by different social performance expectation for girls and boys. As before, the young woman's hormonal changes of puberty are expected to contribute to the rate, especially the rate for major depression. A familial pattern to mood disorders has been identified and should be considered when planning interventions (Kaplan & Sadock, 1988). Whether or not other family members also have mood disorders, working with all family members is essential.

The occupational therapist may encounter children with social and emotional difficulties in all arenas of pediatric practice (see Chapter 31). Because children with atypical development, physical impairment, and chronic illness are at risk for emotional problems, the therapist treating the whole child should consider a child's social and behavioral competencies as a routine part of clinical assessment.

Children brought to clinical services for psychosocial disorders are likely to be preselected for diagnostic persistence and comorbidity (Cohen, Cohen, & Brook, 1993). This means that children with serious, long-standing, and complex problems are those who are likely to have been seen in traditional settings for psychosocial intervention.

Sholle-Martin and Alessi (1990) provided a view of occupational therapy practice in an inpatient unit. They noted that 41% of the children admitted had prior psychiatric diagnoses, many had received intervention before the current hospitalization, and many had multiple diagnoses. The "top ten" discharge diagnoses in their setting (Table 15-3) are consistent with the pattern of disorder persistence described by Cohen, Cohen, & Brook. (1993).

Sholle-Martin and Alessi (1990) demonstrated that many of the children in their clinical setting had adaptive dysfunction that influenced all areas of childhood performance. Reading a description of a diagnostic label does not always prepare the clinician for the types of behaviors seen on a day-to-day basis. Some common patterns of adaptive dysfunction in the areas of emotional and social performance are discussed in the next section.

### Emotional and Behavioral Problems

*Child-environment fit.* Difficult temperament and atypical development place a child at risk for social and emotional problems (Turecki & Wernick, 1994). Being at risk suggests an increased potential for problems. A good child-environment fit, with sensitivity to the child's needs, can successfully accommodate the atypical child. Recognition of a problem in child-environment fit and a preventive focus in intervention can greatly improve the child's ability to cope and adapt to the environment. Support and education of the parents about the child's strengths and liabilities can ease pressures in the parent-child relationship and improve the child's overall social and emotional function.

Children are perpetually learning from and responding to their environment. The influence of the physical and cultural environments are described in this section.

*Physical environment.* The physical environment consists of the near sensory world. It includes the objects, places, and spaces of daily life. This environment begins its influences on the individual at birth.

Clinical experience supports that inaccessibility to the physical environment limits the child's ability to interact

▲ Table 15-3   Discharge Diagnoses in Child Psychiatry

| Diagnosis | Population (%) |
| --- | --- |
| Attention deficit disorder | 37 |
| Oppositional disorder | 25 |
| Conduct disorder | 17 |
| Dysthymic (mood) disorder | 17 |
| Anxiety disorder | 14 |
| Major depressive disorder | 12 |
| Pervasive developmental disorder (including autism) | 12 |
| Mental retardation | 10 |
| Adjustment disorder (all types) | 8 |
| Organic brain syndrome | 6 |

Modified from Sholle-Martin, S. & Alessi, N. (1990). Occupational therapy in child psychiatry. *American Journal of Occupational Therapy, 44,* 874.

and learn spatial and object properties. By 9 months of age, average children have experienced independent mobility and begin to respond to objects in the environment, rather than to themselves, as spatial landmarks (Campos & Berenthal, 1987). Children with spastic cerebral palsy have limited experience exploring their environment. It has been demonstrated that the use of power mobility devices with young children enhances the development of spatial relations, sensory processing, and emotional independence (Butler, 1984; Campos & Berenthal, 1987).

Occupational therapists need to consider the social expectations and social benefits of adaptive equipment, assistive technology, and mobility needs. Traditionally, occupational therapists have believed that a person should do as much as possible without equipment. When responding to the needs of the whole child the therapist needs to be aware of the time the child has to get down the school corridors with his or her class and the time it takes to hand-write an essay for homework. Powered mobility and computer adaptations are adaptations to improve the child-environment fit. The possible impact on the child's motivation and self-esteem make these adaptations crucial, even when the child is able to slowly perform the necessary task independently (see Chapters 17, 20, and 21).

***Cultural and social environment.*** The cultural environment is in some ways similar to the physical environment. It encompasses the cultural expectations about an individual's behavior in a particular setting. Occupational therapists are frequently reminded to be culturally sensitive, but thoughtful effort is required on the part of the therapist to respond to cultural demands that differ from his or her own.

Magill and Hurlbut (1986) studied self-esteem in adolescents with cerebral palsy. They found that the subgroup of teen-aged girls with cerebral palsy had low self-esteem.

[These girls] scored significantly lower than the boys with (cerebral palsy), the nondisabled boys, and nondisabled girls on physical self-esteem. . . . The scores of the boys with (cerebral palsy) were similar to those of the nondisabled groups (p. 402).

This study probably reflects a cultural view of beauty. The abnormal movements and poor control of facial musculature common to cerebral palsy places girls with these problems at odds with cultural values. These young women are likely to stand out among their peers and have fewer opportunities for social and emotional growth because of the societal valuation of women's beauty. Children with disabilities of all types encounter social constraints that limit their active participation in the daily life of our communities, sometimes in subtle ways.

A white middle-class American child with Prader-Willi syndrome inevitably fails to live up to cultural expectations. Compulsive eating, even when it is based in a biologic condition, is considered a character flaw. Compulsive eating in Prader-Willi syndrome does not respond to behavior modification or other social learning strategies. The child with Prader-Willi syndrome is likely to be unfashionably overweight and will never be able to live without another person controlling and limiting their food intake. Although persons with other mental retardation syndromes like Down syndrome or fragile-x syndrome have the possibility of functioning semiindependently in a group home situation, the person with Prader-Willi syndrome is limited to more restrictive living arrangements because of their compulsive eating. This is a poor person-culture fit. The successes and accomplishments of the young adult with Prader-Willi syndrome will always be threatened by his or her compulsive eating.

### Family and Social Risks

Children are better able to adapt positively to stress when there is a positive parent-child relationship. Specific relationship assets include positive parental attitudes, involvement, and guidance (Gribble et al., 1993). The positive parent-child relationship seems to mediate childhood stress, and children from this type of family function with greater resilience. Children seem to be able to adjust more effectively to physical disorders when there is a strong positive parent-child relationship (Lavigne & Faier-Routman, 1993).

In general, when family interactions are positive, the child's health and functional performance are optimized. When family relations are strained, the child is at increased risk for dysfunction (Vessey & Caserza, 1992). It was noted earlier that children of parents with psychosocial problems are at greater risk for these problems themselves. A parent with a depressive mood disorder or substance abuse seems to be the most destructive to the child (Hammen et al., 1987; Olson, Heaney, & Soppas-Hoffman, 1989).

Family socioeconomic and cultural backgrounds affect the child in many ways. When family and community role expectations are inconsistent, the child is at greater risk for emotional problems (Turecki & Wernick, 1994). Parental role expectations about specific types of performance can increase the child's stress. Parents often hope to recreate happy parts of their own childhood for their child. This tendency, although well meaning, can greatly stress the parent-child relationship. For instance, the mother who excelled at gymnastics may push her dyspraxic daughter in gymnastics class.

Sometimes trying to protect their child from remembered hurt can be equally damaging. The father who remembers trying every sport only to be left on the bench may be too quick to pull his own son out of activities that the child enjoys. This man's son may enjoy participating in the activity even though he is not a highly skilled athlete.

### Child Abuse*

The same children who are at risk for psychosocial and emotional difficulties are at risk for child abuse. The occupational therapist needs to support both the child and the family. The therapist also has the responsibility to objectively consider parents' current ability to adequately care for their child. Because of the high-risk nature of the children commonly seen by occupational therapists, it is necessary to understand and evaluate the abuse risk factors as a component of the developmental assessment.

Three factors associated with abuse are (1) the characteristics of the child, (2) environmental stress, and (3) the parents' personality and background. Abuse is most prevalent in preschoolers, especially in those whose cognitive, social, or physical developmental delays extend the child's dependency and demands on their caregivers. Physical abuse has been associated with difficult temperament characteristics and neurologic impairments.

Assessment of the child at risk should include observations of the child's physical appearance and affective and social behavior. Observations documented over time are more reliable and court admissible than those documented only once. Norm-referenced evaluation tools should be used whenever possible because these also provide the most reliable evidence should the case go to court.

Assessment of the home environment and the parent teaching style is valuable in planning all interventions but vital when the child is at risk for abuse. The *Developmental Interview for Parents of Young Children at Risk* (Davidson, 1995) offers an interview format designed to identify problems in the child's home environment. The *Nursing Child Assessment Teaching Scale (NCAST)* (Barnard, 1980) also focuses on the family and home environment. This assessment includes the observation of a parent teaching the child a play activity. By comparing the parent's report of their teaching style with direct observation, the oc-

cupational therapist is able to identify discrepancies and potential problem areas.

The parents' personality and background have been given only cursory attention in the earlier sections of this chapter. This factor is crucial and distinct in families in which physical abuse occurs. Parents who engage in abusive or neglectful parenting often have a history of unsatisfactory relationships with their own caretakers. Abuse and neglect are common features in the histories of these parents. These parents report an absence of personal and social resources that makes them more vulnerable to daily environmental stresses (Davidson, 1995).

Monique (4 years old) was new in the early intervention program. During developmental assessment she maintained a flat affect and had no spontaneous exploratory play. She was compliant and waited quietly for the therapist to direct her. Monique's mother arrived late to pick her up. She appeared stressed and disorganized.

Monique did not acknowledge her mother. Monique's mother abruptly demanded, "Has she been bad again?" After the therapist explained that Monique had worked well, her mother replied, "I've had a headache all day and nothing to eat. Come on, Monique, you can't sit there all day." The family left without further comment.

When working with children at risk for abuse, prevention is best, that is, identifying and supporting families at risk, thus heading off the potential for abuse. If the occupational therapist believes that a family is at risk for abuse, careful observation of the child's behaviors and physical appearance is needed. The therapist following Monique documented the exchange described above, along with other worrisome incidents as they occurred.

In a parent-child teaching activity, Monique's mother was asked to help her daughter string beads for a necklace. Both mother and daughter were enthusiastic with the idea. Given the beads, Monique's mother worried about the aesthetics of the necklace, correcting Monique's choices and undoing her daughter's work. As the interaction progressed, Monique became apathetic and passive.

This type of interaction exemplifies behavioral indicators of risk for child abuse. Monique relates poorly to adults in general and shows limited attachment behaviors toward her mother. Monique's mother appeared overwhelmed and socially limited. She did not interact with her daughter in a nurturant manner. Monique's mother was preoccupied with her own needs, to the exclusion of those of Monique. Continued evaluation of the child and parent is indicated and should be followed by preventive intervention or referral to Child Protective Services.

It is the occupational therapist's responsibility to refer the family to the state Child Protective Services agency if abuse or neglect is suspected. Referrals involve a telephone call, followed by a letter that outlines the client's name, age, address, and a summary of the reasons for concern. Reports are categorized according to severity and type, and investi-

---

*The authors wish to acknowledge Deborah Davidson for her contribution to this section on child abuse.

gations are scheduled accordingly. Repeated reports should be made if continued observations of the problem behavior occur. Multiple referrals are sometimes needed before a case qualifies for an in-depth Child Protective Services evaluation or legal intervention.

Preventative intervention for the family at risk for abuse can be initiated at any point in the therapy relationship. The occupational therapist can assist parents in two major ways: by facilitating the establishment of a social support network and by educating them regarding child development and parenting skills. The development of a support system begins with the parent-therapist relationship. Parent groups and parenting classes also provide valuable information and social contacts. These groups need not be limited to abusive or "at-risk" families. Some facilities routinely offer parenting seminars presented by members of the interdisciplinary team. This approach offers nonjudgmental support that may alleviate the pressure at home and reduce the likelihood of abuse (Davidson, 1995).

***Families with mental health problems.*** When the parents are experiencing mental health problems, their children often have emotional and behavioral disorders (Goodman, 1987; Hammen et al., 1987). Poverty and social stress result in increased mental health problems in adults; the study by Sholle-Martin and Alessi (1990) affirmed that the same pattern is true of children. The families most impaired were those dealing with a depressive disorder, often depression and alcohol abuse. The children of depressed mothers almost always demonstrated less social competence and behavioral problems. Goodman (1987) completed a study of mothers with schizophrenia and depression. The sample consisted primarily of single, low-income black women.

Deficits were found in the child-rearing environment provided by the disturbed mothers. Both schizophrenic and depressed mothers were rated as less affectively involved and less responsive than well mothers. Schizophrenic mothers were rated as providing the poorest overall environment: less play stimulation, fewer learning experiences, and less emotional and verbal involvement (p. 411).

Sensitivity to the home environment in assessing the child is particularly important. In addition to determining how children measure against the test standards, the therapist needs to analyze the child's adaptive behavior in the actual environment in which the child needs to perform. A child may learn behaviors that are inappropriate in society at large but are effective in meeting their needs in a difficult home environment. These issues point to the importance of family-centered intervention if the intervention is to be effective.

## Secondary Emotional and Behavioral Problems

In some cases children are referred to occupational therapy services for the treatment of emotional problems that are secondary to medical illness and long-term hospi-

talization (Cherry, 1989; Frank et al., 1991; Stowell, 1987). Disorders in interests, motivation, and play behavior are common in hospitalized children. Emotional and behavioral problems are often associated with children who have incurred traumatic brain injury or other neurologic (cognitive) impairment. The first noticeable signs of cognitive impairment are often social affective deficits (Table 15-4).

Emotional lability in this case means that moods change abruptly. Emotional response may not be inappropriate to the situation, as in some adult cases of lability, but the children seem to be more sensitive and intense in their reactions. In particular, they are more easily upset when challenged. Perhaps in response to their perception of having little control, children with cognitive problems sometimes become bossy and negative. These children perform poorly in directive environments like most classroom and therapy situations. If the family observes that their child's behavior is fine in some situations but intolerable in others, the child's perception of control may be part of the explanation.

▲ Table 15-4    Early Signs of Emotional Distress

| Problem | Signs |
|---|---|
| Emotional lability | Abrupt mood changes |
| | Sensitive to criticism |
| | Exaggerated emotional outbursts in response to ordinary events |
| Negativity | Finds fault with every suggestion or activity |
| | Refuses to particpate in activity or participates without making any effort to succeed |
| Social withdrawal | "Shuts down" and does not talk to the therapist even in response to direct questions |
| | Poor relatedness to others (even parents) |
| Low frustration tolerance | Throws toys and objects rather than persisting at challenging tasks |
| | Quits working abruptly and does not complete activities |
| Poor task initiation | Does not mentally organize tasks and has difficulty knowing where to begin |
| | Sits and self-distracts without an external prompt to begin a task |
| Oppositional | May become bossy and negative |
| | Argues with the therapist's ideas and plans |
| | Denies that personal behavior is relevant to problems completing tasks |

Chronic conditions in childhood affect the child's overall development. The scope of chronic conditions seen by the pediatric therapist changes with changes in health care delivery and health technology. Stowell (1987) presented a model of psychosocial intervention with pediatric bone marrow transplant patients. This article outlined the social and emotional challenges secondary to a disease process that was once fatal and a treatment process that impairs the child's development.

Another condition increasingly seen in early intervention programs is perinatal human immunodeficiency virus (HIV) infection (Anderson, Hinojosa, Bedell, & Kaplan, 1990). Children with perinatal HIV infection have difficulties in neuromotor, developmental, and psychosocial realms of performance. Interventions should be sensitive to the overall developmental needs of the child and the needs of the caregivers.

With HIV, cancer, and many other childhood conditions, the prognosis affects therapist and caretaker decisions. Children who are expected to have little chance of survival into the adult years are treated differently than other children. Establishing future goals, long-term plans, and skill building for competence help shape developing cognitive skills. A child who is sheltered from his or her potentially limited life span may lose important developmental learning experiences (Vessey & Caserza, 1992).

Atypical development in any performance area places the child at risk for inappropriate expectations (Turecki & Wernick, 1994). The concept of resilience and vulnerability is discussed in the research literature because child and family characteristics are consistently more predictive of problems than the specific disease process (Barkley, Anastopoulos, Guevremont, & Fletcher, 1991; Boyce, Barr, & Zeltzer, 1992; Brunquell & Hall, 1991; Daltroy et al., 1992; Youssef, 1988).

Children who have chronic health problems in addition to problems with cognition or depression are the most likely to have secondary difficulties with psychosocial development (Youssef, 1988; Pollock, 1986). These problems occur more typically in elementary or middle-school–aged children (Barkley et al., 1991; Simmons et al., 1987). Important considerations when treating children and adolescents with chronic health problems include the child's temperament, any medication side effects, and the impact of the disease process on the child and on his or her family. A look at the varied environments in which a child needs to function may help by anticipating problems, especially peer problems that affect the child's social and emotional development (Creer, Stein, Rappaport, & Weiss, 1992; Pollock, 1983).

### Pediatric Pain

Any disorder that causes pain, limits the child's activity, or causes increased dependency on adults has the potential to influence the child's psychosocial function. Childhood pain has only recently begun to be discussed in the scientific literature. Pain in both children and adults is a complex interaction of biologic, psychologic, and sociologic phenomena. Turnquist and Engel (in press) report that

> . . . [i]n children, prolonged pain can contribute to a sense of loss of control. This sense of loss of control may result in a decrease in courage, motivation, and constructive activity. The child may also develop a sense of learned helplessness.

The pain experience is affected by a child's cognition, coping strategies, ability to communicate feelings, and temperament. Schechter, Bernstein, Beck, Hart, and Scherzer (1991) found that parental anticipation of their child's distress greatly influenced the distress level manifested by the child. Social factors, such as the family, culture, and economics, have been shown to influence children's perceptions and reactions to pain (McGrath & McAlpine, 1993).

In their survey of occupational therapists, Turnquist and Engel (in press) found that few therapists were familiar with tools to assess children's pain and that few of the commonly used adult pain treatments are used with children. The therapists surveyed listed burns, cancer and acquired immunodeficiency syndrome, arthritis, orthopedic injuries, and respiratory disease as the pediatric conditions most likely to be painful. It is suggested that the medical community in general, including occupational therapists, underestimates the importance of pain in planning interventions. A child may be taught strategies to self-manage chronic pain and may benefit from pain management protocols similar to those used with adult clients.

Pain clearly affects children's functional performance, and prolonged pain can leave the child at risk for other emotional and social problems. In children with arthritis, disease severity and disease activity were found to be associated with behavioral problems and poor social competence (Daltroy et al., 1992). If therapists include pain assessment and intervention in planning interventions for children with painful conditions, they will be better able to meet the child's needs and enhance the outcome of occupational therapy intervention.

## THEORETICAL APPROACHES AND FRAMES OF REFERENCE APPLIED TO OCCUPATIONAL THERAPY INTERVENTION

By now it should be clear that complex factors contribute to a child's occupational function, social and behavioral vulnerabilities, and areas of dysfunction. Occupational therapy has been involved in child psychiatry almost as long as the profession has existed. As the practice of occupational therapy has grown and changed, so has the role of the occupational therapist in treating children. The early occupational therapy literature describing psychosocial interventions with children reflected the conceptual models of childhood psychopathology of the social science community at large. As the early pediatric occupational therapy literature is reviewed, it is difficult to identify a specialized role for occupational therapy in psychosocial settings. For a long time occupational therapists used concepts and components from a variety of sources and made them occupational therapy in the way the ideas were clinically applied. This approach worked for many therapists in pediatric psychosocial settings, but little information about the structure and successes of therapy were documented. By the early 1980s it was clear that occupational therapists used play, art, exercise, music, horticulture, teaching, and social groups in their interventions. It was less clear what made them distinct from play, art, recreation, music, educational, and developmental therapists.

Recent occupational therapy literature has rectified this problem. Even when the occupational therapist uses an approach originated in another field, the link between the application of this approach and occupational therapy theory is clearly described. It is important to understand the major theoretical models of intervention used in psychosocial intervention. The prevalent conceptual models are (1) developmental theories, including sensory integration and structured sensorimotor therapy, (2) social learning and behavioral approaches, (3) model of human occupation, (4) model of social interaction, (5) cognitive rehabilitation, (6) psychodynamic theory, and (7) family systems analytic theory. Each is presented briefly as a background for the occupational therapist. Specific examples are given of occupational therapy interventions incorporating these models.

## Developmental Theories

Developmental theories provide much of the basis of pediatric occupational therapy practice. Developmental approaches follow the assumption that children follow orderly, predictable patterns of development. This theoretical model posits that atypical development is the result of some unusual occurrence, such as a disabling condition or severe social stress. This approach can be used to determine stage- and age-appropriate behavior expectations and can be used as a guide to direct intervention. Children with significant delays can be directed toward an age-appropriate skill level, and the therapist can assess a child's current strengths and weaknesses to anticipate difficulties as the child progresses through life.

Developmental theories are compatible with many occupational therapy theories, particularly sensory integration theory (which is itself a developmental theory) and Model of human occupation. Frank et al. (1991) described a long-term child-therapist relationship that reflects sensitivity to the developmental process and the use of developmental information to guide therapy and anticipate potential problems for the child. A good interdisciplinary example of this approach is presented by Johnson, Berry, Goldeen, and Wicher (1991) in their discussion of therapy for the young child with a spinal cord injury.

*Sensory integration.* The sensory integration (SI) occupational therapy frame of reference is widely used in pediatric interventions, especially with children having social and emotional problems (see Chapter 13). Disorders of sensory modulation and extreme sensory thresholds are common in children who have difficulty behaving in school. These children seem to perform better in a child-centered atmosphere, where they can have some control of the activity and suspend the pressures of the social world.

SI is one of the most commonly used theories guiding occupational therapy interventions for children with psychosocial settings. The child-centered environment established by the therapist becomes a safe environment for the child to first try challenging social and emotional skills. Outside of the clinical setting, helping parents and teachers understand SI dysfunction, accommodation, and remediation can promote appropriate adaptations at home and school.

*Structured sensorimotor therapy.* The structured sensorimotor therapy category of intervention is intended to include all sensorimotor developmental interventions other than SI, for example, neurodevelopment treatment and perceptual motor training. This approach is described in Chapter 24. Children with social and emotional difficulties come with all varieties of sensorimotor strengths and weaknesses. These need to be both assessed and treated because each area of weakness limits the potential of the whole child. A child with cerebral palsy needs the same consideration of his or her social needs as a child with depression. Likewise, the depressed child needs attention to his or her sensorimotor needs.

The structure of this therapy approach is useful in helping children organize and sequence tasks. It provides easily measured goals and obvious increments of improvement. These observable changes are reinforcing for many families and often influence social-emotional function, for example, in self-esteem and confidence. This approach directly addresses areas of delayed skills and is reinforcing to parents and their children.

## Social Learning and Behavioral Approaches

Social learning and behavioral approaches include a group of theories based on the premise that all behavior is a consequence of learning. Whether a behavior is adaptive or maladaptive depends on the social context. Both adaptive and maladaptive behaviors result from the same basic principles of behavior acquisition and maintenance. A pattern of maladaptive behavior may result when a child fails to learn an important behavior (Kaplan & Sadock, 1988). If Javan, whose mother is hearing impaired, fails to learn to modulate the volume of his voice, he will have difficulty in the structured environment of school. In this case he has not received normal social feedback and will need to learn it to meet social expectations. If Javan himself is hearing

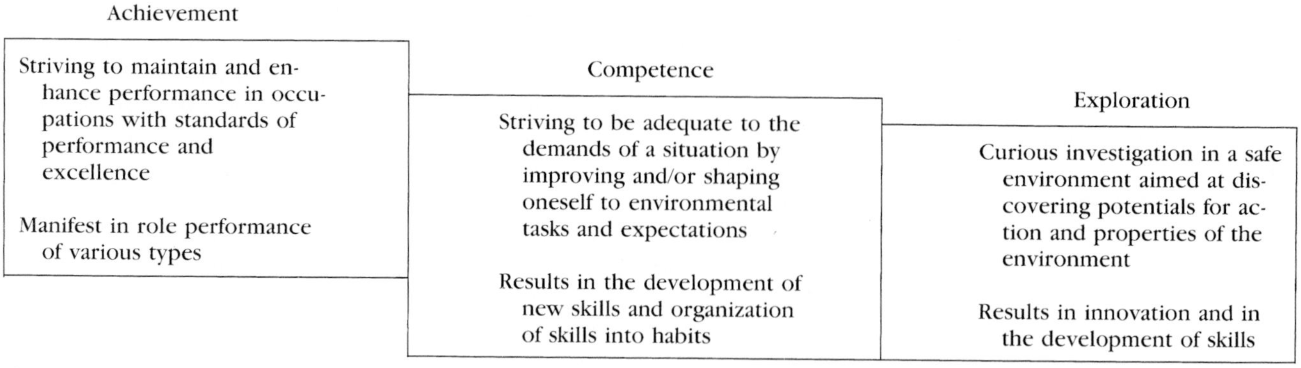

Achievement

| | | |
|---|---|---|
| Striving to maintain and enhance performance in occupations with standards of performance and excellence<br><br>Manifest in role performance of various types | Competence<br><br>Striving to be adequate to the demands of a situation by improving and/or shaping oneself to environmental tasks and expectations<br><br>Results in the development of new skills and organization of skills into habits | Exploration<br><br>Curious investigation in a safe environment aimed at discovering potentials for action and properties of the environment<br><br>Results in innovation and in the development of skills |

**Figure 15-3** Three levels of occupational function. (From Kielhofner, G.S. [1995]. *Model of human occupation.* Baltimore: Williams & Wilkins.)

impaired, the same problem may occur; he may not modulate his voice, but in this case learning to meet expectations is a more difficult process.

Maladaptive behavior also occurs as a consequence of inappropriate learning (Kaplan & Sadock, 1988). As noted earlier, children with a parent who has a depressive disorder are likely to demonstrate poor social competence.

Six-year-old Nikki is the middle child of three children living with her alcoholic mother. Nikki's mother withdraws for days at a time, leaving the children to fend for themselves. Nikki seldom attends school, has poor hygiene, steals, is physically aggressive, and uses inappropriate language at school.

Nikki has learned extreme behaviors, perhaps to earn the attention of her nonresponsive mother. More appropriate behavior can be learned, but ideally the parents should be involved in changing Nikki's environment. Inappropriate learning can be influenced by guiding the child through successive approximations of the difficult skills and modeling the appropriate behavior. Reality testing activities help the older child sort out her personal situation. Another approach would be to reinforce a positive behavior inconsistent with the inappropriate one. Behavior management techniques are common in school and clinical settings. Among the most widely used are time out, performance contracts, self-management and personal responsibility training, and values clarification.

### Model of Human Occupation

The model of human occupation presents adaptive functioning and social competence as the result of efficient, organized occupational behaviors (i.e., play activities, self-care activities, and work). Optimally, these behaviors are organized into patterns or routines that become habit. By relegating everyday behaviors to habit, the child is free to direct more energy to explore, learn, and challenge the environment. The individual is conceptualized as an open system consisting of layers of subsystems. Assessment and treatment planning using the model of human occupation requires consideration of the child's volition (personal causation, values, goals, interests, and personal performance standards), habituation (child's perceived roles, behavior habits, and routines), performance (sensorimotor and cognitive skills), and environment (object, task, interpersonal, and cultural). Patterns of function and dysfunction in each area are noted, and treatment is planned to interrupt dysfunctional cycles and replace them with the performance skills needed to enhance the child's development and adaptive behavior. Especially useful in planning interventions with children are the levels of occupational function presented in Figure 15-3. This provides a framework for assessing the child's social actions as output of the occupational behavior process.

### Model of Social Interaction

A recent addition to occupational therapy theory is the model of social interaction developed by Doble and Magill-Evans (1992). Drawing from the model of human occupation and other sources, this model views the individual as ". . . an open system whose output is socially-oriented occupational behavior" (Doble & Magill-Evans, 1992, p. 143). Figure 15-4 illustrates the components of this model. The *social processing* component is made up of three separate processes: reception, interpretation, and planning. Through social processing the individual makes sense of social information and develops a cognitive plan for response.

The first component, social processing, is the focus of social interaction problems for children with right-hemisphere dysfunction syndrome and who cannot make sense of information. Impulsive children, like those with ADDH or closed-head injury, are likely to have difficulty making a plan.

The next step, motor planning, is the action after the cognitive plan. Children with SI dysfunction or other motor disorders are likely to be limited in motor planning. The observable output of this step is called *social enactment skills.*

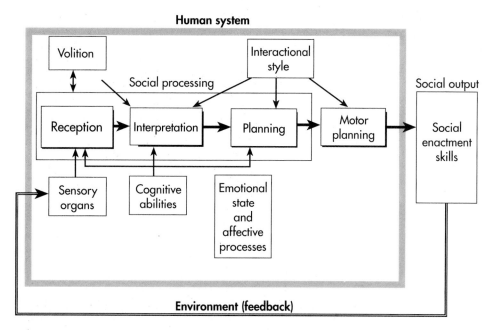

**Figure 15-4**    Model of social interaction. (From Doble, S.E. & Magill-Evans, J. [1992]. A model of social interaction to guide occupational therapy practice. *Canadian Journal of Occupational Therapy, 59*[3], 143.)

As a part of a dynamic open system, the social enactment skills of the individual result in a change in the environment that provides feedback to the individual.

Social enactment skills "enable us to communicate our needs and intentions to others and to respond to the messages of others in a competent manner" (Doble & Magill-Evans, 1992, p. 146). Social enactment skills may be verbal or nonverbal. They include the following major categories of interaction: acknowledging skills, sending skills, timing skills, and coordinating skills (see box on p. 410). This model provides a structured analysis of the social process and grounds intervention in occupational therapy theory.

### Psychodynamic Theory

Psychodynamic theory includes the work of Freud and later clinicians building on his model. Much of this complex model relies on unconscious symbols and free association to uncover suppressed emotions. An important aspect of psychoanalytic theory is the defense mechanism.

[M]aladaptive defensive functioning is directed against conflicts between impulses that are characteristic of a specific developmental phase . . ., or the child's internalized representations of the environment. . . . The result [of this defensive functioning] is difficulty in achieving or resolving developmental tasks (Kaplan & Sadock, 1988, p. 638).

Psychodynamic interventions require extensive specialized training and are beyond the scope of occupational therapy. Occupational therapists have assimilated aspects of

the psychodynamic approach to improve the occupational functioning of children. Intervention usually involves some creative or expressive media that augments the child's ability to express emotion.

### Family Systems Analytic Theory

The family systems analytic theory uses the open system premise for families in much the same way that the model of human occupation uses it for individuals. The focus of this approach is communication and family interaction. Although similar to occupational therapy theory at the conceptual level, this approach is not well suited to occupational therapy. This approach relies heavily on counseling and verbal interaction and is not an activity-oriented intervention process. Effective use of this approach requires specialized training not commonly available to occupational therapists.

An occupational therapist can collaborate with mental health counselors using a family systems approach without special training. The counselor may identify specific functional and performance problems among family members that lead to negative dynamics among family members. These functional and performance problems could then be appropriately addressed by the occupational therapist. An example of this is presented by Olson et al. (1989). These authors described occupational therapy intervention in a community outreach program focused on children at risk for developing psychiatric disorders. This intervention centers on a parent-child activity group emphasizing play and interpersonal communications.

## Examples of Social Enactment Skills

1. Acknowledging skills
   Looks and gazes
   Touches
   Positions
   Gestures (e.g., nods head)
   Says "yes"
2. Sending skills
   Greets
   Initiates
   Asks and inquires
   Accepts
   Encourages
   Refuses
   Reveals
   Disengages and terminates
3. Timing skills
   Initiates without hesitation
   Speaks without unnecessary interruption
   Speaks without repeating information unnecessarily
   Maintains a reasonable pace when speaking
   Ends message without perseverating
   Ends message without stopping prematurely
   Ends message after reasonable period (does not go on and on)
4. Coordinating skills
   Sends message compatible with social partner's abilities (e.g., language comprehension)
   Sends message compatible with social partner's interests
   Sends message compatible with social partner's affective tone
   Sends message compatible with social partner's level of self-revelation
   Sends message compatible with expectations of situations (physical, interpersonal)
   Builds on partner's prior social messages
   Uses variations in message styles (alternates questions with disclosure and information provision)

From Doble S.E. & Magill-Evans, J. (1992). A model of social interaction to guide occupational therapy practice. *Canadian Journal of Occupational Therapy, 59*(3), 147.

## EVALUATION

Occupational therapy evaluation in pediatrics is dealt with at length in Section II of this text. The children seen by occupational therapists that have limitations in the psychosocial and emotional domains of behavior need to be assessed holistically. Sensorimotor and developmental delays are common with this group and may be assessed with the methods used with any other child. Accommodations may be needed when administering standardized tests to children with behavior disorders. For example, shorter sessions may be needed, extra time may be required to persuade the child to attempt items, and rewards such as stickers or food may be required to motivate the child to respond.

In selecting assessments for this population, it is important to remember that a child's function in a particular environment may differ from the skill demonstrated in a controlled test environment. For instance, a child may be independent in eating when tested in the clinic, but the same child may be so distracted and overstimulated in the school lunchroom that he or she does not persist at the activity. His or her distractibility may lead to excess spillage and inadequate food intake. Besides causing social problems, being hungry all afternoon does not improve the child's mood or ability to learn. Assessments that consider parent and teacher reports are especially useful in singling out daily function from abilities that they may have in controlled settings.

Another important consideration is that children diagnosed with psychosocial or emotional conditions may be taking medications to influence their behavior. It is imperative to ask if the child takes medications and if he or she is taking medicine at the time of testing. This is particularly important when children are taking methylphenidate (Ritalin). Methylphenidate is often given on an as-needed basis (i.e., only when the child is in school) and has a short active period in the body. This medication can greatly influence the child's performance. Some well-coordinated children with attention deficits appear clumsy because of impulsiveness and inattention to tasks when they have not taken their medication. These children may appear dyspraxic if they are tested without their medications even though their performance is normal when medicated.

Medications are widely used for psychosis and affective and anxiety disorders. In acute settings children with these problems are often medicated in the manner of adults with the same problem. There continues to be controversy about the long-term use of these medications, and it is clear that medications alone do not remediate the difficulties in social behavior that are so disabling in school and community situations. The occupational therapist needs to know the intended effects of all medications and their side effects to help monitor the drug's effectiveness and safety.

### Naturalistic Observation

A naturalistic assessment may be a simple as a systematic series of lunchroom observations to determine what in the environment is problematic for a particular child. In interventions designed to help the child function in his or her everyday environment, test scores showing how many standard deviations a child is from the mean are not very helpful to planning. Naturalistic observation is most useful when it is conducted in a systematic organized manner. Table 15-5 provides three good examples of this approach.

▲ Table 15-5    Naturalistic Assessments

| Test/Source | Comments | Age (Years) |
|---|---|---|
| Transdisciplinary Play-Based Assessment (TPA)<br>Source: Paul H. Brookes Publishing<br>    P.O. Box 10624<br>    Baltimore, MD 21285 | Provides information on all areas of functional<br>    performance | 0-4 |
| Preschool Play Scale<br>Source: *American Journal of Occupational Therapy, 36,*<br>    783-788 and *American Journal of Occupational*<br>    *Therapy, 40,* 691-695. | Provides information on many areas of functional<br>    performance; simpler but less comprehensive than TPA | 0-4 |
| Ethnographic Classroom Analysis<br>Source: *American Journal of Occupational Therapy, 48,*<br>    397-402. | Provides information about social and environmental<br>    demands in the classroom | 5-18 |

Children with social or behavioral difficulties often perform better in nondirective environments. Allowing 10 or 15 minutes of child-directed play before formal testing provides valuable clinical observations and may greatly improve the child's compliance on structured test items.

## Informal Scales and Structured Observation

Informal scales provide information about a child's awareness of themselves and their social roles. Interviews, such as *The University of Texas Medical Branch—Initial Interview* (Figure 15-5), provide an example of this. These scales provide an organized format but allow therapists to expand the questions at their own discretion. Although several excellent role assessments have been published, it remains difficult to get reliable responses from an unhappy 13-year-old child in the test environment. Open-ended questions that can be expanded based on the child's answers seem to be the best accepted type of question with children and young adolescents.

### Observational Checklist

Another common use for informal scales is to document the quality of a child's performance. *The University of Texas Medical Branch—Task Performance Scale* is an example of this (Figure 15-6). Another example of this type of tool is a group behavior survey that identifies the specific social behaviors in a group situation. This type of tool is especially useful when the child has difficulties with peer relations and social interaction. *Ayres Clinical Observation of Sensory Integration* (Ayres, 1972) is a widely used performance scale to assess basic sensory integrative function. This scale has been widely copied and adapted in pediatric settings.

The *Developmental Interview for Parents of Young Children at Risk* (Davidson, 1995) offers an interview structure to identify problems between the parent, the child, and the environment. This tool provides valuable information about the family environment, daily routines, and the parent's expectations of the child. This instrument was designed to help identify families at risk for child abuse. Because many of the risk factors for child abuse parallel those for children's social and emotional problems, this instrument provides useful insights for all pediatric therapists.

### Interest and Role Checklists

Interest checklists are widely used in clinical settings. This type of scale was originally described by Matsutsuyu (1969). Neville and Kielhofner (1983) developed a modification of the checklist format that includes current interests as well as both historic and current reporting of actual participation in activities. This gives a clearer idea of how the child actually uses his or her time. It identifies discrepancies between interests and activities and helps the therapist review how the child's leisure behavior has changed.

Role checklists have been developed that are appropriate for older adolescents (Florey & Michelman, 1978). Role assessment is an important tool in assessing childhood performance, but children's roles are less discrete than those of adults. Roles can be interpreted from the information collected on many other tests, including play assessments and developmental assessments. Using this information, the therapist can add informal questions directed at both the child and the caretaker to clarify the child's current role function.

### Sensory and Sensorimotor Histories

Sensory histories are important when a child has social or emotional problems because children often have sensorimotor difficulties as well. Sensorimotor or sensory processing problems can exaggerate social problems. Poor sensory processing can lead to disorders of sensory modulation and sensory avoidance behaviors. These disorders are often associated with inappropriate social behavior and sometimes with aggression. Children with either extremely high or extremely low sensory thresholds are likely to have

**INITIAL INTERVIEW**

**Biographic Information**

How old are you?_____     When is your birthday?_____

Where do you live (city)?_____     What is the street address?_____

**Home**

Who lives in your house? (ages of siblings?)

Do you have any pets?

What is your room like?

What chores do you do at home?

Does your mother/father work?     What does your mother/father do at work?

What do you do at home that gets you in trouble?

Who gets mad at you when you get in trouble?     What do they do?

What does your mother/father do that gets you mad?     What do you do?

**School**

What grade are you in school?

What do you like most about school?

What do you like least about school?

**Peers**

Who is your best friend?     What activities do you like to do with him or her?

Who are some of your other friends?

Is there anyone around your house or at school that you do not like?

Why don't you like him or her?

**Figure 15-5**     Child psychiatric initial interview at the University of Texas Medical Branch.

difficulties similar to those associated with sensory modulation disorders. Table 15-6 lists some published instruments for collecting data on the child's sensory function.

*Psychosocial assessments.* Standardized tests that are specifically useful in assessing psychosocial issues include the *Piers-Harris Children's Self-Concept Scale* (Piers, 1984), which is appropriate for children between 8 and 18 years of age. This test provides information about the child's perception of his or her own behavior, intelligence, school performance, physical appearance, anxiety, popularity, and happiness. The *Vineland Adaptive Behavior Scales* (Sparrow, Balla, & Cicchetti, 1987) is an interview-based survey that is administered to parents or caretakers. This provides a general assessment of strengths and weaknesses and an overall measure of social behaviors compared with developmental norms. A similar test, the *Gardener Social Developmental Scale* (Gardener, 1994) compares parent re-

**Work/Play/Leisure**

What do you do after school?                    What kinds of games do you like to play?

What do you do on weekends?

Do you have any hobbies?

**Personal Here and Now Status**

Why are you in the hospital?

What do you want to change while you are in the hospital?

Tell me something good about yourself.

If you could change anything about yourself by wishing, what would it be?

Length of Interview _____

**Observations**

Good/poor eye contact
Cooperative/uncooperative
Appeared comfortable/uncomfortable
Easy/difficult to obtain responses to questions
Direct/rambling responses
Information reliable/unreliable

**Additional Comments/Observations**

**Interviewer** _____

**Figure 15-5, cont'd.**   Child psychiatric initial interview at the University of Texas Medical Branch.

▲ Table 15-6   Sensory Histories

| Instrument/Source | Comments | Age (Years) |
|---|---|---|
| Touch Inventory for Elementary School-Aged Children Source: Royeen & Fortune, 1990 | The child is interviewed | 6-12 |
| Teacher Questionnaire on Sensorimotor Behavior Source: Carrasco & Lee, 1993 | Teacher questionaire that provides teachers perception of the child's sensory reactions in the classroom | 4-12 |
| Sensory History Source: Cook, 1991. | Questionnaire for parents that provides parent's perception of child's sensory experiences. This form includes information about the school-aged child | 0-12 |
| Sensorimotor History Source: Knickerbocker 1980. | Questionnaire for parents that provides parents' perception of child's early sensory experiences | 0-10 |

Project _____

Structure          None          Minimal          Moderate          High

Completed in _____ sessions

**TASK COMPONENTS**

**Type of Directions Used**
— Written
— Verbal
— Demonstrated

**Ability to Follow Direction**
— Unable
— Needed directions at each step
— Needed directions at the beginning of the project with few reminders during process

**Organization**
— No organization; trial and error approach
— Developed a plan with assistance; needed help in breaking task into sequential steps
— Organized task with little or no assistance

**Problem Solving**
— Unable to recognize problems or suggest solutions
— Able to recognize problems but not suggest solutions
— Able to recognize problems and suggest realistic solutions

**Attention Span**
— Less than 15 minutes
— 15 to 30 minutes with few interruptions
— 30 to 45 minutes with few interruptions

**Concentration**
— Worked only when environmental distractions were at a minimum (outside the group)
— Worked when environmental distractions were at a moderate level (in clinic, others doing quiet tasks)
— No problems noticed (in clinic, others doing loud tasks)

**Figure 15-6**    Task Performance Scale. The University of Texas Medical Branch.

ports of a child or client's behavior with a normative sample of behaviors reported by parents. This test questionnaire is completed by the parent and provides standard information on the child's social behavior. The *Social Adjustment Inventory for Children and Adolescents (SAICA),* (John, Gammon, Prusoff, & Warner, 1987) is a semistructured interview schedule that assesses patterns of social function in children and adolescents in school, in leisure activities, and with peers, siblings, and parents.

## PRIMARY INTERVENTION STRATEGIES
### Environmental Adaptation

Many of the occupational therapy approaches described in this chapter use environmental adaptation as a primary strategy. The occupational therapist adapts the child's environment to alter the sensory input, to help the child organize materials, to affect the child's mood and affect, and to encourage specific behaviors. Environmental adaptation re-

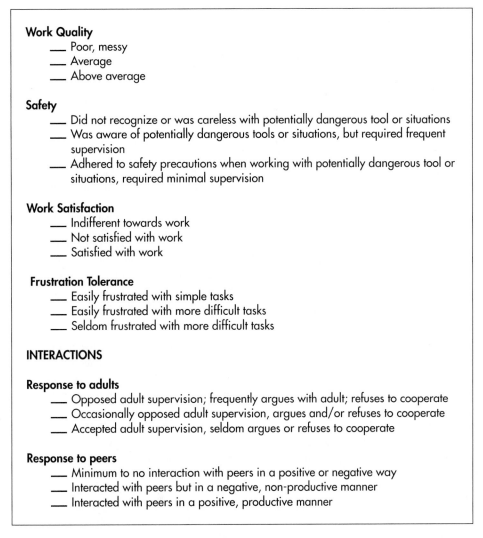

**Work Quality**
___ Poor, messy
___ Average
___ Above average

**Safety**
___ Did not recognize or was careless with potentially dangerous tool or situations
___ Was aware of potentially dangerous tools or situations, but required frequent supervision
___ Adhered to safety precautions when working with potentially dangerous tool or situations, required minimal supervision

**Work Satisfaction**
___ Indifferent towards work
___ Not satisfied with work
___ Satisfied with work

**Frustration Tolerance**
___ Easily frustrated with simple tasks
___ Easily frustrated with more difficult tasks
___ Seldom frustrated with more difficult tasks

**INTERACTIONS**

**Response to adults**
___ Opposed adult supervision; frequently argues with adult; refuses to cooperate
___ Occasionally opposed adult supervision, argues and/or refuses to cooperate
___ Accepted adult supervision, seldom argues or refuses to cooperate

**Response to peers**
___ Minimum to no interaction with peers in a positive or negative way
___ Interacted with peers but in a negative, non-productive manner
___ Interacted with peers in a positive, productive manner

**Figure 15-6, cont'd.** Task Performance Scale. The University of Texas Medical Branch.

quires analysis of the cognitive and psychosocial functions of the individual and then alteration of the environments in which he or she must function to maximize those abilities. In its simplest form, environmental adaptation provides an external device (or place) to organize behaviors. This device may be a notebook with reminders of work and school routines or a designated quiet place where the student can sit when stressed. Other examples of environmental adaptation include organizing a child's work space at school with labeled compartments so he or she knows where to locate and store the tool he or she needs in school or programming a telephone with frequently called numbers. Environmental adaptation can involve assistive technology such as electronic reminders to take medicines, do homework, or walk the dog.

Adapting the sensory environment has long been a component of sensory integrative interventions. Children who have low sensory thresholds or a disorder of sensory modulation may need clothes of only natural fibers or oversized clothes to be comfortable enough to attend to other things in the world. Some easily aroused children may benefit from a noise machine to help them go to sleep. Each of these environmental adaptations compensates for the lack of a particular skill needed in the child's world.

In children with task impersistence, the obvious functional goal is independence in task completion. Attention is an important aspect of persistence. To improve the child's success with tasks, the tasks need to be structured and have clear cues to help the child orient himself or herself as needed. The therapist's job is to organize the task and then teach the child to use cues and self-monitoring strategies. Older children can be taught to organize tasks and cues for themselves.

## Social Behavioral Interventions

The focus of social and behavioral intervention is learning positive, functional-oriented skills. This type of intervention is well suited to occupational therapy and is widely used. The basic tenets of social learning theory dovetail effectively with the model of human occupation (Kielhofner, 1985). Some specific examples of social behavior interventions follow.

Noncompetitive board games can be used in a group situation to demonstrate cooperation and turn taking. A good game for use with adolescents is *The Ungame* (Talicor, 1989). For younger children a variety of noncompetitive games can be adapted for clinical use. The game *Funny Face* (Deacove, 1987) promotes noncompetitive interaction. This game has playing cards requesting specific facial expressions and gestures as the game progresses. It helps children be aware of nonverbal communication in a lighthearted style.

## Self-Management and Values Clarification

Self-management and values clarification discussion groups are used as intervention strategies with adults. The same types of groups have worked well with adolescents, with attention paid to normal developmental issues in adolescence. Self-management remains an important goal with younger children. In children with a neurobiologic basis to their behavior problems (e.g., ADDH or closed-head injury), improvement in self-management may have a highly positive effect on the develoment of social skills.

Self-management interventions with preschool children include modeling and teaching productive peer relations, making the child aware of the behaviors expected in specific environments, and organizing or altering the environment to enable positive performances. By school age, children are often able to articulate concerns, complaints, and fears in a manner specific enough to engage in discussions about hypothetic situations and solutions. Performance contracts are a step toward self-management that can be carried out in all of the child's environments. A successful performance contract must be a collaborative effort. The child and supervising adult (therapist, parent, or teacher) review an area of problem performance, and the child is prompted to describe behaviors that impede progress. The child negotiates the performance standards and consequences of the contract (both rewards and punishments). The following examples describes the use of self-management intervention.

Travis (10 years old) was worried about an upcoming class field trip. He had been suspended from school after the last field trip because of aggressive and disruptive behavior on the school bus. This upcoming trip would involve a total of 5 hours on the bus. He wanted to see the museum but was considering skipping the field trip to stay out of trouble. The occupational therapist led Travis to describe specifically what had happened before and why he thought it was so difficult to ride the bus.

Travis had an intense temperament, a high activity level, and a low sensory threshold. Tactile defensiveness had been observed in the therapy environment. Travis said that the bus was "too loud," he got a headache, and felt "edgy" when riding for even

short periods. Travis also disliked being bumped and stepped on by other kids. Travis was polite and cooperative at home and in occupational therapy sessions. At school he was rude and disruptive. He said he felt "out-of-control" and that the teacher "set him up" for problems. Travis functioned adequately in his expected roles, except the important roles of student, team member, and friend. His intensity and poor impulse control left him at risk for continuing problems in cooperative activity. Travis had difficulty remaining seated for long periods and experienced a low frustration tolerance and high distractibiltiy.

He and the therapist consulted with his family and the teacher as they developed their strategy. Travis would bring his tape player and headphones to cut out some of the bus noise. He would be early so that he could pick a good seat near the front of the bus (he was sure less jostling happened here) and by the window. That way he would not be on an aisle, likely to be stepped on.

Travis had a successful field trip. He also learned that he could think through difficult situations and gain control of them. He gained the respect of his teacher for trying to constructively change his behavior, and his teacher became more sensitive to his needs. Both Travis and his family were excited to have found a way to anticipate and negotiate difficult situations.

Values clarification groups, in their traditional format, are above the developmental levels of most pediatric clients. The idea of using social and personal values can be applied in concrete, functional terms with school-aged children. This is done much in the same way as self-management. Specific places and activities are presented, with leading questions about appropriate and inappropriate behavior. For example, questions like "Do you like going to the grocery store?" "Why?" "What happens when you get in trouble?" "Why did you want to do that?" "Who had to pick up all the cans?" "Did anyone get hurt?" "Could anyone have gotten hurt?" lead the discussion to a responsibility for the safety of others and personal behavior in public places. Following this up with a trip to the grocery store would help the child remember and apply the discussion.

Board games may be used to provide practice for difficult social situations. The structure and format of these games make them accessible to young adolescents. This provides a forum for values clarification with younger clients. Commonly used therapeutic board games are *The Ungame* (Talicor, 1989), which offers a noncompetitive format that prompts the child to express likes, dislikes, and emotions in a group setting, and *Stop, Relax, & Think* (Bridges, 1990), which promotes cognitive strategies to overcome impulsivity and increase prosocial behavior in a variety of situations.

## Interest Groups

Soon after a child begins school their social environment dramatically expands. Middle childhood is the time when children understand that they have different roles in different social environments. As children seek to identify a sense of self, they begin to develop interests or habits. Most school-aged children in North America can tell you what they like about school, about sports, and about music. The acquisition of social and personal values serves as a precursor to adult decision making. Interest groups for children might better be called self-awareness groups because the focus is on "who am I?" "what do I do well?" "what frustrates me?" "what makes a game fun?" From this, children begin to distill personal and social interests. Many children with social and emotional problems have limited social interests, and much of their time is focused on things that frustrate them. This adds to their sense of helplessness and isolation. Identifying and developing interests is a way to interrupt a negative cycle.

In adolescence, interest groups can evolve into vocational interest groups. Children with a history of school failure may not be able to picture themselves in a competent adult role. Children with severe physical disabilities may have a sense of physical helplessness that limits the possibilities they consider. Exploring vocational interests while supporting the development of community skills is an appropriate direction for adolescent interventions.

## Socratic Questioning

Socratic questioning (SQ) is a familiar technique in education and cognitive therapy and is well suited to occupational therapy interventions. This approach is structured and directed by the therapist, yet gives power and responsibility to the child. SQ involves facing a task or activity as a problem. The child is asked something like "What do you need to do first?" Each of the child's responses are guided by further questions such as "Why did you choose that?" "Is there another way to do it?" The child is led through skillful questioning to organize the problem and then come to an answer.

This approach helps the individual sort out and learn to organize his or her thoughts. As they learn foundation skills, like basic social rules, these rules can serve as prompting questions when the children deal with new behaviors. With this approach the children have a growing sense of accomplishment that results from coming to the answers themselves. A strength of this approach is that the learning seems to be more readily internalized so that the child can problem solve independently in new situations.

James loved sports but was not allowed to participate in any after-school programs because of his disruptive behaviors. Playing basketball on the playground in the after-school program was a personal goal of his. The occupational therapist encouraged a dialog with James about this issue, asking this question sequence: "Why won't the teachers let you play?"; "Why do you think they don't like you?"; "Do all the kids think that they are mean, or just you?"; "Why do you think they single you out?"; "Do you like getting into all those fights?"; "Why do you get into so many, then?" This process continues for some time until James comes to state that his behavior has been the reason he was excluded. From that point the questioning can be turned to "What happened before you felt like hitting Bobby?"

In time James can be directed to acknowledge not only his responsibility in the problem, but also some of the precipitating factors and some potential solutions that will allow him to play basketball. As James gained skill in the SQ process, it could be used as a problem-solving tool for difficult school tasks, social problems, and for working things out with his parents.

SQ is a powerful therapy tool and is relatively easy to learn. The difficult part of SQ is persisting with the resistive child long enough to begin to elicit productive responses. This approach is useful in task-focused applications and is more easily accepted by children in that form. A training program like Lindamood's (1981) *Lindamood Visual Conceptual Program* has been used clinically to improve visual perception and handwriting skills while teaching the SQ method. After a task-based introduction, the questioning is easily transferred to more sensitive subjects such as peer acceptance and teacher conflicts that limit the child's ability to perform in the school environment.

## Social Skills Training

Many commercial social skills training programs have been developed for teachers to enhance social behavior in children. These are generally developed for a classroom activity but may be individualized and used successfully by occupational therapists. Occupational therapists should use these programs in conjunction with theory-guided assessment and intervention planning. With a theory-based and developmentally delineated understanding of social behaviors to guide decisions, the occupational therapist may successfully train social and interpersonal skills without a commercial program. In the following description of a young girl, the critical nature of social skills to all functional areas and roles is exemplified:

Sophia was 8 years old when she was referred to occupational therapy at school for sensorimotor delays. At age 5 she was removed from an abusive home, where she had been confined to a small room. Before placement in a foster home, Sophia had never been around other children, had seldom been out in public, and had habitually spent 10 to 12 hours alone daily with the television on. Her medical record indicated a suspicion of fetal alcohol syndrome, and both biologic parents had a history of polysubstance abuse.

After adoption by her foster parents, Sophia participated in intense psychotherapy and was home-schooled for 2 years. Sophia was now entering school as a first grader. She was quiet and withdrawn in the classroom. She was able to do the academic work but did not interact with the teacher or peers in the classroom. She did not consistently speak when spoken to, and in cooperative activities she would pull away from the group.

Sophia has good language comprehension but difficulty in all other cognitive areas associated with interpretation of social information. She has poor awareness of social rules and inferring the meaning of social behaviors based on contextual cues. For example, on the playground several children were playing "freeze tag." Sophia had never seen any sort of tag game before. When a boy ran by her and tagged her roughly, Sophia ran away crying hysterically. She later said she was afraid that he was going to hurt her because she was in the way. Sophia was unaware that her self-imposed isolation punctuated by dramatic outbursts made her classmates uncomfortable. She was fearful and had a highly externalized sense of control. Sophia's usual first response to social overtunes was a failure to acknowledge or respond.

Her occupational therapy program goals focused on sensorimotor delays and teaching basic social rules in therapy (and later playground) situations. Sophia's motor skills improved rapidly, and with it her behavior in occupational therapy began to change. From a quiet withdrawn child, she became physically boisterous and impulsive. Her social interactions were extreme and unpredictable. The intervention team speculated that as Sophia gained skill and confidence in motor skills, she felt secure enough to explore and try new behaviors.

An activity program based on art and handwriting skill training was initiated to capitalize on Sophia's growing social awareness. As she drew, she was drawn into a story-telling game. She and the therapist took turns adding to the story and drawing new aspects to the mural they made. The focus of this intervention was problem solving social situations. Sophia quickly understood and began to use appropriate sending and timing skills. When the therapist included her in a handwriting skills group, Sophia began to demonstrate appropriate acknowledging behaviors and began to learn how to negotiate and coordinate with age-mates.

### Child-Centered Intervention

Child-centered intervention (CCI) activity was first developed as a form of psychotherapy (Guerney, 1983). With this approach, interventions have a flexible sequence, involve exploration and creativity, and are centered in the child's choices and interests. In CCI the child is the initiator of activity, and the adult is the facilitator. The therapy environment for CCI must be organized to make activities available that promote development. Part of the art of this approach is creating an appealing environment that limits inappropriate play choices without adult intervention. CCI is useful in all types of pediatric interventions. It has been used successfully for improvement of sensorimotor problems as well as for enhancing social and behavioral skills (DeGangi, Wietlisbach, Goodin, & Scheiner, 1993) (see Chapter 10).

This approach to the child emphasizes interpersonal interaction by relying on negotiation and flexibility rather than structure and verbal praise. CCI is useful in initial therapy sessions for establishing rapport and a positive environment. As the child recognizes that he or she has some control and that his or her opinion is solicited, antisocial behaviors tend to decrease. CCI often works well with children having difficult temperaments because it seems to disarm their struggle to take control. By allowing them some control, the children accept both the therapist and therapy environment more' readily. Even in situations better suited to structured interventions, CCI is useful as a transition technique. It can be a gentle introduction to therapy and can be used later when inappropriate behavior interferes with therapy progress. CCI is a positive, supportive intervention that helps when the child appears stressed or "down."

Sophia was so withdrawn and passive in her first contact, the occupational therapist decided to use CCI while establishing rapport. In the first session Sophia was given a choice of toys and activities and was warmly invited to play. She sat quietly and did not explore the room. The therapist then walked around the room pointing out the equipment, toys, and art supplies. Shyly, Sophia took a piece of paper and some markers to the table. The therapist mirrored her activity. As Sophia drew, the therapist remarked "I'm drawing too; I want to make a picture like yours," "That is a very pretty cat; I want to try and draw a cat too," "Your picture has a lot of yellow in it; I will put some yellow on my picture." During the entire session, Sophia verbalized very little, but her affect brightened, she made eye contact more often, and she did not demonstrate the avoidance gestures common in the classroom.

Soon Sophia had ideas about what she wanted to do in therapy and requested them. By retaining the CCI approach the therapist could support both social and sensorimotor skill development. When the relationship seemed secure, the therapist began making activity suggestions, although Sophia continued to have veto power. Sophia came to trust that the therapist would choose activities that were fun and not too hard for her. As she spoke more, simple negotiations of play activities began, allowing the presentation of social play rules and allowing Sophia to practice skills she needed in peer interactions.

Child-centered activity was the subject of research by De-Gangi et al. (1993). Their findings with the preschool population are consistent with the clinical experience of this author.

The child-centered activity approach may allow the child to exert autonomy and control over the environment, to organize attention and play schemes, and to seek out environmental stimuli that are more self-organizing (p. 782).

Child-centered activity is also useful in eliciting imaginative play and storytelling. For children with difficulty in appropriately expressing emotions and with poor social skills, this provides a safe, stimulating therapy environment to explore these skills.

### Expressive Interventions

Expressive interventions include diverse activities such as role playing, art and craft projects, and drama. Fraenkel and Tallant (1987) present a structured drawing program as a projective media for school-aged children. The program uses a structured drawing workbook with captions such as "This is me" and "Things that bug me." The following are suggested occupational therapy treatment objectives:

1. To encourage the expression of feelings and conflicts
2. To facilitate the expression of fantasies and wishes
3. To help the child gain insight and self-awareness
4. To encourage the child to become aware of and relinquish their maladaptive defense mechanisms
5. To enhance the development of decision-making skills

Other examples of occupational therapy interventions incorporating expressive aspects in pediatric interventions are Bracegirdle's (1992) analysis of uses of play and Fazio's (1992) application of the therapeutic metaphor. In both of these examples the psychodynamic aspect is only a part of the intervention. These approaches are focused on acquisition of skills and improved daily function. Expressive interventions are also appropriate to both the model of human occupation and the model of social interaction.

### Parent-Focused Therapy

Parents are crucial in the success of any occupational therapy program. Previously it was noted that many children with social and behavioral problems have a parent with similar problems. Involvement of parents in the child's program is discussed at length in Chapter 5. It is often advantageous to teach parents the skills and behaviors that are limiting their child and to provide them with concrete but socially neutral examples. Parent training and social skills training may be combined to encourage the parent to support their child. The following are some suggested parent training goals (Cousins & Weiss, 1993, p. 449):

1. To learn more about the importance of developing social competence and positive peer status
2. To use incidental teaching and self-evaluation strategies
3. To become strategic organizers of the child's social life
4. To become service coordinators to facilitate more consistency between the significant adults in the child's social environment

## ▲ Therapy Considerations to Promote Psychosocial Development in all Children with Disabilities

### SOCIAL VALUES REASONING

Culture is the social background that is learned and then used to evaluate things and behaviors. Culture influences all aspects of human life. Different cultures value possessions, formal education, food, and even time in different ways. The occupational therapist needs to be sensitive to the possibility that certain behaviors, including a family's failure to follow through with the therapist's recommendations, may be attributable to differing cultural values. The role of the occupational therapist is to identify those cultural issues creating conflict. In the case of the uncooperative family, the conflict may be between the goals established by the therapist and the goals valued by the family. Conflict may also be between the values of the family and the values of the community.

When the conflict is between family cultural values and the community values system, the occupational therapist is in the position of mediator. The reason a mediator is needed is that most children must deal with both the culture of their family and that of the community. A warm, supportive home environment that embraces the child's physical disability as a unique aspect of the child is an ideal offered in many homes. This loving nurturance may also be paired with a tendency to exclude the child from social responsibility as he or she reaches adolescence. The rude 3-year-old child with cerebral palsy is cute, but the rude 15-year-old child is disabled physically and socially. Chapter 5 develops the dilemma. There is a fine line between preparing a child to face the adult world and imposing middle-class values on persons from differing cultural backgrounds.

## ESTABLISHING A POSITIVE THERAPY ENVIRONMENT

The first step in managing the child's behavior is to establish a positive and supportive therapy environment. Affirmation and positive reinforcement of behavior help establish appropriate responses. Praising specific appropriate behavior causes that behavior to increase and informs the child about your expectations. It is important to praise specific behaviors. For example, say, "you are aiming those beanbags very carefully" rather than "good boy," and, "I like the careful way you are listening," rather than "nice work."

Another important strategy employed by therapists is intermittent echoing of appropriate speech. Repeating and paraphrasing the child's speech shows respect for the child and his or her ideas. It also indicates to the child that the therapist is listening. This approach has the advantage of improving and increasing the child's verbal communication while modeling appropriate turn-taking in conversation. If the child says, "this is going to be a picture of a spider," the therapist replies, "it is fun to draw interesting things like spiders." When the child says, "I like to go fast on the swing," the therapist replies, "It's really fun to go fast on that swing."

A final and often overlooked part of the therapy environment is the therapist's affect. The therapist should clearly demonstrate that he or she has enjoyed the time with the child. Laughter and clowning convey this impression. The therapist's delight in the interaction helps the child feel valued and over time helps him or her to develop positive feelings about the therapy experience.

## BEHAVIOR MANAGEMENT INTERVENTIONS

Behavior management is based on behavior modification methods and is an effective tool for improving both social and academic behaviors. Behavior management includes both the use of external controls (such as time out) and techniques to teach individuals to control their own behavior (such as performance contracts). The management of behavior is important with all occupational therapy interventions. Inappropriate behavior can limit the child's function and can limit the child's progress on therapy goals.

The therapist expects to manage the behavior of a child who is labeled "emotionally handicapped," but most children seen for therapy need some degree of external behavior control during the course of therapy. Because of different cultural values, guilt, or simply poor understanding of their child's abilities, some parents of children with disabilities do not teach basic manners and social behaviors. These physically disabled or "ill" children, who have no psychosocial disorders, often develop dysfunctional interpersonal behaviors that exaggerate their disability. Their behaviors often limit social interactions more dramatically than their disability ever would.

Rude behaviors are attention getting, even though they isolate the individual. Children with disabilities need to be respected as individuals with feelings, ideas, and emotional needs. Likewise, children with disabilities need to respect other individuals in their world. Manners are a social tool reflecting respect. The occupational therapist needs to model and expect developmentally appropriate social interactions in the therapy session. The theory and intervention models presented in this chapter provide specific approaches to this type of intervention.

Society does not deal well with long-term disability. The individual who has a disability often is allowed to break social rules. Overdependency and passivity may be inadvertently fostered. Parents are often caught up in day-to-day matters and do not see how their child's social behavior will affect them as adults. The occupational therapist needs to discuss these concerns with the parent and include the family in any plan to introduce social skills training. This is a sensitive area because targeting it for intervention is often interpreted by families as a poor reflection on their parenting. Therapists need to be sensitive to this possibility both in describing the problem and in soliciting family input for remediation.

## Routine Behavioral Strategies for Managing Problems in Therapy

Therapists should establish behavior rules early in the therapy relationship and repeat them before "at-risk" activities. When appropriate, rules can be posted. A sign stating "Ask before using the swings" is neutral and lets the child know the rule is for everyone. Rules for intervention groups should be more extensive than those for individual behaviors. Group rules should reflect respect for the rights of others. Obvious rules might be "No physical contact without permission," or "Each person is allowed 2 minutes to talk in circle time." School-aged children can help develop their own group rules and consequences. If children are included in the rule-making process, they are more likely to accept the rules. When group rules are negotiated, the rules need to apply to both children and adults.

Behavior interventions should be carefully graded based on their consequences for others, that is, which ones are irritating or rude and which ones are dangerous or destructive. Many irritating behaviors are attempts at gaining attention, and withholding attention keeps the behavior from increasing. The critical issue is knowing which ones can tolerated. Children can exhibit extremely inappropriate behaviors to disconcert the adults in their world.

*Ignoring* means be silent about the behavior; it is important to not use nonverbal or verbal cues that reveal feelings about the behavior. Although this approach ultimately decreases some behaviors, the behaviors usually get worse before they get better. With a child like Sophia, whose sudden unexpected outbursts disrupt activity, the therapist must keep interactions task focused. If the outburst disrupts the task, the task should be casually changed or the child should deal with the natural consequences of the resultant disarray. This transition is made without comments or offers to clean up the destroyed activity. The child should not be allowed to control the flow of therapy with this behavior. Once the child believes that he or she cannot gain the attention of the therapist, the behavior will discontinue.

As these difficult early stages in the therapy relationship are initiated, the power of praise and imitation should be used. Praise must be given for positive behaviors, especially for those that are incompatible with the problem behavior. The therapist should mirror the child's positive behaviors with his or her own. For example, if the child draws a spider, the therapist compliments the good idea and then proceeds to draw another spider, not competing artistically with the child. If the decision has been made to ignore spitting, the therapist ignores it when the child spits on the floor and instead praises the spider drawing. If the child spits at the therapist, the game stops, without discussion and without bargaining. This is so socially offensive that it cannot be ignored, and the therapist must move to a more serious level of behavior control.

## Establish a Sequence of Behavioral Controls

Therapists should alternate liked and disliked activities whenever possible. This rewards the child with a liked activity as he or she completes a difficult one. In addition, it reminds the child that the difficult one has an end; it will not fill the whole session once the assigned task is completed. This can be combined with a rule that any activity started must be completed. The activity can be shortened or simplified if it appears too challenging for the child. Once the rule is established, if a child procrastinates on a disliked activity, he or she can be reminded that she is losing time at the reward activity.

Establishing simple rules such as those previously described can lead to establishing performance contingencies.

Children need to be given control in the therapy session, and they need to understand what that control means. At first the therapist rewards any approximation of the desired behavior, then he or she increases the standards as the child makes progress. Criticism or commands should be replaced with reminders about rewards and repercussions.

## Organization

Many attention-getting and avoidance behaviors are subtle. The child may leave therapy having accomplished little for no apparent reason. The therapist should develop a behavior recording system to establish or document maladaptive behaviors and should look for antecedent behaviors, such as tapping the pencil on the table, that can indicate the imminence of offensive behavior. Ideally the activity can be changed or the child can be redirected before the offensive behavior occurs.

Recording the child's behavior helps identify behaviors that are not negative in isolation, like telling stories, but that can be effective stalling techniques in the therapy session. Before the therapist can effectively manage behaviors, he or she needs to target the specific problems and deal with them one at a time.

The next thing to organize is the reward system. The therapist should record what the child seems to particularly enjoy. The activities (or objects) may be found both in and out of the therapy environment. Questions such as "If you had $0.50, how would you spend it?" and "If you could do something special in occupational therapy, what would it be?" Parents and teachers can be enlisted in identifying a "menu" of reinforcers. A choice of reinforcing activities is important so that the rewards can be varied. The child who earns a sticker for each completed activity will soon tire of stickers. The menu must be frequently updated because the interests of children frequently change.

## Develop a Coordinated Strategy With Family and Team

Behavior management works best if it is consistently applied. If Joey is spitting in occupational therapy, he is probably spitting in the classroom and at home. All of the adults working to help Joey need to decide as a group what is and is not acceptable. Maybe Joey's occupational therapist can ignore the spitting, but his teacher cannot. If Joey's spitting is ignored in the classroom, other children will begin to imitate the behavior. Behavior management is most efficient when it occurs in all the aspects of a child's day. The same is true of reinforcers. Young children need to be quickly reinforced, and for small successes. An older child can save up points. Ten points may earn him or her 10 minutes on the playground after school or 30 seconds with the can of silly string chasing the therapist. If the family is involved, points may earn a favorite meal, a movie, or cash.

## Behavior-Recording Charts

Well-designed charts make the behavior goals and progress clear to even a young child. They serve as a tool to remind others to praise positive behaviors and to give the child assurance that he or she can succeed. Behavior change is an abstract idea to young children, but stickers on a chart are concrete. Behavior-recording charts can be individualized to the child's level of understanding. As a behavior management program is begun, progress should be rewarded immediately. A coloring chart, such as the ice cream cone in Figure 15-7, is a good reinforcer for short-term goals. Every 5 minutes that pass without whining entitles the child to color a section. The occupational therapist draws the chart to assure that the child can earn the "big" reward in a short time. For example, the ice cream cone in Figure 15-7 has six parts so that a 30-minute session with no whining might earn the child a trip to the ice cream parlor. Once the program is established, sections could be colored every 10 minutes.

A spider chart for 9-year-old Joey might look something like Figure 15-8. For every 10 minutes without spitting Joey gets to put a bug sticker on his chart. In this case the level of compliance that earns a reward can be negotiated. The chart records 2 weeks of therapy behavior. If Joey

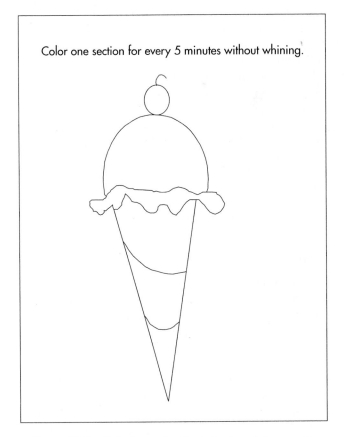

Color one section for every 5 minutes without whining.

**Figure 15-7** Coloring project for behavior reinforcement.

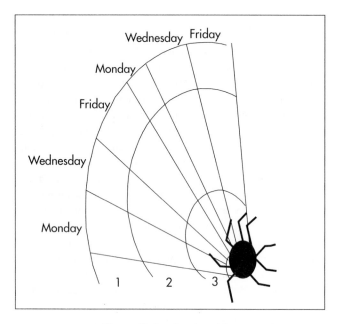

**Figure 15-8** Joey's spider.

earns 10 of 18 possible stickers, he may earn 30 minutes of playing video games. This can be adjusted to 12 then 15 stickers as he begins to control his behavior. With the older child, behavior-recording charts should be focused on self-control of behaviors. When feasible, the child should be in charge of keeping his or her behavior records in therapy.

Older children and teenagers can keep and carry their behavior-recording charts between classes at school and at home. If the child is responsible for keeping a chart and recording his or her performance at regular intervals, he or she is more likely to think about his or her behavior. In this type of self-recording system, both positive and negative behaviors are recorded. Children are less likely to misuse the system if they are documenting progress as well as problems. Self-recording can be followed with self-evaluation and then self-reinforcement, moving the child toward behavior self-management.

### Effective Punishments

Punishment is a last resort. Unfortunately, positive reinforcement and ignoring alone are seldom enough to change established inappropriate behaviors. The approach to punishment should always be a team decision. Time-out is a widely used standard for schools and clinical settings, but time-out is effective in only some instances. For example, time-out does not work with a 13-year-old who wants to be left alone. Likewise, cutting the therapy session short when Joey spits on the floor only works if Joey loves occupational therapy. For punishment to be a positive teaching tool, the child must know the rule that was broken and the consequences for breaking it.

### Time-Out Process

Time-out is a process. It is a widely used punishment in schools and clinical settings because it is relatively effective and involves a minimal amount of physical force. The point of time-out is to exclude the child from attention and liked activity. The first step to using time-out effectively is choosing the time-out spot. It should be a neutral place, boring maybe, but not unpleasant. In the clinical setting it is often effective to be sure the child in time-out can see all of the interesting activities in the room. When the child is the only one in the room, staring at a swing or a piece of equipment that he or she enjoys often motivates good behavior. A chair or carpet square should define the "quiet" or "thinking" place. The use of a timer is important. When the therapist keeps the time, staying in time-out may continue to be a power struggle. The neutral timer takes some of the emotion and control issues out of the situation. The rule is 1 minute of quiet time-out for each year of age (up to 5 minutes).

The timer runs while the child is quiet and cooperative. If the child is uncooperative, the timer does not start until he or she is quiet. Young children may not have a developed sense of time or numbers. Stopping and then resetting the timer is more concrete than adding minutes. Time-out "quiet" times should not exceed 5 minutes. The time-out process may take much longer, with warnings and resetting the timer until a 5-minute quiet time results. Figure 15-9 presents a flow sheet of the time-out process. This model shows how to make time-out a learning time for the child.

Although time-out is used widely, it is still important to teach children the rules in new settings. This can be done informally at first, with appropriate behavior modeled. Praising and allowing the child more control in the therapy setting are good rewards for appropriate behavior. When behavior is not appropriate, the therapist must be certain that the child knows that the behavior is wrong. Before initiating any punishment the therapist explains to the child why the behavior is not acceptable and establishes rules to guide future behavior.

When a behavior is not dangerous or highly offensive, the child should have one warning. If the warning results in improved behavior, focus on the positive behavior. The praise does not need to be qualified by referencing the unacceptable behavior. For some children, any reaction or response to the negative behavior is enough reinforcement to continue the behavior. If the child does not change his or her behavior with the warning, time-out is initiated.

The difficult part of time-out involves the child who refuses to go to or stay in time-out. Because the time-out is to *withdraw* attention, the therapist must maintain a calm, flat affect. If the child must be carried to time-out, it should be done silently. The child's power to control the situation must be removed, at least in appearance. When the therapist is unable to keep the child in time-out, the family and interdisciplinary team should become involved. Children

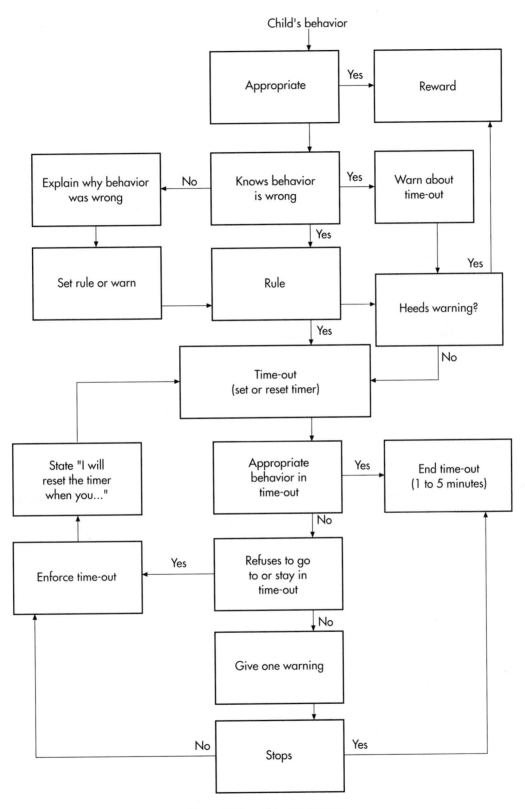

**Figure 15-9**   Time-out process.

can lose television time or other favorite activity for a short time if they resist time-out. Physically holding the child in time-out can be effective but should only be done as a last resort and with the parents' support.

The child's parents should be informed about difficult behavior and the strategies for changing that behavior. The family is encouraged to praise and reward the positive behaviors that are documented. Behavior change takes a long time, and several therapy periods may be devoted to time-out before the child begins to work appropriately. The child's behavior should not excuse him or her from therapy, nor should the parents be made to feel responsible for behavior in the therapy session.

### Performance Contracts

Around the age of 8 time-out often needs to take other forms, like grounding or withdrawal of television privileges. With older children the behavioral consequences need to be negotiated with the family. There are other behavior management techniques that may be used in the therapy setting. Performance contracts (discussed earlier) work well with school-aged children. Both the child and the therapist should sign the contract. The terms of the contract should be made public, either by posting or presenting copies to the child's parents.

### Overcorrection

Overcorrection might be a good approach to Joey's spitting. Overcorrection uses natural consequences to stop inappropriate behaviors. Joey could be required to "undo" the mess he has made by spitting on the floor. When he spits, he must immediately stop and clean not only his spit, but the whole clinic floor. The overcorrection of the damage done should be so unappealing that it discourages future inappropriate behavior. If overcorrection or any type of physical restraint is used, it must be a documented program reviewed by the team and meeting facility standards for review. An occupational therapist should attempt no punishment other than short time-outs without the active cooperation of the family and the intervention team.

## TRANSITION TO ADULTHOOD

The transition to adult lifestyles and adult responsibilities is an important aspect of psychosocial and emotional development. In the child with atypical development, poorly developed personal causation, learned helplessness, and difficult interpersonal skills can contribute to a difficult transition to adulthood. Although successful neuromuscular interventions and technologic aids, such as power wheelchairs, may make the young adult with cerebral palsy or spinal cord injury eligible for a community living placement, the inability to negotiate and cooperate with peers, passive dependence in money management and personal hygiene, and lack of respect for social rules can quickly send

the person back to the safety of his or her family home or an institutional setting.

A critical responsibility of the occupational therapist is to prepare children to be a part of the community. This is not a responsibility limited to those therapists who treat adolescents. Long-term considerations of a child's psychosocial and emotional needs are critical. What types of outcomes can be expected? How will the child's behavior change in 5 or 15 years? The bear hug of a young boy with Down syndrome quickly becomes socially inappropriate as he becomes a young adult. The boy hospitalized for a conduct disorder needs more than a hierarchy of privileges in the hospital setting to develop a sense of control and responsibility for the effects of his or her behavior. Even in the hospital, goals should incorporate skills needed by that child or teenager to be accepted in the society to which he or she will return.

## Interests and Roles
### In Late Childhood

Interest groups were discussed in the section on occupational therapy theory and interventions. Both formally and informally, the development of psychosocial interests should be encouraged in children of all ages. In the elementary school years, interests can be used by the occupational therapist as a theme for activities, to establish rapport, and to help the child build a sense of self as an individual. Children with chronic health conditions or behavior disorders tend to focus narrowly on the present. These individuals do not anticipate or constructively use leisure time. By encouraging interests as constructive leisure skills, the occupational therapist can aid the child's transition to the less structured "real" world.

Much of social and role learning that occurs at this time is from peers. If the child's peer group engages in socially unacceptable behaviors such as substance abuse and physical violence, the child is likely to value those behaviors over those modeled by adults in a clinical setting. To enhance appropriate role learning, the occupational therapist needs both to provide an appropriate model, and whenever possible, to link that model to the individual's interests and values. Group activities and games exploring relationships and friendships are often accepted by children in later childhood.

### In Adolescence

Adolescence is a time of acquiring social and personal values. It is a time when many people begin to work outside of the home. Teenagers in North America are aware of money and the acquisition of things. Money becomes a critical factor in the leisure and work roles of teenagers. Planning for and budgeting money often interests teenagers and is important to establishing self-reliance. Interests can be directed toward careers and leisure time considered as time

STUDY QUESTIONS

1. Review the case study of Derrick (p. 396). Using the examples in the text, consider how Derrick's temperament characteristics are likely to affect his academic performance. What kind of classroom adaptations might make it easier for him to succeed?

2. Robert has difficulty with a sense of mastery in academic work. The therapist's solution to his handwriting remediation was discussed on p. 395 When asked what their biggest concern was about their child, Robert's parents responded, "His inability to make friends and his lack of concern with his schoolwork. He has a lack of self-esteem." Explain mastery motivation in a way that might help Robert's parents understand his behavior and the relationship between mastery, self-esteem, and personal causation.

3. Four-year-old Rex has Down syndrome. He has difficulty imitating sequential behaviors and organizing his play. Consider your early intervention goals for Rex and his family. How do the issues of learned helplessness and locus of control influence your intervention decisions?

4. Review the characteristics of temperament. Do you think your temperament is extreme in any aspect? How do you think your temperament affects your study style? your friendships? or your behavior when you are ill? Answer these questions again while considering a sibling or peer. How does the "fit" between you work (or not work)?

5. Review the case study of Travis (p. 416). Using the examples in the text, what sort of an activity group would you suggest for Travis? Defend your answer with examples of his behavior and the need for specific skill development?

6. Bryce (age 14) arrives for sensorimotor testing. He is rude, offensive, and uncooperative throughout testing. The only way you can finish testing at all is by threatening to end the test session and return him to the classroom. Bryce has some sensorimotor delays, but his behavior is so extreme that it exaggerates his problems and makes him a poor candidate for traditional sensorimotor intervention. What are some additional tests that might be appropriate to understand Bryce's problems? What information will let you know if Bryce needs to be referred for specific psychosocial intervention?

7. Review the characteristics of disruptive behavior disorders. How would your approach to these behaviors change in an early intervention, public school, or acute psychiatric clinic setting? Choose a theoretical model and a therapy format for treatment of a 10-year-old child with conduct disorder in a setting of your choice.

Review the case example of Bryce (age 14) from study question 6. Bryce continues to be rude, offensive, and uncooperative in therapy sessions. His interests are tennis, video games, and skateboarding. He says that he hates school and does not want to do well in any school-related task. Bryce has some sensorimotor delays, but because of his age, he should be looking beyond his school days. He needs to develop work and interpersonal skills to make a successful transition to adult life. Consider the strategies listed in this chapter for maintaining a positive therapy environment and making the transition to adult life. Organize a behavior management program for Bryce that is appropriate for his age and that can be graded toward increasing self-control.

8. Review the case study of Sophia (pp. 417-418). Sophia had a history of fetal alcohol syndrome and physical abuse. Her current home environment is warm and supportive, but she still retains many of the behaviors common to an abused child. The psychotherapist following Sophia has given her a diagnosis of posttraumatic stress disorder (PTSD). Child-centered intervention continued to be used to support social skill development. As Sophia gained skill, however, her behavior became more difficult to manage. She was impulsive and sometimes explosive emotionally. She would be playing on a swing, and then throw herself to the ground, screaming, "I hate her! I hate her!" and pounding her fists. Review the discussions of child abuse, PTSD, and behavior management to develop a strategy to help Sophia and her family.

9. Review the behavioral indicators of risk for child abuse presented in the case of Monique (p. 404). How might these behaviors look in a school-aged child? How is a history of abuse likely to affect development and the transition to adulthood? What type of performance skills would you emphasize in a 15-year-old child with a history of abuse?

to earn money. Teenagers want to be in control of their lives. By helping them understand how their time-use decisions and interests can be channeled to increase their control, caregivers can lead their teenagers toward self-reliance.

Before developing true vocational skills, the teenager needs to develop good interpersonal skills, some form of reliable communication, self-direction in activities of daily living, task orientation, task persistence, and task organization abilities. Each of these areas should be assessed by the occupational therapist, with appropriate interventions planned.

For interests and roles to mature into an adult pattern, the individual needs experience. Most young adolescents have ideas about careers and interests that are based on fantasy rather than experience. The adolescent seen in occupational therapy is likely to have even less experience and less awareness of his or her own abilities than the average teenager. Career awareness programs are available in most public schools, but it may be difficult for a child with an atypical history to see how those potential careers relate to him or her. The following are major career goals of adolescents (Jordan & Heyde, 1979):

▲ Crystallization of interests
▲ Realistic self-appraisal of strengths and deficits in relation to vocational choice
▲ Development of work experience
▲ Acceptance of responsibility in acquiring skills
▲ Self-direction in the development and implementation of a vocational or career plan
▲ Self-reliance in transportation and mobility in the community

The occupational therapist should work with the school or vocational counseling personnel to help the teenager apply interests and career information to their own future planning. The adolescent client may benefit from help appraising work abilities and work demands. The management of personal self-care extends beyond acquiring skills to an awareness of proper grooming and social rules about grooming behavior. Transition services and supported employment programs are presented at length in Chapter 32.

## SUMMARY

The treatment of all children requires an understanding of and sensitivity to the domains of psychosocial and emotional development. Nearly all clients seen by pediatric occupational therapists are at risk for delays in these areas of development. Overlooking critical dimensions of development, such as the development of interpersonal relations, can greatly affect the individuals function and resources as he or she faces adulthood.

Routine assessment should include an overview of the child's or adolescent's function in social performance ar-

eas. Play with family members and peers has an important part in the child's ability to learn and assimilate social behaviors. In addition to measures of the individual's performance, several approaches to family and environmental assessment are included in this chapter. These assessments help develop meaningful goals for the child in his or her own situation. They also can help identify children at risk for abuse and can be used to structure programs that include improving the parents' skills.

Decisions about specific theoretical approaches and interventions should reflect the intervention setting in which the child is seen. Most children seen by occupational therapists are not seen in traditional psychiatric intervention settings. It is important that the therapist understands that assessment and remediation of the psychosocial and emotional domain of behavior is not a specialty area but crucial to all pediatric practice.

## REFERENCES

American Psychiatric Association. (1994). *Diagnostic and statistical manual of mental disorders* (4th ed.). Washington, DC: American Psychiatric Association.

Anderson, J., Hinojosa, J., Bedell, G., & Kaplan, M.T. (1990). Occupational therapy for children with perinatal HIV infection. *American Journal of Occupational Therapy, 44*(3), 249-255.

Asarnow, J.R. (1988). Peer status and social competence in child psychiatric inpatients: a comparison of children with depressive, externalizing, and concurrent depressive and externalizing disorders. *Journal of Abnormal Child Psychology, 16*(2), 151-162.

Atkins, D.M. & Silber, T.J. (1993). Clinical spectrum of anorexia nervosa in children. *Journal of Developmental and Behavioral Pediatrics, 14*(4), 211-216.

Ayres, A.J. (1972). *Southern California Sensory Integration Test.* Los Angeles: Western Pychological Services.

Ayres, A.J. (1989). *Sensory Integration and Praxis Test.* Los Angeles: Western Psychological Services.

Barkley, R.A., Anastopoulos, A.D., Guevremont, D.C., & Fletcher, K.E. (1991). Adolescents with ADD: patterns of behavioral adjustment, academic functioning, and treatment utilization. *Journal of the American Academy of Child and Adolescent Psychiatry, 30*(5), 752-761.

Barnard, K.E. (1980). *Nursing Child Assessment Teaching Scale.* Seattle, WA: NCAST Publications.

Boyce, W.T., Barr, R.G., & Zeltzer, L.K. (1992). Temperament and the psychobiology of childhood stress. *Pediatrics, 90*(3 Pt 2), 483-486.

Bracegirdle, H. (1990). The acquisition of social skills by children with special needs. *British Journal of Occupational Therapy, 53*(3), 107-108.

Brazelton, T.B., Tronick, E., Adamson, L., Als, H., & Wise, S. (1975). Early mother-infant reciprocity. In *Parent-infant interaction:* Ciba Foundation Symposium 33. Amsterdam: Associated Scientific Publishers.

Bretherton, I. & Beeghly, M. (1982). Talking about internal states: the acquisition of an explicit theory of the mind. *Developmental Psychology, 18,* 906-921.

Bridges, B. (1990). *Stop, relax, and think: a game to help impulsive children think before they act*. Fourth Street Company.

Brunquell, D. & Hall, M.D. (1991). Issues in the psychological care of pediatric oncology patients. *Annual Progress in Child Psychiatry and Child Development*, Part IV (27), 430.

Butler, C. (1984). Effects of powered wheelchair mobility on self-initiative behaviors of two- and three- year old children with neuromuscular disorders. In *Proceedings of the 2nd International Conference on Rehabilitation Engineering* (pp. 176-177). Ottawa, Ontario: RESNA.

Butler, R. (1989). Mastery versus ability appraisal: a developmental study of children's observations of peers' work. *Child Development, 60*, 1350-1361.

Campos, J.J., & Berenthal, B.I. (1987). Locomotion and psychological development in infancy. In K. Jaffe (Ed.). *Childhood powered mobility: developmental, technical, and clinical perspectives* (pp. 11-42). Washington, DC: Association for the Advancement of Rehabilitation Technology.

Carpenter, G. (1975). Mothers face and the newborn. In R. Lewin (Ed.). *Child alive*, London: Temple Smith.

Carrasco, R.C. & Lee, C.E. (1993). Development of a teacher questionnaire on sensorimotor behavior. *Sensory Integration Special Interest Section Newsletter, 16*(3), 5, 6.

Cherry, D.B. (1989). Stress and coping in families with ill or disabled children. *Physical and Occupational Therapy in Pediatrics 9*(2), 11-32.

Chess, S. & Thomas, A. (1983). Dynamics of individual behavioral development. In M.D. Levine, W.B. Carey, A.C. Crocker, & R.T. Gross (Eds.). *Developmental-behavioral pediatrics* (pp. 158-175). Philadelphia: W.B. Saunders.

Chess, S. & Thomas, A. (1984). *Origins and evolution of behavior disorders: infancy to adult life*. New York: Brunner/Mazel.

Chess, S. & Thomas, A. (1987). *Know your child*. New York: Basic Books.

Cohen, P., Cohen, J., & Brook, J. (1993). An epidemiological study of disorders in late childhood and adolescence: II. Persistence of disorders. *Journal of Child Psychology and Psychiatry, 34*(6), 869-877.

Cohen, P., Cohen, J., Kasen, S., Velez, C., Hartmark, C., Johnson, J., Rojas, M., Brook, J., & Streuning, E. (1993). An epidemiological study of disorders in late childhood and adolescence: I. Age- and gender-specific prevalence. *Journal of Child Psychology and Psychiatry, 34*(6), 851-867.

Condon, W.S. & Sander, L.W. (1974). Neonatal movement is synchronized with adult speech: interactional participation and language requisition. *Science, 183*, 99-101.

Cook, D. (1991). The assessment process. In W. Dunn (Ed.). *Pediatric occupational therapy service delivery*. Thorofare, NJ: Slack.

Coster, W. & Jaffe, L. (1991) Current concepts of children's perceptions of control. *American Journal of Occupational Therapy 45*(1), 19-25.

Cousins, L.S. & Weiss, G. (1993). Parent training and social skills training for children with attention-deficit hyperactivity disorder: how can they be combined for greater effectiveness? *Canadian Journal of Psychiatry, 38*(6), 449-457.

Creer, T.L., Stein, R.E., Rappaport, L., & Lewis, C. (1992). Behavioral consequences of illness: childhood asthma as a model. *Pediatrics, 90*(5 Pt 2), 808-815.

Daltroy, L.H., Larson, M.G., Eaton, H.M., Partridge, A.J., Pless, I. B., Rogers, M.P., & Liang, M.H. (1992). Psychosocial adjustment in juvenile arthritis. *Journal of Pediatric Psychology, 17*(3), 277-289.

Davidson, D. (1995). Physical abuse of preschoolers: identification and intervention through occupational therapy. *American Journal of Occupational Therapy, 49*(1), 235-243.

Deacove, J. (1987). *Funny face*. Perth, Ontario: Family Pastimes.

DeGangi, G., Wietlisbach, S., Goodin, M., & Scheiner, N. (1993). A comparison of structured sensorimotor therapy and child-centered activity in the treatment of preschool children with sensorimotor problems. *American Journal of Occupational Therapy, 47*(9), 777-786.

Dillard, M., Andonian, L., Flores, O., Lai, L., MacRae, A., & Shakir, M. (1992). Culturally competent occupational therapy in a diversely populated mental health setting. *American Journal of Occupational Therapy, 46*(8): 721-726.

Doble, S.E., & Magill-Evans, J. (1992). A model of social interaction to guide occupational therapy practice. *Canadian Journal of Occupational Therapy, 59*(3), 141-150.

Famularo, R., Kinscherff, R., & Fenton, T. (1990). Symptom differences in acute and chronic presentation of childhood post-traumatic stress disorder. *Child Abuse and Neglect, 14*(3), 439-444.

Fazio, L. (1992). Tell me a story: the therapeutic metaphor in the practice of pediatric occupational therapy. *American Journal of Occupational Therapy, 46*(2), 112-119.

Field, T.M. (1983). High-risk infants "have less fun" during early interactions. *Topics in Early Childhood Special Education, 3*, 77-87.

Field, T.M. & Fox, N.A. (Eds.). (1985). *Social perception in infants*. Norwood, NJ: Ablex.

Florey, L. & Michelman, S. (1978). Occupational role history: a screening tool for psychiatric occupational therapy. *American Journal of Occupational Therapy, 32*, 301.

Fraenkel, L. & Tallant, B. (1987). Mostly me: a treatment approach for emotionally disturbed children. *Canadian Journal of Occupational Therapy, 54*(2), 59-64.

Frances, A.J., First, M.B., Pincus, H.A., Davis, W.W., & Vettorello, N. (1994). Changes in child and adolescent disorders, and the multiaxial system. *Hospital and Community Psychiatry, 45*(3), 212-214.

Frank, G., Huecker, E., Segal, R., Forwell, S., and Bagatell, N. (1991). Assessment and treatment of a pediatric patient in chronic care. *American Journal of Occupational Therapy, 45*(3), 252-263.

Frankenburg, W.K., Dodds, J.B., Fandal, A. (1990). *Denver Developmental Screening Test II*. Denver: LADOCA Project and Publishing Foundation.

Freud, S. (1933). *New introductory lectures in psychoanalysis*. New York: Norton.

Friedman, R. & Doyal, G. (1992). *Management of children and adolescents with attention deficit-hyperactivity disorder* (3rd ed.). Austin, TX: Pro-Ed.

Gardener, M. (1994). *Gardener social developmental scale*. Burlingame, CA: Psychological and Educational Publications.

Goldberg, S. (1977). Social competency in infancy: a model of parent-child interaction. *Merrill-Palmer Quarterly, 23*, 163-177.

Goodman, S.H. (1987). Emory University project on children of disturbed parents. *Schizophrenia Bulletin, 13*(3), 411-423.

Greenspan, S. & Greenspan, N.T. (1985). *First feelings: milestones in the emotional development of your baby and child*. New York: Penguin Books.

Gribble, P.A., Cowen, E.L., Wyman, P.A., Work, W.C., Wannon, M., & Raof, A. (1993). Parent and child views of parent-child relationship qualities and resilient outcomes among urban children. *Journal of Child Psychology and Psychiatry, 34*(4), 507-519.

Guerney, L.F. (1983). Client-centered (nondirective) play therapy. In C.E. Schaefer & K.J. O'Connor (Eds.). *Handbook of play therapy* (pp. 21-64). New York: John Wiley & Sons.

Guralnick, M.J. & Groom, J.M. (1990). The correspondence between temperament and peer interactions for normally developing and mildly delayed preschool children. *Child Development, 16*(3), 165-175.

Hammen, C., Gordon, D., Burge, D., Adrian, C., Jaenicke, C, & Hiroto, D. (1987). Maternal affective disorders, illness, and stress: risk for children's psychopathology. *American Journal of Psychiatry, 144*(6), 736-741.

John, K., Gammon, G.D., Prusoff, B.A., & Warner, V. (1987). The social adjustment inventory for children and adolescents (SAICA): testing of a new semi-structured interview. *Journal of the American Academy of Child and Adolescent Psychiatry, 26*, 898-911.

Johnson, K.M., Berry, E.T., Goldeen, R.A., & Wicker, E. (1991). Growing up with a spinal cord injury. *Spinal Cord Injury Nursing, 8*(1), 11-19.

Jordan, J.P. & Heyde, M.B. (1979). *Vocational maturity during the high school years*. New York: Teachers College Press.

Kaplan, H.L. & Sadock, B.J. (Eds.). (1988). *Synopsis of psychiatry*. Baltimore: Williams & Wilkins.

Kashani, J.H., Soltys, S.M., Dandoy, A.C., Vaidya, A.F., & Reid, J. C. (1991). Correlates of hopelessness in psychiatrically hospitalized children. *Comprehensive Psychiatry, 32*(4), 330-337.

Kaye, K. (1982). *The mental and social life of babies*. Chicago: University of Chicago Press.

Keogh, B.K. (1986). Temperament and schooling: meaning of "goodness of fit"? *New Directions in Child Development, Mar*(31), 89-108.

Keogh, B.K. & Burstein, N.D. (1988). Relationship of temperament to preschoolers' interactions with peers and teachers. *Exceptional Child, 54*(5), 456-461.

Kielhofner, G. (Ed.). (1995). *A model of human occupation: theory and application*. Baltimore: Williams & Wilkins.

Lavigne, J.V. & Faier-Routman, J. (1993). Correlates of psychological adjustment to pediatric physical disorders: a meta-analytic review and comparison with existing models. *Journal of Developmental and Behavioral Pediatrics, 14*(2), 117-123.

Lindamood, P. (1981) *Lindamood Visual Conceptual Program*. San Luis Obispo, CA: Lindamood Language and Literacy Center.

Linder, T.W. (1990). *Transdisciplinary play-based assessment: a functional approach to working with young children*. Baltimore: Brookes.

Magill, J. & Hurlbut, N. (1986). The self-esteem of adolescents with cerebral palsy. *American Journal of Occupational Therapy, 40*(6), 402-407.

Matsutsuyu, J. (1969). The interest checklist. *American Journal of Occupational Therapy, 23*, 323.

McGrath, P.J. & McAlpine, L. (1993). Psychologic perspectives on pediatric pain. *Journal of Pediatrics, 122*(5 Pt 2), S2-S8.

Meltzoff, A.N. & Moore, M.K. (1983). Newborn infants imitate adult facial gestures. *Child Development 54*, 702-709.

National Advisory Mental Health Council. (1990). *National plan for research on child and adolescent mental disorders*. Washington, DC: National Institute of Mental Health.

Neville, A. & Kielhofner, G. (1983). *The modified interest checklist*. Unpublished workbook, National Institutes of Health.

Olson, L., Heaney, C., & Soppas-Hoffman, B. (1989). Parent-child activity group treatment in preventive psychiatry. *Occupational Therapy in Health Care, 6*(1), 29-43.

Piaget, J. (1952). *The origins of intelligence in children*. New York: Norton.

Piaget, J. (1954). *The construction of reality in the child*. New York: Basic Books.

Piers, E.V. (1984). *Piers-Harris children's self concept scale* (Revised manual). Los Angeles: Western Psychological Services.

Pollock, S. (1986) Human responses to chronic illness: physiologic and psychosocial adaptation. *Nursing Research, 32*, 4-9.

Rothbaum, F. & Weisz, J. (1989). *Child psychopathology and the quest for control*. Beverly Hills, CA: Sage.

Rowan, A.B. & Foy, D.W. (1993). Post-traumatic stress disorder in child sexual abuse survivors: a literature review. *Journal of Traumatic Stress, 6*(1), 3-20.

Royeen, C.B. & Fortune, J.C. (1990). TIE Touch Inventory for Elementary School-aged children. *American Journal of Occupational Therapy, 44*, 165-170.

Ruble, D.N. (1983). The development of social comparison processes and their role in achievement related socialization. In E.T. Higgins, D.N. Ruble, and W.W. Hartup (Eds.). *Social cognition and social development:* a socio-cultural perspective (pp. 134-157). New York: Cambridge University Press.

Rutter, M. (1987). The role of cognition in child development and disorder. *British Journal of Medical Psychology, 60*, 1-16.

Schechter, N.L., Bernstein, B.A., Beck, A., Hart, L., & Scherzer, L. (1991). Individual differences in children's response to pain: role of temperament and parental characteristics. *Pediatrics, 87*(2). 171-177.

Schultz, S. (1992). School-based occupational therapy for students with behavioral disorders. *Occupational Therapy in Health Care, 8*, 173-196.

Sholle-Martin, S. & Alessi, N. (1990). Occupational therapy in child psychiatry. *American Journal of Occupational Therapy 44*, 871-882.

Simmons, R.J., Corey, M., Cowen, L., Keenan, N., Robertson, J., & Levison, H. (1987). Behavioral adjustment of latency age children with cystic fibrosis. *Psychosomatic Medicine, 49*(3), 291-301.

Sparrow, S., Balla, D., & Cicchetti, D. (1987). *The Vineland Adaptive Behavior Scales*. Circle Pines, MN: American Guidance Service.

Stowell, M. (1987). Psychosocial role of the occupational therapist with pediatric bone marrow transplant patients. *Occupational Therapy in Mental Health, 7*(2), 39-50.

Szejeres, S.F., Ylvisaker, M., & Holland, A.L. (1985). Cognitive rehabilitation therapy: a framework for intervention. In M. Ylvisaker (Ed.). *Head injury rehabilitation: children and adolescents* (pp. 219-246). San Diego: College Hill Press.

Turecki, S. & Wernick, S. (1994). *The emotional problems of normal children*. New York: Bantam Books.

Turnquist, K. & Engel, J.M. (in press). Occupational therapists' attitudes, perception, and knowledge of pain in children. *Physical and Occupational Therapy in Pediatrics*.

Vessey, J.A. & Caserza, C.L. (1992). Chronic conditions and child development. In P.L. Jackson & J.A. Vessey (Eds.). *Primary care of the child with a chronic condition* (pp. 26-44). St. Louis: Mosby.

Voeller, K.K.S. (1986). Right-hemisphere deficit syndrome in children. *American Journal of Psychiatry, 143*(8), 1004-1009.

Voeller, K.K.S. (1991). Toward a neurobiologic nosology of attention deficit hyperactivity disorder. *Journal of Child Neurology, 6*(suppl 1991), S2-S9.

Wellman, H.M. & Estes, D. (1987). Children's early use of mental verbs and what they mean. *Discourse Processes, 10,* 141-156.

Wichstrom, L., Holte, A., Husby, R., & Wynne, L. (1993). Competence in children at risk for psychopathology predicted from confirmatory and disconfirmatory family communication. *Family Process, 32*(2), 203-220.

Youssef, N.M. (1988). School adjustment of children with congenital heart disease. *Maternal and Child Nursing Journal, 17*(4), 217-302.

Zakich, R. (1989). *The ungame.* Anaheim, CA: Talicor.

Zametkin, A.J., Nordahl, T., Gross, M., King, A.C., Semple, W.E., Rumsey, J., Hamburger, S., & Cohen, R.M. (1990). Cerebral glucose metabolism in adults with hyperactivity of childhood onset. *New England Journal of Medicine, 323,* 1361-1366.

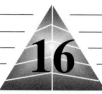

# Feeding and Oral Motor Skills

JANE CASE-SMITH ▲ RUTH HUMPHRY

Eating is an essential daily living skill that requires overall motor ability, specific oral motor function, sensory perception, and social and cognitive skills. Difficulty in eating or feeding affects every aspect of the child's life, including his or her ability to grow and learn and to form relationships with others. Prerequisites to an ability to feed are integrity of the oral structures and intact cranial nerves for the activation of swallowing. At a more sophisticated level, but certainly as important, are the social and cultural aspects of eating and feeding. Eating is a cultural event; the type of food, amount presented, and time of eating are usually a matter of family traditions and values. Feeding is also a critical time of interaction. As one of the most frequent and positive ways of interacting between the parent and child, it is a critical time for the child to learn nonverbal communication and turn-taking skills. The nurturing that occurs during feeding helps the parent bond to the child and the child trust in and rely on the parent to meet his or her needs.

Therefore feeding is both a physical task and a social event during which the child meets nutritional needs and develops oral sensorimotor and social interaction skills. To plan effective interventions in feeding, the child, the family, and the environment must be assessed and addressed. The goodness of fit of these variables is critical to successful feeding and by extension to growth and development.

Feeding skills develop along a continuum that follows the development of oral motor skill and are highly influenced by the child's overall health, the caregiver's relationship with the child, and other psychosocial, economic, and cultural factors in the environment. The first part of this chapter describes oral sensorimotor development as it relates to feeding. A general framework for evaluation is presented. Interventions for specific feeding problems are described. Nutritional aspects of feeding are discussed. In the final section the implications of a feeding problem are examined as they impact on the child and influence the nature of parent-child interactions. In this section the effects of the environment, culture, and the family on the child's acquisition of feeding skill are also considered.

## TYPICAL DEVELOPMENT OF ORAL STRUCTURES

The development of oral motor skills for eating involves the development of discrete but related skills. They include sucking and drinking from a cup, munching and chewing, biting, and coordinating the suck-swallow-breathe sequence. These skills develop concurrently as the child gains control of jaw, tongue, cheek, and lip movement. The coordination of these structures for purposes of feeding is often impaired when the child has a developmental disability.

Table 16-1 shows the oral structures involved in feeding and their function in feeding.

The anatomic structures of the mouth and throat change significantly in the first 12 months of life. The growth and maturation of the oral structures allow for development of more mature feeding patterns.

The neonate has a small oral cavity with fatty cheeks and a tongue that fill it. When the nipple is placed inside the mouth, the tight fit enables the infant to easily compress the nipple and achieve automatic suction. The negative pressure that automatically occurs during sucking movements

of the jaw is sufficient for expressing liquid from the nipple (Morris & Klein, 1987). Therefore the full-term, healthy neonate is successful in sucking from a breast or bottle nipple.

In addition to the close proximity of the structures inside the neonate's mouth, the structures in the throat are in close proximity to each other. The infant's epiglottis and soft palate are in direct approximation. As a result, the liquid from the nipple safely passes from the base of the tongue to the esophagus. During swallow the larynx elevates and the epiglottis falls over it to protect the trachea. Therefore aspiration is unlikely before 4 months, and the infant can safely be fed in a reclined position.

As the infant grows, the neck elongates and the relationship of the oral and throat structures change. The oral cavity itself becomes larger and more open. The fatty tongue becomes thin and muscular, and the cheeks lose much of their fatty padding. With the increase in oral cavity space, the tongue, lips, and cheeks must provide greater control of liquid or food within the mouth. New sucking patterns emerge to enable the infant to effectively handle liquid without the structural advantages of early infancy. These include up and down movements of the tongue to express liquids from the nipple. The increasing oral space also provides room to masticate food and to move the tongue in the rolling patterning required during chewing.

As the infant approaches 12 months of age, the hyoid, epiglottis, and larynx descend, creating space between these structures and the base of the tongue. The hyoid and larynx become more mobile during swallow, elevating with each swallow. Greater coordination of these structures is required during the suck-swallow-breathe sequence. With the elongation of the pharynx, feeding in a reclined position creates a greater possibility of aspiration. The pull of gravity in this position can interfere with the control needed by the infant to move the liquid to the entrance of the esophagus. Figure 16-1 shows the structures of the mouth and pharynx of the infant.

▲ Table 16-1  Functions of Oral Structures in Feeding

| Structure | Parts | Function During Feeding |
|---|---|---|
| Oral cavity | Hard and soft palate, tongue, fat pads of cheeks, upper and lower jaws and teeth | Contains the food during drinking and chewing and provides for initial mastication before swallowing |
| Pharynx | Base of tongue, buccinator, oropharynx, tendons and hyoid bone | Funnels food into the esophagus and allows food and air to share space; the pharynx is a space common to both functions |
| Larynx | Epiglottis and false and true vocal folds | Valve to the trachea that closes during swallowing |
| Trachea | Tube below the larynx and cartilaginous rings | Allows air to flow into bronchi and lungs |
| Esophagus | Thin and muscular esophagus | Carries food from the pharynx, through the diaphragm, and to the stomach; at rest it is collapsed and distends as food passes through it |

Modified from Wolf, L.S. & Glass, R.P. (1992). *Feeding and swallowing disorders in infancy: assessment and management.* Tucson: Therapy Skill Builders.

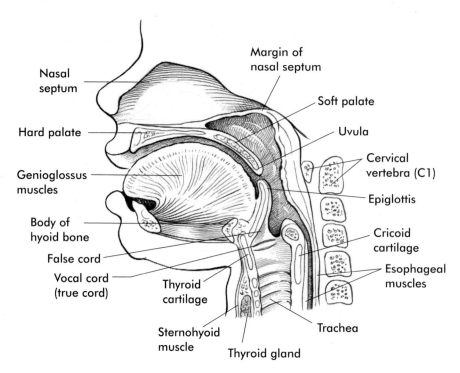

**Figure 16-1**    Anatomic structures of the mouth and throat.

## TYPICAL DEVELOPMENT OF ORAL MOTOR AND FEEDING SKILLS

The development of sucking, drinking, biting, and chewing is highly related to the overall motoric development of the child. The development of more mature oral patterns occurs at the same time the child has changing nutritional needs, demonstrates interest in self-feedings, and expands communication efforts. The changes in jaw, tongue, lip, and cheek movements are described as they are associated with the development of skills in (1) sucking and drinking, (2) biting and chewing, and (3) coordination of sucking, swallowing, and breathing (Morris & Klein, 1987; Wolf & Glass, 1992).

### Sucking and Drinking Skills

The sucking reflex is present in the fetus and predominates as the method of oral feeding through the first 8 to 10 months of life. Sucking patterns differ when the child is sucking on a pacifier (nonnutritive) than when sucking on a nipple of a bottle (nutritive). The nonnutritive pattern is rapid and rhythmic (usually about two sucks per second). The nutritive pattern is rhythmic but is characterized by a burst-and-pause pattern. This pattern allows the infant to breathe and rest between sucking bursts.

When infants are born prematurely, they typically are fed by nonoral means before 33 weeks' gestational age. Before this age the infant demonstrates a rhythmic nonnutritive sucking pattern, but sucking strength and endurance limit

oral feeding. Often by 35 weeks, the jaw and tongue movements are sufficiently strong to allow for oral feeding, at least part of the time. The amount of liquid taken in is determined by the rate of sucking, the force of suction or compression, and the length of time the infant eats. Two characteristics that seem important to feeding efficiency are the rhythm of sucking and the type of suction (i.e., negative pressure for expression of liquid) that the infant is able to achieve and sustain over time (Daniels, Devlieger, Casaer, & Eggermont, 1986). Wolf and Glass (1992) explained that both compression and suction are needed to express liquid. These aspects of feeding are achieved through sucking patterns that include sealing the lips around the nipple and moving the tongue in a simultaneous extension and retraction and up and down movements. By 36 weeks' gestational age the typical premature infant takes all food by mouth and uses a sucking pattern similar to that of the full-term infant.

The full-term infant (born at 40 weeks) has strong oral reflexes that enable him or her to take in liquid nutrition without difficulty. Given tactile stimulation near the mouth, the hungry infant's rooting reflex induces the infant to turn his or her head, thereby allowing him or her to latch onto any potential nutritional source. The sucking reflex is strong and rhythmic, diminishing appropriately with satiation. The infant also exhibits a gag and cough reflex to protect the airway from the intake of liquid.

The sucking pattern of the full-term neonate is rhythmic, sustained, and efficient. The pattern of each infant is unique and varies in efficiency of sucking according to the infant's level of fatigue and hunger. Most infants complete an oral feeding in 20 to 30 minutes.

The infant's first sucking pattern is termed *suckling* (Morris & Klein, 1987). This pattern is characterized by a forward-backward movement of the tongue. Accompanying this rhythmic back-and-forth tongue movement is jaw opening and closing. The tongue typically extends to but not beyond the border of the lips.

Suckling predominates in the first 4 months of life. The pattern may cause slight liquid loss and intake of air and is primarily observed in the second and third months of life, after the infant's physiologic flexion has disappeared and before mature oral motor control has been established. At 4 months the tongue begins to move in an up-and-down direction that characterizes a true sucking pattern. The wide jaw excursions of the young infant are reduced. Less liquid is lost, and suction on the nipple increases.

The 6-month-old infant demonstrates strong up-and-down tongue movement with minimal jaw excursion during sucking. Jaw stability has increased and allows for better control of tongue movement. The lip seal is good, such that the infant does not lose liquid during sucking on a nipple. In many cultures in the United States the cup is introduced at 6 months. Usually a sipper cup with a spout is presented. The infant initially uses a suckling movement with this new stimulus so early cup drinking results in wide jaw excursions and liquid loss. Some coughing may be observed as the infant first attempts this skill.

By 9 months the infant continues to feed from the bottle, using strong sucking patterns. Long sequences of continuous sucks are observed when the infant drinks from the cup. The jaw is not consistently stable on the rim of the cup so the baby is messy drinking from a cup.

At 12 months, many infants make the transition from the bottle to the cup for drinking during mealtime. Often the infant continues to bottle-feed at bed time. When the infant drinks from a cup, the jaw continues to move up and down and the tongue moves in a suckle pattern forward and backward in the mouth. The tongue may protrude slightly beneath the cup to provide some additional stability (Morris & Klein, 1987). For the first time, tongue tip elevation occurs during swallow.

The toddler uses an up-and-down sucking pattern to obtain liquids from a cup by 18 months. He or she bites on the rim of the cup to obtain external jaw stabilization. The upper lip closes on the edge of the cup to provide a seal for drinking. The tongue elevates to bring the liquid into the mouth.

The child at 24 months can efficiently drink from the cup. He or she uses up-and-down tongue movements and tip elevation. Internal jaw stabilization emerges so that the jaw appears still. Therefore the rim of the cup rests on the stable jaw, and biting on the cup's rim is no longer necessary. The child swallows with easy lip closure and does not lose liquids from the cup. Lengthy suck-swallow sequences are observed.

## Biting and Chewing

The first biting or chewing movements of the infant are reflexive. At 4 to 5 months the infant uses a rhythmic, stereotypic phasic bite-and-release pattern on almost any substance placed in the mouth, for example, a soft cookie, cracker, or toy. Jaw movements are up and down rather than diagonal. When the phasic bite-and-release pattern is used in a repeated rhythm, it is termed a *munching pattern*. The munch is characterized by jaw movement in the vertical direction and tongue movement in extension and retraction (lateralization has not yet developed). Therefore the munching pattern is effective with pureed foods or soft foods that quickly dissolve.

By 7 to 8 months of age the infant demonstrates some variability in the up-and-down munching pattern. He begins to use some diagonal jaw movement when the texture of the food requires variation in jaw movement. The infant continues to use the phasic bite-and-release pattern when presented with a cookie, thus the jaw closes abruptly on the cookie and then the infant sucks on it. The jaw holds the cookie but the infant cannot yet successfully bite through it. A bite is obtained by breaking off the piece while the jaw is held closed on the cookie. When food is presented on the spoon, the upper lip actively cleans it from the spoon. The lips become more active during sucking and maintaining the food within the mouth.

By 9 months of age the infant is handling pureed and soft food well. He or she continues to use a munching pattern; however, the vertical up-and-down jaw movements now include diagonal movements. The infant transfers the food from the center of the mouth to the side using lateral tongue movements. These same lateral movements keep the food on the side during munching, making that process effective in mastication of soft or mashed table food. The lips are active during chewing, so they make contact as the jaw moves up and down.

Rotary chewing movements begin at approximately 12 months, made possible as the child gains jaw stability and controlled mobility. This control is also exhibited when the child demonstrates sustained, well-graded bite on soft cookies. The tongue is active in chewing by moving food from the center of the mouth to the sides, licking food from the lips, and demonstrating tip elevation on occasion. The infant is able to retrieve food on the lower lip by drawing it inward into the mouth.

The toddler, at 18 months, demonstrates well-coordinated rotary chewing. He or she is able to chew soft meat and a variety of table foods. Bite is well controlled and sustained, and the child can bite off a piece of a hard cookie or pretzel. The tongue becomes increasingly mobile and efficiently moves food within the mouth.

At 24 months of age the child can eat most meats and raw vegetables. The bite is well graded and sustained, and the child bites on hard foods with ease. Circular rotary jaw movements that characterize mature chewing are present.

The tongue transfers food from one side of the mouth to the other using a rolling movement. The tongue moves skillfully to clear the lips and gums. Lip closure during chewing prevents any food loss.

## Coordination of Sucking, Swallowing, and Breathing

As the infant demonstrates increasing control of jaw, tongue, and lip movement, he or she also learns to coordinate and sequence oral movements into rhythmic patterns of sucking, swallowing, and breathing. The coordination of the oral structures as they work together to prepare and swallow food are perhaps more important to the feeding process than development of control of any one oral structure.

The 1-month-old infant demonstrates one suck to one swallow at the beginning of the feeding. He or she can sequence two to three sucks per swallow after his or her initial hunger has been satiated. By 3 or 4 months of age the infant sequences 20 or more sucks from the breast or bottle before pausing. Swallow occurs intermittently (after four to five sucks) and without pausing. Breathing slows during sucking and occurs within and between sucking sequences. Occasionally the infant may cough or choke when coordination of sucking, swallowing, and breathing is momentarily lost.

As the infant approaches 12 months, these long sequences continue in bottle- or breast-feeding. When the infant begins to drink from the cup, this coordination is lost. At 9 months of age he or she stops to swallow or breathe after one to three sucks from the cup. By 12 months, swallowing follows sucking without pausing and the infant takes three continuous swallows before pausing. Swallowing is efficient (without coughing) when the amount of liquid flow is minimal.

By 15 to 18 months of age the infant has excellent coordination of sucking, swallowing, and breathing. When drinking from a cup, the infant's swallowing follows sucking without pauses. The infant performs at least three suck-swallow sequences before pausing, and the amount of liquid swallowed each time has increased (to at least 1 ounce). Coughing or choking rarely occurs.

It is important for the occupational therapist to understand the sequence of typical oral motor development when evaluating feeding skills. Other aspects of feeding and oral motor skill evaluation are explained in the following section.

## EVALUATION

Comprehensive information is needed to plan feeding interventions. Feeding evaluations should include gathering and synthesizing information from the sources discussed in the following paragraphs.

## Parent Interviews

A discussion regarding the feeding problem from the perspective of the parents is critical for determining its basis and for developing an intervention plan. The parents' primary concerns should become the priorities of the feeding team who work with the child. Are the parents most concerned about weight gain? Is the length of time required for feeding dominating the parent's daily activities? Does the child seem to lose most of the food consumed during feeding (e.g., through vomiting or reflux)? Is the child's behavior during feeding creating havoc for the entire family during mealtime? While the parents' voiced concerns become the focus of intervention, the concerns of the professionals, when these differ from the parents, should be explained and considered in developing the feeding plan.

The parents also provide the team with information about the child's developmental history and feeding history. Obtaining this history helps the therapist identify the basis of the feeding problem (e.g., if long-standing sensory or behavioral issues have influenced feeding performance). By asking about the feeding history, the therapist also obtains a sense of the parents' frustration and ability to cope with the child's feeding issues. The techniques used by the parents and their experiences in feeding the infant are helpful in identifying appropriate intervention strategies. Parents whose children have received therapy services in the past probably have important information to share regarding interventions that worked and those that did not.

Information about the current feeding methods must be obtained. Often detailed information can be gathered by simply asking the parents to describe feeding over the course of a typical day. This open-ended request allows the parent to bring forward their concerns. After this, the therapist can then guide the discussion to obtain comprehensive information. The box on p. 435 provides a list of guiding questions.

## Medical and Development History

All medical records should be obtained and reviewed. Of particular importance are reports of the results of neurologic examinations, including results of computerized tomography scans or brain imaging scans. Documented instances of pneumonia and upper respiratory infections provide critical information for the team and should be analyzed for frequency and course. The results of barium swallow and videofluoroscopic swallow studies (VFSSs), if they have been done, should be carefully read.

Recorded developmental histories supplement the parents' report. The written reports of other occupational and physical therapists, early childhood specialists, and teachers provide foundational knowledge about the child. The developmental progress of the child provides important information for predicting the goals that the child will achieve in the coming months. Understanding the child's develop-

## Questions Regarding Feeding at Home

1. Who feeds your child at home?
   a. Do different caregivers feed your child in different ways (e.g., different positions)?
   b. Does your child seem to respond different to different feeders?
   c. If only one caregiver feeds your child, what is the effect of this total responsibility on this caregiver?
2. Describe your child's problems with feeding.
   a. Does your child have difficulty sucking or drinking?
   b. Does your child have problems biting or chewing?
   c. Does your child cough or choke? When? How often?
   d. What do you think is causing your child's problems with eating?
3. How much help does your child need with feeding?
   a. Do you manually assist your child in chewing and drinking?
   b. Does your child self-feed or do you assist him in self-feeding?
   c. Is your child independent in using a cup or do you have to assist him or her?
4. How do you know when your child is hungry?
5. How do you know when your child has had enough?
   a. Does your child stop eating when satiated?
   b. Can your child's endurance cause him or her to stop eating before he or she is full?
6. When and how often is your child fed and how long does a meal take?
7. How much formula, milk, baby food, or other food does the child consume? Each meal? Each day?
8. If your child gets something other than formula, milk, and baby food, do you do anything special to prepare the food (e.g., mash it or cut it into small bites)?
9. When your child is fed at home, where does he or she sit (e.g., in a regular chair at the table, in a high chair, or in a wheelchair)?
   a. How do you position your child?
   b. Is there anything special that you do to adapt the seating?
10. What bottles, nipples, or spoons are used in feeding? (Explore specific types or shapes)
    a. If adapted equipment is used for feeding, what is it and how is it used?
    b. Have you tried special equipment before and decided it was not working for you and your child?
11. Describe your child's response to feeding. When does your child most enjoy feeding?
12. How does your child react to foods that are new or that have different textures, tastes, or temperatures?
13. Does your child's performance and behavior during feeding differ in the morning, midday, or at night?
14. Who is around during most meals, and what else is going on in the room?
15. Has anyone given you suggestions on how to feed your child? How did these work for you?

mental course across domains is important to making realistic objectives for the child and for selecting appropriate intervention strategies.

## Feeding Observation

The feeding observation should be as naturalistic as possible. Ideally the therapist has an opportunity to play with the child before feeding. During play the therapist can observe overall developmental skills, including cognitive skills, postural stability, gross and fine motor skills, and language skills. This information helps the therapist plan the feeding evaluation, for example, how to position the child, whether self-feeding should be included, and how to communicate with the child during the feeding observation. This play session also helps build rapport between the therapist and the child. The relaxed and positive interaction can influence the nature of the interaction during feeding, given that feeding experiences may have been stressful and uncomfortable for the child.

If the evaluation takes place in a clinic or school, foods that the child typically eats should be used. Parents should help the team select the menu, or they may be asked if they can bring preferred foods from home. The child should be placed in his or her typical feeding position, and feeding utensils and methods familiar to the child should be used. One parent is asked to feed the child a portion of the meal.

The observation of the parent-child interaction helps the therapist understand factors that may promote or inhibit the child's intake. It gives the therapist the everyday context for feeding from which to begin to make recommendations. Does the parent talk to the child? Communication with the child during eating can facilitate the child's participation and foster eating independence. Many children with oral motor problems have difficulty sending clear cues and have limited communication. Parents of children with severe disabilities need a high level of sensitivity and responsivity to successfully foster communication during feeding. It is important to call the parents' attention to times they read the child's cues and attempt to respond.

After observing typical feeding by the caregiver, it is advantageous for the therapist to also feed the child. This gives the therapist additional information about the individual child's responses to new positions and different foods. The outcome of this part of the evaluation can be to assess the potential effectiveness of therapeutic techniques that the therapist postulates will improve oral motor skills. Therefore assessment information is obtained regarding what intervention strategies seem to promote skills and the child's responsiveness to different intervention methods.

The focus of the evaluation is assessment of the child's oral sensitivity; postural control; jaw, lip, cheek, and tongue movements; coordination of those movements; and overall strength and endurance during feeding. A speech pathologist may assist in analysis of oral motor skills. The therapist emphasizes specific oral sensorimotor skills based on the child's primary problem; these are listed under the problems described in the following sections.

## Videofluoroscopic Swallow Study

VFSS has become an important tool in analyzing feeding disorders and is particularly important for children who aspirate or are at high risk for aspiration because of severe motor problems. Factors that suggest swallowing problems may include gagging or choking, repeated ineffective swallows, and reflux. Sometimes the aspiration may be silent, so the only indications are wet, noisy respiration after feeding and the occurance of repeated respiratory infections.

The VFSS is also termed a *modified barium swallow.* A food substance is saturated with barium, then ingestion of the barium is videotaped to show how the food passes from the mouth through the pharynx. The occupational therapist consults with the radiologist so that the infant or child is placed in typical feeding positions or potentially therapeutic positions. The therapist also selects the types of food textures to try based on knowledge of the child's current diet and feeding goals (Fox, 1990; Schuberth, 1994).

In a typical VFSS, liquid barium is mixed with other liquids or pureed foods and barium paste is spread on crackers or cookies. The food may be given using a bottle, cup, or spoon. The purpose of the VFSS is to identify whether the child aspirates and how the child handles different textures in different positions. Because the video record shows how the food travels in the mouth and pharynx, detailed information about the swallow problem is received. After typical feeding procedures have been imaged and studied, therapeutic methods should be tried and videotaped (Logeman, 1983; Wolf & Glass, 1992). For example, the child is fed thickened liquids or is fed in new positions. Swallowing when the child is fatigued can be observed after a variety of foods and liquids have been consumed. The outcome of the VFSS is usually more than a simple recommendation that the child be fed using nonoral methods, but it is a detailed recommendation of the positions and textures to use during feeding that seem to result in optimal swallowing patterns without aspiration. Often a speech pathologist contributes to interpretation of the results (Benson & Lefton-Greif, 1994).

Although the VFSS gives the therapist important information and insight regarding the swallow problem, it is an image of one time and may not be representative of the child's typical feeding in a more natural environment.

Having completed the assessment process, which ideally included several opportunities to interact with the child and family, an intervention plan is designed. Intervention for feeding problems considers the whole child, involves the family, and includes collaboration with professionals of other disciplines. In the following sections, key issues that affect feeding in infants and children are discussed. Al-

though the issues are discussed separately, feeding problems are seldom attributable to a singular cause and usually are the result of delays or impairment in multiple performance areas. For example, children with severe sensory problems generally have oral motor skills delays, and children with swallowing disorders often have motor deficits.

## INTERVENTION FOR SENSORY ISSUES

Young children with feeding problems often exhibit sensory defensiveness in and around the mouth. They demonstrate aversive responses to touch in the mouth and demonstrate extreme responses to textured food within the mouth. Behaviors observed when pureed food on a spoon is placed in the mouth include spitting, choking, or gagging. These behaviors are typical when a new texture is introduced to most children. However, the child with oral tactile defensiveness persists beyond the time usually required to develop tolerance. Sensory defensiveness is a critical problem for the child because it often limits the amount of nutritional intake, limits the variety of foods that are accepted, and creates a negative situation during feeding. Also, increasing the texture of food is important to facilitating higher levels of oral motor skill (that is, chewing and diagonal tongue movements are elicited when the texture of the food requires those movements). Knowing the basis of the child's defensiveness is important to planning an intervention program that helps to resolve the problem. Wolf and Glass (1992) explained that sensory defensiveness may relate to the three causative factors.

First, sensory defensiveness of the oral area is often associated with the early experiences of the child (i.e., as a neonate and young infant). Neonates with medical problems at birth often endure procedures that are noxious to the oropharyngeal area and result in aversive responses to all tactile stimulation of the mouth. Examples of nursing and medical procedures associated with oral tactile defensiveness are mouth and lung suctioning, intubation, and nasal gastric feeding. In each of these procedures, hard plastic tubes are entered into the mouth and throat, almost always causing gagging, coughing, and choking. Over time, when such experiences are repeated, the infant develops defensive responses to all oral-sensory input, perhaps in an attempt to protect that highly sensitive area (DiScipio, Kaslon, & Rube, 1978).

Second, sensory defensiveness also may result in the child who was not fed by mouth for an extended period. When oral feedings are delayed and compensatory oral stimulation is not provided, the child develops hypersensitivity of the oral area. It appears that oral stimulation is critical at certain developmental periods for establishing sensory processing around and inside the mouth. (Handen, Mandel, & Russo, 1986; Illingworth & Lister, 1965). Lack of oral experiences may be the easiest type of sensory defensiveness to overcome.

A third cause of oral-sensory defensiveness may be neurologic impairment that directly affects those sensory tracts. Young infants with neurologic immaturity often have difficulty with sensory modulation and are hypersensitive to tactile input. Children with cerebral palsy or other disorders may demonstrate oral defensiveness as a manifestation of neurologic impairment. A child with cerebral palsy may exhibit general sensory defensiveness and may require a program that addresses overall sensory integration. In children with general sensory defensiveness, hypersensitivity of the oral area may be a long-standing problem.

Sensory defensiveness often is the result of all three causative factors. Infants with neurologic impairment often demonstrate oral motor dysfunction and as a result receive nonoral feedings and invasive oral procedures. Feeding intervention for children whose defensiveness seems to be related to both offensive oral experiences and general sensory impairment is particularly challenging.

## Evaluation

The child's ability to accept a variety of sensory stimuli in his or her mouth should be assessed through a parent or caregiver interview and observation. In the interview the therapist explores the questions outlined in the box on p. 435. The child with sensory defensiveness may accept only one or two food textures, may swallow food without mastication or preparation, may spit out foods on a regular basis, or may exhibit a hyperactive gag and frequent choking that seems unrelated to the amount of food placed into the mouth.

Trial of different textures should be preceded by relaxed play with the child so that he or she becomes comfortable and so that rapport with the therapist is established. To observe the child's sensory responses, a variety of textures should be used and placement of food in different parts of the mouth should be attempted. When the child exhibits aversive responses to food inside the mouth, the therapist asks the parent if the responses are typical or exaggerated because of discomfort with an unfamiliar environment or a different feeder.

## Intervention

Sensory defensiveness can seriously interfere with the nutritional intake and the oral motor skills of the child. It is often a problem that can improve significantly with intervention. At first, intervention activities should be implemented at times other than mealtimes. Because intervention activities are often uncomfortable and challenging for the child, they may best be performed between feedings to not disrupt times of nutritional intake.

First and foremost the therapist must establish a relationship of trust with the child. The child may distrust anyone who attempts to place food in his or her mouth; therefore poor rapport and positive interactions are critical. Activities to desensitize should be placed in the context of play, should be self-guided as much as possible, and should be introduced gradually. Once the therapist begins oral desensitization, the trust relationship can be maintained if the therapist always acknowledges the child's physical cues of discomfort (by at least a verbal response and when appropriate by withdrawal of the oral stimulus). The therapist should also allow turn taking, decision making, and as much active participation by the child as possible.

Oral desensitization should begin by encouraging the child to explore his or her mouth with his or her own hands. The child can begin to suck on his or her hands and fingers with the guidance of the therapist's hand. Rubber toys can be introduced into the oral play. The NUK toothbrush or a regular toothbrush may be used to brush and massage the gums (Morris & Klein, 1987). The therapist can engage in turn-taking games with the child using a rubber toy or toothbrush in a hide-and-seek game. The therapist's goal in this game is to stimulate different areas of the mouth using different degrees of pressure. The parent can rub the child's gums with a warm washcloth, applying firm sustained pressure and allowing the child to chew or suck on the cloth. The texture of the washcloth seems to be easily accepted by children and is helpful in improving sensory tolerance of other textures. For older children with higher-level oral motor skills, blow toys can be used to desensitize the oral area. Blowing bubbles and making sounds are particularly motivating activities.

Desensitization activities between meals should include small amounts of food. Rubber toys can be dipped in pureed food, and toothbrushes can be dipped in fruit juice before entry into the child's mouth. The taste and texture of different foods should be introduced into the oral play as much as possible. Once the child is in preschool, snack time is an excellent time to focus on oral desensitization because it may not be as important to eat a certain amount of food. Turn-taking games and sharing with peers can encourage oral intake and can improve the child's willingness to try new textures.

Oral desensitization is also important immediately before the child's mealtime. A program should be developed that seems to effectively prepare the child for oral intake and requires only a brief amount of time and energy by the caregiver and child. Using a warm washcloth around and inside of the mouth can desensitize this area before feeding. The washcloth may be easier to tolerate than the therapist's finger. The therapist's finger inside a nipple is generally well accepted by the child and can offer some protection to the therapist's fingers as he or she rubs the gums, tongue, and palate. When applying any method of direct oral stimulation, the therapist should wear gloves and follow Occupational Safety and Health Administration (OSHA) guidelines for exposure to body fluids such as saliva. (Federal Register, 56 [235]. December 6, 1991.) These regulations require that "gloves be worn when it can be reasonably anticipated that the employee may have hand contact with blood, other potentially infectious materials, mucous membranes, and nonintact skin" (pp. 64133-64134).

Sensory preparation should be systematically applied, beginning with stroking in body areas where it is tolerated. Firm rubbing and deep pressure are stimuli that seem to desensitize and increase tolerance to touch (Meuller, 1975). Gradually, and based on the child's response, the tactile stimulation is applied to the cheeks, outer lips, inside the mouth, gums, and tongue (Glass & Wolf, 1992). Sustained firm pressure to the upper palate seems to desensitize the entire mouth, enabling the child to accept touch in other parts of his or her mouth. This pressure can produce calming and more organized responses.

In addition to these preparatory activities, adaptations to the child's position and the texture of the food should be considered. The child's trunk and head should be optimally supported so that the child feels secure and stable but not confined. Children who have generalized sensory defensiveness may be more comfortable in a chair or positioner than in the arms of the care provider. Children with concomitant respiratory problems should be positioned to allow for maximum thoracic expansion and optimal respiration during feeding.

Adjusting the texture of the child's food is perhaps the most important intervention the therapist can offer to the child with tactile defensiveness. The box at right provides guidelines for adapting food texture to accommodate and decrease the child's sensory defensiveness.

New textures should be introduced gradually and in a way that makes them palatable to the child and easily consumed. For example, mashed potatoes can be mixed with other vegetables and soft meats to help hold those foods together. This sensory experience may be more acceptable to the child than the new food alone, which may become a collection of discrete bits after chewing. Parents should be encouraged to add the right amount of moisture to food to make it easily manageable in the mouth. Thickening foods becomes important for the child with poor oral motor control because the thicker substance moves more slowly within the mouth and provides more sensory input, making it easy for the child to control.

When changes in the types of food are recommended, for example, more fruits and vegetables, consultation with a nutritionist regarding the effect of the dietary change is important. Children with disabilities are often on high-caloric and high-protein intake, making the balance of nutrients more difficult to achieve. Often children with oral motor problems take medications that interact with nutrient intake. Accordingly, their diet needs to be adjusted with higher or lower daily requirements of certain nutrients to prevent detrimental side effects of the medications.

In addition to adjusting the food texture, the utensils used and the placement of the spoon in the child's mouth should be assessed relative to the child's tolerance. Food placed in

---

## Guidelines for Adapting Food Texture for Children With Sensory Defensiveness

1. Ensure adequate nutritional intake by attending to the nutrient value and amount of food intake when changing the texture of foods consumed.
2. Pureed, smooth foods are the first solid foods to attempt with a child with severe oral-sensory defensiveness. The texture of pureed foods can be gradually increased by adding food with lumps or of more coarse texture.
3. The textures within any one meal should be varied from those least tolerated to those most tolerated. When the child successfully eats a food with strong sensory input, he or she can be rewarded with a spoonful of a favorite food.
4. Soft foods that have cohesion when masticated offer increased sensory experiences. Cheese, chicken, and well-cooked vegetables with no skins increase chewing when placed between the teeth.
5. Graham crackers, butter cookies, and some cereals (e.g., Cheerios) provide discrete bits of food in the mouth that promote desensitization. Soft crackers and cookies promote chewing and at the time dissolve quickly once inside the mouth, presenting less danger of choking.
6. For children who need altered food texture over time, a food grinder to puree the child's food is a useful tool. The food texture can be progressively altered by changing the food grinder setting.
7. Grainy breads provide more texture than soft white breads, which tend to form a ball and adhere to the upper palate.
8. It may be helpful to introduce textured foods that require some chewing by mixing them in foods that are familiar to the child and that add cohesion to the food bolus.
9. The therapist should maintain a pleasant, fun atmosphere during feeding, and when appropriate, use play and verbal interaction to distract the child from focusing attention on the food within his or her mouth. Verbal encouragement and looks of delight are rewarding to the child who has eaten a new food; offering another bite might be frustrating rather than rewarding.

Modified from Case-Smith, J. (1993). Self care strategies for children with developmental deficits. In C. Christiansen (Ed.). *Ways of living: self-care strategies for special needs* (pp. 101-156). Rockville, MD: AOTA.

---

the anterior part of the mouth is better tolerated than food placed on the posterior tongue. It may be better tolerated on the center of the tongue than the sides. However, food placement on the side is often desirable for increasing chewing and tongue lateralization.

Table 16-2 is a chart of food progression from smooth, pureed foods to coarse and chewy foods. The chart lists foods in different nutrient groups in the sequence that a typi-

▲ Table 16-2  Food Progression Based on Texture Consistency*

| Food Group | Food and Food Forms | | | | | |
|---|---|---|---|---|---|---|
| **MEATS AND MEAT SUBSTITUTES** | Strained meats and egg yolk | Commercial junior meats; soft meats ground fine in baby food grinder with liquid added; mashed egg yolk | Ground meats with gravy or other liquid added; soft-cooked eggs | Ground meats without added liquid; scrambled eggs; smooth peanut butter | Well-cooked and soft meats, fish, and poultry; hard-cooked eggs | Cut up meats of increased texture (roast beef and ham) |
| **DAIRY PRODUCTS** | Strained cottage cheese; thinned puddings; plain yogurt; thinned, strained cream soups | Fork mashed cottage cheese; pudding; custard; thickened cream soups | Cottage cheese | Yogurt with soft fruits; ice cream; some soft cheeses (Muenster and American) | Harder cheeses (Swiss and Cheddar) | |
| **BREADS AND CEREALS** | Infant cereal thinned with milk | Thicker infant cereals; Cream of Wheat; Farina | Cooked cereals such as oatmeal or Malto-meal; crackers; toast; plain cookies; bread without crust | Cooked cereals with soft fruits added; bread with crust; well-cooked pasta (noodles and spaghetti) | Dry cereals with milk; sandwiches with smooth filling and cut in small pieces; rice; firmer texture pasta | Sandwiches with a variety of fillings |
| | Strained fruits and vegetables | Junior fruits; applesauce; ripe, mashed bananas; junior vegetables, mashed potatoes | Fork-mashed, soft canned fruits without skins; soft, ripe, mashed fresh fruits (peeled); fork-mashed, well-cooked vegetables without skins; boiled or baked potatoes without skins | Canned fruits (peaches and pears); soft, ripe fresh fruits (peeled); well-cooked vegetables cut in small pieces | Canned fruits of increased texture (fruit cocktail and pineapple); vegetables of increased texture (steamed carrots and broccoli); soups with well-cooked vegetables | Raw or dried fruits; raw vegetables; vegetables with skins (corn, peas and lima beans); chunky soup |

*The suggestions for texture progression is an aid to be used as part of a treatment plan for children with oral sensory or motor problems. It identifies foods and food forms in each food category which may be appropriate in progressing toward a regular diet.

cal child learns to tolerate and handle solid foods. The food groups also follow the progression of oral motor skills achievement.

## INTERVENTION FOR MOTOR IMPAIRMENTS

Children with significant motor impairments often exhibit oral motor delays. Examples of children with motor dysfunctions that can affect feeding are those with cerebral palsy, prematurity, or genetic syndromes such as trisomy 21, 18, or 13. Problems in oral motor control in young infants are often different from those of older children. Delays in feeding skills caused by oral motor dysfunction may not occur until the child moves to solid food and until more sophisticated oral motor responses are required.

Often the muscle tone of children with cerebral palsy in the proximal areas of the face, neck, and trunk is hypotonic, resulting in poor head and trunk stability. The child's jaw tends to move in wide excursions, completely open or clamped shut. The child often demonstrates inability to grade the jaw's movement in the midranges typically observed in sucking and chewing. When the child has low facial muscle tone, the mouth is often open, resulting in excessive drooling and loss of food from the mouth during feeding. An open mouth during feeding also makes swallowing difficult.

In the child with hypotonia, the tongue may be inactive, moving primarily with the lower jaw. The tongue may move only in extension and retraction, or it may move into extreme ranges (e.g., completely retracted into the back of the mouth). Morris and Klein (1987) proposed that these extreme ranges or lack of movement are associated with poor jaw stability such that the jaw does not function as a base for tongue movement. These patterns also seem to relate to the primitive movement patterns exhibited by children with cerebral palsy.

The lips are often inactive and hypotonic. Lip seal on the bottle's nipple, the cup rim, or a spoon is inadequate and results in food loss or air intake. Hypotonic cheeks result in less suction of the nipple and difficulty maintaining food in the tongue's center.

Children with hypotonic oral musculature often have overall postural instability. Postural instability results in poor postural alignment and increased difficulty with oral motor skills. When upright, the child may fall into trunk and cervical flexion. When slightly reclined, his or her head may fall into extension. The child may also elevate the shoulders and retract the arms in an attempt to stabilize the head. When the child's neck is in hyperextension, neck alignment is not appropriate for safe and efficient swallow.

When a child demonstrates hypertonicity in the face and mouth, usually he or she has spastic cerebral palsy. Sometimes a child who initially exhibits low tone may exhibit spasticity as he or she matures and as he or she attempts to assume positions more upright against gravity. Children with hypertonicity tend to exhibit hyperextension of the trunk and neck without reciprocal flexion. They may exhibit tonic oral reflexes or abnormal oral motor patterns that are never observed in a typically developing child. (They differ from children with low muscle tone who exhibit delayed oral motor patterns that could be observed in children who are younger.) The following are examples of oral motor patterns observed in children with hypertonicity:

1. *Tonic bite:* The gums or teeth close or clamp together in a forceful motion. Once closed, the jaw remains clamped and the child may need to be repositioned to open the mouth. The tonic bite occurs more often when the child is inappropriately positioned in some neck extension or when he or she has extreme tactile defensiveness.

2. *Tongue thrust:* In tongue thrust the child completely extends his tongue outside the borders of his lips. The tongue's movement is forceful and is often maintained in the extended position. Tongue thrust also tends to occur more often when the child is positioned in trunk and neck extension. This forceful tongue movement results in loss of food or liquid from the mouth and does not effectively initiate a swallow. Children with severe tongue thrust may lose much of the food presented to them and may be diagnosed as failure-to-thrive. Without knowledge of how much of the food that enters into the mouth is actually swallowed, it is difficult to estimate the amount of food consumed. Jaw thrust, a strong, forceful, downward movement of the lower jaw, may be observed with tongue thrust. This movement is also observed when the child is in a position of extension.

3. *Lip retraction and lip pursing:* Some children with high muscle tone associated with cerebral palsy exhibit lip retraction. The lips pull away from the midline and stay fixed in the retracted position when utensils and food or a cup and drink are entered into the mouth. This stiffening replaces the soft seal of the lips typically observed. Lip pursing is a response in which the lips draw tightly together at midline. Both movement patterns result in food loss and difficulty obtaining the food from the spoon or the drink from the cup. These movement patterns occur most frequently when the neck is extended, and appropriate head and trunk alignment is not achieved. They tend to occur when the child experiences an emotional reaction to a situation.

### Evaluation

Assessment of the child's motor control as it affects feeding includes the following:

1. Overall evaluation of motor patterns, strength, and muscle tone

2. Assessment of postural alignment and postural control, including asymmetries, with a focus on head and trunk stability

3. Evaluation of jaw, tongue, cheek, and lip movement pattern (note typical delayed and atypical patterns)
4. Evaluation of the coordination and sequencing of jaw, tongue, and lip movements during feeding, that is, coordination of suck-swallow-breathe
5. Observation of how oral movement patterns are affected by the child's posture using different external sources of postural support (e.g., in the caregiver's lap versus in a feeder chair or small child's chair)
6. Observation of changes in oral motor patterns when the jaw or cheeks are supported and observation of child's responses to handling around the mouth before and during feeding

The goal of the evaluation is to assess oral motor skills with the child in typical positioning, with optimal positioning and environmental conditions, and during application of intervention strategies. The resulting information provides guidance to the therapist as to the nature of the child's oral motor strengths and problems and the types of intervention that seem to promote improved oral motor control.

## Intervention

### Postural Alignment

The first intervention strategy to implement to help the child gain oral motor skill is to improve postural alignment and stability through good positioning. Some oral motor problems immediately resolve when the child is well positioned in good postural alignment. Appropriate alignment for feeding consists of the following:

1. Neutral pelvic alignment of the trunk. Pelvic alignment is promoted when the child sits well supported against a flat back, on a flat seat, and square on the buttocks with 90 degree of hip flexion and 90 degrees of knee flexion
2. Good head, neck, and shoulder alignment with the head in slight flexion or at neutral
3. Chin tuck with the neck in an elongated position

Correct postural alignment can be achieved in a variety of positions, depending on the size of the child and his or her postural stability. One guideline is to provide the child with more external postural stability than is actually needed. Feeding requires high-level, intricate oral movement and focused concentration; therefore complete postural stability, excellent alignment, and comfort are critical to successful eating.

### Characteristics of Feeding Positions and Positioning Devices

*Infant is held sideways in the feeder's lap.* This position allows for full body contact. It is appropriate for very young children; however, it may be difficult to maintain alignment. This position is fatiguing and is inappropriate for the older child or the child who has poor postural control.

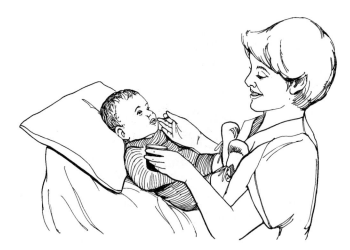

**Figure 16-2** Face-to-face position for feeding.

*Infant is held on caregiver's thighs facing caregiver* (Figure 16-2). With young children this position provides excellent stability and good alignment and promotes midline. It frees both of the caregiver's hands. This intimate position allows for eye contact and therefore promotes communication. It does not work with older, bigger children.

*Child is placed in an infant seat.* The infant seat works well for infants with fair head control who are not yet independent in sitting. It can be adapted with small rolls on the side to maintain a symmetric posture. When the child is placed in the infant seat, the parent's hands are freed and then can be used for support at the chin or chest during feeding. Straps are available with this seat, and the cost is low. It is not an appropriate device for a child with established sitting balance or for the child who weighs more than 25 pounds.

*Cradle bouncer.* This seat is similar to an infant seat. It holds the child in more extension and is inappropriate for a child with increased extensor muscle tone. The bouncing motion of the seat could be used to promote rhythmic movement during feeding, but would be a distraction to the child who has difficulty tolerating vestibular system input.

*Foam-filled feeder seat.* This positioner offers full head and trunk support and promotes good alignment. The feeder seat comes with a strapping system, and different chest straps can be ordered. The curved sides of the chair promote midline and decrease shoulder retraction. The infant seat can be reclined to the angle desired for feeding, that is, the angle at which the head is in an optimal position. The Tumble Forms chair comes in two sizes, is easily cleaned, easily transported, and safe when used on the floor. It is more expensive than an infant seat. It is inappropriate for children who sit independently (Figure 16-3).

*Regular car seat.* The child's car seat has features similar to the Tumble Forms seat. Most car seats provide

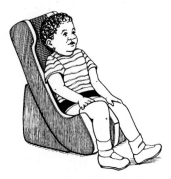

**Figure 16-3** Tumble Forms Feeder Chair offers support and an adjustable feeding angle.

good alignment and postural stability for the infant. Usually adjusting the seat's degree of tilt is more difficult or may not be possible.

*Travel chair.* The Travel chair may be the optimal seating device for feeding a child with severe motor limitations. It is typically the most supportive seating arrangement for the child. Each travel chair is individualized with head support, lateral supports, and trunk straps as needed. Therefore the chair offers optimal external stability of the child's posture. The tray provides an additional truncal support and a surface for weight bearing on arms. A key feature beneficial to children with poor head control is that the chair tilts into a variety of positions while maintaining optimal postural alignment for feeding (neutral pelvis and 90 degrees hip and knee flexion). In some chairs the postural support tilts on a stable base. In others the postural support moves with the base, reclining in increment degrees. The travel chair places the child at a height that makes feeding convenient for the adult. The disadvantage of feeding in the travel chair is that it is a restrictive device that removes the child from peer interaction, as in a preschool setting where the children eat snacks seated at a common table.

*Rifton child's chair.* Once the child has fair to good sitting stability, the Rifton chair is an excellent choice for feeding. The Rifton chair places the child in a completely upright position and requires good head control. This chair has a firm seat and back, adjustable foot rests, arm supports, and pelvic strapping. A pelvic abductor pad can be added to the system. A tray is desirable for weight bearing on arms during feeding and for additional sitting stability. The tray provides a surface for play with food or for self-feeding, should the child have those skills.

*Beanbag chair.* The beanbag chair is a comfortable seating option for the child who otherwise might be in a wheelchair or on the floor. It brings the child into a semiupright position for visualization of the environment and for eye contact with peer or adults. The bean-

bag chair is not the best option for feeding because postural alignment is difficult to control and the child tends to be primarily in extension. The beanbag is particularly inappropriate for children with extensor posturing because it does not successfully inhibit these postures.

*Corner chair.* The corner chair with a seat elevated from the floor level that allows for hip and knee flexion and feet flat on the floor is a good choice for feeding when the child has good head control. The corner chair provides a tray surface for beginning self-feeding, and the 90-degree corner back support promotes midline arm position and inhibits shoulder retraction. The disadvantage of a corner chair is that it cannot be reclined backward for the child with limited head control. Also the height of the corner chair seat and tray cannot be adjusted once the child is seated. The child sits low to the ground, requiring that the feeder sit on the floor.

*Child's high chair.* A regular high chair is standard furniture for many families with young children learning to eat solid foods. It is the positioner of choice if the child has appropriate postural stability and motor control. Minimally, the child should be able to independently maintain a propped sitting position for several seconds.

The high chair provides back support, side rests, pelvic strapping, and a tray. It can easily be adapted to provide foot support and additional lateral support. The high chair places the child at a height that allows him or her to participate in the family's meal. It also provides for the child to sit at a height that is convenient for the feeder. The high chair is desirable because it is readily available and economical; it is especially appropriate for the child who will soon be independent in sitting.

***Summary.*** Parents should be given a range of options for positions; however, certain positioning choices should be discouraged. For example, although holding the child in the caregiver's lap is a comforting position, it does not enable the parent optimal control when the child has poor control of movement. Infants and children with postural instability benefit from placement in a stable seating device that helps the child focus on oral movements and frees the parent's hands for providing manual assistance to the child's oral movements.

## Handling Techniques in Support of Oral Movement

Handling techniques to improve oral motor skills have been described by Morris and Klein (1987), Meuller (1975), and Wolf and Glass (1992), among others. Occupational therapists often collaborate with speech pathologists in developing an intervention program for oral motor skill development. The effectiveness of oral support using the therapist's fingers on the infant's cheeks and under the chin has been investigated in a recent study of premature infants (Einarisson-Backes, Deitz, Price, Glass, & Hays, 1994). The intervention techniques and strategies seem most effective with young children who have not learned abnormal motor patterns. They should always be individualized and adjusted based on the child's responses. The techniques involve touch in and around the mouth; therefore desensitization of the oral area is often a required prerequisite to handling. All of the techniques are applied after the child is positioned in good postural alignment and has optimal postural stability.

***Handling before feeding.*** Certain neuromotor problems are best addressed both before and during feeding. Children with hypotonicity of the oral musculature often benefit from techniques to improve muscle tone. Glass and Wolf (1992) described techniques that improve muscle tone and therefore muscle responsivity during feeding. Tapping or quick stretch of cheeks and lips provides sensory input that increases muscle tone around the mouth. The tapping or stretch should be applied symmetrically and rhythmically, repeating the stimulation several times within a brief period immediately before feeding. Vibration is a stronger stimulus that can effectively increase tone and ready muscles for movement. Children with low muscle tone and sensory defensiveness often benefit from vibration around the mouth.

***Preparation for children with hypertonicity.*** When the child has high muscle tone of the lips, cheeks, and tongue, deep and firm pressure using a downward stroking motion can be applied symmetrically to the cheeks and around the lips. Firm rhythmic sustained pressure can be applied through the lower jaw (chin), facilitating a chin tuck position. Touch pressure can also be applied to the cheeks to inhibit or decrease lip retraction.

In the child with oral hypertonicity, often the tongue is retracted to the back of the mouth or is extended beyond the lips. Good postural alignment often helps inhibit these extreme tongue positions. The therapist can place his or her finger (or the bowl of the spoon) in the middle of the tongue and apply rhythmic, downward pressure. The pressure should be forward for the retracted tongue and backward for the extended tongue. Rhythmic pressure using a downward motion of one beat per second can promote a sucking pattern (Morris & Klein, 1987). Jiggling or lateral movement of the spoon or finger on the tongue can be inhibitory and should be used based on the child's response. Once feeding begins, downward pressure should continue with the use of the bowl of the spoon.

***Techniques during feeding.*** External support of the jaw can be provided by the therapist's fingers under and around the lower jaw. The therapist can apply his or her hand to the child's chin either from the front or from the side (Figure 16-4). One finger places pressure through the front of

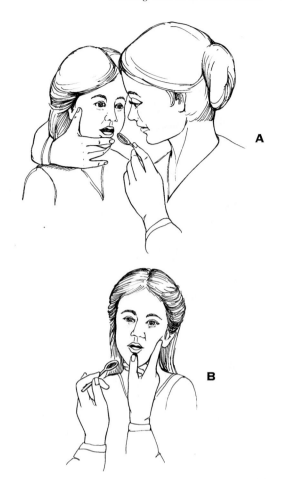

**Figure 16-4** Jaw control and oral support, **A,** from the side and **B,** from the front.

the chin to promote chin tuck, and another provides support under the jaw. The finger under the jaw provides a source of stability, inhibits wide jaw excursions, and provides a support base for tongue movement. Important aspects of successfully using jaw support is use of the flat side of the finger (rather than the fingertip) and use of the finger as a source of support to the child's jaw movement, not to direct the child's movement. Forcefully moving the child's jaw is inappropriate. The therapist's hand should be maintained under and around the jaw during the entire feeding rather than removed and reapplied with each bite. The finger under the chin should be midway between the tip of the jaw and the throat, and caution should be observed not to move the hand's pressure into the throat. This support to the jaw may be particularly critical when the child is drinking from a cup, at which time the jaw's movement may increase. The goal of this activity is for the child to gain adequate internal jaw stability for independent mouth closure during eating and drinking.

***Cheek support.*** In young infants, touch pressure to the cheeks may be applied using the thumb and index finger

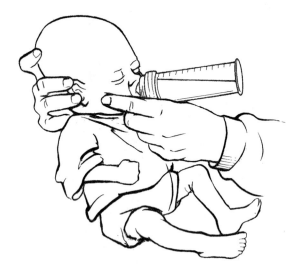

**Figure 16-5** Jaw and cheek support of the young infant during bottle-feeding.

(with the third finger under the jaw). This pressure is appropriate only during bottle feeding as a method to increase negative pressure within the mouth and therefore improve suction on the nipple. The pressure to the cheeks can improve the lip's seal and sucking patterns (Figure 16-5).

***Spoon placement.*** The placement of the spoon can influence the child's oral motor responses. Downward pressure of the spoon on the center of the tongue can facilitate a sucking response. This might be effective for moving the food to the back of the tongue for swallow.

Downward and inward pressure with the spoon (or nipple) can promote the up and down tongue movement observed in mature sucking. This pressure can also inhibit tongue thrust during feeding. Central placement of the spoon is appropriate when the child has only a sucking pattern and the tongue moves in extension and retraction. To encourage tongue lateralization and the beginning of chewing patterns, the spoon should be placed to the side. Food placement between the gums and teeth directly promotes chewing. Consideration should be given to placing the food on alternating sides (to prevent development of skills on one side only) and should remain in the central to anterior part of the mouth. Placement of the spoon or food on the posterior portion of the tongue not only results in gagging, but also does not allow the child to move, chew, and control the food before swallowing.

***Head position.*** A chin tuck position with the head well aligned on the shoulders is generally best for feeding. This head position may require the support of the parent or therapist's arm in back of the neck or under the occipital lobe.

Although complete upright posture allows for correct swallow and helps reduce the possibility of aspiration, a position of slight neck flexion may be needed to help certain children swallow. When the head is slightly forward in neck flexion, the possibility of aspiration is reduced because the distance that the larynx must move upward to initiate the swallow is reduced.

A position of neck flexion should be used with caution because it may interfere with breathing. Some children posture in neck hyperextension despite efforts to hold them in a position of neutral neck alignment. This seems to be the case with children who have difficulty breathing and are seeking a completely open air passageway. A VFSS may help elucidate if aspiration occurs in this position, giving guidance to the therapist as to how important neutral neck alignment is to the child's feeding. A habit of pushing the neck into extension during feeding should be discouraged, by handling the neck at key points to improve neck alignment (e.g., manual pressure on the upper chest).

***Altering the sensory quality of foods.*** The progression of the food textures listed in the chart in Table 16-2 provides examples of food consistencies that require progressively higher-level oral motor skills. Although the therapist and parent use strategies to help the child develop improved oral motor skills, foods selected for the child's diet should accommodate the child's current skill level and should challenge the child to develop higher-level skills. Thin liquids are the most difficult consistency to control in the mouth and should be thickened when the child has poor tongue control and an inefficient suck-swallow pattern.

Eating pureed foods requires no more than a suck-swallow response; therefore giving the child pureed foods elicits sucking. To elicit munching and chewing patterns, soft foods must be given. Increasing the sensory input using highly textured foods facilitates tongue lateralization and tip elevation, active lip movements, and increased chewing responses.

A long piece of vegetable or soft meat can be held between the side teeth to promote graded biting. Strips of soft cheese, chicken, or a long green bean may initially be used. Soft cookies and crackers placed to the side can also promote controlled biting. Pretzels and apple slices require more jaw strength and can be tried as a next step in promoting biting skills.

Certain foods can increase muscle tone and chewing. Fruit Rollups promote rotary chewing and graded jaw movements but at the same time dissolve fairly quickly to minimize the risk of choking. Some dried fruits (e.g., apricots and apples) can be used to increase chewing. Tough or fibrous meats are contraindicated. A list of foods that are indicated and contraindicated for children with immature oral motor skills is provided in the box on p. 445.

## Foods Indicated/Contraindicated for Children With Immature Oral Motor Skills

| Properties of Foods Indicated for Children with Difficulty Swallowing | Properties of Contraindicated Foods |
|---|---|
| Even consistency<br>Increased density and volume<br>Thick liquids<br>Uniform texture<br>Stays together (will not break up in the mouth)<br>Easy to remove and easy to suck | Multiple textures and consistencies (tacos, jello, fruit, vegetable soup, stews, and salads)<br>Sticky (peanut butter)<br>Greasy (fried foods)<br>Tough (red meat, processed meats, and diced fruit)<br>Fibrous and stringy (celery, citrus fruits, and raw vegetables)<br>Skins (raw fruits and peanuts)<br>Spicy (pepper and horseradish)<br>Seeds and nuts (plain or in breads and cakes)<br>Thin liquids (water, carbonated drinks, broth, coffee, tea, and apple juice)<br>Quickly liquefying (jello and watermelon)<br>Foods that break up in the mouth (cottage cheese and flaky pastries)<br>Crunchy (chips and carrots) |

## INTERVENTION FOR SWALLOWING PROBLEMS

### Swallowing and Coordinating the Suck-Swallow-Breathe Sequence

Children with swallowing disorders tend to have severe sensorimotor impairments or physiologic immaturity that interferes with the coordination of the suck-swallow-breathe sequence. To understand swallowing disorders related to neuromotor dysfunction or physiologic immaturity, the normal phases of swallow are briefly described below.

### Oral Phase

In the first phase of swallow, the oral phase, the food enters into the mouth where it is processed. This phase consists of biting, sucking, chewing, or munching. The food is moved side to side for chewing and comes to the center as a bolus for transit to the back of the tongue. In the oral transit phase, the masticated food or liquid is moved to the back of the tongue, where swallow is initiated. Therefore swallow is essentially a reflexive response to the sensory input of the food on the posterior portion of the tongue.

### Pharyngeal Phase

In the pharyngeal phase the bolus moves from the back of the tongue through the pharynx to the opening of the esophagus. The propulsion of the bolus is based on negative pressure; therefore closure of the nasal, laryngeal, and oral openings is important for efficient bolus transit. The larynx is protected by the closure of the epiglottis over the trachea and the contraction of the true and false vocal cords. At the same that time the esophagus opens, the negative pressure propels the bolus through the pharynx to the esophagus opening.

### Esophageal Phase

In the esophageal phase the food or liquid moves through the esophagus using peristalsis. Peristalsis is involuntarily initiated by the swallow itself and the sensation of the food. (Kennedy & Kent, 1988; Wolf & Glass, 1992).

The oral and oral transit phases are the only swallow phases the child controls. These phases establish the timing and coordination of the swallow and are therefore critical to efficient swallow. Therapeutic input to influence swallow is designed to improve the child's control of the initial oral phases.

### Problems

The following problems can affect the child's ability to coordinate sequential swallows without aspiration. When sensory motor problems are severe, the tongue moves primarily in extension or demonstrates minimal movement and tone. Children with severe oral motor dysfunction are often unable to gather the food into a bolus for swallow. The food may trickle over the sides of the tongue and the pharynx without eliciting a swallow. Foods that break apart can scat-

## CASE STUDY #1

Carol was born prematurely at 30 weeks estimated gestational age and had hyperbilirubinemia, respiratory distress, and a grade III intraventricular hemorrhage at birth. A developmental assessment at 12 months indicated mild delays in gross and fine motor skills. Her parents fondly called her their "lazy baby." She was alert and pleasant and had recently begun to babble in long sequences. She had learned to sit independently at 11 months. She rolled from place to place as her form of mobility and did not creep or cruise. She held two objects, one in each hand, waving and banging them. She did not yet combine objects and had limited control of release.

Carol's mother was interviewed at the 12-month assessment. She reported that Carol fed completely from the bottle. Her mother had tried pureed foods on several occasions; however, Carol spit them from her mouth and became upset. These behaviors prevented her mother from continuing to try pureed foods and cereals. Carol demonstrated a strong sucking pattern, but she did not demonstrate tongue lateralization or graded bite. Her jaw was unstable when she attempted cup drinking. Although her weight was appropriate for her age, her mother wanted to introduce new foods and to progress to feeding with a spoon and cup.

### Feeding Evaluation

The therapist's evaluation indicated that Carol was hypersensitive in and around her mouth. Although she exhibited an effective sucking pattern, her tongue and jaw movement were unorganized when pureed foods were introduced. She coughed and choked on pureed food, with loss of most of the food placed on her tongue. Carol's parents were anxious to progress to a variety of foods and a more balanced diet. They were discouraged by the failed attempts to introduce new foods into her diet.

### Intervention

Carol's oral sensory defensiveness was first addressed at times other than feeding. Using a warm, wet washcloth, the therapist began by stroking her face around the mouth and then in the mouth, rubbing the gums and palate. The NUK toothbrush was used to rub her gums. Carol seemed to like this; therefore the NUK toothbrush was used to introduce food tastes and textures. It was dipped into fruit baby food before oral stimulation. A nipple with the therapist's finger inside was then dipped into the baby food and pressed onto the anterior tongue, then lateral tongue and gums.

As Carol's tolerance of the baby food presented on the nipple and toothbrush increased, a latex-covered spoon with pureed food was introduced. Smooth pureed food was used at first; then foods with greater texture were introduced. Jaw support was provided to inhibit her jaw's excessive movement and to promote the tongue's movements. This support was removed as Carol's suck-swallow sequence of pureed foods became efficient.

By 15 months of age Carol's diet included a variety of pureed foods. At this time coarse foods were introduced and the therapist and parent initiated placement of the food on the side of her tongue and between her gums. Jaw support was reintroduced as a support of tongue lateralization. When tongue lateralization was observed, the food was placed completely to the side between the gums.

Cup drinking was introduced at this time because Carol's jaw stability had increased. A small plastic, transparent cup was used. Its transparency helped the parent and therapist regulate the flow of liquid into her mouth. Small, single sips were given at first, then a sequence of suck-swallow movements were facilitated.

By 18 months of age Carol was eating soft foods. Because she was yet unable and unsuccessful in self-feeding with a spoon, she preferred finger foods, such as strips of soft cheese or processed meats such as turkey. Cup drinking remained difficult, although she was learning to bite on the cup for stability. Her mother used thickened liquids, such as milk with yogurt and juice with baby food, to slow the movement of the liquid and give her a better opportunity to control its flow. At this time oral sensitivity was no longer a primary issue, although she exhibited mild discomfort when new foods were introduced. Carol's mother was pleased with the variety of foods she consumed and with her continued weight gain and growth.

ter in the mouth, and bits may fall into the pharynx. When a swallow is not triggered, the protective closure of the epiglottis does not occur, leaving the trachea open, and aspiration becomes highly probable. When liquids and food pool in the pharynx, the child is at high risk for aspiration. When the oral transit phase is slow or is without a rhythmic sequence, the swallow either appears delayed or seems to occur at random. The primary problem created by delayed swallow is that food enters the pharynx before or after the swallow, where it pools or where it may enter the larynx.

The child with respiratory disorder is also at high risk for swallow dysfunction. Although the child typically demonstrates adequate oral motor skills and swallow, the suck-swallow-breathe sequence is poorly coordinated. Typically the infant with respiratory distress syndrome demonstrates rapid and shallow breathing patterns. The infant's oxygen level may plummet when breathing momentarily pauses to allow for swallow. Rapid breathing in an irregular pattern prevents development of a regular, rhythmic pattern of swallowing. The infant who struggles to breathe has increased respiratory difficulty when feeding. He or she may attempt to breathe and swallow at the same time.

## Evaluation

Assessment of swallow disorders or the possibility of a swallowing disorder includes all of the strategies previously described in the chapter, including obtaining the following:
1. A history of feeding from the caregiver
2. A medical history by written or parental report
3. A clinical observation of feeding
4. A VFSS

### Parental Report

First a detailed description of typical feeding is requested of the parent. From the parent's description, the following questions need to be asked regarding feeding at home. These can be asked during or after the parent's narrative description of mealtime.
1. What are your primary concerns about feeding your child and your child's nutritional intake?
2. How, where, and when is the child fed?
3. What kinds of foods are given to the child?
4. How does the child respond during feeding? Does he or she demonstrate aversive responses? Does the child choke, gag, or cough? Is food lost during feeding?
5. Does the child sound raspy during feeding? Does breathing sound noisy (wet) during or after feeding?
6. Does your child have frequent upper respiratory infections?

For the child who is underweight or diagnosed as failure to thrive, a detailed record of the amount of food eaten over a 3-day period is obtained. The nutritionist analyzes this record to develop a comprehensive intervention plan for increased nutritional intake.

### Medical History

All medical records should be obtained, including records of neurologic examination and results of computerized tomography scans and brain imaging scans. Frequently occurring pneumonia and upper respiratory infections are typical in the child who regularly aspirates. Past records of the results of VFSS should be carefully read and considered in the intervention plan. Consultation with a speech pathologist who has completed an evaluation of the child can also help the occupational therapist gain understanding of the child's oral motor function.

### Clinical Observation

The observation should be in the child's natural environment when possible. If the evaluation takes place in a clinic or school, foods that the child typically eats should be used. The child should be placed in his or her typical feeding position, and feeding utensils and methods familiar to the child should be used. After observing typical feeding, new positions and different foods can be attempted as appropriate. The foods and methods tried during the evaluation are techniques that the therapist postulates will improve oral motor skill and swallow. Therefore assessment information is obtained regarding what intervention strategies seem to promote skills and the child's responsiveness to different intervention methods.

As discussed previously, the parent should be asked if the child' behaviors are typical or unique to the stress of the evaluation situation (i.e., interacting with strangers in an unfamiliar setting).

### Videofluoroscopic Swallow Study

The VFSS is an important component of the evaluation process. Often the VFSS provides the most conclusive evidence of the swallowing problem and results in specific recommendations for food consistencies and feeding positions that seem to promote oral motor skill and reduce the possibility of aspiration.

## Intervention

Intervention for swallowing dysfunction relates specifically to the child's unique strengths and limitations as shown in the evaluation. The following techniques were outlined by Glass and Wolf (1992).

### Increase Rhythmic Initiation of Swallow

The muscles involved in swallow can be activated by applying cold stimulation to the tongue and soft palate using a frozen pacifier. When the muscles are readied for action, the swallow reflex is initiated more quickly. Wolf and Glass (1992) also recommend the use of chilled formula to quicken the swallow reflex. In an older child, a popsicle or piece of ice can be used before feeding or can be used intermittently during feeding. As with any technique, the effect of using cold stimulation should be carefully evaluated and adjusted as needed.

### Improve Oral Transit

Many children have swallowing dysfunction associated with poor oral motor control. The food is not efficiently masticated, gathered into a bolus, and moved to the back of the tongue, where the swallow reflex is triggered. This child may benefit by head and jaw support. The jaw support should include facilitation of mouth closure and tongue movement. Jaw support allows the child to focus on moving the tongue within the mouth. Improving mouth closure can increase pressure gradients in the mouth, thereby improving the efficiency of swallow. Thickening liquids is often extremely helpful in improving swallow. The thickened liquid moves more slowly within the mouth, allowing the child to better control it; it also has the characteristic of greater adhesion and therefore tends to remain a bolus. A third benefit of the thickened liquid is that it is heavier and therefore gives more proprioceptive input to the tongue during oral transit.

Position can improve the child's ability to swallow. When the child is positioned in extension, he or she has less control of the food's movement because of the effects of gravity. With the neck extended the child has difficulty with mouth closure and efficient tongue movements. Positioning the child's head in neck flexion can improve closure of the larynx during swallow, therefore decreasing the possibility of aspiration. Good neck alignment increases the child's ability to control the food's movement.

### Coordination of the Suck-Swallow-Breathe Sequence

When children have respiratory disorders, swallowing is problematic as it relates to breathing and the child's coordination of the suck-swallow-breathe sequence. This problem is most typical of premature infants and neonates. Older infants who continue to have difficulty coordinating the suck-swallow-breathe sequence are those with ongoing cardiovascular and respiratory problems. These infants may aspirate because timing of swallow in relationship to breathing is faulty.

### Handling and Intervention During Feeding

In therapy with the infant who remains on some oxygen support, use of a nasal canula or another source of oxygen during feeding is important. With oxygen support, rapid breathing is slowed to a pace that better allows for intermittent swallowing. Slowing of respiration encourages better control of the suck-swallow-breathe sequence.

Placing the child in a full upright position can also improve respiration during feeding and can facilitate coordination of swallow. Often the infant with a respiratory disorder struggles during feeding because he or she initiates a rapid sequence of sucking and is unable to establish an appropriate suck-swallow-breathe sequence. As a result the infant coughs or chokes when the breathing becomes an absolute, immediate necessity. Wolf and Glass (1992) recommended a technique termed *external pacing*. To pace the infant's sucking pattern, the therapist breaks the infant sucking sequence by gently removing the nipple from the mouth. By interrupting an otherwise long sucking sequence, the therapist gives the child an opportunity to breathe and relax. It gives the child an externally imposed pace and suck-swallow-breathe sequence.

### Modifying the Infant's Food

Children with respiratory or cardiac disorders typically have poor endurance and less oral intake than other children. One way to improve their nutrient and caloric intake is to increase the caloric density of their food. Formula is available in different caloric densities, and Karo syrup can be added. For older children, peanut butter, butter, gravies, and powdered milk can be added to foods. These diet changes require consultation and direction by a nutritionist. Any diet change should be discussed with a nutritionist or the physician to ensure that the child's overall nutritional intake is positively affected.

## Nonoral Feeding

A number of methods of nonoral feeding are available to infants with persistent swallowing disorders that result in aspiration, with poor feeding endurance that results in failure to thrive, or with limitations in oral motor function that prevents adequate food intake. Nonoral methods include naso-gastric tubes, oral gastric tubes, gastrostomy tubes, and feeding tubes that extend into the intestines. In any infant or child whose food intake is inadequate for growth or whose lack of oral motor skills and swallow efficiency make feeding unsafe, nonoral feedings should be considered. Nonoral feeding should be viewed as a method to improve the health and developmental status of the child. It should not result in complete removal of oral stimulation or complete removal of the feeding interaction. In many instances the placement of a gastrostomy or the use of other nonoral feeding methods is a temporary measure to promote the child's nutritional status and growth.

Hyperalimentation is a medical procedure that uses a central line to introduce highly nutritional solutions directly into the bloodstream. It provides protein and calorie intake sufficient to sustain life and to promote growth in the absence of adequate gastrointestinal tract function. It is used for children with congenital bowel anomalies or in severe medical crises (Coley & Procter, 1989).

A surgical procedure is required to insert the catheter into a large vein, typically a vein near the heart. The brachial artery may be used. The fluid is pumped into the blood stream, requiring that the child be connected to an intravenous pump at all times (Coley & Procter, 1989). A complication of this form of nutritional intake is yeast and bacterial infection; this can result in death. Although long-term use of hyperalimentation is possible, generally children who cannot make the transition to another form of nutritional intake do not survive beyond infancy.

Use of nonoral feeding should not end the child's oral experiences and the enjoyment of interaction during feeding. When bolus feedings are given, the child can be given oral stimulation. Small amounts of food can be given before the nonoral feeding or during the feeding. Simple tastes and sucking experiences can be implemented during gastrostomy feeding if the child has routine aspiration. The goal is to link a pleasurable oral experience with the satiation of hunger. This type of oral stimulation during nonoral feeding is particularly critical for the child who is expected to return to oral feeding.

## Transition from Nonoral to Oral Feeding

The transition from nonoral to oral feeding is initiated with a physician's recommendation, based on the child's medical status and an evaluation of the child's oral motor skills by an occupational or speech therapist. After considering the health care team's recommendations, the family decides whether a transition to oral feeding is desirable and, if so, when and how they would like to approach this process. Occupational therapists often are instrumental in each phase of the transition.

A program to transition a young child from nonoral feeding typically includes four components (Blackman & Nelson, 1987; Case-Smith, 1993). The first is *oral motor intervention*. The child must demonstrate that he or she is capable of oral feeding. The therapist works with the child to desensitize the areas around the mouth and the structures within the mouth. Specific oral motor skills are facilitated during sensory play (Morris & Klein, 1987). Activities to desensitize include chewing and sucking of rubber toys and textured cloth, described in the section on sensory defensiveness. Small amounts of food textures are gradually offered to the child, usually while he or she is fed through the gastrostomy tube. Other activities that encourage oral motor skill development are making sounds, blowing bubbles, and giving kisses. Toothbrushing and oral play with toys are emphasized. The occupational therapist can point out the small successes that the child makes and can help the parent and child maintain an appropriate perspective on the goals (e.g., enjoyment of oral-sensory experiences). Usually the first food experiences are introduced as play, and whatever the child chooses to do with the food is praised or encouraged.

Often the child vies for control of the oral sensory experiences, perhaps because of the discomfort involved and the association with lack of control of his or her own hunger and satiation because feeding is nonvoluntary. The child's manipulative behaviors during feeding are often rewarded by increased attention from the parent, who has anxiety about the child's achieving oral feeding and successfully making the transition without weight loss or health problems. Approaches to behavior issues are described in later sections of this chapter.

Another component of the transition from nonoral to oral feeding is *manipulation of the gastrostomy feeding* so that bolus feedings are given rather than continuous feeding (e.g., feeding overnight). Bolus feedings are given four to five times per day to emulate a meal schedule. Once the child's digestive tract adjusts to the bolus feedings, health and weight are evaluated to determine if feedings can be reduced. If the child is expected to accept food by mouth, he or she needs to experience hunger; therefore the amount of food given must be reduced. Often children who require gastrostomy feedings are not medically and nutritionally stable enough to reduce their caloric intake; therefore the transition to oral feeding requires a lengthy time. Some weight loss almost always results from this process; therefore children who cannot tolerate any weight loss are not candidates for making the transition.

The therapist's support and encouragement are important to the child's and the parents' success in this process. The longer the child has been on nonoral feeding, the more difficult the transition. *Continual support* to the family is needed, and regular communication with the family is critical. The parents need encouragement for the small increments of progress and the loss of progress that occurs at times. The therapist's encouragement helps the parents maintain the energy and positive attitude needed to successfully reach the goal of oral feeding. Parent who experience feeding problems with their child can provide mutual support and assist each other in problem solving. Parent-to-parent support can strengthen their abilities to cope with stressful problems on a day-to-day basis (Chamberlin, Henry, Roberts, Sapsford, & Courtney, 1991). Parent groups are particularly appropriate when children have difficult feeding problems that include behavioral issues that need to be managed over lengthy periods.

## INTERVENTION FOR ORAL STRUCTURAL PROBLEMS

Children with oral structural problems at birth may have feeding problems that directly relate to the structural deficits. Two structural problems that occur frequently are *cleft lip and palate* and *micrognathia*. These problems often create feeding difficulties, particularly in the perinatal period. The role of the occupational therapist is typically to make recommendations for feeding equipment, adapted methods, and positions to be used until the child undergoes plastic surgery or outgrows the structural problem. Because oral structural problems rarely occur with neurologic impairment, this child typically demonstrates intact oral movement and effective suck-swallow coordination once the structural problems are resolved.

### Cleft Lip and Palate

A cleft is a separation of parts of the mouth usually joined together during the early weeks of fetal development (Morris & Klein, 1987). A cleft lip is separation of the upper lip and often the upper dental ridge. A cleft palate is a separation of the hard or soft palate and occurs with or without a cleft lip. Cleft lips and palates are closed through surgery. Cleft lips can be repaired in the first few months of life; repair of a cleft palate is more extensive, and the surgeon generally waits until the infant reaches a certain weight, usually by 12 or 18 months (Shah & Wong, 1980).

### Micrognathia

Micrognathia refers to a small, receded lower jaw. The mouth and tongue may be of normal size but are posteriorly positioned in relation to the upper jaw and the airway. Children with Pierre Robin syndrome have both micrognathia and cleft palate.

## Evaluation

Evaluation involves inspection of the oral structures and assessment of how the defects limit the feeding process. Evaluation should include observation of feeding to assess how the food travels through the mouth and how well the infant can express liquids from the nipple.

During the evaluation process a number of different feeding devices, methods, and positions should be tried to identify methods that effectively overcome the structural defects and allow safe oral intake. A VFSS may be needed to identify if aspiration occurs or if liquids move into the nasal passageway.

## Intervention

A variety of nipples have been designed to be used with children who have structural problems. These nipples are designed to compensate for lack of negative pressure and for limitations in tongue position and movement.

Squeeze bottles can be used to express liquids into the infant's mouth when suction is limited. Some nipples adjust the flow of the liquid during feeding by turning the nipple's rim. Long thin nipples can be used to carry the liquid to the back of the mouth past the cleft palate to avoid liquid flow into the nasal passageway. Wolf and Glass (1992) suggested that cross-cut nipples be avoided because they create an uneven flow that is more difficult for the infant to control. The therapist must work carefully with the parent so that the liquid flows easily from the bottle but is not excessive, resulting in a flow that the child cannot control. The nipple characteristics in Table 16-3 should be considered when making recommendations to parents or nurses.

The infant with cleft lip and palate or micrognathia benefits from upright positioning. By holding the young infant in a vertical position, the risk of aspiration is reduced. Upright positioning can promote forward movement of a recessed jaw and can prevent nasal and pharyngeal aspiration in the infant with cleft palate.

### Medical Intervention

When the micrognathia is severe, the tongue may actually occlude the airway. When the condition compromises respiration, placement of a tracheostomy and gastrostomy may be indicated. These procedures provide temporary support of respiration and nutrition until the structural problems can be surgically repaired.

The following case example illustrates the role of the occupational therapist with the infant with Pierre Robin syndrome.

Sarah was born with Pierre Robin syndrome and presented with a recessed, small chin and retracted tongue. She also had a deep

▲ Table 16-3   Nipple Characteristics Related to Use with Children Who Have Oral Structural Defects

| Nipple Type | Characteristics |
|---|---|
| Long, thin nipples | Work well when the tongue is recessed, can bring the tongue forward |
| Single nipple hole | Results in a steady liquid stream, which can be easier to handle than bursts of liquid |
| Wide nipple | Can be compressed for liquid expression for the child with a cleft palate |
| Broad-based nipple | Can help the infant with a cleft lip gain suction |
| Nipple with cross-cut hole | Can create an uneven liquid flow or a burst of fluid that is difficult for the infant to control |
| Nipple with enlarged hole | Should be used with great care; when the caregiver enlarges the hole, it is difficult to predict what type of liquid flow will result |
| Soft, pliable nipple | Appropriate for young infants with cleft palates who are unable to achieve suction |
| NUK nipple | Has the hole on top of the nipple and should not be used with children with cleft palates; this nipple may be functional if its position on the tongue is reversed |

cleft in her hard and soft palate. She struggled with her first feedings. On the third day of life, her retracted tongue fell into her airway, completely occluding it. Because Sarah was on a monitor, the medical team immediately intubated her. She then received a tracheostomy and gastrostomy to avoid further complications caused by the position of her tongue.

She was discharged home on continuous feedings and moist air to her tracheostomy. She required respiratory treatment and frequent suctioning to keep her lungs clear.

In the first few months she had frequent pneumonia but became healthy by 3 months. Her growth was adequate although she remained in the fifth percentile of weight for height.

Occupational therapy was ordered to develop an oral motor program to promote development of her oral motor skills while she received gastrostomy feedings and awaited surgery, which was anticipated to occur at 18 months. The occupational therapist provided a program of graded oral input. Initial stimulation included introduction of her hand to her mouth and gum rubbing with the pacifier. The pacifier was used for brief periods, but she was unable to maintain suction on it to independently hold it in her mouth. Her preferred oral stimulus was her mother's finger.

Rhythmic, slow stroking was applied to her tongue to bring her tongue forward. By 5 months she was able to hold the pacifier in her mouth. At this time juice was introduced on the pacifier to introduce tastes. She was mouthing her finger frequently. Sarah's mother began using the NUK toothbrush for additional stimulation. She enjoyed chewing on it. Tolerance of a warm washcloth on her face had increased.

By 7 months of age she had learned to sit upright when supported at the pelvis and to sit at midline in an infant seat. Her increased stability of neck and trunk allowed for more oral motor experiences. Pureed foods were introduced, first on the nipple and NUK toothbrush. Desensitization using stroking with the washcloth was applied first to increase her sensory tolerance. She then began to take two to five spoonfuls of pureed fruits. Downward and forward pressure was applied with the bowl of the spoon. She tolerated this procedure and actually seemed to enjoy it after several weeks. She seemed to develop good suction on the pacifier. At the time, the physician recommended that feedings be given in boluses to emulate oral feedings. When bolus feedings began, oral stimulation was performed immediately before the gastrostomy feeding with the hope that she would be hungry and more receptive to oral stimulation. She was receptive but would not consume more than five spoonfuls. (Because she received total nutrition through the gastrostomy, she was not very hungry.) At this time her suck-swallow sequence was well coordinated, and her tongue was in a forward position.

At 9 months of age Sarah tolerated a wide variety of food textures in her mouth. Oral motor skills had rapidly progressed and were only slightly behind those of her typically developing peers. Her tongue and mandible had moved into a forward position, and the physician recommended that she transition to oral feedings without waiting for repair of the cleft palate, which was 9 months in the future. The occupational therapist and nutritionist met with Sarah's mother to design a diet that would increase oral intake and simultaneously reduce gastrostomy feedings. Because oral sensory issues had been addressed in the occupational therapy program and because her oral motor skills were almost age appropriate, the team thought that the transition would proceed quickly. As the gastrostomy feedings were reduced, her weight was carefully monitored to ensure that her oral intake maintained the nutritional intake required for growth. Although children almost always lose weight in the transition from nonoral to oral feedings, Sarah did not. She and her mother were ready for oral feedings to begin, and Sarah successfully made the transition in 2 weeks.

## NUTRITION

Adequate nutrition is necessary for life. It is critical for growth and development and is of particular concern for children with development disabilities who demonstrate the feeding problems described in this chapter. When the amount or type of food intake is limited, the child is at risk for malnutrition or a failure-to-thrive condition that can actually exacerbate or worsen the developmental condition (Brizee, Sophos, & McLaughlin, 1990). When a child with development disabilities demonstrates feeding difficulties and appears to have limited intake, it is important that his or her nutritional status be evaluated and that the resulting recommendations become integral to the child's daily feeding and occupational therapy program. Nutritional screening can be done by the occupational therapist with guidance by the nutritionist. Problems in the child's nutritional status should be referred to the nutritionist for advice and recommendations regarding dietary changes.

A nutritional screening consists of (1) interviewing the caregivers regarding amounts and types of foods consumed daily; (2) collecting data on height, weight, and weight for height; (3) observing general appearance of skin, hair, and gums; and (4) reviewing medical records. Problems identified in the screening that indicate the need for a more in-depth nutritional assessment and services are as follows (Brizee et al., 1990):

1. Weight for height below the 10th percentile
2. Weight for height above the 90th percentile
3. Height and weight below the 5th percentile
4. Parent's concern about nutrition
5. Behavioral or oral motor problems that result in severe limitations in the types or amounts of food ingested

The following principles apply to the occupational therapist's intervention and its potential affect on the child's nutritional status.

When oral motor intervention is somewhat stressful for the child, for example, trying new textures, the intervention activities should occur at times other than mealtime. Mealtime should be maintained as the time for the child to receive an optimal amount of nutrition and to have the satisfaction of satiation. Challenging oral motor interventions, particularly those that strongly influence the sensory system, may upset or frustrate the child and result in food refusal. Mealtime can then evolve into a battle of the child who exerts control of a situation that creates discomfort or stress and a parent concerned about the amount of foot intake. When oral desensitization and new oral motor skills are addressed at times other than mealtime, the child and the parent or therapist can approach these activities in a more relaxed, playful manner.

Therapeutic strategies to improve oral motor skills should always consider the consequences of food intake and nutrition. When therapists recommend that the parent place less food on the spoon or wait for the child to indicate readiness for the next bite, the impact of those recommendations on the total amount of nutritional intake must be assessed. When therapeutic techniques that promote oral motor skill result in a mealtime that is two times longer, the benefit of those techniques needs to be weighed against the child's endurance and the parent's time. Techniques that extensively lengthen feeding time should be implemented only once a day or only in the beginning of the meal. Techniques to improve oral motor skills should always consider their efficiency in light of whole meal consumption. Perhaps difficult-to-chew food should be given in the middle of the meal after the child's initial hunger is satiated and before fatigue.

Often therapists make recommendations for changes in food texture. When new textures are attempted, the nutrient value should be considered. Use of cookies, candies, puddings, and ice cream can be motivating for the child; however, acceptance of these foods does not translate into a nutritional diet from the child. When attempting new textures of food, the therapist should reinforce the importance of nutrition by selecting foods with high nutritional value. Cheese and fruits should be used to work on chewing rather than cookies.

When the child makes a transition to new textures, either because oral motor skills have improved or because hypersensitivity has been decreased, the types of food ingested should be evaluated for nutritional intake. All major changes in the child's diet should be assessed by a nutritionist. For example, blanket recommendations to use high-caloric foods can be inappropriate, even when the goal for the child is weight gain. Sometimes high-caloric food supplements actually decrease the child's overall appetite and food intake. Increases in the caloric density of foods need to be balanced with increases in fluid intake. The long-term effect of artificially increasing caloric density should be considered.

Collaboration with the nutritionist is essential for children who are underweight, and frequent consultation with the nutritionist is critical to avoiding malnutrition and to improving the child's overall health and development. Often the occupational therapist interacts with the failure-to-thrive child and his or her family more frequently than the nutritionist and is privy to information regarding the child's eating. Food refusal and loss of appetite can be particularly detrimental to these children. The occupational therapists can share insight into the interactional components of the problem. Issues other than failure to thrive warrant referral to the nutritionist. The occupational therapist might recom-

mend that the family consult with a nutritionist in the following instances:

1. When certain medications have been used for long periods
2. When changes in the child's health suggest concern for drug and nutrient interaction
3. When the child gains or loses weight suddenly
4. When major changes in diet occur
5. When conditions such as constipation are long-standing problems

Although these problems do not always require direct intervention and changes in diet, it is important that they are monitored by the nutritionist and that recommendations for management of these situations are followed.

## INTERACTIONAL ASPECTS OF FEEDING

As stated in the beginning of this chapter, eating problems affect many aspects of the child's life. Intervention is guided by knowledge about typical development and feeding problems, assumptions about the nature of a problem (theory), and the information collected about a specific child's problem (evaluation strategies). This section further organizes how the clinician approaches the information collection about and intervention with feeding problems in children by emphasizing an interactional or systems approach. In addition to addressing the child and parent, the effect of cultural, physical, and social environment on feeding is explained.

Figure 16-6 suggests a multisystems approach to the issue of feeding (Humphry, 1995). The figure illustrates three levels of systems the clinician must understand for effective intervention. The child and his or her abilities to eat represent the central issue. Working at this level the occupational therapist examines the oral motor issues discussed in this chapter. The therapist can also identify important developmental experiences that may be changed if there are feeding problems. Successfully feeding an infant or child is a two-person, interactive process, so the feeding dyad is the second level of the model. The child in the partnership must participate by cuing the adult regarding his or her needs and must take in and swallow the food. The parent, caregiver, or teacher in the feeding dyad must prepare and present food in a manner consistent with the child's developmental abilities. The adult must read the child's cues regarding speed, taste preferences, and comfort and adjust the feeding process accordingly. How well the adult participates in the feeding interactions depends on present abilities and how the caregiver feels about past successes or failures in feeding. The feeding dyad is influenced by the cultural, physical, and social context—the third level. To be successful in feeding interventions, the therapists needs to consider the interactive effect of the family system (see Chapter 5).

Using a systems model, such as that suggested here, enables the occupational therapist to address the complex is-

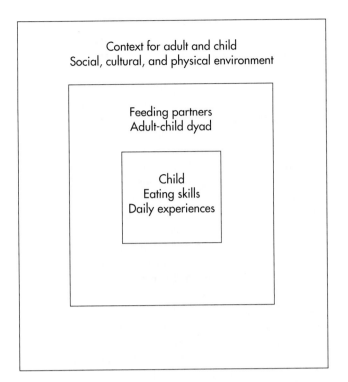

**Figure 16-6**   Ecologic view of feeding problems.

sue of feeding and to focus on more than one aspect of the problem at a time. Using this model helps the therapist understand how a busy, overstimulating environment and a mother pressed for time may negatively influence the child's ability to eat. Conversely, a child who has difficulty feeding and requires continual caregiver assistance may be disruptive to the family's mealtime.

The fact that a single focus is not effective can be seen in work with children who are diagnosed as failing to thrive. In the past when children did not gain weight, the problem was categorized as either organic (a medical problem that led to poor nutrition) or nonorganic (a problem related to factors in the environment). The interactive systems model offers a more complete picture of feeding for understanding problems such as failure to thrive. Children who are diagnosed with nonorganic failure to thrive, where parental neglect and inappropriate feeding practices were identified problems, may also show oral motor delays that affect their amount of nutritional intake and compound the other issues. Regardless of the source of feeding problems, the multilevel systems model leads to considering the quality of the fit between parent and child by enhancing appropriate feeding skill acquisition in the child, parenting practices, and enhancing interaction between the dyad.

## CHILD'S DEVELOPMENT

Because children eat several times a day, meals represent frequent learning opportunities that can influence cognitive and psychologic components of function. The perception of hunger and signaling and receiving adult response are the first contigency-response experiences of many infants. Children, especially babies, create opportunities to interact with the adults in their lives. Once the immediate feelings of hunger are satiated, infants are predisposed to use feeding time to trigger interactions with their parents (Brazelton, 1993). The reciprocity developed during feeding experiences may be a foundation for subsequent communication. The close physical contact during breast-feeding or bottle-feeding also provides a variety of sensorimotor experiences. As the infant gets older, self-feeding is one of the first experiences to negotiate the issue of autonomy between child and parent. For preschool- and school-aged children, verbal interactions of families during meals provide learning experiences that promote language and concepts about the world (Beals, 1993).

When a young child has feeding problems, the occupational therapist and other team members need to consider how to help the family learn to compensate for the secondary effects on parent-child interaction and play. Collaboration with nurses and speech language pathologists who are also interested in parent-child interaction helps the occupational therapist consider how the feeding program assists or at least does not diminish opportunities for psychosocial development. The clinicians, teachers, and parents also can work together to understand the child's typical communicative acts. If the child signals preferences by making faces or looking toward a desired drink, these communications should be recognized and honored, when possible.

One example is an interaction between a teacher and Megan, a 3-year-old girl with spastic cerebral palsy. When the teacher feeds Megan, she implements the occupational therapist's suggestions to promote jaw stabilization by placing her fingers under Megan's jaw as she offers a bite of ground food. The teacher notes that Megan looks at the chocolate pudding on the side of the tray. The teacher can acknowledge Megan's interest in the pudding by naming it and talking about how she will have the pudding after her meal. If Megan's feeders were only concentrating on head position and jaw stability, Megan would learn that her efforts at making her needs known were not worth the effort.

## IMPLICATIONS FOR THE PARENT

For the primary caregiver, feeding an infant can be a warm, positive experience that enhances the bond between adult and child. Many adults think that to nourish the child is one way to nurture. Watching a baby gain weight is visible evidence of success in the caregiver role. When feeding is not pleasurable and becomes a job, significant negative consequences result (Brazelton, 1993). The parent or teacher who approaches interactions with a sense of duty decreases the effectiveness of their efforts and teaches the child that eating is work rather than pleasure.

Parents of children with feeding problems frequently report their difficulties begin at 6 months of age (Ramsay, Gisel, & Boutry, 1993). These early experiences can have a negative effect on parents and caregiving behaviors. Mothers of infants with eating problems feed their babies more frequently, feed them for longer periods, worry more about the baby's health, and experience more isolation from social support systems than mothers of infants with no feeding problems (Hagekull & Dahl, 1987). Among toddlers and preschool-aged children with a history of mealtime problems, the parent is more likely to be coercive and have behaviors that can contribute to or sustain feeding problems in the child (Sanders, Patel, LeGrice, & Shepherd, 1993).

Occupational therapy intervention for feeding problems facilitates behavior change in both the child and the parent. The occupational therapist first considers how to establish a working relationship with the parent and communicate intervention strategies in a way that supports the parent. The therapist recognizes that the parent may feel as if he or she has failed at a primary role in caregiving. Acknowledgment of the legitimate basis for the parent's stress is a first step in the parent being able to articulate his or her needs. Once the therapist and parent establish a collaborative relationship, the therapist can suggest alternative strategies to achieve a feeding goal and ask the parent to select those that he or she feels comfortable implementing. Two important strategies to promote success are to recommend ways that feeding techniques can be incorporated into daily routines and to allow the parent to decide when and how frequently the techniques will be implemented. A parent may determine that working on drinking from a cup is only realistic at night, just before the child's clothes will be changed for bed. Another parent may decide that giving the child time to practice self-feeding may only be possible on weekends.

## CONTEXTS OF FEEDING

All aspects of the environment—cultural, physical, and social—have an impact on feeding. Meals also have a temporal context and must occur within the demands of time for other family or classroom activities. Direct observation is an ideal strategy to understand contextual factors in feeding. When this is not unrealistic, the therapist should ask the parent to describe a typical meal, requesting specific details of the child's behaviors and the environment.

As discussed at the beginning of the chapter, selection and preparation of food and the interactive rituals during mealtimes can be determined by the family's cultural background. The therapist must learn about food-related traditions of families with different ethnic backgrounds. Asking parents about the different foods in their culture helps to build rapport because it shows the therapist's interest in the family's traditions.

Parenting values and family roles also relate to cultural background. Different cultures ascribe different family values to the act of feeding and nurturing the child. For example, in some cultures, affection is expressed by performing daily care activities for a young child. If a grandmother's primary responsibility is to nurture the youngest children in the family, she may want to continue feeding her grandchild past the time when the therapist thinks the child is ready to finger feed. An alternative parenting value may be to promote independence and self-sufficiency. Young infants may be encouraged to hold their own bottle as soon as possible among these families and are described as "lazy" if they do not acquire this skill by 6 months. Another example of how cultural differences can impact on feeding is how much the parent can tolerate a child making a mess during meals. Among some Cuban families adults believe that a clean child reflects good parenting practices. The occupational therapist who tries to implement a self-feeding program that leads to messy attempts to use a spoon meets with resistance because the therapist does not recognize the importance of this cultural value.

Economic resources of the family can have a significant impact on the physical context of feeding. Some families simply put food in the tray of a walker for self-feeding rather than buy a high chair simply because they cannot afford both. Low-income housing and overcrowded conditions may not provide a positive environment that is conducive to special feeding programs. Young children with feeding problems are less likely to be fed in a specific location and are more likely to be fed in noisy surroundings (Heptinstall et al., 1987). Adapting interventions to the socioeconomic backgrounds of families may be more difficult than adjusting to ethnic differences because parents may be reluctant or embarrassed to admit they do not have common furniture such as a kitchen table.

The social context of the family, such as siblings, extended family, and friends, also affects feeding. The nature of social interaction can have both positive and negative consequences for feeding. A child who is easily distracted by interaction with others may eat less food during a meal. At the same time, social context can be a therapeutic tool. The presence of a peer model is sometimes a successful way to address swallowing and food acceptance in young children.

Another component of the social context of feeding is the generally shared assumptions about good parenting and feeding. Even among parents of typically developing children there is confusion about the amount children typically eat at different ages. Occupational therapists are just one of many sources of information on feeding. Information about how and what to feed a baby is acquired from family members, neighbors, texts on child development, and other health professionals. The occupational therapist who asks about what feeding techniques the parent has tried should specifically explore suggestions that have come from relatives and neighbors (see box on p. 435). If the family structure is hierarchic, the therapist may need to discuss feeding alternatives with the family member who has the authority to make decisions, rather than the primary caregiver who is feeding the child. Often meeting with several family members is required to come to a consensus.

The occupational therapist may see the child in a clinic or special part of the classroom where the social and physical context of feeding cannot be directly observed. Questions about meals, listed in the box on p. 435, are important to making effective suggestions. For example, techniques with a lot of tactile input, such as jaw stabilization, that are successful when auditory and visual stimuli are low may be too intrusive for the child when the same technique is tried in a natural meal setting.

## SELF-FEEDING
### Typical Development

Children are often eager to feed themselves. The infant may first initiate self-feeding at 6 months when he or she first holds the bottle. Typically, finger feeding develops quickly and naturally as an extension of the hand-to-mouth behaviors that the child has practiced during the first months. Introduction of finger foods to the infant can be influenced by parental attitudes and cultural practices. In most families the infant accomplishes self-feeding of a cracker or soft cookie by 8 months. By this time the child can sit independently and therefore has the freedom to use his or her arms and hands for reaching, food play, and hand-to-mouth activity. The development of a more refined, precise grasp and release pattern also contributes to the 8-month-old infant's success in finger-feeding. He or she typically exhibits a radial digital grasp, which positions the cookie well for entry into the mouth. From 8 to 12 months of age the infant develops a number of skills that contribute to his or her ability to self-feed. Control of sitting posture and improved sitting balance, development of refined pincer grasp with controlled release, and refinement of isolated forearm and wrist movements result in efficient finger-feeding. The 12-month-old child prehends small pieces of food such as dry cereal, peas, macaroni, and pasta and places them accurately in his or her mouth. At 12 months finger-feeding is generally a preferred and enjoyed activity. The selection of finger foods should match the child's oral motor skills. Nuts, hard candy, popcorn, and grapes are contraindicated because these can occlude the airway if they are aspirated. Soft foods that dissolve in the mouth and require minimal chewing are appropriate for first finger-feeding.

At 12 months the infant may play with a spoon, banging it on the high chair tray, but is not yet able to handle spoon-feeding. The infant plays with the spoon for several months before becoming efficient in feeding with the spoon. The infant practices bringing the spoon to the mouth but does not have adequate control of the wrist and forearm to bring it into the mouth. Independent spoon feeding develops between 15 and 18 months. At this time, adequate shoulder and wrist stability enable the toddler to bring the spoon into his or her mouth with minimal spillage. The child holds the spoon in a pronated gross grasp and brings the spoon to the mouth using exaggerated shoulder abduction. By 24 months the child spoon-feeds without spillage (with more solid foods). He or she holds the spoon in his radial fingers, with the forearm supinated, and is able to obtain the food and efficiently place the spoon into his or her mouth. Between 30 and 36 months the child may begin to prefer a fork for "stabbing" foods and may learn to eat foods that are more difficult to maintain on a spoon (e.g., cold cereal and rice).

### Drinking

The infant may demonstrate interest in the cup as early as 6 months. However, skills in drinking from a cup do not emerge until about 12 months. At that time the infant is better able to correctly orient the cup to the mouth and to tip it to a degree that spillage is not inevitable. A number of cups are available that make learning to drink from a cup an easy transition for the child. The first cup that the infant uses has a lid and a spout. It may have handles or may be a small cup that the infant can hold in one hand. Initially the parent places only a small amount in the cup to decrease spillage and promote the child's success in directing the flow of liquid. The child may begin to use a small (4- to 6-ounce) cup without a lid at 24 months of age; however, spillage is inevitable at that time. The child continues to use a small cup. Straw drinking appears to emerge at about 2 years. It may become a skill before the second birthday if the child is exposed to straw drinking. Use of a straw requires good lip seal and strong suction to bring the liquid into the mouth. It is advantageous in that the child can drink through a straw without handling the cup. In addition to the oral motor skills required to draw the liquid into the mouth, cognitive skills are needed to problem solve how to use the straw. The young infant often bites or blows on the straw before learning how to suck through it.

### Self-Feeding Problems

Delays in self-feeding skills may result when the child has cognitive, behavioral, or motor problems or delays. Occupational therapists most often provide services to children whose self-feeding delay is secondary to motor impairments. Self-feeding involves moving the hand through space toward a target that the child cannot visualize (the mouth). Therefore graded arm control and accurate proprioceptive perception are prerequisites to control the spoon in self-feeding. Children who have poor control of free movement in space (e.g., children with athetosis) and children who overly rely on vision to guide movement have particular difficulty in self-feeding. Children with ataxic cerebral palsy who exhibit tremor in the upper extremity during purposeful fine motor tasks often have great difficulty learning to self-feed. They struggle when attempting to eat spillable foods on a spoon. Stabbing food with a blunt-ended fork may be a more effective self-feeding method.

Children with orthopedic impairments that limit upper extremity range of motion may benefit from using adapted equipment (e.g., bent utensils or long-handled utensils). Children with neuromuscular impairment or disorders who have decreased upper extremity strength may require adaptive equipment (e.g., lightweight utensils, a scoop dish with suction cups, or mobile arm supports). Children with upper extremity weakness of instability may benefit from eating on a raised tray that they can use as a surface for resting their elbows while bringing the hand to the mouth. Behavior issues in self-feeding require a comprehensive team approach. These issues are discussed in Chapter 15.

## Intervention

Occupational therapists implement intervention strategies to improve self-feeding during mealtime and in activities to improve arm strength and control. Mealtime strategies include position of the child, handling techniques, and use of adapted equipment. This section describes mealtime strategies. Other intervention activities to improve arm and hand strength and control are described in Chapter 12.

### Positioning

Correct postural alignment and postural stability are critical to the child's success in self-feeding. Control of the arm in space in bringing the spoon to the mouth requires a stable postural base as a prerequisite. Children with cerebral palsy often lack adequate postural stability as a base of control for smooth, active movement in the arm toward midline. The child must feel secure and relaxed during self-feeding so that his or her endurance is adequate to feed the entire meal. The child's wheelchair may offer ideal positioning and comfort for feeding; it often has a tray to support the plate and cup. Positioning with the head, neck, and trunk in upright alignment is similar to the positioning previously described for feeding the child. Correct posture for self-feeding includes a tucked chin, depressed shoulders, and neutral pelvis. An upright position for feeding can be maintained when the wheelchair has a firm seat and is an appropriate size. Pelvic and hip abductor straps and lateral trunk support help support the position of a neutral pelvis and a symmetric, upright trunk. When the child tends to retract his or her shoulders, padded humeral "wings" on the back of the chair or on the wheelchair tray can maintain the arms in a forward protracted position. These "wings"

help increase arm stability and maintain the child's hands at midline for self-feeding (Bergen & Colangelo, 1985).

A wheelchair tray adaptation that helps increase arm stability and improve the arm's position for feeding is a small (short) bolster that can be placed under the arm. By separating the elbow from the trunk, the shoulder is abducted and the elbow is stabilized at a height that enables the child to scoop food onto the spoon and reach the mouth using a pattern of elbow flexion. The bolster serves as a lever from which the child can efficiently reach both the tray (and food) and his or her mouth.

Another effective intervention strategy to improve control of the hand-to-mouth pattern is to raise the tray or feeding surface. Raising the tray brings it higher on the child's trunk, thereby assisting with trunk stability. A higher tray also holds the arms in greater humeral abduction, which decreases the distance the hand must travel to reach the mouth and can improve control of the hand-to-mouth movement. By stabilizing the elbow on the tray, the child can move in a simple pattern of elbow flexion and extension to self-feed.

## Handling Strategies During Self-Feeding

Self-feeding is a particular challenge for children with poor arm and hand control, such as those with athetoid cerebral palsy. These individuals may benefit by handling during feeding to improve control and to enhance the movement patterns used during feeding. The techniques used often involve facilitation of shoulder depression and protraction and scapular stability to increase the child's control of distal arm movement. The therapist may place his or her hand on top of the child's shoulders or scapula. Support or guidance of the humerus may be needed to establish a smooth hand-to-mouth pattern. The therapist helps stabilize and support the arm as it moves through space rather than forcefully move it through the range. Arm support should be intermittent and as needed based on the responses of the child.

In one recommended technique the occupational therapist holds the spoon handle between the extended index and third fingers. The therapist slips these fingers into the child's palm with a thumb on the dorsum of the child's hand. The child holds onto the fingers and spoon using a palmer grasp, and the therapist facilitates a self-feeding pattern using subtle and natural facilitation from within the child's hand. Morris and Klein (1987) recommended that the therapist hold the spoon in the child's palm by placing one finger in the palm and the thumb on the back of the wrist. Using this handling technique, the therapist can facilitate wrist extension and apply pressure in the palm to encourage sustained grasp. These techniques are particularly successful with a child who has developed a basic hand-to-mouth pattern but has difficulty placing the spoon into his or her mouth (Case-Smith, 1993).

One disadvantage of these handling techniques is that they require the therapist, teacher, or parent to be seated

Jonathan was diagnosed with spastic quadriparesis when he was 6 months old. His lower extremities exhibited high muscle tone, particularly in hip adductors and hamstrings. As a result he demonstrated a scissoring pattern when standing or when held in his mother's arms. At 2½ years old he had many assets; a ready smile, good social skills and responsivity to social interaction, beginning language (about 20 words), and a pleasant affect. He sat with minimal assistance, had begun to crawl on his belly, and rolled segmentally about the room. He required external postural support to play with toys; however, once he had postural stability, he brought his hands to midline, grasped using a radial palmar grasp, released toys in a container, transferred objects, and had begun to fit an object into a precise space. Although eye-hand coordination was emerging, he continued to have difficulty with integrating visual skills with arm and hand movements.

Jonathan ate soft foods and had begun to try some harder foods such as pretzels, ham, and apples. He took the food from the cup or spoon using active lip movements. Lip closure while chewing was fair, but not perfect, as he continued to have some food loss. He used both a munching pattern and some rotary chewing. He reverted to a vertical up and down munching pattern with more difficult foods (e.g., those that are hard or tough). He used a sucking pattern on pureed foods and a diagonal-rotary pattern with soft foods. Jonathon demonstrated a variety of patterns of tongue movement, including tip elevation, lateralization, and beginning rolling. Jaw control was emerging; he exhibited a sustained bite pattern and jaw stabilization had increased on the cup rim. He continued to bite on the cup during drinking. The occupational therapist and Jonathan's parent had implemented a program to continually upgrade the texture of his foods, and he had made continual progress in feeding skills. Drinking thin liquids remained difficult, and his mother managed drinking by providing some manual head and jaw support and by thickening his liquids to a nectar quality. Jonathan handled liquids better when using a straw and when taking small sips of liquid at a time. As his appetite increased and he continued to demonstrate improvements in oral skills, he had shown increasing interest in self-feeding. He began to finger feed bites of sandwiches, crackers, cheese, and strips of ham or chicken.

Jonathan's mother had given him a spoon on several occasions; his first attempts at self-feeding resulted in much more food going on his face and clothes than in his mouth. His mother had tried self-feeding in his high chair using an adult spoon and a bowl of yogurt. Despite his lack of success, Jonathan seemed eager to try to use the spoon and often grabbed it from his mouth during feeding. The occupational therapist evaluated his feeding to help this mother develop a system for self-feeding that would be more efficient and began to address self-feeding as a goal in the intervention program.

**Evaluation**

In the high chair, Jonathan was without foot support and had minimal trunk support. He frequently fell to one side. The self-feeding movements were evaluated; he successfully scooped the yogurt, then fully abducted his shoulder and flexed his elbow to bring the spoon to his mouth. Although this motion brought the food to his mouth, Jonathan was unable to turn the spoon for entry into his mouth. His efforts to get the food resulted in spillage. Although he failed to get food into his mouth, he remained highly motivated and seemed to enjoy the activity.

**Intervention**

The occupational therapist and Jonathan's mother developed a plan to increase Jonathan's fine motor skills for self-feeding and to adapt the feeding position and equipment so that he was more successful. Activities to enhance self-feeding with the spoon included games that required forearm supination with objects held in a radial digital grasp. Examples included placing pegs vertically into a pegboard, placing peg people into a school bus or airplane, and using a toy accordion with vertically oriented handles. These activities were performed with Jonathan in the Rifton chair or corner chair with tray, where he was well supported and posturally stable with feet flat.

The position for self-feeding was adjusted and simple equipment recommended. Instead of feeding in the high chair, the occupational therapist suggested that he sit in the Rifton chair for self-feeding. He was stable in the Rifton chair, which had lateral supports, foot supports, and a tray that was positioned close to his body at a height that enabled solid weight-bearing on elbows. As previously mentioned, he demonstrated his best hand and arm control in this chair (Figure 16-7). A scoop dish was used with suction cups on the bottom. This bowl allowed him to obtain food without holding the bowl with his other hand. A small child's adapted spoon was used. The spoon selected was short, had a bent angle at the bowl, had a flat, small bowl, and a thick handle. The spoon could be easily handled with a radial palmer grasp and could be entered into his mouth without wrist rotation or radial deviation. Initially the therapist provided some support at his hand by entering her index finger into his hand and placing her thumb on the hand's dorsum as he grasped the spoon. The therapist's hand supported his arm and wrist movements, and she only exerted pressure when his arm movement appeared inadequate for entry into his mouth (Figure 16-8). This assistance was soon eliminated. Use of a small padded block under his elbow proved to be helpful as an extra source of stability; Jonathan maintained his elbow on the pad and used elbow flexion to bring food to his mouth.

The occupational therapist suggested that pudding be the first food used in feeding practice because of its cohesive, sticky texture. Yogurt and ice cream were soon added and quickly became Jonathan's favorite treats (Figure 16-9).

With this equipment and position, Jonathan regularly practiced self-feeding. The occupational therapist continued to address oral motor skill and fine motor skill development as important performance components that would contribute to his increasing ability to self-feed.

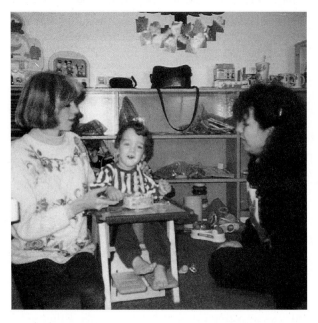

**Figure 16-7** Rifton chair provides a firm base of support to trunk and feet during self-feeding.

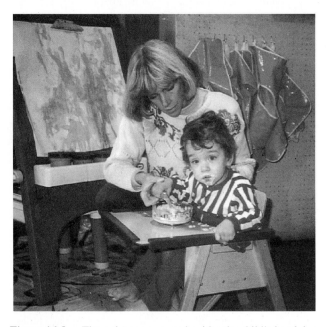

**Figure 16-8** Therapist supports and guides the child's hand during self-feeding using thumb on hand dorsum and finger in his palm.

behind or to the side of the child. This positioning limits eye-to-eye interaction with the child during feeding and can create a barrier to communication. This limitation is not as important in a group situation such as the family mealtime or the school's snack time. Practice of self-feeding using these techniques on an intermittent basis can improve the movement pattern when consistent feedback and reinforcement are provided to the child regarding his or her self-feeding efforts.

In applying these techniques, the goal of the therapist is to facilitate the child's success and to gradually decrease the amount of physical assistance and adaptive equipment required in self-feeding.

## Adaptive Equipment

A variety of adaptive equipment has been specifically designed to accommodate the needs of individuals who experience difficulty in self-feeding. Often the equipment provides simple, yet critical adaptations to the feeding experience that enable the child to be independent in self-feeding. Examples of adapted feeding equipment include adapted

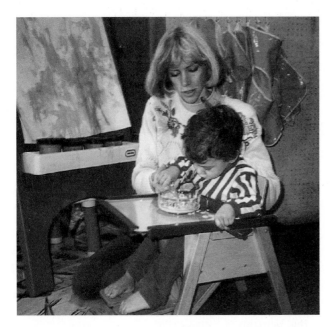

**Figure 16-9**   Foods that are successful when first attempting self-feeding are those that stick together, are easily scooped, hold to the spoon, and taste good!

utensils, plates, bowls, cups, and straws. The child may benefit from utensils with built-up handles that are easier to grasp or straps on the handle to secure it to the hand. Utensil handles that are longer or shorter than standard utensils or that are curved or bent are also available. To scoop food onto the spoon, the child may need a dish with a raised edge. These "scoop dishes" often have suction cups underneath to stabilize them on the tray or table. The high curved side of the dish makes scooping the food more successful when the child is unable to use an assisting hand to obtain the food. Cups with lids reduce spillage by controlling the flow of liquid into the mouth. Lids without spouts are recommended when the child exhibits suckling tongue movement. Straws can promote the child's ability to suck and can allow the child to drink without lifting the cup from the table surface. Straw drinking can also promote a chin tuck position as the child must move forward using active neck flexion to obtain the straw. More sophisticated adapted equipment, such as the electric feeder, may enable a child to self-feed without using the arms. Criteria for selecting adaptive equipment to improve the child's independence in self-feeding include durability, ease of cleaning and use, and developmental appropriateness (Coley & Procter, 1989).

## SUMMARY

Intervention to promote feeding and eating skills is an important role of the occupational therapist. Feeding behaviors are influenced by oral sensory and motor function, physiologic parameters, environmental issues, and the quality of interaction with caregivers. Although these aspects of

## STUDY QUESTIONS

1. You receive a referral for a 9-month-old infant who refuses all attempts to be fed pureed baby foods. She currently takes six bottles of formula per day. Your initial evaluation indicates that she has severe tactile defensiveness of the oral area. Describe the first three activities that your would implement in intervention. Identify two recommendations that you would give to her parents.

2. You are working with a 12-year-old child who has severe motor delays and difficulty feeding. He has fair head control and poor trunk control; he is not a candidate for self-feeding at this time. He demonstrates primitive oral movements; his jaw is unstable and moves in wide excursions, and his tongue moves in extension and retraction. He often loses food from his mouth and frequently chokes and coughs during feeding. Coughing is most frequent during drinking. Describe in detail how you would position him for feeding and what positioning devices you might use. What types of food and drink would you recommend?

3. You are the occupational therapist for a 6-year-old child with feeding difficulties. When you feed her at school, you suspect that she is aspirating some of her food and drink. List two ways that you would pursue investigating this possibility. What are two questions that you would ask her parents? What might you ask of the physician to further investigate the possibility of aspiration?

4. One of the children that you are working with on oral feeding is demonstrating a keen interest in feeding himself. He has poor control of his upper extremities. His shoulder stability is poor, and he exhibits only a gross grasp and involuntary release. He does not yet have the ability to maintain grasp of a utensil while guiding it to his mouth. What activities might you implement to improve his ability to self-feed? What would be the first foods and eating activities that would allow him to succeed in self-feeding?

5. When a child has significant oral motor problems, often drinking is a more difficult skill to achieve than eating solid foods. Given the importance of maintaining hydration, what are three recommendations that you would make for children whose oral motor skills suggest the possibility of aspiration when drinking liquids?

feeding were addressed separately in the chapter, they are interrelated, and feeding interventions involve a holistic approach where multiple aspects of the child's behaviors and the environment are considered. Because of the complexity and critical importance of feeding interaction and nutritional intake, a collaborative interdisciplinary approach is recommended, with the family's concerns and priorities central to the intervention plan. This chapter provides a foundation for occupational therapy practice to help children develop eating skills that allow for good nutritional intake and thus for growth and development. The occupational therapist emphasizes interventions that support positive interactions during the feeding and helps caregivers gain confidence, skill, and enjoyment in feeding their children.

## REFERENCES

Beals, D.E. (1993). Explanatory talk in low-income families' mealtime conversations. *Applied Psycholinguistics, 14,* 489-513.

Benson, J.E. & Lefton-Grief, M.A. (1994). Videofluoroscopy of swallowing in pediatric patients: a component of the total feeding evaluation. In D.N. Tuchman & R. Walter (Eds.). *Disorders of feeding and swallowing in infants and children* (pp. 187-200). San Diego: Singular Publishing Group.

Bergen, A. & Colangelo, C. (1985). *Positioning the client with central nervous system deficits.* Valhalla, NY: Valhalla Rehabilitation Publications.

Blackman, J.A. & Nelson, C.L.A. (1987). Rapid introduction or oral feeding to tube-fed patients. *Journal of Developmental and Behavioral Pediatrics, 8,* 63-66.

Brazelton, T.B. (1993). Why children and parents must play while they eat: an interview with T. Berry Brazelton. *Journal of the American Dietetic Association, 93,* 1485-1387.

Brizee, L.S., Sophos, C.M., & McLaughlin, J.F. (1990). Nutrition issues in developmental disabilities. *Infants and Young Children, 2*(3), 10-21.

Case-Smith, J. (1993). Self-care strategies for children with developmental deficits. In C. Christiansen (Ed.). *Ways of living: self-care strategies for special needs* (pp. 101-156). Rockville, MD: AOTA.

Chamberlin, J., Henry, M.M., Roberts, J.D., Sapsford, A.L., & Courtney, S.E. (1991). An infant and toddler feeding group program. *American Journal of Occupational Therapy, 45,* 907-911.

Coley, I.L. & Procter, S.A. (1989). Self-maintenance activities. In P. Pratt & A. Allen (Eds.). *Occupational therapy for children* (pp. 442-456). St. Louis: Mosby.

Daniels, H., Devlieger, H., Casaer, P. & Eggermont, E. (1986). Nutritive and non-nutritive sucking in preterm infants. *Journal of Developmental Physiology, 8,* 117-121.

DiScipio, W.J., Kaslon, K., & Rube, R.J. (1978). Traumatically acquired conditioned dysphagia in child. *Annals of Otology, Rhinology and Laryngology, 87,* 509-514.

Einarsson-Backes, L., Deitz, J., Price, R., Glass, R., & Hays, R. (1994). The effect of oral support on sucking efficiency in preterm infants. *American Journal of Occupational Therapy, 48*(6), 490-498.

Fox, C.A. (1990). Implementing the modified barium swallow evaluation in children who have multiple disabilities. *Infants and Young Children, 3,* 67-77.

Glass, R. & Wolf, L. (1992). Feeding and oral motor skills. In J. Case-Smith (Ed.). *Pediatric occupational therapy and early intervention* (pp. 225-288). Andover, MA: Butterworth-Heineman.

Hagekull, B. & Dahl, M. (1987). Infants with and without feeding difficulties: maternal experiences. *International Journal of Eating Disorders, 6,* 83-98.

Handen, B.L., Mandell, F., & Russo, D. (1986). Feeding induction in children who refuse to eat. *American Journal of Diseases in Children, 140,* 52-54.

Hanzlik, J.R. (1993). Parent-child relations: interaction and intervention. In J. Case-Smith (Ed.). *Pediatric occupational therapy and early intervention.* Boston: Andover Medical Publishers.

Heptinstall, E., Puckering, C., Skuse, D., Start, K., Zur-Szpiro, S., & Dowdney, L. (1987). Nutrition and mealtime behavior in families of growth-retarded children. *Human Nutrition: Applied Nutrition, 41A,* 390-402.

Humphry, R. (1995). Feeding problems and failure to thrive: literature review and research ideas. Unpublished manuscript. Chapel Hill: Univeristy of North Carolina.

Illingworth, G. & Lister, J. (1965). The critical or sensitive period, with special reference to certain feeding problems in infants and children. *Journal of Pediatrics, 65,* 839-848.

Kennedy, J.G. & Kent, R.D. (1988). Physiologic substrates of noral deglutition. *Dysphagia, 3,* 24-27.

Logemann, J.A. (1983). *Evaluation and treatment of swallowing disorders.* San Diego: College Hill Press.

Meuller, H. (1975). Feeding. In N.R. Finnie (Ed.). *Handling the young cerebral palsied child at home* (2nd ed.) (pp. 113-132). New York: E.P. Dutton.

Morris, S.E. & Klein, M.D. (1987). *Pre-feeding skills.* Tucson: Therapy Skill Builders.

O'Brien, S., Repp, A., Williams, G.E., & Christophersen, E.R. (1991). Pediatric feeding disorders. *Behavior Modification, 15,* 394-418.

Polan, H.J., Leon, A., Kaplan, M.D., Kessler, D.B., Stern, D.N., & Ward, M.J. (1991). Disturbances of affect expression in failure-to-thrive. *Journal of the American Academy of Child and Adolescent Psychiatry, 30,* 897-903.

Ramsay, M., Gisel, E.G., & Boutry, M. (1993). Non-organic failure to thrive: growth failure secondary to feeding-skills disorder. *Developmental Medicine and Child Neurology, 35,* 285-297.

Sanders, M.R., Patel, R.K., LeGrice, B., & Shepherd, R.W. (1993). Children with persistent feeding difficulties: an observational analysis of the feeding interactions of problem and non-problem eaters. *Health Psychology, 12,* 64-73.

Schuberth, L.M. (1994). The role of occupational therapy in diagnosis and management. In D.N. Tuchman & R. Walter (Eds.). *Disorders of feeding and swallowing in infants and children* (pp. 115-130). San Diego: Singular Publishing Group.

Shah, C.P. & Wong, C. (1980). Management of children with cleft lip and palate. *Canadian Medical Association Journal, 122,* 19-24.

Wolf, L.S. & Glass, R.P. (1992). *Feeding and swallowing disorders in infancy: assessment and management.* Tucson: Therapy Skills Builders.

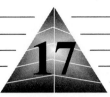

# Self-Care and Adaptations for Independent Living

JAYNE SHEPHERD ▲ SUSAN A. PROCTER ▲ IDA LOU COLEY

## KEY TERMS

▲ Instrumental Activities of Daily Living
▲ Cultural Factors
▲ Grading
▲ Chaining, Forward and Backward
▲ Prompts and Cuing
▲ Adaptive Devices
▲ Adaptive Positioning

## CHAPTER OBJECTIVES

1. Identify the intrinsic and environmental variables that affect a child's abilities in self-care.
2. Heighten awareness of cultural and social factors in the child's performance and parental expectations.
3. Identify assessment procedures and methods in self-care and independent living skills.
4. Describe intervention strategies and approaches, both general and specific.
5. Describe the selection and modification of equipment.
6. Describe adaptations for play, sports, and school activities.

Self-care and instrumental activities of daily living (IADL) tasks are some of the most important tasks learned by children as they mature. Basic self-care tasks include grooming, bathing, toileting, dressing, feeding, and functional mobility and communication. As a child matures, he or she learns to perform these tasks in socially appropriate ways and may perform other self-care tasks such as taking his or her own medications, maintaining health (e.g., exercise, nutrition, and visiting health care professionals),

taking care of personal devices, responding to emergencies, and expressing sexual needs (AOTA, 1994) (see Appendix 8-A).

IADL are more complex ADL needed to function independently in home, school, community, and work environments (Brown et al., 1991; Spencer, Murphy, Bean, & Schelly, 1991). IADL tasks include home management skills such as clothing care, cleaning, meal preparation, shopping, money management, household maintenance, and safety procedures. These are the activities that determine independent living.

The dynamic interaction between child characteristics and the environmental variables as they influence a child's performance in self-care and IADL tasks is discussed in this chapter. Assessment methods, approaches, and strategies for improving performance in self-care and IADL tasks are described. Typical development, problems, and adaptations for toileting, dressing, bathing, grooming, and other related self-care tasks are given. IADL tasks are discussed in relation to performance in community, recreational, and school environments. Examples of adaptations to physical and social environments are given while considering cultural influences.

## IMPORTANCE OF SELF-CARE AND IADL TASKS

The foundations for self-care and IADL tasks begin in infancy and, if given the time and opportunity, are refined throughout the various stages of development. As unique individuals, children develop these skills at varying rates and have occasional regression and unpredictable behaviors. Overall, society and families assume that children develop increasing levels of competence and self-reliance to meet their own self-care and IADL needs. Growth and maturity allow the child to participate within a variety of roles and environments with decreasing levels of adult supervision.

When a child is born with a disability or acquires a disability, parental and child expectations for self-care and daily living independence may need to be modified. Occupational therapists are instrumental in helping parents and children learn how to modify tasks so that self-care and IADL skills are used daily by children. Active participation in a child's own self-care has a number of benefits, including maintaining and improving sensorimotor, cognitive, and psychosocial skills. As the child learns new tasks, he or she develops a sense of accomplishment and pride in his or her abilities. The child can become responsible for developing and maintaining routines that prevent further illness (e.g., checking skin conditions, maintaining cleanliness of self and environment, and cooking nutritious meals) and is able to meet role expectations for community living. This increasing independence also gives parents, teachers, siblings, and other caregivers more time and energy for other tasks.

## FACTORS AFFECTING PERFORMANCE

Both child-related and environmental factors influence the child's achievement of self-care function. The child's sensorimotor, cognitive, and psychosocial performance components determine self-care and IADL ability. Performance variables include the child's chronologic age, developmental stage, disability status, and place in the life cycle within the family (see Chapter 5). Environmental variables include the physical, social, and cultural environments.

### Child Characteristics

Occupational therapy intervention to increase self-care and IADL functions considers the child's sensorimotor, cognitive, and psychosocial skills in relation to the tasks that need to be performed and builds specific skills needed for self-care function (Coster, Haley, & Baryza, 1994).

The child has specific skills and limitations that affect self-care and IADL performance. For example, children with tactile defensiveness may cry during dressing and refuse to dress despite being cognitively and motorically able to dress themselves. They may dislike the textures, or they have learned to cry for Mom's attention (psychosocial). Children with visual impairments may use the sensations in their hands (tactile and proprioceptive) in brushing their hair even though they cannot see it. A child with cerebral palsy may not have the postural control to sit up during dressing but may have the cognitive skills (i.e., problem solving and sequencing), perceptual skills (i.e., right-left discrimination and figure-ground), and gross motor skills to dress in a side-lying position (Case-Smith, 1994).

Interest level, self-confidence, and motivation are strong forces that help children attain levels of performance that are either above or below expectations. Children with men-

tal retardation, traumatic brain injury, or multiple disabilities experience difficulties in coordination, initiative, attention span, sequencing, memory, safety, and the ability to generalize skills across environments. However, with the proper instruction, self-care and IADL tasks are sometimes the tasks these children can perform most competently (Orelove & Sobsey, 1991). In general, children who are highly motivated are able to improve their functional level with adaptations to activities, equipment, and the environment.

### Developmental and Chronologic Age

Self-care and IADL tasks are generally thought to occur in a developmental sequence and to be achievable by certain ages. These sequences help therapists and families form realistic expectations for children and help determine the appropriate timing for teaching tasks. For example, if a 2-year-old child cannot dress independently, intervention would not be appropriate because most children are not independent in dressing until 5 or 6 years of age. By the same token, if a 14-year-old child has never crossed the street alone, the therapist might focus on this community mobility skill as an essential objective.

By considering the child's age, therapists can also determine when it is time to stop working on specific skills. For example, 8-year-old Tilly had occupational therapy for 7 years to increase lip closure and develop a more efficient suck-swallow pattern. If she did not learn this skill in the past 7 years, what are her chances of learning it this year? Instead, it may be time to work on self-feeding strategies or an IADL skill such as operating an appliance with a switch for meal preparation.

Therapists need to be cognizant of the developmental stage of maturation when choosing an activity. Planning self-care and IADL intervention for an adolescent is different than planning for a 2-year-old child. Both children need to be given choices, but the adolescent needs more privacy and autonomy, and self-care and IADL needs will have a different focus. The therapist may intervene for skills in personal grooming, functional graphic communication, community mobility, medication routine, emergency responses, sexual expression, homemaking skills, money management (allowance), and pursuing recreational interests. Intervention for the 2-year-old child may only focus on toileting, feeding, bathing, dressing, and play.

### Disability Status

The disability or health status of the child can affect his or her opportunity and ability to perform self-care and IADL tasks. Children who are acutely ill or who have multiple disabilities with numerous procedures done throughout the day (e.g., tube feeding, tracheostomy care, bowel and bladder care) may not have time or energy to work on self-care and IADL tasks. For example, within a 45-minute period, Jenna, a 10-year-old child with C6 quadriplegia, can dress herself independently, but she and her family decided it was preferable for someone else to dress her so that she has more energy for school tasks. Self-care or IADL tasks may be modified or stopped for children with progressive or terminal diseases (e.g., acquired immunodeficiency syndrome or Duchenne's muscular dystrophy). These children and children with multiple disabilities may physically be unable to do all or any part of self-care tasks, but they can direct others on how to care for them. Children with psychosocial problems may cease doing any normal self-care and IADL routines because of depression or anxiety. Occupational therapists use their medical knowledge and the preferences of the child and family to clinically judge when and what type of intervention is appropriate.

## Family Characteristics

The social enviornment is influential in establishing the role expectations and the routines for the child (Kielhofner, 1995). Parents or other family members are typically the primary caregivers who are responsible for the child's daily living needs and who are with the child most consistently. Families vary in their ability and availability to assist and encourage the child to perform self-care and IADL tasks. This ability is often dependent on where the family and child are in the family life cycle.

Occupational therapists need to be aware of the child's and family's place in the life cycle because self-care and IADL issues change accordingly (Turnbull & Turnbull, 1990). In early childhood (0 to 3 years), feeding is usually of utmost importance because infants are dependent on their parents for nutrition. Parents often seek instruction on how to dress and bathe the baby at this stage. By age 3, self-feeding, dressing, and toileting skills may become issues for parents.

When the child enters school by age 6, self-care issues such as functional mobility within the school environment, dressing (especially outerwear), toileting, socialization with nondisabled peers, grooming (i.e., washing hands and face), and functional communication (e.g., writing, drawing, and expressing needs become increasingly important). Simple household tasks like taking out the trash, setting and clearing the table, making a simple sandwich, washing or dusting countertops, and following safety precautions are appropriate goals. At this stage, parents are often looking for community resources to get children involved in recreational and other extracurricular activities. Older siblings may become more aware of and sensitive to their brother or sister's disability and may be asked to help them learn self-care tasks and perform more household tasks themselves.

During adolescence (13 to 21 years), increasing independence in self-care and IADL skills often determines if a child will "fit in" with peers or be successful in obtaining a job outside of the school environment. Increased responsibility for personal device care, medication routines, and health maintenance routines is given to the child. During this stage, families may further investigate current community resources as they think about future living arrangements, vocational opportunities, and the availability of other recreational activities for their child (Turnbull & Turnbull, 1990). Parent issues may focus on the child's ability to express sexual needs, to be safe within many environments, and to respond to emergency situations appropriately. Additional skills in caring for clothing, preparing meals, shopping, managing money, and maintaining a household may be addressed during this stage. Children with severe disabilities who require maximum physical assistance in activities of daily living become a great concern to parents as they approach adulthood. For the first time, parents may not have the physical strength to handle the daily care needs of their child.

Other characteristics of the family influence the child's development of self-care and IADL skills. These include the number of members in the family and the family expectations, roles, and routines for managing daily living needs (Turnbull & Turnbull, 1990). Large families may assign different members to perform or help with specific self-care tasks for a child with a disability, whereas in other families, the parent may be the sole person responsible for the daily living needs of their child. For example, a child living on a farm may be expected to get up at the crack of dawn, put on overalls and boots, complete chores like feeding the animals, receive home schooling from Mom and an older sister, and help sell eggs to augment the family income. These role expectations, personal preferences, and routines must be discussed by the parents and the therapist so that appropriate and meaningful assessment and intervention strategies may be chosen.

Personal characteristics of family members such as temperament, coping skills, and health status are considered when planning treatment (Turnbull & Turnbull, 1990) (see Chapter 5). Family members' physical, cognitive, and psychosocial abilities influence the kind of assistance they provide, and activities, techniques, equipment, and assistive devices need to be chosen carefully and collaboratively. For example, parents with mental retardation or mental health problems need to see modeling by the therapists and need to practice and learn cuing systems when structuring tasks for their children (Copeland, Ford, & Solon, 1976; Turnbull & Turnbull, 1990). Parents with physical problems may need instructions in using adapted techniques and assistive devices safely.

## Social Context
### Other Caregivers

Children grow up with assistance, support, and guidance of many caregivers. Other caregivers such as teachers, aides, attendants, baby-sitters, and day care staff are part of the social environment. They have short-term involvement, and their role is determined by the nature of the program.

The relationship between the caregiver and the child is affected by the number of caregivers available in a particular environment and the student-teacher ratio. Interventions should be simple in situations where time is at a premium and multiple caregivers are involved. Expectations of parents, teachers, and therapists for the child may vary because each has a different frame of reference. The therapist must collaborate with the family and other caregivers so that expectations can be discussed, brought into perspective, and established on a consistent basis.

### Peers

Peers can positively or negatively influence a child's ability and willingness to perform tasks. For example, peers at school are often fascinated with assistive devices such as adapted spoons, augmentative communication devices, wheelchairs, or computers used by the child with a physical disability. This interest may encourage the child to use the device and may begin friendships. Peers also can make fun of a child's method of self-feeding or of using an adaptive writing utensil. This may discourage the child from using adaptive methods and interacting with peers. Social interactions and networks of peers or friends in school, home, recreational, and community environments can be extremely powerful in the success of an intervention strategy.

### Social Routines

An analysis of social routines helps determine when and how self-care and IADL tasks are taught. Within home, school, community, and recreational environments, routines may differ significantly, and children need to adapt to these differences. The variation in routine may confuse or disorganize children with mental retardation or attention deficit disorders but may be motivating to children without attention or cognitive problems. Therapists need to be aware of the social routines so they can choose appropriate times to teach tasks. When tasks are taught or practiced at times and places where they naturally occur, they more quickly become part of the child's behavior repetoire (Brown et al., 1991). For example, school-based therapists may meet children at the bus to work on functional mobility skills and as the child removes his or her coat to work on dressing skills. When tasks are embedded throughout all environments, children receive multiple opportunities to practice skills and learn how to use the natural cues within the environment to modify their behavior. Social routines and social norms within a community are considered when planning individual or group therapy. Toileting, dressing, and bathing are usually done individually, but children may be able to cook or clean together as a cooperative effort within the school environment.

### Cultural Environment

As therapists work with a variety of children and families in an array of service provision models, they need to be aware of their own and of others' cultural beliefs, customs, activity patterns, and expectations for performance in self-care and IADL tasks (Lynch & Hanson, 1992). Occupational therapists usually become involved with a family because someone else believed that their services were needed. These services may or may not be welcomed as the therapist asks personal questions about a child's and family's self-care and IADL tasks and routines. Lynch and Hanson (1992) have edited a useful guide to help interventionists develop skills in working with families and children from different cultures. Therapists need to ask parents questions and use community resources to better understand the cultural backgrounds of their clients.

Cultural expectations of the family, caregivers, and social group as a whole may determine behavior standards. Family beliefs, values, and attitudes about childrearing, autonomy, and self-reliance influence how self-care and IADL tasks are perceived. In Anglo-European cultures, parents are usually concerned about children meeting developmental milestones (Hanson, 1992), yet other cultures (e.g., Latino) may be more relaxed about milestone attainment (Zuniga, 1992). This basic difference may determine whether parents see the importance of intervention. In some Indian cultures that are adult centered, children are expected to be independent at an early age. They are rewarded by the parents and society for taking the initiative to do chores around the house or community. In other cultures, children may be given more time to be childlike and may not be pushed to do adultlike skills and chores until a later age (Willis, 1992).

Social role expectations and routines are influenced by culture. In general, Anglo-European parents may encourage children to become independent and self-reliant (Hanson, 1992), and Latino (Zuniga, 1992) and Asian (Chan, 1992a) families may encourage dependency or interdependency within the family. Routines for dressing, feeding, bathing, bedtime, and carrying out household tasks vary among cultural groups.

Culture also influences the type and availability of activities, tools, equipment, and materials that are used by a child to perform self-care or IADL tasks. Customs and beliefs may determine how children are dressed, what they eat, what utensils are in the kitchen, how they prepare and store food, what type of bed is used, or how health care needs are met. Economic conditions, geographic location, and opportunities for education and employment can influence what resources and supports are available to families.

### Physical Environment

Children in early and middle childhood often perform self-care and IADL skills in different environments. The four primary environments of children are home, school, community, and play or recreational area. The box on p. 465 gives an example of the typical environments children experience.

Each environment has physical, social, and cultural characteristics. Once the occupational therapist understands

## Environmental Domains and Subenvironments Where Children Perform Self-Care and IADL Tasks

**HOME**

Bedroom
Bathroom
Kitchen
Living room or family room
Laundry room
Backyard
Immediate neighborhood
Garage

**SCHOOL**

Classroom
Bathroom
Resource room (e.g., music, art, or home economics)
Cafeteria
Gymnasium
Library
Auditorium
Playground or athletic field

**COMMUNITY**

Stores (e.g., convenience, grocery, or department)
Mall
Restaurants
Public restrooms
Laundromats
Hairdresser
Doctor's office
Neighborhood
Church

**RECREATION**

Neighborhood
Sports arenas or fields
Park
Organized recreational facilities
Clubs
Sport facility (e.g., bowling alley, minature golf course, skating rink)
Theaters

*IADL,* Instrumental activities of daily living.

these contexts, intervention strategies may be chosen to be congruent with the environment or to change the aspects of the environment that are barriers to the child's performance of self-care and IADL tasks.

A number of barriers within the physical environment may hinder the child's development of self-care and IADL skills. These include building construction, terrain, furniture, and objects within the environment. Inaccessible buildings and rooms crowded with furniture limit how children

in wheelchairs move throughout the environment. Differences in the terrain or the room surface also affect mobility. For example, a child who can run outdoors on the asphalt playground may trip and fall inside when walking on a rug. Other physical characteristics that are assessed relate to what type of furniture, objects, or assistive devices are in the environment—are they usable and accessible? This includes the type of equipment, household items, clothing, or toys.

## ASSESSMENT OF SELF-CARE AND IADL SKILLS

Families and their children have key roles in determining which assessment procedures to use. By collaboratively working with families, therapists learn about the characteristics of the child, the contexts in which task performance occurs, and the expectations and concerns of the family. When children get older and are able to communicate, they too are included in determining what areas of self-care and IADL skills are important to them. When parents and children are given a chance to select or refuse assessments and choose where the assessment will be done, by whom, and when, they are often more vested in the results (Giangreco, Cloninger, & Iverson, 1993). Therapists also have a better understanding of the contexts in which skills must be performed.

### Assessment Procedures

Interviews, inventories, and structured and naturalistic observations are assessment methods typically used to measure self-care and IADL performance in occupational therapy. These methods can be used alone or in combination to develop intervention strategies and measure outcomes of treatment (Snell & Brown, 1993). Table 17-1 lists assessments of self-care and IADL tasks appropriate for use with children.

Self-care and IADL skill independence includes obtaining (setting up) and using supplies to complete a particular task. In general, performance is rated according to the child's ability to set up and complete a task. Performance may be assessed by grading the child's level of independence. Table 17-2 gives one example of how a child's independence in bathing may be rated. A system of grading the child's level of independence can be used with any of the methods or purposes discussed in the following section.

### Assessment Methods
#### Interviews and Inventories

Interviews can be informal or unstructured where the therapist asks the interviewee (e.g., parents, children, teachers, and other significant caregivers) questions about the child's abilities, environmental characteristics, or goals and dreams (Snell & Brown, 1993). Inventories are question-

▲ Table 17-1  Self-Care and Instrumental Activities of Daily Living (IADL) Assessments for Children and Adolescents

| Instrument, Author, Publisher | Direct | Interview and Inventory | Observation | Age Range | Description |
|---|---|---|---|---|---|
| **AAMD Adaptive Behavior Scales (ABS)** (Lambert & Windmiller, 1981) American Association on Mental Deficiency 5201 Connecticut Avenue, NW Washington, DC 20015 | X | X | X | 4 years and up | Standardized, criterion-referenced measure for children with adaptive behaviors in 10 domains with 7 domains related to IADL (independent functioning, economic activity, numbers, time, domestic, self-direction, responsibility, socialization, vocational, and recreational). Maladaptive behaviors measured in 14 domains. School version in development. Useful for children with moderate to severe disabilities. |
| **Assessment of Motor Processing Skills (AMPS)** (Fisher, 1994) Unpublished manual. Dr. Anne Fisher Department of Occupational Therapy 100 Humanities Building Colorado State University Fort Collins, CO 80523 | X | X | X | Adolescent to adult | Criterion-referenced test for IADL tasks; assesses the underlying motor and process skills used to perform the task. Clients can choose two or more IADL tasks they want to do (50 possible) as they are videotaped. Examiners need to be trained; examiner ratings are calibrated. Appears useful for all ages and disabilities. |
| **Battelle Developmental Inventory (BDI)** (Newborg, Stock, Wnek, Guidubaldi, & Szinicki, 1984) Riverside Publishing 8420 West Bryn Mawr Avenue Chicago, IL 60631 | | X | X | 0 to 8 years | Activities of daily living (grooming, toilet hygiene, dressing, and eating) is one of four domains assessed. An in-depth assessment or a screening format can be used. |
| **Callier-Azusa Scale** (Stillman, 1975) Callier Center for Communication Disorders, University of Texas—Dallas 1966 Inwood Road Dallas, TX 75235 | X | | | 0 to adult | Daily living skills (dressing, personal hygiene, eating toileting) is one of five domains, 18 subscales. Used in a classroom with students who have deafness, blindness, and multiple disabilities. Examiner should observe child for at least a 2-week period. Criterion for items is listed. Minimal psychometric testing. |
| **Carolina Curriculum for Preschoolers With Special Needs** (Johnson-Martin, Jens, Attermeier, & Hacker, 1990) Paul Brookes Publishing Co. P.O. Box 10624 Baltimore, MD 21285 | X | X | X | 0 to 3 years | Curriculum-referenced assessment; self-care is one of five domains measured. Includes sequences in responsibility, self-concept, interpersonal skills, and self-help. |
| **Choosing Options and Accommodations for Children** (Giangreco, Cloninger, & Iverson, 1993) Paul Brookes Publishing Co. P.O. Box 10624 Baltimore, MD 21285 | | X | X | 3 to 21 years | Curriculum-referenced, transdisciplinary team assessment and curriculum with four domains: personal management, community, home, and vocational. Skills are scored and given a potential priority and rank by each evaluator. For children with moderate, severe, or profound disabilities; has been used with younger children with mild disabilities. |

▲ Table 17-1   Self-Care and Instrumental Activities of Daily Living (IADL) Assessments for Children and Adolescents— cont'd

| Instrument, Author, Publisher | Direct | Interview and Inventory | Observation | Age Range | Description |
|---|---|---|---|---|---|
| **First STEP (Screening Test for Evaluating Preschoolers)** (Miller, 1992) The Psychological Corporation 555 Academic Court San Antonio, TX 78204 | X | | | 3 to 6 years | Screening measure where self-help is one of five domains assessed within a 15-minute test. Identifies children who are at risk or developmentally delayed. |
| **Functional Independence Measure (FIM)** (Hamilton, Granger, Sherwin, Zielenzny, & Tashman, 1987) The State University of New York University at Buffalo Buffalo, NY 14214 | X | X | X | 8 years to adult | Functional outcome measure for clients with physical disabilities. Six domains assessed: self-care, mobility, locomotion, sphincter control, communication, and social cognition; 18 subdomains. Uses 7-point ordinal scale to measure the level of independence. Norm-referenced test. |
| **Functional Skills Screening Inventory (FSSI)** (Becker, Schur, Paoletti-Schelp, & Hammer, 1986) Functional Resources Enterprises, Inc. 2743 Trail of the Madrones Austin, TX 78746 | | X | X | 6 years and older | Criterion-referenced test of adaptive behavior; self-care, independent living, vocational, recreational, and social-emotional domains are assessed, with five other domains also assessed. Optional computer scoring, visual profiles, and identification of priorities. Appropriate for children with moderate to severe disabilities. |
| **Hawaii Early Learning Profile (HELP)** (Furuno, O'Reilly, Hoska, Zeisloft, & Allman, 1984) VORT Corporation P.O. Box 11132 Palo Alto, CA 94306 | | X | X | Birth to 3 years | Curriculum-referenced assessment; self-care is one of six domains. Inventory of developmental skills, activity guide, and other materials related to parents with disabilities. No psychometric testing. |
| **Pediatric Evaluation of Disability Inventory (PEDI)** (Haley, Coster, Ludlow, Haltiwanger, & Andrellos, 1992) New England Medical Center Rehabilitation Medicine Department Boston, MA 02215 | | X | | 1 month to 7 years | Normative, judgment-based (parent interview) outcome measurement; three domains (self-care, mobility, social function) are assessed using two subscales: functional skills (197 tasks) and caregiver assistance (20 tasks). |
| **Pyramid Scales** (Cone, 1984) Pro-Ed 5341 Industrial Oaks Blvd. Austin, TX 78735 | | X | X | 3 to adolescent | Assesses self-care, independent living, vocational, recreation/leisure, social emotional domains. Appropriate for children with moderate to severe disabilities. |
| **Self-Help Assessment: Parent Evaluation (SHAPE),** Research Ed. (Miller, 1993) The KID Foundation 8101 E. Prentice Avenue, Suite #518, Englewood, CO 80111 | | X | | Birth to 6 years | Assesses activities of daily living (ADL), community functioning, self-control, relationships, and interactions. Uses a pictorial format for parents to rate their own child's abilities. |

▲ Table 17-1   Self-Care and Instrumental Activities of Daily Living (IADL) Assessments for Children and Adolescents— cont'd

| Instrument, Author, Publisher | Direct | Interview and Inventory | Observation | Age Range | Description |
|---|---|---|---|---|---|
| **Vineland Adaptive Behavior Scales** (Sparrow, Balla, & Cicchetti, 1984) American Guidance Service Circle Pines, MN 55014 | | X | | Birth to adult | Norm-referenced evaluation. Assesses social competency with behavioral observations in ADL, communication, socialization, and motor domains. Optional maladaptive behavior domain for children 5 years and older. Three versions are available: interview and survey form; interview and expanded form; and classroom and teacher form (3 years to 12 years, 11 months). Appropriate for students with or without disabilities. |
| **WeeFIM (Functional Independence Measure) for Children** (Hamilton & Granger, 1991) WeeFIM Research Foundation of the State University of New York University at Buffalo Buffalo, NY 14214 | | | | 6 months to 6 years | Functional evaluation for children with physical disabilities. Six domains assessed: self-care (grooming, dressing and feeding), mobility, locomotion, sphincter control, communication, and social cognition; 18 subdomains. Direct adaptation of the Functional Independence Measure (FIM) for adults. Undergoing standardization procedures. |

naires (or they can be administered like an interview) that ask the rater to answer questions about the child's ability to perform self-care and IADL tasks and perhaps about future goals and concerns for the child. Interviewing methods and inventory methods may be used together to give the therapist useful information about how the child performs within different contexts. These assessments are dependent on the ability of the person to answer the questions accurately and honestly.

### Structured and Naturalistic Observation

*Structured observation* occurs when the therapist gives the child a task to do and then rates the child's performance. This testing may be done in any environment with a variety of materials. For example, while receiving occupational therapy as an outpatient, a child with a traumatic brain injury may be taken to the occupational therapy kitchen and asked to make a sandwich. The child's performance on this evaluation may vary significantly because of unfamiliarity of materials and equipment in the occupational therapy kitchen. Structured observation provides information regarding how well the child performs the task in a structured situation, but it does not determine if the child will initiate doing the task at the appropriate time or perform the task

in different envionrments. For example, will the child make a sandwich for lunch when left alone?

In *naturalistic or ecologic observation,* the therapist gathers information in the typical or natural setting that the activity occurs. Usually a task analysis is completed to identify the component processes and subskills of an activity. In a naturalistic task analysis, the therapist evaluates the child's ability to do the task itself, as well as the physical, social, and cultural characteristics of the environment. For example, when observing a child's ability to use the toilet at school, the therapist notes accessibility barriers, typical classroom routines and expectations for toileting, and any cultural aspects of the toileting process (e.g., type of clothing the child is wearing). By understanding these contexts, intervention strategies can be chosen more appropriately. Environmental observations can be time consuming, but when used in a team effort, they provide an abundance of information. The therapist also examines each component or subskill of the task and writes down the observable behaviors or steps it takes to complete the task. Snell (1994) suggested that task analyses are best if steps are sequenced logically and the size of each step is similar in size to the other steps. She also suggested that child behaviors or steps are differentiated from the steps of the caregiver or thera-

▲ Table 17-2   Example of Rating Self-Care Skill Independence Using a Task Analysis

| Levels of Independence | Definition | Bathing Example |
|---|---|---|
| Independent | Child performs all of task, including set up | Child gets out needed supplies and equipment; bathes, rinses, and dries self without assistance |
| Independent with set-up | After someone sets up task, child performs all of task | Bathtub seat placed in tub and bathing supplies organized by mother; child bathes, rinses, and drys self without assistance |
| Supervision | Child performs task on his or her own but is unsafe to be left alone; may need verbal cuing or physical prompts for 1% to 24% of task | Child bathes, rinses, and dries self without assistance but because of balance and judgment, needs monitoring when getting in and out of tub and reaching lower extremities |
| Minimal assistance or skillful | Child performs 51% to 75% of task independently but needs physical assistance or other cuing for at least 25% of task | Child bathes and rinses body parts independently; needs physical assistance getting in and out of tub and is cued to monitor water temperature and dry body parts |
| Moderate assistance or 26% to 50% partial participation | Child performs 26% to 50% of task independently but needs physical assistance or other cuing for at least 50% of task | Child adjusts water temperature, washes and rinses face, torso, and upper extremities independently; needs physical assistance getting in and out of tub and washing and rinsing lower extremities and back |
| Maximal assistance or 1% to 25% partial participation | Child performs 1% to 25% of task independently but needs physical assistance or other cuing for 75% of task | Child independently washes, rinses, and dries face but needs verbal cues to wash torso; needs physical assistance to get in and out of tub and in washing other body parts |
| Dependent | Child is unable to perform any of task | Mother physically picks up and places child in tub and washes, rinses, and dries the child's body parts. Child does not lift body parts to be washed or dried |

Modified from Trombly, C.A. & Quintana, L.A. (1989). Activities of daily living. In C.A. Trombly (Ed.). *Occupational therapy for physical dysfunction* (3rd ed.) (p. 387). Baltimore: Williams & Wilkins.

pist and that the exact wording of instructions for the child be placed directly on the task analysis sheet so the child is not confused by inconsistent directions (Snell, 1994). Data can be collected as part of the task analysis to help therapists modify how the skill is taught, when progress is not observable. Figure 17-1 gives an example of a toileting task analysis data sheet for Sara, a preschooler with right-sided hemiplegia.

Ecologic or environmentally referenced assessments are appropriate for all children and are particularly useful for children with moderate to severe disabilities who have difficulty generalizing tasks from one environment to another (Orelove & Sobsey, 1991; York & Rainforth, 1991). A *top-down approach* considers the contexts in which tasks are performed, not just what skills the child can perform (Bryze & Curtin, 1993). In this approach, the environments where the task occurs, the task components, and the child's skills are considered. Specific areas within the environment are identified. Next, the components of the task are determined. Then the therapist compares the requirements of an identi-

fied task to the child's actual performance on the components of the task. Discrepancies between the child's current abilities and those skills needed to perform in the environment are identified and prioritized. This approach focuses on the child's performance in different contexts and helps the therapist plan strategies to teach the skills directly within the natural environment or to modify the requirements of the task (York & Rainforth, 1991).

## Evaluation for Program Planning

Curriculum-referenced or guided assessments are typically used in settings like early intervention or school system practice by team members who share the responsibility for the assessment process. Self-care is often one area of the assessment. Interview, inventories, direct testing, or environmental observation methods may be used for these assessments. The Carolina Curriculum for Preschoolers with Special Needs (Johnson-Martin, Jens, & Attermeier, 1986) and the Hawaii Early Learning Profile (Furuno, O'Reilly,

**Name:** Sara
**Therapist:** Jayne
**Instructional cue:** "Sara, it's time to go to the potty."
**Program:** Toileting
**Environment:** Preschool classroom
**Objective:** Given a natural opportunity or request to go to the potty, Sara will independently perform at least 10 out of 12 steps of the task analysis for toileting for 3 consecutive days, by March 15, 1995.

| | | Baseline | | | | | Intervention | | | | | | | | | | Reevaluation | | | |
|---|---|---|---|---|---|---|---|---|---|---|---|---|---|---|---|---|---|---|---|---|
| | | 1 | 2 | 3 | 4 | 5 | 1 | 2 | 3 | 4 | 5 | 6 | 7 | 8 | 9 | 10 | 1 | 2 | 3 | 4 |
| 1. | Walks to the bathroom with walker | I | I | I | I | I | I | I | I | I | I | I | I | I | I | I | I | I | | |
| 2. | Pulls down outer clothes over short leg braces | V | V | V | G | G | V | V | I | I | I | V | I | I | I | I | I | I | | |
| 3. | Pulls down underpants | V | V | I | I | I | I | I | I | V | V | I | I | I | I | I | V | I | | |
| 4. | Responds correctly to, "Are your pants wet?" | G | G | G | V | V | I | I | V | I | V | V | I | V | V | V | V | I | | |
| 5. | Sits on toilet | I | I | I | I | I | I | I | I | I | I | I | I | I | I | I | I | I | | |
| 6. | Sits on the toilet for 10 minutes or until she eliminates | P | P | P | G | G | G | G | G | G | V | V | V | V | V | V | V | I | | |
| 7. | Responds to "Did you go pee-pee in the potty?" | I | I | I | I | I | I | I | I | I | I | I | I | I | I | I | I | I | | |
| 8. | Wipes herself (front to back) | V | V | V | V | V | V | V | V | V | V | V | I | V | V | I | V | V | | |
| 9. | Stands up holding grab bar | I | I | I | I | I | I | I | I | I | I | I | I | I | I | I | I | I | | |
| 10. | Pulls up underpants | P | P | P | P | P | G | G | V | V | V | V | I | I | I | I | V | I | | |
| 11. | Pulls up outer clothes | G | G | G | V | V | V | I | I | I | I | V | I | I | I | I | I | I | | |
| 12. | Flushes toilet | G | G | G | V | V | V | I | I | I | I | I | I | I | I | I | V | I | | |

*I,* Independent; *V,* verbal prompt; *G,* gestural prompt; *P,* physical prompt; —, error; *R,* refused.

**Figure 17-1**   Task analysis data sheet for toileting sequence.

Hosaka, Ziesloft, & Allman, 1984) are typical curriculum-referenced assessments used in early intervention. Others are listed in Table 17-1

Giangreco, Cloninger, and Iverson (1993) have developed a useful transdisciplinary, curriculum-based assessment and guide, *Choosing Options and Accommodations for Children (COACH)*. COACH is used to assess school-aged children with moderate to severe disabilities and uses a family prioritization interview and environmental observations to help plan inclusive educational goals. Priorities, outcomes, and needed supports are identified for specific environments and across environments in the areas of communication, socialization, personal management, leisure and recreation, and applied academics. Team members plan goals together, and no discipline-specific goals are written on the child's educational plan.

## Measurement of Outcome

Within the past decade, universal assessments to measure the outcomes of self-care and IADL tasks have been developed in the fields of rehabilitation and occupational therapy. These assessments are in various stages of development because they are being refined and used with different populations of children and adolescents with disabilities. Occupational therapists must continually read the literature to gain information about the development of assessments and their psychometric properties.

The Functional Independence Measure (FIM) and the Assessment of Motor and Processing Skills (AMPS) are two universal assessment tools developed for adolescents and adults, and the Functional Independence Measure for Children (WeeFIM) and the Pediatric Evaluation of Disabilities Inventory are useful with children 6 years of age and younger. (See Table 17-1 for all publishers; also see Chapters 8, 9, and 24.) In the FIM and WeeFIM a global view of a child's self-care and IADL functioning is presented because only 18 subtasks are rated by the rehabilitation team.

Another functional evaluation tool developed by occupational therapist, Anne Fisher (1994), is the AMPS. This tool is still in the development phase and has been used with adolescents and adults with different cultural backgrounds

▲ Table 17-3    Approaches to Improving Self-Care and Instrumental Activities of Daily Living

| Approach | Appropriate Frame of Reference | Problem: Buttoning Buttons Without the Use of Right Hand |
|---|---|---|
| Use a typical developmental sequence | Developmental<br>Visual perceptual<br>Neurodevelopmental treatment | Uses shape-sorting boxes, pegboards, and coins in a piggy bank to work on fine motor skills before beginning with buttons |
| Reduce impairment | Biomechanical<br>Neurodevelopmental treatment<br>Sensory integration<br>Behavioral | Improves range of motion of hand and uses dexterity activities to improve fine motor control; decreases tone in upper extremity and hand; plays with foam or play dough; toys hidden in rice to give hand sensory input |
| Use compensation techniques | Rehabilitation<br>Human occupation | Teaches one-handed buttoning technique |
| Use assistive technologies | Rehabilitation<br>Biomechanical<br>Neurodevelopmental treatment | Uses a button hook; elastic sewn-on buttons; hook-loop tape; positions self and devices for stability during activity |
| Modify task or task expectations | Human occupation<br>Rehabilitation | Uses a pullover shirt so buttoning is not an issue or uses an extra large shirt with buttons already buttoned; wears button shirt overtop of a pullover shirt like an open jacket |
| Use personal assistance | Human occupation<br>Psychosocial<br>Coping | Parent, sibling, or peer is asked to button shirt |

Modified from Smith, R., Benge, M., & Hall, M. (1994). Technology for self-care. In C. Christiansen (Ed.). *Ways of living: self-care strategies for special needs* (pp. 379-422). Rockville, MD: American Occupational Therapy Association.

and an array of disabilities (Bryze & Curtin, 1993; Fisher et al., 1992). In the AMPS, the adolescent is given a list of approximately 50 IADL tasks and chooses two tasks to perform for evaluation purposes. Process and motor skills are assessed and results help predict what other IADL tasks the child may or may not be able to perform. The AMPS tasks use a top-down approach to evaluating skills (Bryze & Curtin, 1993), which gives a comprehensive view of how the child is functioning within performance contexts.

## INTERVENTION STRATEGIES AND APPROACHES

### Critical Questions to Ask Before Intervention

Intervention procedures consider the child's characteristics and performance skills in relation to temporal and environmental contexts. Therapists need to be sensitive to parents and other caregivers needs and concerns. Therapists must listen, give reassurance, involve parents in making observations, and engage them in problem solving. While planning treatment for children with performance problems in self-care and IADL tasks, the therapist needs to answer the following questions:

1. Are the skills **age appropriate** (used by same age peers without disabilities)?
2. Is it **realistic** to expect the child to perform or master this skill? Can they learn it and, if so, how quickly?
3. Will these skills be **useful** in current and future contexts? Are they **functional?**

4. Does this skill **improve the child's health and safety?**
5. What are the **preferences** of the child or the family?
6. Are there **cultural issues** that may influence how tasks are taught?
7. Can this task be assessed, taught, and **practiced in a variety of environments?**

Therapists who can answer "yes" to the above questions have probably chosen meaningful self-care and IADL tasks for treating children with self-care and IADL dependence (Brollier, Shepherd, & Markley, 1994; Snell, 1994).

### Intervention Approaches

Therapists can use a variety of approaches to remediate self-care problems. Smith, Benge, and Hall (1994) identified five ways therapists intervene when there is a problem performing self-care tasks: (1) reduce the disability, (2) teach compensation techniques, (3) use assistive technology, (4) modify the task or task expectations, and (5) use others for assistance. In pediatrics, a developmental approach is also used to intervene with children having problems in self-care. Therapists often use a combination of these approaches and a variety of theoretical orientations to help children achieve the tasks. Table 17-3 gives an example of these six approaches and possible theoretical orientations to use when teaching a child to button his or her shirt. These approaches are discussed throughout each area of self-care and IADL in later sections of the chapter.

## Developmental Approach

A developmental approach may be used to teach self-care tasks to children. Therapists consider the child's developmental and chronologic age and plan treatment according to a typical developmental sequence. This approach helps therapists select some skills for treatment and gives parents some expectations for skill development (Kramer & Hinojosa, 1993). Following the developmental sequence is useful when working with young infants and preschoolers with mild disabilities.

Many children with developmental disabilities do not learn or acquire skills as their same-age peers do, nor do they learn skills in the same typical developmental sequence (Orelove & Sobsey, 1991; Snell, 1993). In fact, their developmental age may be significantly below their chronologic age, yet they are able to perform higher-level skills. For example, 15-year-old Jimmy is functioning at a 3-year-old level in sensorimotor and cognitive skills, but with adaptive aids and techniques, he is independent in bathing, dressing, grooming, toileting, and functional mobility. By considering his chronologic age as well as his developmental age, intervention targeted essential skill components that resulted in increased independence in self-care functions.

## Remediation Approach

After therapists identify gaps in skills, they attempt to remediate the underlying problem, usually using a neurodevelopmental treatment, sensory integration, or perceptual motor approach. For example, before dressing a child with spastic cerebral palsy and tight extensors, the therapist may use handling techniques to inhibit the child's tone. The therapist places the child in a supine position and slowly rolls the child's hips from one side to the other side to reduce the tone, increase range of motion, and encourage trunk rotation (Boehm, 1988). After this preparation, the child's task performance improves and the therapist may then facilitate movement patterns by stabilizing body parts while the child performs the task.

## Compensatory Approach

In the compensatory approach, when a skill is not expected to be remediated, alternative physical techniques or substitute movement patterns are used to complete a task. These techniques are practiced in therapy until they become functional. For example, the child with bilateral upper extremity amputation learns to use his or her feet to write or fold clothes as an adapted physical technique. New movement patterns may be needed to use an assistive device. For instance, the child is taught to hook an arm on the wheelchair push handle to increase stability while learning to fasten his or her pants. Or, the child mentioned previously learns to use existing trunk and shoulder movements to operate a prosthetic arm before learning to type with the device.

## Assistive Technology

Assistive technology assists children in performing many activities independently by changing the physical characteristics of the environment. These devices have low to high complexity. Low-technology devices have few moving parts and are as simple as using a button hook, building up a handle on a brush, or giving a child nonslip matting to hold a plate or toy in place. High technology refers to devices that have greater complexity and may have an electronic component included. Special chairs for bathing, switches for toys or computers, electric page turners, environmental control units, robotics, and electronic spell checkers are examples of high-technology devices.

This myriad of assistive devices is available through equipment vendors, catalogs, and specialty department stores. They are changing constantly. These aids range from simple to complex, inexpensive to costly, and have varying quality. Assistive devices may be commercially available or custom-made by the therapist and skilled craftsmen, orthotists, or rehabilitation engineers. By using local and national data bases and publications on product comparison (e.g., Abledata, HyperAbledata, OT FACT), therapists can keep abreast of new assistive devices to find equipment for unique or specific problems (Smith et al., 1994). The choice of an assistive device is a cooperative decision made by the child, parents, therapists, and other persons who work with the child. Together, they systematically evaluate the child's abilities and limitations, his or her performance contexts, and the capabilities of the device itself. Then they choose the device that has the best "environmental fit." Adolescents who are striving to identify with their peer group tend to reject devices that call attention to their disabilities. Young children are easily frustrated if using the device exceeds their coordination abilities, their attention spans, or gadget tolerances. To be worthwhile, an assistive device should have the following qualities:

1. **Assist in the task** the child is trying to complete without being cumbersome
2. Be **acceptable** to the child, family, and contextual environments in which it will be used (e.g., appearance, functions, upkeep, and storage)
3. Be **practical and flexible** for the environments in which it is used (e.g., dimensions, portability, positioning, and use with other assistive devices)
4. Be **durable** and easy to clean
5. Be **expandable** (e.g., Will it meet the needs for the child now and in 2 years when the child has grown and has more sophisticated skills?)
6. Be **safe** for the child to use (e.g., Will cognitive, behavioral, or physical characteristics such as drooling, throwing, or difficulty with sequencing interfere with using the device?)
7. Have a **system of maintenance or replacement** with continued use
8. **Meet the cost constraints** of the family or purchasing agency

Overall, the child should complete tasks at a higher level of efficiency using this device than without using it. Trial use of a device is highly recommended. This helps determine the feasibility of using the device and demonstrates its value to the child and primary caretakers (Enders, l984).

## Modifying the Task or Task Expectations

By modifying tasks or task expectations, reliance on other persons or impractical assistive devices can be reduced. This search involves creative teamwork between the therapist, the child, and the caregivers. A prompt from the therapist, "Now, how can you do this?..." often taps the child's motivation to find his or her own solution to the problem. The therapist observes and analyzes the child's attempts and then guides and adapts the most promising effort toward success. Therapists and parents collectively agree to change the task or task expectations. For example, elastic waistbands or velcro shoes certainly eliminate the need for assistive devices like zipper pulls or special laces. Sometimes a routine in the social environment needs to be modified to help the child perform a task. For example, a child may have the skills to brush his or her teeth but will not do it after reading a bedtime story. The therapist or parent can change the task expectation by requiring the child to brush his teeth before story reading.

*Grading techniques.* Grading is the adaptation of a task or portions of a task to fit the child's capabilities. By using a task analysis, component skills of the activity are rated and varied according to their degree of ease or difficulty for the child. Those skills that the child is capable of performing are practiced independently. The task may be modified for other difficult skills. Tasks may be graded according to qualities—gross to fine, light to heavy, and simple to complex. Grading of a task may include gradually increasing the number of steps for which the child is held responsible, fading the amount of therapist or caregiver assistance given to the student, or decreasing the amount of time used to complete an activity. The sensory qualities of the environment are also graded to meet the specific sensory processing problems of the child. Developmental approaches also use grading techniques.

## Use of Personal Assistance

*Partial participation.* Each self-care and IADL task involves a series of steps that are performed together in a specific sequence. Through task analysis, the therapist gains an understanding of the sequence of steps involved in each self-care task. The child partially participates in the task by performing some of the steps or part of the steps, and the therapist completes the task. This option of "partial participation" helps the child be part of the activity and use current skills (Ferguson & Baumgart, l991). Backward or forward chaining is used to teach the task and to involve the child in the task. **Backward chaining** occurs when the child performs the last step of a sequence and then receives positive reinforcement for completing the task. Then the child may perform the last two steps of a sequence. New steps are added until the child completes all the steps of the task. This method is particularly helpful for children with a low frustration tolerance or poor self-esteem because it gives immediate success. In **forward chaining** methods, the child begins with the first step of the task sequence, then the second step, and continues learning steps of the task in a sequential order until all the steps in the task can be performed. Forward chaining does not give immediate natural feedback (i.e., completion of the task) but can be helpful for children who have difficulties with sequencing and generalizing skills.

*Prompts or cuing.* Varying amounts of cues or prompts can be given before or during an activity. Therapist or person cues and environment or task cues can occur naturally or artificially within an environment. Therapists use verbal, gestural, or physical cues or a combination of all three (Snell, l994). Environmental or task cues may include picture sequences or checklists, color coding, positioning, or adapting the sensory properties of the environment or materials used in a task. Reese and Snell (l991) described a hierarchic approach to presenting artificial cues from being least intrusive to most intrusive: verbal cues, verbal and gestural cues, verbal and physical cues. In toothbrushing, Reese and Snell (l991) described a hierarchy for physical cues: shadow the child's movements, use two fingers to guide the child, and use a hand-over-hand approach to guide movement. It is best to use the least amount of cues possible and to fade cues as part of the intervention strategies.

Natural prompts or cues are those cues that occur naturally within the environment. They may relate to the people, materials, or the task being performed. For example, if a child observes other family members washing their hands for dinner, he or she is given the cue to wash his or her hands. This cue can be embedded in multiple environments. Before eating a snack at school or eating out at a restaurant, all persons wash their hands.

## Adaptations to the Environment

In all the approaches discussed, the therapist uses the interaction between the child and the environmental contexts to improve performance. Physical environments may be adapted by changing architectural and other physical barriers. To facilitate wheelchair access, ramps may be installed or furniture may be moved. For example, the family computer may be placed on a more usable work surface and moved to a more accessible location so the child that is wheelchair dependent can use it for homework. For some children, therapists minimize stimuli and eliminate both visual and auditory distractions. Other children may require environmental stimulation from color, music, and objects.

▲ Table 17-4   Environmental Adaptations for the Home When Accessibility Is Limited

| Architectural Barrier | Structural Changes | Possible Assistive Devices | Task Modification |
|---|---|---|---|
| Entrances and Exits | Hand rails<br>Hand stairs<br>Ramp<br>Built-up terrain to door height<br>Stair lift<br>In-home elevator<br>Increased door width (33 to 36 inches minimum)<br>Step back hinges<br>Door rehinged to open in or out<br>Pocket door<br>Folding door<br>Electric door openers | Strapping or loop on door handle<br>Lever handles<br>Portable door knob<br>Built-up key holders<br>Combination locks<br>Environmental control unit | Use different entrance<br>Remove inside doors<br>Use curtains for privacy<br>Use hip or wheelchair to open doors |
| Bathrooms | Enlarged room<br>Sink mounted low<br>Open space under cabinet<br>Showers installed with a seat<br>Changed placement of tub faucets<br>Ramped shower stall<br>Toilet bidet installed<br>Linen closet shelves with no door | Safety rails<br>Seat reducer<br>Raised commode seat<br>Wheelchair commode<br>Step placed in front of commode<br>Insulated pipes<br>Single-lever faucets<br>Tub seats<br>Hydraulic lifts<br>Toilet paper tongs<br>Toilet paper mounting<br>Angled mirrors<br>Wall-mounted hairdryer with switch<br>Wheelchair shower chair | Free-standing commode in secluded area<br>Use a urinal<br>Empty leg bag into litter container<br>Bed bath<br>Sponge bath<br>Use liquid soap<br>Soap on a string<br>Shampoo pump<br>Dry shampoo |
| Bedroom | Bedroom on first floor<br>Enlarged space<br>Enlarged closet doors<br>Low closet pole<br>Closet storage system with shelves<br>Built-in bookshelves at low and medium heights<br>Cut holes in work surfaces for holding objects and electrical cords<br>Built-in dressers or dressers bolted to the wall<br>Special glides for wall drawers | Leg extenders<br>Bed rails<br>Firm mattress<br>Straps or rope ladders<br>Mounted shoe rack<br>Environmental control units or switches for television, radio, and light access<br>Enlarge or add loop to drawer handles<br>Positioning devices<br>Adaptive chairs | Place bed on floor<br>Keep most used clothes in accessible drawers<br>Use shelves instead of dresser drawers for clothes<br>Toys stored in shoe bag |
| Kitchen | Enlarged space<br>Lowered countertops<br>Lowered cabinets<br>Sink with no cabinets under it<br>Built-in range top<br>Sliding drawers and organizers in cabinet<br>Wall-mounted oven side by side<br>Dishwasher mounted higher<br>Front-opening washer | Adapted utensils<br>Automated learning devices for appliances turned on by switches<br>Adapted seats<br>Wheelchair laptray<br>Use barstool | Items most used in low cupboards<br>Bowls and pans hang on wall instead of in cabinet<br>Eat on wheelchair laptray instead of table<br>Water kept in insulated bottle with pump on table<br>Most-used items kept on accessible surfaces<br>Stool for washing dishes |

▲ Table 17-5   Stabilization Materials, Procedures, and Applications

| Materials | Application |
|---|---|
| Tape | Generally a temporary solution. Can be applied quickly as need arises; is inexpensive, and readily available in households, schools, and therapy units. Duct tape is sturdy, with good holding power. Masking and cellophane tapes are less sturdy, but widely used. |
| Nonslip pressure-sensitive matting | This can be ordered through therapy supply catalogs in rolls or pads and is becoming available to the public in kitchen stores. Minimizes slipping and sliding of objects with large bases that are placed on it. Small pieces can be glued to small objects to aid stabilization. These products rely on friction between materials for stabilization. |
| Suction cup holders | These holding aids are widely available in both stores and through therapy supply catalogs. Single-faced suction cups are generally permanently applied to a toy or object. Double-faced suction cups can be set up where suction is needed between the object and work surface. |
| C-clamps | These are readily available and suitable for securing flat objects to lay trays, table edges, and other surfaces. |
| Tacking putty | This product is sold for sticking posters onto a wall and is quite useful for holding lightweight objects on tables, lap trays, angle boards, walls, etc. |
| Pressure-sensitive hook and loop tapes (Velcro) | These tapes can be glued to the base of toys and other objects, and to play or work surfaces for stabilization. Soft loop tape can be used on areas that will contact the child's skin or clothing. |
| Wing nuts and bolts | In some cases it is possible to bolt toys and other objects to a table surface through holes drilled through the object and holding surface. This stabilizes objects more permanently. |
| Magnets | Magnets that are affixed to a toy can aid stabilization in metallic surfaces such as refrigerator doors, metal tables, and magnetic play boards. |
| L-brackets | These hardware store items are particularly effective for stabilizing items in an upright plane. Holes are drilled in both the work or play surface and the toy or other object to correspond with the L-bracket holes. Objects are then secured with nuts and bolts. |
| Soldering clamps | Small clamps are mounted to free-standing bases that are weighted, suction-cupped, or use clamps for stability. These are best used to hold small items for intricate play, hobbies, or work. |
| Elastic or webbing straps | Straps can be attached to toys to tie them down, or to play or work surfaces to secure flat objects. |

The physical environment is filled with useful tools, materials, and equipment that can be adapted. Children learn to eat with utensils; sit in chairs; read books, magazines, and newspapers; and write with pen and pencil. Occupational therapists often make adaptations to the tools and hardware within physical everyday environments to enhance a child's function. Typical adaptations include enlarging the object, adding pieces to the object, elongating pieces for better mechanical advantage, and amplifying the characteristic of the object.

Because changes to the physical environment affect other persons and activities and routines that take place in the same space (social environment), the therapist considers these interrelationships to arrive at workable solutions. Modifications to the environment include changes in structures, using assistive technology, and adapting materials or task expectations. Table 17-4 gives examples of how physical and social environments are adapted. This chart should be referred to when considering self-care and IADL activities.

## Work Surface

The work surface is conceptualized as any surface in the immediate environment that supports the child, materials, tools, and assistive devices in an activity (Eriksson et al., 1987). For example, the floor supports the child and toys during play activities. Adding a positioning device changes the orientation of the child to the floor and the toys.

Boundaries of the work space help children keep within usable or safe environments. For example, a play pen, a cut-out surface on a table or games board, or a lip on a wheelchair tray makes boundaries for children. Various textures, colors, and pictures are added to the work surface or play area to give sensory cues about boundaries and to motivate children. Even with these adaptations, some children continue to lose items off the surface. Table 17-5 gives suggestions for stabilizing objects placed on the work surface or when held by the child.

There are many other ways to adapt the work surface to enhance or modify an activity and the child's performance. Characteristics that are amenable to adaptation include

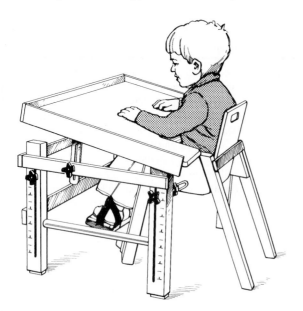

**Figure 17-2**   Commercially available chair with positioning components and a desk with an adjustable height and adjustable inclined work surface.

height, angle of incline (Figure 17-2), size, distance from the body, distance from other work areas, and general accessibility of a work surface. Changes in these characteristics enhance the child's function in varied ways, such as improving arm support, increasing the visual orientation of a task, adapting seat height for transfers, or improving table height for wheelchair access.

The position of the activity depends on the characteristics of the work surface. Activities are placed anywhere on or off a work surface. Positions are modified according to the child's needs. For example, if a child has left hemiplegia and left hemianopsia, placement of the toothpaste and toothbrush on the far right side of the work surface might be needed to cue the child to brush his or her teeth.

In the school environment, the height of tables and desks may need to be adjusted for wheelchair access. If a desk storage compartment interferes with leg clearance, another desk or small table without underneath storage should be provided for the child. If a computer or augmentative communication device is used on top of the desk, additional surface space is often needed. Table height must be adjusted so that the level of the keyboard is appropriate for the child. When several students share a computer, a height-adjustable table is appropriate.

## Positioning

Therapists consider the position of the child and the position of the materials or activity when planning intervention. A change in either position modifies a child's performance. For example, a child with a balance problem cannot put boots on while standing, but if the child sits on a firm bed (the work surface), he or she is independent in the task. If the same child is sitting on the bed, and the posi-

tion of the boots is changed from being placed beside the child to being on a shelf above the child's head, he or she cannot perform the task. Therapists modify where activities and materials are placed to meet different goals.

***Child position.*** Children who have problems with posture and movement often lack sufficient control to assume or maintain stable postures during activity performance and benefit from positioning adaptations. There are a variety of body positions for self-care and daily living tasks, and no one position is best. Lying down, sitting, and standing are the major positions used, with numerous options in each. When possible, the most typical position for a given activity is used, as are the lowest number of restrictions or adaptations to stabilize the body for function (Bergen, Presperin, & Tallman, 1990).

Alternative body positions are extremely helpful to children with disabilities. These changes help compensate for physical limitations in strength, joint movement, control, or endurance and provide relief to skin areas and bony prominences. They also allow children to experience different spatial relationships and thus develop a perceptual set for spatial orientation (Bergen & Colangelo, 1985; Ward, 1983) (see Chapter 14).

Appropriate positioning maximizes symmetric alignment of the skeleton, prepares children for movement, provides support that can free the hands for manipulation, allows participation in activities at a variety of developmental levels, and maximizes access to the environment (Ward, 1983).

External support is provided through the use of standard or special furniture, seating systems for wheelchairs, and use of physical handling techniques. These mechanisms support the child's posture and improve functional potential. Primitive or pathologic postural reflexes and unequal pull of muscles on joints can be mediated. Maximizing the child's ability to balance and shift weight with less effort facilitates a variety of functional movement patterns. More normalized sensory feedback is elicited and aids in learning new patterns of movement.

A therapist considers positions that maximize independent task performance. Key points for stability that enable the child to use available voluntary movement are the pelvis and trunk, the head, and the extremities. When muscle weakness occurs, the therapist determines where support is needed or, for the child with muscle tightness, whether a preferred and comfortable position is contraindicated. Looking carefully at the entire body of the child, the therapist asks the following questions:

1. Is the child **aligned properly?** Where are the hips, shoulders, and head in relation to the trunk? (Figure 17-3)
2. What positions or devices increase **trunk stability?** Inserting lateral supports? A surface for supporting the feet? Widening the sitting base by abducting the legs?
3. Does positioning in **sidelying** or **sitting** allow the

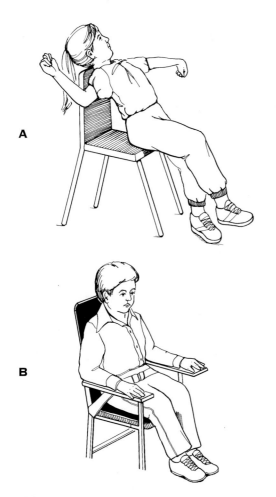

**A**

**B**

**Figure 17-3** Sitting postures. **A,** Incorrect sitting resulting from a massive extension pattern and an asymmetric tonic reflex posture. **B,** Correct sitting posture. Weight equally distributed on the sitting base and feet and elbows supported.

child to use balanced flexion and extension? Does it inhibit flexion patterns that are dominant in the prone position and the extension patterns seen in the supine position? Is adequate anterior, posterior, and lateral support provided?

***Classroom seating.*** In the school environment, sitting and sometimes standing are the most appropriate positions for the child to perform the visual-motor tasks required. In addition to postural alignment, the therapist recommends positions that provide the child with (1) good orientation of his or her body to the work surface and school materials, (2) good body and visual orientation to the teacher, (3) the ability to get to and leave workstations as independently as possible, and (4) physical proximity to other classmates.

Chair height may need to be modified so that the feet are flat to support postural stability and facilitate transfers. If seat height must be raised, a foot rest should be provided. Chair legs can be shortened or lengthened with blocks or leg extenders.

The occupational therapist often fabricates positioning

units for standard classroom chairs to enhance posture, fine motor performance, and the ability to attend. One or more of the following adaptations may be necessary. Seat back height and seat depth can be modified as needed. A seat belt may be added to stabilize the pelvis or chest. If more stability is needed, a wedge cushion or antithrust seat made from high-density foam or ethafoam can be added to the seat base to prevent hip extension. Small foam lumbar pads are useful for children with spontaneous trunk righting. These adaptations encourage a more neutral pelvic position and an erect spine. Lateral trunk supports are often needed for children with impaired trunk righting, equilibrium, and alignment. Lateral hip and thigh pads are helpful in centralizing the pelvis and maintaining a neutral thigh position. Abductor units are useful for limiting hip adduction or asymmetric hip position but should never be used to hold the child back in the seat. Contour seat backs behind the scapula can help mediate spinal hyperextension and shoulder retraction.

## SPECIFIC INTERVENTION TECHNIQUES FOR SELECTED SELF-CARE TASKS

Specific intervention strategies for toilet hygiene, dressing, bathing, oral hygiene, grooming, and functional communication are described in the following sections. Interrelationships between skills and contextual demands are considered. A combination of approaches and strategies described previously are employed to help children become as independent as possible in self-care tasks.

### Toilet Hygiene
#### Typical Developmental Sequence

Independent toileting is an important self-maintenance milestone with wide variation among individual children. It carries considerable sociologic and cultural significance. Self-sufficiency may determine participation in day care centers, school programs, recreational and community opportunities, and in secondary school vocational choices. Like other self-care tasks, toileting is a complex task requiring a series of learning subskills. But before embarking on learning this task, a child must be physically and psychologically ready. Also, parents or caregivers need to be ready to devote the time and effort to toilet training the child. A communication system between caregivers and the child is essential. At birth a newborn voids reflexively and involuntarily. Changes in position, handling by others, and other stimuli can trigger micturition. As the child matures, the spinal tract is myelinated to a level for bowel and bladder control at the lumbar and sacral areas and the child learns to control sphincter reflexes for the volitional holding of urine and feces. Children are often physiologically ready for toileting if they have a pattern of urine and feces elimination.

Bowel control precedes control over the bladder, and

▲ Table 17-6    Typical Developmental Sequence
of Toileting Skills

| Approximate Age | Toileting Skill |
|---|---|
| 10 months | Child indicates when wet or soiled |
| 12 months | Regularity of bowel movements |
| 15 months | Child sits on toilet when placed there and supervised (short time) |
| 18-21 months | Regularity of urination |
| 20 months | Toileting becomes regulated |
| 22 months | Child indicates need to go to the toilet |
| 24 months | Daytime control with occasional accidents Must be reminded to go to the bathroom |
| 30 months | Child tells someone he or she needs to go to the bathroom Child seats self on toilet |
| 34 months | Child goes to the bathroom independently |
| 3-4 years | Child may need help with clothing |
| 4-5 years | Completely independent |

Modified from Orelove, F. & Sobsey, D. (1991). Self-care skills. In F. Ore-love & D. Sobsey (Eds.). *Educating children with multiple disabilities* (2nd ed.) (p. 376). Baltimore: Brookes.

studies indicate that girls are trained an average of 2.46 months earlier than boys (Erickson, 1976). Independence in toileting includes getting on and off the toilet, managing fasteners and clothing, cleansing after toileting, and washing and drying hands efficiently without supervision. Progress is accomplished in sequence, according to each child's unique pace of development. Table 17-6 gives the typical developmental sequence for toileting.

### Typical Problems Interfering with Toileting Independence

***Loss of normal sensation and excretory function.*** Children with spinal cord injury, spina bifida, or other conditions that produce a full or partial paralysis require special management for bowel and bladder activities. Loss of control over these bodily functions can produce embarrassment and decreased feelings of self-esteem. School-aged children are characteristically modest about their bodies, and adolescents are struggling with identity issues and the need to be like their peers.

***Bladder control.*** There are two types of bladder problems. When there is a lesion in the lumbar region or below, the bladder is flaccid. The reflex arc is not intact, and the bladder has lost all tone. Sometimes this is called a lower motor neuron bladder. When an injury occurs higher, above the level of bladder innervation, the reflex arc remains intact. Thus when the bladder is full or its contents reach a critical level, it empties by reflex. In this situation the bladder is said to be a reflex bladder, an automatic bladder, or an upper motor neuron bladder. Training programs are undertaken for the upper motor neuron bladder to develop an automatic response. Children with a flaccid bladder cannot be trained because the bladder has no tone to empty.

Bladder training and management programs are determined after medical testing and collaborative discussions with children and their parents. Depending on medical test results, there are four main methods to manage urine: (1) condom catheterization (for males), (2) indwelling catheters, (3) intermittent catharizations (every 4 to 6 hours), and (4) ileal conduits. Fluid intake is restricted to prevent bladder distention. When there is partial control of bladder function, girls wear disposable diapers or incontinence pants that are available in various styles and sizes.

***Bowel control.*** A basic principle for success in bowel reeducation is to have a regular, consistent evacuation of the bowel. The time for this is a matter of choice, but there should be a schedule that remains constant. In some cases, suppositories and a warm drink are given before evacuation. This stimulates contractions and relaxation of muscle fibers within the walls of the intestine that move the contents onward. Other techniques include digital stimulation, massage around the anal sphincter, or manual pressure by Credé's method on the abdomen. Occasionally, removal of the stool by hand or a colostomy is recommended. Similar to an ileostomy, colostomy collection bags are emptied and cleansed on a regular basis.

***Assistive devices and adapted clothing.*** Although nurses are often the professionals who teach bowel and bladder control methods, the occupational therapist may be asked to get involved to provide assistive devices or to help design adapted methods. Children performing catheterizations or bowel programs may have difficulty in any of the following areas: maintaining a stable yet practical position so they can see what they are doing; hand dexterity; perceptual awareness; strength; range of motion; and stability and accuracy when emptying collection devices. Memory, safety, and sensory awareness are needed to use any of these procedures. Urinals, catheters, leg bag clamps, long-handled mirrors, positioning devices to provide postural stability or to hold legs open; and universal cuffs with a catheter or digital stimulator attached are some examples of assistive devices therapists may provide.

Closely associated with bowel and bladder care is **care of the skin** in the perineal area. Skin should be cleansed thoroughly to protect the tissue against contact with waste matter and to eliminate odor. All children with decreased sensation are susceptible to decubiti. These are pressure sores that occur fairly rapidly when blood vessels are compressed, such as around a bony prominence such as the ischial tuberosity. This can result in ischemia, or lack of tissue nourishment. Self-care of skin for these children includes daily inspection of the skin by mirror and avoiding sitting in one position for long periods. Also, a variety of special cushions designed to prevent tissue trauma are commercially available.

## Children With Limited Motor Skills

Diapering becomes a difficult task when infants or children have strong extensor and adduction patterns in their legs. Mothers are taught therapeutic methods to decrease extensor patterns before diapering, and these methods are incorporated into the diapering routine. For example, the mother may first place a pillow under the infant's hips, flex the hips, and slowly rock the hips back and forth before the legs spread apart for diapering.

Toileting independence may be delayed in children with limitations in tone, strength, endurance, range of motion, postural stability, and manipulation or dexterity. With unstable sitting posture, the child has difficulty relaxing and maintaining a position for pressing down and emptying the bowels. With weakness and limited range of motion, the child may be unable to manage fastenings because of hand involvement or may have problems in sitting down or getting up from the toilet seat because of hip-knee contractions or quadriceps weakness. Cleansing after a bowel movement may be difficult if the child cannot supinate the hand, flex the wrist, or internally rotate and extend the arm to cleanse after a bowel movement. An anterior approach may work. It is important to caution girls against contamination from feces, which can cause vaginitis. If at all possible, girls should wipe the anus from the rear. Solutions to cleansing problems are difficult and often discouraging.

## Children With Cognitive Limitations

Children with mental retardation take a longer period to learn toileting skills, but they often become independent (Orelove & Sobsey, 1991). Problems with awareness, initiation, sequencing, memory, and dexterity in managing their clothes are typical. As with all children, physiologic readiness for toileting is a prerequisite before beginning training programs. The therapist uses task analysis to determine which steps of the process are a problem. He or she then determines what cues and prompts are needed to achieve the child's best performance. Finally, the therapist evaluates which methods work as successful reinforcement (Snell, 1994). Foxx and Azrin (1973) developed a rapid method of training by giving persons with mental retardation multiple opportunities to go to the bathroom and be reinforced. In this procedure, fluid intake was increased and the person with mental retardation and the trainer literally spent the entire day in the bathroom repeating the toileting sequence and dry pants check. This program used behavior modification principles and gave positive reinforcement for toileting success.

## Aspects of the Environment That Influence Toileting Independence

Characteristics of physical and social environments at home or at school influence how a child manages toileting hygiene. Assisting children in determining where to perform the procedure and how to manage it within their home, school, and recreational environments is often a challenge. Social routines and expectations are also important variables to consider when making recommendations for managing toileting. These expectations depend on the child's age and abilities and how the family perceives the child's ability to manage this part of his or her self-care.

### Physical Environment

The bathroom is often the most inaccessible room in the house, yet it is essential that every family member has access to it. The floor space inside is rarely sufficient to permit turning a wheelchair for tub or toilet transfers. Adaptation possibilities include remodeling, selecting assistive devices, or devising alternative strategies to enhance independence. Adaptations to provide privacy are particularly important for the older child and adolescent. Caretaker needs are also addressed, as the child becomes heavier and more difficult to assist with toileting.

### Social Environment

Of all self-care tasks, toileting may require the most sensitive approach on the part of those who work with the child on a self-maintenance program. Children may purposely restrict their fluid intake at school in an effort to avoid the need for elimination. Unfortunately, then they get more infections and have more difficulty regulating the bowel and bladder.

Therapists help children who lack bowel and bladder control to develop routines and health habits that eliminate possible odors. Odors are produced by the collection devices or the collected urine or stool. Regular cleaning and changing of appliances (collection bags for ileal conduits and colostomies) and urine collection bags are learned and incorporated into schedules. Also a good fluid intake is recommended to prevent odors and bacteria growth.

### Adaptations for Unstable Posture

Before children sit independently on the toilet, they need to feel posturally secure. When toilet seats are low enough that the feet rest firmly on the floor, the accessory muscles that normally aid in defecation have the opportunity to fulfill their function.

Small children often need reducer rings to decrease the size of the toilet seat opening and thus improve sitting support. A step in front of the toilet helps small children get onto it. Safety rails that attach to the toilet or wall may assist with balance so that the child is safe to be left in privacy and use their hands freely. Free-standing commodes are used by the child who has outgrown small training potties and may be useful when wheelchair access to the bathroom is impossible. Units that roll into place over the toilet may be an option.

Finnie (1975) offered suggestions for adapting potty chairs and toilet seats for children with poor postural control. For example, she suggested placing the portable potty in a corrugated cardboard or wooden box until the child's balance improves. A bar can be attached across the top of the box for the child to hold onto for added security. Commodes that feature such modifications as adjustable legs, safety bars, angled legs for stability, and padded, upholstered, and adjustable backrests and headrests are available on the market. Commodes are also available with seat reducer rings, seat belts, and adjustable footrests.

### Other Adaptations

Simple, inexpensive aids include various types of toilet paper tongs and toilet paper holding devices. For the child with bilateral upper limb deficiency, a holding device clamped to the toilet seat is an option.

A combined bidet and toilet offers a means for total independence. Several models are available that attach to any standard toilet bowl. A self-contained mechanism spray-washes the perineal area with thermostatically controlled warm water, and dries it with a flow of warm air. Controls can be operated with the hand or foot (Figure 17-4). The unit is expensive but is worth considering, particularly for the sensitive adolescent.

For children who wear diapers, a full-length crotch opening with a zipper or Velcro closure makes changes easier. Girls may wear wrap-around or full skirts because these are easy to put on and adjust for toileting. Leg bags are reached and drained with greater ease when the child's pants have zippers or Velcro closures along the seams. Flies with long zippers or Velcro closures make it easier for boys to urinate when in wheelchairs.

## Menstruation

Menstruation normally begins between 10 and 17 years of age and is an important task for young girls to manage. If young girls are unable to take care of their own needs, the burden of this responsibility is given to the family or caregivers. This task may be aversive to others and embarrassing to the young girls who require assistance. In particular, in male, one-parent families, a daughter's inability to care

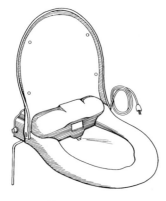

**Figure 17-4** Electrically powered bidet makes it possible to clean the perineal area independently without hands or paper.

for her feminine hygiene may be the reason residential treatment or alternative living arrangements are made.

Therapists need to realize the personal nature of discussing feminine hygiene needs with girls and their families. Based on the family's culture, this topic may be taboo for an outsider or any other family member to discuss. For this reason, families may prefer that therapists practice the techniques on dolls and use other simulated instruction methods instead of working with the adolescent directly (Epps, Stern, & Horner, 1990). The start of menstruation may be distressing to some parents as an indication of their child's puberty, and they may need support and counseling in ways of giving their child reassuring, understandable explanations.

The first experience with menstruation may offer the young woman with a disability an affirmation of equality with her peers (Duffy, 1981). Her body, although different in some ways, is operating normally in an area of particular significance, confirming her identity as a sexual being.

In performing feminine hygiene care, young girls with physical disabilities may have difficulty positioning themselves and the equipment, maintaining their balance, and manipulating materials. Therapists analyze the environments where the task is to occur and then suggest functional positions. For example, some children who are ambulatory may be able to put one leg on the toilet while inserting a tampon, and others function better by lying in bed or scooting down in their chairs. Positioning aids as previously discussed may help provide the support needed for postural control.

Disposable diapers in the toddler size, urinary incontinence pants, stick-on menstrual pads, and underwear with elastic straps to hold a menstrual pad are helpful solutions for manipulating materials. If the adolescent chooses to use tampons, there are a variety of brands to choose from that may work with the dexterity and postural control skills of the child. There are also adaptive devices to assist with insertion. Therapists may provide long-handled or standup mirrors or a universal cuff adaptations to assist in tampon insertion.

Girls with mental retardation have difficulty with judging how and when to perform feminine hygiene tasks and learning the sequence. Task analysis, repetition, and fading prompts are methods used to help adolescents with mental retardation independently perform this task (Epps et al., 1990).

## Dressing

### Typical Development

Independence in dressing usually takes 4 years of practice. Characteristically, learning to undress comes before learning to dress. This is an important guideline in setting expectations. Self-dressing is introduced in a natural way, at bedtime, by allowing the child to complete the final step in pulling off a garment. Similarly, when the child becomes more goal directed and motivated to be independent, he or she is ready to try the more difficult tasks of learning to put on clothing. Again, the caregiver begins by putting the garment on the child and then allowing the child to com-

▲ Table 17-7   Typical Developmental Sequence for Dressing

| Age (Years) | Self-Dressing Skills |
| --- | --- |
| 1 | Cooperates with dressing (holds out arms and feet) |
|  | Pulls off shoes, removes socks |
|  | Pushes arms through sleeves and legs through pants |
| 2 | Removes unfastened coat |
|  | Removes shoes if laces are untied |
|  | Helps pull down pants |
|  | Finds armholes in over-the head shirt |
| 2½ | Removes pull-down pants with elastic waist |
|  | Assists in pulling on socks |
|  | Puts on front-button coat or shirt |
|  | Unbuttons large buttons |
| 3 | Puts on over-the-head shirt with minimal assistance |
|  | Puts on shoes without fasteners (may be on wrong foot) |
|  | Puts on socks (may be with heel on top) |
|  | Independently pulls down pants |
|  | Zips and unzips jacket once on track |
|  | Needs assistance to remove over-the-head shirt |
|  | Buttons large front buttons |
| 3½ | Finds front of clothing |
|  | Snaps or hooks front fastener |
|  | Unzips from zipper on jacket, separating zipper |
|  | Puts on mittens |
|  | Buttons series of three or four buttons |
|  | Unbuckles shoe or belt |
|  | Dresses with supervision (needs help with front and back) |
| 4 | Removes pullover garment independently |
|  | Buckles shoes or belt |
|  | Zips jacket zipper |
|  | Puts on socks correctly |
|  | Puts on shoes with assistance in tying laces |
|  | Laces shoes |
|  | Consistently identifies the front and back of garment |
| 4½ | Puts belt in loops |
| 5 | Ties and unties knots |
|  | Dresses unsupervised |
| 6 | Closes back zipper |
|  | Ties bow now, buttons back buttons |
|  | Snaps back snaps |

Modified from Klein, M.D. (1983). *Pre-dressing skills.* Tucson: Communication Skill Builders.

plete the action. Gradually the child learns to do a little more, eventually accomplishing mastery. Table 17-7 gives the typical development of dressing skills.

It is easy to understand that children need eye-hand coordination for manipulating fastenings and knowledge of their physical selves and how body parts are related (Coley, 1978). They must know where their bodies are in space. They visually attend to arm and leg movements during dressing. Kinesthetically, they feel the position of their body parts, and many even verbalize motor actions aloud. They consciously direct some body movements, whereas other movements are automatic and compensatory, enabling them to maintain equilibrium in the various positions they assume. They are aware of the two sides of their bodies and, because of neurologic integration, are able to use their limbs cooperatively and reciprocally. Balance, range of motion, strength, and control of movement are needed.

Children visually perceive and analyze the clothing they don to distinguish boundaries of the clothing article. Visual scanning, visual discrimination, and figure-ground perception are required. Children also discriminate the form and totality of an article of clothing and categorize it as a sweater, shirt, sock, or other item. This is an extension of the sensory process that involves concept formation. Having identified a clothing article, children maintain a visual form constancy of it, even if it is turned upside down. Through experience they gain understanding of form and space, which is generalized to other activities of daily living, such as assisting with the laundry by folding and sorting clothes.

### Typical Problems and Intervention Strategies

*Perceptual problems.* From the description of the dressing process, some of the problems that may occur with dressing can begin to be predicted. Among those children who have perceptual deficits, difficulties may exist in distinguishing right and left sides of the body, putting a shoe on the correct foot, or turning the heel of a sock. A child may be unable to tell the front of his or her clothing from the back or identify which leg goes with which pant leg or which sleeve goes with which arm. If the child is observed closely, there may be evidence that the child avoids crossing the midline by performing dressing tasks on the right side of the body with the right hand and those on the left with the left hand. At the other end of the spectrum, a child most likely has great difficulty with fastening clothes and tying shoelaces, tasks that require both hands to work together.

*Intellectual limitations.* Children with mental retardation tend to be chaotic in their organization of perceptual stimuli and, in addition to problems with left-right discrimination, may be unable to make connections with words such as *above, behind,* or *in front of* insofar as their own bodies are concerned (Copeland et al., 1976).

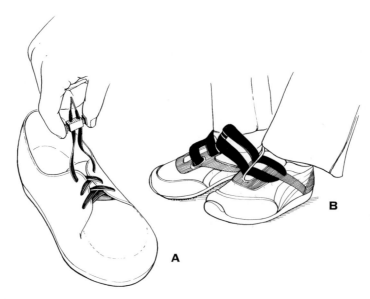

**Figure 17-5**   These shoelace fasteners can be managed with one hand. **A,** Spring tension blocks. **B,** Velcro fasteners.

The child who has intellectual limitations cannot remember instructions and has a short attention span. Behaviorally, there may be a low tolerance for frustration because the child cannot perform and dress as quickly as his or her siblings can. Language skills may be inefficient, which restricts the child's verbal capacity to express frustration. This may increase when the child is faced with tasks that require fine manipulations. Coordination too may be impaired, as shown in attempts to button, snap, zip, or buckle.

To acquire independence, the child may require a special approach. After making a baseline assessment, the therapist carefully analyzes each dressing task into its fine component parts. After determining the task analysis, backward and forward chaining methods are used and reinforcement is given for the correct completion of a task (Copeland et al., 1976).

*Physical limitations.* Children with various conditions find dressing difficult because of the **coordination** and the range and strength required for pulling clothes on and off and connecting fasteners. Youngsters with arthritis who have painful fingers frequently require assistance during a flare-up of their disease. They may be unable to move their arms freely and to reach certain areas of their body. Children with the use of only one hand find it difficult to zip trousers, tie shoelaces, and button shirts or blouses. Dressing is tedious and tiring. In most cases they learn compensatory techniques, often through their own experimentation, or use assistive technology. Children with abnormal muscle tone and retained postural reflexes often have difficulty balancing themselves or positioning their bodies while donning and removing clothing. Limited dexterity may also interfere with dressing. Tasks can be made easier by using simple measures such as proper positioning, dressing the involved extremity first, or by using adaptive aids such as button hooks, rings on zippers, one-handed shoe fasteners, or Velcro closures (Figure 17-5).

## Dressing Infants and Children with Motor Limitations

Although the common approach to dressing an infant is to do so while he or she is lying supine, the supine position frequently increases extensor tone in those infants with neurologic impairment. For that reason, some therapists advocate placing the infant prone across one's knees with the infant's hips flexed and abducted, thus inhibiting the extensor-adduction tone. As soon as the infant gains head and trunk control, he or she can be dressed in a sitting position with his or her back resting against and supported by the caregiver's trunk. In this arrangement the infant has an opportunity to observe his or her body. Knowledge of the physical self is to be encouraged whenever possible. As early as 14 months some infants begin to point to a named body part.

During dressing, the caregiver carefully bends the infant's hips and knees before putting on his or her shoes and socks (Figure 17-6), and brings the infant's shoulders forward before putting his or her arm through a sleeve. Attention is continually directed to positioning and to keeping the body in a symmetric alignment. When a child achieves sitting balance, a good way to proceed with dressing is to place the child on the floor and later on a low stool, continuing to provide support where needed from the back. Orientation to the body and its various parts should remain a focus in the social interaction. The caregiver can help the child understand how his or her body relates to his or her clothes and to the various positions—the arm goes through a sleeve and the head goes through the neck of a garment.

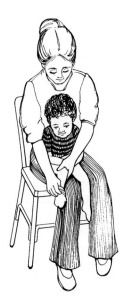

**Figure 17-6** When dressing the child who is hypertonic, the hip and knee should be carefully flexed before putting on socks and shoes.

There are many perceptual concepts to be explored and learned as a part of the dressing procedure.

When the child is older and heavier, there may be no alternative but to dress the child while he or she is sidelying or lying supine. Placing a hard pillow under the child's head, thus raising his or her shoulders a little, will make it easier to bring the child's arms forward and to bend his or her hips and knees. If it is possible to maintain the child in a sidelying position, this posture may make it easier to bring the child's shoulders and head forward, to bring his or her arm forward, and to straighten his or her elbow (Figure 17-7).

## Special Techniques and Adaptive Equipment for Self-Dressing

### Positioning and Support

The child who has hand skills but poor balance may be able to take advantage of the function he or she possesses when in a sidelying position with the effect of gravity lessened. For the child who can sit but is unstable, a corner of two adjoining walls or a corner seat on the floor may provide enough postural support for independent dressing. Finnie (1975) suggested using chairs as supporting devices while the child either kneels on the floor or stands holding on, particularly when balancing on one leg, as when pulling on pants.

Associated reactions may occur as the child starts to use both hands. Thus one hand may be needed for holding on while the other hand performs the task. Many dressing tasks require bilateral use of the hands. Sitting balance is more precarious as one reaches out with the arms, which occurs

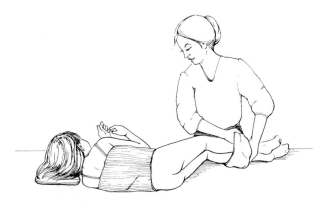

**Figure 17-7** Sidelying may decrease tone and make dressing easier.

frequently when donning overhead garments and reaching to the periphery of the body; therefore additional external support is needed.

The occupational therapist helps improve the child's dressing skills by offering the parent and child a variety of ways to solve problems from which the child and parents may choose. The following outline offers choices in problem solving, either through clothing selection and changes or by use of a technique or adaptive equipment that is feasible for the child.

***Pull-up garments.*** Clothing aids that facilitate independence include loops sewn inside the waistbands of pants and skirts to assist with pulling; elasticized waistbands, provided the bands do not restrict pulling movements; and pressure tape as a substitute for conventional fastenings. If zippers are used, the grasping surface can be enlarged by adding a metal ring or fabric loop. A dressing stick may be used when limited range of motion of the lower extremities or trunk hinders donning pants or other articles of clothing that are pulled onto and up the legs. For the child who is unstable in standing, sitting or lying on the floor is encouraged so that once the feet are through the pant legs or skirt band, the child can roll to either side while pulling up the waistband. If trunk balance allows, the child may kneel to pull up the garment once the waistband is above the knees. Having a chair close by is useful for support.

***Pullover garments.*** The most important feature for ease in donning pullover shirts and sweaters is an easy opening for the head. It should be a neckline that expands, such as one made of rib-knit fabric. In addition, flexible, elasticized waistbands and large sleeve openings are helpful. Stretchy knit fabrics allow children to experiment with movements as they gradually become more efficient in dressing.

For perceptual orientation it is helpful to have the child lay the garment on the lap, floor, or table, front side down. Then, reaching out and opening the bottom of the garment, one arm can be pushed into the corresponding, or ipsilateral, sleeve followed by the arm on the other side. After the arms are in the sleeves, the bottom of the garment can be grasped with one hand and pulled over the head.

If the fabric has sufficient give and the child has adequate trunk balance, an alternate technique is to pull the garment over the head and then hold a sleeve open with one hand while pushing the other arm through. This movement is repeated on the other side. An important point for making dressing easier is to always put clothing on the affected limb first.

***Front-opening garments.*** Selecting clothes with sleeves as loose as possible also applies to front-opening shirts, jackets, and sweaters. Fullness in the back of the garment through pleats, gathers, or gussets allows more freedom in movement. One of the most common techniques used by children with coordination or weakness problems is flipping the garment over the head. This is done by laying the garment on the lap, floor, or table (front side up) with the neck of the garment closest to the body. The child then puts an arm in each sleeve, working each down until the hand is visible. The next step is to duck the head forward while extending the arms over the head. Shrugging the shoulders and pulling down with the arms helps the garment fall down into place.

***Buttons.*** Buttoning can be avoided by selecting pull-over styles or by sewing buttons on the right side of the garment and using hook-loop tape for fastening. When buttoning is introduced, flat buttons large enough to grasp and buttons that are not sewn on tightly are easily manipulated. Buttons with shanks may be easier to grasp. The location of buttons affects the child's success in fastening. To reinforce success, the buttons should be easy to see, possibly of a contrasting color, and easy to reach. The child begins buttoning with the bottom button so that it is possible to see the hands working. Having once secured the bottom button, it becomes easier to line up the others. Clothing adaptations are often helpful. Buttons on sleeve cuffs may be sewn on with elastic thread to allow the buttoned cuff to stretch open enough for the hand to slide through.

***Zippers.*** When possible, parents should test zippers at the time garments are purchased to ensure glides are easy. In general, nylon coil zippers are pliable and less likely to snag than metal ones. The occupational therapist instructs the child in how to make the zipper taut by holding the garment below the zipper with one hand while pulling up the zipper tab with the other. To pull up a side zipper with one hand, the child holds the bottom of the zipper by leaning against a steady table or a wall. Zipper openings may also be adapted with Velcro to minimize the fine dexterity demands of the task. Zipper rings and zipper pull handle devices can facilitate grasp of the tab while working the zipper.

***Socks.*** Children are frequently frustrated when attempting to don socks because the socks may be too tight and unyielding or the tops may be edged with tight elastic. Soft, stretchy fabric and a larger size alleviate strain in pulling. Tube socks eliminate problems with heel placement. Sewing loops on both sides of the socks may make them easier to pull into place. Folding or rolling down the upper part of the sock over the foot of the sock can make sock donning more successful for the child.

If the child wears a brace or cast or if he or she has sensitive feet, footwarmers or boots made of a soft flannel or velour may be practical. These can be made larger than the foot and can be tightened by a single Velcro strap. Slippers with nonskid bottoms should be used.

***Shoes.*** Styles that provide a broad, long opening help children who have limited ankle motion. Tabs at the heel help the child to pull the shoe on. Pressure-sensitive tape closures eliminate lacing and tying. As previously suggested, shoes can be put on more easily if the leg is flexed and toes are pointed down. As the foot slides forward, the child is encouraged to push down at the heel. Loose laces allow wide opening of the shoe. Long-handled shoehorns and tabs on the heels of some sport shoes can be helpful when learning to don shoes.

### Special Considerations in Clothing

***For children sitting.*** Most clothing is made for individuals in a standing position. For those who spend long hours in a wheelchair, the sitting position can cause pulling and strain on some areas of the garment and a surplus of fabric in others. Alterations can be made to provide more comfort in sitting (Kennedy, 1981; Kernaleguen, 1978), for example, pants that are cut higher in the back and lower in the front and cut larger to give additional room in the hips and thighs. A longer inseam also allows the proper hem height for pants when sitting (rests on top of shoe). No pockets are placed on the back because they may cause sheering or skin breakdown with prolonged sitting. Instead, pockets can be placed on the top of the thigh or on the side of the calf for easy access. Front and side seams can be sewn with Velcro fasteners or zippers and wrist loops to pull them up. Pullover tops with raglan and gusset sleeves allow more room when maneuvering the wheelchair. If the shirt is cut longer in the back and shorter in the front, it is easier to keep a neat appearance. Rain capes or winter capes are comfortable in a wheelchair. They are cut longer in the front to cover the child's legs and feet, and shorter in the back so they do not rub against the wheel of the chair.

***For children who wear braces.*** The child who wears a brace may need to have clothing reinforced to protect against rubbing. Ideas include sewing fabric patches inside the garment where friction and stress occur and adapting the pants with side seams and Velcro closures to help get them over the brace.

## Adapted Clothing

Increased attention to the needs of individuals with disabilities has been shown over the last decade, with some adaptive clothing becoming available through catalogue supply companies. Because of marketing volume, there is a limited range of choice and a higher cost-per-item factor, but a beginning has been made to provide attractive, functional clothing.

Parents should be encouraged to purchase attractive, fashionable clothing that meets functional requirements, yet conforms in appearance to the child's peer group standards and fashion trends. Modifications should be inconspicuous, and, in general, the appearance of the clothing should not single out the wearer in any way. When possible, clothing should conceal physical impairments or at least not attract attention to them. The clothing should contribute to the wearer's sense of well-being. Functionally, the design of the clothing should enable the wearer to take care of personal needs as much as possible, help maintain proper body temperature, and provide freedom of movement.

### Selection of Clothing

As community living is considered, independence in dressing involves choosing appropriate styles and color combinations. Confidence in one's appearance is essential to an individual's sense of worth. Good grooming and attractive clothing invite positive responses from others. When children present a pleasant image to their peer group, they receive positive messages of acceptance that help shape a healthy self-concept.

For children who need assistance in this area, others in the environment can assist them by placing clothes together that match on the same hanger or in the same location. Color coding, consistent feedback, and establishing a weekly routine can result in appropriate clothing selection. Self-correction, by looking in the mirror, should also be reinforced.

## Bathing or Showering
### Typical Development

A child's interest in bathing begins before age 2, when he or she begins to wash while in the tub. By age 4, children are able to wash and dry themselves with supervision. It takes another 4 years, until the child is 8 years old, when he or she can independently prepare the bath and shower water (i.e., amount and temperature) and independently wash and dry himself or herself.

Good grooming habits are important for all children but take on added significance for children with disabilities. At an early age the child with a disability needs to be encouraged and helped to achieve cleanliness to maintain his or her health. Bathing should be a pleasurable activity, but for the parent of a child who lacks balance it can be a tedious task that requires constant attention and alertness. The work involved multiplies as the child grows and becomes larger and heavier.

Cultural expectations and social routines for bathing vary immensely and should be considered when assessing a child's independence. Family preferences on how often a person bathes and with whom (e.g., parent and children bathing together) must be respected.

### Adapted Techniques

Finnie (1975) outlined a number of measures to make bathing easier. As has been stressed repeatedly, positioning and handling are prime considerations. The child with a strong startle reaction should receive special mention because triggering the reaction can result in sudden loss of balance. Keeping the child's head and arms forward before lifting and maintaining them there while lowering the child into the tub are advisable. Finnie suggested handling the child slowly and gently, and when the child is old enough, telling him or her what is going to happen next, including turning the water faucets on and off and draining water from the tub. It is a good idea to drain the tub and wrap the child in a towel before lifting him or her from the tub.

### Assistive Technology for Positioning

Making the child feel safe and secure can also be aided by special equipment that gives the support needed. There are bath hammocks that fully hold the body and enable the parent to wash the child thoroughly (Figure 17-8, *A*). A simple, inexpensive way for giving security is to use a plastic laundry basket lined with foam at its bottom (Figure 17-8, *B*). Commercially, a light, inconspicuous bath support (Figure 17-8, *C*) offers good design features. The front half of the padded support ring swings open for easy entry and then locks securely, holding the child at the chest to give trunk stability. Various kinds of bath seats and shower benches are available for the older child to aid bathtub seating transfers (Figure 17-8, *D*).

For the child with severe motor limitations who is lying supine in the tub in shallow water, a horseshoe-shaped inflatable bath collar (Figure 17-8, *E*) serves to support the neck and keep the child's head above water level. A bath stretcher is constructed like a cot and fits inside the bathtub rim level or mid tub level to minimize the caregiver's bending while transferring and bathing the child.

Some parents and children find a hand-held shower useful in removing soap suds. A long-handled bath brush or sponge helps in reaching body parts. Children with limited grasp may be able to wash themselves using a pump soap dispenser and a bath mitt.

### Safety Issues

Nonslip bath mats are essential for safety, both beside the tub and in the tub. Grab bars and their placement require careful thought and planning in each individual case. A rubber cover for the bathtub faucet can prevent injury if the child slips and hits his or her head.

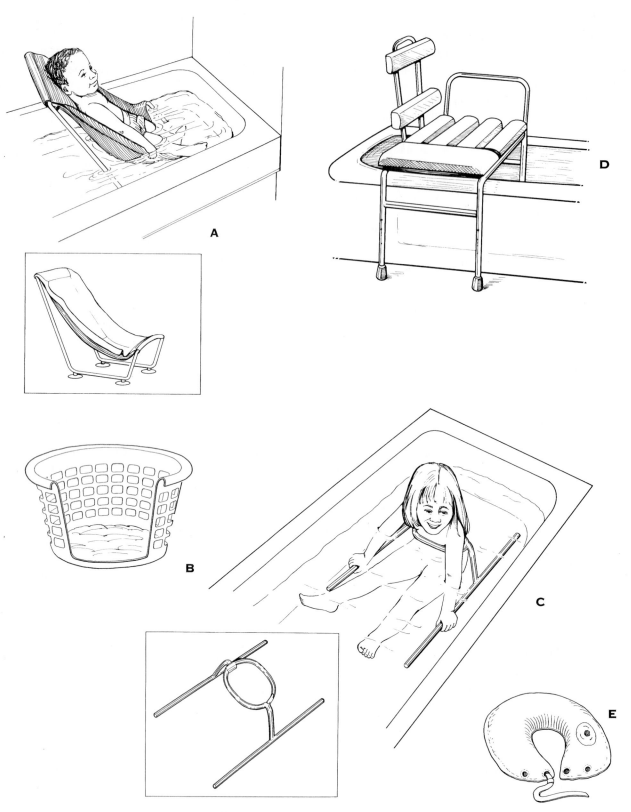

**Figure 17-8** Adapted seating equipment for bathing. **A,** The hammock chair is adjustable and equipped with oversized suction feet. It fully supports the child who has no sitting balance and poor head control. **B,** The front of a plastic laundry basket is cut out to allow room for the child's legs. The basket gives security during first baths in a large tub. **C,** Trunk support is lightweight and compact and fits all bathtubs. **D,** Shower bench aids seating and transfers. **E,** Inflatable bath collar can be used when the child is in either the supine or prone position.

Parents should be taught to use good body mechanics during bathing to prevent back injury. To lessen strain, it is best for the adult to sit on a stool beside the tub or kneel on a cushion. Lifting is done with knees bent and back straight, using legs for power. As children get older and heavier, a hoyer lift or easily accessed shower stall arrangement may be necessary.

## Oral Hygiene
### Typical Development

By the time children are 2, they imitate parents brushing their teeth. Toothbrushing supervision continues until about age 6 when children are able to brush their teeth without adult supervision. By age 9 or 10, some children acquire braces and need to learn a new set of skills related to oral hygiene.

### Problems and Intervention Strategies

Toothbrushing can be especially difficult for the child with oral sensitivity. For that and other reasons, when assistance is given, the teeth should be brushed slowly and gently. This helps prevent fear of the toothbrush. A small, soft brush is easier to move around in the mouth, especially if the child has a tongue thrust or gag reflex. When the gums are tender, a soft sponge tip called a toothette can be substituted for a brush. This is a disposable product.

If a child has problems with a weak grasp, the handle can be enlarged with sponge rubber, or if necessary a Velcro strap can be added. When the difficulty is a matter of wrist coordination and arm movement, an electric toothbrush can be evaluated for use. This proves to be a good solution in some cases, but the unit may be too heavy for certain children to manage. Some electric toothbrushes have dual controls, moving from side to side and up and down, allowing for good cleaning of the teeth and gums. To help with managing toothpaste, a long handle attached to the bottom of the tube helps in squeezing paste onto the brush.

## Grooming
### Typical Development

Face washing, handwashing, and hair care are typical grooming activities. The timing for developing grooming independence is highly influenced by the child's culture, family values, and individual interests. Adolescence begins at the onset of puberty and is a period of remarkable growth toward physical and sexual maturity as well as emotional and social maturity. The physiologic changes that occur at puberty are attributable, in part, to the increased output of hormones by the pituitary gland. For example, body hair grows and the sebaceous glands become more active, producing oily secretions. New self-maintenance tasks emerge with these physical changes.

### Intervention Strategies

*Hair care.* A simple style and good haircut are among the easiest ways to facilitate hair care, but children want to identify with their peers and observe current fads. For a child with incoordination, it is sometimes less tiring and gives greater stability when the child supports both arms or wrists on a table or against his or her body while combing or brushing his or her hair. A large comb or brush with a thick handle may be easier for the child to use. Holding the brush closer to the bristles or on back of the bristles may give more control. A mirror at the proper height and angle should be placed so that progress with personal grooming can be checked (Figure 17-9). When the child is unable to reach his or her head, extended brush handles or a hairdryer firmly attached to a gooseneck can be tried.

Children who are tactilely defensive may hide from the hairbrush or comb or scream during shampooing. They need to have input on what type of hairbrush feels good to them. In general, usually brushes with few flexible, plastic, rubber-tipped bristles are preferred. Before shampooing, remedial techniques such as deep pressure on the body or head may make the child more receptive to tactile input. A hose attached to the faucet helps when washing hair over a basin or tub. If flexibility of the neck is a problem, a plastic shampoo tray can be fitted around the neck to direct water and suds away from the face.

*Fingernail care.* Caring for fingernails is often a trial for any child but is especially difficult when there are coordination problems or when the child has use of only one hand. A child may be able to file his or her fingernails if an emery board is taped to the edge of a table. Fingernail clippers nailed to a board with an elongated handle taped onto it allows one-handed fingernail cutting.

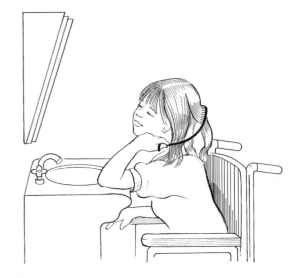

**Figure 17-9** Specially adapted comb and mirror at the proper height and angle can facilitate independence in grooming.

***Hair removal.*** Shaving is often simplified with the use of an electric razor. Although it is heavier, it can be safer and requires less precision. It also eliminates shaving soap and the need to handle blades. Electric razors can be adapted with holders for those with weak or impaired grasp. Lightweight disposable safety razors eliminate blade changing and can be easily adapted with built-up handles to facilitate grasp or with a long handle to accommodate limited reach or range of motion.

***Skin care.*** Regular face washing and bathing are important to manage increased body secretions and skin conditions accompanying adolescence. Use of deodorant, perfumes, and facial ointments for excessive oils or acne become important. Children can be assisted in developing these routines by structuring the environment with natural cues. For example, instead of being put in a closet, cleansing solutions are left out at the sink with a jar of cotton balls. Deodorant kept on the dresser in full view reminds adolescents to put it on before dressing. Choice of containers and types of grooming aids may determine if adolescents can or will use them.

***Make up.*** Girls often become interested in using makeup when they reach adolescence. The therapist often becomes involved in adapting self-care product containers to permit independent use. To accommodate weak grasp, jar lids may be left loose. Transferring ointments to pump containers can reduce the hand dexterity needed to use the product. Lipstick or mascara tubes can be built up with foam rubber tape for ease of handling. Girls with ataxia can prop arms on the counter to give them more stability and accuracy while applying makeup. Modeling and pictorial cues may help with self-correcting behaviors for girls who apply too much makeup.

## Functional Communication

Children learn how to send and receive messages to and from other people through verbal, nonverbal, and graphic communication systems. Children who are nonverbal may use gestures, writing, or assistive devices to communicate their needs. This chapter discusses emergency systems and telephones (see Chapter 19 for improving handwriting skills and Chapter 20 for augmentative communication and computer access).

### Emergency Alert and Call Systems

Children with serious medical problems or with life support systems need more frequent monitoring both day and night. This need becomes more critical when children have impaired mobility, dexterity, or communication skills. Intercom systems assist parents with this responsibility and give the child a way to initiate calls for help or social interaction. Call switches or buzzers that attach to the bed or wheelchair can provide an independent means of seeking assistance from individuals in other rooms. A variety of portable intercoms and inexpensive environmental control units are available at electronic supply stores and children's stores. Sometimes a portable phone is the safest device to have. This phone can be carried with the child around the house and can be used as a telephone or an intercom, depending on the model chosen.

Emergency alert systems, worn as pendants or stabilized on wheelchairs, can be purchased with a service that places emergency calls when the system is activated. Outside alarms that can be heard in the neighborhood can be used to summon assistance. Arrangements and alternatives must be carefully planned and made in advance. An attendant or visiting nurse can come to the house at prescribed intervals to assist with specific functions such as toileting. The ability to get out of the house is most directly influenced by the child's ability to get to the door, open it, and get out.

### Telephones

Changes in telephone design have improved access for children with disabilities. Phones may have large numbers and many features like redial, preprogrammed phone numbers, and built-in intercoms or amplifiers. These features are useful for children with limited dexterity and limited abilities to sequence or remember phone numbers. For children with auditory limitations, special phones with lights and vibration or a telecommunication device for the deaf may be used.

If dexterity or endurance is problematic, phones are mounted on goosenecks or used with an attached universal cuff to hold it. Buttons are dialed with a T-bar or universal cuff with a pencil. Instead of writing messages down, the answering machines can record the messages. Some adolescents record a message asking the caller to "keep on ringing until I can get to the phone!"

### Other Self-Care Skills

Families and therapists encourage children to be responsible for all aspects of self-care. Caring for personal devices (e.g., hearing aids, wheelchairs, or splints), taking medications, and being responsible for health maintenance generally become realistic expectations for children with disabilities as they mature. Children can partially participate in any of these tasks if they cannot perform them independently. The child with motor limitations can learn to direct others on how to change wheelchair batteries or inflate tires. Charts, daily or weekly medicine boxes, or special watches with alarms can cue children with memory problems to take medications. As children make decisions about their health routines, they learn firsthand what happens if they do not follow bowel and bladder programs or develop routines for physical fitness or proper nutrition. Activities that promote the development of problem solving skills and help children gain confidence in their abilities to be self-sufficient are critical to the child's development of self-care independence.

## Home Management Tasks

During childhood, children learn home management tasks that help them contribute to family functioning. Performing these tasks give children a feeling of self-worth and develop skills for independent living and work environments. Home management tasks include cleaning, clothing care, meal preparation and clean up, shopping, money manage-

▲ Table 17-8    Definitions of Home Management Skills for Children*

| Tasks | Typical Activities |
|---|---|
| Cleaning | Picks up and puts away toys and other items; sweeps; mops; dusts; vacuums; cleans tables and other surfaces; empties trash; makes bed |
| Meal preparation and clean up | Plans a meal; sets and clears table; gets utensils and food items; opens containers and makes a food item; uses appliances; cleans up (e.g., washes pots and pans and utensils, uses diswasher); stores food safely |
| Clothing care | Puts clothes in dirty laundry; sorts; folds; uses appliances (washing machine and dryer); irons; puts clothes away; mends |
| Shopping | Makes shopping list; selects, obtains, and purchases items at drug store, convenience store, grocery store, and others; pays for items correctly |
| Money management | Manages allowance; saves to buy special items; budgets for school, recreation, and other needs |
| Household maintenance | Does yardwork and gardening; washes car; cleans appliances (e.g., cleaning heads to video or cassette recorder); cleans refrigerator and oven; makes simple repairs with tools; changes a light bulb |
| Safety precautions | Takes precautions to prevent injuries (knows to pick up toys or other items so others do not fall on them); uses appliances correctly around water |

*Definitions and categories adapted from AOTA Uniform Terminology (3rd ed). 1994.

ment, and household maintenance (AOTA, 1994) (see Appendix 8-A). All of these tasks are done with safety in mind. Table 17-8 gives examples of what activities may be involved in these tasks for children and young adolescents.

### Typical Developmental Sequence

As early as 18 months, children begin to understand what it means to "help out" in performing household chores. As young children observe their parents routinely dust, sweep, set tables, or do laundry, they often initiate doing a task without any cues from a parent (Rheingold, 1982). "Me do it" or "I want to sweep" are typical comments. As children get older, they become more capable of performing household chores, and parents often wish that enthusiasm for helping around the house continued. Instead, adolescents

▲ Table 17-9    Developmental Sequence for Home Management Tasks

| Age | Task |
|---|---|
| 13 months | Imitates housework |
| 2 years | Picks up and puts away toys with parental reminders |
| | Copies parents domestic activities |
| 3 years | Carries things without dropping them |
| | Dusts with help |
| | Dries dishes with help |
| | Gardens with help |
| | Puts toys away with reminders |
| | Wipes spills |
| 4 years | Fixes dry cereal and snacks |
| | Helps with sorting laundry |
| 5 years | Puts toys away neatly |
| | Makes a sandwich |
| | Takes out trash |
| | Makes bed |
| | Puts dirty clothes away |
| | Answers telephone correctly |
| 6 years | Does simple errands |
| | Does household chores without redoing |
| | Cleans sink |
| | Washes dishes with help |
| | Crosses street safely |
| 7 - 9 years | Begins to cook simple meal |
| | Puts clean clothes away |
| | Hangs up clothes |
| | Manages small amounts of money |
| | Uses telephone correctly |
| 10 - 12 years | Cooks simple meal with supervision |
| | Does simple repairs with appropriate tools |
| | Begins doing laundry |
| | Sets table |
| | Washes dishes |
| | Cares for pet with reminders |
| 13 - 14 years | Does laundry |
| | Cooks meals |

become more absorbed in personal grooming or social activities and participate less in household chores (Duckett, Rafaelli, & Richards, 1989). Table 17-9 outlines the developmental sequence for learning to perform home management tasks.

## Contextual Considerations

Participation in home management tasks depends on child's age and capabilities and the temporal and environmental contexts. The size of the family and the accessibility of the environment can encourage or discourage participation in household chores. Age, gender, socioeconomic status, geographic location (Light, Hertsgaard, & Martin, 1985), and customs and values about self-sufficiency (Lynch & Hanson, 1992) may influence when and how chores are performed. Girls often do more chores than boys (Seymour, 1988), and furthermore, they may choose more cooperative, indoor chores than boys, who choose more independent outdoor chores (e.g., washing the car, and lawn care) (Duckett et al., 1988). Children from low socioeconomic environments may be expected to do more chores (Seymour, 1988), and adolescents in rural areas may be expected to perform more farm chores than household chores (Light, et al., 1985). Families may encourage independence or they may promote interdependency among family members. Therapists need to consider these factors when working with children and their families.

The family's modeling behaviors, patience, routines, and expectations as well as the child's preferences influence which chores children do. Children observe others doing chores and are given explanations for what is being done and why. For example, mothers or fathers say, "I'm washing the table because it is sticky." They may further elaborate on this statement by saying, "If I leave it sticky, then your paper and clothes will get sticky when you color." As the child gets older, sanitary and health explanations may be given. This role modeling of chores by all family members is important to establishing household chores are routine and expected. If household chores are done chaotically or rarely, children may not be included in "helping out" roles nor learn the typical routine to complete household maintenance.

When children with or without disabilities first begin to wash tables, dust, or vacuum, extra time and patience from the parent is necessary as well as modified expectations for performance. Instructions may be repeated and tasks often are redone, taking more time than if parents had completed the task themselves. Children are given time to problem solve and ideally should be allowed to learn from their mistakes.

## Performance Problems in Household Tasks

Development of household skills are often overshadowed by the medical-physical or educational needs of a child with a disability. Occupational therapists collaborate with parents to set up routines and modify tasks and environments so the child can perform all or a portion of household tasks.

Children with sensorimotor problems may have difficulty obtaining materials, manipulating and using typical equipment, or completing the entire task. Children with cognitive limitations may have difficulty initiating and terminating the task, following and remembering the sequence, and generalizing the skills to other environments (e.g., differences in cleaning kitchen and living room floors). When a child has a low frustration level and poor impulse control, parents may be fearful to give them tasks that could potentially be unsafe.

## Strategies for Performing Household Tasks

Environmental modifications, assistive technology, task modification, and varying levels of help from others are often the approaches used for teaching home management tasks. Refer to Table 17-4, which gives examples of how various environments in the home may be adapted with structural changes and assistive devices to allow the child to participate in household tasks.

## Transporting, Carrying, and Putting Equipment Away

Household items, toys, or equipment kept on low and open shelves or all in one bucket helps the child obtain and put away supplies. When children can not reach the sink to obtain water from the faucet, they may use a pump beverage dispenser.

Carrying the supplies to the needed location may be accomplished by using lapboards with lips, cut-out holes or "saddle bags"; carts, buckets, or trash cans on wheels; aprons with pockets or fanny packs (i.e., zippered pouch worn around the waist), or divided boxes or utensil drawers with handles. Hook-loop tape, nonslip matting, and other items listed in Table 17-5 can assist the child in stabilizing items.

If memory is a problem, all the needed supplies may be kept near where they are going to be used. For example, the bathroom sponge is placed on the bathroom sink. This natural cue helps the child find the object and might remind him or her to clean the sink after toothbrushing or face washing. Artificial cues such as color coding or labeling shelves, cabinets, and bins with pictures or words also help children locate objects within the environment.

## Selecting and Modifying Equipment

Selecting equipment that is easy to handle and allows the child to perform contextual roles is ideal, but this option is not always available when families already have an array of household equipment. For example, a front-opening washer or double-sided refrigerator may make tasks easier to perform for a child in a wheelchair. A microwave on a countertop can be safer to use than an oven.

Children with range of motion, strength, dexterity, or postural control problems may need equipment modified. When cleaning table surfaces, typical equipment may include: dusting or wiping mitts, crumb sweepers, sponges with plastic handles, and spray bottles with cleaning solutions in them. Long-handled dustpans, dusters, or buckets on wheels with a stick attached may help the child who cannot bend forward. Broom, mop, and vacuum handles can be cut to the child's size, enlarged, or adapted with additional pieces to allow the child to hold them.

## Modification of Task and Task Expectations

Children with intellectual limitations may encounter problems with sequencing, judgment, and performing the tasks on a regular basis (Browder & Snell, 1993). These children may need pictorial cues in the form of a chart on the wall or a flip card book. The charts list the steps of a task or a sequence of tasks (e.g., task analysis), and the child checks off each step or task when it is completed. The picture allows the child to judge if he or she has done the task correctly; for example, the child can refer to a placemat with predrawn plate and utensil on it when setting the table. If these materials have an acetate or plastic covering they can be used routinely with a washable marker. As the child learns the task, pictorial cues are faded.

Regular routines for household tasks are set up according to families' needs and schedules. The child may be more willing when given a choice in what task is done and when (e.g., day of week, time of day) (Browder & Snell, 1993). Realistic routines need to be established or parents may become overwhelmed by their other family roles. For example, if both parents are employed outside the home and there are multiple tasks to be done in the morning, perhaps bedmaking only needs to be done on the weekend when families and their children are not pushed for time.

*Caring for pets.* As children grow, they are given responsibilities for caring for others. This responsibility typically begins with an animal and later may include caring for younger siblings. For a child in a wheelchair or a child with dyspraxia, feeding the family dog or cat is difficult because of inaccessible materials and incoordination in pouring food or water. Greenstein (1993) gives an exceptional example of how to modify this task by building an L-shaped jig out of wood to stabilize the dog bowl. The bottom or horizontal piece holds the dog bowls in place with four small dowels, and the vertical piece has a funnel and an old cut-off milk bottle inverted and positioned over the dog bowls. The child can then pour the water or dog food into the large opening, which then goes into the bowls accurately. Aquariums placed on open tables allow a child in a wheelchair to pull up to it. Fish food placed in a shaker container with a handle and fish nets with enlarged or extended handles may be helpful. Check sheets to determine when the fish or other animal were last fed may help everyone in the family keep track of the feeding schedule.

## Use of Personal Assistance

Most families are interdependent in performing home management tasks. Although independent performance is highly valued, complete self-reliance in a task may not be achievable or even desirable if the task requires too much time and energy, or if it exacerbates abnormal behaviors or movement patterns. Dependency in some tasks is appropriate at times and may permit completion of other, more readily achieved independent living skills.

Verbal, gestural, or physical cues are used when children are first learning a task. Verbal cues may tell the child how many times to "squirt" the solution when cleaning tables or mirrors. Gestural cues may point to bed corners to check if a bed is made properly. Or a hand-over-hand method may help a child with dyspraxia to learn the motor movements to mop the kitchen floor. As the child learns the task, these cues are faded and hopefully the child will remember them for self-correction.

Children with disabilities participate in home management tasks at all different levels. Some may never be independent in cooking, but they can be included in an activity through partial participation. For example, a child with athetoid cerebral palsy may not have the coordination or gross motor control to pick up a beater, but she can participate in the task of making a cake or cutting up vegetables by using an automated learning device (ALD) with an electric mixer (Levin & Scherfenberg, 1987). An ALD is a control unit with a switch that activates an appliance. The ALD reduces the voltage of the appliance to a lower voltage at the switch. It may have a timer that allows the appliance to remain on for a set amount of time without the child activating the switch during this time.

## Safety Within the Household

Many parents fear allowing their children with disabilities to perform household tasks. Safety while using appliances, utensils, and other equipment is of utmost importance. For example, children with myelomeningocele may not have sensation in their lower extremities. They need awareness to potential burns from hot plates or pots carried on their lap or touching a stove, dryer, or other hot items. If an emergency does occur, children need to be ready to respond. Access to the telephone and the ability to get in and out of the house are key skills. An accessible telephone station, combined with knowledge of how to contact emergency services or a designated helper, are of prime importance.

Many parents fear leaving their older children with disabilities alone at home. The fear of fire from which the child cannot escape, the child falling or getting caught in one spot, or having a medical emergency or an urgent personal need (like going to the bathroom) are common concerns. Typical consequences are that either the parents' activities are curtailed or the child is taken everywhere. Children with immature judgment cannot be left unsupervised on life support systems. However, the parents' inability to leave the child is often caused by the fact that effective emergency alert or escape mechanisms have not be established. This is of particular concern with teenagers who want and need the opportunity to be alone at home to develop more independence.

Therapists consider cultural characteristics in relation to safety issues. In some cultures, parents are expected to protect their children until they are married and leave the house (Lynch & Hanson, l992); they may not want children (with or without disabilities) exposed to uncertain or potentially risky situations. In addition, safety knowledge may be lacking for some families. For example, recently immigrated families may not have previously used electricity or plumbing and may not be aware of safety issues with water and electricity (Lynch & Hanson, l992).

# COMMUNITY
## Community Activities and Skills

Shopping, eating in restaurants, banking, and attending sports and recreational events involve many similar skills. These include mobility, communication with strangers, handling money and packages, and functional reading and writing. An ecologic assessment is done to target what tasks and skills are necessary, to identify where adaptations or skill development is needed, and to develop and analyze what instructional strategies will "fit" the environmental demands. Children are then taught these tasks in the actual community site (Falvey, 1986; York & Rainforth, l987). The use of assistive devices in public depends on the degree of portability, ease of use, and attitudes of the child and family.

Managing one's money during shopping tasks is often difficult for the child with physical or cognitive disabilities. Instead of using wallets, small zipper purses (i.e., fanny packs) that go around the waist or can be hooked to the wheelchair are used. These are adapted with a large zipper pull and can be attached with Velcro to a lapboard for stability. The child can hand the fanny pack to the store clerk and ask them to get the money out or put their change in the fanny pack. When purchasing an item, children can also instruct clerks to put their change in the paper bag that is given to them. A calculator can be used to help with the arithmetic. Also cue cards can be carried to remind children of the value of money.

## Community Mobility

Functional mobility in the community is critical to the child's development and to the family's ability to be active outside the home. Community participation ranges from the early stages when the child accompanies his or her parents on errands to the time when the child goes out on his or her own. Transportation of the children with disabilities is

addressed from both functional and safety standpoints. Furthermore, when new equipment is selected for a child, the methods used for home, school, and community mobility are considered to ensure that the device can be used and transported as necessary with the child. For example, a power wheelchair was ordered for a child to maneuver around school and to participate in community outings. This chair gave the child tremendous capabilities when she was at school. However, at home the power wheelchair stayed on the porch as it could not fit inside. Also the family vehicle was inadequate in transporting the chair. If these variables had been considered at the time of assessment, these problems would not have occurred.

### Environmental Factors Affecting Mobility

Factors to consider include other people and crowds, street crossings, use of personal or public transportation and elevators, and architectural barriers. Occupational therapists often are involved with a team to select the most appropriate mobility device for a child. Chapter 21 elaborates on the devices that are available for children. Once problems in mobility are identified, the occupational therapist may consult with or teach the child, parent, and other caregivers techniques for improving mobility in a variety of community settings. The therapist can use their expertise on how to get in and out of doorways and elevators, up and down curbs, and maneuver within tight spots.

### School Mobility

Distances between classrooms and other rooms such as the cafeteria and bathrooms should be evaluated to determine travel time requirements and potential for fatigue. Additional time may be needed for class changes. Appropriate mobility devices such as power wheelchairs permit the student to get about at a functional speed that is commensurate with peers. For an individual student, careful planning of room assignments that are in proximity and avoid stair use is a strategy that also requires the action of school administrators. Mobility expectations within the school environment need to be realistic. At times a child who is capable of independent mobility with a walker or crutches is allowed to use a power or manual wheelchair to transfer between classes. The decision to use an "easier" method of mobility may be made when it is important that student's energy be conserved for schoolwork. In addition, when walking between classroom means that the child is late for class or has no opportunity to interact with classmates, use of power wheelchair becomes the most appropriate method of school building mobility.

### Transportation Safety

*Car seats.* State safety laws requiring children to use restraint systems while traveling in cars vary across the country. Commercial car seats are useful for many children with disabilities who are small enough to fit into them. Other children who have skeletal deformities, poor head or trunk control, spica casts, or abduction braces often need modifications of commercial seats to increase access, support, comfort, and protection. Simple modifications that do not alter the structure of the car seat can be made by the therapist. These might include adding foam or towel rolls to improve lateral control or adding closed cell foam positioning inserts to the inside shell.

The Automotive Safety for Children Program (James Whitcomb Riley Hospital for Children, Indianapolis) has developed a car seat modification for children in hip abduction casts. This adaptation involves cutting away the lower side of the plastic shell, placing a firm pad under and behind the pelvis, and adjusting the harness (Brandenburg & Vanderheiden, 1987). Shaw (1987) recommended that therapists work closely with manufacturers or qualified engineers for structural modifications because such changes always affect the safety features of restraints.

Children who have outgrown standard commercial car seats, yet have not developed adequate sitting balance, may use car seats designed specifically for larger children with disabilities. Transport- or travel-type wheelchairs (see Chapter 21) are designed to be used also as car seats and are an option for some children. Restraint harnesses attach to the regular car seat or school bus seat and help restrain children with postural or behavior problems (Shaw, 1987). Older, heavier children who cannot manage car transfer may benefit from free-standing portable or special car lifters.

***Van or bus transportation.*** Many children with physical disabilities ride vans and buses seated in their wheelchairs. These vehicles are especially helpful for children in power wheelchairs that do not dismantle or fold. This practice is quite common; however, few crashworthiness tests have been performed with all the varieties of mobility devices (e.g., type, size, weight, and construction), and few states keep information on automobile accidents involving wheelchairs (Karge, Yaffe, & Berkowitz, 1994; Sprigle, Morris, Nowachek, & Karg, 1994). If possible, a child should **transfer out of the wheelchair to a seat** in the vehicle and use the already-tested occupant restraining systems. If a child must be transported in a wheelchair, Schneider (1990) recommended the following:

1. **All wheelchairs should be placed rearward or forward but never sideways.** When chairs are placed sideways, they can fold and collapse on impact and potentially cause more injury.
2. Two restraint systems are needed: an **occupant restraint system** and a **wheelchair restraint system.** The occupant restraint system consists of one upper body restraint that is bolted to the vehicle itself and one lower body restraint that is bolted to the chair. Restraints are applied over skeletal regions such as the pelvis and shoulders, rather than over the soft abdominal area. A **wheelchair restraint system** secures the wheelchair frame to the floor of the vehicle. Four-point systems or two separate belts for the front and the back wheels are best.
3. **Rear head restraints** are necessary to prevent backward head excursion (Schneider, 1990).

In addition, Schneider recommends that all hardware and straps used to adapt vans and buses be dynamically tested for strength. Extra padding in the vehicle near the child in the wheelchair is also suggested. **Items attached to the wheelchair need to be removed** and strapped down. For example, on impact in an automobile accident, the lapboard or augmentative communication device could act like a missile and further hurt the child or other occupants in the vehicle.

***School transportation.*** Rules and equipment for transporting children with disabilities and their equipment vary among school bus companies. The occupational therapist's role often involves working with school transportation officials regarding the above safety guidelines and issues and to help solve special problems for individual children. Wheelchairs must offer the child sufficient postural control throughout the bus ride and should have bags or pockets on the back or sides to help safely contain belongings.

***Public transportation.*** With passage of the Americans with Disabilities Act, more communities have accessible public transportation programs for persons with disabilities. *Dial a Ride* type programs that provide door-to-door bus or van service when arranged in advance by telephone are available in many communities. Children who are able to board buses or rapid rail systems must learn important skills such as handling money and tickets, using transit schedules, and identifying correct buses, trains, and stops. For children with memory and sequencing problems, instructional strategies such as partial participation, and graded cuing may assist them with how to sequence the steps of the task.

Large major transportation systems accommodate passengers with disabilities by priority and special seating. Different companies and transportation modes have varying amenities, so it is necessary to compare policies in advance. In most cases, persons with disabilities cannot sit in their wheelchair on planes and trains, making it difficult to use the restroom. Wet cell batteries for power wheelchairs cannot be transported on airplanes. Advance checks on accessibility are advised before traveling by plane or train.

### Independent Driving

The therapist usually consults with adapted driving program specialists unless he or she has had specialized training in driving adaptations and instruction. Strength, range of motion, sensation, coordination, reach, reaction time, balance, and perceptual abilities are considered in functional terms related to driving. Automobile adaptations for the teenage driver with a disability range from simple add-on components to those that convert a car or van permanently. Add-on adaptations that do not affect others' use of the car are preferred when feasible. Steering knobs facilitate grasp and turning the wheel. Built-up brakes and accelerator pedals or left-footed accelerators are useful. Right or left hand controls or relocation of the horn and dimmer switches are examples of other adaptations for the family automobile. For children with quadriplegia or significant upper extremity weakness, zero-effort steering may be useful.

Teenagers may learn to drive with adapted controls, but independence is limited if they cannot transfer themselves and equipment, such as wheelchairs, into and out of the car. Therapists teach a variety of transfer techniques depending on the child's capabilities, especially strength and postural control. Car door openers, enlarged controls (e.g., door locks), transfer boards, webbing loops, modified dressing sticks (to close the door), or wooden jigs to guide wheelchairs into a specific space (i.e., trunk or backseat) are examples of assistive devices that may be used. Teenagers that ambulate for short distances may be able to put a chair into the trunk or side door of a car. Other teenagers who are nonambulatory may also place the chair in the backseat of the car or may get in the front seat on the passenger side of the car and pull the wheelchair in with them. Wheelchair carriers and lifts that go on the rear or top of the car may be another option.

## ADAPTATIONS FOR LEISURE AND RECREATIONAL ACTIVITIES

### Play and Leisure

Therapy objectives for young children differ from those established for older children because of the changes in the child's abilities and interest levels. For example, intervention with the play of the infant or preschooler may be directed toward developing adaptations that enhance exploratory and sensorimotor experiences. In contrast, play intervention with the school-aged child might include adaptations for participation in team sports and board games such as Monopoly.

#### Adaptation for Play Experiences

For many children the ability to enjoy and progress through the various stages of play development depends greatly on the adaptations that can be made. The occupational therapist can help the child, family, and school teachers establish ways of participation in independent and cooperative play through adaptations of positioning, materials, and the environment (Figure 17-10).

#### Positioning to Enhance Independent Manipulation and Exploration

Children play in an interesting and endless variety of positions. Much of early childhood takes place on the floor. Wedges for supine and prone lying, sidelying positioners,

corner chairs, and other floor sitting devices can help the child with poor postural reactions and control. Finnie (1975) and Diamant (1992) have illustrated and described how parents or therapists use their bodies (chest, thighs, abdomen, and lap) to position the child with cerebral palsy for play.

Parents can use other items in the environment to position children during play, by placing the child's back against the wall or base of the sofa, or sitting the child into the corner of a room or contoured area formed by sofa back cushions. Stable seating can be achieved through properly fitted children's chairs, wheelchairs, bolster seats, or chair and table sets that provide full thigh support, back support, and foot support. Additional positioning components may be needed to further enhance posture and control. Play in standing position can be facilitated by use of standing tables, prone standers, and orthotic standers.

Children who require postural support for play typically have difficulty moving into and out of positions for play. If the activity involves movement, consider mobility systems with positioning components (see Chapter 21).

### Toys and Their Adaptations

*Standard toys.* The therapist can help the child and family select standard toys that are appropriate to the child's cognitive level and other performance capacities. The toy should promote the exploratory process so that the sensorimotor, symbolic, and constructive aspects of play are addressed (see Chapter 18). Toy concepts should be simple enough for the child to understand, yet complex enough to provide a challenge and opportunity for achievement. Toy selection guides help the therapist and parent. Sinker (1986) of the national Lekotek Play Library program has compiled a particularly useful resource guide of toys that have been field tested with children who have special needs.

An array of toys available through catalogs or in stores are appropriate for children with disabilities. Video games, battery-operated toys, hand-held games, voice- or noise-activated toys, and computer software programs are a few that are easy to access. More toy manufacturers are using universal design so most children can access them. For example, some of the "pull the string" talking toys are now replaced with large pull-down handles or push buttons.

*Toy and play adaptations.* The occupational therapist is a key professional to make adaptations to toys and locate appropriate adapted toys through special catalogs for the child. The most common needs are stabilization of play materials and facilitation of grasp, manipulation, and access to toys.

Motorically involved children, particularly those with athetoid movements, often displace toys when attempting to manipulate them. Or, when conditions of hemiplegia or quadriplegia are present, one side of the body does not effectively assist in stabilizing toys for play. Examples of techniques and equipment for holding objects are described

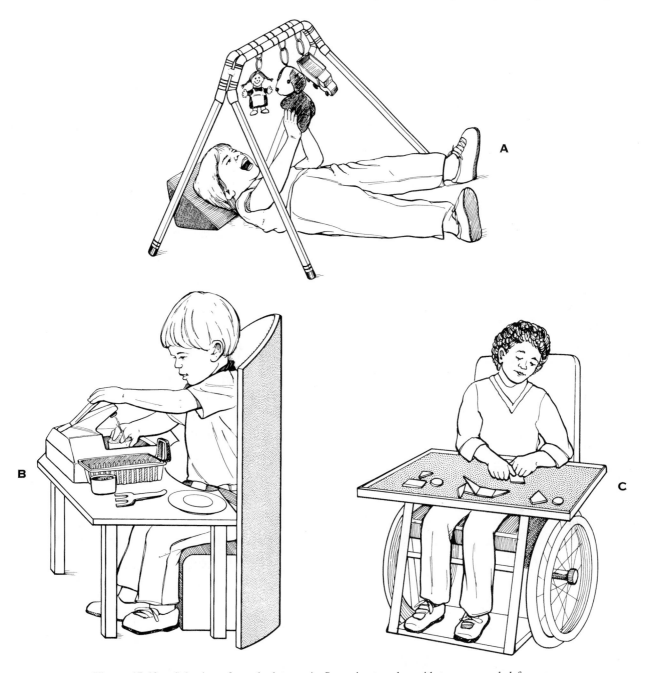

**Figure 17-10**   Selection of standard toys. **A,** Sensorimotor play with toys suspended from an activity frame for a young child with limited upper extremity control and poor sitting posture. **B,** Imaginative play with a sink set, featuring sturdy construction, stable base, and large play pieces that are easy to grasp. **C,** Constructive play at a magnetic play set that permits the child to manipulate pieces by sliding them on the magnetic surface.

in Table 17-5. When grasp or dexterity limitations interfere with play, several adaptations are possible. The addition of handles to toys can permit sustained grasp and orientation of the toy (Figure 17-11, *A*). Extensions made from splinting materials or tongue depressors can help a child operate levers and switches on toys (Figure 17-11, *B*). Straps may be added to attach the toy directly to the hand (Figure 17-

11, *C*). Pressure-sensitive hook-and-loop tapes may help children hold objects in hand mitts (Figure 17-11, *D*). Toys with handles, such as xylophone strikers or hammers, can be built up with small foam balls or cylindric foam padding from therapy supply catalogs to facilitate grasp.

Isolation of the index finger is needed for pressing the keys of toy telephones, pianos, and the wide variety of elec-

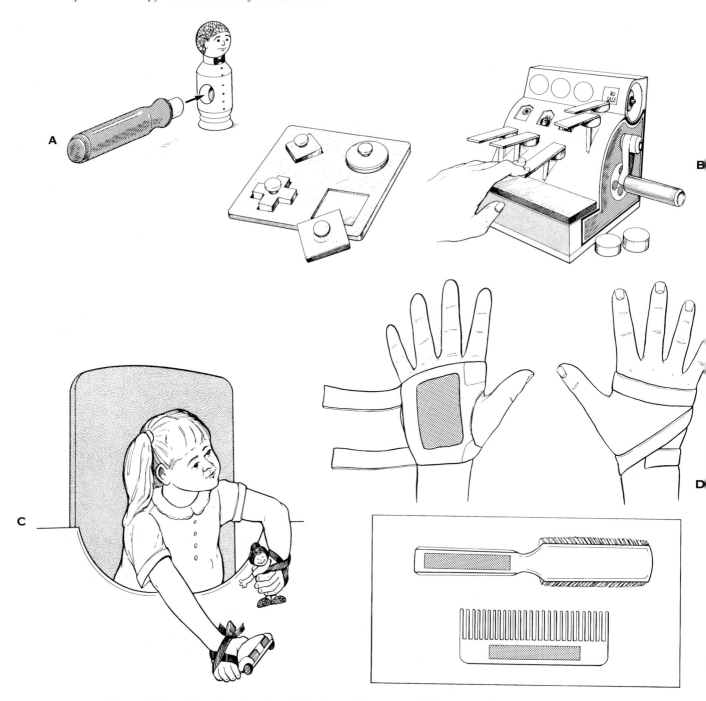

**Figure 17-11**    Adaptations for play. **A,** Handles and knobs can facilitate grasp. **B,** Lever extensions permit operation of the toy with less force and control. **C,** If grasp is nonfunctional, small toys may be strapped to the hand or **D,** a Velcro mitt may be used.

tronic toys with keyboards. Hand-held pointers, including wooden dowels with built-up handles, pencils inserted into universal cuffs, or custom-fabricated hand splints with extensions, can be used.

Carlson (1982) developed a playboard that incorporates some of the adaptations. It was designed for children whose motor problems affect their ability to play. Toys that associate with each other in play schemes are attached to a lap tray. Examples include toy furniture from various rooms in a house or farm sets. Some pieces are bolted down permanently, and other pieces are fixed in routed tracks so that they can be moved around without falling off the board. Other movable pieces are strapped to the child's hand. Such a setup can stimulate imaginative and symbolic play.

Older children develop interests in cooperative and competitive rule games such as cards or checkers. "The combination of pleasure, social skills and learning that these games can promote emphasizes the need for adapting them for children with disabilities who have the mental abilities to participate successfully" (Rast, 1986, p. 39). Card holders and automatic shufflers can be used. Playing cards with extra large markings help the child with impaired vision or visual perceptual deficits. If manipulation of the game materials is impossible, the player can signal to a partner to manipulate the game pieces after the child has decided on a move.

The technology of electronics has dramatically increased play opportunities for the child who has extremely limited motor control. Battery-operated toys, microprocessors, and computers can be adapted for use with special switches and controllers. Many adaptations to meet the needs of this population have become commercially available. Battery-operated toys can be modified to use a remote switch through the addition of a battery adapter or interrupter. Burkhardt (1980, 1982) and Wright and Nomura (1985) present excellent information on how to make or order battery adapters, switches, and toys.

### Adaptations to Play Areas and Surfaces

Accessibility of toys and play experiences often must be structured for the child who has difficulty moving toward toys and playmates. Toys must be moved to the child who is limited in mobility. Presentation of a range of toys in varying locations near the child is beneficial for stimulation of limited movement capabilities. Toys can be placed so that the child can select one and reach it by rolling, crawling, or using a wheelchair, thereby facilatating initiation and self-direction. Keeping toys within reach can effectively prolong independent play and reduce frustration of toys that "get away." One mother discovered that placing a hula hoop around her small son's body and his toys as he played on the floor was a workable solution. Lap trays and tables with rims can also be stabilized. Angle play surfaces can allow gravity to return a toy to a child after it is rolls from him.

*Playground.* Equipment such as swings, slides, and bars are common to community and school playgrounds. Newly constructed playgrounds are adapted with platform swings that accommodate wheelchairs; all public playgrounds must be accessible to children in wheelchairs and those with limited mobility. Often ramps are built up to the slides and the downward grade accommodates children with poor stability. The use of adapted tricycles and bicycles on playgrounds can provide faster mobility in a manner that promotes group and independent play.

### Organized Sports

Sports equipment, performance techniques, and game rules may need to be modified to permit full participation by a child with disabilities. Many sports are learned at home or school. Community agencies such as recreation departments offer integrated programs where children with disabilities are included with children without disabilities. Recreational events such as the Special Olympics and the Na-

tional Wheelchair Basketball Championships take place at regional and national levels as well. Athletic and recreational departments are the primary resources for these programs, but the occupational therapist may assist with individual adaptations.

Many of the recent wheelchair design improvements can be traced to wheelchair sports. Cambered wheels, lighter and stronger aluminum and titanium frame materials, precision wheel bearings, adjustable rear axles, and quick release wheels were introduced to improve athletic performance. Good equipment is essential for participation in all wheelchair athletics, including basketball, track and field, and tennis. National organizations for wheelchair sports can provide information regarding training and competition.

Water sports hold many advantages for children with disabilities. The water allows them to achieve greater freedom and flexibility of movement. Swimming is the skill common to all water sports and recreation. Flotation devices to keep the head above water and other equipment, such as hand paddles and flippers, assist safety and movement. Pool lifts that transfer the swimmer from a wheelchair and ramps that lead to the water promote access. The American National Red Cross and other community organizations (e.g., YMCA, YWCA) have adapted aquatics programs that provide lessons and information about accessible pools.

### Individual Outdoor Sports

Boating requires mastery of swimming and use of a flotation device. Flat-bottom boats are more stable and may even accommodate a wheelchair. Safety harnesses are available for sailing. Children who require cushions for skin protection can often use air-filled pillows in boats. Custom seats can be fabricated for kayaks to stabilize the pelvis of the adolescent with excellent upper body control but impaired hip and low trunk function. Special skis are available for water skiing in the seated position.

For winter skiing, a sled ski resembling a kayak can be used by children with paraplegia or diplegia, provided that upper body control is good. These devices have two runners molded onto the bottom surface and are balanced by the skier by means of short forearm ski poles that have little skis on the end. Beginners are tethered to a ski instructor or parent and guided down the slope until they are sufficiently skilled to ski independently. Skiers with lower-extremity limb deficiency use two forearm-braced outrigger skis to give them a three-point balance (Figure 17-12). Upper-extremity amputees can ski with one or no poles. Blind skiers may be accompanied by a sighted companion who provides directions by verbal command or a tether. Adapted recreational skiing and lessons are now available in more areas with ski programs for the disabled such as Alpine Meadows in California and Winter Park in Colorado. Toboggans can be used just about anywhere in the snow, provided that safety considerations are addressed.

Fishing requires less physical activity than other recreational activities and is therefore a good choice for children

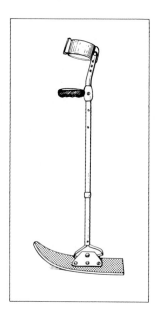

**Figure 17-12** A child with a lower extremity limb deficiency uses an outrigger ski with forearm support for stability and balance.

with motor disabilities. Fishing rod adaptations are made so children with limited dexterity and range of motion can participate in fishing. The reel handle is enlarged by a golf ball and the handle of the fishing net is elongated with a wooden dowel so the child can reach the water from his wheelchair (Greenstein, 1993). Adaptations for stabilizing fishing rods have used PCV pipe as well as commerically available stabilizers that hook onto the side of the wheelchair. Other devices, such as the EZ Cast, attach to the wheelchair arm and assist casting and reeling with limited use of one arm. Lightweight trunk belts and harnesses also are used to mount rods.

Horseback riding has become one of the most popular and enjoyable adapted sports for children with disabilities. Many communities have stables that offer therapeutic riding. Mounting platforms that place the child at saddle level are often equipped with ramps for wheelchairs. Adapted saddles with hand holds, back rests, and harness systems to stabilize the rider are typically found in adapted programs. Fleece-covered or padded seats are available for children with sensory impairment who are at risk of pressure sores. A rein-bar that attaches to the saddle permits control with one hand. Protective helmets and safety stirrups are usually worn.

## Adaptations for the School Environment
### Commercially Available Equipment

Adjustable classroom chairs with positioning components are available, as are tables with cutouts that provide increased arm support and orientation of the trunk. Tables with adjustable-angle tops, such as drafting tables, permit

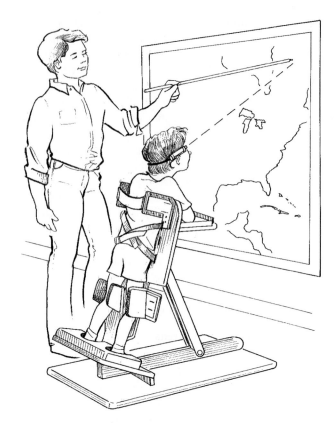

**Figure 17-13** Optical headpointer used for choice-making.

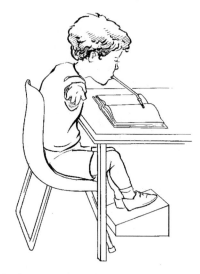

**Figure 17-14** Mouthstick used for turning pages.

further adaptability of the work surface. Children who have their own wheelchairs benefit from seat inserts if they have difficulty maintaining appropriate posture for classwork.

### Adaptive Equipment to Manage Classroom Activities

For children with severe disabilities, Eriksson and colleagues (1987) have published a pamphlet describing the use

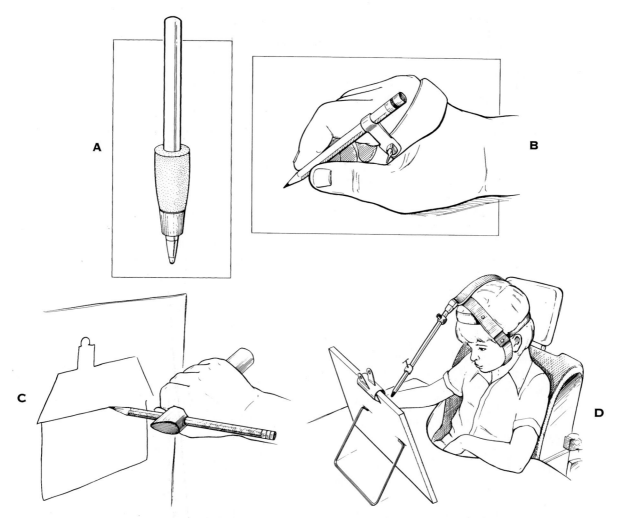

**Figure 17-15**   Adaptations to writing tools. **A,** Foam cylinder can be used to build up grasp surface. **B,** This adaptation encourages the tripod grasp of a pencil. **C,** This adaptation accommodates grasp and wrist position. **D,** Headwand with felt-tip pen attached is used for marking in a workbook that has been clipped to a slantboard.

of headsticks, mouthsticks, and optical pointers in everyday school and home environments. These ideas are particularly useful for school settings because they help children with severe motor involvement to be included in activities with their peers. Optical pointers (from augmentative communication devices) are mounted onto a helmet, eyeglasses, head band, or hat. The pointer is then used for turn taking, decision making, and demonstration of a child's knowledge. Figure 17-13 demonstrates how the child uses the pointer to answer questions about geography. Other activities described by the authors include using the pointer for orientation games ("go here"), hide and seek, I spy, choosing toys, showing others how to draw, and finding objects in a book.

Mouthsticks and headwands are used for reading, math, and art activities (Eriksson et al., 1987). The mouthstick is adapted with a rubber tip to turn pages (Figure 17-14) or to use a calculator with a keyguard on it. Mouthsticks also are

used to activate switches on electrical classroom equipment (e.g., to show slides on a screen). By adapting a headwand with a magnetic stick mounted on a ball joint, children can play games with their peers. The games are modified by recessing the boards and putting paperclips on the game pieces (Eriksson et al., 1987).

## Writing Devices

Grasp can be facilitated by building up handles with foam or rubber materials (Figure 17-15, *A*), or by using large marking pens or primary pencils. The tripod (three-point pinch) position is encouraged by a number of writing aids available from therapy equipment suppliers or can be made by the therapist from thermoplastic materials (Figure 17-15, *B*). The child who cannot use a tripod position can use devices that accommodate wrist and finger positions (Figure 17-15, *C*). Some children must use other parts of their bodies to write. Headwands and mouthsticks can be used

## STUDY QUESTIONS

1. Linda is 2 years old and has high tone with numerous spasms. Her mother has asked for suggestions for dressing and diapering. Linda's mother tells you that she feels like she has a morning struggle pulling her legs apart. What would you suggest?

2. Mark is 7 months old and has Down syndrome and is hypotonic. His mother has just returned to work and his grandmother is taking care of him. She is having difficulty with dressing Mark. She complains that her back is hurting her and that Mark is just like a rag doll. What would you suggest?

3. Hank is 16 years old and has diabetes. He is cognitively intact, but has peripheral neuropathies, low endurance, and poor coordination. He is in a wheelchair and lives in a wheelchair-accessible home. Hank wants to be able to stay by himself when he comes home from school, but his mother is leery. He needs to be able to take his medicine and fix himself a snack. As Hank's therapist, what things will you need to think about? What adaptations may he need?

4. Andy is 2½ years old and has begun toilet training. He has below-average equilibrium reactions for his age and has difficulty with fasteners. What suggestions would you have for his day care providers as they begin to address toilet training?

5. Colin is 5 years old and has been identified with severe perceptual problems as well as low tone and endurance. What do you hypothesize will be his problems with dressing? What can you do to make the task easier?

6. Nine-year-old Jeffrey has poor postural control and is tactilely defensive. Bath time is difficult for his mother; Jeffrey particularly hates to have his hair washed. What suggestions do you have for her?

7. Twelve-year-old Melinda has difficulty with balance, but she is motivated to dress herself. What positions could help facilitate her independent performance in putting on pants, shoes, or a shirt?

8. Mario is an 8-year-old child who has a strong startle reaction and is low tone. His mother is having difficulty getting him into the tub. What positions and equipment do you suggest to Mario's mother once Mario is in the tub?

9. Jay is 3 years old and has myelomeningocele. Mobility is difficult for him. Currently, he scoots himself around the floor. What suggestions would you have to improve functional mobility? What precautions would you need to think about?

10. Your principal has announced that a new elementary school will be built and it is expected to have approximately 20 students who are in wheelchairs. He asks you, "What should I consider for environmental adaptations?" Thinking of this age range, what do you suggest?

11. Gary is 10 years old and was placed in traction for 4 months because of a severe break in the femur. He is modest and wants to be able to wash and dress himself. What suggestions would you give to Gary and his caregivers?

---

to hold writing tools, often in conjunction with angled writing surfaces (Figure 17-15, *D*).

When stabilization of the paper is difficult, some of the methods presented in Table 17-5 may be used. As alternatives, the therapist may recommend clipboards with pressure-sensitive matting on the bottom, use of a writing tablet rather than single sheets of paper, or a one-handed writing board available from therapy suppliers.

### Management of Classroom Materials

Holding, manipulating, or carrying books and papers can be difficult and result in destruction of the materials. Students with severe motor or visual limitations need to have materials set up for them to reduce handling requirements. Bookstands can be used to hold written materials at the proper angle and to hold books open. Page turning can be assisted with the eraser tip of a pencil, a rubber fingertip cover, or a headband or mouthstick with a rubber tip to increase friction. Electric or battery-operated page turners can greatly enhance the independence of severely physically involved students. These devices hold the book open and use a single switch or switch array to turn pages. Backpacks can be used to carry books to free both arms for use in mobility functions. Papers or worksheets can be held on stenographers' stands or easels.

Alternatives to note-taking include photocopying the notes of a classmate or tape-recording lectures. Rather than taping an entire lecture, students can record only pertinent segments by using the switch control on the microphone. Portable electronic typewriters or small augmentative communication devices are also useful for taking notes.

### Adapted Physical Education

The therapist often consults with the adaptive physical education specialist regarding the capabilities of students and activity and equipment adaptations to enhance participation. The adaptive physical education specialist is well versed in adapting sports equipment and games, such as bowling frames and batting tees. However, the therapist is more likely to be called on to address special individual problems, such as adapting a ping-pong paddle to facilitate grasp.

## SUMMARY

This chapter discussed methods of enhancing self-care and independent living skills through adaptation of the activity process, tools, and materials. Adapted techniques and equipment are important tools for the occupational therapist when they are appropriate to the child's developmental level, functional capacity, and life environments, with consideration of parents, other caretakers, and the child's motivation. The importance of positioning and orientation of the child to the work or play surface were stressed. Examples of assistive devices, adapted techniques, and environmental modifications to increase the level of independent functioning were presented. New devices are continually developed and available; it is the occupational therapist's responsibility to be familiar with new technologies and to be aware of the range of current methods and equipment that promote independent function in children with disabilities.

## REFERENCES

American Occupational Therapy Association. (1994). Uniform terminology for occupational therapy—Third edition. *American Journal of Occupational Therapy, 48*(11), 1047-1054.

Becker, H., Schur, S., Paoletti-Schlep, M. & Hammer, E. (1986). *Functional skills screening inventory.* Austin, TX: Functional Resources Enterprises.

Bergen, A.F., Presperin, J., & Tallman, T. (1990). *Positioning for function: wheelchairs and other assistive devices.* Valhalla, NY: Valhalla Rehabilitation Publications.

Bergen A.F. & Colangelo, C. (1985). *Positioning the client with CNS deficits: the wheelchair and other adapted equipment* (2nd ed.). Valhalla, NY: Valhalla Rehabilitation Publications.

Boehm, R. (1988). *Improving upper body control: An approach to assessment and treatment of tonal dysfunction.* Tucson: Therapy Skill Builders.

Brandenburg, S. & Vanderheiden, G. (1987). *Communication, control, and computer access for disabled and elderly individuals. Resource Books 1-3.* Boston: College-Hill Press.

Brollier, C., Shepherd, J., & Markley, K. (1994). Transition from school to community living. *American Journal of Occupational Therapy, 48*(4), 346-353.

Browder, M. & Snell, M. (1993). Daily living and community skills. In Snell, M.E. (Ed.). *Instruction of students with severe disabilities (4th ed.)* (pp. 480-525). New York: Macmillan.

Brown, L., Schwarz, P., Udvari-Solner, A., Kampschroer, E., Johnson, F., Jorgensen, J., & Gruenewald, L. (1991). How much time should students with severe intellectual disabilities spend in regular education classrooms and elsewhere? *Journal of the Association for Persons with Severe Handicaps, 16,* 39-47.

Bryze, K. & Curtin, C. (1993). A top-down approach: relationships to research and occupational performance. *Developmental Disabilities Special Interest Section Newsletter, 2,* 2-4.

Burkhardt, L.J. (1980). *Homemade battery devices for severely handicapped children with suggested activities.* College Park, MD: Linda J. Burkhardt.

Burkhardt, L.J. (1982). *More homemade battery devices for severely handicapped children with suggested activities.* College Park, MD: Linda J. Burkhardt.

Carlson, F. (1982). *Prattle and play.* Omaha: University of Nebraska Medical Center.

Case-Smith, J. (1994). Self-care strategies for children with develomental deficits. In C. Christiansen (Ed.). *Ways of living: self-care strategies for special needs* (pp. 101-156). Rockville, MD: American Occupational Therapy Association.

Coley, I.L. (1978). *Pediatric assessment of self-care activities.* St. Louis: Mosby.

Cone, J.D. (1984). *Pyramid scales.* Austin, TX: Pro Ed.

Copeland, M., Ford, L., & Solon, N. (1976). *Occupational therapy for mentally retarded children.* Baltimore: University Park Press.

Coster, W.J., Haley, S., & Baryza, M. (1994). Functional performance in young children after traumatic brain injury: 6-month follow-up. *American Journal of Occupational Therapy, 48*(3), 211-218.

Diamant, R. (1992). *Positioning for play.* Tucson: Therapy Skill Builders.

Duckett, E., Raffaelli, M., & Richards, M. (1989). Taking care: maintaining the self and the home in early adolescence. *Journal of Youth and Adolescence, 18*(6) 549-565.

Duffy, Y. (1981). *All things possible.* Ann Arbor, MI: A.J. Gavin & Associates.

Enders, A. (1984). *Technology for independent living sourcebook.* Washington, DC: Association for the Advancement of Rehabilitation Technology.

Epps, S., Stern, R.J., & Horner, R.H. (1990). Comparision of simulation training on self and using a doll for teaching generalized menstrual care to women with severe mental retardation. *Research in Developmental Disabilities, 11,* 37-66.

Erickson, M.L. (1976). *Assessment and management of developmental changes in children,* St. Louis: Mosby.

Eriksson, B., Gawell, A., Munthe, K., Riddar, A., Rygaard, K., Windling, U., & Zachrisson, G. (1987). *Activities using headsticks and optical pointers: a decription of methods.* Stockholm, Sweden: Swedish Institute for the Handicapped.

Falvey, M. (1986). *Community based curriculum: instructional strategies for students with severe handicaps.* Baltimore: Brookes.

Ferguson, D.L. & Baumgart, D. (1991). Partial participation revisited. *Journal of the Association for Persons with Severe Handicaps, 16,* 218-227.

Finnie, N. (1975). *Handling the young cerebral palsied child at home* (2nd ed.). New York: Dutton-Sunrise.

Fisher, A. (1994). *Assessment of motor and process skills* (version 8.0).

Unpublished test manual, Fort Collins, CO: Colorado State University.

Fisher, A., Murray, E., & Bundy, A. (1991). *Sensory integration theory and practice,* Philadelphia: F.A. Davis.

Foxx, R.M. & Azrin, N.H. (1973). Dry pants: a rapid method of toilet training children. *Behaviour Research and Therapy, 11,* 435-442.

Furuno, S., O'Reilly, K., Hoska, C.M., Zeisloft, B., & Allman, T. (1984). *Hawaii Early Learning Profile.* Palo Alto, CA: Vort.

Giangreco, M., Cloninger, C., & Iverson, V. (1993). *Choosing options and accommodations for children (COACH).* Baltimore: Brookes.

Greenstein, D. (1993). *Backyards and butterflies: ways to include children with disabilities in outdoor activities.* Ithaca, NY: New York State Rural Health and Safety Council.

Haley, S.M., Coster, W.J., Ludlow, L.H., Haltiwanger, J., & Andrellos, P. (1992). *Administration manual for the Pediatric Evaluation of Disability Inventory.* Boston: New England Medical Center.

Hamilton, B.B. & Granger, C.U. (1991). *Functional Independence Measure for Children (WeeFIM).* Buffalo, NY: Research Foundation of the State University of New York.

Hanson, M. (1992). Families with Anglo-European roots. In E.W. Lynch & M.J. Hanson (Eds.). *Developing cross-cultural competence* (pp. 65-87). Baltimore: Brookes.

Johnson-Martin, N., Jens, K.G., Attermeier, S.M., & Hacker, B. (1991). *The Carolina Curriculum for Handicapped Infants and Infants at Risk.* Baltimore: Brookes.

Karge, P., Yaffe, K, & Berkowitz, D. (1994). Positioning and securement of riders and their mobility aids in transit vehicles: an analytical review. *Assistive Technology, 6*(2), 94-110.

Keith, R.A., Granger, C.V., Hamilton, B.B., & Sherwin, F.S. (1987). The Functional Independence Measure: a new tool for rehabilitation. *Advanced Clinical Rehabilitation, 1,*6-18.

Kennedy, E. (1981). *Dressing with pride: vol. 1.* Groton, CT: PRIDE Foundation.

Kernaleguen, A. (1978). *Clothing designs for the handicapped,* Edmonton, Canada: The University of Alberta Press.

Kielhofner, G. (Ed.). (1995). *A model of human occupation: theory and application (2nd ed.).* Baltimore: Williams & Wilkins.

Kramer, P. & Hinojosa, J. (1993). *Frames of reference for pediatric occupational therapy.* Baltimore: Williams & Wilkins.

Lambert, N.M. & Windmiller, M. (1981). *AAMD Adaptive Behavior Scale, school edition.* East Aurora, NY: Slosson Educational Publications.

Levin, J. & Scherfenberg, L. (1987). *Selection and use of simple technology in home, school, work, and community settings.* Minniapolis: Ablenet.

Light, H., Hertsgaard, D., & Martin, R. (1985). Farm children's work in the family. *Adolescence, 20*(7), 425-432.

Lynch, E. & Hanson, M. (1992). *Developing cross-cultural competence.* Baltimore: Brookes.

Mann, W.C. & Lane, J.P. (1991). *Assistive technology for persons with disabilities: the role of occupational therapy.* Rockville, MD: American Occupational Therapy Association.

Miller, L. (1992). *The first STEP (Screening Test for Evaluating Preschoolers).* San Antonio, TX: The Psychological Corporation.

Miller, L. (1993). *Self help assessment: parent evaluation (SHAPE).* (research edition). Englewood, CO: The KID Foundation.

Newborg, J., Stock, J.R., Wnek, L., Guidubaldi, J., & Szinicki, J. (1984). *Battelle developmental inventory.* Chicago: Riverside Publishers.

Orelove, F. & Sobsey, D. (1991). Self-care skills. In F. Orelove & D. Sobsey (Eds.). *Educating children with multiple disabilities* (pp. 373-406). Baltimore: Brookes.

Rast, M. (1986). Play and therapy, play or therapy? In *Play: a skill for life.* Rockville, MD: American Occupational Therapy Association.

Reese, G.M. & Snell, M.E. (1991). Putting on and removing coats and jackets: the acquisition and maintenance of skills by children with severe multiple disabilities. *Education and Training in Mental Retardation, 26,* 398-410.

Rheingold, H. (1982). Little children's participation in the work of adults: a nascent prosocial behavior. *Child Development, 53,* 114-125.

Sailor, W., Halvorsen, A., Anderson, J., Goetz, L., Gee, K., Doering, K., & Hunt, P. (1986). Community intensive instruction. In R. Horner, L. Meyer, & B. Fredericks (Eds.). *Education of learners with severe handicaps,* (pp. 251-288). Baltimore: Brookes.

Schneider, L.W. (1990). Transportation of wheelchair-seated students. In B.A. Fraser, R.N. Hensinger, & J.A. Phelps (Eds.). *Physical management of multiple handicaps: a professional's guide (2nd ed.)* (pp. 151-164). Baltimore: Brookes.

Seymour, S. (1988). Expressions of responsibility among Indian children: some precursors of adult status and sex roles. *Ethos, 16*(4), 355-370.

Shaw, G. (1987). Vehicular transport safety for the child with disabilities. *American Journal Occupational Therapy, 41,* 35.

Sinker, M. (1986). *Toys for growing: a guide to toys that develop skills.* Chicago: Year Book Medical Publishing.

Smith, R., Benge, M., & Hall, M. (1994). Technology for self-care. In C. Christiansen (Ed.). *Ways of living: self-care strategies for special needs* (pp. 379-422). Rockville, MD: American Occupational Therapy Association.

Snell, M.E. (1994). Principles for teaching self-care skills. In C. Christiansen (Ed.). *Ways of living: self-care strategies for special needs* (pp. 77-100). Rockville, MD: American Occupational Therapy Association.

Snell, M. & Brown, F. (1993). Instructional planning and implementation. In M.E. Snell (Ed.). *Instruction of students with severe disabilities* (4th ed.) (pp. 99-151). New York: Macmillan.

Sparrow, S., Balla, D., & Cicchetti, D. (1984). *Vineland Adaptive Behavior Scales.* Circle Pines, MN: American Guidance Services.

Spencer, K., Murphy, M., Bean, G., & Schelly, C. (1991). Vocational needs assessment: a functional, community referenced approach. In K. Spencer (Ed.). *From school to adult life: the role of occupational therapy in the transition process* (pp. 185-213). Fort Collins: Department of Occupational Therapy, Colorado State University.

Springle, S., Morris, B., Nowacek, G., & Karg, P. (1994) Assessment of adaptive transportation technology: a survey of users and equipment vendors. *Assistive Technology, 6,* 111-119.

Stillman, R. (1978). *Callier-Azusa Scale.* Dallas: Callier Center for Communication Disorders.

Trombly, C.A. & Quintana, L.A. (1989). Activities of daily living. In C.A. Trombly (Ed.). *Occupational therapy for physical dysfunction* (3rd ed.) (pp. 386-410). Baltimore: Williams & Wilkins.

Turnbull, A.P. & Turnbull, H.R. (1990). *Families, professionals, and exceptionality: a special partnership* (2nd ed.). Columbus, OH: Merrill.

Ward, D. (1983). *Positioning the handicapped child for function.* St. Louis: Diane E. Ward.

Willis, W. (1992). Families with African-American roots. In E.W. Lynch & M.J. Hanson (Eds.). *Developing cross-cultural competence* (pp. 121-146). Baltimore: Brookes.

Wright, C. & Nomura, M. (1985). *From toys to computers: access for the physically disabled child.* San Jose, CA: Christine Wright and Mari Nomura.

York, J. & Rainforth, B. (1991). Developing instructional adaptations. In F.P. Orelove & D. Sobsey (Eds.). *Educating children with multiple disabilities* (2nd ed.) (pp. 259-295). Baltimore: Brookes.

Zuniga, M.E. (1992). Families with Latino roots. In E.W. Lynch & M.J. Hanson (Eds.). *Developing cross-cultural competence* (pp. 151-175). Baltimore: Brookes.

## SUGGESTED READINGS

Dunaway, A., & Klein, M.D. (1988). *Bathing techniques for children who have cerebral palsy.* Tucson: Therapy Skill Builders.

Hale, G. (1979). *The source book for the disabled.* New York: Paddington Press.

Jones, M.J. (1981). *Home care for the chronically ill or disabled child.* New York: Harper Row.

Klein, M.D. (1988). *Pre-dressing skills.* Tucson: Therapy Skill Builders.

Lefchaez, R. & Winslow, B. (1979). *Design for independent living.* New York: Watson-Guptill.

Musselwhite, C. (1986). *Adaptive play for special needs children.* San Diego: College-Hill Press.

Russell, P. (1985). *The wheelchair child.* Englewook, NJ: Prentice Hill.

Snell, M.E. (1993). *Instruction of students with severe disabilities.* New York: Macmillan.

Wilcox, B. & Bellamy, G. (1982). *Design of high school programs for severely handicapped students.* Baltimore: Brookes.

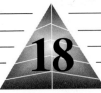

# Play

CHRISTINE DOYLE MORRISON ▲ PEGGY METZGER ▲ PAT NUSE PRATT

## KEY TERMS

▲ Exploratory, Competency, and Achievement Behaviors
▲ Playfulness
▲ Intrinsic Motivation
▲ Internal Reality
▲ Locus of Control
▲ Play Skills

## CHAPTER OBJECTIVES

1. Use the work of major theorists to define play and its development.
2. Use a working knowledge of the pediatric play definition to define the criteria of play.
3. Understand playfulness and how to use the concept when looking at a play situation.
4. Identify the different methods of using play in intervention.
5. Apply the knowledge gained in this chapter to specific children who have been referred to occupational therapy for assessments or intervention.

Because play is the primary occupation of children, occupational therapists who practice in pediatrics need to understand the power of play. In observations of pediatric practice, play can readily be identified as the tie that binds occupational therapy assessment and treatment.

## SCOPE OF PLAY IN OCCUPATIONAL THERAPY

A thorough review of literature on play is impossible within the constraints of this chapter, but the references and suggested readings should be helpful. This chapter presents a background on the developing uses of play in occupational therapy and then describes the scope of play in practice and provides a definition of play as a therapeutic modality and intervention outcome. Assessments that measure (1) play skills, (2) traits of playfulness, and (3) developmental skills in a play environment are described. The role of play and playfulness during therapy sessions is explained, distinguishing between the use of play as a modality to improve skills and therapy focused on improving play skills and interactions.

## Historical Perspective

During the early part of the twentieth century, the perspective of play of diversion was prevalent. Play was viewed as the means of recruiting the mind-body connection in the strive toward wellness. For example, Susan Tracy (1912), in a book designed to train nurses in the treatment of occupation, provided lengthy descriptions for making toys from common objects when working with children who were sick. The goal of this treatment was to alter the environment of the sick room and to divert children from thoughts of illness by engaging them in the occupation of creating toys. Play as diversion was an integral part of occupational therapy (OT) intervention with children during this paradigm.

Kielhofner and Burke (1983) suggested that during the 1940s and 1950s the field of OT entered a period of crisis. Because the medical community of the time was focused on identifying the internal mechanisms that underlie bodily functions, "medicine did not recognize as scientific the holistic concepts which characterized the paradigm of occupation" (Kielhofner & Burke, p. 27). In addition, secondary to advances in medical technology, occupational therapists were working with people with a variety of new and unfamiliar diagnoses (Slagle & Robeson, 1941). The paradigm of occupation could no longer provide OT practitioners with answers to all of their questions. In a search for answers to these questions, competing points of view were prevalent in the literature.

Specific to play, during the beginning of this crisis period, Slagle and Robeson (1941) described play as synonymous with recreation and as a therapeutic modality equal in importance to crafts and habit training. The diversional focus of play and the dominance of the mind over the body were seen in their writings. However, over the next 20 years a subtle shift was seen, and play began to take on the role of a therapeutic modality. Play was described as "activities not only to maintain status quo, but also to serve as a stimulus for normal growth and development" (Richmond & Lis, 1949, p. 186) and as the mechanism through which children develop their muscles and learn to use their bodies (Alessandrini, 1949). Thus play moved from a diversional role in the mind-body connection to healing and began to be viewed as a treatment modality for facilitating development.

Kielhofner and Burke (1983) proposed that by the end of the 1950s OT entered into the second paradigm, which they called the *inner mechanisms paradigm*. Occupational therapists were no longer focused on the ideas of occupation, mind-body unity, and diversion but were focused instead on scientific principles of practice that could explain why the process of treatment worked (Kielhofner & Burke, 1983).

It was during this paradigm that the practice theory of neurodevelopmental treatment (NDT) came into more widespread use and the theory of sensory integration (SI) originated. These theories became the primary focus of pediatric OT. Fiorentino (1966) captured this change when stating that the aim of pediatric OT was "purposeful function; the development and/or restoration of such function to the maximum ability of the child" (p. 251). Occupation was no longer mentioned, and although *function* was the stated endpoint of OT treatment, the goal was to "suppress or inhibit the primitive, abnormal tonic reflexes and facilitate higher, integrated righting and equilibrium reactions" (Fiorentino, 1966, p. 99). By so doing, the child was expected to learn to move using more normal patterns; function was expected to improve automatically. The therapist did not necessarily attend to function during treatment sessions but instead used a strong developmental frame of reference. Thus play was no longer viewed as a relevant focus of pediatric OT.

Kielhofner and Burke (1983) suggested that a second crisis period emerged in the 1970s, which was "precipitated by recognition of the limitations of reductionism for science and of technology for the needs of the chronically disabled and by the internal confusion and incoherence of occupational therapy" (p. 46). During this time play resurfaced as a topic in the OT literature.

## Reilly: Play as Exploratory Learning

Reilly (1974) developed a theory of play that has influenced the course of occupational therapy. She explained that play (1) has an organizing effect on human behavior and (2) is a critical base for adult competence. Reilly proposed that the ultimate service that play provides is to give meaning to the complexities of society (Florey, 1989). Reilly's theory of play consisted of three aspects: (1) an explanatory framework for child behavior, (2) a learning system through which the play process is explained, and (3) a developmental progression through which the changes in the outcome of the play process can be viewed.

Play must be acknowledged as a multidimensional phenomenon. Reilly (1974) stated, "existing theories about behavior are limited in their ability to explain multiple dimensions and integrating mechanisms" (p. 118). She believed that the outcomes of play were learning to symbolize and learning meanings. She defined *learning* as "a product of the interaction of external facts of reality with internal values" (Reilly, 1974, p. 131). The child continually asks "what is it," particularly in the presence of novelty. Hence play is energized by curiosity, and the child explores the environment to learn how objects, people, and events work. Through this exploratory action, the child generates a rule about how to operate a toy or use an object according to its intended or unintended purpose. These learned rules become the child's understanding of the meaning of the world and provide the foundation for the development of competency.

Reilly conceptualized three hierarchic stages of play: (1) exploratory behavior, (2) competency behavior, and (3) achievement behavior. Each stage expresses a higher level of excitement and requires a greater degree of control. Although curiosity is the underlying force that drives the system, each stage is documented by its own motivational force.

*Exploratory behavior* in play is usually seen in early childhood or when an event is new or different. It is a class of behavior that is motivated by "functional pleasure." It is engaged in for its own sake and, therefore, is driven by intrinsic motivation. When the child is anxious or under pressure, he or she is unable to engage in exploratory play. Meeting basic needs is therefore a requisite for the child to explore the environment in free play. This type of play is associated with experiences of art, music, and dance. Exploratory behaviors are done for themselves and generate a feeling of hope and trust in the player.

*Competency behavior* is characterized by a drive to act on and influence the environment. It results in sensory feedback that influences the player. To achieve competence, the child is persistent and concentrates on the activity. Through practice in play, tasks are mastered. At this stage the child may appear to overpractice or overlearn behaviors. The repetition enables the child to develop habits and absolute competency in an activity. Through this practice and resulting mastery, the child gains self-confidence and self-reliance.

*Achievement behavior* is the third stage and focuses on performance. Using the concept of *achievement motive* as defined by McClelland, Atkinson, and Lowell (1953), Reilly described *expectations* that are developed by the child through anticipated or past achievements. As the child plays and acts on the environment, certain results are produced. The feedback from these results is accumulated by the child and becomes the basis for his or her expectations about future performance. The child believes that he or she is capable of achieving certain outcomes, and the child's desire to meet those self-imposed standards becomes the basis of his or her play. The child's own standards of excellence become linked to public standards and whether his or her behavior was acceptable to others. Therefore this stage is characterized by competition, with self or others, and is linked to levels of aspiration. Achievement behaviors strive to increase one's own capability in activities and involve a higher level of excitation than the other two stages. "Danger and risk taking are characteristic of this behavior. The hope and self-confidence generated by the other two stages must . . . be transformed to a state of courage" (Reilly, 1974, p. 148).

Together these stages explain how the child develops rules through sensorimotor exploration. By understanding rules, the child learns appropriate social roles to engage in cooperative and competitive interaction.

Thus the early manipulation of objects and people and engagement in arts, crafts, and games yields the risk-taking behaviors seen in craftsmanship and sportsmanship. The results of engagement in these risk-taking behaviors are seen as necessary preconditions for engagement in adult workmanship (Florey, 1989, p. 39).

Reilly has given the profession of OT an essential understanding about the child's development of play, competency, and achievement that serves as a foundation for facilitation of those goals in intervention. Several of Reilly's colleagues have also contributed to the profession's understanding of play; the work of Florey and Takata is briefly described. The work of other noted play researchers follows.

## Florey: A Classification of Play

Florey (1971) defined play as the action on human and nonhuman objects that is engaged in for its own sake. Florey further described play as a learning process. This concept has been differentiated somewhat by other theorists. Piaget, as cited by Flavell (1977), defined play as those actions of the child that are dominated by assimilation, that is, when the child is able to direct actions with established mental schemes. In contrast, Piaget believed that playful actions that were dominated by accommodation are more properly described as imitation. Hutt (1979) proposed a taxonomy of play that nicely integrates Piagetian theory with the more global view of Florey. Hutt stipulated that there are two major categories of play. *Epistemic play* behaviors are concerned with the acquisition of new information and knowl-

edge. *Ludic play* includes those behaviors that are dominated by use of past experiences. This differentiation can be useful to the occupational therapist for selection and adaptation of activities.

Florey (1971) developed a classification system that organizes the developmental sequence of play behaviors according to variations in actions with human and nonhuman objects. Actions with human objects include play with parents, peers, significant others, and the child's own body. Nonhuman objects are divided into three groups according to the inherent properties of the object that may change as a result of the child's actions. Type I objects include creative and unstructured media that can be directly changed by the playful actions of the child. Objects that can be changed when combined with other objects are classified as type II. Objects that maintain their original form in relatively stable conditions regardless of play actions, such as bicycles and dolls, are referred to as type III. Florey indicated through her classification that differential and preferential engagement in play with human and nonhuman objects vary over the course of time. For example, during the preschool years, play with human objects is often directed toward the self and family. As the child matures, more action is directed toward peers and away from the self and parents. Similarly, involvement with an increasingly broad range of nonhuman objects occurs as the child ages.

## Takata: A Taxonomy of Play

In work that enriches concepts of play that were presented earlier by Florey (1969, 1971), Takata (1974) sought to identify critical patterns and representations of play and related these to age and milieu. This was accomplished through the construction of a two-directional taxonomy that can be used to examine the content of play and to help prescribe areas for intervention. The taxonomy's elements are reviewed here.

Takata proposed that play evolves through a sequence of age-related *epochs*, and Takata characterized these in an integration of concepts developed by Piaget, Erikson, and Florey. Each epoch has representative elements, which Takata identified as materials, actions, people, and setting. The epochs are the following:

1. *Sensorimotor epoch:* During the period from birth to 24 months, the play of the child is characterized by exploration and manipulation of the self, parents, siblings, significant others, and common objects in the environment. The child engages in play for its sensory experience and comes to know the basic actions and sensory properties of people and things.

2. *Symbolic and simple constructive epoch:* Through the emergence and refinement of language, the child develops symbols for the actions and properties that were discovered during the sensorimotor period. The

ability to communicate through symbols, coupled with increasing gross and fine motor capacity, allows the child to construct relationships between objects. Relationships are established through the child's sensorimotor experiences but are extended through the developing imagination of the child.

3. *Dramatic, complex, constructive, and pregame epoch:* The 4- to 7-year-old child learns to act out concepts and experiences through play and begins to put concepts together to form elementary rules of actions. Dramatic play replaces imaginative fantasy because the child now knows better what is likely to happen. The putting together of objects through construction becomes increasingly important as the child's ability to represent reality increases. Peer interaction becomes pivotal as the child begins to test the validity of constructs and skills. This period is transitional from exploratory to competency play as defined by Reilly (1974).

4. *Game epoch:* The elementary school-aged child is driven by the urge to control the actions of objects and events. Occupation in game playing predominates because such activities offer the child increasingly complex variations of rules and thus increase the child's sense of control and mastery. Rules prescribe ways of doing things and show the child a way to increase competence. Competence is measured by the rough competitive play with peers.

5. *Recreation epoch:* The play behavior of the adolescent assumes a more mature form through involvement in recreational activities. The balance of occupational behavior has shifted in the direction of work, and recreation allows the refinement of skills and interactions that relate to or support the youth's performance in adult roles. The games and social activities of recreation demonstrate increasingly sophisticated rules, role functions, and patterns of cooperation with the team or group.

This play taxonomy was originally designed to be used in conjunction with Takata's play history. The play history is an interview of the parents used to gather data on the child's play skills, interests, and preferences and is described in the section on play assessments.

## Characteristics of and Contexts for Play

Rubin, Fein, and Vandenberg (1983) combined the work of their predecessors (Piaget, Smilansky, and Parten) into a definition of play that helps explain the concept of playfulness. They believed that play can be defined three different ways. In the first approach, play is defined by the traits that distinguish it from other types of behaviors. They identified six commonly cited characteristics that distinguish play from nonplay. Each of these characteristics represents a continuum; at one extreme, each is a trait of play; at the other,

each reflects nonplay. The characteristics listed by Rubin and his colleagues are as follows.

1. Play is an intrinsically motivated behavior
2. In play, the player pays more attention to the means than the ends; the process than the product
3. Play is guided by the organism, not the stimulus (i.e., "what can I do with this object?" rather than "what does this object do?")
4. Play comprises nonserious renditions of activities
5. In play, the player is free from externally imposed rules
6. When playing, the player is actively engaged in the play activity and is not a passive participant

A second way that psychologists define play is as observable categories of behavior (Rubin et al., 1983). For example, Piaget, Smilansky, and Parten developed categories of play that define social and cognitive play (Table 18-1).

▲ **Table 18-1**    Theorists and Play Categories

| Theorist | Play Categories |
|---|---|
| Piaget (1962) | Practice play: the play of infants, when a child repeats actions that have been acquired |
| | Symbolic play: involves manipulation of tools |
| | Games with rules: involves practice with rules |
| Smilansky (cited in Rubin, Maioni, & Hornung, 1976) | Functional play: sensorimotor or practice play that consists of simple repetitive movements |
| | Constructive play: manipulation of objects to construct or create something |
| | Dramatic play: recognition, acceptance, and conformity to rules imposed on an activity |
| Parten (cited in Rubin et al., 1976) | Unoccupied play: playing with one's own body; random activity |
| | Solitary play: playing with toys differently from children within speaking distance; interest centered on own play and independent activity |
| | Onlooker play: watching others but not entering into the situation |
| | Parallel play: playing independently beside, not with, others |
| | Associative play: group play with group agreement on common activities and interests. |
| | Cooperative play: the group is organized to achieve some goal; highly organized group activity |

Another approach to defining play is by the context in which the play occurs. Rubin et al. listed five components thought to promote play:

1. An array of familiar peers, toys, or other materials interesting to the child
2. An agreement between the child and adult that the child is free to choose whatever he or she may want to do
3. Adult behavior that is minimally intrusive or directive
4. An atmosphere that makes children feel comfortable and safe
5. Scheduling that reduces the likelihood of the children being tired (p. 701).

Neumann (1971) identified three common themes in the literature that defined play. The common criteria for play were: (1) intrinsic motivation, (2) internal reality (the ability to suspend reality), and (3) internal locus of control. When all three criteria were present the child was engaged in a play interaction.

## Bundy: Playfulness

Based on the work of Rubin and Neumann, Bundy (1987) proposed a definition of play and playfulness to be used by occupational therapists. Bundy's goals were to help therapists effectively evaluate and promote play. Bundy's working definition helps the therapist understand the prerequisites of play and to recognize when the child is engaged in genuine play. She defined play as a continuum:

> Play is a transaction between the child and the environment which is intrinsically motivated, internally controlled, and not bound by objective reality . . . . Acknowledging that it is not always possible for children to be in complete control of their environment or to fully determine their own reality, play is considered to be a continuum of behaviors which are more or less playful depending on the degree to which the criteria are present (p. 16).

To fully understand Bundy's definition of play, it is important to understand the individual criteria present in the definition. These criteria—internal locus of control, intrinsic motivation, and ability to suspend reality—are briefly explained.

### Intrinsic Motivation

There are varied ways to define intrinsic motivation, but most theorists agree that it is an important criterion of play. Neumann (1971) defined intrinsic motivation as the player being self-motivated and concerned with the purpose and process inherent in the activity. Similarly, Levy (1978) defined *intrinsic motivation* as "the drive to become involved in an activity originating from within the person or the activity: the reward is generated by the transaction itself" (p. 6). Rubin et al. (1983) defined intrinsic motivation by contrasting it with what it is not. A behavior that is intrinsi-

cally motivating is not governed by appetitive drives, compliance with social demands, or inducements external to the behavior itself.

Similarly, OT theorists also have defined intrinsic motivation through contrast. Florey (1971) defined an intrinsic motive as one that does not depend on rewards outside the activity. Takata (1974) indicated that play is not associated with a particular end or an eventual gain or profit. The player is more concerned with the process than the product of the transaction. In other words, an intrinsically motivating activity is, in itself, motivating to the child.

A child who is intrinsically motivated is the child who is totally absorbed in an activity, so much so that the child is unaware of the activity going on around him or her. The child is also more involved in the process of the activity than the outcome. For instance, the child who is finger painting and changes the picture continually as he or she adds different colors and strokes to the picture is intrinsically motivated.

### Internal Reality

Internal reality, the second of Bundy's criteria, is defined slightly differently by different theorists. Neumann (1971) defined internal reality as the player's being free to suspend reality to establish the rules, procedures, and content of play. That is, play behaviors are not serious renditions of the activities they resemble (Bateson, 1972). Internal reality also pertains to the individual's being able to do whatever he or she wants with objects (Rubin et al., 1983). Focusing on the imaginative aspect of suspending reality, Levy (1978) defined internal reality as "the loss of the 'real self' and the temporary acceptance of an 'illusory self' or 'imaginative self'" (p. 12).

Bundy (1991) stated that the individual's ability to pretend, internal reality, was only one aspect of a larger construct of play, the suspension of reality. Included in suspension of reality is the elimination of consequences that might normally be associated with the activity if performed in real life (Vandenberg & Kielhofner, 1982). The child may be suspending reality when he or she answers, "whatever I want" to the question, "what can you do with this object?" Because this question (1) guides play, (2) is the basis of internal locus of control, and (3) may reflect suspension of reality, the theoretical link between the ability to suspend reality and locus of control during a play transaction becomes more evident.

A child who is free to suspend reality is the child who creates play situations without needing the structure provided by specific toys or objects. Further, the child's play is fluid and flexible. A child might sometimes use a car as a car, but this child might be just as likely to turn a box into a car or boat. After a time, he or she might turn the same box over and make it into a house or tunnel.

## Locus of Control

Locus of control has also been defined slightly differently by different theorists. Neumann (1971) defined locus of control as the player's determining exactly what occurs during the transaction. Similarly, Levy (1978) defined internal locus of control as "the degree to which individuals perceive they are in control of their actions and outcomes" (p. 15).

Rubin et al. (1983) contrasted internal control with exploratory behavior. When a child is exploring, the child's behavior seems to answer, "I don't know" to the question, "What can you do with this object?" This behavior suggests that the child lacks control over the transaction. Hutt (1976, 1979) and Rubin et al. (1983) agreed that children need to explore objects and environments before they gain control and thus truly play. As the child becomes comfortable with the environment, he or she uses objects in a variety of ways (that is, plays with them). Conversely, the child who is exploring remains focused on obtaining information about the object.

A child who is in control of the transaction is one who is able to decide what and with whom he or she plays. This child is also able to decide what he or she is going to do with either the object or the person. This child is skilled at negotiating steps to accomplish the desired outcome for the transaction.

## Play Transaction as a Continuum

Intrinsic motivation, internal reality, and locus of control are not mutually exclusive, and, as stated previously, they are each on a continuum. No transaction can be totally intrinsically motivating, internally controlled, and free for the suspension of reality. However, every play transaction has a combination of the criteria present to greater or lesser degrees. Depending on the extent to which each of the criteria is present, the transaction becomes more play or nonplay.

Bundy (1991) presented a pictorial scale for examining the relationship between perception of control, source of motivation, and suspension of reality in any given play scenario. Figure 18-1 can be used to conceptualize where a play transaction falls on the continuum of play and nonplay.

Two other important aspects need to be addressed in expanding the play definition: *transaction* and *framing the play, thus giving and reading cues* (Bateson, 1972). This definition of play stated that play is a transaction between the child and the environment. Neumann (1971) defined transaction as a "relationship entered into by the child and his environment . . . during which specific aspects of the environment and of the child are manipulated by the child" (p. 137). This notion of a transaction is also supported by Rubin et al. (1983), who stated that a player must be active for a behavior to be considered play. This active engagement or manipulation of the environment implies a constant awareness of, and response to, the immediate surroundings by the child.

## Prerequisites to Play

When playing, the child communicates a message that "This is play, this is how I am going to act" (Bateson, 1972). Thus the child provides a cue regarding his or her intent to whomever is interacting in or observing the play transaction. Cues are the verbal and, more importantly, the nonverbal messages that the child gives and receives during transactions with others. In play, giving cues that say "I'm playing now" and "This is how you should act toward me" as well as responding appropriately to the cues of those with whom the child is playing are integral to being a successful player. It is proposed that cue giving and reading are a necessary foundation for play. Therefore it is also proposed

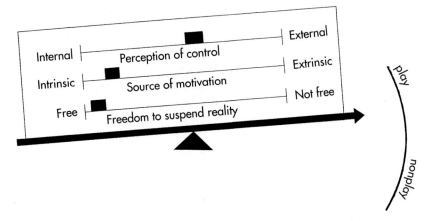

**Figure 18-1**   Elements of play and nonplay. (Modified from Bundy, A.C. [1991]. In A.G. Fisher, E.A. Murray, & A.C. Bundy [Eds.]. *Sensory integration: theory and practice* [p. 60]. Philadelphia: F.A. Davis.)

that helping an infant to give and read cues early on may be an important first step in the development of a playful child. This can be done in infancy by responding to the infant's cues. For example, when an infant pushes with his or her arms and legs and turns his or her eyes away from the adult talking to him or her it generally means that the infant needs a break from the transaction. The adult can respond to those cues by not talking, allowing the infant to look away, and providing the break that the infant is requesting. In the same way, if the infant is rooting toward anything that touches his or her cheek and is beginning to fuss, the infant is probably telling the adult that he or she is hungry. When the adult responds by feeding the infant, he or she has appropriately responded to the infant's cues. In both of these instances the adult is giving the infant the message that his or her cues are valued and that the infant is important and in control.

An infant's cues also provide the adult with information regarding the infant's likes and dislikes in relation to the environment around him or her. For example, the infant who molds his or her body to the mother's body each time the mother picks up the infant may be telling her that physical contact is enjoyable. Conversely, the infant who fusses, squirms, and pulls away each time he or she is touched may be expressing that touch is not pleasant for him or her. So, in addition to telling the infant that his or her cues are valued and that he or she is important, responding to an infant's cues by adapting the environment to minimize those experiences that are unpleasant provides the infant with the message that the environment is a safe and pleasant place to be and, again, that he or she is in control.

Once the infant feels safe and comfortable, he or she can begin to explore the environment around him or her and play. In the development of the Test of Playfulness (ToP), Bundy (in press) and colleagues found that feeling safe is the most basic prerequisite characteristic of play. If the children did not feel safe, they did not play. This feeling of safety also allows the child to explore and gather sensory information that precedes and evolves into play. This is the time during which the child learns everything he or she can about an object or the environment before using that knowledge in play.

These environmental components have been supported by various authors (Cohen, 1987; Hutt, 1976; Rubin, 1977; Schwartzman, 1984), all of whom have suggested that when a child feels comfortable and safe in the environment, he or she will be able to play. Given this definition, how do occupational therapists assess play behaviors? A review of play assessments follows.

## Play Assessments

Several play assessments have been developed by occupational therapists. These include the *Play History* (Takata, 1974), *Guide to Observation of Play Development* (Florey,

1971), the *Play Scale* (Knox, 1974), the *Preschool Play Scale* (Bledsoe & Shepherd, 1982), and the *Test of Playfulness* (Bundy, in press).

In the *Play History,* Takata (1974) used an extensive method of history taking and observation to evaluate the play development of children. The interview also gathers information about the play environment, including what toys the child uses and when, where, and with whom the child plays. The play history shows assets and limitations in the child's ability to play and in the available play opportunities (Takata, 1974). Its five sections gather information regarding (1) general information about the child, (2) previous play experiences, (3) actual play examination, (4) play description, and (5) play prescription. After gathering all of this information the therapist is able to put together a picture of the child's play development, analyze it for any problems, and make a prescription to minimize problems.

The assessment that has been most often used and cited in OT literature is the Play Scale (Knox, 1974), which was revised by Bledsoe and Shepherd (1982) and called the Preschool Play Scale. Knox (1974) intended *The Play Scale* to be used to determine the child's *play age* as well as his or her *play profile.* She used descriptions of normal play behavior of preschool children in yearly increments. Knox divided play development and play characteristics into four dimensions composed of specific categories relating to that particular dimension: *space management* focused on gross motor skills; *material management* was defined as the manner in which the child manipulated objects and materials and the purpose for which the child used them; *imitation* was the manner in which the child demonstrated an understanding of the social environment and feelings; and *participation* examines the degree and manner in which the child interacts with people in the environment. She found the scale to be useful for measuring the everyday play behavior of children and suggested that it be evaluated for validity and reliability. In 1981 Bledsoe and Shepherd revised and renamed the Knox's Play Scale as the Preschool Play Scale and examined it for reliability and validity. The results of their study suggested that the Preschool Play Scale yields objective, stable, and valid measurements of play behavior. However, they recommended that the Preschool Play Scale be used in "conjunction with an assessment of playfulness or degree of involvement in play. This aspect of play is vital to a total assessment of play behavior" (p. 788).

The ToP (Bundy, in press) reflects the criteria of play identified in Bundy's (1987) definition mentioned previously. The three criteria have been defined as elements of playfulness. The ToP also incorporates the aspect of giving and reading cues originally discussed by Bateson (1972) and described previously.

All of the assessments described previously, with the exception of the ToP, assess the child's skills within a play situation and not the play of the child. A comprehensive OT evaluation should include playfulness as well as developmental skills within the context of play.

## Playfulness

Lieberman (1977) was one of the first to define playfulness as a characteristic of the player and to design a measurement tool to capture its essence. Barnett (1990, 1991) continued to explore the playfulness trait posited by Lieberman. She revised the playfulness scale and titled it the *Children's Playfulness Scale (CPS)*.

In a recent study, Knox (in press) explored the play of preschool children using qualitative methods. She visited a child care center in southern California 15 times over a 3-month period and observed children aged 18 months to 3 years and 3 to 5½ years. Some of these children stood out as playful; others seemed to be always "on the fringe" of the activities. In analyzing her observations, as well as the interviews of parents and teachers, Knox identified actions and behaviors that seemed to differentiate more playful from less playful children. She found the more playful children to be more flexible in their play; that is, they often became the center of the action and seemed to be in charge of play situations. They were creative and often elaborated on games or episodes that others started, gradually making them their own. Some of the characteristics she described in the more playful children included curiosity, imagination, joy, physical activity, and social and verbal flexibility.

The less playful children initiated games but retreated to follower or onlooker roles as soon as other children took the lead. These children seemed not to have the spontaneity or flexibility to "go with the flow" of the play episode. Knox described characteristics of less playful children as negative affect or verbalizations, physical or emotional withdrawal, lack of control over a situation, refusal to participate, preference for adults or younger children, and emotional immaturity (Knox, in press).

To summarize, play has been described from within an OT perspective as well as within related fields. Various definitions were reviewed, and a definition believed most appropriate for therapists to use within their practice was given. Three criteria (intrinsic motivation, internal control [locus of control], and freedom to suspend reality [internal reality]) make the transaction either play or nonplay. These criteria can also make the transaction more or less playful. However, all of this discussion has been primarily theoretical. It is time to look at the relationship between play and OT intervention in pediatrics. The following sections describe how the occupational therapist can use playful interactions and play activities to promote the child's developmental and functional skills as well as his or her playfulness.

## INTERVENTION

The earlier discussion regarding cue giving and reading suggested that it is important for the therapist to let the child know that the child is important and in control. This also gives the message that the therapist cares about what the child communicates about feeling safe within the environment. The therapist can do this by responding to the child's cues regarding what he or she likes or dislikes. Once the child learns that the therapist is interested in his or her cues, it is possible to build a trusting relationship with the therapist. From that point it is possible to begin therapy that truly challenges the child (Figure 18-2).

Occupational therapy intervention specific to play has three perspectives:

1. Intervention that uses play as a therapeutic modality when the treatment goals are to improve specific component skills (i.e., fine motor, gross motor, cognitive, and psychosocial skills) (Table 18-2)
2. Intervention focused on improving play skills
3. Intervention focused on facilitating playfulness

## USE OF PLAY AS A THERAPEUTIC MODALITY

Bundy (1991) stated, "If play is the vehicle by which individuals become masters of their environments, then play should be among the most powerful of therapeutic tools" (p. 61). To effectively use play as a therapeutic tool, it is important to remember that play is (1) "a transaction between the child and the environment which is intrinsically motivated, internally controlled, and free from objective re-

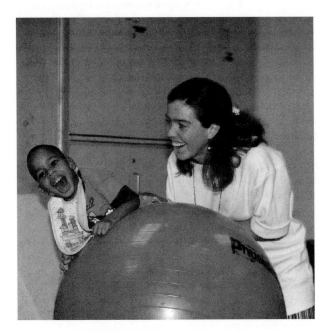

**Figure 18-2** Child demonstrates a sense of control and safety in the therapy environment. Therapy is now able to challenge his motor system.

▲ Table 18-2   Types and Examples of Play Activities

| Category/ Characteristic Age | Description | Properties of Activities | Representative Toys and Activities |
|---|---|---|---|
| Exploratory play/ 0 to 2 years | Play: recreational experiences through which the child develops a body scheme, sensory integrative and motor skills, and concepts of sensory characteristics and actions of human and nonhuman objects | Material and objects: Child's own body Significant others Environmental textures Infant toys with distinct sensory characteristics and actions Everyday household objects Human relationships: Strongest relationships occur through play between child and parents | Auditory toys (rattles, play piano); balls (all sizes and textures); bells, blocks, busy boxes; containers and nesting toys; dolls and stuffed animals; hammer and pegs; imitative hand-body games; inflatables; language play with parents; mirrors; mobiles; pop-up toys; pots and pans; rolling, crawling, and cruising activities; sand and water toys and activities; brightly colored scarves; scooter boards; scribbling with crayons; See 'N' Say, sensory play with parents; shape boxes; empty spice bottles; squeeze toys; teething toys; textured surfaces; 1- to 3-piece puzzles |
| Symbolic play/ 2 to 4 years | Play and recreational experiences through which the child formulates, tests, classifies, and refines ideas, feelings, and combined actions Associated with the development of language Objects are given importance according to the child's ability to symbolize, control, change, and master | Materials and objects: Gross motor play equipment Simple construction toys Simple art materials Toys for fantasy-imaginative play Human relationships: Play with peers begins with parallel imitation and develops into cooperative interaction | Balance-rocker boards, blocks, beads, blowing bubbles, cars, trucks, trains, chalk and blackboard activities, clay, modeling dough, colorforms, construction kits, crayons, paints, paper, dolls and stuffed animals, dollhouses, dramatic songs, "dress up" materials, fingerpaints, hand puppets, household play items, inflatables, magnets, miniature figures, musical instruments, nesting toys, play tunnel, put-together toys, puzzles, records, rocking horse, rolling in the grass, sand and water toys, sewing cards, simple story books, slides, space stations, stacking toys, swings, toy telephone, tricycle riding |
| Creative play/ 4 to 7 years | Play and recreational experiences through which the child refines sensory, motor, cognitive, and social skills; explores combinations of actions on multiple objects; and develops interests and competencies that promote performance of school-related and work-related activities | Materials and objects: Arts and crafts Complex construction toys Dramatic play materials Household activities such as cooking, simple woodwork, pet care, and gardening Human relationships: Play begins in cooperative peer groups with gradual emergence of competitive atmosphere; peer validation of play products becomes increasingly import Parents assist and validate in the absence of peers | Baking cookies, stringing beads, bicycle riding, craft kits, cutting and pasting, finger painting, gardening, origami, painting, paperdolls, play house, simple weaving (placemats and pot holders), simple woodworking, stencils |

Modified from Pratt, P.N. (1989). Play and recreational activities. In P.N. Pratt & A.S. Allen (Eds.). *Occupational therapy for children.* (pp. 295-310). St. Louis: Mosby.

▲ Table 18-2   Types and Examples of Play Activities—cont'd

| Category/ Characteristic Age | Description | Properties of Activities | Representative Toys and Activities |
|---|---|---|---|
| Games/ 7 to 12 years | Play and recreational experiences that have distinct rules and involve skill development and social interaction in a competitive atmosphere<br>Actions and results of actions are compared against those of peers | Materials and objects:<br>Arts and crafts<br>Complex construction toys<br>Dramatic play materials<br>Household activities such as cooking, simple wookwork, pet care, and gardening<br>Human relationships:<br>Play begins in cooperative peer groups with gradual emergence of competitive atmosphere; peer validation of play products becomes increasingly important<br>Parents assist and validate in the absence of peers | Board games, card games, checkers, clubs, collections, computer games, field days (races and tug-of-war), hangman, jacks, marbles, jump rope, organized outdoor games, ping pong, roller skating and ice skating, school plays, performances, scooter board races, team sports, trading cards |

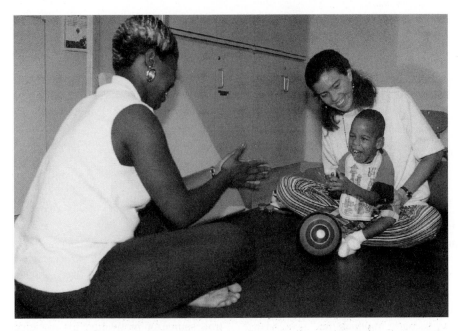

**Figure 18-3**   Therapist uses play as a therapeutic modality to increase child's involvement in a task focused on improving bilateral use of hands.

ality" (Bundy, 1991, p. 59) and (2) a continuum of behaviors from play to nonplay. The therapist can then turn a nonplayful interaction into a playful one by altering the perception of control, the source of motivation, or the need for objective reality in a situation (Figure 18-3).

Jake is a 4-year-old boy who loves to play and is ingenious in persisting with his play despite significant motoric challenges. Jake has spastic cerebral palsy that affects his ability to move both of his legs. Although he has functional use of both arms, active use increases his muscle tone, making it difficult for him to reach for and manipulate toys and objects. This difficulty is manifested in his attempts to play with his action figures (Jake calls them his

"guys") and in his difficulty with lower-extremity dressing. Jake's OT goals are to improve accuracy and range of reach, increase manipulation skills, and improve dressing skills (i.e., don pants, shoes, and socks). Treatment activities that involved hand-over-hand repeated practice of reach to a target were frustrating and demotivating for Jake. His perception of these therapist-designed activities is depicted in Figure 18-4.

Without changing the goals, the occupational therapist decided that the first objective was to engage Jake in play. She set up the environment with a variety of toys and activities then encouraged Jake to actively explore the entire environment and to choose what he would like to do. Jake

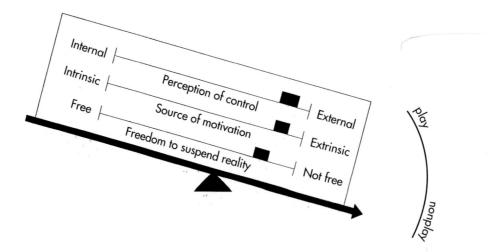

**Figure 18-4** Nonplay transaction. (Modified from Bundy, A.C. [1991]. Play theory and sensory integration. In A.G. Fisher, E.A. Murray, & A.C. Bundy [Eds.]. *Sensory integration: theory and practice* [p. 60]. Philadelphia: F.A. Davis.)

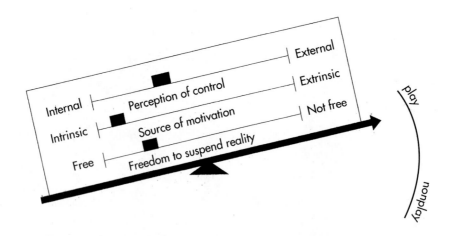

**Figure 18-5** Play transaction. (Modified from Bundy, A.C. [1991]. Play theory and sensory integration. In A.G. Fisher, E.A. Murray, & A.C. Bundy [Eds.]. *Sensory integration: theory and practice* [p. 60]. Philadelphia: F.A. Davis.)

chose to play with his "guys." The therapist and Jake began to engage in a play scenario in which the "guys" visit different planets, each with a variety of objects to explore, successfully changing both the motivation (Jake chose one of his favorite toys and activities) and the reality (different surfaces requiring arm placement to a variety of planes became the planets of the play scenario). Inherent in the above play transaction are many opportunities for practicing arm placement in different planes (planets) and for manipulating different sized and shaped objects (present on the different planets). This therapy session, as depicted by Figure 18-5, is no longer frustrating for Jake, but, in fact, is quite enjoyable.

The therapist has successfully used play in the orchestration of a treatment session that is fun for Jake and allows him to practice difficult arm placement and manipu-

lation tasks. By considering the child's perception of control, source of motivation for participating in a task, and the reality of the situation, it is possible to use play as a powerful therapeutic tool in planning and implementing treatment sessions that not only challenge the child to develop new skills, but also are enjoyable.

Motor impairment may often prevent the child's full participation in play. Through knowledgeable selection of activities, in cooperation with the child's interests and capacities, the occupational therapist can design a treatment program that improves motor function and at the same time promotes continuity in the child's development of play and related skills. The techniques that are used most with children who have motor problems include adaptation of position (of the body and work surface) and adaptation of the tools, material, and equipment that are used for an activity.

# INTERVENTION FOCUSED ON IMPROVING PLAY SKILLS

The second way in which play is important to pediatric OT intervention is apparent when a child demonstrates a play deficit. Because play is the primary occupation of children, it follows that if assessment of a child indicates a play deficit, intervention would then be aimed at improving play skills. Assessment of a child may show play deficits in one or more of the following ways:

1. The child demonstrates play skills that are developmentally immature for his or her chronologic age.
2. The child has a preference for types of play for which he or she does not have the necessary skills. In this situation there is a mismatch between the child's skills and his or her play preferences.

## Child With Immature Play Skills

In 1972 Gray discussed the effects of hospitalization on work-play behavior. She proposed that, to a greater or lesser degree, the medical focus on the individual's disability and related intervention overrides concern for the life that has been disrupted. When a child is hospitalized, family members tend to "do for" the child. In addition, the child is often isolated from the mainstream of childhood play and interactions. Therefore it becomes increasingly important for occupational therapists to provide the types of play experiences that promote skill development in the areas cited by Gray.

Gralewicz (1973) conducted a study that compared the play of small samples of nonhandicapped children and multihandicapped children who were 3 to 5 years old. Observations of play were recorded in the children's homes by their parents. Gralewicz found that the children without disabilities spent significantly more time playing, had more play companions, and engaged in a wider variety of play activities than the children with disabilities. In addition, although data were not statistically significant, the multihandicapped children spent more time engaged in no observable activity at all.

A later study by Kielhofner and others (1983) examined the differences in play of three nonhospitalized preschool children and three hospitalized children of similar ages who had spent more than 60% of their lives in hospitals. The children were videotaped at play in a hospital playroom and in a standardized play environment in which selected play objects were specifically set up before all videotape sessions. The investigators found significant differences in the level of play development and the playfulness of the children. The nonhospitalized children were more advanced. The investigators noted that the hospitalized children used toys more simply, rather than trying out a variety of actions, and that they usually did not engage in symbolic and interconnected play activities (Kielhofner et al., 1983).

These studies indicate that the children who are seen by occupational therapists in both educational and medical settings are likely to demonstrate problems in both quality and quantity of play experiences. Therefore it is important that the therapist provide opportunities for children to engage in play for its own sake, exclusive of objectives for improvement of specific functional correlates.

Treatment is aimed at expanding the child's play repertoire or ability to interact with his or her environment through play. One approach to intervention might be to use a developmental frame of reference and to treat the underlying component skills (e.g., social, fine motor, and gross motor) that impeded the child's performance during play. The underlying assumption to this approach to treatment is that the play skills automatically improve once the child gains skills in the component areas.

## Play to Promote Motor Skills

Donna is an 8-year-old girl with moderate spastic hemiplegia who was referred to occupational therapy for improvement of gross and fine motor skills. Assessment indicated that her typical play behaviors were at the level of symbolic activities, although she was interested in participating in more creative play and games. She was able to use her uninvolved left hand in all fine prehension patterns, but precise manipulative ability was generally poor. Although her involved right hand was used fairly well as a gross assist and was relaxed at rest, she tended to become tight during concentrated efforts. In such instances she became frustrated because she would lose control over her right hand as an assist.

Donna's sensory integrative function appeared slightly depressed. Equilibrium responses were adequate against mild resistance, but she needed support to maintain positions against moderate resistance. Social skills were well developed. Although her articulations were not always clear, her speech and language development were generally age-appropriate. General goals of occupational therapy were to improve performance in schoolwork and age-appropriate play activities. Because of her age, she received her occupational therapy services two times weekly as a member of a group that included three age-mates who had similar problems. As a general rule the group worked on creative activities once a week, with an emphasis on development of fine motor skills. The other weekly session was reserved for gross motor play through competitive activities.

One favorite activity was the puppet show, which was chosen to strengthen fine motor skills and symbolic representation. The therapist prepared two-sided outlines of simple animal shapes for felt hand puppets. The two sides were fastened together with a few paper clips over a slightly smaller cardboard template and set up in a table clamp. Donna sewed her puppet together by using a large needle and yarn in her left hand and by using the right hand to stabilize the edge near her stitches. She then cut out paper patterns for the puppet's facial features using one-handed scissors that roll across the material once it is stabilized on the table surface. When the puppets were completed, the children worked together to develop a skit to present to the rest of their class.

Because each of the children had weak balance and underdeveloped gross motor control, the therapist designed a beanbag toss game that allowed them to compete with each other and strengthen their gross motor skills. With the therapist, the children developed a set of rules that governed the actions and scoring of the game. A rocker board was used for sitting, knee-standing, and standing. Each child was responsible for positioning the rocker board behind the starting line before each throw. Target distances ranged from 5 to 10 feet; the children selected new targets after each turn was completed. Initially, the target was a large square area on the floor that was bordered by masking tape. As the children became more proficient and competitive, they suggested that the target change to a hula hoop and later to a wastebasket. Donna began by using an underhand toss and progressed to an overhand throw. An overriding concern of the group was that each child should compete fairly with the others. Consequently, the children modified the rules according to the performance capacity of each group member. For example, because Donna was the best thrower in the group, her starting line was placed 1 foot behind the others. Each child's positions on the rocker board varied according to his or her postural stability.

## Play to Promote Psychosocial Function

Children who are experiencing emotional difficulty may be characterized by diminished and regressed play behaviors (Llorens & Rubin, 1967). Children who are withdrawn usually withdraw from play as well. Children who demonstrate acting-out behaviors may use play objects in the course of such episodes, but the actions with such objects are not likely to be described as play; their play tends to be perseverative, and the play objects are more appropriate to younger children. Adaptation of play activities for the child with emotional problems is often accomplished through structure of the play environment and therapeutic relationship. Axline (1969) reported on the use of Rogerian form of play therapy with young children. She chose toys that, in general, lent themselves to symbolic play, such as action figures, dolls and dollhouses, and water play items. Toys that did not elicit feelings and expression were not used in the program. As children explored, played with toys, and talked about their play, Axline used nondirective techniques to focus, clarify, and enhance the child's expressive capacity.

Vandenberg and Kielhofner (1982) reported on the OT treatment of a 13-year-old boy with a diagnosis of adolescent adjustment reaction who demonstrated a tendency to withdraw from new situations. The boy resisted initial efforts to participate in a ceramics activity. Subsequently, the occupational therapist began to play with the clay, thus providing a role model for the boy. When the therapist dropped the clay, the situation was handled in a playful manner, subtly indicating to the boy that mistakes in new situations were permissible. Through this experience and subsequent treatment sessions with clay and other craft activities, the boy developed the capacity to approach and explore new situations with a sense of control and satisfaction. In this case the therapist's structure of the interpersonal relationship was subtle. The choice of clay, a medium that lends itself to many different uses and forms, was complemented by the structuring of a playful atmosphere.

Llorens and Rubin (1967) reported on a graded program of play activities that was used by OT for treatment of children with emotional disturbances. The core of the program was the children's involvement in activity groups. The *basic skills group* for children aged 6 to 12 emphasized free exploratory play with sensorimotor toys. When a child chose to play with an unfamiliar toy, the therapist instructed the child in one way to play with it. This technique was used, first, to provide the child with a successful play experience with the new toy and, second, through the success experience to stimulate the child's motivation to explore the toy further and develop additional skills.

The *skill development group* was more structured, with specific training in performance of symbolic and creative activities. The children worked on projects in a large group. Although specific expectations for project completion were established, children were permitted to perform at their own individual rates. Interactive experiences with the other children in the group were fostered by the therapist. The *advanced group* used craft activities and was highly structured. The therapist adopted the role of a teacher. Children were expected to work cooperatively and maintain a level of performance with the rest of the group. Activities ranged from structured kits to materials that demanded original designs. Increasingly complex techniques were taught through units, and children were graded on their productions.

Throughout this program, play progressed from being parallel, to cooperative, to competitive. This program demonstrates how OT can provide a microcosm of developmental play experiences for children.

Many of children's social skills are developed through play experiences. The occupational therapist needs to be alert to this and to structure play situations to provide opportunities for social development. Using the levels of social play developed by Parten (1933), occupational therapists can create play interactions that enhance social interaction skills. The young child's play with a new object is often solitary as the child obtains firsthand knowledge of characteristics and actions of the toy. The child may then imitate behaviors that were recently observed. Social behaviors in relation to sharing and cooperation are developed through parallel play experiences. Modeling and imitation of appropriate social behaviors are important learning methods for young children. The therapist can help by establishing simple rules for behavior and following up with clarification as to whether behaviors are appropriate or not. Children often want to play with a toy that another child is using. The therapist can develop skills of sharing and cooperation by structuring time limits and suggesting ways that two children can play together with the desired toy.

Associative and cooperative play experiences are easily promoted in the OT program. Craft projects and games are well suited to the development of interactive planning, decision making, and role-taking. In addition, children must take turns with tools and materials and develop and follow other cooperative rules. In the clinical example presented previously, a group of children made felt hand puppets. Although adequate tools could have been made available, the therapist structured the situation to promote social skills development by providing a limited number of scissors, needles, and bottles of glue. The children had to pace their own work to share. The subsequent puppet show was written by the children, each taking turns to contribute lines for one's puppet character and offering ideas for each others' characters. Through this process the individual child's involvement was directed from his or her own puppet to the success of the group project.

Another approach to treatment incorporates treatment activities aimed at facilitating the underlying skill deficit and allowing the child to generalize these skills through practice in play.

John is a 5-year-old boy with sensory integrative dysfunction. His difficulty in planning and sequencing unfamiliar motor tasks interferes with his ability to enjoy the playground equipment of his kindergarten class and to play soccer with the other children in his class. Part of John's occupational therapy is aimed at improving his underlying dyspraxia as described in Chapter 13. However, the other part of his treatment focuses on providing him with the opportunity to practice playing soccer and to allow him to practice playing on the playground equipment. The therapy sessions in which John practices his play skills allows him to do so in a safe and positive environment that allows him to fail without any consequences. By working on motor planning skills and simultaneously allowing him to practice difficult play tasks, the sessions build toward improved developmental performance during play. Part of the overall plan for John includes his family taking him to practice climbing on a neighborhood playground known to be safe and to have unusual, motivating climbing structures. Recommendations for safe playground play involve the entire family and help them understand principles for promoting John's skills and confidence.

## Mismatch Between Preference and Skill

To examine the problem of a mismatch between play skills and play preference, it is necessary to first review some of the OT play research. In a study by Clifford and Bundy (1989), the play preferences of two groups of 4- to 6-year-old boys were examined. One group consisted of boys who were typically developing, and one group consisted of boys diagnosed with sensory integrative (SI) dysfunction. Both the typically developing boys and the boys with SI dysfunction expressed a preference for sensorimotor play. However, when the relationship between play skill and play preference was examined for individual boys, many of the boys with SI dysfunction had adapted their preference in play to

reflect their skills. This suggests that, even at a very young age, children's play is influenced by the feedback they get from their environments.

Applying this research to clinical practice, it is suggested that it is important to assess both a child's preference and his or her play skills. Play preferences may be assessed by asking the child about his or her interests, by interviewing the parents, or by observing the child's choice in natural environments (e.g., home and school). It is suggested that children who (1) have the skills to play in the way that they prefer or (2) have altered their preferences for play to reflect their play skills do not have a play deficit and most likely do not require intervention focused on improving either play skills or altering preference.

However, for those children who prefer more complex play for which they do not have the necessary skills, it is suggested that they have a play deficit. For example, Jake, (see p. 513) preferred to play with his "guys" by moving their tiny arms and placing the various tools in their hands. Although he had the skill for imaginary figurine play, he did not have the fine motor skills for precise manipulation or their tiny parts and he often became frustrated when attempting to play.

In this instance, therapy with Jake could take one or more of three approaches. The occupational therapists could (1) focus treatment on improving fine motor skills and hope to improve his ability to play with his "guys" in his preferred manner, (2) expose Jake to a variety of other types of play for which he has the play skills and hope to alter his preference, or (3) alter the environment in some way to facilitate Jake's play with the toys he prefers.

### Focus on Altering Preference

When working with any child whose plays skills are insufficient for his or her preferred type of play (e.g., pretend play, or gross motor play), it is important to explore why the child prefers that type of play. What is it about that type of play that motivates the child? It may then be possible to find other play scenarios that can meet the same need or that are as motivating for the child. Jake, for example, may prefer to play with his "guys" by moving their arms and legs and manipulating the small tools because he likes to play with his older brother and best friend when they play with their toys in this way. The motivating factor for Jake may be the social interaction with his brother and his friend.

In this case it may be possible to include Jake's older brother in the treatment sessions and to explore with both Jake and his brother ways to play with the action figurines that both of the boys are able to master. Another scenario may be to explore with Jake and his brother types of play (e.g., computer games, playing with cars and trucks in the sand box, or playing with playdough) that require less fine motor dexterity than manipulating the tools and extremities of the action figurines. The goal of this type of intervention is to provide Jake with an activity that satisfies his intrinsic motivation but for which he has the skills to be in control.

By exploring with Jake what motivates him about his stated preferred method of play and by exposing both Jake and his brother to a variety of play scenarios in which both of them could still play together (which was the motivating factor), it was possible to help Jake to develop play preferences that reflected his play skills, instead of preferences that were beyond his skill level.

### Altering the Environment to Facilitate a Match Between Preference and Skills

The third approach to treatment when the child's play skills do not match his or her play preferences and interests is to examine the environment in which he or she plays (Vandenberg, 1981). Kielhofner (1995) stated ". . . the environment both affords opportunities for performance and presses for certain types of behavior" (p. 2). Environmental affordance refers to the "possibilities or potentials for achieving various forms of occupational behavior" along with the concept that the environment provides us with a range of opportunities for occupational behaviors" (p. 3). *Press* is defined as "what the environment expects or demands of the individual" (p. 3). Kielhofner (1995) further stated:

> . . . because environments both press and afford, they create a synergy of influences that channel our behavior in the midst of unfolding circumstances. That is, the environment, by simultaneously providing opportunity and constraint, creates behavioral pathways. As with any pathway, certain directions are easier to go by virtue of having the way cleared. However, pathways also imply that alternative routes are constrained, not as easy to traverse, or not accessible at all. By affording and pressing, environments invite and instruct behavior to go in particular directions (p. 6).

Applying this concept to the treatment of play in children, intervention environments are constructed to afford and press for certain play skills in a child. The occupational therapist (1) systematically constructs play environments, (2) facilitates the practice of play skills in the various treatment environments, (3) determines which aspects of the environment are affording or pressing the child to play in the manner in which he or she prefers, and (4) generalizes the characteristics of the treatment environment to other environments in the child's world.

A prerequisite to exploring the environment that challenges or affords the child to play in his or her preferred manner is to construct an overall environment that affords play. As previously described, Rubin and his colleagues (1983) defined a context in which play occurs and listed five components thought to promote play.

Once the general treatment environment has been organized to promote play, it is then necessary to begin systematic exploration of how to promote a child to play optimally. Kielhofner (1995) suggested that the environment consists

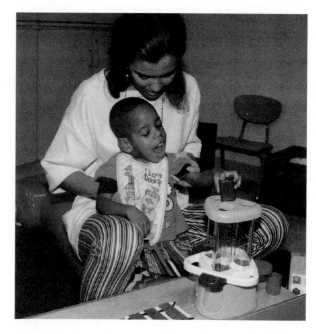

**Figure 18-6**   Therapist's support at child's shoulders and upper trunk enables the child to reach for and play with his preferred toys.

of both a physical and a social environment. It is necessary to explore both of these aspects of the environment to determine which aspects will be systematically altered.

Darrius is a 2-year-old boy with a diagnosis of athetoid cerebral palsy who is playful but who has difficulty playing with all of the toys that interest him. In exploring his environment, it is determined that his social environment is supportive of his play. However, his physical environment requires adaptations for him to play with the toys he prefers. Darrius is unable to sit independently and has difficulty reaching for toys. By having him sit on a bolster and providing him with proximal stability at his trunk, with facilitation at his shoulder while reaching, he is able to reach for and play with the toys he prefers (Figure 18-6).

Equipment and materials are provided to promote his play skills during activity time in preschool. Darrius is placed in a Rifton chair with full back support, arm rests, tray, and foot support. Toys are made available that have physical characteristics that facilitate his control of movement. Heavier toys provide greater proprioceptive input and are used in activities for building and constructing. Toys with magnetic pieces are used so that he can create designs and play scenarios by simply pushing pieces along the surface.

## INTERVENTION TO FACILITATE PLAYFULNESS
### Child Who Is Not Playful

A final way in which a play deficit may be manifested is when a child is not playful. Approaching intervention from this perspective is less familiar to pediatric occupational therapists and should be discussed. Bundy (in press) stated:

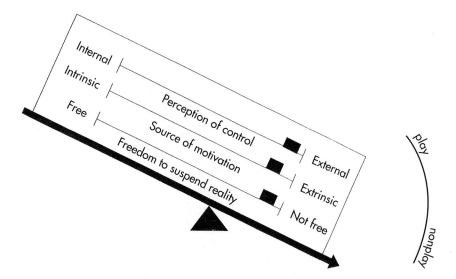

**Figure 18-7**    Alexis' playfulness profile. (Modified from Bundy, A.C. [1991]. Play theory and sensory integration. In A.G. Fisher, E.A. Murray, & A.C. Bundy [Eds.]. *Sensory integration: theory and practice* [p. 60]. Philadelphia: F.A. Davis.)

. . . while it may be perfectly appropriate to evaluate an individual's abilities in self care or work by evaluating their performance of self care or work activities, this approach may not apply well to play. Rather, it may be more important to assess an individual's playfulness than his or her performance of particular play activities (p. 22).

If it is important to assess playfulness rather than particular play activities, it is proposed that intervention should also address aspects of playfulness as well as performance of play skills.

Playfulness describes the quality of a child's play and not just the child's performance of specific play activities. The more playful child may generalize this flexible approach to environmental interaction beyond play and into other aspects of his or her life. For the child with a condition that impedes his or her ability to interact with the social or physical environment, a flexible (playful) approach may enable the child to succeed more frequently in these difficult situations.

The ToP (Bundy, in press) provides a way of examining playfulness in a particular child. The ToP gives therapists information regarding the quality of a child's play. Bundy suggested that after assessing a child with the ToP, a playfulness profile should be constructed for that child. The playfulness profile consists of information regarding the child's intrinsic motivation, internal control, suspension of reality, and framing observed during the play situations. Intervention would then be based on this information.

Alexis, an 18-month-old girl, had a diagnosis of failure to thrive and developmental delay and received weekly occupational therapy. She had followed a fairly typical developmental course with delays in all developmental areas. The occupational therapy

room had a variety of toddler toys arranged in no particular fashion. Each week, Alexis sat in the middle of a therapy mat and did not initiate any movement toward the toys. Her mother continually brought a variety of toys into her immediate environment and put them in her hands. Once the toys were in her hands, Alexis put them in her mouth. Occasionally she waved the toys in the air or banged them against another toy within her reach. Throughout most play sessions Alexis did not make eye contact with her mother, her therapist, or other children or therapists in the treatment room. She did not verbalize through babbling and did not gesture to indicate her wants or make her needs known. Typically, Alexis's mother directed all of the interaction between herself and Alexis. Periodically, Alexis scooted from her mother and the therapist by pulling herself along on her buttocks with her legs straight out in front of her. During these times Alexis either moved into the middle of the therapy room and turned around in circles or left the therapy room and went into the hallway. Once Alexis left the play environment she did not typically return and play with the toys.

Alexis's play profile can be developed by again referring to Figure 18-1 and placing markers along the continuum representing motivation, control, and suspension of reality (Figure 18-7 for specifics to Alexis).

## Intrinsic Motivation

The marker representing Alexis's source of motivation was placed closer to the extrinsic side of the continuum from intrinsic to extrinsic motivation. At times Alexis appeared to be mildly engaged in the process of mouthing and banging toys; however, these behaviors were considered to be primarily exploratory rather than playful. Throughout the play sessions, Alexis's affect was flat; the only occasions during which she manifested any joy was when she left the treatment room and went into the hall. However, it was unclear from observing Alexis exactly what her motivation was during any of these interactions.

## Internal Control

The marker for locus of control was placed closer to the external than to the internal end of the continuum. Alexis initiated little play with the toys in her environment. Alexis' mother appeared to be in control of which toys Alexis played with and when she played with them. The one behavior that Alexis consistently initiated was leaving the treatment environment. When Alexis did interact with the toys, she appeared to be exploring them more than playing with them. As discussed earlier, several theorists have suggested that when the child explores objects instead of playing with them, it is because he or she is not in control of the transaction (Rubin, 1980; Rubin et al., 1983) and is attempting to gain control (Hutt, 1976, 1979). This suggests that Alexis was not operating from an internal locus of control. Finally, Alexis demonstrated minimal modification of her interaction with the toys, again suggesting that she did not feel enough in control of the situation to alter it.

## Suspension of Reality

The marker for freedom to suspend reality was placed almost completely toward the not-free end because all of the interactions observed appeared to be bound by objective reality. There was no apparent pretending noted. The way in which Alexis played with the toys (mouthing and banging) is more typical of a younger child; therefore the lack of pretending could be related to her overall play age.

## Framing, Giving, and Reading Cues

Alexis did not appear to enter into a play frame when observed during therapy. Her activities were primarily exploratory in nature, and she did not appear to make the shift from exploration to playing with the objects. In relation to giving play cues, Alexis provided few cues that indicated that she was playing. In fact, she provided few verbal or nonverbal indications of how one should act toward her at all. The few cues that Alexis did give are not typical of an 18-month-old child (i.e., backing up toward the therapist instead of approaching her with her face forward) and are difficult to interpret as play cues. In addition, her clearest cue was when she completely withdrew from the play environment.

## Profile Summary

Alexis is not a playful child. Although she demonstrated performance during play (approximately 6 to 8 months) that was significantly below her chronologic age and showed some component skill deficits (i.e., difficulty picking up and manipulating toys, poor ideation regarding what she can do with the toys once she grasps them). At this time her most significant play deficit appeared to be related to her low level of playfulness.

## Intervention

*Setting the environment and facilitating internal locus of control.* The first step in intervention for the child whose playfulness profile indicates that she is not playful is to set up the treatment environment to facilitate play. When the environment has been set up to make the child feel safe, it is most likely that the child will initially explore the environment and the toys in the environment before beginning to play. Following Neumann's suggestion (1971) that an internal locus of control is the most important criterion of a play interaction, the next step is to facilitate the child's sense of control over the situation and thus to facilitate the transition from exploration to play. It may be possible to do this by giving the child the verbal and nonverbal cues that he or she is free to choose whatever he or she wants to play with and by determining exactly how the play will unfold. The assumption is that the child will choose toys and play scenarios that are intrinsically motivating, thus incorporating a second criterion for playfulness into treatment.

As the child guides the play interaction, he or she also guides the therapist's role in the play. The therapist enters the play frame only when he or she is invited to enter by the child. The child invites the therapist into the play frame by providing either verbal or nonverbal cues that suggest the therapist's involvement (i.e., eye contact, reaching toward the therapist with toys or arms, or movement of any kind). When the therapist reads and responds to the child's cues, the message is given that the child is important and in control. To substantiate this message, it is important that when the therapist enters the play frame, the child's lead is followed and the child's strengths are emphasized. By consistently doing this, a relationship between the therapist and the child develops that is based on trust.

In the case of Alexis, the therapy room was set up with a variety of infant and toddler toys placed randomly around a therapy mat. The therapist and Alexis's mother sat on the far edges of the mat, and Alexis was placed in the middle of the toys. Several of the toys were within easy reach. After approximately 5 minutes Alexis reached for and picked up a rattle and began shaking it but initiated no interaction with either her mother or the therapist. For this reason both the therapist and the mother stayed on the edges of the therapy mat and did not interact with Alexis. After 10 to 15 minutes more of shaking and mouthing the rattle, Alexis reached for and picked up a bucket of plastic blocks but still did not initiate interaction with the therapist or her mother. Her play with the blocks was also mouthing and banging. This continued for approximately 15 minutes before Alexis scooted to toys that were between herself and her mother. She then proceeded to back up to her mother, to touch her mother's knee briefly, and to scoot quickly away. When Alexis briefly touched her mother, her mother acknowledged the contact by saying "hi," but she did not suggest other play. Alexis then moved toward toys that were closer to the therapist and also backed up toward the therapist and touched a rattle to the therapist's leg. The therapist picked up a rattle and began shaking it in imitation of Alexis's play. Sessions continued in this manner for several weeks, with Alexis guiding how much interaction occurred both with the toys (physical) and with the people (social) in her environment.

*Building trust and challenging the child.* When the therapist responds to the child's cues, the therapeutic relationship that unfolds is based on trust. It is then possible for the therapist to build on the child's strengths and to begin the process of expanding the child's repertoire of playful behaviors. To do this while maintaining the child's trust, the therapist provides the child with the *just right challenge* (Ayres, 1979). The therapist builds the play frame precisely where the child's skills are sufficient to meet the challenge of the activity. It is important throughout all of this that the environment remain safe and that there are no consequences for the child's performance. That is, the child is free to practice activities without fear of failure.

Csikszentmihalyi (1975) suggested that optimal performance occurs at the point where the challenge of the activity is such that the individual must use a significant portion of his or her skill to perform the activity. When the challenge of the activity is higher than the skill of the individual, the situation can cause anxiety. When the challenge is significantly less than the individual's skill, the situation can result in boredom (Csikszentmihalyi, 1975). Therapy that both responds to the child's cues and adapts situations to

---

### STUDY QUESTIONS

1. Describe how you would use the pictorial scale of playfulness to orchestrate a treatment session in which play is used as a therapeutic modality for the following child:
   Susan is an 18-month-old with spastic quadraparesis who loves *Barney*. Occupational therapy long-term goals are for independent feeding from a cup. Component skills impeding this task performance are decreased head and trunk control in sitting and difficulty reaching with both arms simultaneously.

2. Identify which of the following scenarios describes a child(ren) who is (are) more intrinsically motivated and which describes a child(ren) who is (are) more extrinsically motivated:
   a. A group of children running around an open field chasing each other.
   b. A group of children engaged in relay races in the same field.
   c. The child playing with playdough who creates one object after the other with minimal interest in the outcome. The child may even squash the object as soon as he or she completes it and immediately begin making something else.
   d. The child who is making a teapot out of playdough and alters it until she gets it just right before presenting it to the teacher.

3. Identify which of the following scenarios describes a child who is more internally controlled and

which describes a child who is more externally controlled:
   a. The child who decides to play Candy Land, convinces his parents to play with him, then proceeds to decide that instead of using the gingerbread markers that come with the game they will use Teenage Mutant Ninja Turtles as game pieces.
   b. The child who decides to play Barbie dolls and to have the dolls go out to dinner, then go home and feed the baby.
   c. The child who is playing T-ball because mom and dad say he has to.
   d. The group of children on the playground who are playing dodgeball because the gym teacher says it is time to play dodgeball, even though they would rather play kickball.

4. Identify which of the following scenarios describes a child who is suspending reality and which describes a child who is not:
   a. The child who decides that the small child's table is a ship, the chairs that are placed on the table are the captain's chairs, he is the captain, the teddy bear in the chair is the assistant, and the pillows around the table are the water.
   b. The child who insists on keeping the same chairs on the floor next to the table, and uses the table only for coloring.

continually challenge the child's newly acquired skills may facilitate increasingly more playful behaviors.

*Facilitating incorporation of the playful attitude into other aspects of intervention.* Once the child demonstrates playful behaviors during play transactions, therapy sessions may begin to focus on the treatment of other components or developmental play skills and on generalizing this playful approach to other situations. This is done by incorporating the approach of play as a therapeutic modality and by providing the child with the *just right challenge* (Ayres, 1979). In addition, the concepts regarding determination and generalization of aspects of the environment that facilitate the child's optimal performance are relevant.

It is clear that Alexis' play skills and ability to both give and respond to cues were limited. For this reason, therapy sessions progressed slowly both in terms of the cues given to her by the therapist and in terms of challenging her underlying play, fine motor, and praxis problems. When Alexis indicated an activity was too challenging by leaving the play environment, she was allowed to do so. When she returned, the level of challenge was decreased somewhat. In addition, the therapist and her mother often modeled how to play with a variety of simple cause-and-effect toys when Alexis was next to them and made eye contact with them. When Alexis attempted to play in any way, her attempts were encouraged. Any actions that were not completely successful were not acknowledged at all.

## SUMMARY

Key definitions of play from psychology, education, and OT have been presented. Play as a modality is an important and basic component of therapy sessions. Certain criteria must be met to engage the child in a play interaction. A model for using play in intervention was proposed that included three outcomes that may be achieved by using play as a therapeutic modality. An important goal of this chapter is to explain how occupational therapists use play not only as a modality to enhance the developmental and functional skills of the child, but also as an approach for increasing the child's enjoyment of play and playfulness.

## REFERENCES

Alessandrini, N.A. (1949). Play: a child's world. *American Journal of Occupational Therapy, 3,* 9-12.

Axline, V.M. (1969). *Play therapy.* New York: Ballantine Books.

Ayres, A.J. (1979). *Sensory integration and the child.* Los Angeles: Western Psychological Services.

Barnett, L.A. (1990). Playfulness: definition, design, and measurement. *Play & Culture, 3,* 319-336.

Barnett, L.A. (1991). The playful child: measurement of a disposition to play. *Play & Culture, 4,* 51-74.

Bateson, G. (1972). Toward a theory of play and fantasy. In G. Bateson (Ed.). *Steps to an ecology of the mind* (pp. 14-20). New York: Bantam.

Bledsoe, N.P. & Shepherd, J.T. (1982). A study of reliability and validity of a preschool play scale. *American Journal of Occupational Therapy, 36,* 783-788.

Bundy, A. (1987). The play of preschoolers: its relationship to balance, motor proficiency, and the effect of sensory integrative dysfunction. Unpublished doctoral dissertation, Boston: Boston University.

Bundy, A.C. (1989). A comparison of play skills of normal boys and boys with sensory integrative dysfunction. *The Occupational Therapy Journal of Research, 9,* 84-100.

Bundy, A.C. (1991). Play theory and sensory integration. In A.G. Fisher, E.A. Murray, & A.C. Bundy (Eds.). *Sensory integration: theory and practice* (pp. 46-68). Philadelphia: F.A. Davis.

Bundy, A.C. (in press). Play and playfulness: what to look for. In D. Parham (Ed.). *Play in occupational therapy.* St. Louis: Mosby.

Clifford, J.M. & Bundy, A. (1989). Play preference and performance in normal preschool boys and preschool boys with sensory integrative dysfunction. *Occupational Therapy Journal of Research, 9,* 202-217.

Cohen, D. (1987). *The development of play.* New York: New York University Press.

Csikszentmihalyi, M. (1975). *Beyond boredom and anxiety: the experience of play in work and games.* San Francisco: Jossey-Bass.

Fiorentino, M. (1966). The changing dimension of occupational therapy. *American Journal of Occupational Therapy, 20,* 251-252.

Flavell, J.H. (1977). *Cognitive development.* Englewood Cliffs, NJ: Prentice-Hall.

Florey, L. (1969). Intrinsic motivation: the dynamics of occupational therapy theory. *American Journal of Occupational Therapy, 23,* 319.

Florey, L. (1971). An approach to play and play development. *American Journal of Occupational Therapy, 25,* 275-280.

Florey, L. (1989). Reilly: an explanation of play. In P. Pratt & A. Allen (Eds.). *Occupational therapy for children* (2nd ed.). St. Louis: Mosby.

Gralewicz, A. (1973). Play deprivation in multihandicapped children. *American Journal of Occupational Therapy, 27,* 70.

Gray, M. (1972). Effects of hospitalization on work-play behavior. *American Journal of Occupational Therapy, 26,* 180.

Hutt, C. (1976). Exploration and play in children. In J. Bruner, A. Jolly, & K. Sylva (Eds.). *Play and its role in development and evolution* (pp. 202-215). New York: Basic.

Hutt, C. (1979). Exploration and play. In B. Sutton-Smith (Ed.). *Play and learning* (pp. 175-194). New York: Gardner.

Johnson, C.B. & Deitz, J.C. (1985). Time use of mothers with preschool children in a pilot study. *American Journal of Occupational Therapy, 39,* 578.

Kielhofner, G. (1995). *Human Occupation* (2nd ed.). Baltimore: Williams & Wilkins.

Kielhofner, G., Barris, R., Bauer, D., Shoestock, B., & Walker, L. (1983). Comparison of play behavior in non-hospitalized and hospitalized children. *American Journal of Occupational Therapy, 37,* 305.

Kielhofner, G. & Burke, J. (1983). The evolution of knowledge and practice in OT: past, present and future. In G. Kielhofner (Ed.). *Health through occupation: theory and practice in occupational therapy* (pp. 3-52). Philadelphia: F.A. Davis.

Knox, S. (in press). *Play and playfulness of preschool children.* In R. Zemke & F. Clark (Eds.). *Occupational science the past five years.* Philadelphia: F.A. Davis. Philadelphia: F.A. Davis.

Knox, S.H. (1974). A play scale. In M. Reilly (Ed.). *Play as Exploratory Learning* (pp. 247-266). Beverly Hills, CA: Sage.

Levy, J. (1978). *Play behavior.* New York: John Wiley & Sons.

Lieberman, J.N. (1977). *Playfulness: its relationship to imagination and creativity.* New York: Academic Press.

Llorens, L.A. & Rubens, E.Z. (1967). *Developing ego functions in disturbed children: occupational therapy in milieu.* Detroit: Wayne State University Press.

McClelland, D.C., Atkinson, J.W., & Lowell, E.L. (1953), *The achievement motive.* New York: Appleton, Century, Craft.

Neumann, E.A. (1971). *The elements of play.* New York: MSS Information.

Parten, M.B. (1933). Social play among school children. *Journal of Abnormal Psychology, 28,* 136.

Piaget, J. (1962). Play, dreams, and limitation in childhood. New York: Norton.

Pratt, P.N. (1989). Play and recreational activities. In P.N. Pratt, & A.S. Allen (Eds). *Occupational therapy for children* (2nd ed) (pp. 295-310). St. Louis: Mosby.

Reilly, M. (Ed.). (1974). *Play as exploratory learning,* Beverly Hills, CA: Sage.

Richmond, J.B. & Lis, E.F. (1949). Occupational therapy in pediatrics. *American Journal of Occupational Therapy, 3,* 185-189.

Rubin, K., Fein, G.G., & Vandenberg, B. (1983). Play. In P.H. Mussen (Ed.). *Handbook of child psychology* (4th ed.) (Vol. 4). (pp. 693-774). New York: Wiley & Sons.

Rubin, K., Maiono, T.L., & Hornung, M. (1976). Free play behaviors in middle and lower class preschoolers: Piaget and Parten revisited. *Child Development, 47,* 414-419.

Rubin, K.H. (1977). Play behaviors of young children. *Young Children, 32,* 16-24.

Rubin, K.H. (1980). Fantasy play: its role in the development of social skills and social cognition. In K.H. Rubin (Ed.). *Children's play* (pp. 69-83). San Francisco: Jossey-Bass.

Schwartzman, H.B. (1984). Imaginative play: Deficit or difference? In T. Yawkey & A. Pellegrini (Eds.). *Child's play: developmental and applied* (pp.49-62). New Jersey: Lawrence Erlbaum Associates.

Slagle, E.C. & Robeson, H.A. (1941). *Syllabus for training nurses in occupational therapy.* Utica, NY: State Hospitals Press.

Takata, N. (1974). Play as a prescription. In M. Reilly (Ed.). *Play as exploratory learning* (pp. 209-246). Beverly Hills, CA: Sage.

Vandenberg, B. (1981). Environment and cognitive factors in social play. *Journal of Experimental Child Psychology, 31,* 169-175.

Vandenberg, B. & Kielhofner, G. (1982). Play in evolution, culture, and individual adaptation: implications for therapy. *American Journal of Occupational Therapy, 36,* 20-28.

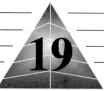

# Prewriting and Handwriting Skills

SUSAN J. AMUNDSON ▲ MARSHA WEIL

## KEY TERMS

- ▲ Domains of Writing
- ▲ Manuscript
- ▲ Cursive
- ▲ Legibility Components
- ▲ Handwriting Evaluation Tools
- ▲ Handwriting Instructional Programs
- ▲ Frames of Reference
- ▲ Pencil Grasp
- ▲ Functional Written Communication
- ▲ Service Provision

## CHAPTER OBJECTIVES

1. Describe the role of the occupational therapist in the evaluation and intervention of children with handwriting dysfunction in educational and clinical settings.
2. Discuss the factors contributing to handwriting readiness for young children.
3. Examine four key aspects critical to examining the child's performance of a handwriting task.
4. Discuss the performance components and the performance context that contribute to a child's handwriting.
5. Develop handwriting intervention programs based on a variety of pediatric occupational therapy frames of reference.

Occupational therapists view the occupational performance of children to be characterized by self-care, work, and play activities. In the area of work, school-aged children's occupational performance includes educational activities such as reading, writing, calculation, and problem solving. Functional written communication is required at school and at home when children compose stories, com-

plete written examinations, copy numbers for calculations, and dictate telephone messages and numbers. Thus learning to write legibly is a critical skill for children to convey to their parents, teachers, and peers knowledge and information and for children to accomplish a variety of sophisticated academic tasks.

Despite the advances of word processors and augmentative communication systems, the task of handwriting consumes much of the school day in a child's life. McHale and Cermak (1992) examined the amount of time allocated to fine motor activities and the type of fine motor activities that school-aged children were expected to perform in the classroom at school. In their study of six classes consisting of two classes from grades 2, 4, and 6 in middle-income public schools, they found that 31% to 60% of the children's school day consisted of fine motor activities. Of those fine motor tasks, 85% of the time consisted of paper and pencil tasks, whereas the remaining fine motor items focused on the children handling manipulatives. Based on the results of this study, children spend a quarter to a half of their classroom time involved with paper and pencil tasks each day at school.

Typically developing children, by the age of 6 or 7 years old, are fairly competent at writing legibly when instructed with a traditional handwriting curriculum (Bergman & McLaughlin, 1988) or *whole language* method (Graham & Miller, 1992). By mastering basic handwriting skills during early elementary school years, children gain an opportunity to progress to higher-level writing tasks, such as, composing, without giving any thought to the mechanics of handwriting (Martlew, 1992). Students with neurologic impairments, learning problems, and developmental disabilities often expend an enormous amount of time and energy learning to write in a legible format while enrolled in a standard handwriting curriculum. Frequently, children who need to pay considerable attention to the mechanical requirements of writing have difficulty with the learning of other higher-order writing processes, such as dictation or story writing, in the school setting (Beringer & Rutberg, 1992). Typical handwriting problems for these children at school are illegibility, inability to keep up with written class assignments, avoidance of writing because of the struggle of forming letters, and the lack of automaticity of handwriting.

*Problems with handwriting performance* is one of the most common reasons for referring school-aged children to occupational therapy (Cermak, 1991; Oliver, 1990). The related role of the occupational therapist includes (1) determining which domains of handwriting (e.g., near-point copying and dictation) are problematic for the student; (2) evaluating the environmental factors that seem to affect the child's ability to write; (3) examining which, if any, underlying sensory, motor, cognitive, or psychosocial deficit is interfering with handwriting production; and (4) providing intervention strategies and approaches focused on the functional performance of handwriting and the performance components or underlying reasons interfering with the child's functional written expression. Another role of the occupational therapist related to handwriting is the evaluation and intervention of children's prewriting and handwriting readiness skills (Oliver, 1990), particularly children of preschool and kindergarten age.

## PREWRITING
### Handwriting Development

Many children begin to scribble on paper shortly after they are able to grasp a writing tool, and if not supervised, will eventually write on any available surface. As children mature, their scribbling evolves into the handwriting skills specific to their culture. Table 19-1 details the development of prewriting and handwriting in children in the United States. Age levels of handwriting progression listed are only approximations because variation in skill development is to be expected among young children.

As for letter copying acquisition, little information has been documented in the literature. One study by Tan-Lin (1981) examined the sequential stages of letter acquisition of 110 children between the ages of 3 and 5 years. Children were observed copying numbers, letters, a few words, and a sentence three times over a period of 4 months. Her findings showed the following sequential stages of prewriting and handwriting: (1) controlled scribbles; (2) discrete lines, dots, or symbols; (3) straight-line or circular upper-case letters; (4) upper-case letters; and (5) lower-case letters, numerals, and words.

### Pencil Grasp Development

The development of pencil grasp in young children follows a fairly predictable course in children who are typically developing. Children commonly begin by holding the pencil with the whole hand, pronating the forearm, and using the shoulder to move the pencil. Later, children use a more mature pencil grasp, holding the pencil between the distal phalanges of the thumb, index, and middle fingers. At this latter stage the forearm is usually supinated, and the intrinsic muscles of the hand move the pencil (Erhardt, 1982; Rosenbloom & Horton, 1971).

### Handwriting Readiness

Some controversy exists as to when children are ready for formal handwriting instruction. Differing rates of maturity, environmental experiences, and interest levels all are factors that can influence children's early attempts and successes in copying letters. Some children may be ready for writing at age 4, and others may not be ready until age 6 (Lamme, 1979; Laszlo & Bairstow, 1984). A number of authors (Alston & Taylor, 1987; Wright & Allen, 1975) have stressed the importance of the mastery of writing readiness skills before handwriting instruction is initiated. These authors contend that children who are taught handwriting before they are ready may become discouraged and develop poor writing habits that later may be difficult to correct.

The readiness factors needed for writing require the integrity of a number of sensorimotor systems. Letter formation requires the integration of the visual, motor, sensory, and perceptual systems. Sufficient fine motor coordination is also needed to form letters accurately (Alston & Taylor, 1987). Donoghue (1975) and Lamme (1979) identified six prerequisites that children must have before handwriting instruction begins. These are (1) small muscle development; (2) eye-hand coordination; (3) the ability to hold utensils or writing tools; (4) the capacity to smoothly form basic

▲ Table 19-1  Development of Prewriting and Handwriting in Young Children

| Performance Task | Age Level |
|---|---|
| Scribbles on paper | 10-12 months |
| Imitates horizontal, vertical, and circular marks on paper | 2 years |
| Copies a vertical line, horizontal line, and circle | 3 years |
| Copies a cross, right oblique line, square, left diagonal line, left oblique cross, some letters and numerals, and may be able to write own name | 4-5 years |
| Copies a triangle, prints own name, copies most lower- and upper-case letters | 5-6 years |

Modified from Bayley, N. (1993). *Bayley scales on infant development.* (rev. ed.). San Antonio, TX: Psychological Corporation, Harcourt Brace; Beery, K.E. (1982). *The Development Test of Visual-Motor Integration.* Cleveland: Modern Curriculum Press; Tan-Lin, A.S. (1981). An investigation into the developmental course of preschool/kindergarten aged children's handwriting behavior. *Dissertation Abstracts International, 42,* 4287A; Weil, M. & Amundson, S.J. (1994). Relationship between visual motor and handwriting skills of children in kindergarten. *American Journal of Occupational Therapy, 48,* 982-988.

strokes such as circles and lines; (5) letter perception, including the ability to recognize forms, notice likenesses and differences, infer the movements necessary for the production of form, and give accurate verbal descriptions of what was seen; and (6) orientation to printed language, which involves the visual analysis of letters and words and right-left discrimination.

Other authors define readiness for writing on the basis of a child's ability to copy geometric forms. Beery (1982) and Benbow, Hanft, and Marsh (1992) suggested that instruction in handwriting be postponed until after the child is able to master the first nine figures in the *Developmental Test of Visual-Motor Integration (VMI)*. The nine figures are a vertical line, a horizontal line, a circle, a cross, a right oblique line, a square, a left oblique line, an oblique cross, and a triangle. Weil and Amundson (1994) performed a study in which they examined 60 kindergarten children who were typically developing (aged 54 to 64 months) and their abilities to copy letter forms on the VMI. The findings indicated that children who were able to copy the first nine forms of the VMI were able to copy significantly more letters than those who were not able to copy the first nine forms, thus providing support for the opinions of Beery (1982) and Benbow et al. (1992). Weil and Amundson (1994) also found that kindergarten children were, on average, able to correctly copy 78% of the letters presented, despite not having received formal handwriting instruction. Based on these results, the authors concluded that most kindergarten children who are typically developing should be ready for actual handwriting instruction in the latter half of the kindergarten school year.

## Activities to Promote Handwriting Readiness

The occupational therapy practitioner can incorporate activities into therapy sessions or the classroom to develop children's handwriting readiness skills. Selected activities should be aimed at improving fine motor control and isolated finger movements, promoting prewriting skills, enhancing right-left discrimination, and improving orientation to printed language (Barchers, 1994; Benbow et al., 1992; Myers, 1992). Some children with significant cognitive or physical impairments may not acquire many of the prerequisite components needed for writing, and their written communication needs may be best met with augmentative communication devices (see Chapter 20). Other children, despite lacking the prerequisite components for handwriting, may be able to learn to write their names with repeated drill and practice. The occupational therapy practitioner must determine when it is appropriate for the child to work on prerequisite handwriting skills, the functional skill of handwriting, or both.

Handwriting readiness can be developed by activities *to improve children's fine motor control and isolated finger movements,* such as (1) rolling ¼- to ⅛-inch balls of clay or Silly Putty between the tip of the thumb and tips of the index and middle fingers; (2) picking up small objects, such as Cheerios and raisins, with tweezers; (3) pinching and sealing a Ziplock bag using the thumb opposing each finger, while maintaining an open web space; (4) twisting open a small tube of toothpaste with the thumb and index and middle fingers while holding the tube with the ulnar digits; and (5) moving a key from the palm to the finger tips of one hand.

*To promote prewriting skills in children,* the following activities may be tried: (1) drawing lines and copying shapes using shaving cream, sand trays, or finger paints; (2) drawing lines and shapes to complete a picture story on chalkboards; (3) drawing pictures of people, houses, trees, cars, or animals with visual and verbal cues from the practitioner; and (4) completing simple dot-to-dot pictures and mazes.

Activities for children of preschool and kindergarten age to *enhance right-left discrimination* include (1) playing "hokey-pokey"; (2) maneuvering through obstacles and focusing on the concept of turning right or left; and (3) connecting dots at the chalkboard with left to right strokes.

*Improving children's orientation to printed language* may be achieved through the following activities: (1) labeling children's drawings based on the child's description; (2) having children make their own books on specific topics, such as favorite foods, the alphabet, and special places; (3) labeling common objects in the classroom or therapy room; and (4) having adults demonstrate the utility of writing in the presence of children, for example, when writing and sending notes between parents and teachers.

## HANDWRITING ASSESSMENT

When a child with poor handwriting has been referred to occupational therapy, the methods to gather assessment information must be carefully selected and sequenced. A comprehensive assessment related to a child's handwriting function includes (1) examining written work samples; (2) discussing the child's performance with the teacher, parent, and other team members; (3) reviewing the child's educational and clinical records; (4) directly observing the child when he or she is writing in the natural setting; (5) evaluating the child's actual performance of handwriting; and (6) assessing any suspected interfering performance components related to handwriting. By assembling data and information from a variety of sources, the occupational therapist can obtain an integrated picture of the difficulty the child is experiencing in written expression in the education setting, along with other areas of school function, such as handling eating utensils and a food tray during lunch time, managing outdoor clothing, or playing with peers in games and on playground equipment during recess. Although poor handwriting is a common referring concern in a classroom, poor performance of other school functions may have gone unnoticed and should receive attention from the occupational therapist administering the assessment.

## Work Samples

Often, the referring person (e.g., the parent or educator) approaches the occupational therapist with the child's handwritten classwork or homework. Written work samples range from spelling lessons to mathematic problems and ideally provide the occupational therapist with a typical performance of the child's handwriting either at school, home, or both. When reviewing the child's written product, a comparison of the writing samples of the child's peers may also be helpful.

## Interviews

Conducting interviews with the child's parents, educator, and other team members serves as a mechanism for building rapport and gathering important data related to the handwriting performance of the child. The educator can describe the specific handwriting curriculum (e.g., Palmer or D'Nealian) or approach toward learning handwriting that is being used, the child's progress within the program, and the child's handwriting background, if any. The standards of the individual teacher, grade level, school, or school district may also be discussed because expectations and handwriting curricula vary widely among educators and school settings. Individual team members' perspectives about the child's handwriting performance in comparison with his or her peers contribute to a comprehensive picture of the child's written communication.

The child's parents may be a valuable resource to provide a different perspective of the child and the child's handwriting abilities at home and at school. Not only can parents relate the child's developmental, medical, and familial background to the educational team, but also they can share invaluable information about the child's interests, social competence, and attitudes toward learning and school (King-Thomas & Hacker, 1987). Discussions with parents related to the child's skills might be facilitated by the following questions: (1) Do parents expect the child to complete school assignments or written work at home? (2) What is the child's response to written homework? (3) How does the child perform his or her written assignments at home and at school? and (4) What other writing tasks are expected of the child at home (e.g., correspondence with relatives or recording of telephone messages)? Parents and other educational team members provide important perspectives to give the occupational therapist a comprehensive view of the child both at home and at school.

## File Review

In the school setting, relevant information regarding the child's past academic performance, special testing, or receipt of special services can commonly be obtained in the referred child's educational cumulative file. Medical or clinical reports related to the child's education may also be located in the child's regular or special education files. For clinic- and hospital-based occupational therapists, the child's parents will be able to share academic records and reports with them. This useful documentation contributes pertinent assessment data related to handwriting that may facilitate further discussion among the child's parents and team members.

## Direct Observation

Observing the child involved in written communication within the classroom or at home is critical. The referral of the child to occupational therapy is commonly made by the teacher or parent observing the child struggling with handwriting performance in the classroom or at home; thus occupational therapists need to examine the child in this similar environment. Figure 19-1 shows a young boy performing his math problems at his school desk. Skilled observation by the examiner usually occurs in the child's classroom and focuses on the task performance, behavior, attention, and frustration tolerance of the child, along with environmental factors that might be contributing to the child's handwriting difficulty. Which writing tasks, for example, copying from the chalkboard or composing a poem, are most problematic for the child? What behaviors are manifested when the child is required to write? For example, does the pupil chew on the eraser of the pencil or construct paper figurines to avoid writing? Can the child engage in the task of writing independently, or are physical and verbal cues needed from the teacher or educational assistant? Is the child easily distracted by visual and auditory stimuli

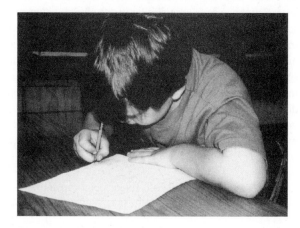

**Figure 19-1** Child completing math calculations using a dynamic tripod grasp in the classroom.

during writing? If the child becomes frustrated during writing activities, when does this occur? In addition, the classroom arrangement, the physical placement of the referred child, other students, and the educator, and the child's social interactions with the teacher and peers may also influence the child's overall academic performance, including handwriting.

## Measuring the Functional Performance of Handwriting

When evaluating the actual task of children's handwriting, the four following areas warrant discussion: (1) domains of handwriting, (2) legibility components, (3) writing speed, and (4) ergonomic factors (Amundson, 1992). The occupational therapist should consider all four aspects to closely examine a child's handwriting in either manuscript (print), cursive (joined script), or both to assist the educational team and parents in identifying the child's problematic areas of handwriting as well as to establish the child's baseline of handwriting function. Accurate and relevant assessment data of the handwriting task are required so that the occupational therapist, the child's parents, and the educational or clinical team can target specific goals and objectives related to the child's handwriting performance in the classroom or at home and later monitor the child's handwriting progress.

### Domains of Handwriting

Handwriting tasks similar to those required of students in the classroom include writing both the alphabet and numerals from memory, near- and far-point copying, manuscript-to-cursive transition, dictation, composition, and endurance. *Writing the alphabet in both upper- and lower-case letters and writing numbers* requires the child to form each individual letter and numeral from memory, to sequence letters and numbers, and to use consistent letter cases. *Copying* is the capacity to reproduce numerals, letters, and words from a similar script model, either manuscript to manuscript or cursive to cursive. *Near-point copying* is producing letters or words from a nearby model, commonly on the same page or on the same horizontal writing surface, such as when an elementary pupil copies the meaning of a word from a nearby dictionary. Copying from a distant vertical model to the writing surface is termed *far-point copying,* demonstrated by early elementary students writing the words "Happy Mother's Day" on construction

paper cards from a model the teacher has written on the class chalkboard. More advanced than copying, *manuscript-to-cursive transition* requires a mastery of letter forms in both manuscript and cursive; the child must transcribe manuscript letters and words to cursive letters and words. A higher-level handwriting task that combines the ability to integrate auditory directions and a motoric response is *dictation.* Writing letters, words, and numerals without a visual model is performed by children when writing dictated words, names, addresses, and telephone numbers. *Composition* is the generation of a sentence or paragraph by the child (demonstrated by writing a poem, a story, or a note to a friend). Educators perceive the composing process to use the cognitive functions of planning, sentence generation, and revision (Beringer & Rutberg, 1992); thus this writing task involves complex integration of linguistic, cognitive, and sensorimotor skills. By evaluating the various handwriting domains, the occupational therapy practitioner can determine in which, if any, particular tasks the child has difficulty and address these performance areas in the team's intervention plan (Amundson, 1992).

### Legibility Components

Legibility is often categorized as components of letter formation, alignment, spacing, size, and slant (Alston, 1983; Ziviani & Elkins, 1984); however, legibility must equate to readability. Whether the child, parent, or teacher can read what was written by the child is of primary importance at home and in school. A child's writing sample may be readable even though a legibility component such as poor letter alignment interferes with its appearance. Legibility, however, is often poor when the child has below-standard performance in two areas. Figure 19-2 illustrates decreased legibility of cursive writing when two legibility components are faulty; letter formation is inadequate, and the size of letters is disproportionate.

For intervention planning and implementation, the components of handwriting legibility need to be evaluated and considered. In *letter formation,* Alston (1983) identified five features that negatively affect legibility: (1) improper letter forms, (2) poor leading in and leading out of letters, (3) inadequate rounding of letters, (4) incomplete closures of letters, and (5) incorrect letter ascenders and descenders. *Alignment,* or *orientation,* refers to the placement of the letters on and within the writing guidelines. The distribution of letters within words and words within sentences is termed *spacing* (Larsen & Hammill, 1989). *Size* of the letter in pro-

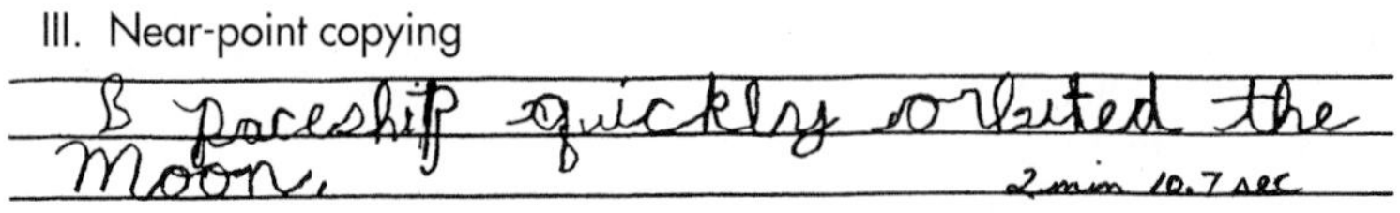

III. Near-point copying

**Figure 19-2**  Cursive handwriting sample exemplifies improper letter forms and disproportionate letter size.

portion to the writing guidelines as well as to the other letters is another component of legibility. Finally, the uniformity, or consistency, of the *slant* or the *angle of the text* should be observed.

## Writing Speed

A child's rate of writing (the number of letters written per minute) along with legibility are the two factors determining whether the child's performance meets the standards of the teacher and the curriculum. The quality of writing may decrease when the amount or complexity of the writing task increases or greater speed is required than the child's natural writing speed (Rubin & Henderson, 1982). Baseline writing speeds of children who are developing typically vary throughout research studies because of the differences in methodologies, subjects, and data collection (Tseng & Cermak, 1991; Ziviani & Elkins, 1984). Table 19-2 displays the writing speeds of children in different studies and lists the methods used to estimate speeds at different ages. When children are initially learning cursive script, their writing speeds often fall below the speed of their manuscript writing.

## Ergonomic Factors

Writing posture, upper-extremity stability and mobility, and pencil grasp are ergonomic factors that must be analyzed as the child engages in writing. Sitting posture in the classroom should be observed. Does the child rest his or her head on the forearm or desktop when writing? Is the child falling from the chair? Does the child stand beside the desk or kneel in the chair? Are the desktop and chair at suitable heights? *Stability and mobility of the upper extremities* refers to the stabilization of the shoulder girdle, elbow, and wrist to allow the dexterous hand to manipulate the writing instrument. Does the child write with whole-arm movements? What is the position of the writing arm? Does the nonpreferred hand stabilize the paper? Does the child apply excessive pressure to the writing tool? Finally, how does the child hold the pencil or what type of pencil grasp is used?

The specific relationship of functional writing and pencil grasp has not been determined. Traditionally, teachers and occupational therapists have stressed the importance of a dynamic tripod pencil grasp (Rosenbloom & Horton, 1971; Tseng & Cermak, 1991). A child exhibits a tripod grasp by resting the writing utensil against the distal phalanx of the radial side of the middle finger and controlling it with pads of the thumb and index finger (Rosenbloom & Horton, 1971). Recent studies have found that adults and children with good handwriting skills use a wide variety of pencil grasp patterns and that an atypical grasp pattern by itself does not necessarily result in handwriting difficulties (Schneck, 1991; Schneck & Henderson, 1990; Ziviani, 1987; Ziviani & Elkins, 1984). Schneck and Henderson (1990), reported in their study of children who were typically developing, that by the age of 6½ to 7 years, 95% of them had adopted a mature pencil grasp, either the dynamic tripod (72.5%) or the lateral tripod (22.5%). Thus the lateral tripod grasp may be considered an acceptable alternative to the traditionally preferred dynamic tripod. A left-handed lateral tripod grasp is shown in Figure 19-3. Ziviani (1987) reported that different grasp variations are expected and that poor writers are more likely to demonstrate a variety of atypical grasp patterns than legible writers. An unconventional pencil grip does not necessarily affect the speed or legibility of a child's handwriting (Tseng & Cermak, 1991).

## Handwriting Evaluation Tools

Formal or standardized tests are critical in the assessment of children because they provide objective measures and quantitative scores, aid in monitoring a child's progress, assist professionals to communicate more clearly, and advance the field through research (Campbell, 1989). A number of standardized handwriting assessment tools are commer-

▲ Table 19-2   Writing Speeds of Children (Letters Per Minute)

| Grade | Ayres (1912)* | Groff (1961)† | Phelps et al. (1985)‡ | Phelps et al. (1987)‡ | Ziviani & Elkins (1984)§ | Larsen & Hammill (1989)‖ |
|---|---|---|---|---|---|---|
| 1 | | | | 32 | | <20 |
| 2 | | | | 35 | | 20-25 |
| 3 | | | 25 | | 32 | 26-33 |
| 4 | 55 | 35 | 37 | | 34 | 34-40 |
| 5 | 64 | 41 | 47 | | 38 | 41-46 |
| 6 | 71 | 50 | 57 | | 46 | 47-55 |
| 7 | | | 62 | | 52 | 56-65 |
| 8 | | | 72 | | | >65 |

*Children were to copy passage until familiar with it; then write for speed.
†Children were to read a passage aloud until familiar with it; then write for speed.
‡Near-point passage presented; children were then to copy passage for speed.
§Near-point symbols, letters, and words presented; children were to copy for speed.
‖Authors do not provide source for writing speeds.

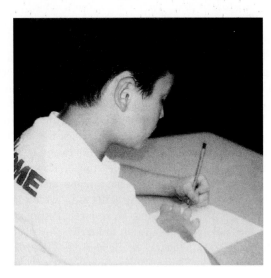

**Figure 19-3** Child uses a lateral tripod grasp to perform written class assignments.

cially available. Instruments commonly used by occupational therapists in the United States include the *Children's Handwriting Evaluation Scale* (Phelps, Stempel, & Speck, 1984), the *Children's Handwriting Evaluation Scale-Manuscript* (Phelps & Stempel, 1987), the *Denver Handwriting Analysis* (Anderson, 1983), the *Test of Legible Handwriting* (Larsen & Hammill, 1989), the *Minnesota Handwriting Test* (Reisman, 1991), and the *Evaluation Tool of Children's Handwriting* (Amundson, in press). Each tool possesses various features regarding domains of handwriting tested (e.g., far-point copying and dictation), age or grade of child assessed (e.g. first and second grades), script examined (e.g., cursive), scoring procedures of the writing performance (e.g., legibility of manuscript), and scores obtained (e.g., percentiles). Typically, the tests measure (1) handwriting legibility by examining the components of handwriting and (2) the speed of handwriting. A description and publication information of the handwriting evaluations commercially available to occupational therapists are listed in Appendix 19-A.

For tool selection, the occupational therapist should keep in mind the characteristics of each instrument as well as the strengths and limitations of the tests regarding normative data, reliability, validity, and other psychometric properties (see Chapter 9). Critiques and lengthier descriptions of handwriting instruments by several authors (Amundson, 1992; Daniels, 1988; Reisman, 1991; Tseng & Cermak, 1991) provide helpful information when selecting a handwriting test. The instrument chosen should match the areas of concern regarding the child's handwriting and should allow for effective intervention planning by the occupational therapist, the child's parents, and other team members.

## Performance Components Related to Handwriting

The last line within the handwriting assessment process is evaluating one or more of the sensorimotor, cognitive, and psychosocial performance components that may be interfering with the child's functional performance to produce text. Applying their clinical reasoning skills, occupational therapists observe a child struggling to write or visually analyze a child's distorted, unreadable handwriting to identify the performance components interfering with written communication. For example, a 9-year-old girl with a traumatic brain injury may have an illegible script marked with overlapping letters and poor use of margins, which may lead the occupational therapist to believe that the child is experiencing a deficit in visual perceptual skills. Hence, the *Test of Visual Perceptual Skills* (Gardner, 1982) may be administered to the child to determine if delays in this area exist and, if so, the extent of the delays. Table 19-3 identifies sensorimotor components that typically influence children's handwriting and their relationship to handwriting performance.

With an emphasis on sensorimotor aspects, the cognitive and psychosocial performance components related to a child's handwriting dysfunction are occasionally overlooked by the occupational therapist. Neglecting these factors may result in an incomplete assessment of the child and, furthermore, an intervention program that is remiss in addressing the cognitive and psychosocial needs of the child that are influencing classroom performance. Cognitive skills required for handwriting include (1) attending to a writing task over time, (2) recalling letter formations and handwriting strategies over periods through visual, verbal, and auditory memories, and (3) generalizing of handwriting from practice in an intervention program to real-life situations, such as performing classroom assignments, copying a recipe, and signing checks. Psychosocial aspects to consider include the child's values and interests, self-regulation, self-concept, and coping skills. For the child who sees his or her handwriting as a continual visual reminder of inadequacy at school, the loss of interest and motivation in producing written text is not surprising (Pasternicki, 1987). Because of the continual criticism and judgment of their handwriting performance by educators and others, some students with poor handwriting tend to feel inadequate and their self-esteem suffers (Bailey, 1988).

## EDUCATOR'S PERSPECTIVE
### Writing Process

When educators speak of the writing or composing process, they view it as a goal-directed activity that uses the cognitive functions of planning, sentence generation, and revision (Hayes & Flower, 1986). The child who needs to pay considerable attention to the mechanical requirements of

▲ Table 19-3   Sensorimotor Performance Components Influencing Handwriting

| Sensorimotor Components | Impact on Handwriting |
|---|---|
| **SENSORY** | |
| Tactile and proprioceptive | Gives information regarding grasp of writing tool, eraser, writing medium, and surface |
| Visual | Allows scanning the printed line, sustaining visual regard, and focusing on stationary text and formation of letters |
| Kinesthesia | Provides feedback related to extent, weight, and direction of movement, allowing appropriate pencil pressure and directing writing tools |
| Form constancy | Enables child to discriminate between numerals, letters, and words that are similar, such as *b/d* and *was/saw* |
| Position in space | Influences spacing between letters, words, and numerals, placing letters on and within writing lines, and using margins appropriately |
| Visual closure | Enables child to identify which letters have been formed completely |
| **NEUROMUSCULAR** | |
| Muscle tone | Allows sustaining of an upright position and upper-extremity stability and mobility |
| Strength | Impacts ability to firmly grasp and maintain positional consistency of the writing tool over time |
| Postural control | Influences ability to make postural adjustments while writing in various positions |
| **MOTOR** | |
| Crossing the midline | Assists to write in a horizontal plane across the midline of the body without interruption or distraction |
| Bilateral integration | Enables child to use symmetric and asymmetric hand movements to hold writing tool and stabilize paper |
| Laterality | Allows consistent and superior use of one hand for writing |
| Praxis | Influences capacity to plan, sequence, and execute letter forms and arrange letters to build words |
| Fine motor coordination, particularly in-hand manipulation | Provides moving pencil from palm to fingers (translation), adjusting pencil shaft in fingers for writing (vertical shift), and turning pencil end-over-end for erasing (complex rotation) |
| Visual motor integration | Impacts ability to reproduce numerals and letters accurately, to color within lines, and to trace |

Modified from Amundson, S.J. (1992). Handwriting: evaluation and intervention in school setting. In J. Case-Smith & C. Pehoski (Eds.). *Development of hand skills in the child* (pp. 63-78). Rockville, MD: American Occupational Therapy Association; Boehme, R. (1988). *Improving upper body control.* Tucson: Therapy Skill Builders; Exner, C.E. (1992). In-hand manipulation skills. In J. Case-Smith & C. Pehoski (Eds.). *Development of hand skills in the child* (pp. 35-45). Rockville, MD: American Occupational Therapy Association; and Price, A. (1986). Applying sensory integration to handwriting problems. *American Occupational Therapy Association Developmental Disabilities Special Interest Section Newsletter, 9,* 4-5.

writing may interrupt higher-order writing processes, such as planning or content generation. Three situations may contribute to this disruption: (1) paying attention to the demands of text production may lead the writer to forget already-developed intentions and meanings, in addition to writing plans; (2) the mechanical demands of writing speed may not be fast enough to keep up with the child's thoughts; and (3) the mechanical difficulties may affect students' persistence, motivation, and sense of efficacy in the writing process, resulting in the avoidance of writing. Hence, most educators view the mechanical requirements of handwriting as an integral subset of the writing process.

## Handwriting Instruction Methods

During the past few years, an educational debate has been focused on teaching handwriting systematically through commercially prepared or teacher-developed programs or learning it through a *whole-language* approach. The whole-language philosophy purports that both the substance (meaning) of writing is addressed as well as the form (mechanics) of writing (Graham, 1992). Thus when using the whole-language method as children are learning and mastering handwriting, advice and practice are given only on an individual, as-needed basis from the teacher. For example, if an educator sees a first-grader struggling to form the letter *n* while writing a story about *monsters,* he or she may instruct the child regarding the correct letter formation of *n* and encourage extra practice of the letter during the story composition period. Conversely, in a traditional handwriting instruction approach, students are introduced to letter formations and practice them outside the context of writing. For children with learning disabilities and mild neuromuscular impairments, regular practice in forming letters is essential in the early stages of handwriting development, and yet handwriting should have a meaningful context. Thus a combination of systematic handwriting instruction and whole-language methods may be most beneficial to this group of children (Graham, 1992).

In the United States, traditional handwriting instruction programs vary among school districts and occasionally among schools and grades. The most common instruction methods include Palmer, Zaner-Bloser, italics, and D'Nealian (Alston & Taylor, 1987; Thurber, 1983). Unlike the United States a few countries such as the United Kingdom and New Zealand have adopted national curricula for handwriting to improve the standards of handwriting assessment and instruction within their school system (Alston, 1991).

## Manuscript and Cursive Styles

A generally accepted sequence for handwriting instruction is manuscript writing for use in grades 1 and 2, with children transitioning to cursive writing at the end of grade 2 or the beginning of grade 3 (Barchers, 1994; Bergman & McLaughlin, 1988). The need for manuscript writing may continue throughout life, when students label maps and posters, adolescents complete job or college applications, and adults complete official or legal forms. By junior high age, many students have blended both manuscript and cursive to form their own style of handwriting. No research has decisively indicated the superiority of one script style over the other (Hagin, 1983).

Both manuscript and cursive styles possess complementary features, and these should be considered when the occupational therapist, child, child's parents, and educational team are collaboratively deciding which style might best serve the child. Manuscript is endorsed for the following reasons:

1. Letter forms are simpler and hence easier to learn.
2. It closely resembles the print of textbooks and school manuals.
3. It is needed throughout adult life for documents and applications.
4. Beginning manuscript writing is more readable than cursive.
5. Ball and stick strokes of manuscript letter formations are more developmentally appropriate than cursive letters for young children.
6. Manuscript letters are easier to discriminate visually than cursive letters. (Barbe, Milone, & Wasylyk, 1983; Bergman & McLaughlin, 1988; Graham & Miller, 1980; Hagin, 1983).

Cursive writing is beneficial for the following reasons:

1. Cursive movement patterns allow for faster and more automatic writing.
2. Reversal of individual letters and transpositions of words are less likely to occur than in manuscript.

3. One continuous, connected line enables the child to form words as units.
4. Cursive is faster than manuscript.
5. It allows the poor printer a new type of written format that may be motivating at the child's current maturity level (Armitage & Ratzlaff, 1985; Bergman & McLaughlin, 1988; Graham & Miller, 1980; Hagin, 1983).

## HANDWRITING INTERVENTION
### Planning

In the school setting, if the referred child's parents and educational team decide that functional written communication with handwriting is a priority for the child's educational program, the occupational therapist may be instrumental in directing and guiding that aspect of the program. Theories, strategies, and approaches of occupational therapy intervention may at first seem unconventional to children, educators, parents, and other school personnel. Therefore the occupational therapist must be able to (1) clearly articulate intervention techniques and environmental arrangements being used, (2) collaborate with the teacher and others to provide service in the least restrictive environment, (3) implement therapeutic strategies for remediating handwriting problems, (4) train others to work with children with handwriting dysfunction, and (5) closely monitor the progress of the child involved with handwriting intervention.

Initially, the child, the child's parents, and the educational team need to achieve consensus regarding the type of script and the method of handwriting instruction (e.g., Zaner-Bloser) that seems most advantageous for the child. Subsequently, the type, frequency, and duration of service delivery as well as the service provider, for example, certified occupational therapy assistant, may be determined within the planning meeting.

Occupational therapy frames of reference that apply to designing handwriting intervention programs include (1) neurodevelopmental, (2) acquisitional, (3) sensory integration, (4) biomechanical, and (5) behavioral. When considering any intervention plan for handwriting, practitioners should consider the far-reaching parameters of each frame of reference along with the overlap and the interplay between them. During the course of an intervention session and sequence of sessions, one frame of reference may dominate as another recedes. The occupational therapist must be skillful in the use of one or several frames of reference concurrently and in teaching others to implement strategies originating from these frames of reference. By remaining focused on the child's goal related to handwriting and by selection of a frame of reference for the child's educational program, the occupational therapist can provide important opportunities for the child mastering the skill of handwriting.

## Frames of Reference to Guide the Occupational Therapist
### Neurodevelopmental

The neurodevelopmental theoretical approach is based on neuromaturation principles and the typical sequence of neuromotor development. It focuses on an individual's ability to execute normal postural responses and movement patterns (Bobath & Bobath, 1972). This frame of reference provides an ideal orientation for addressing problems of children who have inadequate neurodevelopmental organization exhibited by poor postural control, automatic reactions, or arm control. Decreased, increased, or fluctuating muscle tone, inadequate righting and equilibrium responses, and poor proximal stability may interfere with successful performance in fine motor activities, such as handwriting production, at home and in school.

Postural and upper extremity preparation activities are an important component of a comprehensive handwriting program for children with neuromuscular impairments. Preparing the child's body for handwriting should be the preliminary ingredient of handwriting intervention, occurring approximately 5 to 10 minutes before the instructional program begins (Amundson, 1992; Maddox, 1986). Selecting preparatory activities to address each individual child's deficits and carefully analyzing the child's response to the activity are both critical in the preparatory phase of the handwriting intervention program. The remaining paragraphs of this section include postural and upper-extremity activities that help prepare the child to write. Goals of these preparatory activities include (1) modulating muscle tone, (2) promoting proximal joint stability, and (3) improving hand function.

Postural preparation to modulate muscle tone may involve activities to increase, decrease, or balance muscle tone (Maddox, 1986). Activities to increase tone include jumping while sitting on a hippity-hop ball, spinning on a Sit-and-Spin, and jumping on a mini-trampoline. Without leaving the classroom chair, children may increase muscle tone through their arms and trunks by placing their hands on the sides of the chair and bouncing in place for a "popcorn ride" or by performing simple calisthenics such as pushing down on the tops of their heads with their hands. For children whose muscle tone needs to be reduced, slow rocking and rolling are two effective inhibitory influences to the vestibular system (Oetter, 1986). Slow rocking may be achieved by sitting astride a large bolster and slowly rocking from side to side to the rhythm of a child's poem recited aloud. In the class before writing, a child's postural tone may be decreased by rocking in a rocking chair to the beat of a slow, rhythmic instrumental or vocal music from a headset, by snuggling into a beanbag chair, or by participating in a relaxing, visual imagery exercise. Balancing muscle tone may be achieved through activities requiring weight shifting; smooth, repetitive, alternating movements; and controlled rotation. Bending laterally to the right and left while sitting, weight-shifting in half-kneeling, and shifting from side-sitting to kneeling with hands on hips are specific movements to be incorporated into children's games to assist in balancing muscle tone.

Children with poor handwriting frequently exhibit poor proximal stability (Amundson, 1992). To encourage cocontraction through the neck, shoulders, elbows, and wrists, young children may enjoy animal walks such as the crab walk, the bear walk, the inchworm creep, and the mule kick. Figure 19-4 shows three boys engaged in animal walks preparing to write. Older children may prefer calisthenics such as push-ups on the floor or against the wall, resistive exercises with elastic tubing or theraband, or yoga poses requiring weight bearing on the upper extremities. Within the school setting, proximal stability may be improved through cleaning chalkboards and table tops, pushing heavy external doors open, or pushing and moving classroom furniture or physical education equipment.

Some children may also benefit from developing more coordinated synergies of the intrinsic and extrinsic muscles of the hand to improve overall hand function. Prewriting, handwriting, and manipulative activities on vertical surfaces can assist children in developing more stability in wrist extension. A position of wrist extension facilitates balanced use of the intrinsic musculature of the hand (Benbow, 1990b). Activities requiring in-hand manipulation or the adjustment of an object after placement within the hand may be appropriate for children with deficits in this area (see Chapter 12). Moving the writing utensil from the palm to the fingers of the hand, or *translation, shifting* the shaft of the utensil within the hand for proper grasp, and *rotating* the pencil from the writing to the erasing position are all in-hand manipulation skills needed for writing tool manage-

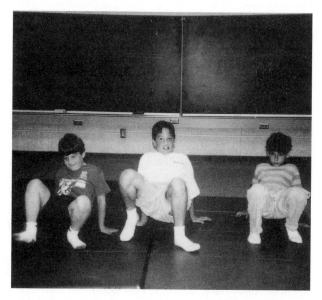

**Figure 19-4**   Postural preparation of three boys performing the crab walk.

ment (Amundson, 1992; Exner, 1992). Boehme (1988) suggested that vertical excursion of the writing line is produced by the flexion and extension movements of the digits, whereas horizontal excursion originates primarily from lateral wrist movements. Hence, the balanced interaction of the intrinsic and extrinsic muscles of the hand is key to the dynamic, efficient, and fluid movements required for handwriting.

## Acquisitional

Handwriting may be viewed as a complex motor skill and, like other acquisitional skills, can be improved through practice, repetition, feedback, and reinforcement (Holme, 1986). Graham and Miller (1980) recommended that instructional guidance in handwriting be (1) taught directly; (2) implemented in brief, daily lessons; (3) matched to individual needs of the child; (4) planned and changed based on evaluation and performance data; and (5) used in a meaningful manner by the child. When therapists and educators employ these conditions in a positive, interesting, and dynamic learning environment, children are more likely to become efficient, legible writers (Barchers, 1994; Milone & Wasylyk, 1981).

For occupational therapists, handwriting as a motor skill relates to theories of motor learning. Learning a new motor skill has been described as progressing through three phases: cognitive, associative, and autonomous (Fitts & Posner, 1967). First, in the cognitive phase, the child attempts to understand the demands of the handwriting task and to develop a cognitive strategy for performing the necessary movements. Visual control of hand movements is thought to be important at this phase. A child learning handwriting in this phase may have developed strategies for writing some of the easier manuscript letters, such as *o, l,* or *t,* but may have more difficulty writing complicated letters, such as *a, q,* or *g.* Next, in the associative phase, the child has learned the fundamentals of performing handwriting and continues to adjust and refine the skill. Proprioceptive feedback becomes increasingly important during this phase, and reliance on visual feedback declines. For example, in the associative phase, a child may have mastered the formations of letters but is engaged in improving the handwriting product, which could be learning to space words correctly, to write letters within guidelines, or to maintain consistent letter slant. Children continue to need practice, instructional guidance, and self-monitoring strategies of handwriting performance. In the final, autonomous phase, the child can perform handwriting automatically with minimal conscious attention. Variability of performance is slight from day to day, and the child is able to detect and adjust for any small errors that may occur during the autonomous phase (Schmidt, 1982). Once the child has reached this level of handwriting, his or her attention can then be expended on other higher-order elements of writing (Graham, 1992) or it can be saved to alleviate fatigue. Implications

and strategies for handwriting instruction and remediation evolve from reviews of handwriting studies (Bergman & McLaughlin, 1988; Graham & Miller, 1980; Peck, Askov, & Fairchild, 1980) as well as motor learning theory (Schmidt, 1982). Many handwriting remedial programs are commercially available (see Appendix 19-B), each composed of a sequence of letter and numeral formations and successive instructional techniques (Graham & Miller, 1980; Taylor, 1985). The scope and sequence of the handwriting program should focus on a structured progression of introducing and teaching letter and numeral forms. Frequently, letters with common formational features are introduced as a group, such as the lower-case letters *e, i, t,* and *l,* which after mastery of letter forms can immediately be used to write the words, *eel, tile,* and *little.* Although the commercially available or teacher- or therapist-prepared handwriting programs describe a sequence for learning letter formation, each child's program should be individualized to consist of those letters and to use them with mastered letters, excluding letters the child is forming incorrectly or ones unknown to the child because this only reinforces unwelcomed perceptual-motor patterns (Ziviani, 1987). Combining newly acquired letters with already mastered letters reinforces learning and expands writing practice from repetition of letter to the formation of words and sentences. This immediate reinforcement of writing words is more powerful and meaningful for the child than repeatedly writing strings of letters.

Instructional approaches of handwriting intervention programs vary but tend to purport a combination of sequential techniques including modeling, tracing, copying, composing, stimulus fading, and self-monitoring (Bergman & McLaughlin, 1988; Milone & Wasylyk, 1981) (See Appendix 19-B). When acquiring new letter forms, initially the child may need many visual and auditory cues; however, the occupational therapist eliminates the cues as soon as the child can successfully form the letter without them. Next the child proceeds to copying letters and words from a model and then to writing letters and words from memory as they are dictated. Finally, the child advances to generating words and sentences for the handwriting group to practice. In each phase, the child should be expected to correct or self-monitor his or her own work. Older children might refer to a written checklist addressing spacing, size, alignment, letter forms, and slant during the self-assessment of their writing; however, younger children may need to verbally evaluate letter formation and overall appearance with the service provider.

When children are learning correct letter forms, other components of legibility are addressed concurrently, such as size, slant, and alignment. Spacing between letters and words often needs direct attention because overspacing and underspacing are common among children with visual perceptual deficits. Larsen and Hammill (1989) recommended that the space between words should be slightly larger than the width of a single lower-case letter. Techniques to assist children with spacing include placing actual objects, such as a pencil shaft or fingers, to form the space width between letters and words; this can later be visualized rather than placed on the writing surface. A clever idea to facilitate spacing is to use a wooden spoon (tongue depressor type) to be "Spaceman." The wider portion (Spaceman's head) is used to space between words, and the narrower shaft of the spoon represents the appropriate space between letters (Cathy Rainey, personal communication, May 14, 1994). Different-sized spoons may be used, depending on the size of the letters and writing lines.

### Sensory Integration

The parameters for this frame of reference include controlling sensory input through selected activities to enhance the integration of sensory systems at the subcortical level. By providing various sensory opportunities, the child's nervous system may integrate information more efficiently to produce a satisfactory motor output, e.g., legible letters in a timely manner. All sensory systems, including the proprioceptive, tactile, visual, auditory, olfactory, and gustatory senses, can be tapped within a handwriting intervention program, which is thought to enhance learning. Incorporating a sensory integrative approach into handwriting intervention equates to the use of a variety of sensory experiences, mediums, and instructional materials. Additionally, providing novel and interesting materials for children to practice letter forms may keep students motivated, excited, and challenged, enhancing student success and learning. Children with handwriting difficulties who have experienced frustration with commonly used paper and pencil drills may be much more amenable to handwriting instruction using this unique multisensory format.

Writing tools, writing surfaces, and positions for writing are all integral parts of a sensory integrative approach in handwriting intervention. Examples of writing tools to be used include felt-tip pens, crayons and "wipe-off" crayons, paint brushes, grease markers, weighted pens, mechanical pencils, wooden dowels, vibratory pens, and chalk. Lamme and Ayris (1983) examined the effects of five different types of writing tools on handwriting legibility. Results indicated that the type of writing tool did not influence legibility, but the educators involved in the study reported that children's attitudes toward writing were more positive when children were able to use a felt-tip pen rather than a No. 2 pencil. This suggests that children's feelings about writing might improve when allowed to use a variety of writing tools. Writing with chalk, grease pencils, or a resistive tool also provides additional proprioceptive input to children because more pressure for writing is required than with the traditional paper and pencil medium. For older children who are learning cursive handwriting, the photoelectric pen or "talking pen" may be met with enthusiasm. This special light-sensitive tool yields auditory feedback when the pen, controlled by the student, goes off-track while tracing over black cursive letter formations.

Writing surfaces may be in a vertical, horizontal, or vertically angled plane. Common vertical surfaces for writing include the chalkboard, painting easels, and poster board and laminated paper attached to the wall. Inclined desktop easels provide a vertically angled plane and facilitate a more mature grasp of the writing tool by placing the child's wrist in extension. A position of wrist extension promotes palmar arch and an open web space between the thumb and fingers (Benbow et al., 1992). An upright orientation may also decrease directional confusion of early writers when learning letter formations (Hagin, 1983). On the vertical plane, *up* means *up* and *down* means *down*, as opposed to working at a desktop, where the direction *up* means *away from the body* and *down* means *toward the body*. Furthermore, standing in front of a chalkboard with the body in full extension and parallel to the writing surface may promote more internal stability of the trunk, increase the child's arousal, provide more proprioceptive input throughout the arm and shoulder, and allow the hands to move independently or dissociate from the arm (Amundson, 1992).

Handwriting practice on a horizontal surface at the table or on the floor might be performed using plastic freezer bags partially filled with colored hair styling gel; trays filled with sand, dry pudding mix, clay, or a light coat of hand lotion; and chalk mats. Writing trays are baking sheets or styrofoam meat packaging trays filled with various substances to provide children additional tactile and proprioceptive input when forming letters, numbers, and words with isolated fingers or wooden dowels. The chalk mat, a portable, foldable chalkboard, can be laid flat on the floor or attached to the wall as another resistive medium. Figure 19-5 shows children engaged in writing activities using

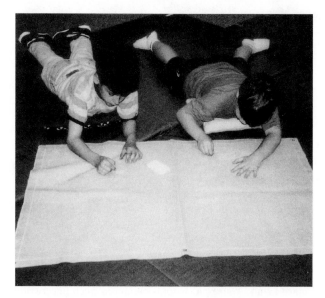

**Figure 19-5**  Children practicing handwriting on the chalk mat.

chalk and the chalk mat. Other writing activities might occur on textured wall paper, nylon netting, finely meshed screen, or indoor-outdoor carpet squares to again provide more proprioceptive input.

An effective writing surface is a color-coded laminated sheet that provides immediate visual cues to the child while learning letter forms, accompanied by verbal cues from the service provider. Beneath the solid red writing baseline, the color brown represents the soil or ground; the space above the solid baseline and dashed black middle guideline is green for the grass; and above the dashed guideline to the top solid writing line is blue for the sky. For example, the letter *h* would start at the top of the sky, head downward, and end in the grass.

Alternate positions to the typical classroom posture of sitting at a chair and desk, such as lying in a prone or sidelying position, can be useful. The prone position requires weight bearing on the forearms for writing, which increases proximal joint stability and disassociation of the hand and digits from the forearm. Because this prone position is difficult to maintain for more than 5 to 10 minutes, students should be encouraged to start the session in this position and then modify their positions to sitting or side-lying on the floor when desired. A young girl practices writing in the prone position with isolated finger movements on a gel bag in Figure 19-6. Alternative writing positions, various writing media, and nontraditional writing tools provide beneficial input for children who struggle with handwriting.

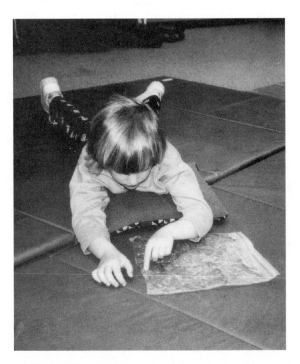

**Figure 19-6** Young girl is softly cushioned when fingerwriting in a prone position.

## Biomechanical

In the truest sense, the biomechanical frame of reference addresses occupational performance in terms of range of motion, strength, and endurance. The following handwriting discussion, however, focuses on the ergonomic factors of sitting posture, paper position, pencil grasp, writing instruments, and type of paper. Compensatory strategies including adaptive devices, procedural adaptations, and environmental modifications to improve the interaction and fit between a child's capabilities and the demands of the handwriting task are discussed as considerations when providing direct intervention or classroom consultation.

***Sitting posture.*** Although standing and lying prone may be encouraged as alternative writing positions, students spend most of the school day seated at a desk; thus the student's seating position while in the classroom must be addressed immediately. Benbow (1990b) suggested that the student be seated with the feet firmly planted on the floor, providing support for weight shifting and postural adjustments while writing. The table surface should be 2 inches above the flexed elbows when seated in the chair. In this position, the child can experience both symmetry and stability while performing written work. The occupational therapist may recommend adjusting heights of desks and chairs, providing needed foot rests for children in their classrooms and arranging a child's desk to face the chalkboard in the classroom to improve the child's posture for handwriting.

***Paper position.*** The position of the paper should be slanted on the desktop so that it is parallel to the forearm of the writing hand when the child's forearms are resting on the desk with hands clasped (Levine, 1991). This angle of the paper enables the student to see his or her written work and to avoid smearing the writing. Right-handed students may slant the top of their paper approximately 25 to 30 degrees to the left with the paper just right of the body's midline. Conversely, a slant of 30 to 35 degrees to the right and paper placement to the left of midline are needed for students using their left hands (Alston & Taylor, 1987). For the student with a left-handed "hooked" pencil grasp lacking lateral wrist movements, slanting the paper to the left as do right-handed students is appropriate (Benbow et al., 1992). The writing instrument should be held below the baseline, and the nonpreferred hand should hold the writing paper (Alston & Taylor, 1987).

***Pencil grasp.*** Benbow (1990b) defined the ideal grasp as a dynamic tripod with an open web space. The open web space in combination with the radial digits enables the thumb, index, and middle fingers to make the longest flexion, extension, and rotary excursions with a pencil during handwriting (Benbow et al., 1992). Variations of grasps exist, with some grips making handwriting more difficult and less functional (Tseng & Cermak, 1991). Educational team members may consider modifying a student's pencil grasp under the following conditions: (1) when muscular tension during handwriting causes fatigue, (2) when grasp seems to negatively influence handwriting proficiency, such as letter formation or writing speed, (3) when the child is unable to use controlled and precise finger and thumb movements of the pencil because of a tightly closed web space, and (4) when the child holds the pencil with too much pressure or exerts too much pencil point pressure on the paper, resulting in breaking the pencil lead, making holes in the writing paper, and shaking out the writing hand repeatedly (Benbow, 1990b; Ziviani, 1987).

When attempting to modify a grip pattern, characteristics of the child are an important consideration. The occupational therapist should encourage a mature grasp in young writers and recognize that the success in modifying a grasp pattern may be better with younger children (Ziviani, 1987). Once grip positions have been established, they are difficult to change (Benbow, 1990b; Ziviani, 1987). In fact, by the beginning of second grade, changing a child's grasp pattern may be so stressful that the effort should be abandoned (Benbow et al., 1992). Therefore the educational team needs to consider a child's age, cooperation, and motivation as well as the child's acceptance of the new grip pattern or prosthetic device before attempting to reposition the child's fingers in grasp of the pencil.

A variety of prosthetic devices and therapeutic strategies are available to assist the child in positioning his or her fingers for better manipulation of the writing instrument. The occupational therapist should be knowledgeable of hand functions to determine which adaptive devices and techniques are most appropriate for each individual child. Tripod grasps may be facilitated by Stetro grips, triangular pencil grips, and moldable grips (Benbow, 1995). Muscle tension and fatigue from writing may be reduced for some children by using a pencil with wide shafts. To gain mobility of the pencil on the paper's surface, children may hold a small eraser against their palms with the ulnar digits, allowing for more dynamic movement of the pencil in their radial digits. For older children with hand hypotonicity, holding the pencil shaft between the web space of the index and middle fingers with thumb opposition may give them a viable pencil grasp. Other techniques to encourage the delicate stability-mobility balance of a functional pencil grasp include the use of external supports such as microfoam surgical tape supports, ring splints, and neoprene splints (Benbow, 1995). These splints should only be applied by the therapist with working knowledge of hand anatomy and kinesiology.

*Writing instruments.* The type of writing instruments children use in the classroom also warrants consideration. In general, children should be allowed to choose among a variety of writing tools so that parents and teachers may help the individual child determine which writing utensil is most efficient and comfortable. Traditionally, kindergarten and primary classrooms have promoted the use of the wide primary pencils for use with beginning writers. A study examining tool usage among preschool children performing drawing, tracing, and writing tasks found that the readability of their written work was not enhanced by the use of a wider diameter pencil (Carlson & Cunningham, 1990). This study suggested that the pervasive use of the primary pencil is probably not warranted for all kindergarten children because some children perform better with a No. 2 pencil whereas others do well with a primary pencil.

*Type of paper.* Various types of writing paper are available in the educational setting. Unlined paper or lined paper that has a dashed middle guideline between the lower baseline and upper line are both commonly used in the early elementary grades. Most of the research confirms that lined paper improves the legibility of handwriting for the majority of children when compared with the use of unlined paper (Pasternicki, 1987). Children typically start out using wide-spaced (1-inch) guidelines, and, as handwriting proficiency improves, transition to narrow-spaced (⅜-inch) lines such as notebook paper, usually occurs in grade 3 or 4 (Barchers, 1994). The occupational therapist and the educator can allow the student the opportunity to experiment with different-lined, sized, and textured paper to determine which offers the child the best medium for handwriting.

### Behavioral

The basic premise of the behavioral frame of reference is that measurable, adaptive behaviors can be learned through interaction with a reinforcing environment (Levy, 1993). For example, a child may produce neatly written text (a measurable and adaptive behavior) when addressing an envelope to his or her own residence, knowing that the occupational therapist will later use the envelope to send the child a small surprise, such as a bookmark, through the mail, which most children would enjoy and find reinforcing. By sharing with children the importance of readable handwriting and the rationale for intervention as well as providing positive, meaningful, everyday experiences using handwriting, children's behaviors to write more legibly may increase. Simple games at school and home such as tic-tac-toe can be played using the newly acquired letter forms rather than the traditional *X* and *O*. Social reinforcement can be provided by parents when a child presents a neatly drawn and written (relative to the child's ability) Thanksgiving Day card at home. Teachers might reward the child with typically poor handwriting with a special certificate for improved handwriting on receipt of a readable spelling paper or written class assignment. By offering children choices, success, and encouragement within an intervention program and the natural setting, handwriting may be viewed and practiced by children as a positive functional skill (Amundson, 1992).

Using the behavioral frame of reference, the occupational therapist can also employ activities to enhance children's social competence while participating in a handwriting intervention group. Poor social performance is common among children with learning disabilities. Examples of behaviors that indicate limitations in social skills are poor eye contact, physical intrusiveness, lack of greeting others, and unawareness of verbal and nonverbal social cues (Williamson, 1993). Helping children learn needed social skills promotes the success of the group. Examples of skills that facilitate the ability of the group to work together include complimenting others, regulating the tone and volume of one's voice, accepting negative feedback, maintaining personal space, and giving and accepting apologies (Williamson, 1993). For example, when children are lying prone while practicing letter forms on a chalk mat, each of them must decide the amount of room that is comfortable between each other as well as the writing space required for individual practice. Aspects of personal space may be introduced by the practitioner, and assistance may be given to the children to aid in this problem-solving process. Another example related to building social skills in a handwriting intervention group might occur during an in-hand manipulation preparatory activity, such as in a competitive game like Kerplunk. While the children remove plastic sticks that support marbles from the game's cylinder, the social skills of taking turns, regulating one's behavioral state during competition, and following the rules of a game can be reinforced by the occupational therapist.

Other strategies to enhance children's social performance within an intervention group may require a proactive role of the occupational therapist. Giving an overview of the intervention session at the beginning of the period and clearly delineating when activities are beginning and terminating may assist children who have difficulty with transitions between tasks and classes. Developing trust and a sense of cohesiveness among the children might be targeted by having the group decide on a special name, logo, or handshake that is used during the handwriting intervention period. When children feel that they are a part of a special group or involved in a special activity, their enthusiasm and interest increase. Finally, the interventionist should establish clear and reasonable rules and consequences, share them with the group members, and consistently and kindly manage each child's behavior. Promoting the child's enthusiasm for handwriting is critical to achieving long-term gains in handwriting skill.

## Functional Written Communication

Some children are good candidates for improving their actual manuscript or cursive handwriting through remediation;

however, other children are not. Compensatory strategies need to be considered by the occupational therapist and the child's team to allow the child with poor handwriting the greatest opportunity of functional written communication. Alternative methods of functional written communication include use of computers and augmentative communication systems, dictating assignments, and having study buddies to assist with written assignments. In school settings, the educational team must determine which type of written communication is or will be most functional for the child and develop both a short-term plan (e.g., learning survival manuscript words) and a long-term plan (e.g., learning word processing with a computer).

As educational and clinical teams develop and implement integrated handwriting intervention programs, the occupational therapists offer unique and creative contributions based on their professional frames of reference. Through the use of techniques, strategies, and methods from the neurodevelopmental, acquisitional, sensory integration, biomechanical, and behavioral theoretical approaches, a comprehensive, challenging, and motivating intervention program is designed and implemented relative to a child's individual needs. When planning any handwriting intervention program, occupational therapists may include any or all of the following: (1) preparing children's bodies for handwriting, (2) providing sequenced handwriting instruction, (3) using various multisensory writing tools, mediums, and positions for writing, (4) recommending that children use practical techniques and approaches for functional handwriting, and (5) offering methods for children to have success, reinforcement, and social competence within the handwriting program.

## Service Delivery

Providing occupational therapy services to children with handwriting dysfunction should be based primarily on the need of the individual child as determined by the educational or clinical team. Occupational therapy service provision in the public schools has typically been implemented with three models: (1) direct, (2) monitoring, and (3) consultation (AOTA, 1989). However, more therapists in school-based practice are using a continuum of service delivery that allows for more flexibility, fluidity, and responsiveness to an individual child's needs (see Chapters 24, 25, and 32). For example, at the beginning of second grade, Matthew, a child with a learning disability, is assessed by the occupational therapist for poor school performance in handling classroom manipulatives (e.g., glue stick, scissors, and computer mouse) and in handwriting. After a comprehensive occupational therapy assessment, Matthew's parents and the educational team decide to have the occupational therapist and the regular education teacher spearhead Matthew's writing program. The therapist and teacher meet to collaborate regarding certain classroom strategies to be implemented, such as facing Matthew's desk directly at the chalkboard, providing him with a taped stencil on his desktop to guide placement of his writing paper, and reducing the length of his written assignments. The educator also requests that the occupational therapist help her with fun exercises to get the entire class "ready to write" before their daily creative writing period. After this collaborative consultation, the occupational therapist initially conducts a handwriting intervention group, which includes Matthew because of the severity of his handwriting dysfunction, in a corner of the classroom for three 25-minute sessions per week for 2 consecutive weeks. During this direct service time, the occupational therapist further assesses and gains familiarity with each individual child while training the educational assistant who will later phase in as the primary service provider of the handwriting group. Later, the occupational therapist returns to the handwriting intervention session once every 2 weeks to supervise the service provider, monitor the children's progress, and modify the programs, if needed. Also, a regular but brief consultation time should be set with the educator to evaluate Matthew's progress in class, to strategize regarding any new situations affecting his handwriting performance, and to write a short note about his progress to his parents.

In Matthew's case, each of the traditional models of service delivery (direct, monitoring, and consultation) were implemented by the occupational therapist during the first 4 weeks after the initial team meeting, but the provision of services was not locked into a set schedule (e.g., two 25-minute sessions per week of direct therapy). Consequently, by tapping into a continuum of service provision, the occupational therapist was able to respond to Matthew's educational needs by initially working with the teacher collaboratively and directly regarding the environmental arrangements, orchestrating an ongoing intervention program implemented by another service provider, and continuing regular contact with Matthew and the educational team members, including Matthew's parents.

Most occupational therapists are comfortable with providing one-to-one or small group therapy sessions but are more challenged when consulting or training and supervising others to implement approaches, strategies, and programs with children with handwriting dysfunction. Often, alternative service providers, comprising educators, educational assistants, volunteers, high school students, and parents, are capable and willing to implement techniques and programs, with the occupational therapists assuming responsibility of organizing and monitoring the methods and programs. First, the occupational therapist must model the role of the service provider during the training, clearly articulate the rationale for the methods and approaches used in the program, and structure the program in an organized fashion for easy use by the service provider. The therapists can supply (1) specific written and oral directions of the program; (2) a container, such as a basket, full of materials for the handwriting intervention program, which might include theraband, in-hand manipulation games, sequenced writing lessons, clay trays, and different writing tools; (3) data management sheets; and (4) a system to provide reinforcement and rewards to make the program more user friendly for the service provider. By making the materials readily available, the service provider is more likely to implement the program or suggestions that the occupational therapist has recommended. Success is promoted when the occupational therapist regularly observes activities or strategies implemented in the classroom, regularly discusses the rationale of methods used, and continually assesses the children's progress and the need for program changes. The handwriting intervention can be beneficial for an individual child as well as for other children in the classroom who may be struggling with handwriting.

## STUDY QUESTIONS

1. If a 5-year-old girl cannot write her own name, is she ready for kindergarten in which the class will be learning letters and letter forms throughout the academic year? Give your rationale.
2. Why is it inappropriate for an occupational therapist to evaluate a child's in-hand manipulation or visual motor integration as the first step of an occupational therapy assessment focusing on handwriting performance?
3. Identify the frame(s) of reference used and the rationale for its selection when a child is involved in the following handwriting intervention activity:
   a. Jason is pressing modeling clay flat on the table top, removing tiny pieces of clay with his fingers, and rolling them into small balls within one hand.
   b. Natasha is straddling a bolster while painting letters from the day's instructional lesson with an adapted-handled paintbrush during the Hangman game with Jesse.
4. Jerod is having difficulty placing cursive letters on the writing line, spacing between words, and using margins properly. Which performance component(s) seem(s) to be interfering with his writing? What are some intervention techniques to be considered?
5. What would be the advantages of implementing a child's handwriting intervention program within the classroom in a small group setting rather than in a one-to-one "pull-out" therapy session?

# SUMMARY

Handwriting is an important academic occupation for children. Children with neuromuscular impairments, learning disabilities, and developmental delays are often referred to occupational therapy with the primary reason for referral being handwriting dysfunction. The role of the occupational therapist includes evaluating a child's functional performance of prewriting and handwriting skills along with the performance components and environmental features interfering with the child's handwriting. It also encompasses assisting the educational or clinical team in determining and planning an integrated approach to promote a functional communication means for the child. Handwriting intervention programs should be comprehensive, incorporating activities and therapeutic techniques from the neurodevelopmental, acquisitional, sensory integration, biomechanical, and behavioral frames of reference in the child's natural setting. Compensatory strategies may also be employed to provide the child a successful and efficient means for functional written communication.

# REFERENCES

Alston, J. (1983). A legibility index: can handwriting be measured? *Educational Review, 35,* 237-242.

Alston, J. (1991). Handwriting in the new curriculum. *British Journal of Special Education, 18,* 13-15.

Alston, J. & Taylor, J. (Eds.) (1987). *Handwriting: theory, research and practice.* London: Croom Helm.

American Occupational Therapy Association. (1989). *Guidelines for occupational therapy services in school systems.* Rockville, MD: American Occupational Therapy Association.

Amundson, S.J. (1992). Handwriting: evaluation and intervention in school setting. In J. Case-Smith & C. Pehorski (Eds.). *Development of hand skills in the child* (pp. 63-78). Rockville, MD: American Occupational Therapy Association.

Amundson, S.J. (in press). *Evaluation tool of children's handwriting.* Homer, AK: OT Kids.

Anderson, P.L. (1983). *Denver handwriting analysis.* Novato, CA: Academic Therapy Publications.

Armitage, D. & Ratzlaff, H. (1985). The non-correlation of printing and writing skills. *Journal of Educational Research, 78,* 174-177.

Ayres, L.P. (1912). *A scale for measuring the quality of handwriting in school children.* New York: Russell Sage Foundation.

Bailey, C.A. (1988). Handwriting: ergonomics, assessment and instruction. *British Journal of Special Education, 15,* 65-71.

Barbe, W.B., Milone, M.J., & Wasylyk, T. (1983). Manuscript is the write start. *Academic Therapy, 18,* 397-405.

Barchers, S.I. (1994). *Teaching language arts: an integrated approach.* Minneapolis: West Publishing.

Bayley, N. (1993). *Bayley Scales of Infant Development.* (2nd ed.). San Antonio, TX: Psychological Corporation, Hartcourt Brace.

Beery, K.E. (1982). *The Developmental Test of Visual-Motor Integration.* Cleveland: Modern Curriculum Press.

Benbow, M. (1990a). *Loops and other groups.* Tucson: Therapy Skill Builders.

Benbow, M. (1990b). Understanding the hand from the inside out. Handout distributed at a workshop, August, 1990.

Benbow, M. (1995). Principles and practices of teaching handwriting. In A. Henderson & C. Pehoski (Eds.). *Hand function in the child: foundations for remediation* (pp. 255-281). St. Louis: Mosby.

Benbow, M., Hanft, B., & Marsh, D. (1992). Handwriting in the classroom: improving written communication. In C.B. Royeen (Ed.). *AOTA self-study series: Classroom applications for school-based practice* (pp.1-60). Rockville, MD: American Occupational Therapy Association.

Bergman, K.E. & McLaughlin, T.F. (1988). Remediating handwriting difficulties with learning disabled students: a review. *Journal of Special Education, 12,* 101-120.

Bergmann, K.P. (1990). Incidence of atypical pencil grasps among nondysfunctional adults. *American Journal of Occupational Therapy, 44,* 736-740.

Beringer, V.W. & Rutberg, J. (1992). *Developmental Medicine and Child Neurology, 34,* 198-215.

Bobath, K. & Bobath, B. (1972). Cerebral palsy. In P.H. Pearson (Ed.). *Physical therapy services in the developmental disabilities* (pp. 31-186). Springfield, IL: Charles C. Thomas.

Boehme, R. (1988). *Improving upper body control.* Tucson: Therapy Skill Builders.

Campbell, S.K. (1989). Measurement in developmental therapy: past, present, and future. *Physical and Occupational Therapy in Pediatrics, 9,* 1-14.

Carlson, K. & Cunningham, J. (1990). Effect of pencil diameter on the graphomotor skill of preschoolers. *Early Childhood Research Quarterly, 5,* 279-293.

Cermak, S. (1991). Somatosensory dyspraxia. In A. Fisher, E.A. Murray, & A.C. Bundy (Eds.). *Sensory integration: theory and practice* (pp. 138-170). Philadelphia: F.A. Davis.

Daniels, L.E. (1988). The diagnosis and remediation of handwriting problems: an analysis. *Physical and Occupational Therapy in Pediatrics, 8,* 61-67.

Erhardt, R.P. (1982). *Developmental hand dysfunction: theory, assessment, treatment.* Tucson: Therapy Skill Builders.

Exner, C.E. (1992). In-hand manipulation skills. In J. Case-Smith & C. Pehorski (Eds.). *Development of hand skills in the child* (pp. 35-45). Rockville, MD: American Occupational Therapy Association.

Fitts, P.M. & Posner, M.I. (1967). *Human performance.* Belmont, CA: Brooks/Cole.

Gardner, M. (1982). *Test of Visual Perceptual Skills.* Burlingame, CA: Psychological and Educational Publications.

Graham, S. (1992). Issues in handwriting instruction. *Focus on Exceptional Children, 25,* 1-14.

Graham, S. & Miller, L. (1980). Handwriting research and practice: a unified approach. *Focus of Exceptional Children, 13,* 1-16.

Groff, P. (1961). New speeds of handwriting. *Elementary English, 38,* 564-565.

Hagin, R.A. (1983). Write right-left: a practical approach to handwriting. *Journal of Learning Disabilities, 15,* 266-271.

Hayes, J. & Flower, L. (1986). Writing research and the writer. *American Psychology, 41,* 1106-1113.

Holm, M. (1986). Frames of reference: guides for action-occupational therapist. In H.S. Powell (Ed.). *PILOT: Project for Independent Living in Occupational Therapy* (pp. 69-78). Rockville, MD: American Occupational Therapy Association.

King-Thomas, L. & Hacker, B.J. (1987). *A therapist's guide to pediatric assessment.* Boston: Little, Brown.

Lamme, L.L. (1979). Handwriting in an early childhood curriculum. *Young Children, 35,* 20-27.

Lamme, L.L. & Ayris, B.M. (1983). Is the handwriting of beginning writers influenced by writing tools? *Journal of Research and Development in Education, 17*(1), 33-38.

Larsen, S.C. & Hammill, D.D. (1989). *Test of legible handwriting.* Austin, TX: Pro-Ed.

Laszlo, J.I. & Bairstow, P.J. (1984). Handwriting: difficulties and possible solutions. *School Psychology International, 5,* 207-213.

Levine, K.J. (1991). *Fine motor dysfunction: therapeutic strategies in the classroom.* Tucson: Therapy Skill Builders.

Levy, L.L. (1993). Behavioral frame of reference. In H.L. Hopkins & H.D. Smith (Eds.). *Willard and Spackman's occupational therapy* (pp. 62-6 5). Philadelphia: J.B. Lippincott.

Maddox, V. (1986). Postural preparation for writing. *American Occupational Therapy Association Developmental Disabilities Special Interest Section Newsletter, 9,* 3-7.

Martlew, M. (1992). Handwriting and spelling: dyslexic children's abilities compared with children of the same spelling level. *British Journal of Educational Psychology, 62,* 375-390.

McHale, K. & Cermak, S. (1992). Fine motor activities in elementary school: preliminary findings and provisional implications for children with fine motor problems. *American Journal of Occupational Therapy, 46,* 898-903.

Milone, M.N., Jr. & Wasylyk, T.M. (1981). Handwriting in special education. *Teaching Exceptional Children, 14,* 58-61.

Myers, C.A. (1992). Therapeutic fine-motor activities for preschoolers. In J. Case- Smith & C. Pehoski (Eds.). *Development of hand skills in the child* (pp. 47-62). Rockville, MD: American Occupational Therapy Association.

Oetter, P. (1986). *Camp Avanti for children with sensory integrative function.* Santa Barbara, CA: Unpublished.

Oliver, C.E. (1990). A sensorimotor program for improving writing readiness skills in elementary-age children. *American Journal of Occupational Therapy, 44,* 111-124.

Pasternicki, J.G. (1987). Paper for writing: research and recommendations. In J. Alston & J. Taylor (Eds.). *Handwriting: theory, research and practice* (pp . 68-80). London: Croom Helm.

Phelps, J. & Stempel, L. (1987). *The children's handwriting evaluation scale for manuscript writing.* Dallas: Texas Scottish Rite Hospital for Crippled Children.

Phelps, J., Stempel, L., & Speck, G. (1984). *The children's handwriting evaluation scale: a new diagnostic tool.* Dallas: Texas Scottish Rite Hospital for Crippled Children.

Price, A. (1986). Applying sensory integration to handwriting problems. *American Occupational Therapy Association Developmental Disabilities Special Interest Section Newsletter, 9,* 4-5.

Reisman, J. (1991a). *Minnesota handwriting test (pilot version).* Unpublished manuscript.

Reisman, J. (1991b). Poor handwriting: who is referred? *American Journal of Occupational Therapy, 45,* 849-852.

Rosenbloom, L. & Horton, M.E. (1971). The maturation of fine prehension in young children. *Developmental Medicine and Child Neurology, 13,* 3-8.

Rubin, N. & Henderson, S.E. (1982). Two sides of the same coin: variations in teaching methods and failure to learn to write. *Special Education: Forward Trends, 9,* 17-24.

Schmidt, R.A. (1982). *Motor control and learning.* Champaign, IL: Human Kinetics.

Schneck, C.M. (1991). Comparison of pencil-grip patterns in first graders with good and poor writing skills. *American Journal of Occupational Therapy, 45,* 701-706.

Schneck, C.M. & Henderson, A. (1990). Descriptive analysis of the developmental progression of grip position for pencil and crayon control in nondysfunctional children. *American Journal of Occupational Therapy, 44,* 893-900.

Stott, D.H., Moyes, F.A., & Henderson, S.E. (1984). *Diagnosis and remediation of handwriting problems.* Burlington, Ontario: Hayes.

Tan-Lin, A.S. (1981). An investigation into the developmental course of preschool/kindergarten aged children's handwriting behavior. *Dissertation Abstracts International, 42,* 4287A.

Taylor, J. (1985). The sequence and structure of handwriting competence: where are the breakdown points in the mastery of handwriting? *British Journal of Occupational Therapy, 48,* 205-207.

Thurber, D. (1983). *D'Nealian manuscript: an aide to reading development.* (No. Report No. CS 007 057). ERIC Document Reproduction Services No. ED 227 474.

Tseng, M.H. & Cermak, S.A. (1993). The influence of ergonomic factors and perceptual-motor abilities on handwriting performance. *American Journal of Occupational Therapy, 47,* 919-926.

Weil, M. & Amundson, S.J. (1994). Relationship between visual motor and handwriting skills of children in kindergarten. *American Journal of Occupational Therapy, 48,* 982-988.

Williamson, G.G. (1993). Enhancing the social competence of children with learning disabilities. *American Occupational Therapy Association Sensory Integration Special Interest Section Newsletter, 16*(1), 1-2.

Wright, J.P. & Allen, E.G. (1975). Ready to write! *Elementary School Journal, 75,* 430-435.

Ziviani, J. (1987). Pencil grasp and manipulation. In J. Alston & J. Taylor (Eds.). *Handwriting: theory, research and practice* (pp. 24-39). London: Croom Helm.

Ziviani, J. & Elkins, J. (1984). Effect of pencil grip on handwriting speed and legibility. *Educational Review, 38,* 247-257.

## SUGGESTED READINGS

Amundson, S.J. (1992). Handwriting: evaluation and intervention in school settings. In J. Case-Smith & C. Pehoski (Eds.). *Development of hand skills in the child* (pp. 63-78). Rockville, MD: American Occupational Therapy Association.

Benbow, M. (1995). Principles and practices of teaching handwriting. In A. Henderson & C. Pehoski (Eds.). *Hand function in the child: foundations for remediation* (pp. 255-281). St. Louis: Mosby.

Benbow, M., Hanft, B., & Marsh, D. (1992). Handwriting in the classroom: improving written communication. In C.B. Royeen (Ed.). *AOTA self-study series: classroom applications for school-based practice* (pp. 1-60). Rockville, MD: American Occupational Therapy Association.

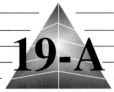

## Commercially-Available Handwriting Evaluations

### CHILDREN'S HANDWRITING EVALUATION SCALE FOR MANUSCRIPT WRITING (CHES-M)

Description: Norm-referenced test that examines rate and quality of children's handwriting within a near-point copying task. Children's handwriting in Grades 1 and 2 are examined qualitatively by letter forms, spacing, rhythm, and general appearance.

Authors: Joanne Phelps & Lynn Stempel (1987)

Publication Information: CHES
6031 St. Andrews
Dallas, TX 75205

### CHILDREN'S HANDWRITING EVALUATION SCALE (CHES)

Description: Norm-referenced tool that assesses cursive writing of children in Grades 3 through 8. Task consists of near-point copying of short paragraphs. Similar features of CHES-M.

Authors: Joanne Phelps, Lynn Stempel, & Gail Speck (1984)

Publication Information: CHES
6031 St. Andrews
Dallas, TX 75205

### DENVER HANDWRITING ANALYSIS

Description: Criterion-referenced tool that evaluates cursive handwriting of students in Grades 3 through 8. Each of the following tasks has a time limit per grade: near-point copying, writing the alphabet from memory, far-point copying, manuscript-cursive transition, and dictation.

Author: Peggy L. Anderson (1983)

Publication Information: Academic Therapy Publications
20 Commercial Boulevard
Novato, CA 94947-6191

### DIAGNOSIS AND REMEDIATION OF HANDWRITING PROBLEMS

Description: Criterion-referenced test with detailed instructions and scoring criteria that requires child to generate a fable, guided by a series of three pictures. No age range is given, except children must have had at least 2 years of manuscript or cursive writing.

Authors: Denis Stott, Fred Moyes, & Sheila Henderson (1985)

Publication Information: DRAKE Educational Associates
St. Fagans Road
Fairwater, Cardiff CF5-3AE WALES

### EVALUATION TOOL OF CHILDREN'S HANDWRITING (ETCH)

Description: Criterion-referenced test that measures a child's legibility and speed of handwriting in Grades 1 through 6. Domains tested in either manuscript or cursive include alphabet writing of lower- and upper-case letters, numeral writing, near-point copying, far-point copying, manuscript-to-cursive transition, dictation, and sentence composition.

Author: Susan J. Amundson, MS, OTR/L (in press)

Publication Information: O.T. KIDS
53805 East End Road
Homer, AK 99603

### MINNESOTA HANDWRITING TEST—RESEARCH VERSION

Description: Norm-referenced test that looks at quality and speed of manuscript handwriting in either Zaner-Bloser or D'Nealian script of children in Grades 1 and 2. Domain tested is near-point copying.

Author: Judith Reisman, PhD, OTR (1987)
Publication Information: Judith Reisman, PhD, OTR
Program in Occupational Therapy
University of Minnesota
Box 388 UMHC
Minneapolis, MN 55455

Authors: Stephen Larsen & Donald Hammill (1989)
Publication Information: PRO ED
8700 Shoal Creek Boulevard
Austin, TX 78758

## TEST OF LEGIBLE HANDWRITING

Description: Examines manuscript or cursive handwriting samples derived from the student's creative story. Norm-referenced tool that examines handwriting with overriding consideration of legibility.

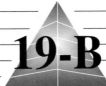

## Handwriting Intervention Programs

## CALLIROBICS

Description: A program that sets paper and pencil exercises within writing guidelines to children's songs in preparation for both manuscript and cursive handwriting. Program cassette tapes accompany the student's workbook and can be implemented either individually or in groups.

Author: Liori Laufer

Publication Information: Callirobics
P.O. Box 6634
Charlottesville, VA 22906
(800) 769-2891

## DYNAMICS OF SENSORY HANDWRITING: CURSIVE OR MANUSCRIPT

Description: A program that provides a structured multisensory approach to handwriting achievement. The program blends letter analysis, visual and verbal instructions, and kinesthetic experiences. Children learn the perception of the letter through sensory experiences before conceptualizing the letter form on paper.

Author: Sarah K. Dyer

Publication Information: Rinehart Incorporated
Allen Drive
P.O. Box 441
Barre, MA 01005

## HANDWRITING WITHOUT TEARS

Description: A comprehensive set of manuals that addresses general handwriting remediation in *Handwriting Without Tears,* manuscript writing instruction in *Printing Power* and *My Printing Book,* and cursive writing in *Cursive Handwriting.* Visual and verbal cues accompany lessons and word and sentence writing is encouraged throughout each program.

Author: Janet Z. Olsen, OTR

Publication Information: Handwriting Without Tears
8802 Quiet Stream Court
Potomac, MD 90854
(301) 983-8409

## LOOPS AND OTHER GROUPS: A KINESTHETIC WRITING SYSTEM

Description: This system has been developed to enable second-grade children to learn the formations of all cursive lowercase letters in 6 weeks. Students learn four groups of letter that share common movement patterns. Children visualize and verbalize the movement patterns while experiencing the "feel" of the letter.

Author: Mary Benbow, MS, OTR

Publication Information: Therapy Skill Builders
3830 East Bellevue
P.O. Box 42050
Tucson, AZ 85733
(602) 323-7500

## SENSIBLE PENCIL

Description: A handwriting program that is designed to teach young children and children with special needs the skills necessary to write in manuscript. Students learn 11 basic lines in the prewriting phase and then progress to writing upper-case letters, lower-case letters, and numerals.

Authors: Linda C. Becht

Publication Information: EBSCO Curriculum Materials
P.O. Box 1943
Birmingham, AL 35201
(205) 991-6600

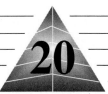

# Augmentative Communication and Computer Access

MIRIAM STRUCK

## KEY TERMS

▲ Assistive Technology
▲ Augmentative Communication
▲ Communication Impairments

## CHAPTER OBJECTIVES

1. Understand the role of the occupational therapist in providing assistive technology services.
2. Describe legal provisions for assistive technology through the Technology Related Assistance Act, 1988, and the Individuals with Disabilities Education Act, 1991.
3. Describe evaluation for assistive technology and augmentative communication devices.
4. Describe training of the child who uses assistive technology, his or her family, and the educational team.
5. Describe input methods using indirect and direct methods for accessing augmentative communication devices and computers.
6. Describe computer output methods and displays.
7. Apply knowledge about augmentative communication devices and assistive technology to children with communication impairments.

The children introduced in Case Studies 1 to 3 are experiencing communication impairments. Communication, in its broadest sense, includes verbal expression, written expression, and physical cues such as gestures and facial expressions that have social meaning. It enables social interaction that is essential for human life.

## CASE STUDY #1

Ben is an eighth grade student with a learning disability. He attends regular education classes and receives special education services from a resource teacher on a daily basis. He is experiencing difficulty keeping up with the written work in his English and Social Studies classes. *(Continued on p. 557.)*

## CASE STUDY #2

Kim is a 6-year-old girl with cerebral palsy who attends a regular first grade class. She receives speech-language therapy, physical therapy, and occupational therapy in addition to special education services. She is unable to express herself verbally or in writing.
*(Continued on p. 558.)*

## CASE STUDY #3

Linda is a high school sophomore with arthrogryposis. She is interested in becoming a journalist and is in the process of exploring this career path. Handwriting and typing are laborious because of limited range of motion of her upper extremity.
*(Continued on p. 559.)*

For children with communication impairment, augmentative and alternative communication (AAC) systems and adapted computer access systems can provide the means to interact and control their own lives. The Augmentative and Alternative Intervention Consensus Statement (NIDRR, 1992) stated the following:

> [Augmentative and alternative communication] AAC refers to all forms of communication that enhance or supplement speech and writing. AAC intervention fosters functional spoken and written communication across all of an individual's environments and throughout life (p. 1).

AAC systems provide the child with adapted methods for communicating both orally and in writing. These methods include a range of available assistive technology (AT), from low technology (nonelectronic aids such as therapist-made communication boards) to high technology (electronic devices such as "dedicated" devices or microcomputers).

Occupational therapists recognize communication as an important performance area for daily living. With their commitment to building competence in tasks of daily living and with their skills in activity adaptation, occupational therapists hold instrumental roles in assisting children with communication impairments to access and use augmentative communication devices (Cummings, 1989).

This chapter provides descriptive information on AAC devices and adapted computer access systems that are available to children with communication impairments. The role of the occupational therapist in providing services in assistive technology is discussed. It is important for occupational therapists working with children who have communication impairments to be knowledgeable about access methods and devices. Selecting the device or system that best meets the child's needs is a challenging task that requires knowledge about availability and appropriate applications of devices.

## WHO BENEFITS FROM AAC TECHNOLOGY

As in the examples of Ben, Kim, and Linda, children with a variety of disabilities can benefit from AAC and adapted computer access systems. Some children require assistance with written language because of a learning disability or physical impairment. Some children are unable to express themselves verbally or in writing because of neurologic impairments.

Children with severe physical disabilities, such as Kim, have limited speaking and writing abilities. The common cause for these difficulties include cerebral palsy or traumatic brain injury. Other children, like Linda, may have muscular or orthopedic impairments that prevent the use of standard computer equipment.

Speech is a primary means of social interaction. Children with oral communication impairment are at a great disadvantage in their development and learning. They have limited ability to communicate their wants and needs. They

have difficulty expressing what they know and have learned and are handicapped in establishing social relationships (Alm, 1993). Without the ability to speak, one's social image as an effective competent person is severely compromised. Nonspeakers are often thought of to be cognitively and intellectually impaired. They are also at a social disadvantage in not being able to participate in the rapid give and take of conversations (Figure 20-1).

## LEGAL PROVISIONS FOR AUGMENTATIVE COMMUNICATION DEVICES AND ASSISTIVE TECHNOLOGY

Federal laws that were passed in the late 1980s and early 1990s have improved accessibility to AT services and devices. There is increased awareness of the potential role of AT among providers and consumers.

The Technology Related Assistance for Individuals with Disabilities Act (Tech Act, 1988) provides a comprehensive definition of AT services and devices. The intent of the Tech Act is to make AT services and devices available by assisting states in implementing consumer-driven services. The law gives a broad definition of services in AT.

Assistive Technology service is any service that directly assists an individual with a disability in the selection, acquisition, or use of an assistive technology device. Included are evaluation services; purchasing, leasing, or otherwise acquiring devices; selecting, designing, fitting, customizing, adapting, applying, maintaining, repairing or replacing assistive technology devices; coordination and using other therapies, interventions, or services with assistive technology devices, such as those associated with existing education and rehabilitation plans and programs; training or technical assistance for an individual with disabilities or family members; and training or technical assistance for providers and employer (Tech Act, 1988).

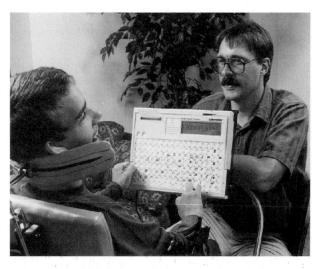

**Figure 20-1** Young man communicates by means of an augmentative device. (Photo courtesy of Prentke Romich Co., Wooster, OH.)

The Individuals with Disabilities Education Act (IDEA) of 1990 provided occupational therapy as a related service to assist children 0 to 21 years of age to benefit from their special education program. Likewise, AT, whether "high" or "low" tech, increases the benefits of special education by providing access to materials and enabling students to participate more fully in their educational programs. AT also supports the legal provisions of IDEA because it can be used to support children in the least restrictive environment (LRE). Inclusion of AT on the Individual Educational Plan (IEP) is a decision to be made by the educational team. The legal definition of AT in IDEA is broad:

Assistive technology devices are any item, piece of equipment or product system, whether acquired commercially off the shelf, modified or customized, that is used to increase, maintain, or improve functional capabilities (IDEA, 1990).

AT enables an individual to function more independently or replaces a function; for example, electronic AAC devices allow an individual who is unable to speak to participate in conversation. AT for AAC needs can include low- and high-technology devices, custom-made or commercially manufactured devices and tools. *Low tech* generally refers to nonelectronic devices and aids. Examples of low-tech devices include head sticks and mouth sticks that are used to access keyboards, communication boards, or electronic aids. Manual communication boards with line drawings or photos are also an example. Low-tech aids are considered by some speech pathologists as the first type of intervention to be tried with individuals who are unable to speak (Beukelman & Mirenda, 1992). Certain low-tech devices, such as the head stick or mouth stick, may be used to access computer keyboards, environmental control systems, and devices that use more sophisticated technology.

*High-tech* aids include both dedicated electronic AAC-systems that serve only as communication aids and computers with communication capability (i.e., with speech output). Almost all children use computer programs at schools, and students with physical disabilities may require adaptations to access the same computer programs. Adapted peripherals such as keyboard emulators, single and multiple switches, and expanded keyboards provide access for children with physical limitations. Certain methods of adapted access require software programs that run concurrently with the primary program. The adapted software can give additional time for responses, allow the child to hold down the keys for a longer time, provide additional auditory or visual input, or allow different types of input to operate the program.

## SERVICE DELIVERY
### Members of the Assistive Technology Team

Teams that provide comprehensive AT services consist of professionals from a variety of disciplines. Cohesive collaboration teams provide optimal AT services, particularly to children (Beukelman & Mirenda, 1992; Church & Glennen, 1992; Swinth, 1994). Because application of AT requires a thorough understanding of the child's function and knowledge of AT, the expertise of professionals of different disciplines is required. In delivering school-based AT services to children, educators, speech-language pathologists, occupational therapists, and physical therapists are core team members (Struck & Corfman, 1994; Swinth, 1994). In a medical or rehabilitation setting or an AT center, team members include occupational therapists, physical therapists, speech-language pathologists, computer or rehabilitation technologists, rehabilitation engineers, vocational counselors, social workers, doctors, and nurses. Parents are an essential member of the team in both settings and play a key role in helping the child incorporate AT into daily use. Table 20-1 illustrates the roles and tasks of AT team members.

▲ Table 20-1   Typical Tasks for Assistive Technology Team Members

| Team Member | Tasks |
| --- | --- |
| Administrator | Administers the team and coordinates services |
| Funding specialist or social worker | Secures funding for devices |
| Occupational therapist | Assesses functional needs in daily living, physical, and environmental needs; adapts and positions adaptive control systems; trains clients in use of equipment |
| Parent | Advocates for their child and provides follow-through at home |
| Physical therapist | Assesses mobility, seating, and positioning as it relates to the use of assistive devices |
| Physician or nurse | Manages medical needs |
| Rehabilitation engineer | Designs, constructs, fits, and customizes devices and systems |
| Special educator | Teaches academic and vocational skills, matches software to curriculum requirements |
| Speech-language pathologist | Assesses receptive and expressive needs and abilities, determines appropriate symbol systems techniques and strategies, manages communication interventions |

Modified from Beukelman, D.R., & Mirenda, P. (1992). *Augmentative and alternative communication: management of severe communication disorders in children and adults.* Baltimore: Brookes; Church, G. & Glennen, S. (1992). Assistive technology programs. In G. Church & S. Glennen (Eds.). *The handbook of assistive technology* (pp. 1-26). San Diego: Singular Publishing Group.

## Settings for Assistive Technology Teams

The structure of an AT service delivery program is influenced by the services that team members provide, the type of facility, the funding sources, and sometimes by the particular disabilities specified in the agency's mission statement. Beukelman and Mirenda (1992) identified three categories of programs for children with communication impairments: hospital-based services, regional centers, and school-based services. Occupational therapists are employed in all of these settings.

### Hospital

Some AT teams are based in hospitals that primarily serve children. In these settings, children may come in on an outpatient basis for a series of assessments by the AT team. The assessments may be completed in one or two visits, or they may require an extensive stay of 2 to 3 weeks. Referrals and recommendations for specific equipment may be made to other agencies or third-party payers. After the initial assessment, team members often have limited access to the child for follow-up and training and they have limited opportunities to consult with the teachers and parents (Beukelman & Mirenda, 1992).

### Regional Agencies

Some regional centers have AT lending libraries. Equipment may be borrowed on a short-term basis by the child, the child's school, or the professionals working with the child in the community. The strengths of regional centers include their ability to serve as an umbrella agency, assuring access to services and devices. The team also has broad-based experience with a variety of diagnoses, resources for obtaining equipment, types of AT, and adapted methods of technology use. Regional centers, like hospital-based services, often have limited follow-up once the child has received the devices and may have minimal input into training the child, family, and educational team to use the device (Beukelman & Mirenda, 1992).

### Public Schools

Schools are becoming the most widely used setting for providing AT services for children (Beukelman & Mirenda, 1992; RESNA, 1992). The demand for school occupational therapists to evaluate AT needs and to help students learn to use AT has become a common feature of school-based practice (Figure 20-2). The large-scale growth of AT services in the school environment has occurred as part of the evolution of special education practices after the enactment of federally mandated programs, as well as electronic and cybernetic development. In school, daily problem solving related to equipment use can occur and the child can receive support in using the device in the setting where its use is most natural and important. Children are expected to attend school every day, thus practice and training in using the AT device can occur on a daily basis. Although the school-based team members have easy access to the child

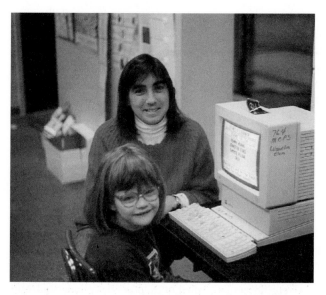

**Figure 20-2** Occupational therapist and student work on a writing activity using a computer and simple modifications of the keyboard.

and the best understanding of the educational curriculum, they do not always have expertise or experience in AT. For this reason, it is important for the school-based team to collaborate with the regional AT teams. Because school-based team members may not all have time to keep abreast of new developments in computer adaptations or AAC devices, often one or two therapists on the team become the technology experts and take responsibility to learn about new developments.

## ROLE OF THE OCCUPATIONAL THERAPIST

As an important and effective member of an AT team, the occupational therapist must gain competence in several areas. These include knowledge of AT devices, working knowledge of and literacy in the technical language of AT, understanding of what AT can and cannot do, and evaluation skills to match technology to individual human needs (Smith, 1991). Hammel and Smith (1993) suggested that accessing and using technology are basic survival skills in today's information age.

Occupational therapists are often called *interface specialists* because their training in the use of adaptive devices and task analysis enables them to identify and customize appropriate devices. They also recommend strategies that increase the child's independence in using AT. Evaluations, equipment acquisition, fitting and adaptation, and coordination and training of the AT user and family members and other professional staff are all within the purview of the occupational therapist on the AT team. Occupational therapists have traditionally used and will continue to use the technology of the day to promote the function of the child (Hammel & Smith, 1993).

In the school setting, the teacher is the curriculum expert. The occupational therapist is the access expert. Collaboration is essential for the child to successfully use AT throughout the student's day. Occupational therapists can serve as consultants to the classroom teacher and the educational team regarding motor control skills, placement of equipment, positioning needs of the child, and relevant mobility issues. Occupational therapists provide valuable information on adapting materials or the classroom environment and can evaluate and train in the use of input controls and writing systems.

## ASSISTIVE TECHNOLOGY SERVICES FOR CHILDREN WITH COMMUNICATION IMPAIRMENTS

### Evaluation

The evaluation provides the baseline information needed to develop a comprehensive training plan. As a dynamic and ongoing process, assessment of needs and responses to training must occur on a regular basis. This assures effectiveness and satisfaction with intervention (NIDRR, 1992).

As in other areas of pediatric practice, evaluation calls for collaboration with other team members such as teachers, speech-language pathologists, physical therapists, parents, and instructional assistants.

The evaluation provides information in three areas: attributes and needs of the child that technology use may help with, attributes of the technology solutions that match the child's needs and strengths, and requirements of the expected environment in which the device needs to be used. In the educational setting, curriculum requirements (educational tasks) such as literacy needs must be considered for technology solutions (Struck & Corfman, 1994).

A profile of the child's cognitive, physical or motor, and sensory abilities, academic skills, motivation, interests, and judgment provides information on functional skills underlying the child's ability to communicate and access a computer. Questions to be answered include the following:

I. Motor
   A. What body parts are capable of reliable, accurate, and controlled movement?
   B. Can the child be positioned adequately in an upright seating posture and maintain it?
   C. Does the child have sufficient range of motion, finger dexterity, strength, and endurance?
   D. What is the child's overall endurance and strength?
   E. What is the child's level of independence in daily living skills?
   F. Can the child access low-technology devices?
II. Sensory and Perceptual
   A. Can the child attend to visual feedback on the monitor?
   B. Can the child respond to auditory feedback?
   C. What are the child's strengths and limitations in visual perception and visual motor skills?

III. Cognitive and Communication
   A. What are the child's face-to-face and written communication needs?
   B. Does the child have a general idea about computer operations?
   C. Can or does the child use low-technology devices?
   D. Can the child sequence multiple-step directions to use the device? What is the cognitive level?
IV. Psychosocial
   A. Does the child seem motivated to use technology and to try alternative methods for communicating?
   B. What activities does the child enjoy?

In evaluating for use of AAC and adapted computer systems, specific performance areas are emphasized. An assessment of postural alignment and control is essential. Proper seating and positioning of the child in relation to the AAC equipment and computer access interface devices is critical to successful use of the technology. Occupational therapists, in coordination with physical therapists, often evaluate and prescribe seating and positioning systems needed for AT access. The seating position must be secure, stable, and upright to allow optimal visual-hand function for operating AAC systems and computer platforms. The position should include an "erect spine over a pelvis perpendicular to the support surface, a chin tuck with neck elongation, and the ability to maintain the arms free and forward for function" (Harryman & Warren, 1992).

The evaluation should include assessment of the child's interest in and motivation to use technology solutions. The child must think that it is rewarding and meaningful to use the device; otherwise, he or she risks frustration and abandonment of the technology (Phillips & Zhao, 1993).

After evaluation of the child, the therapist considers the attributes of devices to match the characteristics of the technology to the child's needs and skills. Aspects of the device to considered include availability, portability, ease of use, maintenance, flexibility, reliability, and cost (Struck and Corfman, 1994). Characteristics of AT devices are discussed later in this chapter.

The therapist also considers physical and social aspects of the child's environments, or settings, where the device will be used:
   1. Where will the device be used?
   2. How can the device or interface be positioned for optimal use?
   3. Do classroom and home environments allow for safe and easy access to educational materials and use of the devices?

Specific short- and long-term educational objectives must also be considered:
   1. What is the focus of the educational program (e.g., academic or functional)?
   2. What performance strengths and limitations should be considered and will relate directly to AT use?
   3. What are the child's educational goals and objectives?
   4. What school district requirements must be addressed?

## Intervention: Selection and Training in Use of Assistive Technology

The intervention plan includes selecting the appropriate AT device, helping the child effectively use the device in his or her everyday environments, and teaching others to support the child's use of AT. *Selecting the most appropriate device* is critical to enable the child to attain optimal functional outcomes. *Training* of support personnel, teaching staff, and other team members, including the parents, is also essential to ensure that the device is well used and integrated into the child's life.

### Selection

Selection of AAC devices and computer interfaces needs to be a team effort. Properties of devices need to fit the child's abilities, desires, and needs. Important questions to ask when selecting a device include the following:

1. What AT is readily available in the child's current setting?
2. Are the features of the device easy to learn and understand?
3. Can the device grow with the child?
4. Is it easy to maintain and repair?
5. Can an inexpensive low-tech device serve the child's needs?
6. Is it portable?
7. Can it be mounted on a power wheelchair if needed?
8. Can it be accessed using a variety of methods (e.g., by direct or indirect selection methods)?

Angelo and Smith (1989) identified six functional areas that occupational therapists are involved in when selecting AAC systems. These include seating and positioning of the child with interface devices, mobility, conversational systems, input method and interfaces, output methods or display methods, and writing systems. Seating and positioning influence the choice of both input and output methods. Often, children with communication impairments have severe disabilities that include difficulty maintaining a proper seating position in association with abnormal postural tone and instability. An optimal seating system should offer postural support and stability in the least stressful and most comfortable manner possible. It should also assure that the child be able to visualize the monitor, keyboard, and other input or output devices. The child's method of mobility also needs to be considered.

Occupational therapists collaborate with physical therapists on where and how the AAC device and switches should be mounted so that they do not interfere with mobility. Through collaboration, the team can design a system of integrated control. Integrated controls make it possible to use one input device to operate several devices such as power mobility, augmentative communication, and an environmental control system. The final sections of this chapter describe some of the devices and technology available and explain how these are used to increase the child's ability to communicate.

### Training

Training of both the child and staff are intimately linked, and both are required to gain optimal benefit of technology use. *Staff training* is important to implementing the intervention plan. Before training others to help the child use AT, the occupational therapist determines successful methods for the child to access the device, analyzes which steps are required to operate the device, adjusts the access methods when needed, and develops a positioning system for the child. The occupational therapist designs and implements the training program, determines how success of the program will be evaluated (including expected child outcomes and timeline for evaluation), and then monitors the child's progress according to that schedule.

The therapist also provides general training in device capability and problem solving, should the device malfunction. Group inservice with hands-on experiences is a useful method to help staff develop skills in using AT. Individualized tutorials are another training method. Often the instructional assistant and educator are the focus of training because they are responsible for the child on a daily basis. The child's instructors need to learn how the equipment and software work and how to problem solve when the system does not work. Therefore the occupational therapist provides information and resources that help staff and parents find solutions when problems in use of the equipment or software occur. Providing step-by-step written instructions and keeping them in a convenient location (e.g., taped to the side of the monitor) are easy methods to use. Typically, this includes a sequential list of instructions (e.g., what to turn on first) and how to operate equipment and software (Struck & Corfman, 1994).

***Training the child.*** During the training, the therapist collects data through observation of the child that then are used to make decisions about equipment selection and set up. Training sessions should be structured to ensure successful experiences. Through practice, the child gains an understanding of how the device operates. Use becomes second nature and automatic. Monitoring the child's performance and use of the technology are important components of a training program. The core team members need to develop a monitoring plan that involves all concerned, including the parents and the child, and is supportive of integrating technology use.

***Parallel training model.*** Angelo and Smith (1989) suggested that as the child practices the skills needed to operate a communication system, his or her need for and use of the system often change. As the child practices using a simple system, the therapist should modify the tasks to accommodate the child's increasing skills. Therefore the therapist has two goals for the child: to efficiently use the equipment and to enable the child to use more sophisticated technology. For example, practice in switch activation of a battery-operated toy can increase the child's skills in single-switch operation of an AAC device or a computer system. Overriding goals for occupational therapy are improved motor and cognitive skills so that the child is less dependent on technology and can function more independently with less use of technology.

Struck and Corfman (1994) identified useful training strategies for educational settings to be performed by the therapist:

1. Conveniently set up the equipment to ensure easy access
2. Select training tasks and activities that emphasize educational priorities
3. Plan and task analyze one or two simple activities that assure the child's success
4. Use nontimed and open-ended activities that do not have "right" or "wrong" responses
5. Use a variety of experiences to develop motor control
6. Create an environment where the child exercises self-directed choices
7. Choose activities that enable the child to become a self-directed learner

## AAC SYSTEMS

Occupational therapists must have a working knowledge of AAC systems to evaluate the child's need and potential use of such systems. The greater the occupational therapist's knowledge of available AAC systems, the more choices he or she can offer the child and family. AAC systems typically use two types of symbols systems: unaided and aided. *Unaided symbols* includes facial expressions, vocalizations, mime, gestures, pointing, and American Sign Language (ASL) (Beukelman & Mirenda, 1992). *Aided symbols* include tangible symbols and representational symbols. *Tangible symbols* consist of real objects, miniature replicas, parts of the object, and artificial association symbols. Real objects are the first symbols children come to understand (Beukelman & Mirenda, 1992; Glennen, 1992). Using *representational symbols* requires more cognitive skill. These symbol systems represent objects and language concepts and include photographs, line drawing systems (Figures 20-3 and 20-4), and orthographic symbols. Orthography refers to written characters that are used to represent a lin-

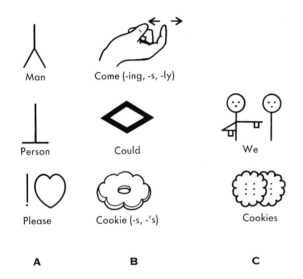

**Figure 20-3**  Examples of symbol systems. **A,** Bliss. **B,** Rebus. **C,** Picsyms.

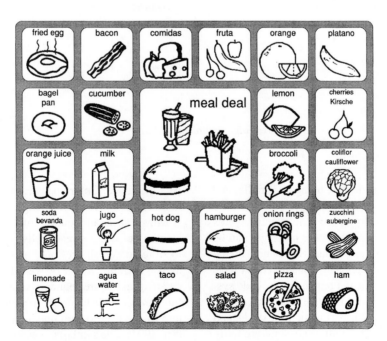

**Figure 20-4**  Personal computer software (PCS) symbols. (Photo courtesy of Mayer-Johnson Co., 1981-1993.)

| | | | | |
|---|---|---|---|---|
| A | \* – | | U | \*\* – |
| B | – \*\*\* | | V | \*\*\* – |
| C | – \* – \* – | | X | – \*\* – |
| D | – \*\* | | Y | – \* – – |
| E | \* | | Z | – – \*\* |
| F | \*\* – \* | | 1 | \* – – – |
| G | – – \* | | 2 | \*\* – – – |
| H | \*\*\*\* | | 3 | \*\*\* – – – |
| I | \*\* | | 4 | \*\*\*\* – – – |
| J | \* – – – | | 5 | \*\*\*\*\* |
| K | – \* – | | 6 | – \*\*\*\* |
| L | \* – \*\* | | 7 | – – \*\*\* |
| M | – – | | 8 | – – – \*\* |
| N | – \* | | 9 | – – – – \* |
| O | – – – | | 0 | – – – – – |
| P | \* – – \* | | Period | \* – \* – \* – |
| Q | – – \* – | | Comma | – – \*\* – – |
| R | \* – \* | | ? | \*\* – – \*\* |
| S | \*\*\* | | ! | \*\* – \* |
| T | – | | | |

**Figure 20-5**    International Morse code.

guistic system, such as icons, letters, numbers, Braille, and Morse Code (Figure 20-5).

Systems that use symbols to represent letters and words are often termed *encoding systems*. Entire messages can be encoded in simple symbols to produce efficiency in the child's ability to express that message. The child must have the cognitive capability to learn and remember the code system being used. Encoding strategies include alpha (letter), alpha-numeric, icons, VOIS-shapes (Phonic Ear, 1991), and color coding. Alpha-numeric and numeric systems are fairly self-explanatory; they use combinations of letters and num-

bers as a code. Color codes combine color with letters and numbers to convey a meaning.

Minspeak is an example of an encoding system. It is a "method of using semantically meaningful picture symbols to store and recall prestored messages" (Baker, 1994). The message *Hello, how are you?* might be stored using the meaningful picture sequence of a *waving hand* plus a *question mark*. More than one meaning is assigned to the picture by the user to gain maximum use of the system (Glennen, 1992). The symbolic meanings change according to the sequence in which they are selected. An advantage to this

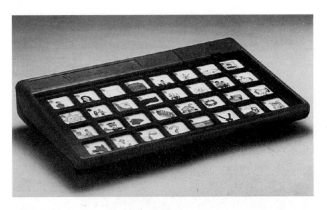

**Figure 20-6** This dedicated augmentative and alternative communication device uses Minspeak on its keyboard. (Photo courtesy Prentke Romich Co., Wooster, OH.)

system is that it allows a child to select complex messages from a small set of symbols (Figure 20-6).

## Types of AAC Devices

There are two categories of electronic AAC devices: dedicated systems and adapted microcomputer systems with communication capabilities (Glennen, 1992).

*Dedicated systems* operate primarily as electronic communication aids. They are portable and can be mounted on wheelchairs. Many can be operated by more than one input method. Speech is the primary output method, although many also have print output or can be used in conjunction with a computer as an alternative keyboard.

*Adapted computers* can include laptops, notebook computers, or standard platforms with central processing units (CPUs), a monitor, and a printer. Adapted computers with communication capability generally have more versatility than dedicated devices. Adapted computers can be used for many purposes and tasks, particularly in the school environment.

*Communication software applications* enable these devices to perform diverse functions. These software programs use the message encoding systems described previously. The applications include prestorage or message prediction methods designed to speed up the communication rate and minimize keystrokes (Glennen, 1992). It is important to remember that it takes more time to converse using a device than speaking. When using a message prediction system the child begins to spell a word (for example, types in *se*), and the computer completes the word automatically (showing a list of words that begin with *se* on the screen, for example, *see, seat, secret*.) These words are based on the working vocabulary of the child. Some systems predict an entire message given one or two words. For example, the child keys in *how* and the computer shows a set of choices that begins *are you?* Many of the programs operate

using rules of syntactic word ordering. These programs are efficient for individuals with severe motoric limitation but require high-level cognitive skills.

The software applications for augmentative communication have either fixed or open memory systems for message storage needs (Glennen, 1992). Fixed memory is preprogrammed by the manufacturer and does not allow the user to program custom messages. They are helpful for communicating routine needs (e.g., "I want a drink" and "I am tired"). This software is also advantageous for training children to first use AAC devices. The disadvantage is that these fixed systems cannot grow with the child as new skills and vocabulary are learned. Open memory allows the user to alter and increase program messages according to their individual needs.

## Input Methods and Interfaces

Input methods refer to the way devices are accessed. School-aged children without disabilities can use conventional computers, keyboards, and software. Children with communication impairments, who often have physical impairments as well, often need alternative access methods to use devices. The occupational therapist evaluates the need for an interface device or alternative input selection method. The type of selection method helps determine the appropriate input device. Potential input methods and interfaces include regular keyboards, touch pads, and alternative and expanded keyboards.

*Direct selection* is a straightforward method of entering desired information into a communication device or computer. In general, letters, words, or phrases are selected by touching or pointing to the desired key or key area. Direct selection is the preferred method if the child is able to perform fine or gross motor pointing functions. It requires less cognitive skill than indirect methods and is therefore easier to learn. Direct selection can offer more choices to the child. Pointing aids to access input devices include head sticks, mouth sticks, hand splints, and high-tech devices such as optical pointers and eye gaze monitors. Many of these are commercially available or can be custom made by the therapist. Whether the child needs to use a pointing aid is determined through evaluation of three motor components required for pointing: range of motion, accuracy, and speed of the extremity that is activating the device (Glennen, 1992).

Selection also can be achieved by voice, eye gaze, or any body part with reliable movement and controlled movement. Figure 20-7 shows a young man using a mouse emulator worn on his head with a sip and puff switch. He makes letter selections by controlling a curser that scans a keyboard, which is exhibited on the screen. Standard keyboards can be made more accessible by adding low-tech aids such as moisture guards, enlarged letter stickers, and key guards (Figure 20-8). Redefinition software allows reconfiguration

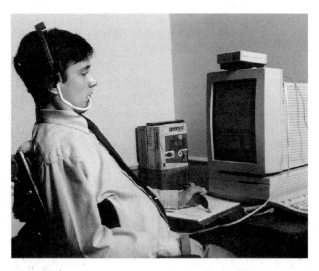

**Figure 20-7** Young man using a mouse emulator on his head with sip and puff switch. (Photo courtesy of Prentke Romich Co., Wooster, OH.)

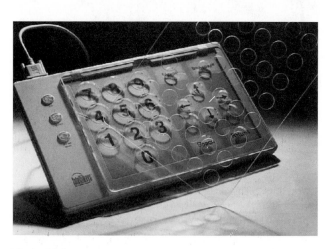

**Figure 20-8** A low-tech aid, IntelliKeys, with numbers overlay and clear acrylic keyboard. (Photo courtesy IntelliTools, Richmond, CA.)

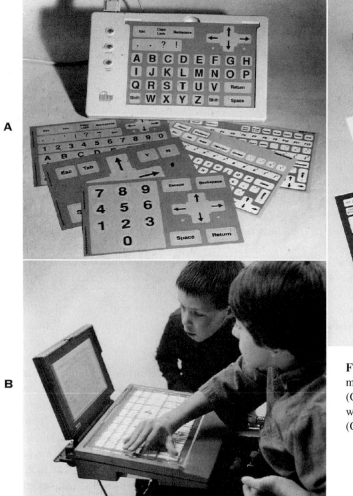

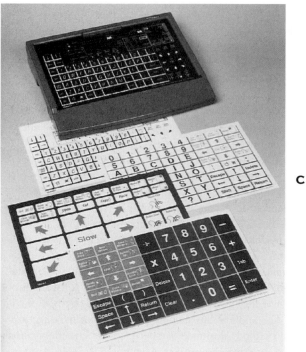

**Figure 20-9** Expanded keyboards with touch-sensitive membrane surfaces. **A,** IntelliKeys with alphabet overlay. (Courtesy of IntelliTools, Richmond, CA.) **B,** Keyboard with overlay. **C,** Alternative keyboard with powerbook. (Courtesy Don Johnston Inc., Wauconda, IL.)

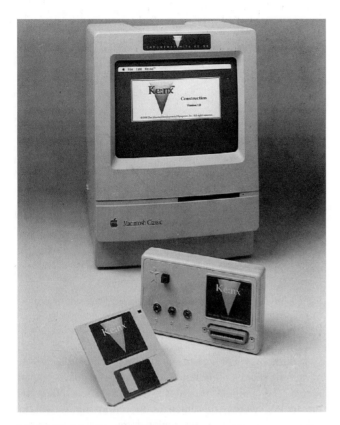

**Figure 20-10** Keyboard emulator device. (Photo courtesy Don Johnston Inc., Wauconda, IL.)

of the standard keyboard keys so that a child with limited range of motion can more easily access the most frequently needed keys. Some features include sticky key functions, which replace the need to hold down two keys simultaneously. Instead keys are hit sequentially and to achieve the same function (e.g., the child sequentially strikes the shift key and a letter to capitalize). Mouse key functions can be converted to the number pad or arrow keys on the keyboard for children who have difficulty controlling the movement of the mouse.

In addition to standard keyboards, other devices can be used. These include track balls, joysticks, a mouse, touch pads, and alternative and expanded keyboards. A track ball is an upside-down mouse and is used in much the same way except the ball is moved directly by the body part. Joysticks and mice are common and familiar equipment to move the cursor on the screen to the desired location.

*Touch pads* are input devices that are activated by the touch of a finger or stylus. Overlays of pictures, words, or phrases can be used with them. They replace the keyboard, mouse, or joystick. Touch pads can be mounted on the monitor or used in the same position as a keyboard.

*Alternative keyboards* replace standard keyboards (Church, 1992). Generally, they offer adaptable key or in-

put space sizes and must be chosen carefully to match the needs of the child. Some use standard keyboard design, and others are entirely different and can be uniquely set up for a child. *Expanded keyboards* are a type of alternative keyboard. Many have a touch-sensitive membrane surface that uses overlays such as the keyboards shown in Figure 20-9. Some of these boards plug directly into the keyboard port of the computer. Others require a keyboard emulator such as the one shown in Figure 20-10 to transfer the information directly into the microcomputer. Church (1992) defined the keyboard emulator as a hardware device "that connects to the computer and allows input from a source other than the standard keyboard" (p. 140). Keyboard emulators can also be used with switch input for scanning.

## Indirect Selection

Indirect selection techniques allow the child to use an intermediate step when sending commands to the computer (Church, 1992). Scanning is a common indirect method. It allows selection by single-switch activation; therefore the child can select different letters or words using a single simple movement. Typically, items to be scanned (letters, words, or symbols on the screen or on the device) are highlighted in an automatic manner until the child presses a switch to indicate a choice. Timing can usually be adjusted to meet the needs of the child. Scanning to assemble messages is slower than direct selection, requires closer attention, and is more cognitively challenging. An advantage to scanning is that it enables even the child with severe physical impairments to use a computer or communication device.

Types of scanning patterns include *circular scanning,* which uses a clocklike display; *linear scanning,* which highlights one item at a time; and *group-item scanning,* which highlights row by row or column by column. Scanning techniques include *automatic,* in which the cursor moves automatically and selection is made by pressing a switch when the item is highlighted, *direct or inverse scanning,* in which the cursor advances when the switch is held down and released, and *step scanning,* in which the cursor moves each time the switch is pressed.

*Single switches* are common interface devices that allow a child with minimal reliable movement to operate a computer and dedicated communication device. Switches can be plugged into the input/output (I/O) port of the microcomputer or a keyboard emulator. Almost any body part capable of movement can be used for direct selection, including legs, arms, fingers, feet, toes, knees, eye blinks, chin, tongue, head, elbow, and wrist. The body part selected to activate the switch must produce reliable movement and have endurance sufficient to move repeatedly. The switch is mounted or placed within easy access of the body part that will activate it (e.g., if the switch is placed at the side of the head, head movement is used to press the switch).

Switches are secured or mounted using a variety of commercially available articulated arms and clamps. The interface or type of switch chosen varies according to the motor skills of the child. Switches come in a variety of shapes and sizes, require varying force, pressure, and positioning. For example, mercury switches activate from any movement that the child can produce that results in some mercury bead movement.

Once the appropriate switch is found and the anatomic site for activation is determined, the child's ability to use the switch is monitored and placement may be adjusted. Optimal placement of the switch can make a tremendous difference in performance. The occupational therapist is often the team member who selects the type of switch mounting and position. The occupational therapist is also instrumental in helping the child learn to use the switch. Using a game format is less demanding and more rewarding at first than practice of switch activation to scan and select letters and words.

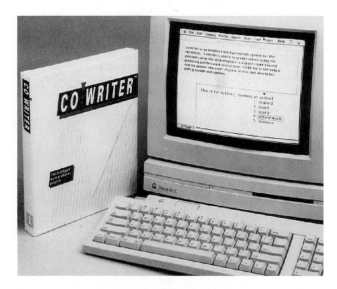

**Figure 20-11** Talking word processing software with word prediction. (Photo courtesy Don Johnston Inc., Wauconda, IL.)

## Output Methods and Displays

In addition to the range of options in computer input methods, a wide range of output methods are available. The individual needs of the child determine the specific output method selected. Choices of output methods include taped, synthesized, or digitized speech, visual displays on computer monitors and screens of AAC devices, and printed text. Sensory abilities and attending skills play a significant role in choosing an output method. Children with visual impairment require screen magnification systems to enlarge characters on the computer monitor. The position and orientation of the screen or display can be adjusted to accommodate the child's visual skills. The screen or visual display should be angled and mounted to reduce physical stress and strain.

Auditory output is important when the child uses the AAC device for conversational use. Auditory output can be used to augment visual output for children with learning disabilities who do not adequately comprehend written text. Speech output can be achieved by software applications and speech synthesis interface cards and peripherals.

Printed output may be desired if a permanent record of speech is needed. In the educational setting, printed copies are usually necessary and can replace handwritten assignments or written tests.

## Writing Systems

Occupational therapists have important roles in evaluating handwriting systems and alternative methods for producing written work (see Chapter 19). For children with severe handwriting deficits, word processing with adaptive input devices or specific software applications can make the difference in achieving academic success.

Talking word processors are common adaptive writing systems used by children with written language impairments. The computer provides synthesized speech output of the letters, words, or sentences the child inputs. Talking word processors have two major components: specifically designed application software and speech synthesis either built into the computer or added with an interface card.

Some word processing software also has word prediction, spell check, and grammar check features. Word prediction helps reduce key strokes and increase the rate of typing. As the child types letter by letter, words are presented, usually in numbered order, on the screen. These words may be commonly used by the child or common in the English language. For example, the child presses *t* and the following words are listed: *the, to, that,* and *there.* The child can either press a number to indicate a choice or press another letter to get more choices until the desired word is on the screen (Figure 20-11). A basic reading level is needed to use these features successfully.

On-screen keyboards are another method for accomplishing word processing. These are software applications that replace the standard keyboard. A keyboard is displayed on the monitor, and the cursor is moved by using an electronic pointing device, typically worn on the head. This method enables children with limited hand and arm movements to perform word processing tasks.

Voice recognition is a software application that also bypasses the standard keyboard and enables the child to perform word processing tasks. The programs "learn" to recognize the voice patterns and enunciations of the child. The child uses a microphone headset much like the one telephone operators use. These applications are most appropriate for children with good speech and cognitive ability, but who also have limited movements.

## CASE STUDY #1—CONT'D

Ben's resource English teacher, speech pathologist, and occupational therapist met to discuss the difficulties he was experiencing in keeping up with written work. He had received occupational therapy intervention since the fourth grade for handwriting needs. Accommodations included use of a tape recorder to record his assignments, increasing the length of time for taking tests, and a peer note taker in class.

He continued to experience great frustration with expressing his thoughts in writing and in producing written papers of acceptable length. His teacher thought he should be more independent with written work and needed to write papers of acceptable length for an eighth grader. His speech pathologist suspected that his difficulty could be language based. His occupational therapist determined that he had fine motor skills and bilateral skills satisfactory for keyboarding. The team believed that his language-based needs might be supported with keyboarding instruction. They agreed that he might benefit from the use of software that reinforced his keyboard input with speech output. They believed that aides in spelling and grammar might help him focus on the content of his written work. The team developed the following written language goals:

*Goal 1:* Using a keyboarding software program, Ben will activate all keys in the correct sequence with 90% accuracy.

*Goal 2:* Using a talking word processing program, Ben will write a paragraph with appropriate spelling, punctuation, and grammar with 90% accuracy.

The team recommended that Ben enroll in a keyboarding class to gain basic skills. His progress was monitored by the resource teacher and occupational therapist. The team chose a number of features to improve the efficiency of his word processing. A talking word processing program with word prediction, spell check, and grammar check features was selected. The program was installed in the computer in the English resource room. His written work and performance using the program were closely monitored by all team members through weekly observations and conferences. As he practiced and gained proficiency with the software program, he increasingly experienced academic successes.

## Resources

Examples of types of devices and software applications have been given previously. At first glance it may seem an impossible task to keep up with innovations in technology. Fortunately, resources are available to occupational therapists who are searching for devices. It is critical that therapists stay abreast of new technology so that optimal options are made available to the child.

AT manufacturers and vendors are a primary source of information. Attending technology fairs and workshops and visiting exhibit halls at conferences is one way to learn about devices. Some manufacturers loan equipment and distribute demonstration software. State technology assistance programs may have demonstration centers or loan closet programs available to children and their families. Regional and national conferences and newsletters from specialty organizations also provide information to learn about technology (Appendix 20-A).

## Procurement

Occupational therapists can be instrumental in securing funding for both AAC devices and computer access devices. Assembling all necessary documentation and using appropriate terms to show the necessity of the devices is critical.

The wording used to request reimbursement can mean the difference between acceptance and rejection by funding sources. All possible funding sources must be identified as well (RESNA, 1991).

Local education agencies (LEAs) are one source for funding and purchasing AT devices for children with disabilities (RESNA, 1992). Provisions in IDEA (1990) support costs of AT devices, provided they are necessary for the child to benefit from their special education program. The LEAs purchase devices for individual children when they are required to meet educational goals; they may also purchase an AT device that remains in the classroom and is used by a number of students over a several-year period.

Third-party payers are another source of funding. The major third-party payer is Medicaid (RESNA, 1991). AAC devices and computer access may be covered by Medicaid if it is prescribed by a physician or other licensed health care provider. Children from low-income families and those receiving Aid for Families with Dependent Children (AFDC) or Supplemental Security Income (SSI) may be eligible to have their devices funded by Medicaid as durable medical equipment (DME). To be funded as DME, the device must meet a medical need. For example, AAC devices may be funded if it is shown that it is necessary

## CASE STUDY #2–CONT'D

Kim had minimal ability to use her hands and to speak. She used a power wheelchair with a contoured seating insert. She communicated with eye gaze, vocalizations, gestures, and gross pointing with her right arm to indicate her needs. Since she began attending regular first grade with nondisabled peers, her motivation had increased. Kim's frustration at not being able to get her meaning across was increasingly noted by her peers, teacher, parents, and therapists. Her core team at school, which included her classroom teacher, instructional assistant, speech pathologist, physical therapist, and occupational therapist, met to discuss her educational program. The team and her parents identified communication needs as primary to her educational program. Her teacher shared test data and observations that indicated that Kim appeared to have academic skills within grade level. The instructional assistant described her as bright and responsive in class. The speech pathologist found her receptive language within the average range. However, her expressive language was severely limited because of her oral-motor impairment. Kim's mother shared with the team that she and Kim used eye pointing and "twenty questions" for communication at home. The occupational therapist found that her physical skills were severely limited. Head movement was her most reliable movement pattern for switch activation. Although she tried to use her right arm, her limited control was not adequate for reliable switch use or direct access of a keyboard. The physical therapist focused on her postural alignment in sitting. The team developed goals for Kim in the areas of expressive and written communication and reading. Below are examples of her goals.

*Goal 1:* Using an augmentative communication device, Kim will indicate her choice for lunch four of five times.

*Goal 2:* Using an augmentative communication device, Kim will indicate her personal needs four of five times.

*Goal 3:* Using a single switch and scanning array, Kim will operate a book software program with 90% accuracy.

*Goal 4:* Using a single switch and scanning array, Kim will write words using inventive spelling independently.

*Goal 5:* Using a single switch, Kim will operate a battery-operated toy with her right arm four of five trials.

Proper mounting of systems and switches and a consistent training program were critical aspects of Kim's program. Operating switches at the head site poses two problems: increased risk of fatigue and compromised visual attending to the monitor or display because of the head's movement in switch activation. Signs of fatigue were monitored closely. She used a soft neck brace when using the switches mounted at the head to prevent fatigue. The AAC device that was chosen had a combined fixed and open memory, scan mode with switch attachment, and an icon display so that it could grow with Kim. Switches of varying shapes and pressure sensitivity were tried until the one best for her was chosen and mounted to her wheelchair.

The same switch was also used to operate the classroom computer. The computer was equipped with an on-screen scanning system and speech synthesis. Kim uses exploratory, beginning literacy, and talking word processing software programs.

The team established a monitoring program with the special educator in charge of curriculum needs and daily use of the equipment. The speech-language pathologist monitored and implemented communication methods. The physical therapist adapted and monitored her seating and positioning. The occupational therapist monitored positioning of her switches and devices and developed a training program to improve right arm and hand control. The team met regularly to discuss Kim's progress and needs.

---

for the child to communicate his or her medical need (RESNA, 1991).

Private third-party payers may also pay for devices. The family's insurance policy should be checked. The key terms to look for are *durable medical equipment* and *therapeutic and prosthetic services and supplies.* In general, a physician's prescription for devices is required, as is a well-documented statement of need.

## Coordinating Use

Coordinating use of AT requires teamwork. Collaboration by team members is essential for integrated use of AAC and computer access devices in all areas of the child's life. The following stories about Ben, Kim, and Linda demonstrate the occupational therapist's role as a team member in enabling each to integrate technology into his or her everyday life.

CASE STUDY #3—CONT'D

Although Linda exhibited multiple deformities in her arms and legs from the arthrogryposis, she was independent and participated in all school activities. She was motivated to succeed and planned to attend college. She had recently joined the school newspaper staff but had difficulty completing assignments because of her physical limitations. Accommodations in place for her included note takers in her regular classes, untimed tests, and use of a tape recorder. Linda and her resource teacher, guidance counselor, and occupational therapist met to discuss additional accommodations so that she could participate on the school newspaper staff. Deadline requirements could not be adjusted for her. Computer access was discussed as a possibility. Linda agreed to work with the occupational therapist to explore various options.

Linda had the ability to use both arms, but her physical impairment prevented isolated movement of fingers. Hand splints that served as dowel holders were made for her by the occupational therapist. She successfully used them to activate the keyboard. She used a software program with word prediction and spell and grammar check to reduce the number of keystrokes. Her computer also had built-in keyboard reconfiguration features that included sticky keys and mouse keys. Linda instructed her journalism and resource teacher on the functions and options of the software programs so that they could make modifications for her if necessary. The occupational therapist monitored Linda's program on a monthly basis and found that she continued to develop her skills and independently tried new options in computer access.

STUDY QUESTIONS

1. List and describe tasks of core team members on an augmentative and alternative communication (AAC) team.
2. Compare and contrast the advantages and disadvantages of direct and indirect selection input methods.
3. List and describe four components in evaluating a child's potential use of assistive technology.
4. List and describe two methods of increasing the rate of communication when using electronic AAC devices.

## SUMMARY

AAC and adapted computer access gives children with severe problems in oral and written communication the ability to communicate; improve social relationships; improve their ability to attend to health and safety needs; enable greater self-determination and control; enable participation in education, family life, and the community; and increase independence (NIDRR, 1992).

Providing technology services requires a collaborative team approach. Occupational therapists are key team players in evaluating and training children in use of appropriate technology. Occupational therapists provide expertise in access methods and training strategies. As use of AT rapidly grows and changes, it is critical for all team members to seek knowledge of AT and to work collaboratively to help children apply technology to reach meaningful, functional, and realistic goals and objectives. Appropriate use of AT is critical to enabling the child with disabilities to participate more fully in tasks of daily living in school, at home, and in the community and to develop personal independence.

## REFERENCES

Alm, N. (1993). The development of augmentative and alternative communication systems to assist with social communication. *Technology and Disability, 2*(3), 1-18.

Angelo, J. & Smith, R.O. (1989). The critical role of occupational therapy in augmentative communication services. In AOTA (Ed.). *Technology review 89: perspectives on occupational therapy practice*. Rockville, MD: American Occupational Therapy Association.

Baker, B.R. (1994). Translating an augmentative communication language system. *Tapping Technology,* June, 14-15.

Beukelman, D.R. & Mirenda, P. (1992). *Augmentative and alternative communication: management of severe communication disorders in children and adults.* Baltimore: Brookes.

Church, G. (1992). Adaptive access for microcomputers. In G.Church and S. Glennen (Eds.). *The handbook of assistive technology* (pp.123-177). San Diego: Singular Publishing Group.

Church, G. & Glennen, S. (1992). Assistive technology programs. In G. Church & S. Glennen (Eds.). *The handbook of assistive technology* (pp. 1-26). San Diego: Singular Publishing Group.

Cumming, F.J. (1989). Children with communicative impairment. In P. Pratt & A. Allen (Eds.). *Occupational therapy for children (2nd ed.).* St Louis: Mosby.

Glennen, S. (1992). Augmentative and alternative communication. In G. Church & S. Glennen (Eds.). *The handbook of assistive technology* (pp. 93-122). San Diego: Singular Publishing Group.

Hammel, J.M. & Smith, R.O. (1993). The development of technology competencies and training guideline for occupational therapists. *American Journal of Occupational Therapy 47*(11), 970-979.

Harryman, S.E. & Warren, L.R. (1992). Positioning and power mobility. In G. Church & S. Glennen (Eds.). *Handbook of assistive technology* (pp.55-92). San Diego: Singular Publishing Group.

*The Individuals with Disabilities Education Act (1990) (P.L. 101-476)* 20 USC 1401.

National Institute on Disability and Rehabilitation Research. (1992). Augmentative and alternative communication intervention consensus statement. *NIDRR, 1*(2).

Phillips, B. & Zhao, H. (1993). Predictors of assistive technology. *Assistive Technology, 5*(1), 36-45.

Phonic Ear (1991). *VOIS shapes*. Petaluma, CA: Phonic Ear.

Rehabilitation Engineering Society of North America (RESNA). (1991). *Assistive technology: a funding workbook*. Washington, DC: RESNA Press.

Rehabilitation Society of North America (RESNA). (1992). *Assistive technology and the individualized education program*. Washington, DC: RESNA Press.

Smith, R.O. (1991). Technological approaches to performance enhancement. In C. Christiansen & C. Baum (Eds.). *Occupational therapy: Overcoming human performance deficits* (pp. 746-786). Thorofare, NJ: SLACK.

Struck, M. & Corfman, S.K. (1994). Strategies for integration of adapted computer use. *School System Special Interest Section Newsletter, 1*(3), 3-4.

Swinth, Y. (1994). The role of the special education team in selecting and implementing assistive technology. *School Systems Special Interest Section Newsletter, 1*(3), 1-2.

*The Technology Related Assistance for Individuals with Disabilities Act. (1988).* (P.L. 100-407) 29 U.S.C. 2202, S 3 (1).

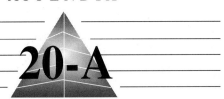

## Sources for Information on Assistive Technology and Augmentative Communication

American Speech-Language-Hearing Association (ASHA)
10801 Rockville Pike
Rockville, MD 20852
(301) 897-5700
  Publishes journals and books on augmentative and alternative communication.

Communication Aids Manufacturers Association (CAMA)
518-26 Davis Street, Suite 211
Evanston, IL 60201-4644
(800) 441-2262
  Distributes a free packet of materials and list of member manufacturers. CAMA also holds workshops that feature AAC devices.

Closing the Gap (CTG)
P.O. Box 68
Henderson, MN 56044
(612) 248-3294
  Publishes a bimonthly newspaper. The February/March issue contains a resource directory on hardware, software, and organizations. CTG also holds an annual conference.

RESNA
1700 Moore Street Suite 150
Arlington, VA 22209-1903
(703) 524-6686
  Provides technical assistance to state technology assistance programs (TAP), publishes a monthly newsletter, quarterly journal, and books on assistive technology and holds an annual conference.

Foundation for Technology Access
2173 E. Francisco Boulevard, Suite L
San Rafael, CA 94901
  Provides a list of Alliance for Technology Access centers in the United States and distributes a newsletter.

International Society for Augmentative and Alternative Communication (ISAAC)
P.O. Box 1762 Suite R
Toronto, Ontario, Canada M4G 4A3
(416) 737-9308
  Provides information on AAC, publishes a journal and newsletters, and holds an annual conference.

Trace Research and Development Center
Room S-151 Waisman Center
1500 Highland Avenue
University of Wisconsin
Madison, WI 53707
(608) 262-6966
  Provides information on communication and microcomputer technology. Publishes information in printed and electronic form.

Technology Special Interest Section
American Occupational Therapy Association
4720 Montgomery Lane
P.O. Box 31220
Bethesda, MD 20824-1220
(301) 652-2682
  Publishes a quarterly newsletter and sponsors the Assistive Technology Lab at the annual American Occupational Therapy Association conference.

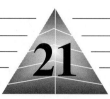

# Mobility

CHRISTINE WRIGHT-OTT ▲ SNAEFRIDUR EGILSON

## KEY TERMS

▲ Developmental Theory of Mobility
▲ Augmentative Mobility
▲ Mobility Assessment Models
▲ Alternative Powered Mobility Devices
▲ Manual Wheelchairs
▲ Power Wheelchairs
▲ Positioning and Seating

## CHAPTER OBJECTIVES

1. Understand the importance of mobility to development.
2. Apply a mobility assessment model to children with different levels of motor function.
3. Identify alternative methods of mobility appropriate to meet the child's developmental and functional needs.
4. Describe wheelchair features and designs that meet the needs of children with various levels of motor control.
5. Explain the biomechanical principles important to positioning and seating.
6. Identify power mobility devices currently available for children.
7. Describe power mobility assessment and intervention.
8. Describe new technology in assessing seating and positioning and new equipment available to children with unique seating and positioning needs.

The information in this chapter is intended to clarify the importance of mobility for growth and development and the responsibilities of the occupational therapist in recommending appropriate mobility devices. Implications of impaired mobility are discussed. Guidelines and criteria for selecting mobility equipment are defined, and descriptions of mobility devices are provided. The importance of positioning and

other factors that influence successful use of assistive devices are emphasized.

Functional mobility is listed in the Uniform Terminology—third edition as one of the occupational performance areas of activities of daily living. The definition of functional mobility includes moving from one position or place to another, such as in bed mobility, wheelchair mobility, transfers (wheelchair, bed, car, tub or shower, toilet, or chair), performing functional ambulation, and transporting objects (AOTA, 1994) (see Appendix 8-A). As described, this chapter primarily addresses mobility as a means of locomotion, with an emphasis on evaluation and intervention principles.

## DEVELOPMENTAL THEORY OF MOBILITY

The neonate has little independent control of any part of the body. Gradually, symmetry and midline orientation begin, followed by controlled purposeful movements and the beginning of alternating coordinated movements. The first form of mobility the infant experiences is by rolling, first from side to supine and then prone to supine, followed by rolling in either direction. The 6-month-old baby achieves mobility by pivoting in the prone position. The infant continually becomes more active against gravity (Figure 21-1). Most 8-month-old babies creep and move from sitting to quadruped and back. By the ninth to tenth month the infant experiences a strong desire to move upward. First, they pull to stand and cruise along furniture, then they hold on to someone or something as they take their first steps. According to Bly (1994), the average age of independent walking is 11.2 months.

Among developmental theorists, it is accepted that physical and psychologic development are interrelated and that early experiences influence subsequent behavior. "Through their motor interactions infants and toddlers learn about things and people in their world and also discover they can cause things to happen" (Butler, 1988, p.18). During the

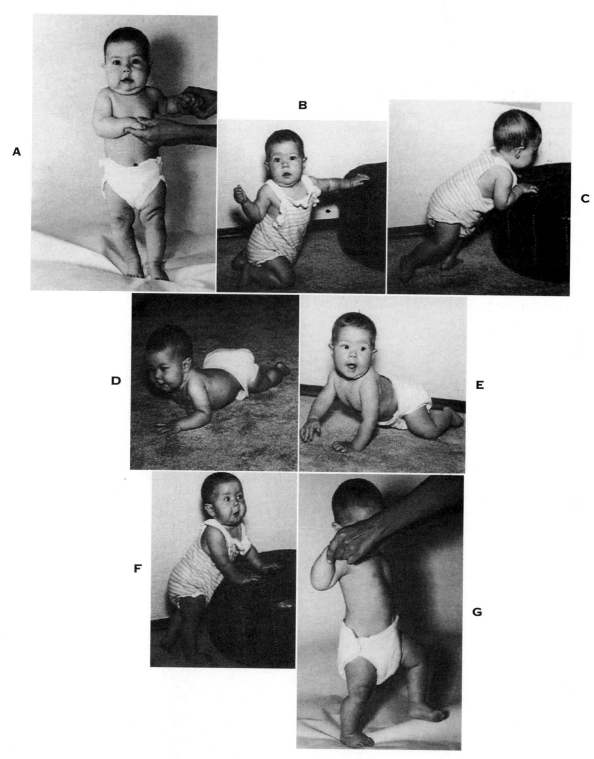

**Figure 21-1**  Development of locomotion. **A,** Infant bears full weight on feet by 7 months. **B,** Infant can maneuver from sitting to kneeling position. **C,** Infant can pull self to standing position. **D,** Infant crawls with abdomen on floor and pulls self forward. **E,** Infant creeps on hands and knees at 9 months. **F,** Infant can stand holding onto furniture at 9 months. **G,** While standing, infant takes deliberate steps at 10 months. (From Wong, D.L. [1995]. *Whaley and Wong's essentials of pediatric nursing* [4th ed.] [p. 274]. St. Louis: Mosby.)

first months of life, children seek physical control of their environment and continue to do so by building and enhancing their motor skills day by day.

During the first 4 years of life, the child gains independence through mastery of important life tasks such as locomotion, ability to manipulate, bowel and bladder control, language development, and social interactions. The most fundamental of these, with the widest influence in all spheres of development, are learning to move about the environment and to use language as a communicative and information processing system.

As they move about, children gain various learning experiences. Locomotion and other motor skills, which develop rapidly during the first 3 years of life, become the primary vehicles for learning and socialization and for the healthy growth of a sense of independence and competence. Piaget (1954) viewed self-produced movement as a crucial building block of knowledge. He theorized that the intercoordination of vision and audition with movements (including locomotion) laid the basis for the child's understanding of space, objects, causality, and the self. The ability of children to influence their environment and to affect or alter it through their own actions is intrinsically motivating. Early experiences are believed to foster curiosity, exploration, mastery, and persistence and therefore are important for later intellectual functioning.

Campos and Bertenthal (1987) called attention to the fact that despite theoretical agreement about the significance of locomotion, little empirical research has been done on the psychologic processes affected by the development of self-produced movement. They claimed that the psychologic domains most likely to be influenced by the development of crawling, creeping, and upright locomotion include the "development of fear of heights, changes in spatial search skills and spatial coding by the infant, and appearance of new forms of emotional communication" (p. 16). These authors stressed that locomotion may be neither necessary nor sufficient for the development of other skills. However, they believe it to play at least a facilitative role as a mediator of development (Bertenthal, Campos, & Barrett, 1984).

## IMPAIRED MOBILITY

"When development along any line is restricted, delayed, or distorted, other lines of development are adversely affected as well" (Butler, 1988, p. 66). Young children with physical disabilities who have difficulty achieving independent motor control are often deprived of self-initiated mobility experiences. Because they lack the necessary movements to engage in and act on their environment, important learning opportunities are also hindered. Restricted experiences and mobility during early childhood can have a diffuse and lasting impact.

According to Becker (1975), long-term physical restriction during the neonatal, infancy, or early childhood period

can significantly alter and disrupt the entire subsequent course of emotional or psychologic development in the involved child. Such deprivation of physical and social contingencies can lead to secondary developmental problems, which are motivational. As stated by Brinker and Lewis (1982), "handicapped infants may begin to lose interest in a world which they do not expect to control" (p. 113). Seligman (1975) characterized this motivational effect as learned helplessness, a condition in which the child gives up trying to control his or her own world because of motor disability and diminished expectations of caregivers. Butler (1988) found that children whose mobility is limited during early childhood, for whatever reason, develop a pattern of apathetic behavior, specifically a lack of curiosity and initiative. These character traits are believed to have a critical influence on intellectual performance and social interaction as already described.

Douglas and Ryan (1987) described the positive effects of newly gained independent mobility on the emotional, social, and intellectual state of a severely physically disabled boy. Paulsson and Christoffersen (1984) found that children with disabilities using mobility devices became less dependent on controlling their environment through verbal commands, more interested in all mobility skills, and more active in peer activities. Butler (1986) suggested that increased independence through locomotion may reduce the need to use language as a control method and improve psychosocial behavior. Teachers at the Blair Learning Center in Bakersfield, California discovered that children who had some means of ambulation could and would make choices, but those who did not ambulate were much less likely to exercise any options that were available. It was concluded that the lack of ambulation severely restricted the opportunities for the children to practice decision making, thus giving them no reason to express an opinion or desire.

Occupational and physical therapists often contribute to decision making on *whether* to introduce mobility devices to children with developmental delays, and if it is determined that a mobility device is important, *when* it should be considered and *what kind* of mobility is appropriate.

*Whether* a child should use a mobility device continues to be controversial. Introduction of mobility aids to children with physical disabilities at early ages appears to facilitate psychosocial, language, and cognitive development. However, professionals seem to lack agreement regarding use of support walkers and powered devices. A support walker provides moderate to maximum support at the pelvis, trunk, and sometimes the head. If the walker does not fit properly, the child may use abnormal movements to propel it. Reinforcement of abnormal movement patterns contradicts therapy goals and may delay or impair the quality of motor development. Most support walkers are now designed with a variety of adjustments and features that provide more desirable positioning than has been available in the past (Figure 21-2).

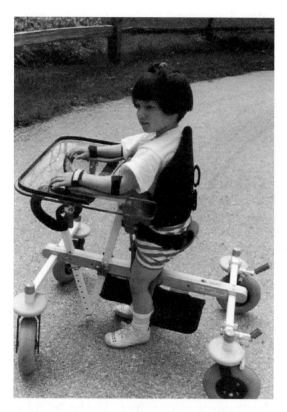

**Figure 21-2**   Prone Support Walker with accessories, manufactured by Consumer Care Products, Inc.

Research has not demonstrated that using powered mobility prevents or delays the child's acquisition of motor skills. On the contrary, improved head control and trunk stability, as well as increased motivation during mobility training and more self-confidence in movement, are common findings (Butler, 1988). Several professionals have also reported improvements in other areas of development (Paulsson & Christoffersen, 1984).

*When* should a child start using mobility devices? The current trend is for devices to be recommended at young ages, when typical children are first attaining mobility. Many professionals believe that if self-initiated mobility does not occur in the first year, the use of devices for mobility should be considered. "Clinical experience and research projects have established that powered mobility devices offer children at least as young as 17 months a safe and efficient method of independent locomotion" (Butler, 1988, p. 18).

It is at times a challenge for the therapist to suggest consideration of a mobility device, particularly a wheelchair, to the family of a young child with a disability. Many care providers consider the suggestion as a symbol of giving up hope for independent ambulation. It is important to convey the concept that all children need a means of mobility and that the mobility device is intended to assist the child in achieving more independence and function until and if another method is acquired.

Several factors need to be considered when deciding *what type* of mobility device is appropriate for a child. These factors include physical and psychosocial abilities and limitations, the environment for intended use, the thoroughness of the assessment process, considerations of all the advantages and disadvantages of a device, effect on treatment goals, and an understanding of the cost versus the benefits. Ideally a mobility-impaired child should have more than one type of mobility device for use in indoor and outdoor environments. Whatever methods are chosen for mobility, all require close cooperation between all professionals working with the child and family.

## AUGMENTATIVE MOBILITY

Butler (1988) introduced the term *augmentative mobility,* referring to all mobility that supplements or augments ambulation.

Given augmentative mobility, disabled children can experience more success in directly controlling their environment, thereby reducing or avoiding secondary social, emotional and intellectual handicaps (p. 18).

The authors of this chapter recommend that the concept of augmentative mobility be expanded to include transitional as well as functional mobility. Transitional mobility allows the child to use a device to experience self-initiated movement without the expectation that it must be functional. The child may not be able to move the device in a desired direction but uses it as a means for exploring the effects of movement and learning how to move. Transitional mobility is best provided by allowing the child to move the device in a large room with open space where the child is free to explore. These experiences may then help the child make the transition to a more functional level of purposeful mobility. Not all children are able to achieve functional mobility; in these instances, transitional mobility remains an important means for the child to explore the environment.

## ASSESSMENT AND INTERVENTION
### Classifying Mobility Skills

Children's mastery of functional mobility skills has been classified and categorized in a number of ways. Hays (1987) examined current existing diagnostic conditions of children without locomotion and divided them into four functional subgroups:

1. Children who will never ambulate. This includes children with cerebral palsy with severe involvement and spinal muscular atrophy types I and II. Generally, these children have no opportunity for independent mobility unless a power wheelchair is prescribed.
2. Children with inefficient mobility, who ambulate but are unable to do so at a reasonable rate of speed or

with acceptable endurance. This includes children with cerebral palsy with less involvement and myelomeningocele with upper-extremity involvement. For these children the power wheelchair may provide an efficient means of mobility above that which they are capable of producing themselves.

3. Children who have lost their independent mobility. This includes victims of trauma and children with progressive neuromuscular disorders. Here the developmental implications may be less critical than in the first two groups, and the issue is acceptance of assisted mobility as an adaptation to the acquired disability.

4. Children who temporarily require assisted mobility and often progress to independent mobility with age. This includes many children with osteogenesis imperfecta and arthrogryposis. Functional considerations in this group are both developmental and practical.

Clearly, there are great differences among these groups that may have implications for mobility and its integration into the child's overall concept of disability, as well as for assessment and intervention.

## Functional Assessment

The purpose of the mobility assessment is to evaluate the child's strengths, concerns, and weaknesses. It should include consideration of all functional needs of the child and the possible technical devices that might be of assistance (Trefler, Hobson, Taylor, Monahan, & Shaw, 1993). Compiling comprehensive information about a child's strengths and needs is generally best met by a team of knowledgeable professionals with participation by the child and family. To evaluate the performance area of mobility, the assessment must include the components of performance (such as neuromotor status, orthopedic condition, and psychosocial considerations) and the performance context (temporal aspects such as chronologic and developmental age and environmental issues). Few standardized instruments address the motor, perceptual, and cognitive factors that influence mobility control, and hence reliable assessment is of concern to therapists. In addition, the tasks that are most relevant for daily independence in mobility function have not been well defined in traditional developmental milestone tests. The Pediatric Evaluation of Disabilities Inventory (Haley, Coster, Ludlow, Haltiwanger, & Andrellos, 1992) is a judgment-based, standardized measure of a child's functional performance that is more objective and comprehensive than previously developed scales. It yields normative scores along two dimensions of performance: the capability for discrete functional skills and the amount of caregiver assistance needed. The authors have defined two basic elements for functional mobility: basic transfer skills and body transport activities.

## Mobility Assessment Models

Selecting the most appropriate positioning and mobility device requires the skills of a therapy team working in close collaboration with the school team, prescribing physician, child, parent or care provider, and rehabilitation technology supplier (RTS). The RTS is a specialist who is trained and experienced in providing durable medical rehabilitation equipment and is certified through the National Association of Medical Equipment Suppliers. It is the therapist's responsibility to identify the needs of the child, recommend features of a mobility device that assists function for both the child and care provider, and assist the family in setting appropriate goals and expectations for using the mobility device. The RTS is responsible for maintaining updated knowledge of available equipment and assisting in identifying choices of mobility devices according to the features the child needs to use it optimally. Once the mobility device is selected and provided to the client, the therapists are responsible for reassessing the fit and function of a device to determine if it meets the stated goals and objectives. Most funding agencies will not approve replacement of a mobility device, such as a wheelchair, within 3 to 5 years of the purchase date. If the equipment is not appropriate, the child and family may not have another option for several years. The limitations in reimbursement become critical when a misunderstanding during the evaluation or ordering process results in a device that does not meet the predetermined outcomes. It is imperative that the therapists, RTS, and family immediately decide on how to best resolve these issues.

There are several approaches for assessing children for mobility devices. The most common is for the therapists to request a local supplier of durable medical equipment or RTS to bring the device under consideration to the therapy session. The RTS offers input as to what features and options are available on the device and how to properly adjust it. The difficulty encountered with this model is that one supplier typically has a limited selection of devices available for demonstration purposes, so only one device may be evaluated at each session. Therefore the therapist does not have the opportunity to compare the child's performance in various types of mobility devices. Without direct comparison of the mobility devices, decisions about which device is optimal for the child are difficult to make. The decision making is less risky when side-by-side comparisons are possible with the devices available during the evaluation. This method enables comparison of performance of each mobility device under consistent child and environmental conditions.

A number of assistive technology centers and rehabilitation engineering centers throughout the country use a multidisciplinary team approach and side-by-side evaluation methods to assess seating and mobility needs, particularly with individuals who have severe disabilities. The teams consist of occupational therapists, physical therapists, rehabilitation engineers, speech pathologists, and RTSs working with the child's therapy team, school team, physician, and family. These centers offer the advantage of being able to consider all the needs of the child and offering a concentrated level of expertise.

## MOBILITY DEVICES

Selection of a specific type of a mobility device depends on several factors: the purpose for using the mobility device, the indoor and outdoor environments in which it will be used, the effort required by the individual to use the device, and positioning needs. The team also considers specific features and device adaptations for optimal use in functional activities such as eating, transfers, augmentative communication, personal hygiene, and school activities. Finally, the needs and concerns of the care provider who will be using, transporting, and maintaining the equipment and costs versus benefits are considered.

The occupational therapist must use the skills of an investigator during the mobility assessment process. Thoughtful planning and careful analysis of person-device-environment fit are needed to ensure that the child and family receive the optimal device. A wheelchair that will not fit into the family van, tips over when the augmentative communication device is mounted on it, or cannot be propelled outside because the family lives in a hilly area are common problems that are experienced when a device is ordered without comprehensive mobility assessment.

### Scooters

*Prone scooters* (Figure 21-3) require use of the arms and the ability to lift the head while moving. The advantages include that the child has greater access for playing on the floor, some children might be able to get on and off independently, and turning is easier than in other types of mobility devices. Disadvantages include fatigue from maintaining neck and back extension, the head is more vulner-

able to hitting objects, hands may get caught in the casters or rubbed on rough surfaces, and it is difficult for the child to view the environment above the ground level. Children with spina bifida may find the prone scooter most functional because they have the upper-extremity function to propel it, and their legs can be supported.

*Caster carts* offer children with upper-extremity function, such as those with spina bifida, another means of mobility (Figure 21-4). Caster carts can be used either indoors or on flat outdoor surfaces, such as playgrounds. Some children may be able to transfer on and off independently because of the close proximity to the floor. The device requires a considerable amount of energy expenditure for propelling long distances because of the small diameter of the wheels. Children with lower-extremity muscle contractures or tightness such as in the hamstring muscles may find it difficult to sit comfortably and securely because they are often unable to tolerate long leg sitting. These children may do better with a triangular-shaped wedge placed under the knees to support their legs in knee flexion.

The *aeroplane mobility device* was designed for children with cerebral palsy who can move their legs but need support of the upper body (Figure 21-5). The device provides developmentally appropriate positioning, particularly for children with spasticity, because the child is positioned with hip abduction and extension and knee flexion and the upper extremities are in a weight-bearing position. This position often reduces muscle tone and abnormal posturing in children who have cerebral palsy. Other advantages include ease in viewing the environment, the device can be handmade, and parents often like the fact that it looks like a toy rather than an assistive device. It is not yet commercially available but can be fabricated from wood. Disadvantages include lack of adjustability for growth, difficulty turning and moving backwards, and that it is heavy to transport.

If a child has upper-extremity function to push and maneuver wheels, a *mobile stander* may provide another means for mobility. These devices allow the child to experience

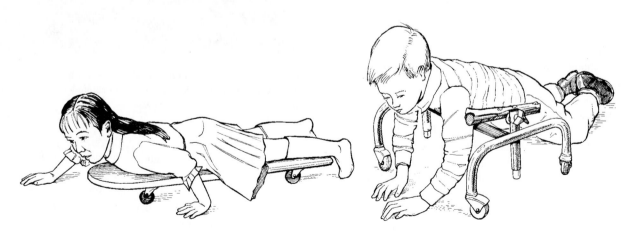

**Figure 21-3** Prone scooter mobility devices.

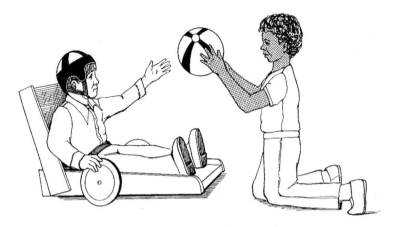

**Figure 21-4**  Caster cart mobility device.

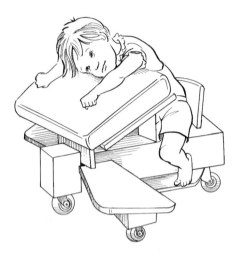

**Figure 21-5**  Aeroplane mobility device can be hand made and is designed for children younger than 3 years of age.

lower-extremity weight bearing in a standing position. Indoor mobility is achieved using large hand-held wheels for self-propulsion (Figure 21-6).

## Walkers

Children who have the ability to pull to a standing position and maintain a grip may be able to use a *hand-held walker.* These walkers are designed for use either in front of or behind the child (reverse walker) (Figure 21-7). Children with mild to moderate cerebral palsy or lower levels of spina bifida with leg bracing most commonly use hand-held walkers. Walkers can have three or four wheels and come in a variety of wheel sizes. The smaller the caster, the more difficult it is for use outdoors and over uneven surfaces. Reverse walkers are available with a feature in which the casters lock when the walker is pushed backwards, such as when a child leans into it. This feature enables the child to stand and lean against the walker for rest periods; however, it makes maneuvering the walker backwards more difficult.

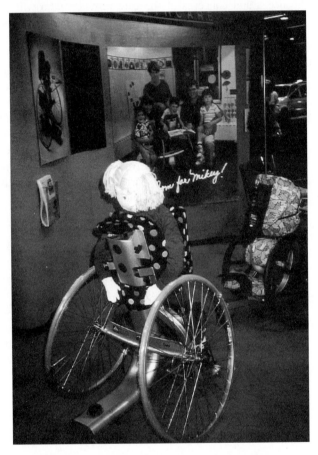

**Figure 21-6**  Mobile prone stander provides mobility for children who can propel the wheels. Manufactured by Taylor Made Inc.

*Support walkers* are designed for children who have some ability to move their legs reciprocally but need support at the pelvis, chest, and possibly the upper extremities (see Figure 21-2). Critical to functional use of these types of walkers is selecting appropriate features and making adjustments that provide optimal positioning for the child. Sup-

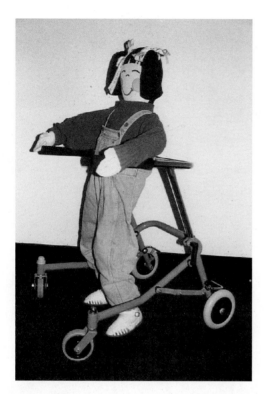

**Figure 21-7** Bugsy Walker is a reverse-style walker manufactured by Taylor Made Inc.

port walkers that provide abduction between the legs tend to reduce muscle tone in children with spasticity, making it more efficient for the child to propel the walker. Another desirable feature in support walkers is adjustable pitch. This feature allows the child to lean forward, placing the feet behind the pelvis and trunk, thereby making it easier for the child to initiate forward movement. Other useful features include adjustability for growth and brakes on the wheels for stability during transfers. Walkers with optional trays may be appropriate for children who need upper body support, such as those with muscle weakness or low muscle tone, but trays often interfere with the child's ability to get close to objects for reaching (Figure 21-8).

Support walkers can provide some children the opportunity to explore their environment in an upright, hands-free position while providing weight bearing and stretching in the hips and knees (Figure 21-9). However, support walkers have limitations in maneuverability and are difficult for some children to turn in a limited space or move backwards.

## Alternative Powered Mobility Devices

Adapted motorized toy vehicles, such as the Big Foot (Figure 21-10), are available for young children to provide early mobility experiences using either a joystick or up to four switches. The greatest advantage for using these toy vehicles from the care provider's perspective is that they look like a toy any other child would use rather than an assis-

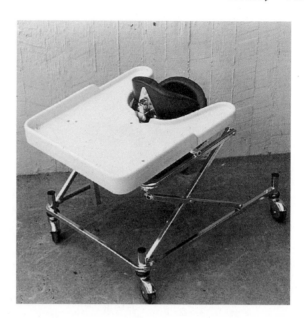

**Figure 21-8** Pommel Walker can be used with a tray to provide support of the upper body. Manufactured by the Special Services Dept., Rehabilitation Centre for Children, Winnipeg, Manitoba, Canada.

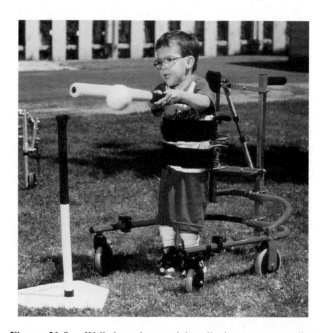

**Figure 21-9** Walkabout is a weight-relieving support walker manufactured by Mulholland Positioning Systems, Inc.

tive device. They are also an option for providing a child with the opportunity to learn how to drive a motorized device in preparation for using a power wheelchair. Disadvantages include difficulty using these vehicles indoors because of limited maneuverability, their large size, and noisy operation.

A new concept in mobility, the Transitional Powered Mobility Aid (TPMA), has been recently developed at the Rehabilitation Engineering Center, Lucile Packard Children's

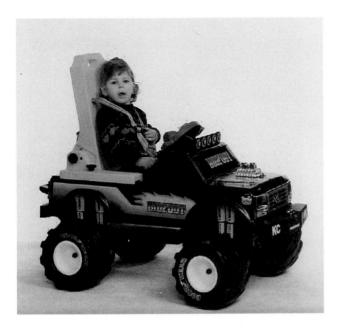

**Figure 21-10** Big Foot powered mobility vehicle can be maneuvered using a joystick or switches. Manufactured by Innovative Products Inc.

Hospital at Stanford (Figure 21-11). The TPMA is designed to enable young, physically challenged children from 12 months to about 6 years of age to move and explore their surroundings in an upright position. The TPMA positions the child in a standing, semi-standing, or sitting position. A joystick or multiple switches can be positioned at any location where the child can reach the controls for driving the device. It is designed for use on level surfaces either indoors or outdoors. It is not a power wheelchair; rather it is a transitional device meant to provide developmental opportunities equivalent to those experienced by able-bodied peers. Problem-solving opportunities; learning how to move through space; hands-free exploration; pushing, pulling, or kicking objects; and the sensation of running are examples of potential experiences. The TMPA is intended for children who would otherwise spend their early developmental years passively sitting in a stroller or manual wheelchair.

## WHEELCHAIRS

Wheelchairs are either manual or powered. Manual wheelchairs depend on the user or an assistant for propulsion, whereas powered devices depend on a motorized unit that the individual accesses using a joystick or alternative controls such as switches.

Wheelchairs are available in standard or custom sizes as measured by the seat width and depth, height of the seat from the floor, and the backrest height. Features and options on wheelchairs must be carefully considered and selected to accommodate the child's growth and physical and functional needs as well as the needs of the care providers.

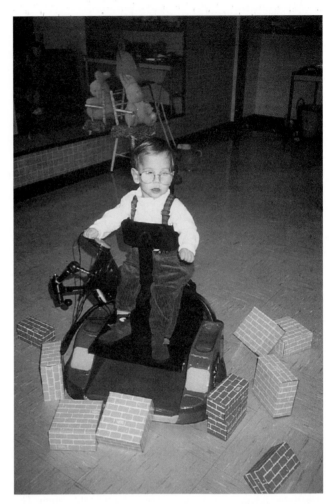

**Figure 21-11** A 20-month-old boy with cerebral palsy who just knocked down blocks during exploratory play while using the Transitional Powered Mobility Aid. He operates it using switches under his right hand. Manufactured by Innovative Products, Inc.

Selection of a wheelchair should begin by assessing and documenting the child's current physical and functional abilities, any changes that might occur in the near future, the positioning and mobility goals, the environments in which the chair will be used, how it will be transported by the care providers, and the sources of funding. The child's mobility needs are then matched to the specific features available in a wheelchair. For example, if a child cannot shift weight independently and is at risk for developing pressure-related problems, then a wheelchair with either a manual or powered tilt-in-space feature may be necessary to shift weight from under the buttocks to the back (Figure 21-12). The manual tilt-in-space feature allows the care provider to press two levers, which tilt the frame of the wheelchair back in space while maintaining the same seat-to-back angle. This differs from a reclining wheelchair, which opens the seat-to-back angle so that the person is lying supine with hip extension. Powered tilt-in-space is an option available on power wheelchairs.

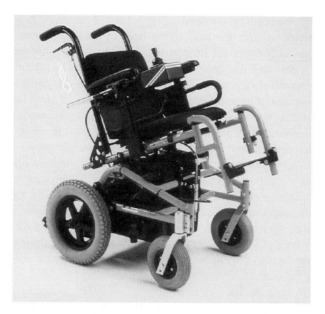

**Figure 21-12**  Zippie P500 power wheelchair features a programmable controller that adjusts to meet each child's ability, a tilt-in-space option, and multiple adjustments to grow with the child. Manufactured by Quickie Designs, Inc.

## Manual Wheelchairs

A manual wheelchair is appropriate for a child who either has the ability to functionally and efficiently propel it or uses it as a means of transport by others. Great strides in manual wheelchair design have resulted in lighter-weight wheelchairs that provide higher performance during propulsion.

Features that need to be considered include style of frame (folding or nonfolding), tilt-in-space, recline, type of footrest (single plate or double plate, fixed or swing away, or multiposition adjustability), angle of footrest (standard, 70 degrees, 90 degrees, or less than 90 degrees), armrest style (tubular, desk arm, height adjustable, or swing away), height of backrest, floor-to-seat height, height of push handles for the adult pushing the wheelchair, style and location of brakes, type and size of tires and casters, and an adjustable axle plate for placement of the wheel. Wheelchairs with large rear tires are most common, but models with large front tires and small back casters are available (Figure 21-13). Propelling a wheelchair with large front tires may be more efficient for the child because more surface area of the tire is exposed when gripping the wheel and pushing. However, the large front tires can limit access to the environment, such as when transferring and sitting at tables. It is also more difficult to push the wheelchair up curbs and over uneven surfaces.

If a child will be independently propelling the wheelchair, it is critical that the equipment allow the child to use proper biomechanics for more efficient propulsion. This is achieved by selecting the proper size of wheelchair frame

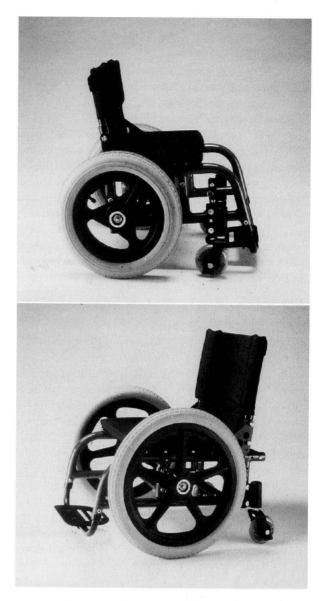

**Figure 21-13**  Quickie Kidz manual wheelchair features wider rear wheels for maximum pushing surface as well as standard or reverse wheel configurations so the chair can be propelled with either a push or pull motion. Manufactured by Quickie Designs, Inc.

and an appropriate seating system. A wheelchair that is too wide is more difficult to push. If the seat is too deep, the child tends to sit with a rounded back and slide out of the seat. The therapist simultaneously considers what type of seating or positioning system is needed and how it will interface with the mobility base for optimal function and performance. For example, a seat cushion may be acquired without considering the frame size of the manual wheelchair. When the cushion is placed on top of the wheelchair frame, it may position the child too far from the wheels for reaching and propelling them efficiently. Had the height of the wheelchair seat been considered when ordering the cushion, alternatives could have been used to prevent this situation (for example, a narrower cushion to recess into the wheelchair frame).

Another common situation that reinforces the need to assess seating and mobility simultaneously is acquiring a backrest cushion for a child after selecting the manual wheelchair. It may position the child too far forward of the axle's wheel. If an individual's center of gravity is forward of the rear wheels, instead of being directly over the rear wheel axle, propulsion is more difficult and inefficient. Many wheelchairs have a standard axle plate where the hub of the wheel is mounted to the frame and the wheels cannot be relocated within the child's reach. However, if an adjustable axle plate on the wheelchair is ordered in combination with the appropriate front caster size, the wheels can be relocated and mounted in the best location for the child to reach the wheels for propulsion.

## Power Wheelchairs

If a child cannot propel a wheelchair long distances at the same speed and efficiency as the average person walks, then a power wheelchair should be considered to increase independence and function. The advantages of a power wheelchair over a manual are increased speed capability, ease of maneuvering, and less energy expenditure required for moving. Some children have both a power wheelchair and a manual wheelchair to use in environments that are not accessible to a power wheelchair or for times when it is being repaired. When possible, assessment of the home environment should be included to ensure that the home can be made accessible for the power wheelchair. The need for two wheelchairs may change because one company recently designed a power wheelchair that converts to a manual wheelchair by replacing the rear wheels and removing the controls and batteries.

Power wheelchairs are available in several styles with various options. The most common approach to selecting a power wheelchair begins by determining which make and model offers the type of electronic controls the child needs to operate the wheelchair. Most wheelchair manufacturers provide a choice of several types of wheelchair models that are intended for joystick operation and models that include sophisticated microcomputer electronics for alternative control methods such as sip-and-puff breath control. Different models offer a variety of features to accommodate the needs of each user. Such features include adjustments for torque, tremor dampening for children experiencing difficulty directing the joystick, short-throw joystick option for users with muscle weakness who do not have the strength to push the joystick to its end range, speed adjustments, and acceleration settings so the wheelchair can be set to increase speed rapidly or gradually.

A joystick is the standard and preferred method for the individual who can efficiently and accurately maneuver it.

Joysticks can be operated using a hand, foot, chin, head pointer, or even the back of the head by using an adaptation that connects the joystick to a bracket which is attached to a moveable headrest. Some children may find it difficult to accurately use a joystick with a hand when the joystick is located in its traditional placement at the front end of the armrest. These children may have better motor control if the joystick is placed inside the armrest, in midline, or rotated toward their body several degrees. A remote joystick may be necessary for these types of situations and is an option with most power wheelchairs. This small joystick is easier to position in midline or under the chin. During the assessment for joystick operation, it is important to consider the positioning needs of the child, placement of the joystick, the type of joystick, the type of joystick knob, and the desired location of the on/off switch for independent access by the user.

A proportional joystick allows the driver to increase acceleration speed of the wheelchair in relationship to the distance the joystick is moved. The further the user pushes the proportional joystick, the more rapidly the wheelchair moves. A nonproportional joystick (digital or microswitch) does not affect the wheelchair's speed; any amount of force used to push the joystick results in the same speed.

Joystick knobs come in a variety of styles, shapes, and sizes to accommodate various hand and arm positions. The most common shapes are round, T-shaped, and I-shaped joysticks. A child with weakness of the upper extremities may find it more efficient to use a U-shaped joystick so that the hand is supported in the palm and at the sides. Selection of the most appropriate style of joystick and its placement directly affect the ability to accurately and efficiently drive a power wheelchair.

Children with severe physical disabilities may be able to operate a power wheelchair but often are not given the opportunity because they are physically unable to operate a joystick. Alternative controls are available for individuals. These controls include sip-and-puff, which is most frequently used by individuals with spinal cord injuries and is activated by gently inhaling or exhaling into a strawlike device held in the mouth. Another alternative is the head switch sensing array, which consists of switches embedded into a headrest that move the wheelchair by detecting head movements. A tongue touch keypad has been recently developed. This keypad is a custom-made retainer in which small switches have been imbedded. The user activates each switch by touching it with the tongue. Multiple switch access is available in which push switches are placed around the body part able to reach the switches. The wheelchair is driven in one of four directions, depending on which switch is activated. It is even possible to drive a power wheelchair with as few as two switches; one switch operates a scanning display, and the other activates the power.

Matthew is 14 years old and has severe spastic cerebral palsy (Figure 21-14). He uses a custom seating system comprising an antithrust seat cushion and lateral hip and trunk pads. This position has increased his ability to activate a push switch placed on the right side of his head. He operates his power wheelchair by using special electronic controls in his wheelchair that are connected to the switch and a small scanning light box mounted in front of him. When he presses the switch, the light begins to scan in one of four directions. Another press of the switch stops the light on the arrow indicating the direction of the desired movement. A third press of the switch stops the wheelchair.

Switches can be placed around any part of the body, such as the hand, head, elbows, or feet, where the child has the most reliable, accurate, and efficient movements. The quality of motor control and accuracy, however, is directly dependent on the child's position and the extent to which the position influences stability, mobility, muscle tone, and energy expenditure. Therefore the assessment of power wheelchair mobility control must include assessment of body position as it influences head and extremity motor control. Positioning is discussed later in this chapter.

There are several other features available on power wheelchairs that are intended to increase a child's function and level of independence. Technology-dependent children who require continuous oxygen support can become mobile by using portable ventilator carts attached to their

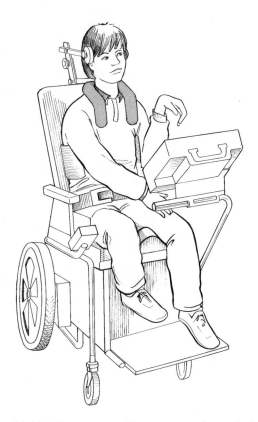

**Figure 21-14** Young man with severe spastic cerebral palsy drives a power wheelchair using a switch mounted at each side of his head to operate the scanning display.

wheelchair. Another recently developed feature enables the child to independently move from a sitting to a standing position and drive around while standing. Other available features include an option for a powered elevating seat that raises the individual to various heights for reaching or moving close to objects such as tables. Additional features include power tilt-in-space, which tilts the seat backwards while maintaining the same seat-to-back angle, and power recline, which places the child in the supine position by reclining the back of the chair. These two features are useful for individuals who need independent and frequent relief of pressure on their buttocks, such as those with spinal cord injury and muscle weakness.

A manual wheelchair can be converted to a power wheelchair by purchasing an add-on unit that includes two motors that are placed on the tires to rotate them, batteries, an electronic control unit, and a joystick. The electronic controls for the add-on units are not as sophisticated or adjustable as those found on standard power wheelchairs. This makes it more difficult for some children with impaired motor responses to accurately operate an add-on unit. They are also not highly recommended for individuals who use their wheelchairs outdoors and over rough terrain because they are not designed to withstand the forces a power wheelchair must endure.

Three wheeled scooters are another option for powered mobility. The individual who uses a scooter typically has good sitting balance, requires minimal positioning adaptation, and can understand and physically operate the tiller handle bar controls.

## POWER MOBILITY ASSESSMENT AND INTERVENTION

The therapist, child, and care provider define the goals for using the powered mobility device. Are the goals to provide transitional mobility so that the child may have new opportunities to learn how to move, explore, and interact within the environment? Is functional mobility appropriate, and what are the desired outcomes? Will the child's mobility needs be met by one device or several, and in which environments will they be used?

The most common method for evaluating a person's ability to use a power mobility device is to actually have the device available for the individual to use during the assessment. A facility typically cannot afford to purchase power wheelchairs for evaluation purposes. However, many rehabilitation technology suppliers will loan a power wheelchair to a clinical therapy unit for short-term assessment purposes. Both the positioning and mobility equipment with the specific features the child will need to use the device should be available during the evaluation. Equipment used during an evaluation should be in optimal working condition. The therapist should begin the evaluation by test driving the equipment to learn the forces and movements required to drive it, select the best speed for the client, and set any other adjustments such as sensitivity of the controls.

A control assessment can begin once the individual is seated in a positioning system or simulator that optimizes motor function. Because a joystick is the preferred means of access for powered mobility, evaluations typically begin with assessing the child's ability to manipulate this control. Several strategies are available to improve the ability of an individual to use a joystick. If the child has difficulty moving the joystick in the desired direction, a template with a cross shape cut out can be placed inside the control box to limit deviation of the joystick to the desired directions. The joystick can also be positioned with proper hardware to another location where control might be enhanced.

Erin, a 4-year-old child who is unable to communicate, was experiencing difficulty driving the power wheelchair using a joystick placed at the end of her right armrest. The teacher questioned Erin's ability to drive safely and accurately, believing that bumping into objects was purposeful. The occupational therapist observed Erin's arm and hand movements and noted that she seemed to have difficulty pushing the joystick forward and to the right side. She tended to internally rotate her arm and pull it toward her body. The joystick was mounted on an adjustable bracket that positioned it in midline, close to her chest. It also enabled the joystick box to be rotated about 30 degrees toward her body. After several more attempts at driving, her accuracy immediately improved. Once the most reliable placement was located, she became a functional driver.

If an individual does not have the physical ability to control a joystick with either the hand, foot, or head, alternative means such as switch operation may be considered. Several types of switches are available, but a simple push switch with auditory feedback to assist the child in understanding when the switch has been activated is sufficient to use during the initial evaluation. It may be helpful to evaluate switch placement by allowing the child to first use switches to operate modified battery-operated toys (Wright & Nomura, 1991). First the therapist identifies the most consistent and efficient movements the child can voluntarily use to operate switches. The child needs to maintain contact on the switch long enough to move the wheelchair in a desired direction. To control the chair, ability to access and use switches in three locations is needed (i.e., for propelling forward and turning). If the child can successfully operate only two switches, use of a scanning device may be considered, but it is more complicated for the child to understand and time consuming to use for driving a power wheelchair.

Switch placement should begin at the hands and proceed to the head, elbows, feet, and any other location determined appropriate. An adjustable mounting bracket, such as that available through AbleNet Incorporated, is extremely helpful for positioning a switch in multiple locations. Once an accurate and reliable motor response has been determined, the switch can be assessed on a powered mobility device.

Several factors can interfere with a person's ability to drive a powered mobility device. If a child has difficulty, the therapist first evaluates whether the type or placement of the controls is appropriate. Second, the therapist evaluates the child's position to determine if changes in the child's posture may influence motor control. Other considerations include undetected visual and perceptual difficulties, impairment in response time, seizures, motivation, and behavior.

Many children may not initially be successful using a power wheelchair because of the overwhelming amount and degree of sensory input. Imagine being a young child with a severe disability who has difficulty with motor planning, coordination, visual perception, and communication and who is experiencing movement in a powered device for the first time. It would, no doubt, be overwhelming to experience the excitement and vestibular sensation of moving while trying to view the surroundings, which are quickly passing by, and simultaneously listen to an adult telling you how and when to move.

It is recommended, whenever feasible, to assess a young child for powered mobility by providing a method that promotes exploration and self-learning for the child. Such a method requires an open space with activities and toys strategically placed around the room to facilitate experiences in movement and exploration. The therapist should "limit physical and verbal commands as much as possible to avoid sensory overload on the part of the child" (Taylor & Monahan, 1989, p. 85). For example, if a child is trying to move toward an object, the trainer should simply state the desired outcome, such as "come closer," rather than specific commands such as "push the joystick left or push the red switch and come over here." Feedback should also be positive, such as "you found the wall," rather than "oops, you crashed again." If further assistance is needed to help the child understand the operation of the control, the trainer can facilitate the proper response by physically guiding the child's movements for the desired response.

It may also be beneficial to loan or rent a power wheelchair to children and their families for an extended evaluation. This allows more time for the child to learn how to use the controls and for the family to become familiar with the features of a power wheelchair to assist them in becoming more informed consumers. It also provides an opportunity for the family to experience the responsibilities of maintaining and transporting a power wheelchair.

Computer programs are also available for powered mobility assessment and training (Taplin, 1989). The program displays a power wheelchair on the screen that the user must navigate through a maze or room. This may be useful for training purposes, but the effectiveness of this teaching method compared with practice in driving a power wheelchair has not been researched.

In most recent years the use of virtual reality for assessing and training powered mobility skills has been explored

(Trimble, Morris, & Crandall, 1992). The user wears a helmet that has a screen display of a three-dimensional room through which the person must navigate by using a joystick. More research is needed to determine if this is an effective means for assessing and training powered mobility skills.

## POSITIONING CONSIDERATIONS

Positioning is critical to the successful use of any mobility device. How an individual is positioned in a mobility device, whether it be in standing or sitting, can have an effect on several physiologic factors: motor performance, postural control (Myhr & Wendt, 1991), ranges of movement, muscle tone (Nwaobi, 1986), endurance, comfort, respiration, and digestion. These factors can then affect functional performance activities such as hand function (Nwaobi, 1987), levels of independence in mobility, self-care, activities of daily living such as transfers, and social interaction with others (Hulme, Poor, Schulein, & Pezzino, 1983).

### Understanding the Biomechanics of Seating

To identify the positioning needs of a child, the occupational therapist must first have a thorough understanding of the biomechanical forces and physiologic factors that can influence posture and movement. Biomechanical considerations are critical to obtaining proper alignment of the pelvis, spine, and head. The position and stability of the pelvis is critical to movements that occur above and below the pelvis. The box at right presents exercises to help the reader understand the importance of good alignment in sitting.

### Seating Guidelines

The goal of seating is to place the pelvis and spine in a position that inhibits abnormal muscle tone, reduces undesirable biomechanical forces, and accommodates stiff postures that are no longer flexible. While accommodating these postural problems, the positions should provide maximum weight distribution for stability, comfort, and skin integrity. Stability at the pelvis can be achieved by providing support at three contact points. First, the type of support underneath the pelvis is assessed. Can the child sit on a flat surface or would more stability be obtained by using a contoured, antithrust seat (a recessed seat that provides a pocket for the pelvis and blocks forward movement of the ischial tuberosities)? Some individuals require supports at the sides of the pelvis to maintain a more symmetric position and to reduce pelvic shift to one side. Support at the sides of the pelvis can be contoured into the seat or added as lateral hip guides. Stability can be provided above the pelvis to reduce sliding in an upward and forward direction. This is typically accomplished by placing a positioning belt at a 45-degree angle to the seat or placing it closer to the thighs.

### Exercises to Understand the Biomechanics of Seating

1. *Sitting in Posterior Pelvic Tilt.* While in a sitting position, place your hands on the anterior crest of your pelvis (the two hip bones). Bend forward by rounding your back. You will feel your pelvis rolling backwards into a posteriorly tilted position. Hold your pelvis in this position and try to sit upright by extending your back. You might be able to move your head upright, but moving the trunk into a vertical position is dependent on placing your pelvis in a neutral or anteriorly tilted position. To view your environment with your pelvis in the posteriorly tilted position, you would either need to hyperextend your neck (an undesirable position), or slide your pelvis forward in the seat until your head achieved an upright position. Try maintaining a rounded or kyphotic back position and slide your pelvis forward in the seat. Feel the excessive pressure at the cervical and upper thoracic levels as well as the coccyx. Imagine being positioned like this for hours at a time and experiencing the discomfort, fatigue, and limited range of your upper extremities if you were in a wheelchair without a proper positioning system to improve or accommodate your posture.

2. *Asymmetric Pelvic Position.* Place your buttocks at the edge of your seat, lean only onto one side of your pelvis, and lift your feet so they are unsupported. Hold your pencil at its top edge and try to write. It is difficult to have accurate and efficient movements of your arm and hands because you do not have a stable base for the movements to occur. Imagine trying to accurately and safely operate the joystick of a power wheelchair in this position.

Stability can also be improved by assuring that the femur is properly supported along its entire length, from the back of the pelvis to approximately 1 inch from the popliteal area under the knee. The pelvis should be supported posteriorly from the back cushion, which assists in maintaining a neutral or anteriorly tilted position. Other components, such as foot plates, lap trays, arm troughs, and neck supports, provide additional support.

There are several areas to consider when evaluating what type of seating system an individual needs in a wheelchair.

These are: (1) the angle between the seat and the back surfaces, (2) the tilt of the system in space (orientation), and (3) the type of surface the person will be seated on (Bergen, Presperin, & Tallman, 1990, p. 17).

Seating surfaces fall into three categories: planar, contoured, and custom molded. Planar seating consists of flat surfaces, with no contours. This type of seating may be more appropriate for individuals with mildly affected development who require only minimal body contact with the support surfaces of the seat. Contoured seating systems allow the body to have more contact with the support surface because its shape conforms to the curves of the spine, buttocks, and thighs. A contoured seat can be accomplished by layering various densities of foam, which respond to the height and weight of the person, thereby contouring around the bony prominences and other body curves. A contoured cushion can be either purchased from a manufacturer in standard sizes or custom made to fit the child. It is often more advantageous to select a contoured cushion that can be opened and adjusted by adding or removing padding to fit a child's individual needs. Custom-molded seat cushions are designed specifically for an individual by taking an impression of the body and making a mold, which is sent to the manufacturer for fabrication of the cushions. Another method uses a computer-generated graphic picture taken from the impression, which is sent to the manufacturer, who then uses a computer-assisted milling machine to fabricate the cushions. Cushions can also be custom molded using foam-in-bag technology in which liquid foam is poured into an upholstered bag that is positioned around the person's body, providing a molded and finished cushion. This technique is more difficult to use because the individual's position must be held in place while the foam is being formed. If the child moves, the quality of the foam is negatively affected.

The use of orthotics or bracing of the extremities or body may also assist in achieving optimal positioning in the seated and standing positions. Ankle foot orthoses are most commonly recommended to align the foot and ankle and assist in either reducing muscle tone or supporting a weak limb. A Thoracic Lumbar Sacral Orthosis (TLSO), or body jacket, may be another alternative for individuals with scoliosis to use for support in the seated position.

## METHODS FOR ASSESSING SEATING AND POSITIONING

The initial assessment should begin by observing the child using the mobility system to note posture, movements, comfort, and other factors that may affect function. The child should then be positioned on a low mat table so the therapist can complete a postural assessment to determine if any limitations in ranges of movement exist that might interfere with the upright seated position. Further information is obtained by positioning the child in sitting while the therapist uses his or her hands to support the child to identify key points of control and positions that provide a desirable change in posture, muscle tone, and control. These key points become the necessary components of the seating system. The positions, such as the angle of hip flexion and the orientation in space of the child, become the pitches and angles of the components necessary in the seating system.

Once information is gathered from the postural assessment, other methods are also available that use evaluation equipment for assessing a child's position to determine what components, angles, and sizes are needed in a seating system. Simulators are self-contained, adjustable fitting chairs that can be adjusted to fit a child or adult. The simulator allows the therapist to "evaluate the client in the system, alter angles of the seat to the back, try varying positions in space, and determine component sizes and accessories that are required before making recommendations for a particular system" (Trefler et al., 1993, p. 73).

Simulators can be used to assess planar, contoured, and molded seating. The evaluator first completes a postural assessment of the individual to determine which seating components are necessary and then adjusts the simulator to the individual's size. Angles, which include seat to back and tilt, are selected. Further adjustments can be made to determine how position influences movement and function. The advantages of using a seating simulator include (1) it stands as a single evaluation tool for a variety of ages, sizes, and diagnoses, (2) it provides information about the various types of seating systems such as planar versus molded, and (3) options are available to motorize simulators to evaluate powered mobility access and the effect of positioning on motor control. The problem often encountered by the assessment team when using simulators is difficulty in transferring the information from the simulator into an actual seating system and knowing how that system will integrate into a mobility base. Another disadvantage occurs when the seating system will be used in a manual wheelchair; the biomechanics of propelling the wheels while positioned in the simulator cannot be assessed. Young children may experience a negative response to the simulator because they may be intimidated by its mechanical appearance and large size.

Another method for assessing seating and positioning is to use a modular "mock up" or adjustable evaluation seat system that can be placed in a mobility base. These are typically available in planar or contoured seating devices rather than in custom-molded devices. The advantages of using this method include the ability for the child to use the mobility device while seated in the mock-up seat. This is particularly important because positioning can influence body movements and therefore functional outcomes. The disadvantage is that more equipment must be available to fit a range of individuals, and pitches and angles cannot always be accurately assessed.

Children with hypotonia, such as those with muscle diseases or cerebral palsy, have specific needs. A useful positioning system includes a back design that supports the sacrum in a neutral position but angles about 15 degrees away from the back at the posterior superior iliac spine. This provides a resting position of the trunk and accommodates the forces of gravity in the upright position. Consideration of a tilt-in-space feature in the mobility base may also provide

CASE STUDIES

The case studies include comprehensive information about the children's equipment and adapted environments. These descriptions demonstrate how mobility equipment is integrated with other assistive technology and environmental adaptations to best meet the children's functional needs.

### David and Eric

David is 11 years old. At the age of 4 he was diagnosed with Duchenne's muscular dystrophy. Shortly afterward, his little brother, Eric (at 5 months), was also diagnosed with the same condition. The two brothers and an older sister live with their parents in a small town.

Duchenne's muscular dystrophy is an inherited x-linked disease that affects the voluntary skeletal musculature with progressive weakness and degeneration of the muscles that control movement. The muscle weakness begins in the proximal and axial musculature and slowly progresses distally. Frequently a wheelchair is needed by age 12. Breathing becomes affected during the later stages of the disease, leading to severe respiratory problems. Respiratory infections commonly claim the patients' lives during their early twenties.

When receiving David's diagnosis, the family was introduced to a team of professionals that specialize in different aspects of musculoskeletal weaknesses. Here they received support to help them deal with the initial shock, as well as necessary information about the disease. Twice a year the family continues to meet with the team for medical and orthopedic evaluations. Social and psychologic concerns are also addressed.

Last year David had an achilles tendon lengthening to release a tight heel cord. Today he walks with a long leg orthosis. It is considered extremely important to lengthen the walking phase in boys with Duchenne's muscular dystrophy to delay hip and knee flexion deformities and equinovarus deformity of the foot and ankle. For two years David used a standard lightweight manual wheelchair for long distance or when he was fatigued. Currently, a power wheelchair is being considered for David to allow him to conserve energy for social and educational activities. Spinal stabilization is planned when David's scoliosis exceeds 25 degrees and normal forced vital capacity (FVC) pulmonary function drops below 50%.

Eric is now 7 years old. The progression of his disease is following the same course as David's, although somewhat slower. The early signs of Duchenne's muscular dystrophy are becoming prominent, such as the waddling gait, tendency to fall, and difficulty rising from a sitting or lying position.

At the time of Eric's diagnosis, the family lived in an apartment but soon decided to build a house. The occupational therapist provided recommendations for designing the house for wheelchair accessibility to maximize function and independence.

The family has been living in the house for two years and are pleased with the features that enable the boys to be independent. The outdoor surfaces (sidewalks and ramps) are firm, stable, and slip resistant. The floor plan is spacious, doorways are wide, and there are no thresholds. A few sliding doors have been installed to allow maximum door width and to eliminate floor swing space requirements. Controls, levers, and switches are placed low to be within reach from a wheelchair. The window's lower edge is only 20 inches above the floor for the same reason. The bathrooms are spacious, and there is a bathtub and a shower. The boys love taking baths because they stay warmer and move more freely in the water. The sink is free-standing so the boys can get close to the sink. An automatic faucet has been installed, which is turned on when the hands are placed under the faucet. A full-length mirror is placed on the wall.

The family continues to need a lot of support and assistance to adjust to new challenges. In addition to direct service to the family, the occupational therapist continues to work closely with the schools to assure that accessibility is available at school.

### Jason

Jason is a 7-year-old boy with cerebral palsy, which has affected his ability to speak, move his body with control, and eat. Although he demonstrates severe delays in his motor skills, he appears alert and attentive and understands what was said to him. From his early days, his family was motivated to assure that Jason have a childhood as normal as possible. They were creative in designing simple devices and tools to accomplish these goals. His grandfather designed the first mobility device for him. It was a push cart used to hold golf clubs, but he mounted a car seat to the frame and placed foam pieces in the seat to help align Jason's body and prevent him from leaning over. His mother would use it to push him around the neighborhood during her daily jogging routine. He also used a standard stroller but required a positioning system to assist him in sitting upright by providing sup-

# CASE STUDIES–CONT'D

port at the pelvis, trunk, and head. The first seating system was made of triwall, a three-layer thickness cardboard that can be used to fabricate temporary seat inserts for young children. Another seat insert was fabricated from triwall, but this one could be placed on the dining room chair so he could eat at the family table instead of a high chair.

By the time he was 12 months, his family built him an aeroplane mobility device (see Figure 21-5) to use at home. When he outgrew this by the age of 2 years, he was evaluated for a support walker and could effectively use the Walkabout by Mobility Plus. He continued to use this not only for indoor mobility, but also for playing in little league for special needs children when he was 5 years old. He and his teammates used an automatic device to hit the ball, and Jason ran around the diamond field using his walker.

At 2½ years the family decided his mobility needs were not being adequately met by the walker alone. He was evaluated for a power wheelchair and could operate the joystick once he was positioned with maximal support at his feet, pelvis, trunk, and head. His therapist and family determined what features he needed to use a power wheelchair. They determined that a molded seating system was needed for support and alignment. To increase independence, the system needed to include the ability to elevate the seat from the floor to various heights. A power wheelchair with these features was provided, along with a custom-molded seating system.

The family made the home environment accessible to Jason in many ways. When he was 2 years old they decided it was important for him to roll out of bed in

the morning and try to roll on the floor. They placed a low-height mattress on the floor in the corner of his bedroom and made it his bed. They lined the sides of it with his stuffed toys to protect him from unintentionally hitting his arms against the walls. This arrangement allowed him to get out of bed on his own. The light switch in his room was also extended so he could reach it from his walker or wheelchair.

Positioning in the bathtub when he was a toddler was a challenge, but his mother made a bath seat for him from a milk crate. Foam was placed around the edges and the seat for comfort. When he outgrew this, his family acquired a bath seat designed for children with disabilities. An adapted toilet seat with a high backrest was recommended by his occupational therapist. It provided the ability to begin toilet training at the age of 2. His family also installed a flip-down bar in front of the toilet so Jason could stand at the toilet "like his Dad."

During these early years, Jason was also introduced to augmentative communication symbols and aids. By the time he was 12 months old he could point to symbols in his communication book and soon progressed to using an augmentative communication device with voice output by accessing it with a light pointer on his head. The communication device was mounted on his power wheelchair. Today Jason is fully included in a second grade class. He uses assistive technology to do his schoolwork and has an attendant with him throughout the day. Both simple and sophisticated assistive technology devices have enabled him to function within a regular education classroom, participating in most of the activities of his typical peers.

the hypotonic or weak child with greater tolerance for sitting upright.

Children with increased muscle tone and spasticity who tend to adduct their legs and extend their hips and spine are often more difficult to position. It is particularly important to identify key points of control for positioning these children. For example, the occupational therapist determines the desired degree of hip and knee flexion, hip abduction, and reduction of asymmetric positioning that positively influences muscle tone and control of extremity movement. These children may also have better postural control in the upright position rather than reclined or tilted (Nwaobi, 1986).

A child's position, particularly in a seated mobility device, must be frequently reevaluated to accommodate pos-

tural, developmental, and growth changes. Once a child receives a seating mobility system, the fit and function should be reassessed within 6 months. Positioning and mobility literature and support materials are available, and it is suggested to the reader that more specific information and techniques on positioning be acquired through additional reading and workshops.

## FACTORS THAT INFLUENCE SUCCESSFUL USE OF MOBILITY DEVICES

As previously mentioned, several factors influence successful use of powered mobility devices. In recent years, studies have shown a significant relationship between certain standardized tests of cognition and perception and use of powered mobility. Some studies have indicated that certain functional performance tasks may correlate to power wheelchair driving. Preliminary findings indicate a relationship between specific cognitive scales and readiness for powered mobility (Tefft, Furumasu, & Guerette, 1993; Verburg, Field, & Jarvis, 1987).

Another factor that can influence a child's ability to use a powered device is the ability of the professional or care provider to determine the most accurate and efficient means for the child to operate the device. If a child is having significant difficulty successfully maneuvering a powered mobility device, the control method must first be assessed to determine if it is the most effective means. Then the child's positioning needs must be considered. The longer it takes a child to successfully demonstrate use of a control, the more likely it is that either the access method or position is inappropriate. The following example best describes this type of situation.

Stephanie is a 15-month-old girl with cerebral palsy who successfully used a switch-operated toy vehicle to maneuver and explore her surroundings. It took her about 5 hours to become proficient at using a system of four hand-activated press switches and to understand the relationship to directionality. However, when she entered another therapy program, the information on her ability to use switches for driving was not considered. Instead, she was placed in a wheelchair training program using the only equipment available, a joystick-operated power wheelchair. After 6 months of training for 3 hours each week, she demonstrated no improvement in her ability to drive the power wheelchair. Had she been provided with the appropriate control method, four switches placed at her hand instead of a joystick, which she could not operate because of her impaired motor function, she might have demonstrated the ability to use the power wheelchair in significantly less time.

Changes the child may be experiencing in the future, both unexpected and expected, must be considered when recommending equipment. Can the system be readily changed as the child gains new skills, grows, or experiences other physical changes? This is particularly important to consider when ordering a power wheelchair. For example, a child with a progressive disability may be able to operate a joystick at the time the chair is ordered. However, as the child's strength diminishes, can the power wheelchair be economically reconfigured to operate using another method such as head switch control? Several options may need to be included in the wheelchair, such as the ability to readily change the control method. It is more economical in most cases to initially order options on equipment rather than reorder the equipment at a later date.

Another issue to consider when recommending mobility and positioning equipment is where and how augmentative communication equipment is mounted to the child's wheelchair. Selection of the appropriate mounting bracket depends on the tube size of the wheelchair frame and locations on the wheelchair where it can be attached. A prob-

## STUDY QUESTIONS

1. What questions should be answered before selecting a mobility device?
2. A young child with cerebral palsy (spastic diplegia) uses a push walker but needs a manual wheelchair for mobility in the community and at school. He is expected to learn how to transfer in and out of it in the future. What features will be needed on his manual wheelchair for optimal independence?
3. What type of wheelchair control would an individual with a spinal cord injury at the C3 level be most likely to use?
4. If a child has less than 90 degrees passive range of movement in knee extension because of tight hamstring muscles, explain how this would affect his ability to sit upright in a wheelchair using standard footrest hangers (60-degree angle).
5. Why is it important to simultaneously consider a child's positioning needs when assessing a mobility device?

lem often encountered with manual wheelchairs is positioning the child or rear wheels too far forward of the center of gravity in the wheelchair, which often causes the wheelchair to tip forward when the communication device is mounted. The most frequent problem encountered with power wheelchairs is the communication device's interference with the field of vision required for driving.

It is the responsibility of the therapy team and RTS to assist the family and child in selecting the most appropriate device by presenting several alternatives. It is the family's role to make a final decision on the specific type of mobility device, after considering the options presented by the therapy team. The most important and significant contribution the occupational therapist can make is to reassess the equipment's fit and function once the child has received it. At times it becomes evident that the device does not and probably will not meet the needs of the child. It is the therapist's responsibility not only to assist the family in making a final decision on choosing equipment by providing a thorough evaluation and information, but also to intervene if the equipment is not meeting the needs of the child by returning equipment to the supplier or obtaining resources to improve the child's ability to use the equipment.

## SUMMARY

The literature indicates that independent mobility plays a facilitative role in cognitive and social development. Hence, when mobility is severely delayed or restricted, emotional and psychosocial development are affected. Augmentative mobility devices can provide either functional or transitional mobility. These devices can provide children with physical disabilities greater opportunities to develop and the ability to become initiators and active participants in daily activites and experiences.

Successful use of a mobility device depends on several factors: the therapist's ability to identify a positioning system for the child that enhances motor performance, comfort, and function; a mobility assessment process that efficiently and positively provides desired results; and the ability to identify the features of the mobility device the child needs for optimal function. It is the occupational therapist's responsibility to ensure that all children with physical disabilities are provided with opportunities for mobility at the earliest age possible to promote development more equal to that of their able-bodied peers.

## REFERENCES

American Occupational Therapy Association (1994). Uniform terminology—third revision. *American Journal of Occupational Therapy, 48,* 1047-1054.

Becker, R.D. (1975). Recent developments in child psychiatry. The restrictive emotional and cognitive environment reconsidered: a re-definition of the concept of the therapeutic restraint. *Israels Annals of Psychiatry and Related Disciplines 13,* 239-258.

Bergen, A., Presperin, J., & Tallman, T. (1990). *Positioning for function: wheelchairs and other assistive technologies.* New York: Valhalla Rehabilitation Publications.

Bertenthal, B.I., Campos, J.J., & Barrett, K.C. (1984). Self-produced locomotion: an organizer of emotional, cognitive, and social development in infancy. In R.N. Emde & R.J. Harmon (Eds.). *Continuities and discontinuities in development.* New York, Plenum Press.

Bly, L. (1994). *Motor skills acquisition in the first year.* Tucson: Therapy Skill Builders.

Brinker, R.P. & Lewis, M. (1982). Making the world work with microcomputers: a learning prosthesis for handicapped infants. *Exceptional Children, 49,* 163-170.

Butler, C. (1986). Effects of powered mobility on self-initiated behaviors of very young children with locomotor disability. *Developmental Medicine and Child Neurology, 28,* 325-332.

Butler, C. (1988). High tech tots: technology for mobility, manipulation, communication, and learning in early childhood. *Infants and Young Children. 2,* 66-73.

Butler, C. (1988). *Powered tots: augmentative mobility for locomotor disabled youngsters.* American Physical Therapy Association Pediatric Publication. *14,* 472-474.

Campos, J.J. & Bertenthal, B. I. (1987). Locomotion and psychological development in infancy. In K.M. Jaffe (Ed.). Childhood powered mobility: developmental, technical, and clinical perspectives. *Proceedings of the RESNA First Northwest Regional Conference* (pp. 11-42). Washington, DC: RESNA Press.

Dietz, J. & Swinth, Y. (1994). Effects of power mobility on preschoolers with disabilities. Annual Conference of the American Occupational Therapy Association and the Canadian Association of Occupational Therapists, Boston.

Douglas, J. & Ryan, M. (1987). A preschool severely disabled boy and his powered wheelchair: a case study. *Child Care, Health and Development, 13,* 303-309.

Haley, S.M., Coster, W.J., Ludlow, L.H., Haltiwanger, J., & Andrellos, P. (1992). *Administration manual for the Pediatric Evaluation of Disability Inventory.* (PEDI) Boston: New England Medical Center.

Hays, R. (1987). Childhood motor impairments: clinical overview and scope of the problem. In K.M. Jaffe (Ed.). Childhood powered mobility: developmental, technical, and clinical perspectives. *Proceedings of the RESNA First Northwest Regional Conference.* Washington DC: RESNA Press.

Hulme, J., Poor, R., Schulein, M., & Pezzino, J. (1983). Perceived behavioral changes observed with adaptive seating devices for multihandicapped developmentally disabled individuals. *Physical Therapy, 62*(4), 204-208.

Myhr, U. & Wendt, L., (1991). Improvement of functional sitting position for children with cerebral palsy. *Developmental Medicine and Child Neurology, 33,* 246-256.

Nwaobi, O. (1986). Effects of body orientation in space on tonic muscle activity of patients with cerebral palsy. *Developmental Medicine and Child Neurology, 28,* 41-44.

Nwaobi, O. (1987). Effect of unilateral arm restraint on upper extremity function in cerebral palsy. *Proceedings of the Annual RESNA Conference,* San Jose, CA, 311-313.

Paulsson, K. & Christoffersen, M. (1984). Psychological aspects of technical aids: how does independent mobility affect the psychological and intellectual development of children with physical disabilities. *Proceedings of the Second Annual Conference on Rehabilitation Engineering,* 282-286.

Piaget, J. (1954). *The construction of reality in the child.* New York: Basic Books.

Seligman, M. (1975). *Helplessness: on depression, development, and death.* San Francisco, W.H. Freeman.

Taplin, C.S. (1989). Powered wheelchair control, assessment, and training. RESNA '89, *Proceedings of the 12th Annual Conference, 9,* 45-46.

Taylor, S. & Monahan, L. (1989). Considerations in assessing for powered mobility. In C. Brubaker (Ed.). *Wheelchair IV, Report of a Conference on the State of the Art of Powered Wheelchair Mobility,* December 7-9, 1988. Washington DC: RESNA Press.

Tefft, D., Furumasu, J., & Guerette, P., (1992). Cognitive readiness for powered mobility in the very young child (Unpublished manuscript). Downey, CA: Rancho Los Amigos.

Trefler, E., Hobson, D., Taylor, S., Monahan, L, & Shaw, C. (1993). *Seating and mobility.* Tucson: Therapy Skill Builders.

Trimble, J., Morris, T., & Crandall, R. (1992). Virtual reality: designing accessible environments. *Team Rehab Report, 3,* 8-12.

Verburg, G., Field, D., & Jarvis, S. (1987). Motor, perceptual, and cognitive factors that affect mobility control. *Proceedings of the 10th Annual Conference on Rehabilitation Technology,* Washington, DC: RESNA Press.

Wright, C. & Nomura, M. (1991). *From toys to computers, access for the physically disabled child,* San Jose, CA: Author.

**IV**

# Arenas of Pediatric Occupational Therapy Services

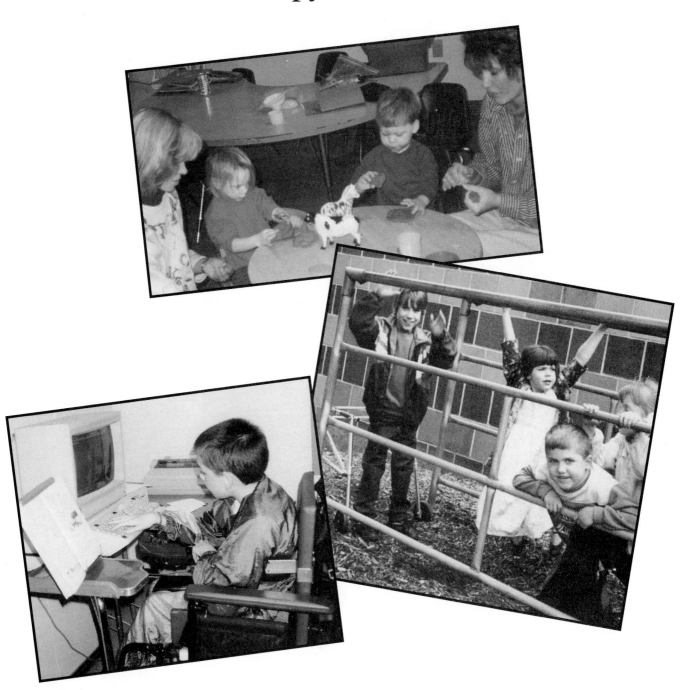

CHAPTER

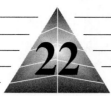

22

# The Neonatal Intensive Care Unit

JAN G. HUNTER

## EVOLUTION OF NEONATAL INTENSIVE CARE

The neonatal intensive care unit (NICU) is a complex and highly specialized hospital unit designed to care for infants who are born prematurely or critically ill (Figure 22-1). Being a newly born preterm infant in a modern NICU has been compared with being abducted from a warm comfortable home by "aliens" or "terrorists," then subjected to an overwhelming barrage of continuous bright lights and jarring noises while having fruitless attempts at sleep repeatedly interrupted with frequent invasive and painful procedures by "huge creatures" (White & Newbold, 1995). A respected neonatologist and a hospital president and chief executive officer explained that there is enough truth in this tongue-in-cheek description of current neonatal units to be sobering. State-of-the-art NICUs today bear little resemblance to the "Special Department for Weaklings," the first special care unit for preterm neonates established by Dr. Pierre Budin in 1893, when medical care for this population emphasized provision of warmth, small feedings, and protection from infection (Hodgman, 1985).

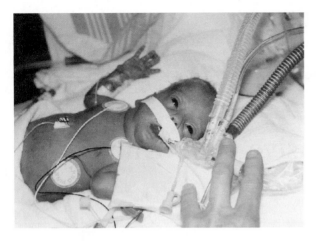

**Figure 22-1**    Preterm infant receiving mechanical ventilation in neonatal intensive care unit. Three cardiorespiratory leads and temperature probe are visible; a percutaneous catheter for intravenous infusions is in right arm. (Courtesy of the Infant Special Care Unit, University of Texas Medical Branch, Galveston, TX. Photograph by Candy Cochran.)

## Nursery Classifications and Regionalization of Care

Advances in medical technology and specialized nursing care for preterm and high-risk infants have skyrocketed since the early 1960s. Neonatal respirators, intravenous (IV) feedings, special laboratory tests, noninvasive monitors, and "rescue" technology such as high-frequency ventilation (HFV) or extracorporeal membrane oxygenation (ECMO) are examples of this progress. The spiraling expense and complexity of care created a growing discrepancy between neonatal mortality rates of major medical centers and smaller hospitals.

In the early 1970s, the concept of regionalization of perinatal care emerged to provide advanced levels of health care to all patients regardless of geographic factors (AMA, 1971). Optimal care was planned to make all levels of care available to any mother or infant within that perinatal region while avoiding unnecessary duplication of services. Hospitals within the area were designated by the level of care provided. Patient care was generally provided at the nearest hospital, with transfer to a higher-level facility occurring as needed for more complex problems.

A level I nursery, such as might be found in a small community hospital, manages uncomplicated pregnancies with expected normal deliveries and well babies. Level II nurseries are able to handle both well newborns and neonates requiring some additional medical management, such as phototherapy for jaundice or IV antibiotics. A neonatologist is usually on staff, but these units typically lack the equipment and additional expertise, such as a pediatric surgeon or cardiologist, to care for all medical emergencies and severe neonatal problems. Level III nurseries have available all the equipment and trained personnel, both in the nurs-

ery and in related disciplines, necessary to care for all potential neonatal conditions and emergencies (Korones, 1985).

Traditional concepts of regionalization of care have been compromised by economic forces of an increasingly competitive health care market since the 1980s (Pettett, Buser, & Merenstein, 1993). The growth of managed health care and the availability of neonatal technology and specialists have encouraged many hospitals to expand their perinatal services. Fragmentation of perinatal services with a wide disparity in level of care provided has resulted (Pettett et al., 1993). Achieving a balance between cost control and universal patient access is the current dilemma and necessity facing organizers and providers of perinatal health care.

## NICU Outcome Indicators: Mortality and Morbidity

Innovations in medical science, technology, and caregiving skills that greatly increased the survival rate of younger, smaller, and sicker infants have also prompted concern over the methodology and outcome of neonatal intensive care (Allen & Jones, 1986; Ellison, 1984). A neonatologist and a researcher, both nationally respected, stated the following:

> Technology has enormously increased our life support systems but has not told us how to avoid rescuing badly damaged survivors. Our facility in caring for the heart and lungs has not been matched by our ability to give intensive care and support to the brain. Intensive care nurseries have become temples of technology, with brightly gleaming hardware, bristling energetic adult caretakers, ringing telephones, and flashing and beeping alarms. Sometimes lost in the transaction is the essential fragility of the tiny, immature human beings who are struggling for life and for normal integration and growth in the midst of this harsh and unnatural setting. The time has come to return to a more gentle and nurturing nursery environment without sacrificing our valuable lifesaving tools (Avery & Glass, 1989, p. 204).

Emerging concerns about the effects of the NICU on preterm infants and about the long-term outcome of NICU survivors have resulted in increased attention to developmental considerations (Als et al., 1986; Gottfried & Gaiter, 1985; Gardner, Garland, Merenstein, & Lubchenco, 1993; VandenBerg, 1995). These issues facilitated the entry of occupational therapists (and other health professionals interested in infant development) into the critical care arena of the NICU (Vergara & Angley, 1992). Preterm infant development, effects of acute and chronic illness, animate and inanimate environmental factors, family dynamics of NICU infants, ultimate outcome of NICU survivors, and increasingly NICU cost containment and use of resources continue to be explored (Affleck, Tennen, & Rowe, 1991; Allen & Alexander, 1994; Blackburn, 1995; Davison, Karp, & Kanto, 1994; Mouradian & Als, 1994; VandenBerg, 1994).

# EVOLUTION OF OCCUPATIONAL THERAPY IN THE NICU

## Changing Focus of Neonatal Occupational Therapy

The parameters of occupational therapy in the NICU have greatly expanded. Traditional occupational therapy 10 to 15 years ago was largely based on a *rehabilitation* model. Infants were identified as appropriate for occupational therapy referral by specific risk factors (e.g., very low birth weight or prenatal drug exposure), by documented pathologic conditions (e.g., congenital anomaly or intraventricular hemorrhage), or by performance indicators (e.g., tone abnormalities or poor feeding). Therapy goals targeted specific problems (such as limited range of motion, high or low muscle tone, extreme irritability, or poor feeding), and intervention activities provided graded sensory stimulation to facilitate normal development in older chronically ill infants (Rapport, 1992). A rehabilitation approach continues to be an appropriate option for a select group of medically stable NICU infants with diagnoses such as arthrogryposis multiplex congenita or myelomeningocele.

The work of Heidelise Als, with its profound influence on environmental and caregiving factors in the NICU, facilitated the move of occupational therapy beyond rehabilitation services into individualized developmental care (Gorga, 1994; Mouradian, in press). Dr. Als' synactive theory of development has emerged as the state-of-the-art transdisciplinary approach to recognizing and meeting developmental needs of each infant and family in the NICU (Als, 1982; Blackburn & VandenBerg, 1993; Creger & Browne, 1989). Within this framework, occupational therapists recognize that all neonates requiring intensive care have vulnerabilities from immaturity or illness that must be addressed for optimal developmental outcomes. Individual infant behaviors indicating stress or adaptation serve as guidelines to modify caregiving practices and to reduce the pervasive effects of environmental sensory stimuli on sensitive infants (Glass & Wolf, 1994; Mouradian & Als, 1994, Vergara, 1993). Inclusion of families in planning and providing care is advocated (Holloway, 1994; Olson & Baltman, 1994). This approach is further discussed in the sections on preterm infant development (synactive theory of development) and intervention.

As the neonatal therapist expands beyond the rehabilitation model to include the practice of individualized developmental care, closer working relationships result with NICU medical staff. Trust and acceptance in the NICU must be earned by the competent therapist over time (Hunter, 1993; Hyde & Jonkey, 1994). It can be reassuring to understand the transitional stages in developing collaborative partnerships between therapists and neonatal nurses during the therapist's process of moving from "guest" to "family" in the NICU (Sweeney, 1993).

Professional guest
- Stage 1: Independent consultation with minimal interaction
- Stage 2: Competitive or protective posturing while evaluating coworker competence

Integrated NICU team member
- Stage 3: Building trust and mutuality in joint caregiving and problem solving
- Stage 4: Committed partnership with peak creative experiences

## Training and Competencies for the Neonatal Therapist

Practice standards to promote relevant competencies for NICU developmental specialists have been documented (AOTA, 1993; Scull & Deitz, 1989; VandenBerg, 1993). Occupational therapy in the NICU is now considered a high-risk and specialized area of practice requiring advanced knowledge and skills.

The specialized knowledge required for practice in the NICU includes familiarity with relevant medical conditions, procedures and equipment; an understanding of the unique developmental abilities and vulnerabilities of the infant; an understanding of theories of neonatal behavioral organization; family systems; NICU ecology; and the manner in which these factors interact to influence behavior. The occupational therapist develops the necessary skills through supervised clinical experience in assessment and intervention specific to the NICU (AOTA, 1993, p.1101).

These standards are essential for safe and effective intervention with the NICU population, but many occupational therapists continue to begin a neonatal practice without adequate preparation (Dewire, White, Kanny, & Glass, in press; Hyde & Jonkey, 1994). This situation creates an ethical dilemma to which occupational therapy educators, administrators, and clinicians must jointly commit to resolve (Anzalone, 1994). NICU competency requires broad-based knowledge and skills that increase in depth and in scope over time. Potential training options ranked as most useful by a surveyed group of neonatal occupational therapists include mentored NICU experience, on-the-job training, pediatric work experience, extended continuing education classes, and formal internships (Dewire et al., in press). Structured self-study can also be a valuable adjunct to supervised NICU training.

# SPECIALIZED KNOWLEDGE FOR NEONATAL THERAPY

## Classifications for Age and Birthweight
### Age

Gestational age (GA) refers to the total number of weeks the infant was in utero before birth. Determination of gestational age may be based on dating the last menstrual period (LMP) either by ultrasound (USG) or by physical examination of the infant (Clopton, 1993). The range used for a full-term pregnancy is 38 to 42 weeks in some hospitals and 37 to 42 weeks at others. An infant born before 37 to 38 weeks is considered preterm; the infant born after 42 weeks is postterm. Once the baby has been born, the GA always remains the same. An infant born 27 weeks into the pregnancy has a gestational age of 27 weeks at birth, at the expected due date, and on the first birthday.

Postconceptional age (PCA) refers to the baby's age in relation to when conception occurred, and thus continually changes over time. PCA is obtained by adding the weeks since birth to the baby's gestational age. The infant born at 27 weeks also has a PCA of 27 weeks at birth (27 weeks' gestation plus no additional weeks since birth). At this baby's expected due date, however, the PCA is 40 weeks (27 weeks' gestation, plus 13 weeks since birth to the original term due date). PCA is commonly used until 40 to 44 weeks, equivalent to term or 1 month corrected age, respectively.

Chronologic age refers to the baby's actual age since birth. Chronologically, the baby born at 27 weeks' gestation is 3 months old on the expected due date and 12 months old 1 year after birth.

Chronologic age of preterm infants is usually "corrected for prematurity" to better correlate with developmental expectations and performance; the baby born at 27 weeks' gestation will not developmentally look the same at 3 months chronologic age as the baby born at term. Corrected age refers to how old the baby would be if born full term rather than prematurely. The number of weeks of prematurity is first determined (subtract GA from the term equivalent of 40 weeks) and then subtracted from the chronologic age. The infant born at 27 weeks' gestation was born 13 weeks prematurely (40 weeks − 27 weeks GA = 13 weeks early). The corrected age of this baby on the first birthday would be 9 months because the actual birth was 3 months earlier than the expected due date. Corrected age is typically used until 2 years of age when assessing developmental status.

### Birth Weight

Infants born above 2500 g (5.5 pounds) are considered average in size. A birth weight of 1500 to 2500 g is termed *low birth weight*. *Very low birth weight* is 1000 to 1500 g, and *extremely low birth weight* is under 1000 g.

Birth weight between the 10th and the 90th percentile on a standardized growth chart is appropriate for gestational age (AGA). Birth weight below the 10th percentile is small for gestational age (SGA), and birth weight above the 90th percentile is large for gestational age (LGA). These categories apply equally to preterm, term, and postterm infants. Any infant growing normally will be AGA. An infant of a mother with severe pregnancy-induced hypertension may have experienced intrauterine growth retardation and may be born SGA, whereas the infant of a mother with diabetes is often LGA.

## Developing a Medical Foundation
### Abbreviations

Learning the language of the NICU is essential for the neonatal occupational therapist. Documentation typically contains many abbreviations, as illustrated by this medical summary:

Cody is a 39 wk pca wm born at 27 wks GA by SVD to a 18 y/o now $G_2P_1Ab_1$, A+,VDRL- mom with hx of IVDA, smokes 1 PPD, PIH and PTL tx'd with $MgSO_4$, SROM 21° PTD. Pt. had CAN x1 (reduced PTD), was SGA at 505 gm, Apgars $1^1,3^5,6^{10}$. Significant medical complications have included RDS, BPD, PIE, PDA (ligated), hyperbilirubinemia, anemia, A's & B's, B gr. 3 IVH, PVL, ROP stage III OD (regressing) and stage III+ OS (s/p laser OS), MRSE sepsis, and NEC (Ø surgery). Pt. was on SIMV for 41 days, NCPAP for 32 days, and remains on $FiO_2$ 1.0 at .5L by NC.

Understanding abbreviations and the terms they represent is obviously a prerequisite to beginning a neonatal practice. Appendix 22-A lists some common NICU abbreviations.

### Medical Conditions and Equipment

Learning NICU medical terminology is an ongoing process that progresses from knowing definitions to gradually understanding the pathophysiology of diseases and biomechanics of equipment. Medical complications and technology both have profound effects on preterm and high-risk infants, with subsequent implications and precautions for neonatal therapists. Development of a basic medical foundation is essential to safely address an infant's developmental needs. Appendix 22-B summarizes selected maternal conditions that may have significant effects on the baby; this list is not all inclusive but serves to illustrate how this information is relevant to the occupational therapist. Appendix 22-C reviews common neonatal medical complications encountered in the NICU.

Table 22-1 lists common medical equipment in the NICU. In addition to the life support technology that is listed in the table, other equipment is used to monitor the physiologic status of the neonate. The pulse oximeter and cardiorespiratory monitor should also be mentioned. Pulse oximetry is a noninvasive method of continually assessing blood oxygen saturation with a sensor wrapped around an infant's hand or foot. False alarms of low oxygen saturation are common; the pulse rate on the oximeter must approximate the heart rate on the cardiorespiratory monitor for the alarm to be considered valid. The cardiorespiratory monitor provides a visual tracing and numerical correlate of heart and breathing rate, as well as an auditory alarm if these rates are not within a preset range (Figure 22-2).

▲ Table 22-1   Common Medical Equipment in the Neonatal Intensive Care Unit

| Equipment | Description | Purpose |
|---|---|---|
| **THERMOREGULATION EQUIPMENT** | | |
| Radiant warmer | Open bed with an overhead heat source | Typically used during medical workup of a new admission or for critically ill infants requiring easy access for frequent or complicated medical care |
| Incubator (isolette) | Clear plastic heated box enclosing the mattress and infant | Used to provide warmth so available calories can be used for growth and healing; infant may or may not be dressed, depending on specific NICU's protocol; access is typcially by opening portholes or a door |
| Open crib | Bassinet-style bed; no additional heat source is provided; infant is dressed and swaddled in blankets | Used for larger and more stable infants; caregivers (including occupational therapist) must be careful to avoid cold stress during baths, assessments, and procedures |
| **OXYGEN THERAPY WITH ASSISTED VENTILATION** | | |
| Bag and mask ventilation | A bag attached to a face mask is rhythmically squeezed to deliver positive pressure and oxygen | Used for resuscitation of an infant at delivery or during acute deterioration and to increase oxygenation if necessary after an apneic spell |
| Continuous positive airway pressure (CPAP) | A steady stream of pressurized air is given through an endotracheal tube, a nasopharyngeal tube, or nasal prongs; supplemental oxygen may or may not be used | Positive pressure is used to keep the alveoli and airways from collapsing (i.e., to keep them open) in an infant who is breathing spontaneously but has a disorder such as respiratory distress syndrome, pulmonary edema, or apnea |
| Mechanical ventilation | A machine controls or assists breathing by mechanically inflating the lungs, increasing alveolar ventilation, and improving gas exchange | Used for infants with depressed respiratory drive, pulmonary disease with increased work of breathing and suboptimal oxygenation and ventilation (i.e., MAS or RDS), and frequent apnea despite CPAP; infant is usually orally or nasally intubated, but may on occasion have a tracheostomy |
| Extracorporeal membrane oxygenation (ECMO) | A sophisticated life-support system that uses a modified heart-lung bypass to provide nearly total lung rest and minimize barotrauma (lung damage that can occur with prolonged high ventilator settings) | Used as "rescue" technology for qualifying infants in neonatal respiratory failure who are unresponsive to conventional medical management or at times for perioperative support during cardiac surgery; these infants meet medical criteria for a ≥80% mortality risk; more than 80% survive with ECMO. Most do well developmentally; school-aged sequelae may occur |
| **OXYGEN THERAPY WITHOUT ASSISTED VENTILATION** | | |
| Oxygen hood (oxyhood) | A plastic hood with a flow of warm humidified oxygen placed over the infant's head | Used for infants who are breathing independently but need a higher concentration of oxygen than the 21% room air |
| Nasal cannula (NC) | Humidified oxygen delivered by a flexible cannula with small prongs that fit into the nares | Used for infants requiring low concentrations of supplemental oxygen (22% to 30%), or when oxygen will be needed for a long period; handling and portability are easier with an NC than with an oxyhood |

*NICU,* Neonatal intensive care unit; *MAS,* meconium aspiration syndrome; *RDS,* respiratory distress syndrome.

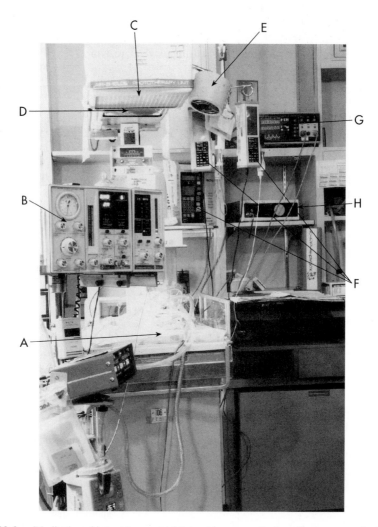

**Figure 22-2** Medical equipment in neonatal intensive care unit. *A,* radiant warmer (bed); *B,* mechanical ventilator; *C,* phototherapy lights (may also be free standing); *D,* radiant heat source; *E,* procedure light; *F,* infusion pumps for fluids and medications; *G,* cardiorespiratory monitor; *H,* pulse oximeter. (Courtesy of the Infant Special Care Unit, University of Texas Medical Branch, Galveston, TX. Photograph by John Glow.)

### Thermoregulation

Preterm infants are predisposed to excessive heat loss and are vulnerable to cold stress from several causes. Extended posture, thin skin, and reduced insulating subcutaneous fat in very premature infants allow heat to transfer from the body to the air. A special *brown fat* used by neonates to metabolize heat is not produced until the last trimester of gestation. Pulmonary dysfunction, central nervous system immaturity, and frequent caregiving interventions may also contribute to heat loss.

The infant may lose heat by convection, conduction, radiation, and evaporation. Convection refers to heat loss from the infant's body to cooler surrounding air. Conduction refers to heat transfer that occurs when the infant's body is in contact with a cooler solid object, such as the therapist's hands. Radiation refers to heat loss from the infant's body to a cooler solid surface not in direct contact

with the infant, such as incubator walls. A major source of heat and water loss in small infants is evaporation, or heat loss that occurs when liquid from the infant's respiratory tract and permeable skin is converted into a vapor.

Radiant warmers, incubators, and swaddling in open cribs are used to conserve heat in NICU infants (Figure 22-3). The neonatal therapist must diligently protect NICU infants from heat loss during all evaluations and intervention (Hunter, Mullen, & Dallas, 1994). Cold stress can burn calories needed for growth and healing, create behavioral and physiologic complications, and in severe cases may result in death.

### NICU Environment

Sensory components of the extrauterine environment in neonatal intensive care are obviously different from the

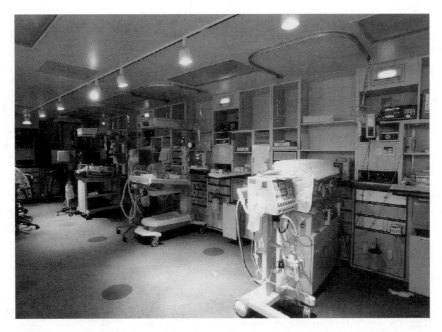

**Figure 22-3** Overview of neonatal intensive care unit. Incubator and mechanical ventilator are in forground; radiant warmers are in background. Track lighting allows option of turning off overhead ceiling lights to reduce room light levels. (Courtesy of the Infant Special Care Unit, University of Texas Medical Branch, Galveston, TX. Photograph by John Glow.)

▲ **Table 22-2** Comparison of Intrauterine and Extrauterine Sensory Environments

| System | Intrauterine | Extrauterine |
|---|---|---|
| Tactile | Constant proprioceptive input; smooth, wet, usually safe and comfortable | Often painful and invasive; dry, cool air; predominance of medical touching versus social touching |
| Vestibular | Maternal movements, diurnal cycles, amniotic fluid creates gently oscillating environment, flexed posture | Horizontal, flat postures; Influence of gravity, restraints, and equipment |
| Auditory | Maternal biologic sounds, muffled environmental sounds | Extremely loud, harsh, mechanical, and constant noise |
| Visual | Dark; may occasionally have very dim red spectrum light | Bright fluorescent lights Often no diurnal rhythm |
| Thermal | Constant warmth, consistent temperature | Environmental temperature variations, high risk of neonatal heat loss |

womb that recently housed the baby (Table 22-2). Before birth the fetus is in a warm, snug, dark world where basic needs are automatically met. After birth, demands are suddenly made on the neonate to breathe, regulate body temperature, move against the effects of gravity, adjust to bright light and unmuffled noise, and cope with invasive or painful procedures and frequent sleep deprivation. The preterm infant's immature central nervous system is competent for intrauterine life but not sufficiently developed to adjust to and organize the overwhelming stimuli and demands of the NICU; this creates a "mismatch" of the neonate with the high-tech world now necessary for survival (Als, 1985, 1986).

Several researchers have suggested the continual overwhelming stimuli created by the NICU environment and caregiving practices stress the highly sensitive preterm infant's already vulnerable disorganized central nervous system. Excessive sensory stimulation may cause insults to the still-developing brain (i.e., from repeated hypoxic episodes related to stress) and can create maladaptive behaviors that contribute to later poor developmental outcome even in the absence of overt central nervous system pathology (Als, 1986; Als et al., 1986; Gorski, Davidson, & Brazelton, 1979; Long, Lucey, & Phillip, 1980). Striving for an appropriate level of stimulation that the infant can tolerate and integrate should be a caregiving priority (Brazelton, 1985).

Neonates with extreme prematurity, critical illness, and major anomalies often have extended hospitalizations with prolonged exposure to potential environmental hazards in the NICU. A joint committee with members from the American Academy of Pediatrics, the National Perinatal Association, and the National Association of Neonatal Nurses was formed to address the impact of NICU environment and interventions on infants (Graven et al., 1992). This group agreed that (1) NICU environmental and caregiving practices create infant stress that contributes to physiologic instability and may hinder subsequent recovery, growth, and development; (2) many NICU factors interfere with the development of parent-infant attachment and optimal parenting; and (3) more sophisticated study and longer follow-up are necessary to clarify relationships between environmental factors and infant neurologic outcome.

Early in 1995 the first of planned annual national conferences on the physical and developmental environment of the high-risk infant affirmed trends of protecting NICU infants from stressful environments but reinforced the lack of current "bottom-line" conclusions and recommendations. National study groups continue to address light, sound, sleep, and sleep deprivation; additional areas of focus will include care issues related to position and motion, pain, smell, taste, oral motor function, family needs, and transitional environments (Graven, 1995). Informed and visionary neonatal occupational therapists should participate in these efforts.

Environmental modifications may contribute to a demonstrated increase in stability and facilitation of recovery in very preterm infants, with improved long-term neurodevelopmental outcome (Als et al., 1994; VandenBerg, 1994). Potential environmental modifications are summarized on pp. 612-615.

### Light in the NICU

The infant's visual system continues to develop during the last trimester of gestation, with significant maturation and differentiation in the retina and visual cortex (Glass, 1993). Concern has been expressed about the exposure of immature infants to frequent or continuous bright light from ceiling and procedure lights, phototherapy, heat lamps, sunlight, and opthalmoscopic examinations (Graven et al., 1992) (Figure 22-4). In contrast to the dark womb and compared with standard adult office lighting of 40 to 50 footcandles, the ambient lighting of modern NICUs ranges from 30 to 150 footcandles, with peaks exceeding 1500 footcandles from sunlight (Glass, 1993). Continuous intense white fluorescent ambient light has been linked to chromosomal damage, disruption of diurnal biologic rhythms, changes in endocrine glands and gonadal function, and alteration of vitamin D synthesis in humans and other mammals (Wurtman, 1975). Small preterm infants exposed to bright NICU lights may suffer retinal damage (Glass et al., 1985). Overstimulation of the immature central nervous system with resultant physiologic instability and subsequent potential effects on developmental outcome has also been suggested (Gorski, Davidson, & Brazelton, 1979; VandenBerg, 1995).

The level of lighting necessary to balance caregiving safety with protection of the developing visual system has

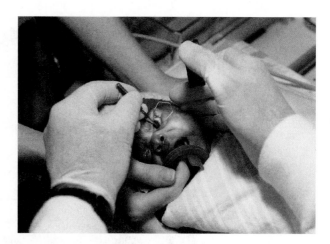

**Figure 22-4** Neonatal intensive care unit infant receiving eye examination by opthalmologist to check for development of retinopathy of prematurity. Nurse provides comfort measures for baby during examination. (Courtesy of the Infant Special Care Unit, University of Texas Medical Branch, Galveston, TX. Photograph by John Glow.)

not been determined. While awaiting definitive studies, it seems prudent to protect premature infants from bright lights in the NICU. Methods to provide this protection are included on p. 612.

### Sound in the NICU

Environmental noise in the NICU is a frequent concern among caregivers and researchers. Hearing threshold has been reported as 40 decibel (db) in the 28- to 34-week gestation infant, 30 db at 35 to 38 weeks' gestation, and <20 db at term; these thresholds are greatly exceeded in the NICU (Lary, Briassoulis, de Vries, Dubowitz, & Dubowitz, 1985). Typical NICU sound levels of 50 to 90 db (comparable to street traffic and light machinery, respectively) with peaks to 120 db (comparable to heavy machinery) have been documented (Gottfried & Hodgman, 1984; Long, Lucey, & Philip, 1980; Thomas, 1989; Weibley, 1989). The limit imposed in industrial standards by the Occupational Safety and Health Administration (OSHA) as the highest safe level for adult workers is 90 db for 8 hours (Lotas, 1992). Safety standards for sound exposure have not been established for infants (Brown & Glass, 1979; Thomas, 1989). Some researchers have speculated that effects of environmental noise might be magnified by risks from ototoxic drugs and prolonged hyperbilirubinemia, thus contributing to the increased incidence of hearing loss in preterm infants (Bhattacharyya, Vijay, & Doyal, 1986). Loud or prolonged sounds can produce hearing loss, affecting the frequency range that corresponds to the frequency of the damaging sound. Preterm infants are at risk for hearing loss in both low-frequency (speech) and high-frequency ranges (Thomas, 1989).

Noise can be highly arousing for preterm and ill infants

in the NICU, causing agitation and crying, which decreases oxygenation and increases intracranial pressure, heart rate, and respiratory rate (Long, Lurey, & Phillips, 1980). Noise may disrupt the sleep state and sleep-wake cycle and may adversely affect the neonate's recovery and growth (DePaul & Chambers, 1995). In a typical NICU, environmental noise is constant throughout the day and night, mechanical versus social, and noncontingent to individual infants. Sound inside the isolette is characterized by continuous white noise and nonspeech sounds; harsh mechanical noises penetrate clearly, while speech sounds are indistinct (Newman, 1981).

Even caregivers who typically habituate to the unit's sound levels on occasion experience irritation from NICU noise, possibly when tired, tense, or ill. Stress associated with noise has been linked to job-related illness (headaches and muscle tension), lowered productivity, increased errors, poor concentration, and job turnover (Suedfield, 1985). Adult caregivers have opportunities to escape the NICU; the babies always remain. Methods to reduce NICU environmental noise are included on p. 613.

### Caregiving in the NICU

NICU caregiving patterns differ significantly from the fetal intrauterine environment or the normal home atmosphere of term infants. Touch in the NICU is usually related to medical care rather than being social in nature, with interventions constant throughout a 24-hour span (Gottfried, 1985). Examples of medical touching include a physical examination, blood drawing, applying or removing tape, taking measurements (temperature, blood pressure, weight, and circumference of head or abdomen), stethoscopic examination, IV insertion, gavage feeds, transfusions, injections, tube adjustments, repositioning, chest percussion, suctioning, bag and mask breathing, and resuscitation efforts. A 28-week gestation infant can differentiate between touch and pain (Beaver, 1987); light touch increases motor movement, and painful touch causes the infant to cry and attempt to withdraw. Caregiving procedures have been related to hypoxemia (Gorski, Hole, Leonard, & Martin, 1983; Long, Alistar, & Phillip, & Lucey, 1980). Even social touch can be arousing and ultimately stressful to immature infants.

Caregiving based on external criteria such as fixed schedules for vital signs and feeding often ignores or delays the caregiver response to the infant's cues indicating care is needed. Caregiving thus becomes noncontingent to the infant's efforts to communicate. Eventually this may discourage the infant's efforts to communicate needs, lead to emotional detachment from the sensation of needs, and contribute to the development of distrust (Gardner et al., 1993).

Infants on intensive care status receive less social contact and contingent caregiving than recovering infants in step-down units (Gottfried, 1985). Preferred babies, described as those infants with long-term NICU status, presence of a devoted family, and potential for successful outcome, tend to experience more social contact than other infants; the initiation of oral feeds also correlates with increased personal attention and social stimulation (Jones, 1982).

Sleep deprivation of NICU infants has been recognized (Lawhon, 1986). The 29- to 32-week gestation fetus sleeps 80% of the time in utero (Dreyfus-Brisac, 1974, 1979). Sleep cycles of prematurely born infants are less organized and of shorter duration (30 to 40 minutes) than the 50- to 60-minute sleep cycles of term infants (Anders & Keener, 1985; Dreyfus-Brisac, 1974). In addition, the NICU infant may be disturbed 80 to 132 times per day, with average undisturbed sleep periods of approximately 4 to 10 minutes (Gottfried, 1985; Korones, 1976). Because secretion of human growth hormone is associated with regular recurrence of sleep-wake cycles and peaks during active sleep (REM sleep), sleep deprivation in the NICU may interfere with optimal growth and development (Gardner et al., 1993).

There are obvious implications for developmental specialists in the data on NICU caregiving patterns. Education and collaboration with staff, encouragement and facilitation of family presence, training and collaboration with families, and direct services by the therapist are valid options. An occupational therapist might "float" in the intensive care area to respond to infant cues as they occur, provide parent support and training, and assist medical staff as situations arise (e.g., supporting the infant during procedures and repositioning or calming as needed). Presence of a developmental specialist in the NICU throughout all shifts 7 days a week would be ideal.

## Preterm Infant Development
### Theories of Neurobehavioral Organization

*Synactive theory of development.* The work of Heidi Als and colleagues has provided a theoretical basis for understanding preterm infant behaviors, including infants' efforts to cope with stresses of the extrauterine environment and to maintain homeostasis in the NICU (Als, 1982, 1986). The fetus is not a deficient organism but is fully competent within the intrauterine environment that should rightfully be home for several more weeks or months. Preterm birth, however, can create a mismatch as the "displaced fetus" now has to function within a different and more complex extrauterine environment (Als, 1986).

Als has proposed a model for understanding the emerging capabilities of preterm infants to organize and control their behavior as they are continually affected by and responsive to environmental influences. The synactive theory of development identifies five separate but interdependent subsystems (autonomic, motor, state, attention-interaction, and self-regulation) within the infant that are in constant interaction with each other and with the environment. Figure 22-5 illustrates the unfolding of these subsystems as the infant continues to mature before and after birth. It is

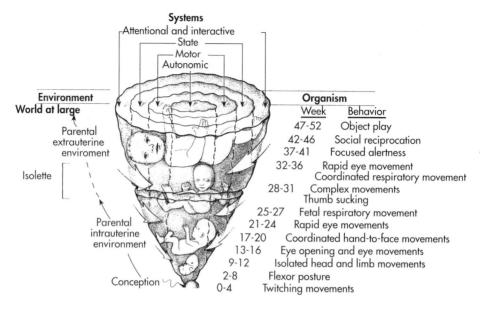

**Figure 22-5**   Beginning at conception, emerging and expanding capabilities of developing infant are illustrated in this model of synactive organization of behavioral development. (From Als, H. [1982]. Toward a synactive theory of development: promise for the assessment and support of infant individuality. *Infant Mental Health Journal, 3,* 229-243.)

through recognizable approach and avoidance behaviors occurring in these subsystems that infants continually communicate their level of stress and stability in relation to what is happening to and around them (Table 22-3; Figures 22-6 and 22-7). Maturation and improved (or declining) health are reflected in sequential observation of subsystem development.

*Synaction* refers to the process by which stable functioning or decompensation in one subsystem can affect the organization and integrity of other subsystems (Als, 1982). For example Marissa, who is now physiologically and motorically stable and able to maintain quiet alertness for about 10 minutes, can reasonably be expected to attend to and interact with specific social stimuli. If, however, the caregiver simultaneously smiles and nods while talking to and stroking her, Marissa may become overwhelmed by the effort required to integrate all these incoming stimuli and respond with avoidance and stress behaviors such as gaze aversion, motor flaccidity, and possibly apnea (Figure 22-8).

Synactive theory forms the basis for individualized developmentally supportive and family-centered care. Caregivers are trained to be sensitive to each infant's fragility and stress versus robustness and stability behaviors. These observations are then used to promote modification of the immediate environment and caregiving practices to facilitate the infant's organization and well-being. The infant's attempts to maintain or return to a calm organized state are also noted and facilitated. The infant and family are seen as an integral unit, with parents supported in assuming an active role with their infant in the NICU. The Neonatal Individualized Developmental Care and Assessment Program

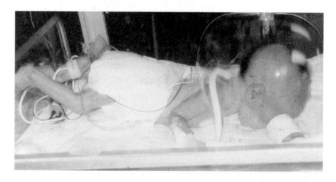

**Figure 22-6**   Preterm infant demonstrating stress with arching and agitated movements of extremities. (Courtesy of the Infant Special Care Unit, University of Texas Medical Branch, Galveston, TX.)

(NIDCAP) provides training and certification in this approach for clinical and research use; additional information is included in the section on neonatal assessment. Clinical application is included in the section on intervention.

Medical, developmental, and financial gains have been attributed to provision of developmentally supportive care (Als et al., 1986; Als et al., 1994; VandenBerg, 1994). Benefits cited include the following:

▲ Decreased incidence of intraventricular hemorrhage
▲ Decreased severity of bronchopulmonary dysplasia, with significant decrease in duration of mechanical ventilation and supplemental oxygen
▲ Better weight gain and faster transition to oral feeds
▲ Increased family involvement and confidence

▲ Table 22-3    Synactive Theory of Development: Neurobehavioral Subsystems, Signs of Stress and Stability

| Subsystem | Signs of Stress | Signs of Stability |
|---|---|---|
| **AUTONOMIC** | **Physiologic instability** | **Physiologic stability** |
| Respiratory | Pauses, tachypnea, gasping | Smooth, regular respiratory rate |
| Color | Changes to mottled, flushed, pale, dusky, cyanotic, gray or ashen | Pink, stable color |
| Visceral | Hiccups, gagging, spitting up, grunting, straining (as if producing bowel movement) | Stable viscera with no hiccups, gags, emesis, or grunting |
| Motor | Tremors, startles, twitches, coughs, sneezes, yawns, sighs, has seizures | No sign of tremors, startles, twitches, coughs, sneezes, yawns, sighs, or seizures |
| **MOTOR** | **Fluctuating tone, uncontrolled activity** | **Consistent tone, controlled activity** |
| Flaccidity | Gape face, low tone in trunk, limp lower extremities and upper extremities | Muscle tone consistent in trunk and extremities and appropriate for postconceptional age |
| Hypertonicity | Leg extensions and sitting on air; upper-extremity salutes, finger splays, and fisting; trunk arching; tongue extensions | Smooth controlled posture<br>Smooth movements of extremities and head |
| Hyperflexions | Trunk, lower extremities, upper extremities<br>Frantic, diffuse activity extremities | Motor control can be used for self-regulation (hand and foot clasp, leg and foot bracing, hand to mouth, grasping, tucking, sucking) |
| **STATE** | **Diffused or disorganized quality of states, including range and transition between states** | **Clear states; good, calming, focused alertness** |
| During sleep | Twitches, sounds, whimpers, jerky movements, irregular respiratory rate, fussy, grimaces | Clear, well-defined sleep states<br>Good self-quieting and consolability<br>Robust crying |
| When awake | Eye floating, glassy eyed, staring, gaze aversion, worried or dull look, hyperalert panicked expression, weak cry, irritability<br>Abrupt state changes | Focused clear alertness with animated expressions (e.g., frowning, cheek softening, "ooh" face, cooing, smiling)<br>Smooth transition between states |
| **ATTENTION-INTERACTION** | **Effort to attend and interact to specific stimulus elicits stress signals of other subsystems** | **Responsive to auditory, visual, and social stimuli** |
| Autonomic | Irregular respiratory rate, color changes, visceral responses, coughs, yawns, sneezes, sighs, straining tremors, twitches | Responsivity to auditory and visual stimuli is clear and prolonged |
| Motor | Fluctuating tone, frantic diffuse activity | Actively seeks out auditory stimulus; able to shift attention smoothly from one stimulus to another |
| State | Eye floating, glassy eyed, staring, worried or dull look, hyperalert panicked expression, gaze aversion, weak cry, irritability<br>Abrupt state changes<br>Becomes stressed if more than one type of stimulus is given simultaneously | Face demonstrates bright-eyed purposeful interest varying between arousal and relaxation |

**SELF-REGULATION:** Infant's efforts to achieve, maintain, or regain balance and self-organization in each subsystem as needed. Examples include motor strategies (e.g., foot clasp, leg and foot bracing, finger folding, hand clasping, hand to mouth, grasping, tucking, sucking, postural changes); state strategies (e.g., lowers state of arousal or releases energy with rhythmic, robust crying) and attention and orientation strategies such as visual locking. The success of various strategies may vary among infants.

Modified from Als, H. (1982). Toward a synactive theory of development: promise for the assessment and support of infant individuality. *Infant Mental Health Journal, 3,* 229-243; Als, H. (1986). A synactive model of neonatal behavior organization: framework for the assessment of neurobehavioral development in the premature infant and for support of infants and parents in the neonatal intensive care environment. *Physical and Occupational Therapy in Pediatrics, 6,* 3-55.

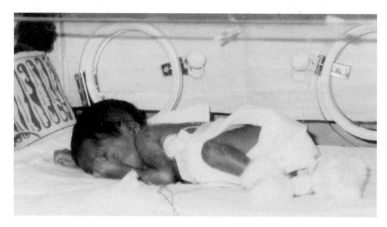

**Figure 22-7**  Preterm infant using motor strategies of hand-to-face, extremity tucking, and foot bracing on mattress surface to maintain calm, organized state. (Courtesy of the Infant Special Care Unit, University of Texas Medical Branch, Galveston, TX.)

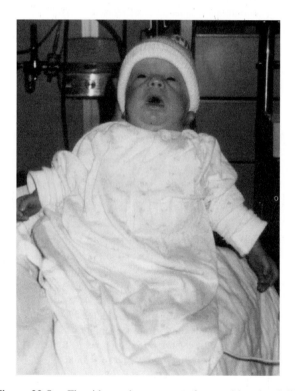

**Figure 22-8**  Flaccid muscle tone, gape face, and low-level diffuse alertness are signs of stress in this preterm infant. (Courtesy of the Infant Special Care Unit, University of Texas Medical Branch, Galveston, TX.)

▲ Shorter hospital stays with significant financial savings

▲ Improved cognitive and motor development as compared with controls (followed to 3 years of age)

*Preterm neurobehavioral organization: in-turning, coming-out, and reciprocity.* Another description of preterm infant behavioral organization was developed by col-leagues of Als and correlates closely with the synactive theory of development. Table 22-4 summarizes and compares the stages and characteristics of preterm behavioral organization as described in these theories.

### Neuromotor

Hypotonia is present but normal for a 28-week infant; immaturity is not the same as pathologic condition (Figure 22-9). Muscle tone in preterm infants develops in a caudo-cephalic (feet to head) direction. Flexor tone develops gradually, beginning in the lower extremities and progressing to the arms. A preterm infant at term equivalency, however, will not demonstrate the same degree of physiologic flexion as a full-term infant. Tables 22-5 and 22-6 provide summaries of preterm neuromotor development.

### Therapeutic Positioning

Therapeutic positioning has consistently been a goal of occupational therapy in the NICU (Updike, Schmidt, Macke, Cahoon, & Miller, 1986). Pioneering neonatal thera-pists frequently received referrals for infants with neuromo-tor problems and implemented therapeutic handling and po-sitioning to normalize tone and increase functional move-ment (Rapport, 1992). Abnormal postures and movement patterns were often already established before occupational therapy was consulted, reinforcing the need to use a reha-bilitation approach. Earlier involvement of therapists in neonatal units and growing awareness of positional defor-mities that premature infants typically develop have resulted in a greater emphasis on preventive positioning measures employed for all infants by all NICU staff (Creger & Browne, 1989; Fay, 1988; Gardner et al., 1993).

*Positional deformities.* Common positional deformities of NICU graduates have been identified and related to in-appropriate nursery positioning (Desmond, Wilson, Alt, & Fisher, 1980; Semmler, 1989; Updike et al., 1986). Dolio-cephaly refers to progressive head flattening that can result

▲ Table 22-4    Stages and Characteristics of Behavioral Organization in Preterm Infant

| Als | Gorski, Davidson, & Brazelton |
|---|---|
| Physiologic homeostasis—stabilizing and integrating temperature control, cardiorespiratory function, digestion, and elimination. Characteristics: becomes pale, dusky, cyanotic; heart and respiratory rates change—all symptoms of disorganization of autonomic nervous system. | "In turning"—physiologic stage of mere survival characterized by autonomic nervous system responses to stimuli (rapid color changes caused by swings in heart and respiratory rates); no or limited direct response; inability to arouse self spontaneously; jerky movements; asleep (and protecting the central nervous system from sensory overload) 97% of the time. Preterms (<32 weeks) are easily physiologically overwhelmed by stimuli. |
| Motor development may infringe on physiologic homeostasis, resulting in defensive strategies (vomiting, color change, apnea, and bradycardia). | "Coming out"—first active response to environment may be seen as early as 34 to 35 weeks (provided some physiologic stability has been achieved). |
| State development becomes less diffuse and encompasses full range: sleep, awake, crying. States and state changes may affect physiologic and motor stability. | Characteristics: remains pink with stimuli; has directed response for short periods; arouses spontaneously and maintains arousal after stimuli ceases; if interaction begins in alert state: maintains quiet alert for 5 to 10 minutes, tracks animate and inanimate stimuli; spends 10% to 15% of time in alert state with predictable interaction patterns. |
| Alert state is well differentiated from other states; may interfere with physiologic and motor stability. | "Reciprocity"—active interaction and reciprocity with environment from 36 to 40 weeks. Characteristics: directs response; arouses and consoles self; maintains alertness and interacts with both animate and inanimate objects; copes with external stress. |

Modified from Als, H. (1986). A synactive model of neonatal behavior organization: framework for the assessment of neurobehavioral development in the premature infant and for support of infants and parents in the neonatal intensive care environment. *Physical and Occupational Therapy in Pediatrics, 6,* 3-55; Gorski, P.A., Davidson, M.F., & Brazelton, T.B. (1979). Stages of behavioral organization in the high-risk neonate: theoretical clinical considerations. *Seminars in Perinatology, 3,* 61-72.

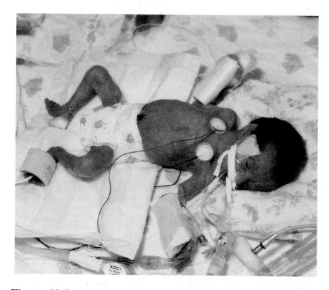

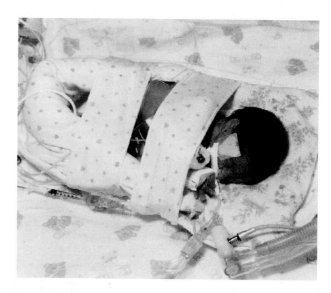

**Figure 22-9**    Hypotonic posture of premature infant. Without therapeutic positioning, "W" configuration of arms, "frogged" posture of legs, and asymmetric head position may lead to positional deformities. Tiny premie diaper ("Wee-pee," Children's Medical Ventures) prevents forced hip abduction from diaper bulk. (Courtesy of the Infant Special Care Unit, University of Texas Medical Branch, Galveston, TX. Photograph by John Glow.)

**Figure 22-10**    Small preterm infant (same baby as Figure 22-9) supported in sidelying position with midline orientation and flexion of extremities. Snuggle-Up bunting maintains the contained posture; Squishon I gel pillow under head facilitates comfort and minimizes head flattening. (Snuggle-Up and Squishon, Children's Medical Ventures). (Courtesy of the Infant Special Care Unit, University of Texas Medical Branch, Galveston, TX. Photograph by John Glow.)

▲ Table 22-5   Preterm Neuromotor Development

| Age | Development (Creger and Browne) |
|---|---|
| 27 to 28 Weeks | **RESTING POSTURE**<br>Generalized hypotonia<br>**RESPONSE TO HANDLING**<br>Full range of motion without resistance is demonstrated by heel-to-ear maneuver<br>When both arms are extended parallel to the body, no attempt is made to recoil arms into flexion<br>When pressure is placed on the ball of the foot, the infant makes no attempt to grasp with toes<br>Placing response is absent<br>Infant makes no attempt to align head and body when pulled to sitting position<br>**ACTIVE MOVEMENT**<br>Movements are spasmodic and involve total extremity |
| 29 Weeks | **RESTING POSTURE**<br>Capable of more variety in posture when compared with earlier hypotonia<br>**RESPONSE TO HANDLING**<br>Continues to demonstrate little resistance to passive movements, but manipulation of one extremity is more likely to elicit a response in the opposite extremity<br>Moro response is incomplete but symmetric<br>In prone position, infant shows some attempt to pull body into flexion using legs<br>Shows some knee flexion in one leg in response to traction of the other leg<br>Extreme head lag in pull-to-sit but attempts to right head anteriorly once in sitting position<br>Some active flexion at the knee is seen with attempts to elicit placing response<br>Minimal attempt to assume an upright posture in supported standing, but a stepping response is seen<br>**ACTIVE MOVEMENT**<br>Movements remain jerky<br>Movements continue to be a reflexive response to handling<br>Movements are predominant in the legs |
| 30 Weeks | **RESTING POSTURES**<br>Shows some beginning flexion in lower extremities<br>**RESPONSE TO HANDLING**<br>Arm recoil is seen, grasp now involves some arm flexion, grasp and traction may begin to lift infant's body from supporting surface<br>Head lag remains extreme, but once in sitting position, the infant can right head anteriorly and posteriorly with head position maintained only momentarily<br>No attempt is made to bear any weight on legs in supported standing position but does exhibit some resistance to supporting surface with feet; still little attempt to assume upright posture<br>**ACTIVE MOVEMENTS**<br>Although active movement still involves the total extremity, movement has become more purposeful and controlled |
| 31 Weeks | **RESTING POSTURES**<br>Displays increased flexor tone in lower extremities when compared with more premature infants<br>**RESPONSE TO HANDLING**<br>More resistance to passive movements is seen in legs than in arms, exhibited by the heel-to-ear maneuver<br>Recoil and traction are more pronounced in lower extremities as compared with upper extremities<br>Shows some attempt to maintain head in alignment with body while being pulled to sitting position; able to right head anteriorly and posteriorly once in the sitting position<br>Still no attempt to bear weight on legs in supported standing; may flex knees and show some resistance to the surface with feet; makes no attempt to align head with body<br>**ACTIVE MOVEMENTS**<br>Flexes arms and legs against gravity; these movements are not always smoothly coordinated as tremors and are commonly observed in preterm infants |

From Creger, P.J. (1989). *Developmental interventions for preterm and high-risk infants: self-study modules for professionals.* Tucson: Therapy Skill Builders.

▲ Table 22-5   Preterm Neuromotor Development—cont'd

| Age | Development (Creger and Browne) |
|---|---|
| 32 Weeks | **RESTING POSTURE**<br>Continues to develop lower extremity flexion<br>**RESPONSE TO HANDLING**<br>Decreased lower extremity range of passive movement<br>Rights head consistently and smoothly in a pull-to-sit position<br>Shows more ability to maintain head aligned with body in supported sitting position compared with younger infants<br>Supported stand: places some weight on feet, begins to right head, has some knee extension with some effort to extend trunk<br>Moro: complete arm extension and abduction; no flexion and adduction component evident<br>**ACTIVE MOVEMENTS**<br>Infant more active with smoother and more purposeful movements<br>Brief periods of hand-to-mouth activity appear |
| 33 Weeks | **RESTING POSTURE**<br>Displays increasingly stronger flexion of lower extremities<br>**RESPONSE TO HANDLING**<br>Heel-to-ear maneuver shows increasing resistance to passive knee extension<br>Recoil and traction responses of upper and lower extremities are stronger and more consistent<br>Infant shows stronger attempts to align head with body in pull-to-sit; able to right head anteriorly and posteriorly in supported sitting position but cannot maintain head upright<br>When held in supported standing position, infant makes some attempt to bear weight on legs; tries to extend trunk and align head with body<br>Palmar and plantar grasps are quickly and easily elicited<br>**ACTIVE MOVEMENTS**<br>Spontaneously flexes and extends arms and legs; movements are becoming smoother and more purposeful |
| 34 Weeks | **RESTING POSTURE**<br>Displays development of hip flexion by assuming froglike resting posture<br>**RESPONSE TO HANDLING**<br>Able to grasp and maintain traction with upper extremities<br>Traction continues to be demonstrated in the lower extremities; infant resists passive knee extension<br>Attempts to extend the hips and knees and right head when in supported sitting position<br>Placing response is now demonstrated<br>Ventral suspension: maintains some flexion in elbows and knees, makes an effort to lift head<br>Moro: extends and abducts arms, followed by partial flexion and adduction<br>**ACTIVE MOVEMENTS**<br>Vigorously kicks during more prolonged awake states. These movements are progressively more purposeful and reciprocal and involve flexion of trunk |
| 35 Weeks | **RESTING POSTURE**<br>More consistent flexion in prone position<br>**RESPONSE TO HANDLING**<br>Resistance to passive movements of knees and hips<br>When prone with head placed in midline, infant will purposely turn head to either side<br>In pull-to-sit maneuver, infant rights head and attempts to maintain it in alignment with body<br>Supported stand: attempts to bear weight on legs and feet and to align head with upright body<br>**ACTIVE MOVEMENTS**<br>May begin to have definite alert periods<br>Movements of head and eyes appear less random and more purposeful |
| 36 Weeks | **RESTING POSTURE**<br>Wide variety of resting postures<br>Flexor tone dominates in trunk and extremities |

▲ Table 22-5    Preterm Neuromotor Development—cont'd

| Age | Development (Creger and Browne) |
|---|---|
| | **RESPONSE TO HANDLING**<br>All newborn primary reflexes can be elicited; Moro is complete; leg recoil is brisk<br>Resists knee extension and hip adduction<br>Tries to align head with body during pull-to-sit maneuver<br>In prone position, infant pulls into flexion with trunk and legs<br>Demonstrates stepping and placing responses<br>**ACTIVE MOVEMENTS**<br>Wide variety; movements becoming more smooth and purposeful |
| 40 Weeks | **RESTING POSTURES**<br>All four extremities are held in flexion; flexor tone of preterm infant who has reached the equivalent of full-term infant is never as good as that of the term infant<br>**RESPONSE TO HANDLING**<br>Preterm infant now resists full extension of knees, hips, and shoulders<br>Preterm infant recoils arms within 2 to 3 seconds after release by examiner, flexing them at elbows at an angle of $< 100$ degrees<br>Preterm infant lacks shoulder muscle tone of the full-term infant, thus may be unable to maintain head alignment with body when pulled to sitting position<br>In supported standing position, preterm infant can usually bear weight on legs but may not yet be able to reciprocally step like the full-term infant<br>**ACTIVE MOVEMENTS**<br>Active movements become smooth and purposeful<br>Neonatal primary reflexes have become consistent and complete in the preterm infant<br>Preterm infant who has reached the equivalent of a full-term infant generally moves in greater ranges than the full-term infant because the preterm infant has less flexor hypertonicity |

in a narrow and elongated "premie-shaped" head. Head flattening has implications for infant attractiveness and may affect social attachment (Semmler, 1989). Shoulder retraction and scapular adduction are common upper-extremity external rotation deformities. A persistent "W" arm position can interfere with forearm propping in prone position, affecting subsequent prone skills and development of shoulder cocontraction necessary for distal fine motor control, as well as reaching against gravity and midline hand play in supine and sitting positions. Lower-extremity external rotation deformities, common when legs rest on the surface in a "frogged" or "M" shape, can produce a significantly outtoeing gait. External tibial torsion, or rotation of the tibia, and decreased depth of the rib cage have also been noted in NICU graduates.

***Positioning considerations.*** Medical and developmental advantages and disadvantages of various positioning options are summarized in Table 22-7; direct citations are included because medical staff have requested references for positioning recommendations. General positioning goals remain essentially unchanged since positioning guidelines were described for preterm infants (Case, 1985), as listed below:

*Young preterm infants* (28 to 35 weeks postconceptional age) (Figure 22-10)

▲ To use proprioceptive input to provide a sense of containment and security

▲ To assist or facilitate a flexed posture and flexor movement in the extremities

▲ To assist in calming and organizing the disorganized infant

▲ To assist in developing hand-to-mouth movements, which are helpful for self-calming

▲ To offer the infant the experience of a variety of well-supported positions

▲ To assist the infant in temperature regulation because a flexed and contained posture reduces exposed body surface

▲ To prevent skin breakdown and maintain skin integrity

▲ To provide vestibular input using a device that is reactive to the infant's own movement, such as a waterbed

*Older preterm infants* (Near term or older postconceptional age) Applicable goals listed for younger infants, plus:

▲ To facilitate movement and to allow activity. Swaddling time can be decreased as containment becomes less important and organized midrange movement is more emphasized

▲ To implement periods of upright positioning in a semiflexed position as an alternative posture, for additional proprioceptive experiences, and for increased visual stimulation

▲ Table 22-6   Neurobehavioral Development of Preterm Infants by Gestational Age

| Neurobehavioral System | Developmental Behaviors |
| --- | --- |
| **INFANTS AT ≤30 WEEKS' GESTATION** | |
| Autonomic | Breathing is irregular and mainly abdominal |
| | Eyelids flutter; limbs twitch and tremor in jerky movements |
| Motor | Reflex smiling and startle response are present |
| | Muscle tone is flaccid. Infant has little head control or back support. Movements are jerky |
| | Infant is unable to coordinate sucking, swallowing, and breathing |
| State | Little state differentiation. Alert or drowsy states are fleeting and not robust |
| | Sleep states predominate, with sleep frequently in a restless undifferentiated state |
| | Rapid eye movement (REM) is apparent as well as continuous tonguing and mouthing |
| | Waking periods occur only in brief intervals |
| Attention/interaction | Visual acuity is poor, with little accommodation |
| | Infant can fixate and follow face, but this is not a common occurrence |
| | When visual stimuli are intense, apnea may result |
| | Hearing is well developed. Preference for mother's voice is possible |
| Self-regulation | Infant may be easily stressed by environmental stimuli |
| **INFANTS AT ≤ 32 WEEKS' GESTATION** | |
| Motor | Overall increase in motor tone with more flexion is apparent |
| | Smooth motor movements are evident |
| | Improved head control is evident |
| State | Regular episodes of active and quiet sleep occur |
| | Active sleep decreases while quiet sleep increases |
| | Movements are sporadic in active sleep |
| | Increase in alert awake time occurs with a decrease in drowsy state |
| **INFANTS AT 34-36 WEEKS' GESTATION** | |
| Autonomic | Color changes accompany most stimulation |
| Motor | Beginning coordination of sucking, swallowing, and breathing is apparent |
| | Head control is not complete |
| | Beginning of leg and trunk support can be noted when infant is held upright |
| State | Quiet sleep is distinguished by slow, regular respiration and little body movement |
| | Overall, less random activity occurs |
| | Active sleep and quiet sleep are clearly defined and alternate regularly |
| | Infant will awaken to stimulation, but awake state is brief |
| | Crying states are more frequent in response to discomfort, pain, or hunger |
| Attention/interaction | Infant can fixate up to 15 seconds on a visual stimulus |
| | Infant may respond briefly to auditory stimulation by turning or widening eyes |
| Self-regulation | Infant may become overaroused when stimulated |
| | Infant can be consoled by swaddling or stroking |
| | Infant may perform hand-to-mouth maneuvers |
| **INFANTS 37 TO 40 WEEKS' GESTATION** | |
| Motor | Infant may support himself or herself when placed upright |
| State | All states of consciousness are evident |
| | Quiet sleep increases with equal periods of active sleep |
| | Crying more closely approximates that of the term infant |
| Attention/interaction | Infant may maintain longer periods of alertness and shows alertness to sound |
| | Infant displays preferences for visual stimuli and tracks objects |

Modified from Yecco, G.J. (1993). Neurobehavioral development and developmental support of premature infants. *Journal of Perinatal and Neonatal Nursing, 7,* 56-65.

▲ To give more consideration to improving neck stability and upper thoracic extension; positioners should have a firmer surface under the upper back to facilitate a neutral trunk as an alternative to the previous total body flexion

▲ To provide a variety of proprioceptive, vestibular, tactile, and visual experiences for the infant
▲ To facilitate symmetry in the infant, particularly the infant who frequently demonstrates asymmetric posturing

▲ Table 22-7  Medical and Developmental Considerations of Positioning Options

| Medical Factors | Developmental Factors |
| --- | --- |
| **PRONE** | |
| **Advantages** | |
| Improved oxygenation and ventilation (despite increased total "work" of breathing) in infants with and without ventilatory support[1,8,16,18,23] | Facilitates development of flexor tone |
| Better gastric emptying than in supine or on left side (unless feeds pool regardless)[25] | Facilitates hand-to-mouth pattern for self-calming |
| Less reflux—especially if head of bed is elevated 30 degrees[3,19,20] | Facilitates active neck extension and head raising |
| Decreased risk of aspiration[11] | Improved coping with extrauterine environment (i.e., if sleep more, cry less)[4] |
| Term and preterm infants sleep more and cry less when prone rather than supine[4,6] | May decrease persistent head turning to the right and skull asymmetry |
| Less energy expenditure when prone rather than supine[17] | |
| Less sleep apnea in prone than in supine in term infants[12] | |
| Best position to expose diaper rash to air or heat lamp | |
| **Disadvantages** | |
| Access for medical care is more difficult | Visual exploration more difficult for baby |
| Agitated or active infant may self-extubate | Face-to-face social contact more difficult |
| **SUPINE** | |
| **Advantages** | |
| Easier access to infant for medical care | Easier visual exploration by infant |
| Supine (in hammock) increases sleep time for preterm infants (vs. "flat" supine)[5] | Supine (in hammock) may facilitate midline position |
| | Easier to position head in midline (than in prone) |
| **Disadvantages** | |
| Decreased arterial oxygen tension, lung compliance, and tidal volume than in prone[1,16,23] | Encourages extension rather than flexion (increased muscle tone with hyperextension of head, neck, and shoulders)[2] |
| More reflux than in prone at any time, or than in upright sitting if infant is awake[19,20] | Encourages external rotation positional deformities of arms and legs (with later delayed hands-to-midline or out-toeing gait) |
| Greater risk of aspiration than in prone or right sidelying[11] | |
| Term and preterm infants sleep less and cry more in supine than prone[4,6] | |
| Supine in hammock may decrease respiration if infant had decreased lung compliance (i.e., respiratory distress syndrome)[5] | |
| Greater energy expenditure in supine than prone[17] | |
| **SIDELYING** | |
| **Advantages** | |
| Right side: better gastric emptying than in supine or left sidelying (about same as prone)[25] | Encourages midline orientation of head and extremities |
| Infant with unilateral lung disease has better oxygenation with good lung positioned uppermost[10] | Counteracts external rotation of limbs; promotes flexion and extremity adduction |
| | Facilitates hand-to-mouth pattern for self-calming |
| | Facilitates hand-to-hand activity |
| **Disadvantages** | |
| Left side: decreased gastric emptying than in prone or right sidelying[25] | May be difficult to maintain flexed position with irritable or hypertonic extended infant |
| **SITTING** | |
| **Advantages** | |
| Alternative position (for variety and skin integrity) | Upright is an alerting posture |
| | Encourages infant visual exploration |
| | Encourages social interaction |
| | May allow use of swing for older neonatal intensive care unit infants |
| | May help temporarily "break up" (relax) high tone |

▲ Table 22-7  Medical and Developmental Considerations of Positioning Options—cont'd

| Medical Factors | Developmental Factors |
|---|---|
| **Disadvantages** | |
| Infant seat or car seat elevated 60 degrees increased frequency and duration of reflux[20] | May be difficult to properly position baby without slumping or slouching of head and trunk[22] |
| More upright (90 degrees) position increases heart rate and mean arterial pressure in preterm infants[22] | |
| Semireclined position may decrease oxygen saturation in some preterm infants[24] | |

**HEAD POSITION AND MIDLINE POSITION**
**Advantages**

| | |
|---|---|
| Head in midline seems to decrease intracranial pressure/intraventricular hemorrhage[9] | Head in midline may improve head shape |
| Elevation of head of bed 30 degrees may reduce intracranial pressure[9] | Midline positioning reduces asymmetry and encourages development of flexion |
| | Waterbeds (and water pillows) may reduce head flattening[7,13,15,21] |

**Disadvantages**

| | |
|---|---|
| May create pressure sore if too long on firm surface | Head midline positioning is difficult in prone |

1. Alastair, A.H. Ross, K.R., & Russell G. (1979). The effect of posture on ventilation and lung mechanics in preterm and light-for-date infants. *Pediatrics, 64,* 429-432.
2. Anderson, J. & Auster-Liebhaber, J. (1984). Developmental therapy in the neonatal intensive care unit. *Physical and Occupational Therapy in Pediatrics, 4,* 89-106.
3. Blumenthal, I. & Lealman, G.T. (1982). Effect of posture on gastroesophageal reflux in the newborn. *Archives of Diseases of Childhood, 57*(7), 555-556.
4. Bottos, M. & Stafani, D. (1982). Letter. Postural and motor care of the premature baby. *Developmental Medicine and Child Neurology, 24,* 706-707.
5. Bottos, M., Pettenazzo, A., Giancola, G., Stefani, D., Pettena, G., Viscolani, B., & Rubaltelli, F.F. (1985). The effect of a containing position in a hammock versus the supine position on the cutaneous oxygen level in premature and term babies. *Early Human Development, 11,* 265-273.
6. Brackbill, Y., Douthitt, T., & West, H. (1973). Psychophysiologic effects in the neonate of prone versus supine placement. *Journal of Pediatrics, 82,* 82-83.
7. Fay, M.J. (1988). The positive effects of positioning. *Neonatal Network, 8,* 23-28.
8. Fox, M. & Molesky, M. (1990). The effects of prone and supine positioning on arterial oxygen pressure. *Neonatal Network, 8,* 25-29.
9. Goldberg, R.N., Joshi, A., Moscoso, P., & Castillo, T. (1983). The effect of head position on intracranial pressure in the neonate. *Critical Care Medicine, 11*(6), 428-430.
10. Heaf, D. et al. (1983). Postural effects of gas exchange in infants. *New England Journal of Medicine, 308,* 1505-1508.
11. Hewitt, V. (1976). Effect of posture on the presence of fat in tracheal aspirate in neonates. *Australian Paediatric Journal, 12,* 267.
12. Hoshimoto, T. et al. (1983). Postural effects on behavioral states of newborn infants: a sleep polygraph study. *Brain Development, 5,* 286-291.
13. Kramer, L.I. & Pierpont, M.E. (1976). Rocking waterbeds and auditory stimuli to enhance growth of preterm infants. *Journal of Pediatrics, 88*(2), 297-299.
14. Mansell, A., Bryan, C., & Levison, H. (1972). Airway closure in children. *Journal of Applied Physiology, 33,* 711-714.
15. Marsden, D.J. (1980). Reduction of head flattening in preterm infants. *Developmental Medicine and Child Neurology, 22,* 507-509.
16. Martin, R.J., Herrell, N., Rubin, D., & Fanaroff, A. (1979). Effect of supine and prone positions on arterial oxygen tension in the preterm infant. *Pediatrics, 63*(4), 528-531.
17. Masterson, J., Zucker, C., & Schulze, K. (1987). Prone and supine positioning effects on energy expenditure and behavior of low birth weight neonates. *Pediatrics, 80*(5), 689-692.
18. Mendoza, J., Roberts, J., & Cook, L. (1991). Postural effects on pulmonary function and heart rate of preterm infants with lung disease. *Journal of Pediatrics, 118,* 445-448.
19. Meyers, W.F. & Herbst, J.J. (1982). Effectiveness of position therapy for gastroesophageal reflux. *Pediatrics, 69*(6), 768-772.
20. Orenstein, S., Whitington, P., & Orenstein, D. (1983). The infant seat as treatment for gastroesophageal reflux. *New England Journal of Medicine, 309,* 760-763.
21. Schwirian, P., Eesley, T., & Cuellar, L. (1986). Use of water pillows in reducing head shape distortion in preterm infants. *Research in Nursing and Health, 9,* 203-207.
22. Smith, P. & Turner, B. (1990). The physiologic effects of positioning premature infants in car seats. *Neonatal Network, 9,* 11-15.
23. Wagaman, M.J., Shutack, J.G., Moomjian, A.S., Schwartz, J.G., Shaffer, T.H., & Foz, W.W. (1979). Improved oxygenation and lung compliance with prone positioning of neonates. *Journal of Pediatrics, 94*(5), 787-791.
24. Willett, L. et al. (1986). Risk of hypoventilation in premature infants in car seats. *Journal of Pediatrics, 109,* 245-248.
25. Yu, V.Y.H. (1975). Effect of body position on gastric emptying in the neonate. *Archives of Diseases in Childhood, 50,* 500-504.

## Feeding

Term neonates are generally robust infants with well-developed central nervous systems and strong physiologic flexion that allow them to adjust to the demands of oral feeding (breast or bottle, nipple type, differences in caregivers or surrounding environment). Preterm infants in the NICU, however, may experience feeding difficulties from a variety of causes (Hunter, 1990b). Neurologic immaturity may reduce the infant's ability to adapt to extrauterine demands and to coordinate suck, swallow, and breathing. Central nervous system insults, such as from intraventricular hemorrhage or repeated hypoxic incidents, may cause neurologic damage that presents as feeding dysfunction. Acute or chronic illness may result in feeding or digestive problems, especially if respiratory or gastrointestinal function is compromised. Low–birth-weight infants often lack fatty sucking pads that contribute to sucking efficiency and may have lower energy reserves to complete oral feeds. Oral hypersensitivity may develop because of aversive caregiving tasks such as frequent oral suctioning or insertion of orogastric tubes. NICU environments and routines that disturb or ignore individual infant biorhythms may also negatively impact feeding performance.

Nonnutritive sucking (NNS), or "dry" sucking such as on a fist or pacifier, is present but disorganized in infants younger than 30 weeks; sucking rhythm generally improves by 30 to 32 weeks postconception. NNS has been described as a self-soothing activity that improves state control, reduces stress, promotes weight gain, improves oxygenation, and increases arousal (Kimble, 1992; Pickler & Frankel, 1995). NNS is frequently used to support and calm an infant during stressful procedures, although it has been suggested that perhaps the pacifier should not be given until after the painful part of the procedure has been initiated so the baby does not learn to associate the pacifier with "pain is coming" (D'Apolito, 1993). NNS during gavage feedings has been recommended to increase maturation of the sucking reflex, decrease intestinal transit time, improve weight gain, and facilitate transition from gavage to oral feeds (Bernbaum, Pereira, Watkins, & Peckman, 1983). A recent study, however, showed no weight gain with NNS during gavage feeds (Ernst et al., 1989).

Some preterm infants do well with feeding by mouth from the beginning, and many of the remainder have only transient feeding difficulties that improve with maturation. A transitional pattern of shorter sucking bursts (3 to 10 sucks per burst, as compared with a mature pattern of 10 to 30 sucks per burst), pauses of equal length, and apneic episodes after the longer bursts have been reported in preterm infants (Meier & Anderson, 1987; Palmer, 1993). This disorganized transitional pattern results from the immature infant's inability to coordinate respiration with sustained sucking and swallowing (Glass & Wolf, 1993; Palmer, 1993; VandenBerg, 1995). Disorganization often persists in the infant with chronic respiratory illness because

the need to breathe supercedes the infant's efforts to suck.

Autonomic, motor, and state stability are also important prerequisites for oral feeding (Glass & Wolf, 1994). The infant with hypotonia or hypertonia and the infant who has difficulty maintaining an awake, alert state display feeding problems rooted in neurobehavioral disorganization, not in actual sucking mechanics. There is increasing evidence that infant neurobehavioral control improves when individualized developmental care is provided throughout the NICU stay and that this increased organization helps the infant to orally feed more successfully (Als et al., 1986; Als et al, 1994).

## Families

The admission of a neonate to the NICU usually puts that family in crisis. Intense and confusing emotions can result from many factors (Shellabarger & Thompson, 1993). The delivery was often unexpected, and the family unit is now separated. Some mothers have continued physical complications or illness from the pregnancy or delivery. Parental shock, denial, and grief over loss of the ideal birth and perfect baby are compounded by concerns for the recovery of a critically ill infant. The appearance of the baby and of the NICU can be frightening. Unknown staff and unfamiliar terminology can hinder communication. Many areas of control are relinquished to medical staff.

The new mother and father are unprepared and uncertain how to parent an infant in the NICU. The primary roles of the occupational therapist are to support these families throughout the hospitalization, to promote attachment between infant and family, and to facilitate effective parenting within the NICU and after hospital discharge. Methods to address these goals are included on p. 622.

The many facets of understanding and working with families who have an ill or special needs child are discussed in depth in Chapter 5. Guidelines for family-centered neonatal care developed by parents are presented in the box on p. 603. The authors of the guidelines are a group of articulate parents of former NICU infants with varying problems and outcomes; not all infants survived. Their guidelines provoke thought, agreement, and controversy among NICU staff.

## NEONATAL EVALUATION IN THE NICU
### General Guidelines

As in all practice areas of occupational therapy, a good evaluation facilitates appropriate intervention. In the NICU, however, special caution must be exercised to avoid harm to fragile infants. The following general guidelines help the neonatal therapist begin an evaluation in a positive framework.

1. Safety for the infant takes priority over convenience for the therapist in all aspects of initial and ongoing evaluation.
2. A new evaluation tool should be learned by reading

## Principles for Family-Centered Neonatal Care

These principles were developed by a group of parents of former neonatal intensive care unit (NICU) infants to encourage families to participate as fully as possible in caring for and making decisions for their hospitalized newborns, to help caregivers respect the diversity of family values and beliefs, and to help parents and professionals form mutually beneficial and supportive partnerships in the NICU and beyond. Neonatologists, pediatric surgeons, and others who care for imperiled newborns must recognize the life-long impact of their treatment decisions on their patients and their patients' families.

1. Family-centered neonatal care should be based on open and honest communication between parents and professionals on medical and ethical issues.

2. To work with professionals in making informed treatment choices, parents must have available to them the same facts and interpretation of those facts as the professionals, including medical information presented in meaningful formats, information about uncertainties surrounding treatments, information from parents whose children have been in similar medical situations, and access to the chart and rounds discussions.

3. In medical situations involving high mortality and morbidity, great suffering, or significant medical controversy, fully informed parents should have the right to make decisions regarding aggressive treatment for their infants. Supportive care provided by family and staff should be recognized as a valid and humane alternative to aggressive treatment when the benefit of aggressive treatment is in doubt.

4. Expectant parents should be offered information about adverse pregnancy outcomes and be given the opportunity to state in advance their treatment preferences if their baby is born extremely premature or critically ill.

5. Parents and professionals must work together to acknowledge and alleviate the pain of infants in intensive care.

6. Parents and professionals must work together to ensure an appropriate environment for babies in the NICU.

7. Parents and professionals should work together to ensure the safety and efficacy of neonatal treatments (advocates research to distinguish harmful from beneficial treatments).

8. Parents and professionals should work together to develop nursery policies and programs that promote parenting skills and encourage maximum involvement of families with their hospitalized infants.

9. Parents and professionals must work together to promote meaningful long-term, follow-up care for all high-risk NICU survivors.

10. Parents and professionals must acknowledge that critically ill newborns can be harmed by overtreatment as well as by undertreatment and must insist that laws and treatment policies be based on compassion. They must work together to promote awareness of the needs of NICU survivors with disabilities to ensure adequate support for them and their families and to decrease disability through universal prenatal care.

Modified from Harrison, H. (1993). The principles for family centered neonatal care. *Pediatrics, 92,* 643-650.

---

(and rereading) the manual, observing a colleague evaluate appropriate infants of varying ages and medical status, practicing on a doll, and then on healthy term infants before actually evaluating a premature infant.

3. Baseline information can be gathered before the evaluation. This may include the following:
   a. General information
      (1) Demographics: names of baby and parents, home address, and telephone
      (2) Socioeconomic and family history: married or single, age and sex of other children, availability of family support, potential obstacles to successful parenting in NICU (distance, finances, illness, emotional or cognitive status, language barriers, other responsibilities)
   b. Medical history
      (1) Pertinent maternal/prenatal history: maternal age, previous pregnancies, prenatal care, history of substance abuse, pregnancy complications, medications before or at time of delivery
      (2) Birth history: date of birth, gestational age, resuscitation efforts required, Apgar scores, birth weight
      (3) Subsequent significant medical history: postnatal medical complications, surgeries, necessity for prolonged intubation or nasal continuous positive airway pressure, nutritional support, feeding tolerance, congenital anomalies, known or suspected genetic abnormalities
   c. Current status
      (1) Unresolved medical complications, recent medical procedures, medical equipment in use, feeding method and schedule, current medications
      (2) Level of physiologic homeostasis: vital signs, medical support, reported and observed tolerance to caregiving, current state

4. Observations should be used extensively, including routine astute clinical observation of the baby and surrounding environment, before the infant is touched.

5. The value of the evaluation procedures should be weighed against any potential stressful effect on infant: what is truly necessary and important?

6. The bedside nurse knows recent or upcoming stressful events of which the therapist may not be aware (e.g., placement of intravenous line or eye examination). The role of the nurse in protecting the baby should be appreciated and clearance obtained for evaluation if the baby will be handled.

7. The evaluation should be scheduled according to the infant's sleep cycle, feeding schedule, caregiving routine, and medical status.

8. Unnecessary duplication of any evaluation procedures that require handling should be avoided. If more than one professional is active as a developmental specialist (i.e., child psychologist, occupational or physical therapist, or speech pathologist), a joint evaluation can be performed.

9. Infant signs of stress during handling must be respected. If the baby has difficulty returning to a calm organized state even with caregiver assistance, the assessment should be completed at a later date.

10. Performing the evaluation is often easier than accurately analyzing the results; overinterpretation and mistaking immaturity for a pathologic condition are frequent errors among new therapists. Routine ongoing reassessment in the NICU and in a follow-up clinic as infants mature and heal is essential for developing sound clinical judgment on the meaning of early clinical findings.

## Potential Evaluation Components

### Environment

*Macro environment.* General lighting, noise, and activity level of the room should be noted. The number of babies and the severity of their illnesses can affect these environmental factors as well as the stress level of the NICU staff.

*Micro environment.* The therapist notes where the infant is located (e.g., in a high-traffic area, near sinks or telephones, near frequently sounding alarms or crying infants, or by a window). The therapist also asks questions such as the following: Is the bed space protected from excessive light and sound? Are positioning aids available and being used consistently and effectively? Are personal items such as a family photograph, drawing by a sibling, quilt, or special toy present? Is there room for the family to visit comfortably and with any privacy?

### NICU Staff Concerns

The current caregiving priorities of NICU physicians and nurses are important to recognize and follow. The therapist

may be eager for results of a needed neurology or orthopedics consult, but medical staff may defer writing the consults until the infant is stable after surgery. The occupational therapist may have scheduled a feeding evaluation for noon, but the nurse is concerned because the infant has had increased apnea since a medical procedure that morning. Staff might appreciate intensive therapist involvement with one family, but on occasion request that information only be given through a few key people with another family because of evident confusion or manipulation. The competent neonatal occupational therapist does not work in isolation but collaborates and supports the team's agenda for the infant's benefit.

### Neurobehavioral Organization

*State.* State refers to the degree of consciousness or arousal (Figure 22-11). In a preterm infant, the state significantly affects other areas such as muscle tone, feeding performance, or reaction to stimuli. State is most frequently classified into six categories (Als, 1982):

*State 1:* Deep sleep. Eyes are closed with no rapid-eye movement (REM). Breathing is regular. Movement is absent except for isolated startles.

*State 2:* Light sleep. Eyes are closed; rapid eye movements may be observed under the eyelids. Breathing may be irregular. Movements are more frequent. There is increased responsivity to external stimuli.

*State 3:* Transitional state of dozing or drowsiness. Eyes open and close, appearing heavy-lidded. Activity level is variable. The infant in a transitional state either returns to deeper sleep or becomes increasingly alert

*State 4:* Quiet alert. Eyes are open and movement is minimal. Quality of the quiet alert state is important. An infant with bright-eyed "robust" alertness is in an optimal state to attend and interact with specific environ-

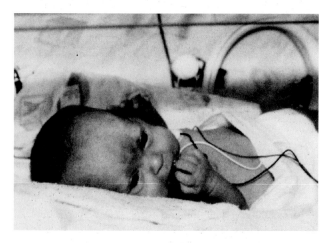

**Figure 22-11** This calm and alert preterm infant is in appropriate state of arousal for therapist to assess her ability to attend and interact with specific environmental stimuli. (Courtesy of the Infant Special Care Unit, University of Texas Medical Branch, Galveston, TX, photo by Dottie James.)

mental stimuli. Conversely, an infant may be in state 4 but unavailable for interaction if the alertness is of poor quality. This is generally noted as a diffuse, low-level alertness with a dull glassy-eyed gaze or a hyper-alertness with a wide-eyed stare that makes the infant appear somewhat panicked (Als, 1982).

*State 5:* Active alert. Eyes are open, and motor activity is increased. The infant may be fussy without really crying and often is unable to focus and interact with specific stimuli.

*State 6:* Crying. Eyes may be open or closed, motor activity is increased, and the infant is obviously distressed. The cry may be lusty with a stable or larger infant, weak in a preterm infant, or inaudible in an intubated infant. Autonomic and motor stress signals are common (Table 22-3).

The therapist should also note the infant's transition between states both spontaneously and with handling. The infant who cannot be aroused, who is excessively irritable, or who swings abruptly between sleep and crying states with no alert periods may be demonstrating immaturity or a pathologic condition. A gradual awakening with smooth transition from sleep to alertness and eventually back to sleep is one sign of maturation and neurologic integrity. This is especially true if accomplished by the infant without excessive facilitation by the caregiver. (Note: Individual temperament may be a variable; some infants are simply more demanding, and others are more relaxed.) Neurobehavioral evaluations are often initiated during sleep to allow observation of the infant's transition between states as the infant is handled.

Noting (or charting over time) the infant's sleep-wake cycles can give important information for planning caregiving. As previously mentioned, however, caregiving frequently interrupts the sleep of an NICU infant and may interfere with development of a consistent sleep-wake cycle.

***Neurobehavioral subsystem maturation.*** Signs of stress and stability in the infant's autonomic, motor, state, and attention-interaction subsystems can be observed while the baby is alone or during any type of caregiving. It is helpful to watch the baby after caregiving is completed because signs of stress may be delayed for 5 to 10 minutes. The infant's efforts and degree of success with self-regulation strategies (Table 22-3) should be noted at the same time, as well as how much assistance the caregiver must provide to help a disorganized infant settle down. These observations can be informal as occasions arise or structured within a formal neonatal assessment; they should also be incorporated into all occupational therapy services for ongoing evaluation. Assessment of an infant during a parent's caregiving is generally best if done subtly and unobtrusively to avoid increasing parental anxiety. A collaborative approach in which an informed parent and therapist watch the infant together to learn more about that baby's communication may be helpful. Correlation of these observations with

stages of neurosocial development (Table 22-4) may help clarify the status of a particular infant regarding availability for interaction.

***Response to stimuli.*** Assessing response to stimuli is multifaceted. Habituation in preterm infants is usually tested while the infant is asleep, with maturation improving the infant's ability to tune out repetitive stimuli of light or sound. A flashlight is shined into the baby's eyes or a rattle is sharply shaken by the baby's ears once every 5 seconds for 10 repetitions or until responses (e.g., changes of facial expression, startles, or squirming) stop.

Sensory threshold refers to the level of stimuli the infant can tolerate and respond to appropriately. When this threshold is exceeded, the infant becomes overstimulated and shows signs of stress and fatigue (Witt & Rusk, 1993). Preterm infants typically tolerate a single stimulus better than several types of stimuli simultaneously applied.

The tactile system is functional in preterm infants, who may respond to stimuli positively or negatively (approach or avoidance). The therapist evaluates the infant's responses to various tactile stimuli. The same infant who responds with stress to light stroking may relax as the caregiver's hands gently contain his or her body or when cuddled on his or her parent's chest.

The vestibular system is constantly activated in the fluid intrauterine environment. Preterm birth dramatically changes this movement experience. The immaturity of the motor system and decreased muscle tone combine with the effects of gravity to reduce the infant's ability to produce smooth movements and position changes. The therapist notes what types of handling (e.g., with extremities con-

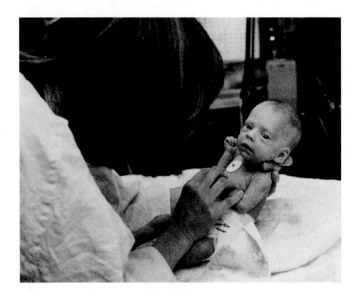

**Figure 22-12** Assessment of preterm infants includes evaluation of neuromotor and neurobehavioral functioning. (Courtesy of the Neonatal Intensive Care Unit, University of Connecticut Health Center's John N. Dempsey Hospital, Farmington, CT. Photograph by Gregory Kriss.)

▲ **Table 22-8** Reflex Development in Preterm Infants

| Reflex | Gestational Age (in Weeks) | | | | | | | |
| --- | --- | --- | --- | --- | --- | --- | --- | --- |
| | 23 to 24 | 25 to 26 | 27 to 28 | 30 | 32 | 35 | 37 |
| Palmar grasp | Slight, latent | Improving | Localized | Less latency, vigorous in fingers and wrists | Stronger traction begins | Firm, effective; head does not follow traction | Vigorous except for neck |
| Galant | Strong | Strong | Strong | Strong | Strong | Strong | Strong |
| Rooting | Incomplete | Slight, yawn, upper lip and sides | Yawn, 3 phases, no lower lip | Incomplete fourth phase, poor head extension | Complete, intense, long lasting | Perfect, head extension still weak | Perfect, weak head extension |
| Sucking | Arrhythmic, brief | Improving | Chewing motions | Better synchrony | Active, good | Better, expresses hunger | Like full-term |
| Gag and swallow | Absent | Absent | Tongue protrusion | Suck and swallow not coordinated with breathing | Active, fair | Better | Like full-term |
| Moro | Minimal (hand only) | Better, slight upper extremity extension | Present, upper extremity extension, no abduction | Vigorous, easily elicited | Complete abduction/ extension upper extremities | Complete, brisk | Perfect |
| Plantar grasp | Absent | Constant | Constant | Constant | Constant | Constant | Constant |
| Automatic walking | Absent | Trace | Improving | Improving | Present, tiptoes | Present, not sustained | Automatic, full plantar support |
| Crossed extension | Absent | Questionable | Contralateral defense reaction | Improving | Flexion/extension good, abduction beginning | More like full-term | Complete, begins toe fanning |
| Doll's eye | Absent | Absent | Absent | Absent | Beginning | Present | Present |
| Placing | Absent | Absent | Absent | Absent | Absent | Weak | Appears |

Modified from Dargassies, S.S. (1977). *Neurological development in the full-term and premature neonate.* New York: Excerpter Medica.

tained or movements slow and gentle) reduce the infant's stress responses to caregiving that involves vestibular stimuli.

Once an infant has autonomic, motor, and state stability with good quality alertness, attention and interaction capabilities can be assessed (Figure 22-12). The preterm infant can visually focus and track by 32 to 33 weeks but may become stressed by the effort. Auditory responses may be a primitive startle, an alerting response without orientation (i.e., eyes widen or shift), or a more mature head turning toward the sound. Auditory response may be dampened in a noisy NICU. Social stimuli are frequently multimodal, meaning multiple types of simultaneous input. A mother might have eye contact (visual) and be singing (auditory) while holding (tactile) and rocking (vestibular) her baby. The infant's tolerance and response should be closely monitored, with adjustments made as needed to avoid exceeding the baby's threshold for stimuli.

### Neuromotor

***Reflex development.*** Reflex testing is one method for therapists to assess an infant's maturation and nervous system integrity (Table 22-8). Generalized reflex testing can be extremely stressful for NICU infants, however, and must be approached cautiously. Unless an infant has a known or suspected neuromuscular pathologic condition (e.g., severe perinatal asphyxia, periventricular leukomalacia, spina bifida, or congenital hypotonia), full reflex testing is probably unnecessary. The benefit of the information to the therapist must be weighed against the potential "cost" to the infant. The decision always favors the baby. Partial reflex assessment, such as grasp, suck, or head righting, can often be completed within the context of normal handling. Responses that are absent, hyperactive, or asymmetric should be noted.

***Muscle tone.*** Muscle tone must be evaluated within the contexts of postconceptional age, distribution of tone, state of arousal, medical status, and function. Muscle tone increases with age and in a foot-to-head direction; this is true both for passive flexor tone seen at rest and the active tone elicited by righting reactions when the baby is handled (Amiel-Tison & Grenier, 1986). State is a significant variable; a premature infant may be active and feisty when awake but appear hypotonic if assessed in deep sleep. Muscle tone cannot be accurately assessed in an acutely ill infant except for that point in time; the underlying muscle tone usually changes as the infant recovers. The influence of muscle tone on resting posture and quantity or quality of movement is an extremely important observation and has implications for positioning and caregiving needs. Atypical findings inconsistent with the factors listed previously, or asymmetric responses should be noted and monitored. Often unusual patterns resolve with maturation and physical recovery.

***Need for therapeutic positioning.*** All NICU infants can benefit from therapeutic positioning, as per the positioning guidelines listed on pp. 618 to 620. The therapist should check for the presence or absence of common premature infant deformities, such as lateral skull flattening (dolio-cephaly), shoulder retraction and external rotation, hip abduction and external rotation, and ankle eversion, are evaluated. When correctly positioned, extremities generally should be gently flexed with midline orientation within surrounding boundaries (e.g., those created by blanket rolls or Bendy bumpers). The therapist determines whether positioning aids are available and used correctly.

Positioning may need modification to accommodate medical equipment or conditions. Conventional phototherapy requires more exposed body surface, unless a fiberoptic "bili blanket" is available. The multiple lines and needs for caregiver access to a supine infant may restrict positioning options during extracorporeal membrane oxygenation (ECMO) (Figure 22-13). An infant with severe chest retractions from respiratory distress is often more stable in prone position. Generalized edema may limit flexion of the extremities. The small jaw and recessed tongue of an infant with Pierre-Robin syndrome may result in airway obstruction if that infant is placed in a supine position. The prone position is not an optimal position for an infant with significant abdominal distention or who has recently had abdominal surgery, and the supine position is not an option for an infant with a newly resected myelomeningocele. Extremity contractures associated with arthrogryposis multiplex congenita can make any therapeutic positioning a challenge, although use of gravity and body weight for gentle sustained stretch can make positioning a treatment option with some of these infants.

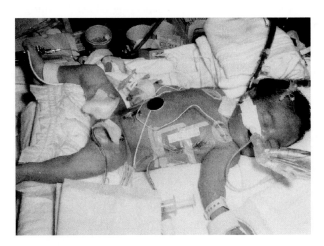

**Figure 22-13** Critically ill infant on extracorporeal membrane oxygenation (ECMO). Medical considerations may supercede positioning goals during critical periods of care. (Courtesy of the Infant Special Care Unit, University of Texas Medical Branch, Galveston, TX.)

## Feeding

Evaluation and management of feeding dysfunction is addressed in Chapter 16. Wolf and Glass (1992) presented a structured format for evaluating feeding in young infants. Another feeding evaluation appropriate for the NICU population is the Neonatal Oral-Motor Assessment Scale, or NOMAS (Palmer, Crawley, & Blanco, 1993). The NOMAS classifies characteristics of jaw and tongue movement into categories of normal, disorganized, and dysfunctional. Disorganization is associated with age and generally improves with maturation; dysfunction has not correlated with gestational or postconceptional age. The NOMAS can help distinguish disorganization from dysfunction during early feeding and measure intervention effectiveness with poor feeders in the NICU. Disorganized and dysfunctional neonatal sucking patterns have correlated with later speech and language delays (Crawley, Lindner, & Braun, 1987).

### Family

Evaluation of family concerns and priorities is primarily to establish how the therapist might best offer support and facilitate a successful infant-parent relationship. Families are in crisis; judgmental opinions are inappropriate. Effective and satisfying parenting of an infant in the NICU is not an easy task; the occupational therapist has an ideal role and unique skills to help parents succeed. The following factors should be evaluated:

▲ Resources and concerns of the parents as related to successful and satisfying NICU parenting. This may include such issues as maternal health, attachment, relationships with NICU staff, active involvement in the infant's care plan and caregiving, availability and strength of support systems, availability of transportation or housing near the baby, and additional job or family responsibilites

▲ Parents' coping mechanisms and learning styles relevant to fostering successful and satisfying NICU parenting

▲ Parents' understanding and skill in recognizing and appropriately responding to their infant's neurobehavioral cues

▲ Parents' understanding and skill in providing therapeutic positioning, developmentally supportive handling, appropriate sensory modulation and stimulation, and nurturance

▲ Parents' understanding and skill in facilitating functional oral feeding by the infant

▲ Parents' understanding and skill in meeting the infant's long-term developmental needs. The therapist identifies if additional assistance is likely to be required after hospital discharge

### Neonatal Assessments

Although usually containing the above components, occupational therapy neonatal assessments may differ somewhat among institutions. Many therapists use a structured assessment that is supplemented with data gathering and clinical

observations relevant to occupational therapy. There are several structured neonatal evaluations from which to choose, some that require specialized training and others that may be learned independently (see box, p. 610, and Table 22-9).

## INTERVENTION IN THE NICU
### Environmental Modifications

The small sick infant experiences significant physiologic stress (e.g., agitation, autonomic instability, and excessive use of calories) when incoming stimuli exceed the immature nervous systems ability to respond. A primary intervention goal for this infant is to avoid costly stress and promote more stable calm states. This is achieved by modifying environmental light and sound, by reducing handling, and by altering caregiver techniques so that the infant is protected from stressful stimuli and allowed to remain quiet and inactive.

The process of recommending and implementing environmental modifications is obviously expedited if change is a physician mandate. Nursing-driven efforts may take somewhat longer if physician acceptance is not initially present, but can also be highly successful. Visions of change held primarily by developmental therapists generally require the most time, patience, and staff-education efforts, but have led to significant improvements in many NICUs.

### Light

NICU lighting must provide protection to the infant without compromising safety. The optimal lighting levels that provide this balance have not yet been determined. Current NICU lighting levels differ significantly among institutions and even among shifts in the same hospital, often reflecting the habits and preferences of individual nurses and doctors and sometimes producing great potential for conflict.

General lowering of ambient room light and shielding of each infant's bed space are recommended practices. (NANN, 1993; Oehler, 1993; VandenBerg, 1995) (Figure 22-3). Day and night cycles of light, noise, and caregiving may have implications for physiologic gains (longer sleep, less time feeding, and better weight gain) and earlier synchronization of behavioral rhythms with the environment (Mann, Haddow, Stokes, Goodley, & Rutter, 1986; Sisson, 1990). The ability to visually attend emerges at 32 to 34 weeks postconception and is enhanced in low lighting. Providing opportunities for spontaneous eye opening in dim or dark conditions might be advantageous after this age (Glass, 1993). Specific modifications to protect NICU infants from excessive bright light are discussed in the box on p. 612.

### Sound

Theoretically, sound in the NICU should be fairly easy to reduce. Information is available on sound levels of some NICU equipment and events; individual units can monitor to locate their specific sources of noise. Use of available

▲ Table 22-9  Neonatal Assessments Requiring Certification for Administration

| Assessment | Contact |
|---|---|
| **NATURALISTIC OBSERVATIONS OF NEWBORN BEHAVIOR (NONB)**<br>Based on Als' Synactive Theory of Development<br>For preterm and term infants too fragile for handling<br>Structured observations of specific behaviors are repeated at 2-minute intervals before, during, and after routine caregiving. Assesses the maturation and interplay of infant neurobehavioral subsystems (autonomic, motor, state, attention and interaction, and self-regulation) as evidenced by behavioral cues to environmental and caregiving events over time. Signs of stress and stability can be catalogued as avoidance or approach behaviors, and attempts at self-organization (including failure, success, and cost of the effort) are noted. The degree of caregiver facilitation required to promote infant neurobehavioral organization may be observed if developmentally supportive care is being provided<br>Neonatal Individualized Developmental Care and Assessment Program (NIDCAP) Level 1 | Heidelise Als, PhD<br>Enders Pediatric Research Laboratories<br>320 Longwood Avenue<br>Boston, MA 02115 |
| **ASSESSMENT OF PRETERM INFANT BEHAVIOR (APIB)**<br>Based on Als' Synactive Theory of Development<br>For stable preterm (> 30 to 32 weeks) and term infants<br>Complex assessment that provides an integrated subsystem profile of the infant, identifying current level of functioning with varying environmental demands. The therapist handles the infant in a stuctured progression of test items to assess neurobehavioral organization and methods of attaining self-regulation, as well as the type and amount of caregiver support needed for the infant to achieve and maintain organized behavior<br>Used more as a research tool than for everyday clinical purposes<br>NIDCAP Level II | Heidelise Als, PhD<br>Enders Pediatric Research Laboratories<br>320 Longwood Avenue<br>Boston, MA 02115 |
| **NEONATAL BEHAVIORAL ASSESSMENT SCALE (NBAS)**<br>For term healthy infants (used in 36- to 44-week range)<br>Evaluates infant neurobehavioral capabilities within the context of a dynamic relationship with the caregiver. Supplemental items can be used with high-risk infants<br>Provided the model for the Assessment of Preterm Infant Behavior<br>Used more as a research tool than for everyday clinical purposes | J. Kevin Nugent, PhD<br>300 Longwood Avenue<br>Boston, MA 02115 |
| **INFANT BEHAVIORAL ASESSMENT (IBA)**<br>From birth to 6 months of age; can be used for follow-up<br>Evaluates infants within the synactive theory framework to sensitize parents or caregivers to the infant's behavioral states and organizational abilities so caregiver interactions can be modified accordingly | Rodd Hedlund, MEd<br>Mary Tatarka, MS, PT<br>Child Development and Mental Retardation Unit<br>WJ-10 University of Washington<br>Seattle, WA 98195 |

Note: Each certification process requires formal training and assessment of rater reliability.

acoustic materials provides benefits with minimal staff effort. Staff-generated, high-frequency noise from laughter and conversation requires only staff restraint for instant reduction but may be surprisingly difficult to change. Staff education, unit policies, peer pressure, and patience may all prove helpful. Modifications to protect NICU infants from excessive sound levels are described in the box on p. 613.

### Caregiving

*General principles for individualized caregiving.*
Timing and technique of all caregiver interventions should

strive to minimize avoidable stress to the infant and assist the baby in self-regulation efforts. Table 22-10 summarizes considerations for caregiving planning related to infant state of arousal. The following general principles of individualized developmental care provide clinical guidelines for caregiving:

▲ Interventions must consider how each infant is affected by and responds to environmental factors such as light, noise, touch, movement, position, sleep interruptions, and family presence.
▲ The individual infant (rather than nursery routines)

## Structured Neonatal Assessments That Do Not Require Certification for Administration

### NEUROLOGIC ASSESSMENT OF THE PRETERM AND FULL-TERM NEWBORN INFANT (NAPFI)
#### Description

For preterm and term infants who can tolerate handling. Administered as per Dubowitz manual; can give partial or total assessment based on infant's specific situation.

Designed to record the functional status of an infant's nervous system by assessing habituation, posture, muscle tone, head control, spontaneous movements, abnormal movements, selected reflexes, state transition, level of arousal and alertness, auditory and visual orientation, irritability, consolability, and cry. Provides a baseline at initial assessment to which continued developmental maturation and progression can be compared during sequential assessments.

#### Reference

Dubowitz, L. & Dubowitz V. (1981). The neurological assessment of the preterm and fullterm newborn infant. *Clinics in Developmental Medicine,* No. 79. Philadelphia: J.B. Lippincott.

### NEONATAL NEUROBEHAVIORAL EVALUATION (NNE)
#### Description

For preterm and term infants who can tolerate handling.

Closely resembles the Dubowitz, but can establish quantifiable indicators of the infant's neurobehavioral maturation over time in the areas of tone and motor patterns, reflexes, and behavioral responses. Standardization was done on term infants at 2 days of age and on preterm infants around term equivalency. Training is recommended but not mandatory; contact
Vicky L. Lee, MA, PT
University of Illinois College of Medicine at Peoria
Department of Pediatrics
320 East Armstrong Avenue
Peoria IL 61603

#### Reference

Morgan, A.M., Koch, V., Lee, V., & Aldag, J. (1988). Neonatal neurobehavioral examination: a new instrument for quantitative analysis of neonatal neurological status. *Physical Therapy, 68,* 1352.

### NEUROBEHAVIORAL ASSESSMENT FOR PRETERM INFANTS (NAPI)
#### Description

For medically stable preterm infants functioning in range of the 32 to 42 weeks postconceptional age. Test items were selected from existing evaluations of Amiel-Tison, Brazelton, Dubowitz, and Prechtl. Neurobehavioral areas evaluated include motor development and vigor, scarf sign, popliteal angle, alertness and orientation, irritability, vigor of crying, and percent of time sleeping.

To assess neurobehavioral maturity of infant over time and to detect neurologically suspect performance.

#### Reference

Korner, A.F., Constantinou, J., Dimiceli, S., & Brown, B.W., Jr. (1991). Establishing the reliability and developmental validity of a neurobehavioral assessment for preterm infants: a methodological process. *Child Development, 62,* 1200.

### NEONATAL NEUROLOGICAL EXAMINATION (NEONEURO)
#### Description

For normal and abnormal term infants during the first week of life only; cannot be used with infants born at less than 37 weeks' gestation.

Examines posture, tone, reflexes, and auditory/visual orientation to assess infant's neurologic integrity.

#### Reference

Sheridan Pereira, M., Ellison, P.H., & Helgeson, V. (1991). The construction of a scored neonatal neurological examination for assessment of neurologic integrity in fullterm neonates. *Journal of Developmental and Behavioral Pediatrics, 12,* 25.

▲ Table 22-10   Newborn States and Considerations for Care Giving

| Newborn State | Comments |
|---|---|
| **SLEEP STATES** | |
| Deep sleep (non–rapid eye movement (REM) <br>   Slow state changes <br>   Regular breathing <br>   Eyes closed; no eye movements <br>   No spontaneous activity except startles and jerky movements <br>   Startles with some delay and suppresses rapidly <br>   Lowest oxygen consumption | Baby is very difficult if not impossible to arouse. Baby will not breastfeed or bottle-feed in this state, even after vigorous stimulation. Baby is unable to respond to environment; frustrating for caregivers. <br> Term babies may exhibit a "slow" heart rate (80 to 90 beats per minute), which may trigger heart rate alarms and result in unnecessary stimulation by neonatal intensive care unit staff. <br> At birth, preterm infants have altered states of consciousness: Early dominant states are light sleep, quiet, and active alert. "Protective apathy" enables the preterm to remain inactive, unresponsive, and in a sleep state to conserve energy, grow, and maintain physiologic homeostasis. |
| Light sleep (REM sleep) <br>   Low activity level <br>   Random movements and startles <br>   Respirations irregular and abdominal <br>   Intermittent sucking movements <br>   Eyes closed, rapid eye movement <br>   Higher oxygen consumption | Full-term infants begin and end sleep in active sleep; preterm infants are more responsive (than term infants) to stimuli in active sleep. <br> Babies may cry or fuss briefly in this state and be awakened to feed before they are truly awake and ready to eat. <br> Lower and more variable oxygenation states. |
| **AWAKE STATES** | |
| Drowsy or semidozing <br>   Eyelids fluttering <br>   Eyes open or closed (dazed) <br>   Mild startles (intermittent) <br>   Delayed response to sensory stimuli <br>   Smooth state change after stimulation <br>   Fussing may or may not be present <br>   Respirations—more rapid and shallow | Baby may awaken further or return to sleep (if left alone). <br> Quietly talking and looking at the baby, or offering a pacifier or an inanimate object to see and listen to may arouse the baby to the quiet alert state. <br> Less mature infants (30 weeks) demonstrate a more drowsy than quiet alert state than older infants (36 weeks). |
| Quiet alert, with bright look <br>   Focuses attention on source of stimulation <br>   Impinging stimuli may break through; may have some delay in response <br>   Minimal motor activity | Immediately after birth, term newborns exhibit a period of quiet alertness, their first opportunity to "take in" their parents and the extrauterine environment. Dimmed lights, quiet talking, and stroking optimize this time for parents. <br> Best state for learning to occur, because baby focuses all of attention on visual, auditory, tactile, and sucking stimuli; best state for interaction with parents—baby is maximally able to attend and reciprocally respond to parents. |
| Active alert—eyes open <br>   Considerable motor activity—thrusting movements of extremities; spontaneous startles <br>   Reacts to external stimuli with increase in movements and startles (discrete reactions difficult to differentiate because of general higher activity level) <br>   Respirations irregular <br>   May or may not be fussy | Baby has decreased threshold (increased sensitivity) to internal (hunger, fatigue) and external (wet, noise, handling) stimuli. Baby may quiet self, may escalate to crying, or with consolation by, caretaker may become quiet alert or go to sleep. <br> Baby is unable to maximally attend to caretakers or environment because of increased motor activity and increased sensitivity to stimuli. |
| Crying—intense and difficult to disrupt with external stimuli <br>   Respirations rapid, shallow, and irregular | Crying is infant's response to unpleasant internal and/or external stimulation—infant's tolerance limits have been reached (and exceeded). Baby may be able to quiet self with hand-to-mouth behaviors; talking may quiet a crying baby; holding, rocking, or putting baby upright on caretaker's shoulder may quiet infant. |

From Gardner, (1993). The neonate and the environment: impact on development. In G.B. Merenstein & S.L. Gardner (Eds.). *Handbook of neonatal intensive care* (p. 570). St. Louis: Mosby.

## MACRO ENVIRONMENT: UNIT-BASED MODIFICATION OPTIONS FOR NICU LIGHT

1. Rheostats allow lighting to be dimmed or brightened as needed.
2. Installation of track lighting can allow area illumination with overhead lights dimmed or turned off (see Figure 22-3).
3. Removal of one lighting tube from each bank of fluorescent lights can reduce brightness without compromising visibility when overhead lights are on.
4. Lighting level can be regulated to create day and night cycles, allowing infants longer periods of uninterrupted rest and helping them establish diurnal (day and night) rhythm.
5. If remodeling or designing a new unit is in progress, consider both individual bedside lighting (decreases dependence on room overhead lights), indirect and deflected lighting, and use of natural light from windows.

## MICRO ENVIRONMENT: BEDSIDE MODIFICATION OPTIONS FOR NICU LIGHT

   Protection for individual infants can be achieved at the bedside.
1. Although shielding infants on radiant warmers from light has been attempted by hanging linen from the overhead warming unit, concerns exist about the potential fire hazard from this practice. Safer protection has been provided by draping a blanket over a frame easily fashioned from the moldable rod core removed from the foam body of a Bendy Bumper, available from Children's Medical Ventures; this method does not create a fire risk and does not interfere with ventilator tubing or infant visibility by staff.

2. The oxyhood can be draped with a blanket to protect the infant from light.
3. An isolette cover, thick blankets, or a quilt can be used to partially cover an incubator. Complete covering of the incubator is usually not recommended, especially with unstable infants. Monitors are useful adjuncts in tracking a baby's physiologic status; however staff must be able to see the baby to monitor his or her behaviors (Figure 22-14).
4. If the room is not dim, an infant's eyes can be shielded when the isolette is opened or uncovered and when the baby is removed from the isolette.
5. The infant's eyes should be shielded during tasks and procedures that require increased light.
6. The eyes of an infant undergoing phototherapy are routinely covered, but staff need to routinely check whether eye shields are in place. Neighboring infants should also be protected from this intense light source (Figure 22-15).
7. Eye covers, necessary during phototherapy, are not recommended for routine use in shielding infants from light because preventing eye opening is not normal at any stage of development. A fetus in utero demonstrates eye opening and closing once eyelids are no longer fused.

Modified from Als, H., Lawhon, G., Brown, E., Gibes, R., Duffy, E., McAnulty, G., & Blickman, J. (1986). Individualized behavioral and environmental care for the very low birth weight preterm infant at high risk for bronchopulmonary dysplasia: neonatal intensive care unit and developmental outcome. *Pediatrics, 78,* 1123-1132; Lawhon, G. & Melzar, A. (1988). Developmental care of the very low birth weight infant. *Journal of Pediatric and Neonatal Nursing, 2,* 56-65.

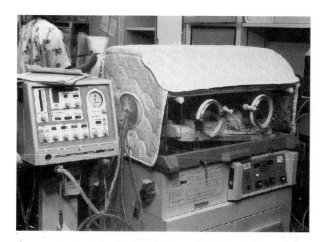

**Figure 22-14**   Isolette cover (Children's Medical Ventures) provides infant protection from room light without eliminating visibility of the infant by neonatal intensive care unit staff. (Courtesy of the Infant Special Care Unit, University of Texas Medical Branch, Galveston, TX. Photograph by John Glow.)

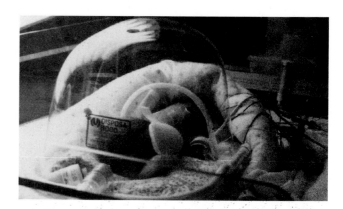

**Figure 22-15** · Preterm infant with protective eye shields during phototherapy for jaundice. Oxygen hood is large enough to encompass upper body and allow hand-to-face (or hand-to-mouth) movement for self-calming. Also, Snuggle-Up provides boundaries for foot bracing but is left open to allow maximal skin exposure to bili lights. (Courtesy of the Infant Special Care Unit, University of Texas Medical Branch, Galveston, TX. Photograph by Al Romeo.)

## Environmental Interventions: Modifying Sound in the NICU

### MACRO ENVIRONMENT: UNIT-BASED MODIFICATION OPTIONS FOR NICU SOUND

1. Installation of bacteriostatic carpet greatly reduces noise level without increased risk of infection. Use of carpet squares can allow area replacement if needed.
2. Acoustic ceiling tiles, soundproof or sound-absorbing building materials, and "pods" that divide space for use by individual or a small number of infants should be considered in remodeling and new unit design.
3. Telephones should be located away from infant care areas. The unit clerk area can be insulated with soundproof walls. The volume of telephone ringing near infants can be lowered.
4. Radios should not be used.
5. Lower levels of lighting seem to automatically reduce the NICU noise level.
6. Staff should be encouraged to lower their speaking volume and tone.
7. A quiet hour can be implemented. During a quiet hour, staff whisper at the bedside, make special efforts not to produce noise, do not allow large equipment to enter the unit, respond quickly to alarms and crying infants, and rearrange caregiving activities to minimize infant disturbances. (Strauch, Brandt, & Edwards-Beckett, 1993). Caution must be taken that the activity level and caregiving after a quiet hour are not so intense and disruptive that the benefits of a quiet hour are negated; some units believe that a quiet hour is not necessary if 24-hour developmental care is well implemented (not a universal reality at present).
8. Instructional parent and staff videos can be viewed away from patient areas.
9. Environmental sound levels in the unit must be monitored to determine noise levels and their sources to help identify successful modifications and additional interventions needed.

### MICRO ENVIRONMENT: BEDSIDE MODIFICATION OPTIONS FOR NICU SOUND

1. The infant's isolette can be located away from sinks, telephones, and high-traffic areas.
2. The monitors and pumps should be positioned an optimal distance from the infant's head.
3. The volume of alarms can be reduced.
4. Alarms should be silenced as quickly as possible to reduce exposure to noise; remote control devices may be available in some NICUs.
5. Respiratory tubing and water traps should be positioned to promote drainage. Accumulated water should be frequently drained to prevent bubbling.
6. Incubator covers may also have sound-absorbing qualities.
7. The front opening and portholes of incubators should be gently closed.
8. Conversations, including medical rounds, should be held away from bedside.
9. Plastic rather than metal trash cans should be installed. Trash can lids can be padded (e.g., with foam-backed temperature probe cover at each end of contact edge).
10. Musical toys and tape recordings can reverberate inside the isolette; the volume should be low.

Modified from Als, H., Lawhon, G., Brown, E., Gibes, R., Duffy, E., McAnulty, G., & Blickman, J. (1986). Individualized behavioral and environmental care for the very low birth weight preterm infant at high risk for bronchopulmonary dysplasia: neonatal intensive care unit and developmental outcome. *Pediatrics, 78,* 1123-1132; DePaul, D. & Chambers, S.E. (1995). Environmental noise in the neonatal intensive care unit: implications for nursing practice. *Journal of Perinatal and Neonatal Nursing, 8,* 71-76; Lawhon, G. & Melzar, A. (1988). Developmental care of the very low birth weight infant. *Journal of Pediatric and Neonatal Nursing, 2,* 56-65.

should determine timing and sequencing of caregiving. Does the baby tolerate and benefit from caregiving procedures that are clustered together (allowing longer undisturbed periods for rest and sleep), or should caregiving procedures be interspersed because of low stress tolerance and prolonged recovery times?

▲ Caregivers must be sensitive and responsive to each infant's ongoing behavioral cues of stress, modifying caregiving pacing and techniques as necessary to facilitate infant stability and efforts at self-regulation.

▲ The necessity and frequency of all procedures and interventions should be reassessed based on each infant's age and medical status (e.g., must weights and baths be done daily, can some vital signs be taken from monitors, can suctioning be on an "as needed" basis, does the baby really need an occupational therapy evaluation requiring handling now?). Unnecessary handling and movement to prevent physiologic instability, frenzied activity, or other withdrawal behaviors should be avoided. Sick infants should be handled as little as possible.

See the box on p. 614 for a listing of specific suggestions for caregiving modifications.

### Sensory Stimulation

Functional maturation of sensory systems occurs first in the tactile and vestibular systems, followed by auditory, then

## Environmental Interventions: Modifying Caregiving Routines and Procedures in the NICU

1. Refer to the boxes on p. 612 and 613 for bedside environmental modifications of light and sound and to general principles listed on p. 615.
2. The infant's deep sleep should not be interrupted for routine caregiving. Nonurgent interventions should be postponed until the baby is in a higher state of arousal.
3. All necessary supplies should be gathered before disturbing baby.
4. An infant can be prepared for touch or movement by speaking softly first and containing extremities during movement and lifting.
5. Bathing by immersion is more soothing than sponge bathing if the water is warm and the infant's body is well supported with extremities contained (Figure 22-16).
6. Even noninvasive caregiving procedures can disturb and stress vulnerable infants, requiring caregiver efforts at consoling and facilitating infant recovery. An infant may be supported during routine manipulations and painful procedures in the following ways:
   ▲ Containing extremities (using Snuggle-Up, blanket swaddling, or hands of parent or second caregiver) (Figure 22-17)
   ▲ Sucking on thumb, fist, or pacifier
   ▲ Grasping blanket edge or finger of parent or caregiver
   ▲ Bracing feet against nest boundaries or caregiver's hand
   ▲ Shielding eyes from bright procedure light
   ▲ Temporarily stopping the procedure to allow a stressed infant to reorganize before proceeding
7. After stressful procedures, caregivers should facilitate recovery and stay with the infant until he or she is stabilized. Each individual infant has preferred recovery methods (e.g., head and extremities cupped within firm but gentle caregiver hands, prone position, sucking or grasping, or removing extraneous stimuli)
8. Parent involvement with caregiving should always be encouraged and supported.

Modified from Als, H., Lawhon, G., Brown, E., Gibes, R., Duffy, E., McAnulty, G., & Blickman, J. (1986). Individualized behavioral and environmental care for the very low birth weight preterm infant at high risk for bronchopulmonary dysplasia: neonatal intensive care unit and developmental outcome. *Pediatrics, 78,* 1123-1132; Shannon, J.D. & Gorski, P.A. (1994). Health-care professionals attitudes toward the current level and need for developmental services in neonatal intensive care units. *Journal of Perinatology, 14,* 467-472.

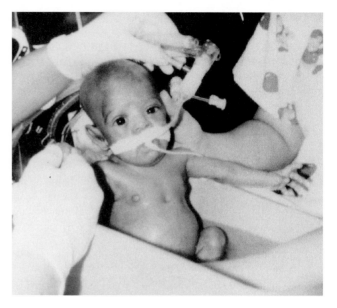

**Figure 22-16** Orally intubated infant on mechanical ventilator receiving tub bath. This infant was 500 g at birth but is now past term equivalency. (See Case Study #1.) (Courtesy of the Infant Special Care Unit, University of Texas Medical Branch, Galveston, TX. Photograph by Jackie Lohner.)

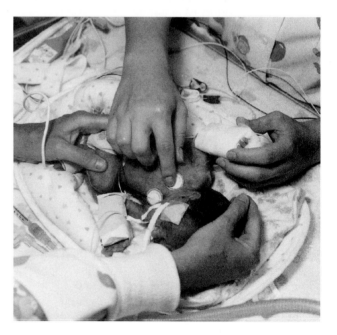

**Figure 22-17** Second person helps minimize stress in this preterm infant by providing containment during caregiving procedure. (Courtesy of the Infant Special Care Unit, University of Texas Medical Branch, Galveston, TX. Photograph by John Glow.)

# General Precautions and Stimulation Guidelines for the Preterm Infant

1. Intervention studies with preterm infants have come from a variety of theoretical as well as atheoretical approaches, sometimes with conflicting results. It cannot be overemphasized that neither short-term nor long-term effects have been adequately demonstrated and that the mechanisms by which the techniques are thought to work are often not understood. There is a strong need for interdisciplinary research to define more accurately specific subgroups of preterm infants and to understand their course of development; the physical, physiologic, and neurophysiologic basis of their development; the effects of the social and physical ecology of the special care nursery on development, and the mechanisms by which stimulation affects short-term and long-term development.

2. Preterm infants are differentially sensitive to stimulation depending on their conceptional age, illness, and individual make-up. The physiologic homeostasis and immature brain of the preterm infant may be more vulnerable to excessive inappropriate, or mistimed stimulation. The immature infant should be protected from stimulation that could destabilize physiologic homeostasis.

3. As the healthy preterm infant becomes less fragile and approaches term, the issue of what is appropriate stimulation can be considered. Stimulation could be related to the developmental level, the needs of the individual infant, and the specific purpose for which the intervention is intended.

4. Infant behavioral cues can be used to determine appropriate interventions for the individual infant. Signs of stress or avoidance behaviors indicate that the stimulation should be terminated. Positive behaviors indicate when stimulation is appropriate.

5. Stimulation is not a unitary concept and, when it is used, the various parameters of stimulation need to be considered. These include the amount, type, timing, patterning, and quality of the stimulation. In addition, the choice of modalities and the number of modalities stimulated are important. Multimodal stimulation may be more stressful to the infant than stimulation in a single modality.

6. Stimulation may have both short-term and long-term effects on development, both of which need to be studied. Short-term effects may include changes in the infant's clinical course, physiologic functioning, sleep-wake behavior, and interactive behavior. It is recommended that physiologic monitoring that could indicate signs of stress (heart rate, respiration, and $pCO_2$) accompany stimulation. Long-term outcome should be evaluated with measures of personality, affect, and temperament in addition to traditional measures such as morbidity, physical growth, and mental and cognitive function.

7. From a developmental perspective, once physiologic homeostasis is stabilized, the organization of state is the next critical step as the healthy preterm infant approaches term age. State organization includes both sleep states and awake states (alertness and crying), which are thought to be fundamentally different. State organization implies the ability to remain in a well-defined state for significant periods and the smoothness of transition from one state to the next. Effective interventions should be aimed at facilitating the infant's control of state organization.

8. The next developmental step after the control of state organization is the infant's ability to engage the social and inanimate environment. The step may not occur until after the infant reaches term age. The stimulation that is provided should support information-processing abilities. At the same time it should be recognized that earlier accomplishments may still be fragile. As intervention strategies are implemented, attention should be paid to possible vulnerabilities in the infant, as indicated by changes in state, motor, and posturing behavior. These behavioral cues should be taught to caregivers and parents to aid their implementation of these strategies without stressing the infant.

9. Intervention with the preterm infant should be organized in the form of an individualized developmental plan to parallel the pediatric plan. The developmental plan should be constructed as a psychosocial intervention to include the parents and other immediate family members and to acknowledge the socioeconomic, cultural, and home environmental factors that will determine the family context in which the infant will be reared. The developmental plan should include assessment of the infant's behavior, working with parents around the infant's medical and behavioral status, and helping the parents to deal with their own feelings, as well as discharge planning and follow-up. The developmental plan should involve an interdisciplinary team that includes input from medicine, nursing, psychology, physical and occupational therapy, child life, and social work.

From Lester, B.M. & Tronick, E.Z. (1990). Introduction. *Clinics in perinatology: stimulation and the preterm infant, 17,*(1), xv-xvii.

visual; logically, sensory stimulation should begin with the most mature system (Glass, 1993). In general, an infant is not ready for "extra" stimulation until autonomic stability is present; motoric and state subsystem stability should be emerging intrinsically (i.e., under the infant's control) but may be facilitated by the caregiver during the transitional "coming-out" stage (see Table 22-4). For example, providing postural security (i.e., swaddling for limb containment and trunk support) and looking quietly at the infant without facial animation may help maintain infant alertness and minimize stress related to the sensory input at this stage.

The box on p. 615 provides general precautions and guidelines for stimulation in the NICU from the viewpoint of neonatologists. The following information on stimulation should be used within this context.

Early stimulation may be safest if it replicates normal social activities such as being held, gently rocked, listening to the caregiver's voice (possibly with eye contact to add meaning to the sound if this is not overwhelming to the infant), or looking at the caregiver's face. This stimulation should be timed and titrated according to when the infant indicates readiness to respond to the environment and tolerance for the stimulation offered. Even though a 32- to 35-week-old infant may be able to respond to visual, auditory, and social stimuli, there is generally a physiologic cost to the effort at that age. Generally speaking, 36 weeks is a safer and more realistic time to consider attention and interaction as possible goals. Infants do vary significantly; therefore sensitivity to each baby's cues is needed. Ideally family members provide this contact; the therapist can substitute if family is absent.

Stable infants approaching term may demand more attention with varying success; it is worrisome if prolonged crying is ignored. For these infants, the occupational therapist may provide mobiles, mirrors, or toys for visual stimulation and musical toys or tape recorders (e.g., with lullabies or tapes of family singing or reading stories) for auditory stimulation. Baby swings or bouncy infant seats can provide vestibular input and a different view of the world. Even the variety of being placed in a standard infant seat may calm some infants (see Figure 22-18). Portable infant carriers may be occasional options for stable infants who can be temporarily separated from their medical equipment. Again, supporting families to be available, involved, and knowledgeable is the best way to meet the baby's developmental and emotional needs, both in the NICU and after discharge.

Glass (1993) raises several issues regarding visual stimulation for preterm infants:

1. An infant's ability to respond to a stimulus does not necessarily mean that stimulation at that level is beneficial. An immature infant may stare at a stimulus because of his or her inability to break away; obligatory visual attention is not a preferred behavior.

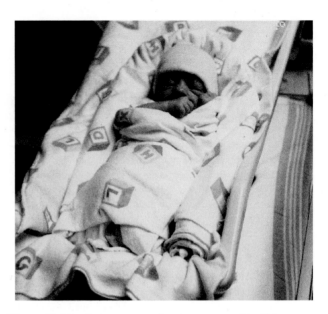

**Figure 22-18** Infant seats and swings can provide different perspectives of the room. This infant calmed and fell asleep after being swaddled with hands by his face and being placed in infant seat. (Courtesy of the Infant Special Care Unit, University of Texas Medical Branch, Galveston, TX.)

2. Increased attention to high-contrast (black and white) stimuli does not mean that infants cannot see pastel colors. The stronger response to black and white may be obligatory and probably is not better.

3. The human face is the most appropriate visual stimulus in early infancy and bears no resemblance to black and white patterns. A face is three-dimensional; has some contrast at the hairline or at features; provides slow, contingent movement around the eyes and mouth; is situated at variable distances from the infant; changes to arouse or quiet the infant; and is not always present.

4. Inanimate visual stimulation should follow this model (Figure 22-19). Softer, simpler forms and three-dimensional objects are preferred to high-contrast designs. Placement of a visual stimulus that the infant cannot escape should be avoided. The infant should have opportunities for hand regard; these may be provided through supportive positioning.

5. The incubator has edges and contrasts that provide visual input. The interior of the isolette cover should be plain; a plain blanket should probably be placed under a brightly colored quilt brought from home.

6. Black and white patterns should be reserved for infants after term who are visually impaired, who are unable to attend to a face or a toy, and who have already received other forms of sensory intervention. As soon as a visual response can be elicited with the high-contrast pattern, the transition should be made to more normal ones.

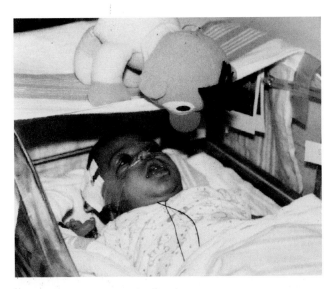

**Figure 22-19**   Softer, three-dimensional objects may be a more appropriate visual stimulus for preterm infants than high-contrast designs. Even though this competent infant could look at or away from "Ernie" at will, doll was removed after 2 to 3 minutes. Avoid placement of visual stimulus that infant cannot escape. (Courtesy of the Infant Special Care Unit, University of Texas Medical Branch, Galveston, TX. Photograph by Candy Cochran.)

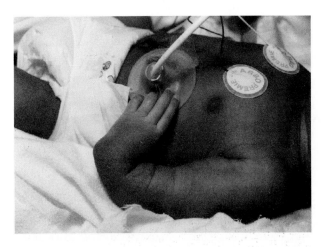

**Figure 22-20**   Term infant with multiple congenital anomalies that require rehabilitation approach, including passive range of motion and splinting. Gastrostomy feeding tube is visible. (Courtesy of the Infant Special Care Unit, University of Texas Medical Branch, Galveston, TX. Photograph by John Glow.)

## Neuromotor

### Range of Motion and Splinting

Passive range of motion (PROM) is primarily indicated for diagnoses that would benefit from a rehabilitation approach because of structural or neuromuscular limitation of movement, or for infants who are demonstrating abnormal tone. PROM incorporated into therapeutic handling is preferable to conventional ranging techniques for most infants. Examples might include congenital malformations and deformations (Figure 22-20), trauma such as a brachial plexus injury during delivery (Hunter, 1990a), or hypertonicity associated with intraventricular hemorrhage or severe bronchopulmonary dysplasia. PROM might occasionally be appropriate for an infant who is sedated or chemically paralyzed for prolonged periods. However, some experience suggests that prevention of positional deformities with therapeutic positioning may be sufficient intervention for infants whose movement is temporarily restricted (Case Study #1). Range of motion that is unnecessary and may be stressful to the infant should be avoided. PROM is usually not needed after osteomyelitis because infants begin to spontaneously move the affected extremity once pain and swelling subside (Hunter, 1990a).

Splinting is sometimes necessary but often difficult. Neonatal extremities are small, making precise fit of the splint difficult. Skin can be fragile and prone to irritation or breakdown. Intravenous lines may preclude wearing a needed splint. Certain splint materials may soften somewhat under a radiant warmer. Multiple caregivers greatly increase the probability of incorrect application of the splint.

Splinting is not the best option if the infant has some spontaneous movement that would be prevented by splinting and if PROM could achieve the same goal. If splinting is indicated, the therapist should anticipate and try to avoid potential problems. For example, pressure areas and slippage might be minimized if the splint is made using neoprene instead of thermoplastic splint material. An outside webbed "pocket" could hold a reinforcing thermoplastic strip, if needed, with the neoprene diffusing the contact.

A photograph of proper splint application should accompany bedside instructions. Posted written directions, wearing schedule, and precautions should be large enough to read and easy to understand. Staff and family education is essential, but does not replace careful monitoring by the therapist. An infant going home with a splint must have well-trained parents and follow-up arrangements for splint changes to accommodate growth and improving function.

### Positioning

Therapeutic positioning is typically a skill learned in the NICU by nurses and refined in the NICU by therapists; everyone can improve and learn from each other. The availability of quality commercial positioning devices can significantly reduce variability among caregivers while improving the ease and consistency of providing therapeutic positioning (Figures 22-21 and 22-22). Positioning aids offer direct medical benefits and thus eventual cost savings. Therefore, in some NICUs, neonatal positioning aids are available either by unit purchase or by billing the equip-

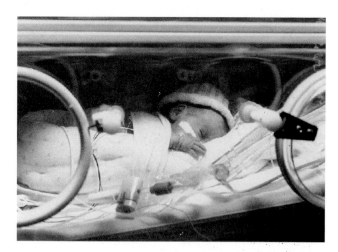

**Figure 22-21** Commercial positioning devices such as the Snuggle-Up (Children's Medical Ventures) have made therapeutic positioning easier for staff, more secure for infant, and much more consistent among caregivers in many neonatal intensive care units. (Courtesy of the Infant Special Care Unit, University of Texas Medical Branch, Galveston, TX. Photograph by John Glow.)

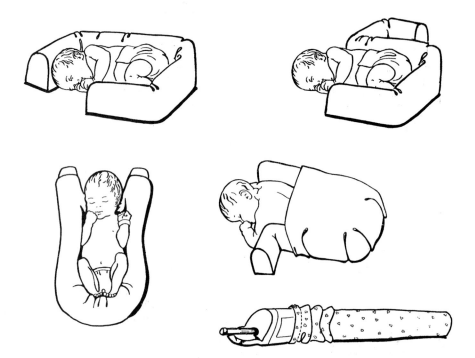

**Figure 22-22** Flexible reusable rod allows Bendy-Bumper to be molded into various shapes to facilitate therapeutic positioning. The rod may also be removed, bent as a freestanding frame over infant, and used to support blanket (for shielding the infant's face from light) or plastic wrap (to minimize heat loss from evaporation). (Courtesy of Children's Medical Ventures Weymouth, MA.)

ment to the patient. Washing machines are available in some units; either parents or staff may be responsible for laundering appropriate positioning items.

Because commercial devices may be unavailable in every NICU and because even the best equipment can be used effectively or ineffectively, positioning guidelines are described as follows below. It is assumed that the reader is aware of relative advantages and disadvantages of each position (Table 22-7). The following suggestions consider practical application of positioning techniques only. Gener-

ally speaking, if the infant looks so comfortable that the caregiver would like to crawl right in and join the baby in bed, positioning has been done correctly.

### *Therapeutic positioning*
#### *General guidelines*
1. A sheepskin or warm water mattress and "nesting" with boundaries somewhat simulate the intrauterine environment and may help the infant "settle in" to rest more peacefully.

2. Motor disorganization is generally most pronounced in supine and unsupported sidelying, especially if limbs are not contained.
3. Motor organization may be improved by
   ▲ Prone positioning because of increased physiologic stability from improved oxygenation and ventilation and from increased postural security with trunk and extremity flexion facilitated.
   ▲ Sidelying. This position is easiest to support with swaddling (Snuggle-Up, blanket nest, or wrapped in blanket); a single blanket roll behind the infant's back is usually inadequate. Hands should be together in midline, preferably up by the face unless there is danger of self-extubation.
   ▲ Swaddling to facilitate extremity flexion and containment.
4. Infants should be repositioned at least every 2 to 3 hours or when behavioral cues suggest discomfort that may be relieved by a position change.
5. Infant individuality and emerging capabilities must be respected (e.g., the occasional baby who seems to fight efforts at containment and rests better when allowed to "sprawl" or the maturing infant who can maintain a flexed posture without firm swaddling).
6. The infant should be gently handled with extremities contained during and after position changes.

*Supine*
1. Head should be supported in midline; ventilator tubing may also need to be secured to avoid pulling the infant's head to one side.
2. Unless the infant is on a waterbed, use of a gel pillow under the head is strongly recommended; subjectively, the author's NICU has essentially eliminated doliocephaly since routine use of gel pillows was begun several years ago. Nurses in some NICUs make water pillows for the infant's head, although often with expressed safety concerns.
3. When using a gel or water pillow with a supine infant, excessive neck flexion that can cause airway occlusion should be avoided and a small roll under the neck may be necessary.
4. With micro premies, the gel pillow may be used as a mattress under the head and body, which generally eliminates excessive neck flexion as a potential problem. The pillow should be warmed before use and placed inside the Snuggle-up or other boundary.
5. Upper extremities should be tucked in by the body with elbows in flexion; this position is supported by surrounding boundaries. (Elbow flexion past 90 degrees may cause occlusion of some percutaneous lines.)
6. Hips should be partially flexed and adducted to near midline (*not* medial to neutral alignment, as adduction with internal rotation places the neonate's hips in an unstable position).

7. Knees should be partially flexed with feet *inside* surrounding boundaries (versus boundary under thighs with lower part of legs dangling over, which can compromise circulation and does not provide a support for the infant to use foot bracing as a self-regulation strategy).

*Prone*
1. Unless on a waterbed, the infant's head should be supported on a gel pillow and rotated to the right and left during position changes by the caregiver (see Figure 22-10).
2. When using a gel pillow, placement of the infant that creates excessive neck extension and shoulder retraction should be avoided. Placement of the gel pillow lengthwise as a mattress under a micro premie may be a solution if the softer surface does not compromise respiratory function. Folding a cloth diaper that is placed perpendicular to the gel pillow (forming a "T", with the pillow as the top bar) is another option; the infant's trunk lies on the folded diaper, and the extremities straddle and flex around it. Stable external boundaries (e.g., Snuggle-Up, custom-bent Bendy-Bumper, stable blanket nest) are generally needed to help the infant maintain a balanced and flexed position on the folded diaper; shoulder protraction and hip flexion in prone are improved with this positioning.
3. Hip flexion may be facilitated by a small roll placed under the lower pelvis. Many infants may also benefit from lower boundaries against which the feet can brace.

*Sidelying*
1. Some neonatologists do not advocate sidelying for micro premies (except in treatment of specific air leaks, such as pulmonary interstitial emphysema, [PIE]), because of concern that prolonged time in this position may promote atelectasis of the dependent lung (lung on the underneath, weight-bearing side). Policy in each NICU and among attending neonatologists should be checked.
2. When positioned appropriately, sidelying decreases the extensor effects of gravity, facilitates midline orientation of the head and extremities, and encourages hand-to-hand, hand-to-mouth, or hand-to-face activity (see Figure 22-10). To maintain sidelying (and to avoid extremity extension and retraction, as well as increased infant stress from positional instability), the infant's top hip and shoulder must be securely positioned forward of the weight-bearing hip and shoulder. This can be achieved with blanket rolls (firmly behind the infant, loosely between the legs, and up along the baby's front to encourage forward tucking around the roll) but is often more secure within a Snuggle-Up (can still use small rolls as needed). A Bendy-Bumper should be custom bent (not just

loosely curved in a "U" or "J" shape) if used for side-lying support.

## Feeding the Preterm or High-Risk Infant in the NICU

Feeding the preterm and compromised infant has been previously discussed in both therapy literature (Case-Smith, Cooper, & Scala, 1989; Harris, 1986; Hunter, 1990b; Wolf & Glass 1992) and nursing literature (Kennedy & Lipsett, 1993; Palmer, 1993; VandenBerg, 1990). This section briefly discusses some considerations in facilitating oral feeding with preterm infants. Two case vignettes that illustrate feeding situations encountered by the NICU therapist are also presented. The reader is referred to sources listed previously for managing specific feeding dysfunction.

### Considerations in Facilitating Oral Feeding

Caregiver sensitivity to infant signs of readiness to feed and nursery flexibility concerning feeding schedules may be beneficial. In one study, young preterm infants at 32 to 33 weeks postconceptional age were found to show cues of being ready to eat during 92% of recorded trials, but 70% of the time these cues did not coincide with a scheduled feed (Cagan, 1995). Readiness cues were summarized as fussiness without crying, associated with hand-to-mouth activity, rooting, or hiccups. Infants who were fed on cue had fewer gavage feeds and less hiccups.

Feeding preterm infants "on demand" is a new concept in many NICUs and may not be appropriate for all infants, but it is beginning to receive consideration as awareness increases of the communication abilities of preterm infants and the benefits of individualized care. In some NICUs nurses attempt to time feed with the infant's natural cycles (rather than by absolute time intervals) by gavage feeding sleeping infants and limiting oral feeds to when the infant is awake and active. Prolonged vigorous crying before feeds should be avoided.

Traditional techniques remain appropriate. Sucking on a pacifier during (and between) gavage feedings should be encouraged. Perioral and intraoral stimulation before oral feeds has been shown to benefit feeding performance (Case-Smith, 1988; Gaebler & Hanzlik, in press). Some infants demonstrate significantly improved sucking organization when given the opportunity to hold on (e.g., to the caregiver's finger) during feeding. If excessive caregiver facilitation is required to elicit nutritive sucking, it may be prudent to temporarily defer oral feeding expectations; maturation is often more beneficial than "extra practice" in immature infants. Many premature infants benefit from external buccal (cheek) and submandibular (chin) support during the transition to becoming efficient and competent feeders (Einarsson-Backes, Deitz, Price, Glass, & Hays, 1994) (Figure 22-23). Warm formula may facilitate feeding (Gonzales, Duryes, Vasquez, & Geraghty, 1995).

The infant's ability to focus on oral feeding can be assisted by swaddling (provides postural stability and increases motoric stability), by shielding from light (facilitates alertness), and by avoiding talking or eye contact during the feed (effort to attend while eating may overwhelm infant and promote decompensation). If apnea and cyanosis persist, externally pacing the infant (i.e., caregiver removing the nipple after a few sucks or controlling the flow of formula) has been suggested to facilitate regular breathing and limit bolus size (Lewallen-Matthews, 1994; Palmer, 1993).

### Feeding Vignettes

*Darian.* Darian was born at 36 weeks' gestation with initial respiratory depression from maternal medications and a right cleft lip that extended through the alveolar (gum) ridge but not into the palate. He was admitted to a level II nursery and was under an oxygen hood for 48 hours and in an incubator for 8 days. Oral feedings were begun on the third day of life with good results; all feeds were taken by

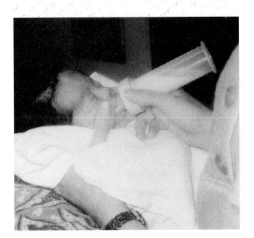

**Figure 22-23** Therapist providing buccal (cheek) and submandibular (chin) support to facilitate feeding efficiency in preterm infant. (Courtesy of the Infant Special Care Unit, University of Texas Medical Branch, Galveston, TX.)

mouth with a regular nipple that was placed to occlude the cleft in his lip.

Occupational therapy was contacted on the tenth day of life because of an acute decline in oral feeding. He had taken less than 30 cc in the last several oral feeds, and gavage feeds had been started. Darian was lethargic and difficult to arouse, which nurses reported as a change. The baby showed no signs of illness other than lethargy and poor feeding, but a complete blood count had been done that morning with normal results and a sepsis workup was being considered.

A trial feed by an occupational therapist showed normal suck-swallow-breathing coordination but extremely low arousal with no active feeding effort after the first 2 minutes. His nurse related that Darian had been awake and active for about 20 minutes, 1½ hours before this scheduled feed. Review of medical records showed two caregiving changes just before the decline in feeding performance; Darian's feeding schedule had been changed from every 3 hours to every 4 hours, and he also had been weaned from his isolette to an open crib.

Collaboration with the nurse and physician produced a consensus that even though Darian was "old enough and big enough," he was possibly not ready for all our changes and "demands." It was decided to place him back in the isolette and let him rest. Oral feedings were offered whenever Darian was awake and appeared ready to eat, with gavage feed supplements as needed for 24 to 48 hours. Oral feeds were then advanced according to his performance. Darian was back on all oral feeds within 4 days and weaned from the incubator 2 days later. In the interim, his mother had made care arrangements for her other children and was able to to stay at the nearby Ronald McDonald house. She expressed a desire to breastfeed Darian, and this transition was successfully made before his discharge on the seventeenth day of life. Darian's feeding problem was real but was related to autonomic and state factors rather than to feeding mechanics; oral stimulation and specialized feeding techniques would not have been the most helpful approach.

*Emile.* Emile was born at 29 weeks' gestation with a birth weight of 1030 g (2 pounds, 4 ounces). Medical complications included a patent ductus arteriosus, respiratory distress syndrome that progressed to bronchopulmonary dysplasia, severe apnea, a bilateral grade I intraventricular hemorrhage, suspected sepsis, retinopathy of prematurity, and feeding intolerance. As she approached term equivalency, her occupational therapist was also concerned about Emile's fluctuating muscle tone, persistent tremors, irritability, and low responsiveness to auditory and visual stimuli even when held and calm.

At 39 weeks' postconceptional age, oral feeds were attempted once a day. Emile demonstrated intermittent and inefficient sucking effort; maximal caregiver support and facilitation were required to complete the feed. A deep midline ridge in her palate was diagnosed as a submucous cleft but was not believed to be the cause of her feeding difficulty. As frequency and volume of oral feeds were slowly advanced, Emile began to desaturate during feeds.

A modified barium swallow was requested. Emile's disorganized suck expressed only small amounts of liquid from a regular nipple, so a Haberman feeder was used to complete the study. Emile demonstrated (1) oral disorganization, as observed clinically; (2) incomplete elevation of the soft palate with occasional regurgitation of barium into the nasopharynx, possibly related to the submucous cleft; (3) a prompt swallow reflex with complete clearance of barium from the pharynx, even when "challenged" with large or continuous boluses squeezed from the Haberman; (4) one or two incidences of threatened airway penetration (trace amount of barium entered the opening of the larynx, but cleared immediately during a subsequent swallow); (5) a significant fatigue factor with increasing need for longer rest periods to allow for extra breathing and recovery of energy, and (6) no significant gastroesophageal reflux.

Feeding recommendations included continuation of oral feeds with gavage supplements as needed, decreasing work of feeding by use of the Haberman feeder, allowing feeds to continue 20 to 30 minutes if rest periods were needed, a trial of supplemental oxygen during feeds if desaturation persisted, and consideration of formula additives to increase calories with less volume (deferred initially because of recent feeding intolerance). Her improvement was slow, but feeding was functional and weight gain occurred.

Emile's teenaged married mother visited frequently and was loving with her daughter but had difficulty with caregiving. She appeared mentally slow to the staff, required repetitive explanations and demonstrations of all aspects of care, and needed structure and encouragement to implement Emile's program. At 1 month corrected age, Emile was transferred to an extended care unit where her mother could be eased into full responsibility for the baby's care under supervision. Because concerns still existed at discharge, plans were made for the husband to drop Emile and her mother off at the grandmother's house on his way to work each morning for continued assistance and support. A check 1 week after hospital discharge showed excellent weight gain. Feeding and developmental progress were monitored at follow-up clinics, and the submucous cleft was managed by the Cleft Palate team, which included a speech pathologist.

## Intervention With Families
### Parent Perspective

Medical care and concerns, the complexity of high-tech NICU environments, and the neurobehavioral immaturity of preterm infants predispose the role of families in the NICU to be undermined. Providing the knowledge and fostering the skills necessary for parents to confidently nurture and care for their infant is the best contribution the therapist can make to any baby's development.

An experienced NICU nurse whose own daughter was born at 26 weeks' gestation shares her experience and offers suggestions to help staff deal with the emotional issues of parents in the NICU (Maroney, 1994). Some ideas with practical applications include the following:

▲ Babies should be made comfortable and as "normal" looking as possible. Such efforts as dressing the infant in baby clothes or a hair bow, providing a cute name tag or soft music, and using the infant's name and correct gender acknowledge that this is a real person, not just a sick premie.

▲ Staff should routinely ask the parents how they are feeling, and validate their response. "At least" statements (e.g., "At least you have two other kids at home") are not empathetic or validating, and may trigger anger.

▲ Parents should have as much control as possible. They are an integral part of the team and should be involved in caregiving as much as possible (this may require teaching). Staff should ask for their opinions and insights; call them at home with an update when they cannot come in.

▲ Staff must recognize that the baby is part of a family unit with a distinct set of dynamics. Parents may need help to overcome intimidation of the NICU so they can participate in their child's life. The father, as well as the mother, should be encouraged to participate in discussions and caregiving.

## Collaboration With Families

Similar to community-based early intervention, the shift in the NICU has been away from "therapist as expert, child as client, parents as students" to family-centered mutual collaboration. Ideal occupational therapy services with families in the NICU are based on relationship; the therapist talks *with* rather than *to* the parents, and acknowledges the family's role on the team. Holloway (1994) provided the following guidelines for parent-therapist collaboration:

▲ Opportunities should be created for a two-way dialogue between parent and therapist.

▲ The therapist should respond to the parents' concerns in addition to the occupational therapist's concerns.

▲ Methods of sharing information that value the parent as a person should be selected; the therapist should avoid being judgmental and acknowledge that the parent has the infant's best interests at heart.

▲ Individual differences should be valued not only in each infant's development and temperament, but in parents' views of their roles and involvement.

▲ The parent and therapist should observe and follow the infant's behavior together.

▲ Parent skills and successes should be acknowledged.

▲ The therapist should watch for and respond to parent reactions to occupational therapy interventions.

▲ The therapist should be sensitive to possible hidden messages in parent-professional communications.

▲ The parent's expertise should be facilitated. One parent's comment: "Seeing others follow through on our suggestions . . . bolstered our confidence in our parenting skills, knowledge of our baby, and ability to develop a closeness with him" (Holloway, 1994, p. 537).

▲ The importance of parent-infant nurturing activities as activities of daily living should be supported, and the therapist should facilitate the NICU environment so that parents feel welcome to engage in them.

When parents make requests that are unusual or differ from what NICU staff might prefer, the NICU caregiver needs to remember that parents have emotional and legal rights to make decisions on behalf of their infant. Baker (1995) suggested a four-question approach to handling conflicts that allows both parents and staff to feel respected: (1) What is the staff goal? (2) What is the parent's goal? (3) Will the parent's request harm the infant? (4) What options are available to meet both goals? In most cases, the parent's choice will achieve the same outcome and staff can maintain their standards for safe, effective, quality care.

The box on p. 623 summarizes principles and practice of family-centered neonatal care.

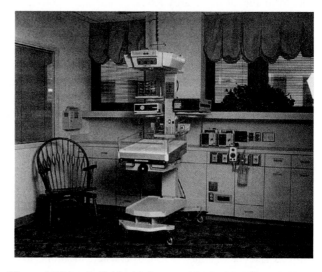

**Figure 22-24** Individual infant "pods" provide infant protection from many environmental stressors of crowded neonatal intensive care units and facilitate development of parent-infant relationship. (Courtesy of the Neonatal Intensive Care Unit, Baptist Medical Center of Oklahoma, Oklahoma City, OK.)

# FUTURE DIRECTIONS

Those who have been involved in neonatal care realize the only constant has been change. Unit designs, technology, and caregiving will continue to evolve as research clarifies how we can improve neonatal morbidity as well as mortality.

## NICU Ecology

A thoughful article, *Reinventing the Newborn ICU* (White & Newbold, 1995), predicts the following trends will reduce environmental hazards and improve the nurturing, healing potential of newborn intensive care units:

▲ Flexible lighting that allows for general dimming, day-night cycles, and task lighting for use with individual infants that will not disturb nearby babies

▲ Improved architectural designs that minimize previous problems of infant chilling or overheating by windows will allow natural light to be used with psychological benefits for caregivers

▲ Durability and improved bacteriostatic features of carpet and other sound-absorbing materials will increase their use in NICUs, with resultant sound reduction

▲ Visual alarms, personal communication devices, and quiet technology will further reduce noise

---

## Family-Centered Neonatal Care

1. Parents are considered and included as integral members of the NICU care team from the very beginning. (See p. 603.) The therapist should seek and value parents' opinions and insights.

2. "Visiting" is an outdated concept; assisting parents to be available to help care for their infant and to experience success with parenting in the NICU should be priorities.

3. Parents should be encouraged to ask questions. Questions should be asked about what the parents feel, what they understand, and what they want to know. Parents are frustrated by information that appears contradictory; much of their anxiety stems from a lack of truth or full information (Shellabarger & Thompson, 1993).

4. Parents can and should learn therapeutic positioning and handling techniques, (e.g., contain extremities in flexion, cup baby's head and lower body in parent's palms, let baby hold onto parent's finger, . . . ) as well as sensory input to avoid (e.g., lightly stroking infant's back, giving too many kinds of stimulation at the same time, . . . ). The therapist should encourage availability of Kangaroo care, which is skin-to-skin holding of the infant on the mother's or father's chest (Anderson, 1991; Gale, Franck, & Lund, 1993; Luddington-Hoe, Thompson, Swinth, Hadeed, & Anderson, 1994).

5. A behavioral and developmental assessment of the infant should be demonstrated to parents. The therapist should help parents learn to observe, interpret, and respond appropriately to their infant's unique behaviors. Fostering this constructive parental sensitivity to the infant's behaviors should be considered as important as other baby care skills in discharge planning.

6. As much as possible, feeding schedules and other caregiving should be arranged to accommodate parents' schedules.

7. The inclusion of siblings during the baby's NICU stay should be encouraged.

8. If parents cannot come frequently to the NICU, the therapist can make or encourage daily phone calls, send frequent photographs or notes sharing significant events or behaviors, or keep a bedside journal in which staff can record thoughts or progress for parents to read when they do arrive.

9. The therapist can facilitate transition to discharge by:
   ▲ Beginning discharge planning on day 1
   ▲ Including and supporting parents throughout hospitalization
   ▲ Considering many factors when planning discharge. Discharge currently occurs earlier from NICUs because of cost-containment mandates in health care reorganization. Transition to home will be improved, however, if the infant's behavioral stability, sleep-wake cycle organization, and self-regulation capacities are considered when planning discharge
   ▲ Providing accommodations for parents to stay with the baby overnight before discharge
   ▲ Providing information about community resources and parent support groups. Referring the infant for local early childhood intervention services if indicated. If possible, the therapist should arrange for parents to meet community resource personnel before hospital discharge.
   ▲ Following up with a telephone call from NICU staff after discharge

---

Modified from Hiniker, P.K. & Moreno, L. (1993). The care and feeding of the low-birth-weight infant. *Journal of Perinatal Neonatal Nursing, 6,* 56-58; Shannon, J.D. & Gorski, P.A. (1994). Health-care professionals attitudes toward intensive care units. *Journal of Perinatology, 14,* 467-472; Shellabarger, S.G. & Thompson, T.L. (1993). The critical times: meeting parental communication needs throughout the NICU experience. *Neonatal Network, 12,* 39-44.

CASE STUDY #1

## Medical history

Elizabeth was born at 27 weeks' gestational age to a 27-year-old married, now $G_2P_2$, mother. Maternal prenatal history was significant for oligohydramnios and severe pregnancy-induced hypertension (PIH); the mother received betamethasone the day of delivery to facilitate infant lung maturity. Delivery was by repeat cesarean section (C/S) secondary to breech presentation and fetal distress.

Elizabeth demonstrated intrauterine growth retardation (IUGR), possibly caused by maternal PIH and oligohydramnios; her birth weight was 500 g. Apgar scores were $8^1/9^5$ (8 at 1 minute and 9 at 5 minutes). She was orally intubated and transferred to the NICU.

Elizabeth's hospital course was complicated (Figure 22-25). She received three doses of surfactant but developed respiratory distress syndrome (RDS), which progressed to bronchopulmonary dysplasia (BPD). Hyperbilirubinemia required the initiation of phototherapy the day after birth and eventually a double-volume exchange blood transfusion. Thrombocytopenia, hypocalcemia, and electrolyte imbalances were medically managed.

A right atrial mass thought to be a thrombus was discovered by cardiac ECHO 6 weeks after birth but resolved spontaneously during the next several weeks. Elizabeth received several transfusions for anemia and multiple rounds of antibiotics for suspected sepsis during her hospitalization. She developed stage 3 zone I retinopathy of prematurity (ROP), undergoing successful laser surgery of both eyes to prevent retinal detachment.

Elizabeth developed abdominal distention and demonstrated feeding intolerance to enteral feeds, but her clinical picture and radiographs were not consistent with necrotizing enterocolitis (NEC). She required long-term total parenteral nutrition (TPN), which contributed to progressive cholestatic jaundice and subsequent ascites and hepatosplenomegaly. The ascites resolved, but feeding intolerance persisted; the impression from a barium enema 5 months after birth was partial obstruction caused by scarring or global dysfunction compatible with prematurity. Advancement of enteral feeds by continuous drip progressed at a conservative rate; concerns existed about possible bone demineralization because of compromised nutritional status from severe and prolonged illness.

Elizabeth remained ventilator dependent because of severe BPD and bilateral atelectasis, which was possibly caused in part by internal compression from continued abdominal distention. Weaning from the ventilator was finally successful 6.5 months after birth, with rapid subsequent medical progress and discharge to home 7 weeks later with an apnea monitor and oxygen by nasal cannula (NC). Chronologic age was 8 months, (corrected age, 5 months) at time of discharge.

## Occupational therapy intervention

**First 6½ months: orally intubated and ventilator dependent.** Elizabeth's medical status and neurobehavioral needs directed occupational therapy services throughout her hospitalization. Her extreme prematurity and immature central nervous system severely compromised her ability to cope with the extrauterine environment of the NICU. This situation was complicated by prolonged critical illness that necessitated intensive nursing care and aggressive respiratory treatments.

NIDCAP observations by occupational therapy during Elizabeth's early life documented frequent physiologic and motoric stress signals in response to both direct caregiving and indirect environmental stimuli (e.g., alarms, telephones). Her care plan emphasized protection, including efforts at modifying caregiving practices and her immediate environment. Nursing care was provided with attention to both Elizabeth's decreased tolerance to any stimulation and the need to protect her sleep; this balance was sometimes elusive as medical priorities emerged. She was shielded from continuous bright light, and attempts were made to reduce nearby noise. She was transferred to an incubator, but soon returned to a radiant warmer because of suspected sepsis. Elizabeth was eventually moved to a small glass-enclosed room that allowed significantly greater flexibility in protecting her from excessive traffic and environmental stresses; she remained in "Elizabeth's room" for several months.

Therapeutic positioning was provided to reduce stress from postural insecurity, minimize positional deformities, facilitate development of extremity flexor tone, and encourage midline orientation. Elizabeth was often placed prone during her first few months of life, but developed an increasing tendency to self-extubate in this position as her energy and ability to move gradually improved. Sidelying, supine, and reclining in a bouncy infant seat were her primary positions for the next several months. Elizabeth was typically swaddled in blankets within a Snuggle-Up to conserve heat and facilitate growth, to prevent self-extubation without use of arm restraints, to facilitate flexion, and for its calming effect. Spontaneous movement was consequently restricted during this period, prompting OT and other caregivers to unwrap Elizabeth for supervised "exercise" periods of free movement. As corrected age approached 3 to 4 months, fine motor activites were added to this free play time to encourage reach, grasp, hand-to-hand, and supervised hand-to-mouth activities.

State regulation, initially marked by diffuse sleep or frequent irritability when disturbed, gradually improved. As awake periods increased, Elizabeth became very responsive to auditory and visual stimuli. She appeared to recognize favorite caregivers and calmed to a human voice or soft music. Toys were changed frequently to provide novelty of visual and auditory stimuli. The bouncy infant seat was used more frequently to give a different view of her world; ventilator tubing was taped to the chair for security.

Elizabeth demonstrated very low tolerance and significant stress to any tactile input, including social touch. Probable causes included months of necessary medical procedures and constant swaddling that provided proprioceptive input but minimal tactile variety. This problem was approached slowly, first giving gentle pressure or patting through the swaddling, and having her hold onto the adult's finger. When Elizabeth was unswaddled for "exercise time," the therapist initially contained the extremities to prevent a startle response then slowly removed this support. Holding was provided by OT, nurses, and parents as possible.

Elizabeth became more tolerant of touch, but did not accept a pacifier readily. She exhibited tongue thrusting with no sustained or rhythmical nonnutritive suck. Prefeeding oral stimulation and pacifier sucking were complicated by prolonged oral intubation for mechanical ventilation, by an indwelling orogastric feeding tube for drip feeds, and by the tape securing these tubes. It was anticipated that eventual transition to oral feeds would be slow.

Elizabeth's family was very "attached" to her, but was unable to come to the hospital as often as they wanted because of transportation difficulties. Phone calls between parents and staff were frequent, and pictures of Elizabeth were taken regularly.

**From 6½ months to hospital discharge: off the ventilator.** She received supplemental oxygen by an oxyhood for 4 days and then by nasal cannula. She was still on continuous drip feeds of Pregestamil with additives to increase caloric density of the formula.

Elizabeth's developmental progress and paucity of anticipated problems during this stage were impressive to the occupational therapist, staff, and family. She tolerated handling without difficulty. She was still provided with loose boundaries, but seemed to enjoy the new freedom to move. Although OT had been concerned about the potential effect of prolonged swaddling, the "imposed" flexion had prevented typical premie deformities and now seemed to facilitate motor skill development. Elizabeth had normal tone with good midline orientation. In supine she demonstrated upper-extremity antigravity flexion in midline, hand-to-hand play, mouthing of hands, and visual observation of hand movements. Leg lifting into the air developed within a month; she also had no head lag in pull-to-sit at this time. Initially Elizabeth would tolerate prone only while sleeping, but by time of discharge 7 weeks after extubation she was propping on forearms, lifting her head consistently to 45 degrees (to 90 degrees with visual stimuli), and rolling purposely prone to supine with appropriate quality and components of movement.

Surprisingly, Elizabeth had minimal aversive behaviors to oral stimulation. She mouthed her hands frequently, willingly mouthed toys when assisted with taking toy-in-hand to mouth, and accepted oral stimulation with a round NUK toothbrush that was used to decrease her tongue thrust and increase tongue shaping (midline grooving). Her tongue thrust was typical of a habitual pattern often developed by infants with prolonged oral intubation as they lick and push against the endotracheal tube; this is different from the neurologically based tongue thrust seen in cerebral palsy. Her nonnutritive suck on a pacifier remained poor because of the tongue thrust.

Oral feeding, begun less than 2 weeks after extubation, was initially difficult because of her thick protruding tongue. Within a week of beginning oral feeds, the therapist was able to intermittently inhibit tongue thrust and elicit sucking bursts of 10 to 12 sucks with good rhythm and efficient stripping. Because these sucking bursts were not consecutive, feeding time was long (40 cc in 20 minutes). Within 2 to 3 weeks, Elizabeth began her oral feeds eagerly, but would abruptly stop and fight nipple insertion. The neonatologist agreed to a trial switch from Pregestamil to stock formula (initially diluted until tolerance was established); that feed was completed in 5 minutes. Elizabeth's feeding resistance vanished, suggesting taste as a factor. She continued to feed with good coordination, taking 90 cc in ≤ 20 minutes when discharged.

## CASE STUDY #1—CONT'D

Although many BPD infants tend to be irritable, Elizabeth had a delightful personality. She loved to be held or just talked to, and would generally only fuss if left to entertain herself for longer than 20 to 30 minutes. She was frequently carried around to visit staff in other nursery areas, and was even taken outside to see a Christmas tree in this subtropical climate. Smiles initially had to be elicited, then became spontaneous and frequent—especially for her family and favorite staff. Vocalizations remained very soft and infrequent.

Transfer to a step-down unit before hospital discharge was initially anticipated, but Elizabeth progressed so rapidly that the decision was made to keep her in the NICU. After nearly 8 months, a transfer for 2 to 3 weeks was not considered in everyone's best interests. The entire family of mother, father, and brother came to the hospital more often as discharge approached and assumed Elizabeth's care. A pictorial "biographical poster" had been assembled by staff and went home with Elizabeth.

Because of Elizabeth's increased risk for developmental delay secondary to prematurity and severity of illness, she was referred to a local Early Intervention Program for developmental follow-up after discharge. She is still considered one of the miracle babies by staff in "her" NICU.

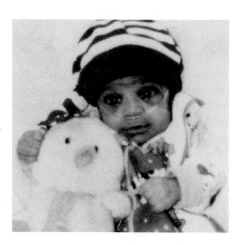

**Figure 22-25** Elizabeth, weighing 500 g (1 pound 1½ ounces) at birth, is finally ready to go home after 8 months in neonatal intensive care unit. Development was nearly appropriate for corrected age at time of discharge. (Courtesy of the Infant Special Care Unit, University of Texas Medical Branch, Galveston, TX. Photograph by Jackie Lohner.)

▲ Computerized information systems will streamline documentation
▲ Continuing increase in parental involvement, perhaps including some "rooming-in" options (Figure 22-24)

Occupational therapy has been increasingly involved in workplace ergonomics with the adult population; it is conceivable that occupational therapists can also make important contributions in creating the ideal NICU.

## FUTURE OF OCCUPATIONAL THERAPY IN NICU

A recent study involving 14 level III nurseries in Illinois had a descriptive survey returned by 530 multidisciplinary health care professionals regarding current level of and need for developmental services in the NICU (Shannon & Gorski, 1994). An overwhelming 86% of respondents stated there was a need for a developmental specialist in their units, 8% were unsure, and only 6% saw no need for a developmental specialist, with many of these comments seeming to reflect a view of developmental intervention as "stimulation" that is not wise or proven with fragile infants. All of 46 potential items listed in a developmental intervention protocol in the survey were rated as more important in an "ideal" unit than in current practice, indicating there is still much progress to be made. Further confirmation that a place for occupational therapy will remain in the NICU is the proliferation of articles on developmentally supportive care in neonatal literature during recent years.

Emerging changes in health care, however, emphasize a bottom line of cost containment and savings. Neonatal therapists are generally convinced that developmental care

## STUDY QUESTIONS

1. Using the description of Cody on p. 586 and Appendixes 22-A, B, and C define the medical terms for each of the abbreviations. Explain the implications of each medical condition that represents a potential threat to Cody's development.

2. Explain how lighting levels pose a threat to the vulnerable neonate. What are two intervention strategies that create more appropriate light input for an individual infant?

3. Explain how sound levels pose a threat to the development of the preterm infant. What are two specific ways to modify the auditory input to individual infants?

4. For each general positioning goal listed below, describe how to meet the goal using a prone, supine, or sidelying position.
   a. To provide proprioceptive input to increase the infant's sense of containment
   b. To increase postural flexion
   c. To promote calming and behavioral organization
   d. To assist in development of hand-to-mouth movements

5. Describe published assessments and informal methods for evaluating each of the following aspects of infant function and behavior.
   a. Neurobehavioral organization
   b. Habituation to sensory stimulation
   c. Neuromotor development

6. Define the precautions that need to be observed when positioning the neonate in supine, prone, and sidelying positions.

is both beneficial and cost effective, and that savings appreciated from a therapist's services are many times greater than the salary expended. Data collection and research studies that document positive outcomes may become increasingly important to the long-term future of occupational therapy in the NICU.

Occupational therapy is ideal for the varied roles appropriate within the NICU because of our unique blend of psychosocial and neurophysiologic training, but occupational therapy is not the only profession that currently fulfills the role of NICU developmental specialist. As a profession of clinicians, educators, and administrators, we must develop a more efficient system to provide training to aspiring neonatal therapists that will assure both baseline and advanced competencies. Concensus exists that training is essential; a way must be found for it to become available.

## REFERENCES

Affleck, G., Tennen, H., & Rowe, J. (1991). *Infants in crisis: how parents cope with newborn intensive care and its aftermath.* New York: Springer-Verlag.

Allen, M.C. & Alexander, G.R. (1994). Screening for cerebral palsy in preterm infants: delay criteria for motor milestone attainment. *Journal of Perinatology, 14,* 190-193.

Allen, M.C. & Jones, M.D., Jr. (1986). Medical complications of prematurity. *Obstetrics and Gynecology, 67,* 427-437.

Als, H. (1982). Toward a synactive theory of development: promise for the assessment and support of infant individuality. *Infant Mental Health Journal, 3,* 229-243.

Als, H. (1985). Patterns of infant behavior: analogues of later organizational difficulties. In F. Diffy & N. Geschwind (Eds.). *Dyslexia.* Boston: Little, Brown.

Als, H. (1986). A synactive model of neonatal behavior organization: framework for the assessment of neurobehavioral development in the premature infant and for support of infants and parents in the neonatal intensive care environment. *Physical and Occupational Therapy in Pediatrics, 6,* 3-55.

Als, H., Lawhon, G., Brown, E., Gibes, R., Duffy, F., McAnulty, G., & Blickman, J. (1986). Individualized behavioral and environmental care for the very low birth weight preterm infant at high risk for bronchopulmonary dysplasia: neonatal intensive care unit and developmental outcome. *Pediatrics, 78,* 1123-1132.

Als, H., Lawhon, G., Duffy, F.H., McAnulty, G.B., Gibes-Grossman, R., & Blickman, J.G. (1994). Individualized developmental care for the very low-birth-weight preterm infant. *Journal of the American Medical Association, 272,* 853-858.

American Medical Association. (1971). *Centralized community or regionalized perinatal intensive care* (Report J). Adopted by the AMA House of Delegates, June 1971.

American Occupational Therapy Association. (1993). Knowledge and skills for occupational therapy practice in the neonatal intensive care unit. *American Journal of Occupational Therapy, 47,* 1100-1105.

Amiel-Tison, C. & Grenier, A. (1986). *Neurological assessment during the first year of life.* New York: Oxford.

Anders, T.F. & Keener, M. (1985). Developmental course of nighttime sleep-wake patterns in full term and preterm infants during the first year of life. *Sleep, 8,* 173.

Anderson, G.C. (1991). Current knowledge about skin-to-skin (Kangaroo) care for preterm infants. *Journal of Perinatology, 11,* 216-226.

Anzalone, M.E. (1994). Occupational therapy in neonatology: what is our ethical responsibility? *American Journal of Occupational Therapy, 48,* 563-566.

Avery, G.B. & Glass, P. (1989). The gentle nursery: developmental intervention in the NICU. *Journal of Perinatology, 9,* 204-205.

Baker, J.G. (1995). Commentary: parents as partners in the NICU. *Neonatal Network, 14,* 9-10.

Bartram, J., Clewell, W.H., & Kasnic, T. (1993). Prenatal environment: effect on neonatal outcome. In G.B. Merenstein & S.L. Gardner (Eds.). *Handbook of neonatal intensive care* (pp. 21-37). St. Louis: Mosby.

Beaver, P.K. (1987). Premature infants' response to touch & pain: can nurses make a difference? *Neonatal Network, 6,* 13-17.

Bernbaum, J.C., Pereira, G.R., Watkins, J.B., & Peckman, G.J. (1983). Non-nutritive sucking during gavage feeding enhances growth and maturation in premature infants. *Pediatrics, 71,* 41-45.

Bhattacharyya, T., Vijay, S., & Doyal, M. (1986). Age related cochlear toxicity from noise and antibiotics. *Journal of Otolaryngology, 15,* 15-20.

Blackburn, S. (1995). Problems of preterm infants after discharge. *Journal of Obstetric, Gynecologic, and Neonatal Nursing, 24,* 49.

Blackburn, S.T. & VandenBerg, K.A. (1993). Assessment and management of neonatal neurobehavioral development. In C. Kenner, A. Brueggemeyer, & L.P. Gunderson (Eds.). *Comprehensive neonatal nursing: a physiologic perspective* (pp. 1094-1130). Philadelphia: W.B. Saunders.

Borland, M. (1989). Neuromotor development. In C.J. Semmler (Ed.). *A guide to care and management of very low birth weight infants* (pp. 216-250). Tucson: Therapy Skill Builders.

Brazelton, T.B. (1985). Commentary three. In A. Gottfried & J.L. Gaiter (Eds.). *Infant stress under intensive care: environmental neonatology* (pp. 279-284). Baltimore: University Park Press.

Briggs, G.G., Freeman, R., & Yaffe, S.J. (1986). *A reference guide to fetal and neonatal risk: drugs in pregnancy and lactation* (2nd ed.). Baltimore: Williams & Wilkins.

Brown, A.K. & Glass, L. (1979). Environmental hazards in the newborn nursery. *Pediatric Annals, 8,* 689-705.

Cagan, J. (1995). Feeding readiness behavior in preterm infants (abstract). *Neonatal Network, 14,* 82.

Case, J. (1985). Positioning guidelines for the premature infant. *Developmental Disabilities Special Interest Section Newsletter,* Vol. 8, No. 3. Rockville: American Occupational Therapy Association.

Case-Smith, J. (1988). An efficacy study of occupational therapy with high-risk neonates. *American Journal of Occupational Therapy, 42*(8), 499-506.

Case-Smith, J., Cooper, P., & Scala, V. (1989). Feeding efficiency of premature neonates. *American Journal of Occupational Therapy, 43,* 245-250.

Chasnoff, I.J. (Ed.). (1991). *Clinics in perinatology: chemical dependency and pregnancy* (Vol. 18). Philadelphia: W.B. Saunders.

Clopton, N.C. (1993). Musculoskeletal and growth measures. In I.J. Wilhelm (Ed.). *Physical therapy assessment in early infancy* (pp. 105-132). New York: Churchill Livingstone.

Cox, J.M., Oliva, M.M., & Perman, J.A. (1993). Nutritional and gastrointestinal problems. In F.W. Witter & L.G. Keith (Eds.). *Textbook of prematurity.* Boston: Little, Brown.

Crawley, K., Lindner, L.G., & Braun, M.A. (1987). Follow-up investigation of speech/language functions in high-risk infants. Presented at American Speech-Language Association meeting, New Orleans, November, 1987.

Creger, P.J. & Browne, J.V. (1989). *Developmental interventions for preterm and high-risk infants: self-study modules for professionals.* Tucson: Therapy Skill Builders.

Daberkow, E. & Washington, R.L. (1993). Cardiovascular diseases and surgical interventions. In G.B. Merenstein & S.L. Gardner (Eds.). *Handbook of neonatal intensive care* (3rd ed.) (pp. 365-398). St Louis: Mosby.

D'Apolito, K. (1993). *Infant developmental care guidelines* (pp. 1-14). Washington, D.C.: National Association of Neonatal Nurses.

D'Apolito, K. (1993). Use of pacifiers. *Neonatal Network, 12,* 61-62.

Dargassies, S.S. (1977). *Neurological development in the full-term and premature neonate.* New York: Excerpta Medica.

Davison, T.H., Karp, W.B., & Kanto, W.P. (1994). Clinical characteristics and outcomes of infants requiring long-term neonatal care. *Journal of Perinatology, 14,* 461-466.

DePaul, D. & Chambers, S.E. (1995). Environmental noise in the neonatal intensive care unit: implications for nursing practice. *Journal of Perinatal and Neonatal Nursing, 8,* 71-76.

Dewire, A., White, D., Kanny, E., & Glass, R. (in press). Education and training of occupational therapists for neonatal intensive care units. *American Journal of Occupational Therapy.*

Desmond, M., Wilson, G., Alt, E., & Fisher, E. (1980). The very low birth weight infant after discharge from intensive care. *Current Problems in Pediatrics, 10,* 5-59.

Drake, E. (1995). Discharge teaching need of parents in the NICU. *Neonatal Network, 14,* 49-53.

Dreyfus-Brisac, C. (1974). Organization of sleep in preterms: implications for caretaking. In M. Lewis & L.A. Rosenblu (Eds.). *The effect of the infant on its caregiver.* New York: John Wiley & Sons.

Dreyfus-Brisac, C. (1979). Ontogenesis of brain bioelectric activity and sleep organization in neonates and infants. In F. Faulkner & J.M. Tanner (Eds.). *Human growth* (Vol. 3). New York: Plenum Publishing.

Ellison, P. (1984). Neurologic development of the high-risk infant. *Clinics in Perinatology, 11,* 41-58.

Einarsson-Backes, L.M., Deitz, J., Price, R., Glass, R., & Hays, R. (1994). The effect of oral support on sucking efficiency in preterm infants. *American Journal of Occupational Therapy, 48,* 490-498.

Ernst, J.A., Rickard, K.A., Neal, P.R., Yu, P., Oei, T.O., & Lemons, J.A. (1989). Lack of improved growth outcome related to nonnutritive sucking in very low birth weight premature infants fed a controlled nutrient intake: a randomized prospective study. *Pediatrics, 83,* 706-716.

Fay, M.J. (1988). The positive effects of positioning. *Neonatal Network, 8,* 23-29.

Felix, J.K. (1991). Screening for hearing loss. In M.D. Jones, C.A. Gleason, & S.U. Lipstein (Eds.). *Hospital care of the recovering NICU infant* (pp. 177-186). Baltimore: Williams & Wilkins.

Finnegan, L.P. & Weiner, S. (1993). Drug withdrawal in the neonate. In G.B. Merenstein & S.L. Gardner (Eds.). *Handbook of neonatal intensive care* (3rd ed.) (pp. 40-54). St. Louis: Mosby.

Flandermeyer, A. (1993). The drug-exposed neonate. In C. Kenner, A. Brueggemeyer, & L.P. Gunderson (Eds.). *Comprehensive neonatal nursing: a physiologic perspective* (pp. 997-1033). Philadelphia: W.B. Saunders.

Flynn, J.T. (1990). Retinopathy of prematurity. In J.W. Eichenbaum, A. Mamelok, R.N. Mittl, & J. Orellana (Eds.). *Treatment of retinopathy of prematurity* (pp. 81-117). Chicago: Year Book Medical Publishers.

Gaebler, C.P. & Hanzlik, J.R. (in press). The effects of a prefeeding stimulation program on preterm infants. *American Journal of Occupational Therapy.*

Gale, G., Franck, L., & Lund, C. (1993). Skin-to-skin (Kangaroo) holding of the intubated premature infant. *Neonatal Network, 12,* 49-57.

Gardner, S.L., Garland, K.R., Merenstein, S.L., & Lubchenco, L.O. (1993). The neonate and the environment: impact on development. In G.B. Gardner & S.L. Merenstein (Eds.). *Handbook of neonatal intensive care* (3rd ed.) (pp. 564-608). St. Louis: Mosby.

George, D.S., Stephan, S., Fellows, R.R., & Bremer, D.L. (1988). The latest on retinopathy of prematurity. *American Journal of Maternal Child Nursing, 13,* 254-258.

Glass, P. (1993). Development of visual function in preterm infants:

implications for early intervention. *Infants and Young Children, 6,* 11-20.

Glass, P., Avery, G.B., Subramanian, K.N.S., Keys, M.P., Sostek, A.M., & Friendly, D.S. (1985). Effect of bright light in the hospital nursery on the incidence of retinopathy of prematurity. *The New England Journal of Medicine, 313,* 401-404.

Glass, R.P. & Wolf, L.S. (1993). Feeding and oral-motor skills. In J. Case-Smith (Ed.). *Pediatric occupational therapy and early intervention* (pp. 225-288). Stoneham, MA: Butterworth-Heinemann.

Glass, R.P. & Wolf, L.S. (1994). A global perspective on feeding assessment in the neonatal intensive care unit. *American Journal of Occupational Therapy, 48,* 514-526.

Gonzales, I., Duryes, E.J., Vasquez, E., & Geraghty, N. (1995). Effect of enteral feeding temperature on feeding tolerance in preterm infants. *Neonatal Network, 14,* 39-43.

Gorga, D. (1994). Nationally speaking: the evolution of occupational therapy practice for infants in the neonatal intensive care unit. *American Journal of Occupational Therapy, 48,* 487-489.

Gorski, P.A., Davidson, M.F., & Brazelton, T.B. (1979). Stages of behavioral organization in the high-risk neonate: theoretical clinical considerations. *Seminars in Perinatology, 3,* 61-72.

Gorski, P.A., Hole, W.T., Leonard, C.H., & Martin, J.A. (1983). Direct computer recording of premature infants and nursery care: distress following two interventions. *Pediatrics, 72,* 198-202.

Gottfried, A.W. (1985). Environment of newborn infants in special care units. In A.W. Gottfried & J.L. Gaiter, (Eds.). *Infant stress under intensive care* (pp. 23-54). Baltimore: University Park Press.

Gottfried, A.W. & Gaiter, J.L. (1985). *Infant stress under intensive care.* Baltimore: University Park Press.

Gottfried, A.W. & Hodgman, J.E. (1984). How intensive is newborn intensive care? *Pediatrics, 74,* 292-294.

Graven, S.N., Bowen, F., Brooten, D., Eaten, A., Graven, M., Hack, M., Hall, L., Hansen, N., Hurt, H., Kavavhuna, R., Little, G., Mahan, C., Morrow, G., Oehler, J., Poland, R., Ram, B., Sauve, R., Taylor, P., Ward, S., & Sommers, J. (1992). The high-risk environment. Part I. The role of the neonatal intensive care unit in the outcome of high-risk infants. *Journal of Perinatology, 12,* 164-172.

Graven, S.N. (1995). Future areas of study to be undertaken by the National Resource Center. Presented at The Physical and Developmental Environment of the High-Risk Infant Conference in Orlando, Florida, January 1995.

Hagedorn, M.I., Gardner, S.L., & Abman, S.H. (1993). Respiratory diseases. In G.B. Merenstein & S.L. Gardner (Eds.). *Handbook of neonatal intensive care* (pp. 311-364). St. Louis: Mosby.

Harris, M.B. (1986). Oral-motor management of the high-risk neonate. *Physical and Occupational Therapy in Pediatrics, 6,* 231-253.

Harrison, H. (1993). The principles for family centered neonatal care. *Pediatrics, 92,* 643-650.

Hill, A.S. & Rath, L. (1993). The care and feeding of the low-birth-weight infant. *Journal of Perinatal Neonatal Nursing, 6,* 56-58.

Hiniker, P.K. & Moreno, L. (1993). *Developmentally supportive care. Theory and application: a self-study module.* South Weymouth, MA: Children's Medical Ventures.

Hodgman, J.E. (1985). Introduction. In A.W. Gottfried & J.L. Gaiter (Eds.). *Infant stress under intensive care* (pp. 1-6). Baltimore: University Park Press.

Holloway, E. (1994). Parent and occupational therapist collaboration in the neonatal intensive care unit. *American Journal of Occupational Therapy, 48,* 535-538.

Hunter, J.G. (1990a). Orthopedic conditions. In C.J. Semmler & J.G. Hunter (Eds.). *Early occupational therapy intervention: neonates to three years* (pp. 72-123). Gaithersburg: Aspen Publishers.

Hunter, J.G. (1990b). Pediatric feeding dysfunction. In C.J. Semmler & J.G. Hunter (Eds.). *Early occupational therapy intervention: neonates to three years* (pp. 124-184). Gaithersburg: Aspen Publishers.

Hunter, J.(1993). Therapist acceptance and credibility in the NICU. In E.R. Vergara, (Ed.). *Foundations for practice in the neonatal intensive care unit and early intervention: a self-guided practice manual,* (pp. 255-258). Rockville, MD: The American Occupational Therapy Association.

Hunter, J., Mullen, J., & Dallas, D.V. (1994). Medical considerations and practice guidelines for the neonatal occupational therapist. *American Journal of Occupational Therapy, 48,* 546-560.

Hyde, A.S. & Jonkey, B.W. (1994). Developing competency in the neonatal intensive care unit: a hospital training program. *American Journal of Occupational Therapy, 48,* 539-545.

Jones, C.L. (1982). Environmental analysis of neonatal intensive care. *Journal of nervous and mental diseases, 170,* 130-142.

Kennedy, C. & Lipsitt, L.P. (1993). Temporal characteristics of nonoral feedings and chronic feeding problems in premature infants. *Journal of Perinatal and Neonatal Nursing, 7,* 77-89.

Kimble, C. (1992). Nonnutritive sucking: adaptation and health for the neonate. *Neonatal Network, 11,* 29-33.

Korones, S.B. (1976). Disturbance and infants' rest. In T.D. Moore (Ed.). *69th Ross Conference on Pediatric Research: Iatrogenic Problems in Neonatal Intensive Care.* Columbus, OH: Ross Laboratories.

Korones, S.B. (1985). Physical structure and functional organization of neonatal intensive care units. In A.W. Gottfried & J.L. Gaiter (Eds.). *Infant stress under intensive care* (pp. 7-22). Baltimore: University Park Press.

Korones, S.B. & Bada-Elizey, H.S. (1993). *Neonatal decision making.* St. Louis: Mosby.

Lawhon, G. (1986). Management of stress in premature infants. In D.J. Angelini, C.M. Whelan Knapp, & R.M. Gibe (Eds.). *Perinatal/neonatal nursing: a clinical handbook* (pp. 319-328). Boston: Blackwell Scientific Publications.

Lawhon, G. & Melzar, A. (1988). Developmental care of the very low birth weight infant. *Journal of Perinatal and Neonatal Nursing, 2,* 56-65.

Lary, S., Briassoulis, G., de Vries, L., Dubowitz, L., & Dubowitz, V. (1985). Hearing threshold in preterm and term infants by auditory brainstem response. *Journal of Pediatrics, 107,* 593-599.

Lester, B.M. & Tronick, E.Z. (1990). Introduction. *Clinics in perinatology: stimulation and the preterm infant; 17,* 1, pp. xv-xvii.

Lewallen-Matthews, C. (1994). Supporting suck-swallow-breathe coordination during nipple feeding. *American Journal of Occupational Therapy, 48,* 561-562.

Long, W.A. (1990). *Fetal and neonatal cardiology.* Philadelphia: W.B. Saunders.

Long, J.G., Alistar, G.S., Phillip, A.G.S., & Lucey, J.F. (1980). Excessive handling as a cause of hypoxemia. *Pediatrics, 65,* 203-207.

Long, J.G., Lucey, J.F., & Phillip, A.G.S. (1980). Noise and hypoxemia in the ICN. *Pediatrics, 65,* 143-145.

Lotas, M.J. (1992). Effects of light and sound in the neonatal intensive care unit environment on the low-birth-weight infant. *NAACOG's Clinical Issues, 3,* 34-44.

Luddington-Hoe, S.M., Thompson, C., Swinth, J., Hadeed, A.J., & Anderson, G.C. (1994). Kangaroo care: research results, and practice implications and guidelines. *Neonatal Network, 13,* 19-27.

Mann, N.P., Haddow, R., Stokes, L., Goodley, S., & Rutter, N. (1986). Effect of night and day on preterm infants in a newborn nursery: randomized trial. *British Medical Journal, 293,* 1265-1267.

Maroney, D. (1994). Helping parents survive the emotional "roller coaster ride" in the newborn intensive care unit. *Journal of Perinatology, 14,* 131-133.

Meier, P. & Anderson, G.C. (1987). Responses of small preterm infants to bottle and breast feeding. *American Journal of Maternal Child Nursing, 12,* 97-105.

Miller, M.Q. & Quinn-Hurst, M. (1994). Neurobehavioral assessments of high-risk infants in the neonatal intensive care unit. *American Journal of Occupational Therapy, 48,* 506-513.

Mouradian, L.E. (in press). Implementing individualized developmental care in the NICU. *American Journal of Occupational Therapy*

Mouradian, L.E. & Als, H. (1994). The influence of neonatal intensive care unit caregiving practices on motor functioning of preterm infants. *American Journal of Occupational Therapy, 48,* 527-533.

Newman, L.F. (1981). Social and sensory environment of low birth weight infants in a special care nursery: an anthropological investigation. *Journal of Nervous and Mental Disease, 169,* 448-455.

Nora, J.G. (1990). Prenatal cocaine use: maternal, fetal, and neonatal effects. *Neonatal Network, 9:* 45-52.

O'Donnell, J.P. & Merenstein, G.B. (1993). Infection in the neonate. In G.B. Merenstein & S.L. Gardner (Eds.). *Handbook of neonatal intensive care* (3rd ed.) (pp. 287-310). St. Louis: Mosby.

Oehler, J.M. (1993). Developmental care of low birth weight infants. *Nursing Clinics of North America, 28,* 289-299.

Olson, J.A. & Baltman, K. (1994). Infant mental health in occupational therapy practice in the neonatal intensive care unit. *American Journal of Occupational Therapy, 48,* 499-505.

Palmer, M.M. (1993). Identification and management of the transitional suck pattern in premature infants. *Journal of Perinatal and Neonatal Nursing, 7,* 66-75.

Palmer, M.M., Crawley, K., & Blanco, I.A. (1993). Neonatal oral-motor assessment scale: a reliability study. *Journal of Perinatology, 13,* 28-35.

Pettett, G., Buser, M., & Merenstein, G.B. (1993). Regionalization and transport in perinatal care. In G.B. Merenstein & S.L. Gardner (Eds.). *Handbook of neonatal intensive care* (pp. 6-20). St. Louis: Mosby.

Pickler, R.H. & Frankel, H. (1995). The effect of non-nutritive sucking on preterm infants' behavioral organization and feeding performance (abstract). *Neonatal Network, 14,* 83.

Platzker, A.C.G. (1988). Chronic lung disease of infancy. In R.A. Ballard (Ed.). *Pediatric care of the ICN graduate* (pp. 129-156). Philadelphia: W.B. Saunders.

Rapport, M.J.K. (1992). A descriptive analysis of the role of physical and occupational therapists in the neonatal intensive care unit. *Pediatric Physical Therapy, 4,* 172-178.

Ryan, J. (1988). Hearing and speech assessment. In R.A. Ballard (Ed.). *Pediatric care of the ICN graduate* (pp. 111-120). Philadelphia: W.B. Saunders.

Sapire, D.W. (1991). *Understanding and diagnosing pediatric heart disease.* Norwalk: Appleton & Lange.

Sarnat, H.B. & Sarnat, M.S. (1976). Neonatal encephalopathy following fetal distress: a clinical and electroencephalographic study. *Archives of Neurology, 33,* 696-705.

Scull, S. & Deitz, J. (1989). Competencies for the physical therapist in the neonatal intensive care unit (NICU). *Pediatric Physical Therapy, 1,* 11-14.

Semmler, C. (1989). Positioniing and deformiities. In C. Semmler (Ed.). *A guide to care and management of very low birth weight infants: a team approach.* Tuscon: Therapy Skill Builders.

Shannon, J.D. & Gorski, P.A. (1994). Health-care professionals attitudes toward the current level and need for developmental services in neonatal intensive care units. *Journal of Perinatology, 14,* 467-472.

Shannon, L. (1995). Clinical perspectives and current trends of HIV infection in the newborn and child. *Neonatal Network, 14,* 21-34.

Shellabarger, S.G. & Thompson, T.L. (1993). The critical times: meeting parental communication needs throughout the NICU experience. *Neonatal Network, 12,* 39-44.

Sisson, R.C. (1990). Hazards to vision in the nursery. *The New England Journal of Medicine, 313,* 444-445.

Strauch, C., Brandt, S., & Edwards-Beckett, J. (1993). Implementation of a quiet hour: effect on noise levels and infant sleep states. *Neonatal Network, 12,* 31-35.

Suedfield, P. (1985). Stressful levels of environmental stimulation. *Issues in Mental Health Nursing, 7,* 83-104.

Sweeney, J.K. (1993). Assessment of the special care nursery environment: effects on the high-risk infant. In I.J. Wilhelm (Ed.). *Physical therapy assessment in early infancy* (pp. 13-34). New York: Churchill Livingstone.

Thomas, K.A. (1989). How the NICU environment sounds to a preterm infant. *American Journal of Maternal Child Nursing, 14,* 249-251.

Updike, C., Schmidt, R., Macke, C., Cahoon, J., & Miller, M. (1986). Positional support for premature infants. *American Journal of Occupational Therapy, 40,* 712-715.

VandenBerg, K.A. (1985). Revising the traditional model: an individualized approach to developmental interventions in the intensive care nursery. *Neonatal Network, 5,* 32-38.

VandenBerg, K.A. (1993). Basic competencies to begin developmental care in the intensive care nursery. *Infant and Young Children, 6,* 52-59.

VandenBerg, K.A. (1994). Individualized developmental care: the Stanford experience. Presented at Developmental Intervention in Neonatal Care Conference. November, Washington, DC.

VandenBerg, K.A. (1995). Behaviorally supportive care for the extremely premature infant. In L.P. Gunderson & C. Kenner (Eds.). *Care of the 24-25 week gestational age infant (small baby protocol).* Petaluma CA: Neonatal Network.

Vergara, E.R. & Angley, J.C. (1992). The occupational therapist's roles in working with infants with life-threatening disorders: an NICU perspective. *Occupational Therapy Practice, 4,* 75-83.

Vergara, E.R. (1993). *Foundations for practice in the neonatal intensive care unit and early intervention: a self-guided practice manual.* Rockville, MD: The American Occupational Therapy Association.

Weibley, T.T. (1989). Inside the incubator. *American Journal of Maternal Child Nursing, 14,* 96-100.

White, R. & Newbold, P.A. (1995). *Healthcare Forum Journal,* March/April, 30-33.

Wilhem, I.J. (1993). Neurobehavioral assessment of the high-risk neonate. In I.J. Wilhelm (Ed.). *Clinics in physical therapy: physical therapy assessment in early infancy* (pp. 35-69). New York: Churchill Livingstone.

Witt, C. & Rusk, C. (1993). Behavioral assessment. In E.P. Tappero & M.E. Hongfield (Eds.). *Physical assessment of the newborn: a comprehensive approach to the art of physical examination* (pp. 139-146). Petaluma: NICU Ink.

Wolf, L.S. & Glass, R.P. (1992). *Feeding and swallowing disorders in infancy: assessment and management.* Tucson: Therapy Skill Builders.

Wurtman, R.J. (1975). The effects of light on the human body. *Scientific American, 233,* 68-77.

Yecco, G.J. (1993). Neurobehavioral development and developmental support of premature infants. *Journal of Perinatal and Neonatal Nursing, 7,* 56-65.

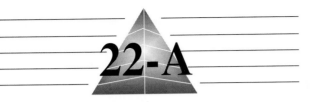

## Common Medical Abbreviations in the Neonatal Intensive Care Unit

### A

A: apnea
Ab: abortions (includes spontaneous)
ABG: arterial blood gas
AEP: auditory evoked potential
AGA: appropriate for gestational age
A-line: arterial line
AROM: assisted rupture of membranes
A's & B's: apnea and bradycardia
ASD: atrial septal defect

### B

B: bilateral, or bradycardia
BAEP: brainstem auditory evoked potential
BAER: brainstem auditory evoked response
BPD: bronchopulmonary dysplasia
BPM: beats per minute (pulse)
BSER: brainstem evoked response (same as AEP, BAER, or BAEP)
BW: birth weight

### C

CAN: cord around neck (nuchal cord)
CBC: complete blood count
CDH: congenitally dislocated hip
CHD: congenital heart disease
CHF: congestive heart failure
CLD: chronic lung disease
CMV: cytomegalovirus
CNS: central nervous system
CPAP: continuous positive airway pressure
CPT: chest physical therapy
C/S: cesarean section
CSF: cerebrospinal fluid
CXR: chest x-ray

### D

$D_5W$: 5% glucose solution
$D_{10}W$: 10% glucose solution
DIC: disseminated intravascular coagulation
DTGV: transposition of the great vessels

### E

ECMO: extracorporeal membrane oxygenation
ELBW: extremely low birth weight (<1000 g)

### F

FEN: fluids, electrolytes, nutrition
FHR: fetal heart rate
$FiO_2$: fraction inspired oxygen (percentage of oxygen concentration)
FT: full term

### G

G: gravida (pregnancies)
GA: gestational age
GER: gastroesophageal reflux

### H

HC: head circumference
HIE: hypoxic-ischemic encephalopathy
HMD: hyaline membrane disease
HR: heart rate
HFV: high-frequency ventilation
HFJV: high-frequency jet ventilation
HFOV: high-frequency oscillating ventilation
HSV: herpes simplex virus
HTN: hypertension

### I

ICH: intracranial hemorrhage
IDM (or IODM): infant of a diabetic mother
IDV: intermittent demand ventilation
IMV: intermittent mandatory ventilation
I/O: intake/output
IPPB: intermittent positive pressure breathing
IRV: inspiratory reserve volume
IUGR: intrauterine growth retardation
IVDA: intravenous drug abuse
IVH: intraventricular hemorrhage

### K

Kcal: kilocalories

### L

L (or LC): living children
LA: left atrium
LBW: low–birth-weight infant (< 2500 g)
LGA: large for gestational age
LMP: last menstrual period
L/S ratio: lecithin/sphingomyelin ratio
LTGV: physiologically corrected transposition of the great vessels
LV: left ventricle

## M

MAS: meconium aspiration syndrome
MCA: multiple congenital anomalies
MRSA: methicillin-resistant *Staphylococcus aureus*
MRSE: methicillin-resistant *Staphylococcus epidermidis*

## N

NB: newborn
NC: nasal cannula
NCPAP: nasal continuous positive airway pressure
ND: nasoduodenal
NEC: necrotizing enterocolitis
NG: nasogastric
NGT: nasogatric tube
NICU: neonatal intensive care unit
NNS: nonnutritive sucking
NP: nasopharyngal
NPCPAP: nasopharyngal continous positive airway pressure
NPO: nothing by mouth
NS: nutritive sucking
NTE: neutral thermal environment

## O

$O_2$ sats: oxygen saturation
OD: oral-duodenal, or right eye
OG: oral gastric
OGT: oral gastric tube
OS: left eye

## P

P: pulse, or para (births)
$P_1$: primipara (first birth)
$PaCO_2$: arterial partial pressure of $CO_2$ (concentration of $CO_2$ in peripheral arteries)
$PaO_2$: arterial partial pressure of $O_2$ (concentration of $O_2$ in peripheral arteries)
PCA: postconceptional age
PDA: patent ductus arteriosus
PEEP: positive end expiratory pressure
PerQ cath: percutaneous catheter
PFC: persistant fetal circulation (more correctly called persistant pulmonary hypertension of the newborn, PPHN)
PIE: pulmonary interstitial emphysema
PIH: pregnancy-induced hypertension (preeclampsia, eclamsia)
PIP: pulmonary insufficiency of the premature
PO: by mouth
PPD: packs per day (refers to smoking)
PPHN: persistant pulmonary hypertension of the newborn
PROM: premature rupture of membranes
PS: pulmonic stenosis
PT: preterm
PTL: preterm labor
PVL: periventricular leukomalacia

## Q

q: every
qh: every hour
qid: 4 times a day

## R

RA: right atrium
RBC: red blood cell
RDS: respiratory distress syndrome
ROM: rupture of membranes
ROP: retinopathy of prematurity (formerly called retrolental fibroplasia, RLF)
RPR: rapid plasma reagin (can be used to test for syphillis)
RRR: rate, thythm, respiration
RV: right ventricle

## S

"sats": refers to oxygen saturation levels
SGA: small for gestational age
SIMV: synchronized intermittent mandatory ventilation
s/p: status post
SROM: spontaneous rupture of membranes
SVD: spontaneous vaginal delivery

## T

TA: trucus arteriosus
TAPVR: total anomalous pulmonary venous return
TCM: transcutaneous monitor
$TcPO_2$: transcutaneous oxygen pressure
TLC: total lung capacity
TOF: tetrology of Fallot
TORCH: congenital viral infections (toxoplasmosis, rubella, cytomegalovirus, or herpes)
TPN: total parenteral nutrition
TPR: temperature, pulse, respiration
TRDN: transient respiratory distress of the newborn
TTN: transient tachypnea of the newborn

## U

UAC: umbilical artery catheter
UAL: umbilical artery line
URI: upper respiratory infection
USG: ultrasound
UTI: urinary tract infection
UVC: umbilical venous catheter

## V

VEP (VER): vision evoked potential (response)
VDRL: Venereal Disease Research Laboratory
VLBW: very low birth weight (< 1500 g)
VSD: ventricular septal defect

## W

WBD: weeks by dates (for gestational age)
WBE: weeks by examination (for gestational age)

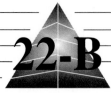

▲ Table 22-B1   Maternal Medical Complications and Associated Infant Risk

| Maternal Condition/Complication | Risk to Infant |
| --- | --- |
| **ABRUPTIO PLACENTAE (PLACENTAL ABRUPTION)** | |
| Separation of the placenta from its uterine implantation site after the 20th week of gestation but before delivery of the fetus; most abruptions occur in the third trimester. Severity ranges from marginal separation to life-threatening complete detachment; majority of cases are mild to moderate. If separation is more than 50%, the fetus usually dies. | Fetal risk is also dependent on the severity of placental separation and degree of bleeding with resultant decrease in oxygen perfusion to the fetus. Marginal abruptions may cause minimal fetal distress; marked detachment may cause severe fetal distress, irreversible neurologic damage, or fetal death. Anemia from fetal blood loss is common. |
| **DIABETES MELLITUS (INSULIN-DEPENDENT)** | |
| Complex, chronic metabolic disorder in which insulin is either secreted or used insufficiently by the body. The most significant complications affect the infant rather than the mother, because glucose easily crosses the placenta and stimulates a corresponding fetal response. Medical management tries to lessen or prevent fetal complications by maintaining the maternal blood sugar at normal levels. Gestational diabetes differs in that it first appears (or is initially diagnosed) during pregnancy and is sometimes controlled by diet alone; insulin may be offered prophylactically to gestational diabetic mothers as one option to better reduce the perinatal risks associated with a large infant. | Problems may occur before, during, or after birth. Fetal macrosomia is common, but placental insufficiency may also retard fetal growth. Additional antenatal complications may include congenital anomalies, premature delivery, or stillbirth. Birth problems from macrosomia may include shoulder dystocia or cephalopelvic disproportion during delivery, birth trauma, and asphyxia. Immature lungs with postnatal respiratory distress may occur in large preterm infants born to mothers with less severe diabetes, whereas chronic intrauterine stress of more severe maternal diabetes may accelerate lung maturation. Metabolic difficulties with transition to extrauterine life may include hypoglycemia, hypocalcemia, and hyperbilirubinemia. Infants of diabetic mothers (IDM) may be unusually prone to infections. |
| **HELLP SYNDROME** | |
| Acronym for a serious pregnancy-related maternal condition. H, hemolysis; EL, elevated liver enzymes; LP, low platelets. HELLP syndrome, believed by some to be a variation or more severe form of pregnancy-induced hypertension, requires intensive medical management before and after delivery; maternal death is a possibility. | Produces an increased risk of intrauterine growth retardation (with corresponding fetal compromise and complications, such as metabolic acidosis) and an increased risk of placental abruption. Because treatment of HELLP includes delivery of the fetus, there is also a higher incidence of preterm infants with variable complications related to prematurity. |
| **OLIGOHYDRAMNIOS** | |
| Too little amniotic fluid may result from fetal urinary tract anomalies (fetus does not excrete expected volume of urine), or chronic leakage of amniotic fluid. | Possible renal agenesis, renal hypoplasia, polycystic kidneys, or obstruction of lower urinary tract. Can also be associated with other body deformities from fetal compression or with intrauterine growth retardation. |

Modified from Bartram, J., Clewell, W.H., & Kasnic, T. (1993). Prenatal environment: effect on neonatal outcome. In G.B. Merenstein & S.L. Gardner (Eds.). *Handbook of neonatal intensive care* (pp. 21-37). St. Louis: Mosby; Korones, S.B., & Bada-Elizey, H.S. (1993). *Neonatal decision making.* St. Louis: Mosby.

▲ Table 22-B1    Maternal Medical Complications and Associated Infant Risk—cont'd

| Maternal Condition/Complication | Risk to Infant |
| --- | --- |

## PLACENTA PREVIA

Refers to a placenta with a low uterine attachment, over or near the internal cervical os (opening). May be termed marginal, partial (incomplete), or complete (central). Nearly half of placentas are low-lying during the second trimester, but few remain a placenta previa at term because of lengthening of the lower uterine segment during the third trimester. Placenta previa usually manifests in the second trimester with painless vaginal bleeding; a few are asymptomatic. Cesarean sections are generally recommended.

Preterm birth, fetal distress related to uteroplacental insufficiency.

## POLYHYDRAMNIOS

Abnormal accumulation of excessive quantities of amniotic fluid (more than 2 liters). Etiology may be unknown, or may be related to maternal diabetes, fetal congenital malformation, Rh incompatability, or multiple gestation. Acute onset of polyhydramnios has a less favorable prognosis than chronic onset, and the probability of a fetal anomaly increases with the severity of polyhydramnios.

Dependent on the etiology. See maternal diabetes and Rh incompatibility for associated problems. Congenital malformations are usually of the central nervous system (anencephaly, encephalocele, myelomeningocele, Werdnig-Hoffman syndrome) or gastrointestinal tract that interferes with the swallowing or absorption of amniotic fluid (atresias, gastroschisis).

## PREGNANCY-INDUCED HYPERTENSION (PIH)

Also called toxemia of pregnancy, PIH is a potentially life-threatening complication that develops in about 7% of pregnancies. Symptoms include high blood pressure, proteinuria, fluid retention, and edema. Preeclampsia varies in severity but always refers to the nonconvulsive form of PIH. Eclampsia is more severe, with all the symptoms of preeclampsia plus convulsions and possibly coma.

Infant small for gestational age, with or without hypolglycemia or hypocalcemia, fetal distress, abruptio placentae, perinatal asphyxia, meconium aspiration syndrome, hypermagnesemia, hypotension, neutropenia, thrombocytopenia, and increased perinatal mortality.

## PREMATURE RUPTURE OF MEMBRANES (PROM)

Spontaneous rupture of the membranes at any gestational age before onset of labor contractions. PROM occurs in 5% to 10% of all deliveries; preterm PROM at <36 weeks' gestational age is associated with one third of all preterm deliveries. The primary maternal complication with PROM is infection.

Risk factors depend on gestational age at PROM.
Term: labor usually proceeds uneventfully; maternal infection and perinatal mortality increase after 24 to 48 hours of ruptured membranes
Preterm: Dangers of prematurity must be weighed against dangers of infection. Risk of infection often believed to outweigh danger of lung immaturity at ≥33 weeks' gestation, with labor encouraged. The risk of pulmonary immaturity is usually considered more important at ≤32 weeks, with attempts to stop labor. Prognosis is extremely poor if PROM occurs before 24 weeks' gestation; severe pulmonary hypoplasia and orthopedic deformities from oligohydramnios, intrauterine death, or very preterm birth are common.

## PRETERM LABOR (PTL)

Refers to the onset of the first phase of labor after fetal viability (20 weeks' gestation, before which loss of the fetus constitutes a spontaneous abortion) but before fetal maturity (38 weeks' gestation). Potential precipitating factors may include:
Maternal complications: PROM, PIH, chronic renal or cardiovascular disease, incompetent cervix, diabetes, uterine anomalies, abdominal surgery, trauma, poor nutrition, infection.
Placental factors: placenta previa, abruptio placentae.
Fetal complications: multiple pregnancy, hydramnios, fetal anomaly or infection, death.

Preterm birth, fetal distress, perinatal asphyxia, hypoglycemia, hypocalcemia, respiratory distress secondary to immature lungs, other organ system immaturity, intraventricular hemorrhage, patent ductus arteriosus, infection, side effects of maternal medications (i.e., beta-adrenergic stimulants given to reduce uterine contractility may cause fetal tachycardia; magnesium sulfate given to relax the myometrium may cause fetal/neonatal depression of the central nervous system, including breathing and sucking. Indomethicin given to facilitate fetal lung maturation may be related to premature closure of the ductus arteriosus).

| Maternal Condition/Complication | Risk to Infant |
| --- | --- |

## PROLAPSED UMBILICAL CORD

An obstetrical emergency that occurs when the umbilical cord is displaced and becomes compressed between the fetal presenting part and the maternal bony pelvis. Treatment may involve (1) sterile vaginal examination, with manual release of cord compression (i.e., lift or move presenting part) and maintaining position until an emergency delivery can be performed, (2) patient placed in knee-chest or Trendelenburg position, and (3) maternal supplemental oxygen.

Fetal hypoxia from cord compression, asphyxia if compression is prolonged, and fetal death if the the condition is not immediately corrected. Half of the deaths from cord prolapse are stillborn. The surviving newborn is given antibiotics after delivery because of the high risk of infection.

## Rh ISOIMMUNIZATION

Refers to an antigen-antibody sensitization response that occurs when the mother develops antibodies to the Rh antigen of fetal blood cells; maternal exposure may occur with transplacental hemorrhages during the current or prior pregnancy, abortion, or ectopic pregnancy. Maternal antibodies can then be transferred through the placenta to the fetus, where they destroy the fetal red blood cells.

Severity of involvement varies; better identification and pharmocologic management greatly reduce current infant morbidity and mortality. Typical complications include hemolytic anemia and hyperbilirubinemia; untreated cases may result in fetal or neonatal death, erythroblastosis fetalis, choreoathetosis, or neurologic and sensory deficits.

# Maternal Life-Style Risk Factors (Substance Abuse and Sexually Transmitted Diseases) and Associated Infant Complications

## ALCOHOL
### Neonatal Risk

Low birth weight may occur with as few as 2 drinks/day (1 oz absolute alcohol) in early pregnancy, and 4 to 5 drinks/day may produce the characteristic anomalies of fetal alcohol syndrome (FAS). A safe level of maternal alcohol consumption during pregnancy has not been determined.

### Neonatal Withdrawal

Symptoms begin 6 to 12 hours after birth and may include tachypnea, irritability, hypertonicity, hyperreflexia, jitteriness, tremulousness, seizures, and weight loss.

### FAS

Diagnosis requires a history of excessive maternal alcohol consumption and at least one abnormality in each of three categories:
1. Growth retardation: before and after birth (length more affected than weight)
2. Dysmorphic features: particularly craniofacial (small eyes, short palpebral fissures, small nose with a low nasal bridge, flat or long philtrum, thin upper lip, and small chin) but may include limb anomalies and joint contractures
3. Central nervous system (CNS) abormalities: microcephaly, mild to moderate mental retardation with an average IQ of about 70

Cardiac, renal, and genital anomalies may also occur in conjunction with FAS.

The degree of involvement in FAS varies according to the precise maternal drinking history:
Mild: Intrauterine growth retardation (IUGR), microcephaly, no characteristic facies or organ malformations, and 50% have slight retardation
Moderate: IUGR, microcephaly, hyperactive or hypertonic, some facial anomalies, organ malformations rare, and mental retardation (not pronounced)
Severe: IUGR, microcephaly, FAS facies, organ malformations, severe retardation, and neurologic disturbances

### Later Infancy and Childhood

Slow development, poor coordination, learning problems, hyperactivity, attention deficit disorder, or memory problems.

## COCAINE
### Neonatal Risk

Cocaine passes thorugh placenta, directly exposing infant to the drug in utero. Placental abruption, stillbirths, spontaneous abortion, and preterm labor and delivery occur frequently. Increased risk for IUGR, microcephaly, malformations of the genitourinary tract, ileal atresia, neural tube defects, electroencephalogram abnormalities, seizures, and intrauterine cerebral vascular accident. Higher risk for sudden infant death syndrome.

### Neonatal Withdrawal

Although no predictable withdrawal pattern has been documented, neonates exposed to cocaine in utero have been reported to exhibit tachycardia, tachypnea, muscular rigidity, decreased tolerance for oral feedings, poor state organization, disturbed sleep patterns, excitement, irritability, poor consolability, tremulousness, startles, visual dysfunction, and depressed interactive behavior.

### Later Infancy and Childhood

The traits previously described have been noted to persist for at least 4 months, with recovery then progressing and the infant often apparently developmentally normal at 8 to 12 months except for a possible language delay. Latent difficulties with reasoning, judgment, memory, attention, and behavior are suspected but not yet proven in the school-aged child.

## HEROIN
### Neonatal Risk

Significant fetal risk occurs from complications of the mother's life-style (poor nutrition, prostitution, promiscuity with increased incidence of sexually transmitted diseases), aseptic drug use techniques with infectious complications, and the pattern of drug use. Specifically, the baby has increased risk for placental insufficiency, IUGR, premature delivery, spontaneous abortion, and stillbirth. Physical malformations are not typically associated with maternal heroin abuse, although narcotic abuse early in pregnancy or use of impure street drugs may have teratogenic effects.

### Neonatal Withdrawal

Symptoms generally appear within the first 3 days of life but may be delayed until 2 to 4 weeks of age in methadone withdrawal. Heroin use just before delivery delays the onset and increases the severity of symptoms. Methadone, substituted for improved addiction control in some pregnant women generally produces stronger neonatal withdrawal symptoms that require longer postnatal pharmocologic control. Duration of withdrawal symptoms is from 1 to 3 weeks; these infants are easily aroused, difficult to console, and have frequent gastrointestinal disturbances and CNS dysfunction. Withdrawal is termed *Neonatal Abstinence Syndrome (NAS);* symptoms include the following:

Neurologic: Restlessness, irritability, excessive crying, tremors, jitteriness, altered sleep, exaggerated Moro, hyperreflexia, hypertonia, and seizures
Autonomic: Mottling, flushing, diaphoresis, temperature instability, fever, and nasal stuffiness
Gastrointestinal: Vomiting; diarrhea or loose stools, disorganized suck, sensitive gag, poor feeding, poor weight gain, and appears very hungry
Respiratory: Tachypnea, apnea, and hyperventilation—respiratory alkalosis

In addition to drug therapy, measures to help the infant with NAS include decreased environmental stimulation (i.e., quiet and dimly lit room), swaddling to decrease flailing, smaller and more frequent feedings to minimize gastrointestinal distress, and gavage feeding supplements with pacifier sucking if suck and swallow disorganization is problematic during withdrawal. Subacute withdrawal symptoms may persist in the infant for 6 months after delivery, with disturbances in sleep organization and state changes frequently noted.

### Later Childhood

Long-term deficits implicated in children exposed to heroin or methadone prenatally include decreased growth (in height and weight), impaired cognition, poor attention (but not clinically significant attention deficit disorder), distractibility, unpredictability, increased incidence of language learning disabilities, somewhat decreased motor coordination and visual-motor-perceptual function, poor work habits (such as disorganization), attachment difficulties, and decreased self-confidence. Although socioeconomic and environmental factors (e.g., maternal nurturing, parent availability, child-rearing practices, poverty, nutrition, and violence) also influence these behavioral and school-related problems (confounding direct cause-effect relationships), the mother's continued addiction appears to be the most pervasive and devasting legacy of maternal prenatal heroin addiction. Continued addiction commonly results in neglect, abuse, and abandonment of the child who remains with the natural mother.

## HUMAN IMMUNODEFICIENCY VIRUS INFECTION
### Neonatal Risk

Vertical transmission (mother to child) of human immunodeficiency virus (HIV) from women infected with this sexually transmitted, bloodborne virus accounts for nearly 90% of known HIV-infected children. Mode of transmission is believed to be either in utero transplacental transmission, perinatal contact with maternal blood during delivery, or postnatally through breast milk. Nearly all infants born to HIV positive mothers initially test positive for HIV, but only 25% to 40% are actually infected; infant infection rate was lowered to less than 10% in recent trials with maternal azidothymidine (AZT) treatment during pregnancy. Accurate diagnosis of infant infection in the absence of overt symptoms is complicated by presence of maternal antibodies for 18 to 24 months. In addition to physical symptoms (i.e., bacterial and opportunistic infections, CNS disorders, failure to thrive, pulmonary disease, cardiomyopathy, and renal disease), HIV-infected infants are often in situations complicated by maternal illness, poverty, and drug abuse. Of HIV-infected infants, 50% become symptomatic in the first year (usually 4 to 6 months); 75% to 80% die by 2 years (Shannon, 1995).

# Maternal Life-Style Risk Factors (Substance Abuse and Sexually Transmitted Diseases) and Associated Infant Complications–cont'd

## SYPHILIS
### Neonatal Risk

The incidence of syphilis, a sexually transmitted disease, has increased significantly in recent years. Intrauterine fetal death may occur. Of infants born to mothers with syphilis, 60% to 70% are asymptomatic at birth but typically receive medical care as if infected. Clinical signs of congenital syphilis are variable but may include IUGR, hepatosplenomegaly, hemolytic anemia, hydrops fetalis, bone lesions, nephrotic syndrome, pneumonia, rash, and neurosyphilis (CNS involvement).

## HERPES SIMPLEX
### Neonatal Risk

This viral infection is usually transmitted intrapartum, with three classes of infant manifestations:

1. Disseminated disease: 30% to 50% of herpes-infected infants will have involvement of nearly all body organs, encephalitis (90%), and high mortality.
2. CNS disease: Limited to encephalitis and possibly lesions of the skin, eye, and mucous membranes.
3. Localized: Third category of herpes infection involves localized lesions of the skin, mouth, and eyes; approximately one third of these infants will develop neurologic abnormalities during the first year of life despite no apparent CNS involvement initially.

Specific symptoms of herpes infection in the neonate may include microcephaly, hydrocephaly, skin lesions, bleeding, coagulopathy, various eye infections, and cataracts.

---

Modified from Briggs, G.G. Freeman, R., & Yaffe, S.J. (1986). *A reference guide to fetal and neonatal risk: drugs in pregnancy and lactation* (2nd ed.). Baltimore: Williams & Wilkins; Chasnoff, I.J. (1991). *Clinics in perinatology: chemical dependency and pregnancy* (Vol. 18). Philadelphia: W.B. Saunders; Finnegan, L.P. & Weiner, S. (1993). Drug withdrawal in the neonate. In G.B. Merenstein & S.L. Gardner (Eds.). *Handbook of neonatal intensive care* (3rd ed.) (pp. 40-54). St. Louis: Mosby; Flandermeyer, A. (1993). The drug-exposed neonate. In C. Kenner, A. Brueggemeyer, & L.P. Gunderson (Eds.). *Comprehensive neonatal nursing: a physiologic perspective* (pp. 997-1033). Philadelphia: W.B. Saunders; Nora, J.G. (1990). Prenatal cocaine use: maternal, fetal, and neonatal effects. *Neonatal Network, 9,* 45-52; O'Donnell, J.P. & Merenstein, G.B. (1993). Infection in the neonate. In G.B. Merenstein & S.L. Gardner (Eds.). *Handbook of neonatal intensive care* (3rd ed.) (pp. 287-310). St. Louis: Mosby; Shannon, L. (1995). Clinical perspectives and current trends of HIV infection in the newborn and child. *Neonatal Network, 14,* 21-34.

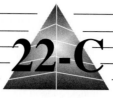

# APPENDIX

## 22-C

▲ Table 22-C1  Common Respiratory Complications of Preterm and High-Risk Infants

| Diagnosis | Description | Implications for Occupational Therapists |
|---|---|---|
| **Transient respiratory distress of the newborn (TRDN)** | Also called transient tachypnea of the newborn (TTN), TRDN refers to delayed resorption of fetal lung fluid. It usually occurs with a term or near-term infant who has undergone a rapid delivery or cesarean section or who has neonatal depression. The baby breathes rapidly to clear excess fluid, and may require oxygen initially. | Infant typically is receiving oxygen ≤ 40% from an oxyhood. TRDN generally resolves within 24 to 48 hours and is not usually associated with lasting complications. |
| **Respiratory distress syndrome (RDS)** | Also called *hyaline membrane disease (HMD)*, RDS is an acute lung disease of primarily preterm infants in which the lungs cannot inflate or function correctly because of a lack of surfactant. Chronic intrauterine stress may facilitate lung maturation and decrease RDS severity; female and black infants may also be less affected. Atelectasis (incomplete expansion of lungs at birth) and collapse of lungs after expiration are primary problems. Typical symptoms of respiratory distress (tachypnea, nasal flaring, grunting, chest retractions, apnea, and cyanosis), poor air entry, and right-to-left shunting often worsen for 36 to 48 hours. RDS may plateau then improve, or it may progress to bronchopulmonary dysplasia. | Surfactant replacement therapy is common. Supplemental oxygen can be given with or without assisted ventilation. Physiologic instability is apparent; protection is indicated to facilitate recovery (Als, 1986). |
| **Pulmonary insufficiency of the preterm (PIP)** | Lung immaturity that results from extreme prematurity. The lungs are underdeveloped and need assistance to provide adequate oxygenation and ventilation for the infant. | Generally denotes an extremely premature infant, often < 1000 g. May be ventilated mechanically or under oxyhood. Protect from avoidable stress. |
| **Meconium aspiration syndrome (MAS)** | Meconium, the fecal matter passed by neonates in early bowel movements, may be released into the amniotic fluid before delivery under certain conditions of stress (e.g., postterm or IUGR infant, complicated delivery, fetal hypoxia, and acidosis). A baby may be "meconium-stained" without aspirating the tarlike substance into the tracheobronchial tree. Not all infants who aspirate meconium are symptomatic. MAS most accurately refers to those infants with meconium found below the vocal cords and typical changes on x-ray films. MAS complications may include pulmonary hypertension, need for mechanical ventilation, secondary bacterial infection, and pulmonary or cerebral hemorrhages. | Symptomatic MAS infants can be critically ill. Mechanical ventilation is required for symptomatic infants; large infants who "fight the vent" may be sedated or chemically paralyzed. Mortality increases if persistent pulmonary hypertension (PPHN) occurs; less severe cases may improve within a week. Progression to chronic lung disease is not uncommon. Acutely ill MAS infants need to be protected from avoidable stress. |

▲ Table 22-C1   Common Respiratory Complications of Preterm and High-Risk Infants—cont'd

| Diagnosis | Description | Implications for Occupational Therapists |
|---|---|---|
| Persistent pulmonary hypertension (PPHN) | Also called *persistent fetal circulation (PFC)*. When respiratory distress (from any cause) and the resultant hypoxia or acidosis leads to constriction of pulmonary vasculature, the increased resistance to pulmonary blood flow allows the ductus arteriosus to remain functionally open or to reopen. As blood is shunted away from the lungs, right-to-left shunting through the foramen ovale and ductus arteriosus continues and the fetal pattern of circulation persists. | Infant ventilation and oxygenation are severely compromised. This is a potentially life-threatening complication; these critically ill infants are typically on minimal stimulation protocols. Strict protection from avoidable environmental and caregiving stressors should be attempted. |
| Bronchopulmonary dysplasia (BPD) and chronic lung disease (CLD) | BPD was originally referred to as the x-ray progression of lung changes in preterm infants with HMD. CLD includes BPD but also recognizes that chronic lung problems can occur from other causes (e.g., heart defects, diaphragmatic hernia, and MAS) The primary source of injury is barotrauma from positive pressure ventilation and prolonged high oxygen concentration.<br><br>Classification of chronic lung disease:<br>  Stage I: Tachypnea<br>  Stage II: Airway obstruction: upper airway (i.e., tracheal stenosis) or lower airway<br>  Stage III: Pulmonary interstitial edema: free air from ruptured alveoli seeps into interstitial lung tissue; this may further compromise the pulmonary vascular supply and ventilation<br>  Stage IV: Hypoxia and hemoglobin desaturation (prolonged oxygen saturation less than 90%, as per oximetry)<br>  Stage V: Cor pulmonale (cardiac right ventricular hypertrophy resulting from CLD) and hypercapnia (carbon dioxide retention). May eventually be fatal. (Platzker, 1988) | Chronic pulmonary compromise, often with prolonged mechanical ventilation (intermittent mandatory ventilation [IMV] or synchronized intermittent mandatory ventilation [SIMV]) or nasal continuous positive airway pressure. Oxygen supplements by nasal cannula may be required for months or years. Prone to recurrent respiratory infections and asthma.<br>CLD infants are often irritable and demonstrate increased muscle tone (aggravated by frequent agitation).<br>Difficulty with oral feeds may occur, especially if the infant remains tachypneic, has excessive secretions, or has developed oral hypersensitivity. Infant usually needs extra calories for growth.<br>Increased risk of long-term neurodevelopmental sequelae. |
| Apnea | Cessation of breathing occurs for more than 20 seconds.<br>Etiology may be central (i.e., related to nervous system immaturity in preterm infant or CNS damage after asphyxia); obstructive (e.g., tracheal stenosis from repeated or prolonged intubation, micrognathia, and posterior tongue placement in Pierre-Robin sequence); associated with illness (e.g., RDS, infection, anemia, cold stress, and reflux), related to stress (e.g., after eye dilation and examination caused by hypermagnesemia or oversedation or idiopathic (cause unknown). | Infant may require prolonged mechanical ventilation or continuous positive airway pressure.<br>Apnea medication is common.<br>Severe apnea has increased risk of CNS damage from hypoxia and increased risk of necrotizing enterocolitis (NEC) from disturbed perfusion of intestine.<br>May go home on apnea monitor. |

▲ Table 22-C1    Common Respiratory Complications of Preterm and High-Risk Infants—cont'd

| Diagnosis | Description | Implications for Occupational Therapists |
|---|---|---|
| Pneumonia | Infectious exposure to various organisms across the placenta or during the delivery; nosocomial infection (hospital-acquired infection, i.e., transmission from inadequate hand washing); or may occur in association with sepsis or meningitis.<br><br>Clinical presentation may include signs of respiratory distress (grunting, flaring, retractions, tachypnea, or cyanosis), shock, and signs of sepsis (temperature instability, apnea, hypoglycemia, lethargy, poor feeding, or seizures). | Seriously or critically ill infant requires mechanical ventilation and intravenous antibiotics. Enteral feeds may be temporarily discontinued. Protect from avoidable stress. |

Modified from Hagedorn, M.I., Gardner, S.L., & Abman, S.H. (1993). Respiratory disease. In G.B. Merenstein & S.L. Gardner (Eds.). *Handbook of neonatal intensive care* (pp. 311-364). St. Louis: Mosby; Korones, S.B. & Bada-Elizey, H.S. (1993). *Neonatal decision making.* St. Louis: Mosby.

▲ Table 22-C2    Common Neurological Complications of Preterm and High-Risk Infants

| Diagnosis | Description | Implications for Occupational Therapists |
|---|---|---|
| Brachial plexus injuries | Transient or permanent upper-extremity paralysis may result from damage to the brachial plexus during a difficult birth. Nerve roots and trunks of the plexus may be bruised, stretched, or torn. | Treatment in the acute stage is primarily aimed at preventing further damage to traumatized structures and preventing contractures of involved joints. |
| Erb's palsy | Damage to the upper trunk of the brachial plexus at the junction of nerve roots C-5 and C-6. Most common brachial plexus injury, best prognosis. | Caregivers are taught positioning and handling techniques that protect the extremity, as well as passive range of motion that emphasizes absent movements (Hunter, 1990a). |
| Erb-Duchenne-Klumpke's palsy | C-5 to T-1. Next most common injury to brachial plexus; generally good prognosis. | |
| Klumpke's palsy | C-8 to T-1. Least common; often less recovery. | |
| Intraventricular hemmorhage (IVH) | Infants <1500 g and < 30 weeks' gestation are at highest risk. Most occur within the first week of life. Causes may be intravascular factors (i.e., fluctuating or increased cerebral blood flow, increased venous pressure or blood flow, platelet and coagulation disturbances); vascular factors (fragile capillaries and immature vascular network is vulnerable to rupture); extravascular factors (poor structural support of capillary bed; fibrinolytic activity extends bleed).<br><br>Grades of IVH<br>  Grade I: Subepyndemal germinal matrix bleed<br>  Grade II: Bleeding extends into the ventricle<br>  Grade III: Ventricles are so full of blood they become dilated<br>  Grade IV: Bleeding extends beyond the cavity of the ventricle into the surrounding parynchema; hydrocephalus is typical | Symptoms may include apnea, temperature instability, poor suck or feeding, vomiting, lethargy, irritability, pallor or mottling, hypotension or shock, bulging and tense fontanel, and seizures.<br><br>Stress and improper handling may precipitate an IVH in a vulnerable infant (e.g., elevating hips with diaper change for a micropremie can elevate intracranial pressure).<br><br>Infants with grade I or II IVH usually do well developmentally, and infants with grade III or IV IVH are more likely to have developmental problems, especially if there is associated periventricular white matter destruction (periventricular leukomalacia [PVL]) or posthemorrhagic hydrocephalus. |

From Hunter, J.G. (1990a). Orthopedic conditions. In C.J. Semmler & J.G. Hunter (Eds.). *Early occupational therapy intervention: neonates to three years* (pp. 72-123). Gaithersburg: Aspen Publishers; Korones, S.B. & Bada-Elizey, H.S. (1993). *Neonatal decision making.* St. Louis: Mosby; Sarnat, H.B. & Sarnat, M.S. (1976). Neonatal encephalopathy following fetal distress: a clinical and electroencephalographic study. *Archives of Neurology, 33,* 696-705.

▲ Table 22-C2    Common Neurological Complications of Preterm and High-Risk Infants—cont'd

| Diagnosis | Description | Implications for Occupational Therapists |
|---|---|---|
| Periventricular leukomalacia (PVL) | PVL is a widely recognized ischemic brain lesion that occurs in 15% to 20% of preterm infants; it may happen in utero. PVL literally means the loss of white matter around the ventricles; it is characterized by necrosis and residual scarring of the white matter, and may be responsible for extension of an IVH into a grade IV bleed. | Areas of increased echodensity on head ultrasound that resolve over time are not true PVL. Repeat ultrasounds of PVL typically show cystic formation from white matter destruction. Developmental sequelae are seen in most (but not all) PVL infants. |
| Hydrocephalus Posthemorrhagic hydrocephalus | Inflammation from blood in the ventricles may impede the normal circulation and reabsorption of cerebrospinal fluid (CSF); fibrin or other debris may occlude the pathways for CSF drainage and thus lead to hydrocephalus. | May need ventriculoperitoneal shunt to allow drainage of CSF. If infant is too small or blood protein is too high for immediate surgery, baby may have frequent lumbar or ventricular taps to relieve accumulating pressure. |
| Congenital obstructive hydrocephalus | Aqueductal stenosis: obstruction of the aqueduct of Sylvius before the fourth ventricle occludes CSF flow, causing lateral and third ventricles to dilate. Arnold-Chiari malformation: medulla is displaced inferiorly through the foramen magnum into the cervical spinal canal (type I), at times with the fourth ventricle (type II, the classic form of ACM associated with spina bifida) or the cerebellum (type III). Obstructive hydrocephalus results. | Infant may be irritable or lethargic. Brainstem dysfunction may occur with Arnold-Chiari malformation, especially after repair of the myelomeningocele and possibly several months after birth. May have silent aspiration with feeds; surgical decompression may relieve pressure on brainstem. Developmental sequelae common. |
| Hypoxic-ischemic encephalopathy (HIE) | Numerous maternal, placental, obstetric, and fetal and neonatal factors can decrease oxygen transfer to the baby. HIE is the neurologic syndrome resulting form perinatal asphyxia. Clinical manifestations and prognosis depend primarily on the severity and duration of asphyxia. The Sarnat classification is a common prognostic indicator, with higher staging and longer duration associated with poor outcome. | Infant may initially be on minimal stimulation protocol. Monitoring of early presentation and subsequent changes is recommended. Irritability, hyperactive tendon reflexes, and no seizures indicate mild asphyxia. Infants with moderate asphyxia show hypotonia, increased tendon reflexes, weak suck, and seizures with an abnormal EEG. Severely asphyxiated infants are unconscious with absent reflexes and unreactive pupils; prognosis is poor. Infant may show signs of more than one stage and may progress to another stage, indicating recovery or deterioration. |

▲ Table 22-C3   Hemolytic and Infectious Complications in Preterm/High-Risk Infants

| Diagnosis | Description | Implications for Occupational Therapists |
|---|---|---|
| Anemia | Refers to low hemoglobin content of the blood. In the neonatal intensive care unit (NICU), anemia most commonly results from blood loss (i.e., frequent intermittent blood sampling or perinatal or postnatal hemorrhage) or from hemolysis (breakdown of red blood cells). Immune hemolytic disorders (e.g., ABO incompatability or Rh incompatability) or hereditary red blood cells disorders are among other causes. | Mild anemia is common; severe anemia can be life-threatening. Infant should not be disturbed during blood transfusions because of large-bore catheter in small fragile veins. Pallor is common; jaundice may occur with hemolytic anemia (i.e., bruising from delivery causes hemolysis and may subsequently result in hyperbilirubinemia). Increased lethargy is common; cardiorespiratory distress is possible. |
| Disseminated intravascular coagulation (DIC) | DIC is an acquired pathologic process that occurs when various underlying disorders or disease processes trigger intravascular clot formation. This clot formation consumes platelets and plasma clotting factors; additional biochemical mechanisms contribute to platelet and red blood cells destruction. DIC usually results in generalized bleeding from puncture sites, the gastrointestinal tract, the central nervous system, and skin. Anticoagulant measures to prevent major vessel thrombus or skin necrosis from thrombi can complicate medical management. | An infant with DIC is seriously or critically ill. Bruising or petechiae (tiny hemorrhages within the skin or subcutaneous layers that appear as small flat red or purple spots) are warning signs; oozing from puncture sites or hemorrhage is a definite red flag. The infant is typically on a minimal stimulation protocol to protect from avoidable stress. |
| Hyperbilirubinemia | Physiologic jaundice resulting from an excess of the bile pigment bilirubin in the blood. Immaturity of the liver and destruction of fetal red blood cells are common causes. Jaundice may resolve spontaneously if mild, require phototherapy if moderate, or need phototherapy and exchange blood transfusions if severe. Phototherapy converts bilirubin into a form that can be excreted; in severe cases exchange blood transfusions may be indicated to reduce blood levels of bilirubin or to correct severe anemia. In some infants, bilirubin levels may rebound after phototherapy is discontinued, and the infant is put back under the bili lights. Untreated severe neonatal hyperbilirubinemia may lead to a condition called kernicterus, which can produce mental retardation as well as sensory and motor disturbances. | Hyperbilirubinemia requiring phototherapy is common in the NICU. An infant under bili lights may appear lethargic or irritable. Unless a fiberoptic bili blanket is available to provide phototherapy when swaddled, the infant will be positioned for maximal skin exposure to the bili lights. Eyes are patched for protection (also need to protect neighboring infants from this light source). An oral feeder can generally be removed from the lights during feeds, but must remain under phototherapy the rest of the time. |
| Sepsis | Bacterial sepsis in neonates is characterized by systemic signs of infection associated with bacteria in the blood (bacteremia); multiple organisms can be responsible. NICU infants are susceptible to infection because of prematurity, immature immune systems, stress, medical complications, and surgical procedures. Bloodborne bacteria can localize and produce focal disease (i.e., osteomyelities or bone infection); pneumonia, meningitis may also result from neonatal sepsis. | Inadequate hand washing is the primary cause of nosocomial infection (infection acquired during hospitalization). Symptoms vary according to severity of the disease but may include sudden deterioration, metabolic acidosis, temperature instability, apnea, and seizures. Protect from avoidable stress. |

From Korones, S.B. & Bada-Elizey, H.S. (1993). *Neonatal decision making.* St. Louis: Mosby; O'Donnell, J.P. & Merenstein, G.B. (1993). Infection in the neonate. In G.B. Merenstein & S.L. Gardner (Eds.). *Handbook of neonatal intensive care* (3rd ed.) (pp. 287-310). St. Louis: Mosby.

▲ Table 22-C4  Vision and Hearing Complications in Preterm/High-Risk Infants

| Diagnosis | Description | Implications for Occupational Therapists |
|---|---|---|
| Retinopathy of prematurity (ROP) (*termed retrolental fibroplasia [RLF] until mid-1980s*) | ROP designates a pathologic condition that occurs primarily (not exclusively) in preterm infants when injury to the still-developing blood vessels of the retina cause subsequent abnormal vascular formation. ROP is described based on location (Zone 1, innermost circle with the optic disc at its center; Zone 2, doughnut-shaped circle surrounding Zone 1; and Zone 3, crescent-shaped outer zone); on extent (retina is divided into clock hours to help describe extent of the disease); and by stage (indicates severity of vascular abnormality from least severe stage 1 to partial or total retinal detachment in stages 4 and 5). *PLUS* disease refers to increasingly dilated, tortuous peripheral retinal vessels. Prematurity with low birth weight, oxygen toxicity, vitamin E deficiency, high light intensity, blood transfusions, and infant medical complications that affect oxygen perfusion or vascular constriction and dilation have all been mentioned as potential factors in ROP. | At least 90% of infants with ROP have spontaneous regression, minimal scarring, little or no visual loss but a high incidence of subsequent refractive errors (astigmatism, myopia, or asymmetric refractive errors), amblyopia, and strabismus (i.e., esotropia and exotropia). Of the 10% that progress to fibrous scar tissue formation, about one fourth will be blind and the rest will have some degree of significant vision impairment. In general, the prognosis for vision worsens with the more posterior the location (i.e., Zone 1), the more clock hours involved (extent), and the higher the stage. |
| Hearing loss | The incidence of confirmed hearing loss in NICU graduates has been reported as 2% to 10%. Medical risk factors include birth weight less than 1500 g, congenital infection (cytomegalovirus, rubella, herpes, toxoplasmosis, and herpes), severe sepsis, bacterial meningitis, severe asphyxia, persistent pulmonary hypertension of the newborn, anatomic malformations of the head and neck, severe hyperbilirubinemia, and prolonged hospitalization. Certain medications can damage inner ear structures, causing permanent sensorineural hearing loss. Family history of childhood hearing impairment or parent consanguinity are additional risk factors for some infants. | Hearing screening is now routinely completed in most NICUs, often by a noninvasive technique that measures brainstem auditory pathway response to sound. Decreased infant responsiveness to auditory parental stimulation may affect optimal parent-infant relationship. Even an intermittent hearing loss (i.e., from fluid accumulation in the middle ear) or a mild hearing loss can adversely affect later speech and language development. |

From Avery, G.B. & Glass, P. (1989). The gentle nursery: developmental intervention in the NICU. *Journal of Perinatology, 11,* 216-226; Felix, J.K. (1991). Screening for hearing loss. In M.D. Jones, C.A. Gleason, & S.U. Lipstein (Eds.). *Hospital care of the recovering NICU infant* (pp. 177-186). Baltimore: Williams & Wilkins; Flynn, J.T. (1990). Retinopathy of prematurity. In J.W. Eichenbaum, A. Mamelok, R.N. Mittl, & J. Orellana (Eds.). *Treatment of retinopathy of prematurity* (pp. 81-117). Chicago: Year Book Medical Publishers; George, D.S., Stephan, S., Fellows, R.R., & Bremer, D.L. (1988). The latest on retinopathy of prematurity. *American Journal of Maternal Child Nursing, 13,* 254-258; Ryan, J. (1988). Hearing and speech assessment. In R.A. Ballard (Ed.). *Pediatric care of the ICU graduate* (pp. 111-120). Philadelphia: W.B. Saunders.

▲ Table 22-C5    Nutritional or Gastrointestinal Complications Encountered in the NICU

| Diagnosis | Description | Implications for Occupational Therapies |
|---|---|---|
| Rickets of prematurity (osteopenia) | Preterm infants (especially those with very low birth weight) miss the period of most rapid intrauterine accumulation of calcium and phosphorus, which cannot be duplicated in parenteral nutrition because of insolubility. Some medications also increase urinary calcium losses. For these reasons, preterm infants are at risk for metabolic rickets of prematurity secondary to poor bone mineralization. | May be a cause of fractures in some infants, especially those with bronchopulmonary dysplasia. Caregivers must handle the infant gently and be alert for signs of possible fractures (e.g., bruising, swelling, and tenderness). |
| Necrotizing enterocolitis (NEC) | NEC occurs primarily (90%) in preterm infants, and is a major cause of mortality in the NICU. The exact cause and pathogenesis of NEC is still unknown; infection, enteral feedings, and local vascular compromise (ischemia, e.g., secondary to cold stress or persistent apnea) of the gastrointestinal tract have all been implicated in the resultant mucosal injury. Bacterial invasion and formation of gas bubbles in the intestinal linings are common. Some cases respond to medical management, although sequelae may still occur. Surgery is indicated if the intestine ruptures or if portions of the intestine become gangrenous. | "NEC watch": Enteral feeds will be stopped; antibiotics and total parenteral nutrition (TPN) are started. The infant is positioned for comfort if abdominal distention is present. Comfort measures with gentle handling are appropriate. An infant with actual NEC will stop enteral feeds, have continuous gastric suction, be on TPN and antibiotics, and may be on a vent. Functional or structural obstruction may occur with or without surgery. Short bowel syndrome with failure to thrive may result, depending on amount and location of bowel surgically removed. |
| Gastroschisis | Results from a defect in the abdominal wall of the embryo, usually on the right side near, but not involving, the umbilicus. The intestines and possibly other abdominal organs (stomach, liver, and spleen) develop outside the body and are exposed at birth with no membranous covering. Gastroschisis often has an associated intestinal malrotation and occasionally there are atretic portions of the externalized bowel but not typically malformations of other organ systems. | Surgery is usually done on day of birth but may be "staged" if not all the organs can fit inside the abdominal cavity immediately (i.e., remainder is sterilely wrapped and suspended above supine infant in a "silo"; gravity and manual manipulation gradually reduce contents, with final surgical repair around 1 week of age). Increased risk of infection. Residual problems with gastrointestinal motility or absorption may affect feeding. |

From Cox, J.M., Oliva, M.M., & Perman, J.A. (1993). Nutrition and gastrointestinal problems. In F.W. Witter & L.G. Keith (Eds.). *Textbook of prematurity.* Boston: Little, Brown; Korones, S.B. & Bada-Elizey, H.S. (1993). *Neonatal decision making.* St. Louis: Mosby.

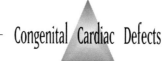

## Congenital Cardiac Defects

### REVIEW OF NORMAL HEART ANATOMY AND PHYSIOLOGY

The normal heart consists of two upper chambers (right and left atria) and two lower chambers (right and left ventricles) divided by septums into right and left sides, along with outflow arteries and inflow veins for both pulmonary and systemic (body) circulation. Blood flow progression is as follows:

1. From the body, returns through the inferior and superior vena cava to empty into the right atrium
2. Passes through the tricuspid valve to the right ventricle
3. Leaves the right ventricle through the pulmonary semilunar valve to the main pulmonary artery
4. Is oxygenated in the lungs and returns to the left atrium of the heart through four major pulmonary veins
5. Passes from the left arium through the mitral valve to the left ventricle
6. Leaves the left ventricle through the aortic semilunar valve to the ascending aorta
7. Travels through the systemic vasculature network

### Congenital Heart Disease

Congenital cardiovascular malformations occur in 8 per 1000 live births. Most of these defects are simple left-to-right shunts that are acyanotic and pose relatively low risk to the infant, such as a patent ductus arteriosus or ventricular septal defect. Approximately 25% of congenital heart disease is serious enough to require cardiac catheterization and other medical diagnostic procedures during the first year. Early surgical intervention is typically more common (and sometimes imperative) with cyanotic congenital heart disease.

### ACYANOTIC CONGENITAL HEART DEFECTS
#### Aortic Stenosis

The aortic valve (or areas immediately above or below the actual valve) is stenosed, with resultant obstruction to outflow from the left ventricle to the aorta. Degree of stenosis is progressive (from fibrin deposits, fibrosis, and calcification) and tends to recur even after surgical correction.

#### Atrial Septal Defect (ASD)

Defect in the septum separating the right and left ventricles. Size and site of the lesion may vary. Spontaneous closure is rare unless defect is small; surgical sutures or patch is typical.

#### Atrioventricular (AV) Canal: Endocardial Cushion Defect

Refers to a spectrum of malformations that includes defects in the lower part of the interatrial septum, the upper part of the interventricular septum, and the portions of the AV (tricuspid and mitral) valves closest to the atrial and ventricular septa. AV valve regurgitation differentiates this anomaly from a simple ventricular septal defect or an ASD. Large defects require surgery.

#### Coarctation of the Aorta

Narrowing or constriction of a portion of the aorta that causes elevated blood pressure proximal to the stricture and decreased blood flow or blood pressure distal to the obstruction. Surgical repair is indicated but may not be urgent.

#### Partial Anomalous Pulmonary Venous Return

One, but not all, of the pulmonary veins does not empty into the left atrium. The pulmonary veins on the right may connect directly to the superior vena cava, or the pulmonary veins on the left may communicate with the inominate vein. This defect may occur in isolation or in conjunction with an ASD. Usually requires surgical correction if at least 2 veins are involved.

#### Patent Ductus Arteriosus (PDA)

A PDA is a short fetal blood vessel that connects the main pulmonary artery to the decsending aorta. It is a normal component of fetal circulation, but failure of the PDA to close soon after birth allows direct shunting of blood between the main pulmonary artery and the aorta. This shunt will be right-to-left if the infant is in respiratory distress or left-to-right with potential congestive heart failure if no significant respiratory illness exists. PDA may close spontaneously or may require medication or surgical ligation.

#### Physiologically Corrected Transposition of the Great Vessels (LTGV)

Origins of the great vessels are reversed (aorta from the right ventricle, pulmonary artery from the left ventricle), but discordant atrioventricular and ventriculoarterial connections result in misalignment such that the right atrium drains into the left ventricle and the left ventricle drains into the right pulmonary artery. Thus systemic blood still returns to the lungs for oxygenation. Oxygenated blood proceeds to the left atrium through the right ventricle and out the aorta back into systemic circulation. LTGV frequently occurs in combination with more complex lesions. Need for surgical intervention is variable.

#### Pulmonic Stenosis

Constriction of pulmonary artery or pulmonic semilunar valve can result in obstructed outflow from the right ventricle through the pulmonary arteries to the lungs. Stenosis is not progressive. Severe cases may need surgical intervention.

## Congenital Cardiac Defects—cont'd

### Ventricular Septal Defect (VSD)

Defect in the septum separating the right and left ventricles. A VSD may be an isolated defect or it may occur as part of complex heart disease; size and exact location of lesion can vary. Most VSDs close spontaneously; some require surgery.

### CYANOTIC CONGENITAL HEART DEFECTS
### Double Inlet Ventricle Also Called Single Ventricle

Either the right or left ventricle is incompletely formed and the remaining ventricle is dominant; the connection is described as double inlet when one, and at least 50% of the other, atrioventricular valve feeds into the dominant ventricle. Although rare, a single primitive ventricle with no dividing septum may occur.

### Double Outlet Right Ventricle

Both the aorta and the main pulmonary artery originate from the right ventricle; a VSD and varying degrees of cyanosis are always present. Surgical repair is necessary.

### Ebstein's Anomaly

Involves a malformation of the tricuspid valve in which leaflets of the valve are displaced downward and adhere to the inflow portion of the right ventricle. This incorporates a portion of the right ventricle into the right atrium; the remaining ventricular cavity may be small. Tricuspid insufficiency is present in varying degrees. May eventually require surgery.

### Hypoplastic Left Heart

Left ventricle and ascending aorta are underdeveloped; mitral and aortic valves are atretic or stenotic. Multistaged surgery may be attempted (10% survival), but this defect is usually fatal without a heart transplant.

### Interrupted Aortic Arch

The aortic arch is interrupted at some point between the inominate artery and the left subclavian artery; a VSD is typically present. Severe congestive heart failure, cyanosis, and respiratory distress appear early. Classic clinical findings are a strong pulse in the right upper extremity but weak or absent pulses from lower extremities and left upper extremity. The lower body becomes hypoxemic and acidotic; subsequent organ damage and death result if surgical repair is delayed.

### Pulmonary Atresia with Intact Ventricular Septum

Forward flow through the usually hypoplastic right ventricle is not possible because of agenesis of the pulmonary valve. Blood returning from the body is shunted from the right to left atrium and mixed with whatever blood is returning from the lungs. Blood then passes into the left ventricle and back into systemic circulation. Surgical intervention is required.

### Tetrology of Fallot (TOF)

Consists of a constellation of defects including a large VSD, right ventricular outflow obstruction (pulmonary stenosis), aorta overiding the VSD, and right ventricular hypertrophy. The degree of pulmonary stenosis typically dictates the severity and course of TOF. *Tet spells* refer to hypoxic episodes of suddenly increasing cyanosis and agitation that are usually associated with arising, eating, activity, or crying. Surgical intervention is usually required, although timing can vary significantly.

### Total Anomalous Pulmonary Venous Return (TAPVR)

None of the four pulmonary veins empties into the left atrium; drainage occurs indirectly through various routes into the right atrium. An ASD must always be present to permit function of the left side of the heart. Early surgical correction is usually required.

### Transposition of the Great Vessels (DTGV)

Origins of the aorta and main pulmonary artery are reversed from a normal presentation; the aorta arises from the right ventricle, and the pulmonary artery arises from the left ventricle. DTGV may occur in an isolated form or with complex heart disease. Early surgery is required.

### Tricuspid Atresia

The tricuspid valve between the right atrium and right ventricle is either absent or not patent, obstructing blood flow into the right ventricle. The right ventricle may be fully formed if a VSD is present, or it may be hypoplastic. Surgical repair is required.

### Truncus Arteriosus: Types I-IV

When normal separation of the aorta and main pulmonary artery do not occur during fetal development, both the right and left ventricles empty into a single large vessel. Types I and IV are common; types II and III are not. The pulmonary arteries are connected to the aorta in Types I, II, and III. In Type IV the pulmonary arteries have no connection to the common trunk (single large vessel), and pulmonary perfusion occurs from collateral circulation. A VSD is always present. Surgical repair is required.

From Daberkow, E. & Washington, R.L. (1993). Cardiovascular diseases and surgical interventions. In G.B. Merenstein & S.L. Gardner (Eds.). *Handbook of neonatal intensive care* (3rd ed.) (pp. 365-398). St. Louis: Mosby; Long, W.A. (1990). *Fetal and neonatal cardiology.* Philadelphia: W.B. Saunders; Sapire, D.W. (1991). *Understanding and diagnosing pediacric heart disease.* Norwalk: Appleton & Lange.

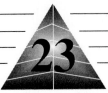

# Early Intervention

LINDA C. STEPHENS ▲ SUSAN K. TAUBER

## KEY TERMS

▲ Early Intervention
▲ Part H of the Individuals With Disabilities Act
▲ Family Centered
▲ Team Models of Interaction
▲ Developmentally Appropriate
▲ Service Coordination

## CHAPTER OBJECTIVES

1. Describe the early intervention legislation and program regulations.
2. Explain family-centered early intervention philosophy and principles.
3. Define the components of an Individual Family Service Plan.
4. Explain models of assessment and typical infant evaluations.
5. Describe developmentally appropriate and family-centered intervention approaches.
6. Define areas of emphasis in occupational therapy.
7. Explain strategies and activities used by occupational therapists in work with infants and young children.

## WHAT IS EARLY INTERVENTION?

The term *early intervention* connotes different meanings to different professionals. In this chapter, *early* refers to that most critical period of a child's development between birth and 3 years of age. *Intervention* refers to program implementation designed to maintain or enhance the child's development in natural environments and as a member of a family. *Early intervention* also is used here to describe children from birth to 3 years who have an established risk, a developmental delay, or are considered to be environmentally or biologically at risk. Intervention strategies and programs are intended to prevent or ameliorate developmental delays and deformities, maximize each child's potential, and assist the family in adjusting to the challenges of daily living both in the home and in the community.

## LEGISLATION RELATED TO EARLY INTERVENTION

The past decade has brought widespread acceptance and support for family-centered care for children with special needs. It is based on the principle that a baby is dependent on his or her mother and other family members for daily care and meeting his or her physical and emotional needs. At the same time, the birth of a baby with special health care needs affects the entire family in many ways: emotionally, socially, and economically. Since the late 1960s, public policy has evolved that paved the way for family-centered care and resulted in legislation specific to children from birth through 2 years of age with or at risk for developmental disabilities.

Shonkoff and Meisels (1990) described the history of early intervention services and emphasized that PL 99-457, the Education of the Handicapped Act Amendments of 1986, was the most important and influential piece of legislation for young children with disabilities and their families. Part H of this piece of legislation established services for children from birth through 2 years of age with disabilities. Part B defines services for children 3 to 21 years of age and is described in Chapters 24 and 25, on school-based practice. Recent amendments to that law, the Individuals with Disabilities Education Act of 1990 (IDEA; P.L. 101-476), strengthened the incentives for establishing early intervention services and further defined how these services are to be implemented. In addition to its strong emphasis on family-centered intervention, IDEA strengthens the importance of prevention rather than remediation (Johnson,

1994) and promotes well-planned and coordinated transitions from Part H (early intervention) to Part B (preschool or school) programs.

## Early Intervention Entitlements and Guidelines Under Part H

Part H and Part B of IDEA differ in their definitions of occupational therapy. In Part B, occupational therapy is defined as a *related service* that the child can have access to when receiving other special education services. In Part H, occupational therapy is a *direct service,* and can be the primary or only service the child receives. Table 23-1 summarizes the differences in Part H and Part B.

Part H is an entitlement program, and Part B defines mandated services. An entitlement simply acknowledges one's rights to something; a mandate is obligatory by law. This means that states do not have to participate in the Part H program; but if they have chosen to receive Part H funds, they must follow the accompanying regulations.

### State Responsibilities for Administering a Program (34 CFR 303.1)

The purpose of IDEA, Part H, is to:

1. Develop and implement statewide comprehensive, coordinated, collaborative multidisciplinary interagency early intervention services for children with disabilities from birth through 2 years of age and for their families
2. Facilitate coordination of funding sources among federal, state, local, and private sectors (including public and private insurance)
3. Enhance each state's capacity to provide quality services by improving and expanding existing programs through public and private partnerships

4. Facilitate state and local providers' ability to serve underrepresented populations, for example, minority, low-income, inner-city, rural populations

It is implied in the legislation that these services are to be of high quality; yet Safer and Hamilton (1993) pointed out that it neither defines *quality of service* nor indicates how states are to assure quality standards. The authors of the law imply that services are to be of high quality, but the determination of providing quality services depends on one's frame of reference on values, philosophy, and knowledge of *best practice*. Safer and Hamilton (1993) suggested measuring quality by considering six dimensions:

1. Timeliness: How quickly are children and families identified, assessed, and provided with the necessary early intervention services?
2. Effectiveness: Do the early intervention services meet the family's desired outcomes and allow each child to meet his or her maximum potential?
3. Individualization: Are the services responsive to each child and family's needs, circumstances, and location? Are they socially, culturally, and linguistically sensitive?
4. Transitions: Is there a written plan in place that details a continuum of services?
5. Child- and Family-Centered: Do services reflect inclusion of the child and family within the community, considering their priorities and their concerns as a family? Are services provided in environments and at times convenient to the family?
6. Coordination of Services: Are services nonfragmented and coordinated among all those who provide services for the child and family?

In addition to these six points listed, the legislation states that evaluation and assessment procedures must be appropriate for infants from birth through 2 years of age.

▲ Table 23-1  Comparison of Legislative Provisions by Age Group

| Issue | 0 to 2 Years | 3 to 5 Years | 6 to 21 Years |
|---|---|---|---|
| Legislation | P.L. 101-476 Part H<br>Early Intervention—medical model<br>Entitlement | P.L. 101-476 Part B<br>Special education—model<br>Mandate | P.L. 94-142<br>Special education—model<br>Mandate |
| Eligibility | Noncategorical | Categorical | Categorical |
| Services | 16 Primary services, including occupational therapy, physical therapy, speech therapy, and special instruction | Related services only as support to special education | Related services only as support to special education |
| | Multidisciplinary and transdisciplinary assessment | Discipline-specific assessment | Discipline-specific assessment as related to education |
| | Individualized Family Service Plan | Individual Educational Plan | Individual Educational Plan |
| | Family-focused | Family-focused in theory, child-focused in practice and therapy | Child-focused and educational |
| | Service coordination | Service coordination recommended but not mandated | Service coordination recommended but not mandated |
| Location | Natural settings | Home-, center-, or school-based | School-based |

## Eligibility for Part H

Specific eligibility criteria are left to state discretion and are not specified in federal regulations (Federal Register, 34 CFR 303.300). Eligibility for early intervention is non-categorical and is designated for infants and toddlers from birth through 2 years of age with the following criteria:

*Established risk:* Children with established risk are those who have been diagnosed with a physical or mental condition that is known to have a high probability of resulting in a developmental delay such as Down syndrome and cerebral palsy.

*Developmental delay:* Developmental delay, measured by an "appropriate" diagnostic instrument or procedure or informed clinical opinion, indicates delay in one or more of the following developmental areas: cognitive, physical (includes vision and hearing), communication, social or emotional, and adaptive. States differ in the criteria chosen to determine "appropriate" instruments or procedures.

*At risk:* This category is included at state discretion and refers to a child who is considered to be *at risk* for the occurrence of a substantial developmental delay unless early intervention services are provided. Causation may be a result of environmental or biologic risk factors, for example, infants born to teen mothers or drug- or alcohol-addicted mothers and very low–birth-weight (VLBW) or failure-to-thrive (FTT) babies.

## Required Services

There are 16 early intervention services that are to be provided under public supervision by qualified personnel and in conformity with the Individual Family Service Plan (IFSP). Services should be family-centered, inclusive, and culturally sensitive. The 16 services include the following:

Assistive technology devices and services
Audiology
Family training, counseling and home visits
Health services
Medical services for diagnostics and evaluation only
Nursing
Nutrition
Occupational therapy
Physical therapy
Psychological services
Service coordination
Social work
Special instruction
Speech and language therapy
Transportation
Vision services

## Identification

The first step in the early intervention process is public awareness and a viable Child Find system under IDEA, Part B. This system must include standard referral procedures to be used by all primary referral sources and assignment of a service coordinator for the child and family as soon as possible after receiving the referral.

## Evaluation Process

Evaluation is the step that determines the eligibility of a child for initial and continuing early intervention services. The child must be evaluated by a multidisciplinary team that includes the professionals listed previously whose services seem warranted or are desired by the family. Parental permission must be obtained before the evaluation. Assessment is the ongoing procedure used during the child's eligibility to determine his or her needs, strengths, necessary services, family concerns, priorities, and resources. The evaluation process must be completed within 45 days of identification (Federal Register, 34 CFR 303.322[e]).

## Evaluation Requirements

The service coordinator is responsible for assuring that the evaluation process (1) is conducted by trained personnel; (2) is based on the state's adopted criteria of standard deviations or informed clinical opinion; (3) includes child's medical and health history; and (4) includes levels of functioning, unique needs, and recommended services related to the five developmental areas (cognition, physical, communication, social and emotional, and adaptive).

Family resources, priorities, and concerns as they relate to their child's development are documented. Collection of this information is family directed and voluntary. Finally, the evaluation procedures must be nondiscriminatory as to race, ethnicity, and socioeconomic background and in the family's native language or mode of communication to the best extent possible.

## Individual Family Service Plan

The IFSP is the third step in the early intervention system. It is a written plan that delineates all the services the child will need. For all eligible children, this plan is developed with the family and must identify the family's desired outcomes as they relate to their child. The IFSP must be written within 45 days after the referral. It is a map of the family's services and informs anyone who will be working with the child and family which services will be provided, where they will be provided, and by whom they will be provided. The IFSP also identifies the service coordinator who will be responsible for working with the family.

The role of a service coordinator is a unique Part H provision of the IFSP. The service coordinator is the designated person who assists the family in accessing information and resources. The box on p. 651 lists the required components as they are stated in IDEA.

If the child requires preschool special education or other services, the services must be written into the IFSP's transition procedures. This step requires contact with the Local Education Agency (LEA) and requires parental consent to

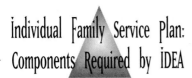

## Individual Family Service Plan: Components Required by IDEA

1. Statement of present levels of function in the five developmental areas.
2. Family information, which includes resources, priorities, and concerns related to child's development.
3. Outcomes to be achieved for child and family with stated criteria, procedures, and timelines to assess progress and necessary changes.
4. Early intervention services are those deemed necessary to meet the specific needs of the child and family and include the following:
   a. Frequency, intensity, duration, and method for service delivery
   b. Natural environments where services will occur
   c. Location of services
   d. Payment arrangements, if necessary
   e. Other services appropriate for child and family, for example, medical care (other than those required by Part H); funding sources to access public or private resources
   f. Dates and duration of services
   g. Service coordinator, who can be from the profession most relevant to child or family's needs or otherwise qualified (specific description of service coordinator's requirements can be found in Part H regulation Section 303.22)
   h. Transition planning for exit from Part H to Part B services, which occurs on the child's third birthday

*IDEA*, Individuals with Disabilities Education Plan.

▲ The right to a timely, multidisciplinary assessment
▲ If eligible under Part H, the right to appropriate early intervention services
▲ The right of refusal to evaluations, assessments, and services
▲ The right to written notice before provider or agency proposes or refuses identification, evaluation or placement of the child, or provision of services to child and family
▲ The right to confidentiality (in compliance with the Family Educational Rights and Privacy Act)
▲ The right to review and, if appropriate, to correct records
▲ The right to be invited, to attend, and to participate in all meetings where a decision will be made in the determination of change in identification, evaluation or placement of the child, or the provision of services to the child and family
▲ The right to legal counsel as pertinent to the early intervention system
▲ The right to an impartial hearing to resolve complaints *(Babies Can't Wait,* 1993)

### Transition Into Preschool Services (Part B)

A transition plan should be identified in the IFSP as soon as possible and as soon as relevant. Referral to the LEA should be made 6 months before the child's third birthday or at 30 months of age. This helps the school system analyze all existing evaluation and assessment information and determine if further testing or information is necessary. It also enables the LEA to determine eligibility under Part B (which in some cases may differ from Part H eligibility) and, if eligible, plan for appropriate placement. When referral is made on a child who is already 3 years old, the LEA has 60 days to complete the evaluation and eligibility process. Once the child is determined eligible for services under Part B, an Individual Education Plan (IEP) is written.

### Funding

Each state that chooses to participate in the Part H program receives federal funds based on a census of infants and toddlers in the state's general population compared with the total number of infants and children nationally. Part H funds are used as the "payor of last resort" for services for eligible children when there are no other available funds through another federal, state, local, or private source. The lead agency is responsible for identifying and coordinating all funding resources and must enter into formal interagency agreements with other state agencies that provide services to young children and their families. Families are entitled to the following services at no cost: Child Find, evaluation and assessment, service coordination, and administration and coordination of IFSP activities and procedural safeguards.

provide records to the LEA for continuity of services and evaluation and assessment information. The IFSP is reviewed every 6 months, with an annual reevaluation.

The IFSP is *not* a treatment plan. Occupational therapy services, for example, may be listed on the IFSP as it relates to the desired outcomes identified by the parents. Specific occupational therapy treatment goals, objectives, and procedures are to be specified on the occupational therapy treatment plan, which is a separate document from the IFSP and should be written by the occupational therapist using acceptable occupational therapy procedures and terminology.

### Procedural Safeguards

Parents must be informed of their rights that underlie the early intervention process. All states that use federal funds for early intervention services have specified procedural safeguards that protect the rights of parents and infants. As an example, the Part H Program Standards in Georgia include the following:

### Interagency Coordinating Council

The role of the Interagency Coordinating Council (ICC) is to advise and assist the lead agency in the implementation of a statewide early intervention system. The system is to be a "comprehensive, coordinated, collaborative, multidisciplinary, program for infants and toddlers with disabilities and their families." The ICC assists the lead agency and the State Education Agency (SEA) coordinating Part H and Part B of IDEA. Members of the state ICC are appointed by the governor. Membership of the ICC consists of parents (at least 20% of total membership), public and private providers (at least 20%), at least one member of the legislature, a representative from personnel preparation, one member from each State agency involved with payment for early intervention services who has authority to participate in policy planning and implementation, one member from the SEA who has authority to participate in policy planning and implementation, one member from the state governance of insurance, for example, Medicaid, and others selected by the governor. Meetings must be held at least quarterly, with prior public notice and invitation for public attendance. Interpreters must be provided as necessary. In addition to the State ICC, each district has a local ICC (LICC), which includes public and private providers as well as parents. Each LICC is responsible for identifying and coordinating services within its geographic area.

## IMPLICATIONS OF LEGISLATION FOR THE OCCUPATIONAL THERAPIST

The practice of occupational therapy in early intervention has been influenced by public legislation in the following ways:

1. Team coordination and interagency communication: The occupational therapist practices as part of a team, rather than in isolation, and contributes occupational therapy findings and suggestions to the IFSP. With parental permission and with confidentiality observed, therapy reports are shared with other agencies that are delivering services to the family.
2. Family service plan versus child-centered treatment plan: The occupational therapist provides services to the child and the family with consideration of total family priorities rather than providing services to the child only.
3. Indirect versus direct treatment: The occupational therapist may consider a variety of service delivery models, including those that may be transdisciplinary or consultative in nature. The model of direct, individual, child-centered services often is not the most appropriate one in early intervention.
4. Concern with generalization of skills: The occupational therapist is concerned with the functional use of skills in the child's natural environment rather than the development of skills in isolation.
5. Ability to practice role release: Professionals in early intervention often find it advantageous to use role release in the provision of services. In this way one professional may be trained to take over functions that traditionally have been performed by another professional.
6. Variety of settings: A major philosophy of early intervention is that services should be provided in those environments that are most natural for the child. Occupational therapists are more likely to provide services in community settings, such as the home or a child care center, than in medical settings.
7. Wide range of disabilities: As state lead agencies and Child Find services identify children who qualify for services, the occupational therapist is expected to work with children with a variety of special needs. These may include biologically or environmentally at-risk populations that traditionally may not have received intervention.
8. Work in small groups: Traditional methods of individual, or one-on-one, treatment are often replaced by the delivery of services to small groups of children or small parent-infant groups.
9. Knowledge about the educational model and educational objectives: Occupational therapists must be competent in working outside the traditional medical model and need to understand educational and family-centered models of practice.
10. Addressing family concerns and priorities: The occupational therapist must be sensitive to family needs and have respect for the parents' priorities. For example, the parent who is homeless or jobless may not be concerned about occupational therapy for the child. Another parent may believe that certain skills or goals are more important than those identified by the therapist. The occupational therapist should also be cognizant of the effect of limiting factors, such as insurance coverage or Medicaid maximum units.

## FAMILY-CENTERED PROGRAMS

Early intervention legislation mandates that the family be included in the planning and implementation of services for the child. This mandate recognizes families as knowledgeable consumers as well as effective change agents for the child. It also acknowledges that families have specific needs related to a child with disabilities and that families also may be the recipients of services. The family's early intervention service coordinator is required to help each family identify its unique strengths, needs, priorities, and concerns. Outcomes and goals are then identified that enable the family to function more effectively and help the child as a member of the family unit. The two primary forms of involvement are the family as a participant in services or the family as a client of intervention services.

Simeonsson and Bailey (1990) identified four different ways in which intervention could be provided for infants with special needs and their families:

1. Therapy administered to the infant, with the parent as a passive bystander
2. Parents involved as members of the intervention team, participating in the planning process and involvement in the child's program
3. Parents trained to carry out therapeutic activities as co-therapists or as the primary intervention agents
4. Families viewed as important recipients of services in their own right

The nature and extent of family involvement may vary and depends on family needs, values, and life-styles as well as variables within the structure of the early intervention program itself. The degree of family involvement may fluctuate and change in response to external or internal factors that affect family functioning and coping. Some examples are degree of acceptance of the child's disability, job status of one or both parents, a new baby in the family, or changes in the family's support networks, such as grandparents, friends, or church groups. Simeonsson and Bailey (1990) have identified a hierarchy of family involvement in early intervention (Table 23-2).

The occupational therapist who works within a family-centered model develops goals collaboratively with parents or primary caretakers. Bailey et al. (1986) identified some skills necessary for the therapist in collaborative goal setting. One skill important to family-centered intervention is to view the family from a systems perspective. In this viewpoint the therapist recognizes the influence and interrelationships of the family within various systems such as extended family, neighborhood, and early intervention programs. The second skill needed is the ability to assess the family's needs as well as the child's needs. The therapist should be skilled in effective listening and interviewing and in negotiating differences in values and priorities. It is important to recognize that differences in values exist and to help the family explore a variety of strategies to reach mutually agreed on functional goals. Featherstone (1980) stated that there are four ways in which professionals can assist families who have children with special needs: providing information, respecting the child and family, providing emotional support, and providing services.

There are eight principles that have been generally accepted in the implementation of family-centered care (Shelton, Jeppson, & Johnson, 1987, 3-44):

1. Recognition that the family is the constant in the child's life, whereas the service systems and personnel within those systems fluctuate
2. Facilitation of parent and professional collaboration at all levels of health care
3. Sharing of unbiased and complete information with parents about their child's care on an ongoing basis in an appropriate and supportive manner
4. Implementation of appropriate policies and programs that are comprehensive and provide emotional and financial support to meet the needs of families
5. Recognition of family strengths and individuality and respect for different methods of coping

▲ Table 23-2   Hierarchic Dimensions of Family Involvement in Early Intervention: Family and Interventionist Roles

| Level | Dimensions of Involvement | Family Role | Interventionist Role | Example |
|---|---|---|---|---|
| O | Elective noninvolvement | Rejects available services | Informs and offers available services | Family elects not to be involved |
| I | Passive involvement | Acknowledges but does not use services | Tracks and advises families | Family allows tracking |
| II | Consumer involvement | Consumer of child-related services | Provider or broker of child-related services | Provision of developmental stimulation and allied therapies |
| III | Involvement focusing on informational and skills needs | Information seeking; acquiring teaching and management skills | Consultant and teacher role in information sharing | Provision of anticipatory guidance for families |
| IV | Personal involvement to secure or extend personal or social support | Seeking support to build or strengthen formal or informal resources | Advocacy and relationship building | Identification of informal or formal support network |
| V | Behavioral involvement to define and deal with reality burdens | Partnership to identify, prioritize, and implement interventions | Goal setting to develop interventions | Coordination of services to facilitate family coping |
| IV | Psychologic involvement to define and deal with value conflicts | Client role in seeking psychologic change at family or personal level | Therapist or counselor role to help with psychologic or existential issue | Provision and coordination of comprehensive therapeutic services |

From Simeonsson, R.J. & Bailey, D.B. (1990). Family dimensions in early intervention. In S.J. Meisels & J.P. Shonkoff (Eds.) *Handbook of early childhood intervention*. Cambridge: Cambridge University Press.

6. Understanding and incorporating the developmental needs of infants, children, and adolescents and their families into health care systems
7. Encouragement and facilitation of parent-to-parent support
8. Assurance that the design of health care delivery systems is flexible, accessible, and responsive to family needs

## EARLY INTERVENTION TEAM

The success of an early intervention program depends largely on the integration of the child's individual program components into a comprehensive system carried out by a cooperative team of professionals. Teamwork is critical because of the interrelated nature of the problems of the developing child and the need for skills and resources from many professionals to meet the needs of both the child and family. The emphasis of intervention should be the child within the family unit, rather than the child alone, and should be carried out through collaboration among all professionals involved. This teamwork may take on a variety of configurations; the most common are multidisciplinary, interdisciplinary, and transdisciplinary.

### Team Approaches
#### Multidisciplinary

The multidisciplinary approach evolved from the medical model in which multiple professionals evaluated the child and made recommendations (Peterson, 1987). In this type of approach, several professionals may be directly or indirectly involved with the child and family but do not necessarily consult or interact with each other. Assessment, goal setting, and direct intervention may be carried out by each professional with minimal integration across disciplines (Bruder & Bologna, 1993). Often services are provided in several locations, with one person, such as the parent or the physician, acting as the case manager.

#### Interdisciplinary

The interdisciplinary approach to treatment is a more cooperative and interactive approach that consists of a team comprised of professionals from several disciplines involved with the child, often at the same location. These professionals have continuing direct involvement with the child and collaborate with each other in carrying out the child's program. Although evaluations are performed independently by each discipline, program planning occurs as a result of group consensus and goals are set collaboratively with professionals and parents. With this approach the child and family can receive coordinated services and are able to benefit from the expertise of professionals from several disciplines who are directly involved (Case-Smith & Wavrek, 1993).

Each member of an interdisciplinary team is accountable to the team as a whole, although the degree and amount of involvement may vary and change depending on the child and family needs. The family's service coordinator is usually the person responsible for the coordination of team members to avoid fragmentation or duplication of services. To ensure the success of this approach, the team members must respect each other's roles, develop effective formal and informal communication patterns, and be flexible in response to family needs and preferences. This requires a willingness to share expertise and knowledge and to assume responsibility to be accountable for intervention procedures.

#### Transdisciplinary

In the transdisciplinary approach, various disciplines interact as a team but one member is usually designated to provide direct intervention with other team members who act as consultants. This approach is based on the belief that the family benefits from having intervention primarily from one professional rather than multiple interventions from a number of professionals. All team members contribute to assessment and program planning, and then the designated person implements the plan with consultation and training from other members of the team. Therefore the transdisciplinary model enables each professional to perform functions that are normally outside the scope of practice of his or her discipline. Implementation of this model requires *role release,* or the relinquishing of some or all of one professional's functions to another professional. This has been defined as a process of sharing and the exchange of certain roles and responsibilities among team members (Lyon & Lyon, 1980).

The transdisciplinary approach is described by Giangreco (1986) as "indirect, integrated, and decentralized; it limits the number of people carrying out a program but makes use of the expertise of a variety of professionals" (p. 9). However, this approach was not intended to promote a team in which each professional developed the same skills across discipline lines, but rather was intended to promote frequent and regular sharing of knowledge and skills.

For example, a 2-year-old child with spina bifida was evaluated by a transdisciplinary team. It was determined that the home was the preferred location for treatment and that the physical therapist would act as the direct service provider. The occupational therapist, speech pathologist, and early childhood specialist taught the physical therapist certain techniques to use for feeding, language stimulation, and cognitive development. As a result, the physical therapist was able to provide a wide variety of intervention strategies on her weekly visits, with periodic monitoring and consultation from the other professionals on the team.

Successful functioning as a transdisciplinary team takes commitment and willingness to cross traditional discipline boundaries as well as effective communication and consultative skills. To implement this approach, the therapist must be "highly skilled in analyzing the child's developmental function and synthesizing the family and home situation given a limited amount of information" (Case-Smith & Wavrek, 1993, p. 144). Although the transdisciplinary model may seem to be the most appropriate in early intervention, several barriers or obstacles have been identified in this approach (Orlove & Sobsey, 1991; Ottenbacher, 1983). These obstacles include philosophic and professional differences, legal liabilities and licensure limitations, variable background education of designated service providers, and inconsistent mastery of skills practiced through role release. In addition, reimbursement from third-party payers may dictate intervention based on a medical model with direct provision of services by each professional.

Regardless of which approach is used, effective teamwork does not come easily. It requires a flexible administration based on a sound philosophic framework and honest, hard work on the part of each team member.

## EVALUATION OF INFANTS AND TODDLERS
### Developmental Approach

Teti and Gibbs (1990) traced the interest in infancy and infant assessment back to the 1800s and the Child Study Movement and the efforts of Stanley Hall, founder of normative study of child development. This is the basis for norm-referenced assessment, which assesses a particular behavior or attribute of children of a particular age-group, establishing a mean age of development and an accompanying developmental curve with which other children can be compared.

An assumption of the developmental theory is that there is continuity of function from the infancy stages of sensorimotor development through the early childhood stages of verbalization and representational functioning. Environmental and physiologic factors, however, influence this development. The knowledge that environmental factors influence the infant's development and the belief that neurodevelopment of the infant is plastic and malleable supports the concept of early intervention (Teti & Gibbs, 1990).

The developmental approach to infant assessment involves a multidimensional, holistic method in which each developmental domain is individually examined, and then the influence the domains have on each other and on the child as a whole is assessed. For example, infants with motor impairments are restricted in their ability to explore their environment, a critical component to sensorimotor development, which in turn can affect other developmental areas of cognition, language, and socialization.

### Components of the Evaluation Process

Early intervention evaluation consists of a series of steps and is an ongoing, collaborative process of collecting, analyzing, and gathering information about the child and the family to identify specific needs and develop goals in the IFSP (Case-Smith, 1993a; Greenspan & Meisels, 1994). The evaluation, combined with a treatment program and ongoing reassessment, is a problem-solving process that continues throughout the period the child is eligible for Part H services.

Developmental evaluations can be used for screening, diagnosing or evaluating, and program planning. These processes are defined in Section II of this book. Family involvement with the evaluation varies and depends on each member's knowledge and comfort level with the process.

### Screening

Children may be identified as appropriate for early intervention based on the presence of established risk factors, for example, a child with Down syndrome or with limb deficiency. Often, the first step in identification is administration of a screening evaluation. Screening instruments should demonstrate high validity and reliability; accurately identify appropriate infants; include comprehensive health, social, behavioral, and environmental components; and involve the family as an equal partnership with professionals (Hanson & Lynch, 1989). Screening tools measure quantitative performance (e.g., the child does or does not do a particular behavior) and do not consider the quality of that performance (e.g., how the child approaches a task).

One of the most basic and widely used screening tools in medical and early intervention programs is the Denver Developmental Screening Test (DDST) II (Frankenburg et al., 1990), which looks at behaviors in four developmental areas: gross motor, fine motor, personal-social, and language. DDST II can be used for children between 2 weeks and 6 years of age.

The Battelle Developmental Inventory/Screening Test (BDI/S) (a subsection of the Battelle Developmental Inventory that is discussed in the evaluation section) assesses five developmental domains: personal-social, adaptive, motor (gross and fine), communication (receptive and expressive), and cognitive (Newborg, Stock, Wnek, Guidubaldi, & Svinick, 1988) The BDI/S can be used for children between 6 months and 8 years of age and can be adapted for children with special needs. It takes about 30 minutes to administer, which is somewhat longer than the DDST II.

### Evaluation

The process of evaluation is the gathering and interpreting of information on the child's health status and medical background, current developmental levels of functioning, and family resources to maximize the child's development.

#### Eligibility Determination

Part H legislation states that the evaluation must be timely and comprehensive and must include the input by a multidisciplinary team. It should be responsive to the family's needs and desires when determining the time and location of the evaluation and which individuals should be present. The family's involvement is central to the evaluation process and should validate parental choices. The focus of the evaluation should be on the process itself rather than on the final product, such as test scores or a list of strengths and weaknesses (Miller, 1994).

The developmental areas to be evaluated to determine eligibility are cognition, communication, motor, social-emotional, and adaptive. Play is another area of importance to assess and that often is not part of most assessment instruments, yet is the foundation for each of these domains. The following are some of the most frequently used instruments for the team assessment approach: Bayley Scales of Infant Development, 2nd Edition (BSID-II) (Bayley, 1993); Battelle Developmental Inventory (BDI) (Newborg et al., 1988); Gesell Developmental Schedules (Knobloch, Stevens, & Malone, 1980).

Standardized assessments should never be the sole source for determining eligibility for early intervention services (McLean & McCormick, 1993). Furthermore, there are few reliable, comprehensive standardized assessments available for children from birth through age 2. Professional judgment, therefore, is a critical element of this process.

### Intervention Planning

Once a child has been declared eligible for early intervention services, further assessment occurs that establishes the outline for the IFSP and determines the intervention strategies and services. At this point, evaluation becomes a comprehensive decision-making process to identify social-emotional, cognitive, motor, and communication problems and define early intervention program planning and monitoring. Any specific assessment approach is merely a sampling of a child's abilities and behaviors observed at a particular time and situation, from a particular perspective, and with a particular instrument (Greenspan & Meisels, 1994). Assessment results that do not reflect the child's typical functioning or behavioral characteristics are neither meaningful nor accurate.

Miller (1994) made the following recommendations for assessment of infants and young children:

1. Assessment must be based on an integrated developmental model. Parents and professionals must observe the child's range of functions in different contexts in an effort to identify how the child can best be helped, rather than just coming up with a grade or score.
2. Assessment involves multiple sources and multiple components of information. Parents and professionals contribute to forming the total picture of the child.
3. An understanding of typical child development is essential to the interpretation of developmental differences among infants and young children.
4. The assessment should emphasize the child's functional capacities such as attending, engaging, recipro-

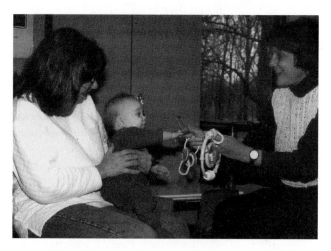

**Figure 23-1** Parent's presence supports the child during assessment and begins the parent-professional collaborative process.

cating, intentional interacting, organizing patterns of behavior, representational or symbolic understanding of his or her environment, and abilities for problem-solving (Greenspan, 1992).

5. The assessment process should identify the child's current abilities and strengths, as well as areas of need, to attain desired developmental outcomes.
6. Young children should not be challenged during the assessment by being separated from their parents or caregivers. The parents' presence supports the child and begins the parent-professional collaborative process (Figure 23-1).
7. Young children should not be challenged by being assessed by an unfamiliar examiner. Time should be allowed for a "warm-up" period. Assessment by a stranger when the parent is restricted to the role of a passive observer represents an additional challenge.
8. Assessments that are limited to easily measurable areas, such as certain motor or cognitive skills, should not be considered complete.
9. Formal or standardized tests should not be considered the determining factor of the assessment for the infant or young child. Most formal tests were developed and standardized on typically developing children and not on those with special needs. Furthermore, many young children have difficulty attending or complying to the basic expectations of formal tests. Formal test procedures are not considered to be the best context in which to observe functional capacities of young children. Assessments that are intended for intervention planning should use structured tests only as part of an integrated approach.

### Assessment and Team Processes

It cannot be overemphasized that early intervention assessment is a collaborative, cooperative, and coordinated process that involves multiple professional disciplines as well

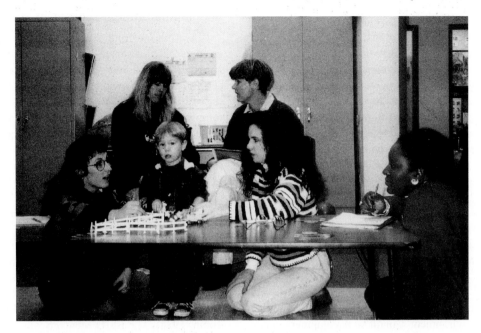

**Figure 23-2**    Transdisciplinary team uses play activities in an arena assessment.

as the parents or primary caregivers and includes information from multiple formal and informal assessment sources. Two of the most common early intervention assessment approaches are the interdisciplinary and transdisciplinary team models, which were discussed previously in this chapter.

There are several assessment tools that are recommended for use as a "core" assessment, that is, one to which all members of the team can contribute discipline-specific perspectives. Using developmental curricula such as the BDI and the Hawaii Early Learning Profile (HELP), each team member can evaluate certain domains of performance and contribute information about that domain to the team's planning process.

One way to implement the transdisciplinary model is through the use of an arena assessment. The concept of an arena assessment is to have an integrated and collaborative understanding about the child's behaviors, accomplishments, and areas of concern. The format of the assessment typically consists of situations that allow for both unstructured and functional play as well as structured and interactive play. One member of the team assumes the role of play facilitator with the child while another facilitates the parent participation (Figure 23-2). The remaining team members are observers, but they can make comments or suggestions during the session. All members contribute to the interpretation of the results, including planning and recommending goals and objectives for intervention. The transdisciplinary model allows for most pertinent information to be gathered, but it does not preclude specific evaluation by individual disciplines if further information is needed. It often is necessary for the occupational or physical therapist to do a more "hands-on" evaluation to assess muscle tone, movement patterns, or handling techniques. Additional information about arena assessment is found in Chapter 8.

Toni Linder (1990) has developed a play assessment process called the *Transdisciplinary Play-Based Assessment (TPBA)*. She also has developed an accompanying intervention guide called *Transdisciplinary Play-Based Intervention (TPBI)* (Linder, 1993). The TPBA includes guidelines that list the normal developmental sequence of skill acquisition in the areas of cognition, social-emotional, communication, and sensorimotor and describes procedures for conducting a transdisciplinary arena-type assessment of the child that uses a play-based format and involves the entire team of professionals and family members. Observation of peer interactions is recommended. Linder's TPBA includes a preassessment and postassessment meeting, sharing observations and identifying needs, priorities, and concerns for the child and family.

Advantages of this model are that it allows for functional play interactions with the child in a natural environment and that it includes parent participation. In addition, the testing activities are flexible and can be adapted to meet the special needs of each child. Linder's TPBA also allows for professionals to contribute their own hands-on or discipline-specific evaluations as part of the TPBA process. The TPBA is an excellent form of evaluation for children who do not comply with standardized evaluation, have difficulty managing behaviors, or demonstrate inconsistent or widely scattered skills.

An example is a 2-year-old boy with an autistic spectrum disorder who has little expressive language, has advanced gross motor skills for his age but is clumsy and fearful of movement (postural insecurity), does not like being touched by others, and is sensitive to certain textures (tactile defensiveness). He also has poor eye contact and does not socially interact with his peers or most adults and often seems unaware of their presence in the same room. Yet, he is able to put together complex puzzles, knows the letters of the alphabet, and can repeat whole parts of video tapes. If the BSID-II were administered, this child would not have related to the materials nor to the examiners and, therefore, would have passed few, if any, items. The score obtained would be an unreliable reflection of his ability and, if presented to parents, would serve no purpose and may be discouraging. A more appropriate assessment for a child with autism would be a play-based approach such as Linder's TPBA.

## Areas of Assessment

The primary developmental domains evaluated are cognitive, social-emotional, audiology and communication, and adaptive or self-help skills.

### Cognitive Development

Cognition is the ability to acquire, store, and use information from the environment. Cognitive development in the infant includes the ability to problem solve; to understand object and person permanence, spatial and timing relationships, and cause-and-effect relationships; to imitate gestures and communication and social-emotional development. Standardized assessments frequently used include the BSID-II Mental Scales and the BDI, Cognitive Domain. Often it is necessary to use nonstandardized procedures. Valuable information can be obtained with the use of Piagetian instruments such as the scales developed by Uzgiris and Hunt (1975) and the accompanying clinical manual developed by Dunst (1980). These tools are useful in identifying cognitive stages of functioning rather than ascertaining a specific age-equivalent score.

### Social-Emotional Development

Social-emotional development is the ability to regulate responses to stimuli from people and the environment. Included within this domain are behaviors that indicate the child's temperament, ability to interact with adults and peers, activity level, attending skills, and coping strategies. It is particularly difficult to obtain reliable information in this area because of the relatively few available tools. Greenspan's Functional Emotional Assessment Scale (1992) looks at six levels of a child's functional capacity such as attending, engaging, reciprocating, intentional interacting, organizing behavior patterns, understanding representational relationships, and skills for problem-solving.

The BSID-II Behavior Rating Scale (Bayley, 1993) looks at five areas: attention and arousal, orientation and engagement, emotional regulation, motor quality, and additional items (soothability, hypersensitivity, adaptation to test materials and stimuli, and tremulousness). It is meant to be used in conjunction with the BSID Mental and Motor Scales but can be used independently. The BDI also includes a Social Domain.

### Communication Development

A hearing screening always should be done as a first step to any speech-language assessment. If a hearing problem is suspected, an audiologic evaluation should be done. The second step should include evaluating the oral motor structure as well as oral motor skills (suck-swallow patterns, tongue movements, and chewing patterns). Oral motor assessment can be done by either an occupational therapist or a speech-language pathologist.

Formal speech-language evaluations consist of assessing both receptive language skills (what the child understands) and expressive language skills (how the child expresses himself). Use of gestures as well as sounds or words is assessed.

Communication assessments include the BDI—Communication Domain, Preschool Language Scale—3 (Zimmerman, Steiner, & Pond, 1992), The Rossetti Infant-Toddler Language Scale (Rossetti, 1990), and the Sequenced Inventory of Communication Development (Hedrick, Prather, & Tobin, 1984). The BSID Mental Scale includes many items that assess the child's receptive and expressive language skills. Speech-language pathologists often include a natural language sample obtained from the parents as well as through observation during the assessment process.

### Sensorimotor Development

Children younger than 2 years of age learn through an interactive process of sensory and motor exploration (Figure 23-3). The subdomains of sensorimotor development include the integration of primitive reflexes and development of movement responses and balance and equilibrium reactions, muscle tone, eye-hand coordination, grasping and

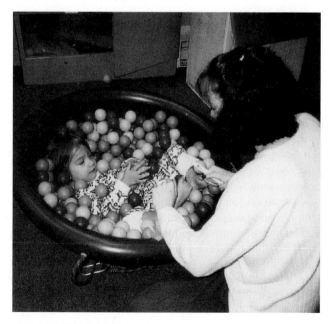

**Figure 23-3**   Occupational therapist helps young child learn through an interactive process of sensory and motor exploration.

reaching patterns, and manipulation of objects. These areas can be assessed with formal or standardized instruments such as the Milani-Comparetti Developmental Examination, the Peabody Developmental Motor Scales (PDMS), the Motor Assessment of Infants (MAI), the Motor Domain of the BDI, and the BSID Motor Scale and informal observation (see Appendix 8-B). Within this domain, the occupational therapist further examines performance in the specific areas of fine motor skill and sensory integration.

*Fine motor skills.* Early movements of the upper extremities are reflexive and random. Primitive reflexes, such as hand grasp and asymmetric tonic neck reflex, dominate arm movements of the very young infant. Once these reflexes become integrated, voluntary patterns of movement emerge. Typically, reflexes become integrated by 6 months.

Evaluation of fine motor skills includes assessing reaching patterns (stability of arm in space), prehension patterns (grasp and release), and manipulation skills. In addition, muscle tone and strength, cocontraction, and motor planning are contributing factors in the development of fine motor skills (see Chapter 12).

A standardized instrument that measures fine motor skill is the PDMS (Folio & Fewell, 1983). The Fine Motor Scale includes items for children from birth to 83 months of age and allows the therapist to rate key motor milestones. Certain items rate qualitative differences. The PDMS can become the foundation for goal setting and communicating with the family about the child's abilities and areas of need.

Identifying the child's sensorimotor and fine motor skills is the first step in the occupational therapist's evaluation. Once an overview of the child's functional status is obtained, the focus becomes the child's quality of movement and posture; response to tactile, vestibular, and proprioceptive input; and ability to integrate sensory and motor systems into a purposeful, coordinated skill (Case-Smith, 1993a).

*Sensory integration.* An infant's ability to respond to his or her environment depends on his or her ability to perceive sensory input. Infants and young children who have decreased responses or have a heightened arousal level to sensory input usually have difficulty regulating and organizing appropriate responses to environmental stimuli.

Because infants and young children often are unable to verbally communicate their perceptions and preferences of sensory information, the occupational therapist's evaluation is based on observation of the child's body language and responses to sensory stimulation. The occupational therapist administers or presents a variety of auditory, visual, and tactile stimuli. The occupational therapist also assesses the child's reactions to rotational and linear movement in various positions (e.g., prone, supine, and sitting).

One tool for evaluating sensory processing in the young child is the Test of Sensory Functions in Infants (Degangi & Greenspan, 1989). The Response to Sensory Input (Ayres & Tickle, 1980) can also yield information about responses to various types of sensory input. However, the most valuable information is that contributed by the parent in the sensory history. An interview guide specifically developed for parents of children younger than 3 years old is useful in assisting parents to identify problem areas related to sensory processing (Jirgal & Bouma, 1989).

### Adaptive or Self-Help Skills

The development of self-help or adaptive skills includes feeding, toileting, and dressing behaviors as well as the ability to be aware of environmental dangers and self-preservation skills. Frequently used assessment instruments include the BDI, Adaptive Domain, and the Vineland Adaptive Behavior Scales (Sparrow, Balla, & Cicchetti, 1984).

Infant feeding and oral motor skills are areas frequently addressed by the occupational therapist. Infants and toddlers with or at risk for developmental disabilities frequently have problems with feeding and oral-motor control. These problems can include atypical or poor suck and swallow patterns, sensory deficits, oral-motor structural deformities such as cleft lip or cleft palate, or increased or decreased behavioral responses (see Chapter 16).

## Role of the Occupational Therapist in the Assessment Process

Occupational therapists are actively involved in all levels of the evaluation process, from diagnosis to program planning and intervention. When working in the area of early intervention, it is essential for the occupational therapist to use a holistic perspective as opposed to a single-discipline or domain-specific perspective. The occupational therapist may administer a core developmental assessment for diagnostic purposes or assume the leadership role in an arena assessment. Occupational therapists bring to the assessment process a unique understanding of the interdependence and relationship between the child's functional and developmental skills and of sensory perception, behavior, and neurodevelopmental processes (Case-Smith, 1993a).

During a *diagnostic evaluation,* the occupational therapist may use informal measures and observations to assess muscle tone, strength, coordination, motor planning, and sensory processing. This can be accomplished by direct handling of the child, if appropriate, or by observing the child's reactions to being handled by his or her parent or a familiar adult. *Evaluation to develop a program plan* emphasizes discipline-specific areas and enables the occupational therapist to suggest appropriate goals and objectives and strategies for meeting them. Other areas such as social-emotional, cognitive, and communication development are assessed from the perspective of how the parents interrelate or influence the child's ability to engage in functional play, move through the environment, or interact with others.

## OCCUPATIONAL THERAPY INTERVENTION

Occupational therapists are important members of the early intervention team and can provide services in a variety of settings using one of several models of intervention. The contribution of occupational therapists is described as follows:

Occupational therapists promote a child's independence, mastery, and sense of self-worth and self-confidence in their physical, emotional, and psychosocial development. These services are designed to help families and other caregivers improve children's functioning within their environments. Therapists use a developmental framework in assessing the following domains: play, adaptive skills, sensorimotor, posture, fine-motor manipulation, and oral-motor feeding. Purposeful activity is then used to expand the child's functional abilities in these areas (Brown & Rule, 1993, p. 254).

General goals of occupational therapy intervention with infants and toddlers have been identified by Case-Smith (1993b). They are to facilitate change in the child's developmental function, to interpret and redefine behavioral responses, to compensate for and adapt to the effects of a disability, and to provide support to family members. Occupational therapy is provided in collaboration with other members of the team and is specified as part of the IFSP. The parent is recognized as the decision maker, and it is this informed decision making that drives the implementation of the IFSP and the extent to which the family is involved in intervention (Dunst, 1991).

### Settings

Early intervention legislation specifies that services should be provided in the child's natural environment to the "maximum extent appropriate to the needs of the child" (Federal Register, 34 CFR 303.12[4][b]). To enable the child to remain an integral part of the family and for the family to be integral parts of the neighborhood and community, services should be community based and in locations convenient to the family (Dunst, 1991). Ideally, a range of options should be offered to the family so they can choose those that best fit their priorities, life-style, and values. These options should include those that provide the least restrictive settings in situations that would be natural environments for a normally developing child of the same age. Some examples are a play group, mother's morning out program, child care center, or Sunday School class.

One philosophy that has gained favor in the 1990s is that of *inclusion*. The Division of Early Childhood of the Council for Exceptional Children supports this philosophy with the following statement (DEC, 1993):

Inclusion, as a value, supports the right of all children, regardless of their diverse abilities, to participate actively in natural settings within their communities. A natural setting is one in which

the child would spend time if he or she had not had a disability (p. 4).

Key components include physical inclusion, social inclusion, and emotional inclusion (Turnbull et al., 1994). The implications for the occupational therapist are that these services should be provided within the natural setting (e.g., the home or child care center) rather than in an outpatient center, hospital, or rehabilitation center.

The inclusion model has many advantages. When the young child attends the community child care program, he or she gains opportunities for interaction from typically developing peers (Figure 23-4). Participation in the community programs gives the family common experiences for relating to friends and neighbors. It helps them view their child as one with differing abilities, rather than one with disabilities. To be successful, the inclusion program should assure that (1) the child's individual needs are met with appropriate aids and support services, (2) the child with special needs benefits from the typical program, and (3) the needs of the typical children are not compromised.

Several obstacles can negatively influence the benefits of placing a child in an inclusive program. The child who needs intense, specialized intervention may be unable to develop his or her potential to the greatest extent because the needed individualization is not possible in a community program. A toddler with significant acting-out behaviors, for example, may require far more attention from the teacher than the teacher is able to provide because of his or her responsibilities to the many other typical children in the group. In addition, personnel may not have adequate training to provide the intervention needed. For some children, inclusion programs must provide a great deal of on-site support to facilitate interaction or to provide adaptations for function. This may not be cost-effective when only one or

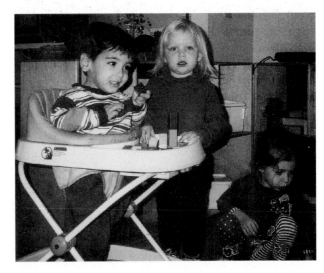

**Figure 23-4**   A child who attends a community child care program benefits from interaction with typically developing peers.

two children are in one location. In areas that have shortages of occupational therapists to provide intervention, it may be impractical for the therapists to spend a great deal of travel time to provide services in the home or in child care centers.

Occupational therapy services can be provided in a variety of settings that represent a continuum from the most restrictive (e.g., residential care facility) to the least restrictive (e.g., inclusion programs). The setting should reflect family preferences and should be consistent with the needs of the child and the goals identified on the IFSP. For example, one child with significant and acute medical problems might be best served in the hospital-based program, whereas another with similar problems may be best served in the home. One toddler with Down syndrome might function best in a mother's morning out program with normally developing peers, and another with the same diagnosis would be more responsive in a center-based early intervention program. Early intervention legislation provides for interagency cooperation, thus families can choose the most appropriate settings and services from either private or public providers.

## Cultural Diversity

To provide appropriate intervention within the family-focused model, the occupational therapist must be aware of and respect differences in beliefs and values based on culture. "Perhaps no set of programs or services interacts with cultural views and values more than early intervention because of the focus on the very young child with a disability and the family" (Hanson, 1990, p. 116). The therapist who provides intervention in the home has an intimate view of such things as customs, eating habits, and child-rearing practices that may vary among cultures. The family's beliefs and views of disability and its cause, their view of the health care system, and their sources of medical information affect their attitude toward early intervention. Based on individual cultural backgrounds, the family may view the therapist either as a helper or as one who interferes.

Many of the areas in which occupational therapists provide intervention and suggestions are those that involve caretaking and those that are closely tied to values and beliefs about parenting and cultural views of children. Practices regarding feeding, toileting, and bathing may vary among cultures. The practitioner is urged to evaluate various health beliefs to determine if the effects are beneficial, harmless, harmful, or uncertain before making recommendations for change (Johnston, 1980).

Early intervention legislation requires that assessments be administered in the family's native language if feasible and that evaluation procedures be conducted in a manner that is not racially or culturally discriminatory (IDEA, 1990). Intervention methods and procedures should recognize and be sensitive to cultural differences. Some suggestions for the therapist are as follows (Vohs, 1989, p. 3):

1. Learn about other cultures.
2. Learn how other cultures view children with disabilities.
3. Invite members of minority cultures to become involved with your organization.
4. Learn at least a few words of different languages.
5. Become familiar with your community and the cultures represented.
6. Examine ways to remove barriers to accessing services for minority groups.
7. Recognize that all of us have prejudices and believe that our values are right.
8. Be sensitive to problems of being a member of a minority.

## Planning

Occupational therapy intervention, as with other early intervention services, is based on identified needs and expected outcomes in the IFSP. This document specifies various services to be provided; who the provider will be; the location of the services; frequency, intensity, and duration of services; and the funding sources (see p. 651).

An IFSP outcome is usually stated in broad terms and reflects family priorities. A definition of outcome is that it is a statement of changes desired by the family that can focus on any area of the child's development or family life as it relates to the child (Kramer et al., 1991). Some examples of outcomes that relate to occupational therapy are as follows:

"Heidi will learn to eat more easily and will eat a greater variety of foods."

"Heidi will use her hands to play with toys."

The occupational therapist's treatment plan identifies the goals and objectives related to the outcomes that will be addressed by activities and strategies developed by the therapist in collaboration with the family. For example, the occupational therapy goals for Heidi include the following:

1. Increase oral-motor functioning for eating
2. Provide adaptations for positioning and increased function in eating and play activity
3. Increase function through developmentally appropriate sensorimotor activities

The objectives for Heidi specifically state what is expected by the end of the time period.

1. Heidi will tolerate textures provided through food or oral-motor facilitation as shown by eating food of various textures with appropriate chewing and swallowing.
2. Heidi's mother will be taught strategies for oral-motor facilitation to be implemented at home at mealtimes.
3. Heidi will drink liquids independently when provided with an adapted cup.

4. Heidi will be provided with seating adaptations at home and in her child care center that will position her appropriately for feeding.

Occupational therapy goals and objectives in early intervention need to be functional in nature and should be addressed in a developmentally appropriate way in consideration of the child's function within her family and her environment.

## Approaches

### Developmentally Appropriate

Occupational therapy for the infant and young child is planned and carried out within the framework of developmental needs rather than the acquisition of isolated skills. For example, it would be inappropriate for the occupational therapist to concentrate on the development of precise fingertip prehension without consideration of how this skill contributes to the overall function of the child in the environment or how it fits into the developmental needs of the child.

Developmentally based curricula such as the HELP, the Early Learning Assessment Profile (E-LAP), or the Carolina Curriculum for Infants and Toddlers with Special Needs provide activities matched to the developmental sequences within each domain. The therapist, however, should guard against using a "cookbook" approach in intervention for specific developmental deficits.

Developmental needs can be effectively addressed by a team whose members have overlapping functions (Figures 23-5 and 23-6). When a need is identified in a specific domain, for example, fine motor skills, activities that require a child to use fine motor skills can be implemented. To promote generalization of the fine motor skills practiced in therapy, it is best to employ play activities that involve the "just right" challenge to the child across domains, that is, activities that include skill building in the cognitive and social domains. For example, stacking rings on a stick is a motor task but also involves cognitive skills such as concept of size and color. It also could involve social interaction, including give and take with the adult, eye contact, praise, and delight at successful attempts.

### Family-Centered Intervention

In family-centered intervention the occupational therapist addresses the needs of the entire family rather than only concentrating on specific deficits in the child. The therapist should be guided by family concerns and the amount of involvement various family members choose to have in the child's intervention program (Figure 23-7) (see p. 663). One important way to increase the effect of therapy is to recommend that therapy activities and exercises be implemented at home. When activities are practiced daily at home, it is much more likely that the child will learn the targeted skill. However, parents may vary as to the amount of therapy they can do between sessions at home.

Sometimes it is more important to support the role of parent rather than make the assumption that the parent can take on the role of the therapist. One mother stated,

There are times when even an acceptable amount of therapy becomes too much—when your child needs time just to be a child, or when you need time to be with the rest of the family. It's OK to say 'no' at those times, for a while. Your instinct will tell you when (Simons, 1985, p. 51).

Daily routines in a family with a child who has a disability can take an excessive amount of time and energy, which

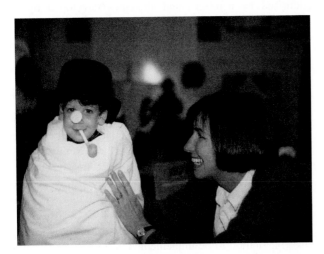

**Figure 23-5** Music therapist's activity of "Frosty the Snowman" (complete with button nose!) helps meet occupational therapy goals of providing tactile input.

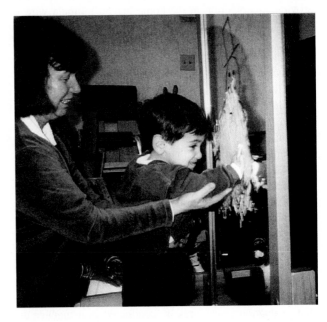

**Figure 23-6** Physical therapist helps a child with his standing balance while the child is involved in an activity that requires tactile input and hand function.

does not allow for carrying out a therapy home program. Suggestions that can be incorporated into the daily routine are the most successful. For example, tactile stimulation and range of motion can be done at bath time; an older sibling can encourage the baby to reach for toys while their mother cooks dinner.

Occupational therapists can provide support for families by listening to them, giving positive feedback regarding parenting skills, encouraging recreational activities for the family, and helping them access community resources (Case-Smith, 1993b). Often the therapist can help the family by providing intervention to make daily routines go more smoothly. Examples are suggestions for positioning and handling to make feeding more efficient or an adapted bath seat to make bathing less taxing.

### Areas of Intervention

Hanft (1989) applied five practice perspectives to occupational therapy with infants and young children: prevention, habilitation, remediation, compensation, and maturation (Table 23-3). These various perspectives may be used at different times, depending on the child's needs and development. The therapist must determine the appropriateness of an approach at any given time. Regardless of the

▲ Table 23-3   Occupational Therapy Intervention for a 5-Month-Old Boy

| Practice Perspective | Examples of Occupational Therapy Goals and Activities |
|---|---|
| Prevention (check the negative effect of developmental problems on future abilities) | Develop awareness of body parts through sensory input to prevent spatial orientation problems |
| | Increase attention and eye contact to enhance interaction with others |
| Habilitation (promote developmental acquisition of future skills) | Develop child's head control through movement, neuromuscular facilitation, and positioning |
| | Enhance basic oral-motor functions of breathing, sucking, and swallowing in preparation for speech |
| Remediation (attempt to diminish dysfuntion) | Decrease drooling through neuromuscular facilitation to mouth |
| | Enhance interaction through alerting techniques before play |
| Compensation (substitute different skills for delayed ones) | Encourage mother and father to carry in baby carrier ("snugli") until child can move on his or her own |
| | Position child so pacifier remains in mouth |
| Maturation (utilize child's own developmental schedule) | Provide appropriate toys to enhance visual attention in crib and play areas |
| | Offer finger foods during meals as child develops pincer grasp |

From Hanft, B. (1989). The changing environment of early intervention services: implications for practice. In B. Hanft (Ed.). *Family-centered care: an early intervention resource manual.* Rockville, MD: American Occupational Therapy Association.

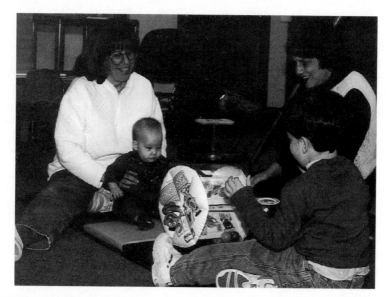

**Figure 23-7**   The older brother participates in the therapy session and learns how to play with his baby sister at home.

CASE STUDY #1

## Background

Alex was referred to occupational therapy by his pediatrician at 11 months of age because of suspected sensory integrative problems. He had a diagnosis of developmental delay and had been receiving physical therapy because of gross motor delays. Alex cries often in a distressful manner. Problem areas for Alex, as reported by his mother, include uncooperative behaviors, rages or temper tantrums, whining and fussing, feeding problems, fearfulness, poor balance, and a dislike for being on his tummy. Although he sat independently at 6 months, he did not reach and grasp an object until 8 months. He rolled from back to stomach at 9 months, and at 11 months, he was not yet crawling.

## Assessment

Alex was a pleasant baby who preferred not to be touched or held. He interacted with the examiner with caution after a brief period of ignoring her. His mother remained in the room and participated in the assessment. A sensorimotor history was obtained by interview with Alex's mother. In the tactile area she had noticed difficulty and pulling away when touched, stiffness, and lack of molding when held. Alex's mother reported that he is irritable when held and resists having his hair or face washed. Alex seemed oversensitive to noises and was bothered by such things as a vacuum cleaner and hair dryer. Although he is better now, he seems apprehensive of toys with noises. Alex seemed to be fearful in situations with auditory and visual stimulation, such as a shopping mall. It was reported that Alex enjoyed swinging and other movement stimuli.

The Test of Sensory Functioning in Infants (Degangi & Greenspan, 1989), standardized for infants up to 18 months of age, was administered to Alex. Results showed deficiencies in reactivity to tactile deep pressure and adaptive motor functions, at-risk response to visual-tactile integration and ocular-motor control, and normal response to vestibular stimulation. Specifically, Alex had a mildly defensive reaction to touch. He was not effective in his motor responses to tactile input, such as removing a mitt on his foot or a piece of tape on the back of his hand. He was more efficient using his right hand than his left. Visual-tactile response was better because he was able to locate the stimulus visually, although he could not motor plan the movement to remove it. However, visual tracking was delayed and inconsistent. Alex enjoyed the vestibular input as he was held and moved up and down or in circular motions. He also enjoyed upside-down positions.

Alex was observed to avoid and resist changing his body position (e.g., going from sitting to quadruped), and he resisted the proprioceptive input of weight bearing on his upper extremities. Extensor muscle tone was increased with lower-extremity weight bearing, so much so that it was difficult to flex his hips passively for sitting. Alex was observed to go into plantar-flexion and lower-extremity extension when bounced on his bare feet.

At a chronologic age of 11 months, Alex received an age equivalent of 9 months on the fine motor subtest of the Peabody Developmental Motor Scales. He used his right hand more efficiently than his left but was able to bring his hands to midline to bang cubes. However, it was reported that he resisted clapping his hands. Alex removed pegs from a pegboard and briefly manipulated a piece of paper. He was able to transfer a cube from his left hand to his right when the cube was placed in his left hand. Alex had difficulty removing rings from a stand. He also displayed difficulty in deliberately releasing cubes to give to the examiner or to put them in a cup.

## Summary and interpretation

Alex was a delightful baby who experienced significant difficulties in receiving and modulating sensory information. This was evident particularly in his irritability and intolerance to touch and auditory stimulation. His responses indicated tactile defensiveness with inadequate adaptive motor function. Alex's tactile defensiveness probably contributed to his fine motor delays. Given his defensiveness, it is understandable that he was limited in his abilities to explore and manipulate objects, especially those that were new to him and in an unfamiliar environment.

## Intervention

Weekly occupational therapy was recommended for Alex. Center-based programming was chosen with involvement of the parent in the sessions and follow-through with daily home programming. A sensory integrative approach was used with developmentally appropriate play with emphasis on increased functional hand use. Intervention included frequent brushing of the extremities and the back with a soft surgical brush followed by deep proprioceptive input. This followed recommended procedures developed by Wilbarger (Wilbarger & Wilbarger, 1991). Treatment sessions included vestibular input, which Alex tolerated well, and proprioceptive and tactile input as tolerated. Alex was encouraged to play with textured toys, use both hands for midline activities, and bear weight on his upper extremities. Alex's mother participated actively in each session and created additional opportunities for tactile exploration and play at home. She was provided with reading material and a videotape to help her learn about sensory integration and the theoretical framework for intervention.

Alex responded well to the treatment approach and began to show indications of more efficient sensory processing and the ability to modulate sensory input.

Within a few weeks, Alex began to mold to his mother when she held him and was less irritable and more relaxed in situations with auditory stimulation. After a month of therapy, Alex's mother reported increased cuddling and noticeable improvement in eating. He attempted a greater variety of foods with fewer aversions, feeding time was shorter, and it was no longer necessary to use the television as a diversion to get him to eat. Alex was interacting more with his siblings and exploring his environment. Best of all, he no longer had temper tantrums when his mother left the room. The occupational therapist reported that Alex was tolerating the prone position and weight bearing on his hands; he had recently begun to crawl. Play skills and hand use had increased significantly and were close to age level.

perspective, the therapist works in collaboration with the family and other professionals to develop functional abilities. The child is viewed in a holistic manner in enhancing development; however, there are certain areas that have traditionally been emphasized more by occupational therapists.

***Fine motor development and manipulative hand function.*** The occupational therapist is often concerned with delayed function or atypical function of those skills that are loosely referred to as *fine motor skills*. They may include grasp and release of objects, bilateral manipulation, in-hand manipulation, hesitancy to touch and explore with the hands, lack of hand-to-mouth pattern, and other skills. Intervention begins with analyzing the quality of movement and determining underlying factors, such as tactile discrimination and kinesthetic awareness.

The therapist notes the influence of muscle tone and proximal stability when the child attempts the task, for example, stacking 1-inch cubes. Is there increased muscle tone, spasticity, tremor, associated movement (mirroring), or total body tone changes with effort? Can the child do it while sitting, unsupported, on the floor? Is there slumping or lack of postural stability? Can the child easily disassociate the movement of the arm from the body? Are there primitive reflexes such as a grasp reflex or asymmetric tonic neck reflex that interfere with movement? Does there seem to be lack of eye-hand coordination, inattention, or lack of understanding of the task? Does the child have difficulty with the motor planning needed for precise release of one block on top of the other? Does there seem to be tactile defensiveness that causes the child to be reluctant to handle

the block or results in flinging or throwing any object in his or her hand?

A child with autistic spectrum disorder or other dysfunction that interferes with the child's ability to interact with persons and things in the environment may be unable to imitate or follow directions for a task. Therefore inability to stack blocks may not reflect a deficit in fine motor ability, but rather inexperience or disinterest in the activity. The best indication of the child's fine motor abilities may be through observation of spontaneous activity.

Stacking blocks is not an important functional skill, but it is important for developing sufficient hand skill for manipulating, placing, and releasing objects. These skills enable the child to use tools with control and with their arms unsupported. The occupational therapist uses a wide variety of age-appropriate toys, games, sensorimotor experiences, and other strategies with the young child to remediate underlying factors that interfere with the development of fine motor skills (Figure 23-8).

## Development of Play

One of the most important areas of a young child's development is the involvement in play. Play is open-ended, self-initiated, self-directed, and unlimited in its variety. It gives the child the opportunity to develop and practice skills that will be the foundation for later occupational tasks such as the ability to manipulate objects, to problem solve, and to attend to the task (Burke, 1993). Play can be exploratory, symbolic, creative, or competitive in nature (see Chapter 18).

Sometimes therapists are so intent on remediating certain deficits that they ignore the importance of play. A toy

CASE STUDY #2

Jeremy, age 18 months, was referred for a transdisciplinary assessment by his pediatric neurologist because of motor delays caused by his mitochondrial encephalopathy. He was assessed in an arena assessment by an early intervention team, which consisted of an occupational therapist, a physical therapist, a speech-language pathologist, and an early childhood interventionist. Both parents participated in the assessment. Although Jeremy had received both occupational therapy and physical therapy since he was 6 months old, his parents thought he would benefit from a small group in which he could receive his therapies and special instruction in an integrated manner.

## Assessment

The team chose to administer the Milani-Comparetti Neuromotor Screening Test, the Bayley Test of Infant Development, and the Battelle Developmental Inventory (BDI). The latter was administered through observation, direct administration of test items, and interview with the parents. Portions were modified to accommodate for Jeremy's physical limitations. Most importantly, the therapists engaged him in play activities and used their interpretation of his interactions and movements to estimate his functional abilities.

Overall, Jeremy had very low muscle tone and poor physical endurance. He needed support for sitting and could only bear some of his weight when supported in standing. He was unable to roll or to crawl. Head control was poor with head stacking in supported sitting and lack of head righting in prone. He used his left hand very well to play with toys when he was positioned appropriately but did not use the right hand and protested when the therapist attempted to evaluate passive range of motion. Jeremy was alert and interested but was reluctant to leave his mother's lap. Communication skills and cognition appeared to be on age level, whereas social skills seemed immature.

## Intervention

Jeremy started in the summer session of a center-based early intervention program as part of a group of six children who met twice a week. He received occupational therapy, physical therapy, speech therapy, and special instruction in a small group format with close coordination and carry-over of all skills throughout the 4-hour session. All therapies and special instruction were aimed at helping Jeremy use his good cognitive and communication abilities in a functional manner to improve social interaction with peers, improve self-help skills, and develop physical abilities to the greatest extent possible. Adapted seating and eating utensils were obtained for him, and group activities were modified to enable him to participate actively and as independently as possible. Meanwhile, Jeremy continued with individual occupational and physical therapies as an outpatient at a nearby hospital.

## Individual Family Service Plan review

After 6 months, the service coordinator, the intervention team, and the family met to review the goals on Jeremy's Individual Family Service Plan (IFSP) and to update and modify it as needed. The family and the team were pleased with Jeremy's progress and thought that he was benefiting from his intervention program. However, they also discussed Jeremy's need to be around his normally developing peers and to participate in community-based activities. Jeremy was gaining confidence in a small group, developing good social and communication skills, and no longer tiring as easily. He was now over 2 years old and the team decided to add an inclusion program to his early intervention services.

Jeremy's service coordinator arranged for him to participate in a special grant program at a local child care center. He was enrolled in a class for 2-year-old children that met just a few hours a week and had the support of an assistant who had been trained to facilitate the inclusion of children with special needs in the typical child care setting. Although this facilitator had several other children to work with and was not in Jeremy's class all the time, she was available at any time he needed help or the teacher had a question or concern. After a few months Jeremy started attending this program two times a week; meanwhile, he continued to attend the early intervention program and receive his therapies.

## Annual reassessment

After 1 year the intervention team reassessed Jeremy in preparation for the development of a new IFSP. This assessment was not done in a formal testing session but was done over a period of weeks as Jeremy participated in a variety of activities with the group. In addition to the BDI, Jeremy's team also updated the Hawaii Early Learning Profile, which they had used throughout the year in planning Jeremy's intervention.

## CASE STUDY #2—CONT'D

Results of the reassessment indicated a bright, happy, verbal 2-year-old child. Although he had gained some in physical abilities, Jeremy needed a stroller-type wheelchair with special inserts for appropriate seating. The removable seat also acted as a floor sitter so Jeremy could be close to the same level as his peers when they played on the floor. The teacher observed that Jeremy had shown considerable improvement in his play skills and that they were definitely more appropriate when he was positioned upright rather than lying on the floor. He now has spontaneous interactions with his peers, takes turns with little prompting, and is beginning to share toys.

Jeremy continued to participate in the class at the child care center, although the grant had ended and the facilitator was no longer there. Initially, the child care center believed that they would be unable to take Jeremy without the support of the facilitator. The occupational therapist and the physical therapist provided on-site consultation. Through a problem-solving approach with close cooperation among the family, child care personnel, and therapists, strategies were developed that made it possible for Jeremy to remain in the class. These strategies included providing wheelchair access to the playground (they had been carrying him), teaching principles of lifting and carrying, and making the stroller available to transport him from room to room so the teacher had her hands free to keep up with other active 2-year-old children.

### Summary

Jeremy is an example of a child who was able to benefit from a combination of programming that included hospital-based therapy, center-based early intervention, and inclusion in a typical child care setting. This required close cooperation among the family, early intervention personnel, and community resources. As Jeremy grows and develops, his parents plan to place him in a total inclusion program, but they believe that, at age 2½, he still needs the intense intervention he gets in the center-based program. Meanwhile, they look forward to his graduation to the class for 3-year-old children and increasing his typical class time to 3 days a week. They have already visited the neighborhood school and hope that he will attend a regular kindergarten class when he is 5 years old and will be supported by therapies at school. Jeremy is bright and, with the right kind of support and technology, he should be able to grow up in the mainstream of society. That's what early intervention is all about!

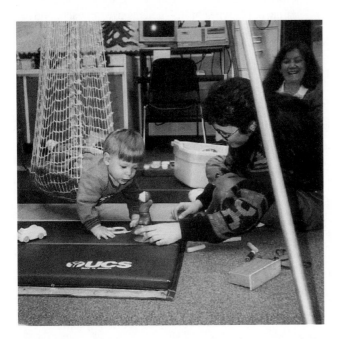

**Figure 23-8** Occupational therapist uses various toys and sensorimotor experiences to achieve desired results.

becomes only a motivator, or a diversion, so that the therapist can elicit a certain movement pattern (Burke, 1993). Although this may sometimes be necessary, it is also important to facilitate play skills in the child and to use play as a way of enabling the child to gain function and enhance development. To use play as intervention the occupational therapist must be playful in interactions with the child. Whether it is a game of peek-a-boo or knocking down a pretend wall when pushed on a scooter board, the activity should elicit a sense of enjoyment and fun.

Children with special needs may have not developed play skills because of long hospitalizations or medical treatments or because of the limitations imposed by a physical impairment. Other children may experience deficits in play because of cognitive limitations or difficulties in social interactions. Use of a play-based assessment can enable the occupational therapist to define the problem areas and plan intervention (see p. 657).

### Sensory Integration

Sensory integration has been defined as "the ability to organize and process information from the different sensory channels and to interrelate and synthesize these inputs in order to emit an adaptive motor response" (Degangi & Greenspan, 1989, p. 2). Infants who have difficulty processing sensory information lack the ability to cope with environmental demands or achieve internal control. These infants may be irritable, may cry frequently, may be difficult to comfort, or may have difficulty with changes in routine. The ability to cope "requires the ability to modulate incoming sensory information while engaged in feeding, face-to-face interactions with family, bathing, and diapering, or just being held" (Stallings-Sahler, 1993, p. 327).

It is important to recognize and address sensory integrative dysfunction in the young child because of its pervasive influence on all areas of development. Appropriate tactile, vestibular, and proprioceptive input should be used that elicit organization and simple adaptive responses on the part of the child. For example, it was determined that a 1-year-old child displayed tactile defensiveness. He refused to hold toys, refused to bear weight on his arms, was irritable when held, pulled away from touch, and avoided exploring his environment. The occupational therapist planned intervention that included proprioceptive and tactile input and midline play with textured toys. She instructed the mother to provide additional tactile stimulation at bath time with water play, foamy soap, and terry cloth rubs. Soon the child was clapping his hands spontaneously—a skill he had not attempted before and a nice adaptive response! (see Case Study #1).

### Oral-Motor Function and Feeding

Occupational therapists who work with infants and toddlers often are called on to address problems in eating and

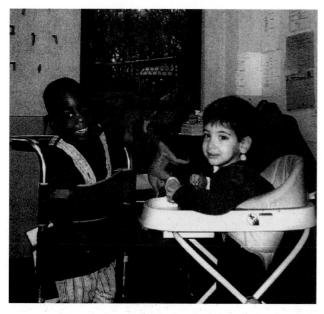

**Figure 23-9**    Use of adapted equipment enables these children to be positioned for play.

feeding. Problem areas may include inadequate intake, excessive time for feeding, or oral-motor problems associated with sucking, swallowing, and chewing (Glass & Wolf, 1993). For the toddler, additional problems may center around behavioral issues such as refusals, overactivity, or messiness. Other concerns are in the area of self-feeding and drinking from a cup.

Addressing concerns in the area of feeding is important not only for food intake, but also for mother-child bonding. Glass and Wolf suggest three guiding principles of treatment for the infant: (1) proper alignment of the trunk and neck; (2) providing proximal stability, especially in the head and jaw; and (3) facilitating appropriate oral-motor patterns through inhibitory and facilitory techniques (see Chapter 16).

### Adapted Equipment and Positioning

The occupational therapist in early intervention can make an important contribution to the overall functioning of young children through the recommendation and provision of appropriate adapted equipment (Figure 23-9). A floor sitter may enable the child with cerebral palsy to play on the

---

## STUDY QUESTIONS

1. Briefly describe the potential roles of the occupational therapist in (1) developing and writing the IFSP and (2) planning the child's transition into preschool.

2. Compare the screening process with the evaluation process. Include a comparison of the (1) purpose of each, (2) types of instruments used in each, and (3) outcomes of each process.

3. Describe developmentally appropriate and family-centered intervention approaches.

4. You are the therapist of a 2-year-old boy with severe cognitive and motor delays. The child is not yet sitting and has limited range of movement in extremities. He eats pureed food and requires thickened liquids because of delays in oral motor skills. Manipulation skills are limited to grasp and release and waving and banging. He is visually alert and seems to enjoy visual stimuli. He has no independent mobility. His family is supportive and caring. His parents have been actively involved with the occupational therapist. Describe appropriate goals and activities for (1) enhancing the child's play (see also Chapter 18), (2) improving sensory integration, (3) improving his fine motor skills, and (4) increasing the variety of food textures consumed (see Chapter 16).

floor near his or her typically developing peers. An adapted insert for a chair may make it possible for a child to begin to use his hands for an art project or to self-feed. As the neurologically involved toddler approaches preschool age and is not yet ambulating, the parents may have to face the prospect of the need for a wheelchair. The occupational therapist can assist not only in recommending appropriate equipment, but also in being sensitive to the effect that envisioning their child in a wheelchair may have on the family. The child with a neurologic impairment who can stay in a baby stroller or a high chair does not appear as "different" as the 3-year-old who must have a wheelchair and special equipment.

## REFERENCES

Ayres, A. & Tickle, L. (1980). Hyper-responsivity to touch and vestibular stimuli as a predictor of positive response to sensory integrative procedures by autistic children. *American Journal of Occupational Therapy, 34*(6), 375-381.

*Babies can't wait: early intervention program standards.* (1993). Atlanta: Georgia Department of Public Health.

Bailey, D.B., Simeonsson, R.J., Winton, P.J., Huntington, G.S., Comfort, M., Isbell, P., O'Donnell, K.J., & Helm, J. (1986). Family-focused intervention: a functional model for planning, implementing, and evaluating individualized family services in early intervention. *Journal of the Division for Early Childhood, 10,* 156-171.

Bayley, N. (1993). *Bayley Scales of Infant Development* (2nd ed.). San Antonio, TX: The Psychological Corp.

Brown, W. & Rule, S. (1993). Personnel and disciplines in early intervention. In W. Brown, S.K. Thurman, & L.K. Pearl (Eds.). *Family-centered early intervention with infants and toddlers & innovative cross-disciplinary approaches.* Baltimore: Brookes.

Bruder, M. & Bologna, T. (1993). Collaboration and service coordination for effective early intervention. In W. Brown, S.K. Thurrman, & L.K. Pearl (Eds.). *Family-centered early intervention with infants and toddlers & innovative cross-disciplinary approaches.* Baltimore: Brookes.

Burke, J. (1993) Play: the life role of the infant and young child. In J. Case-Smith (Ed.). *Pediatric occupational therapy and early intervention.* Boston: Andover Medical Publishers.

Case-Smith, J. (1993a). Assessment. In J. Case-Smith (Ed.). *Pediatric occupational therapy and early intervention* (pp. 81-126). Boston: Andover Medical Publishers.

Case-Smith, J. (1993b). Defining the early intervention process. In J. Case-Smith (Ed.). *Pediatric occupational therapy and early intervention* (pp. 31-61). Boston: Andover Medical Publishers.

Case-Smith, J. & Wavrek, B. (1993). Models of service delivery and team interaction. In J. Case-Smith (Ed.). *Pediatric occupational therapy and early intervention.* Boston: Andover Medical Publishers.

DEC position statement on inclusion. (1993). *DEC Communicator, 19,* 4.

DeGangi, G.A. & Greenspan, S.I. (1989). *Test of Sensory Functions in Infants manual.* Los Angeles: Western Psychological Services.

Dunst, C.J. (1980). *A clinical and educational manual for use with the Uzgiris and Hunt Scales of Infant Psychological Development.* Austin, TX: Pro Ed.

Dunst, C.J. (1991). Implementation of the Individualized Family Service Plan. In M. J. McGonigel, R. Kaufmann, & B. Johnson (Eds.). *Guidelines and recommended practices for the Individualized Family Service Plan* (2nd ed) (pp. 67-78). Bethesda, MD: Association for the Care of Children's Health.

Featherstone, H. (1980). *A difference in the family.* New York: Basic Books.

Federal Register. (May 1, 1992). Title 34, Code of Federal Regulations, Part 303, Early intervention program for infants and toddlers with disabilities (Vol. 57), No. 85.

Folio, M.R. & Fewell, R.R. (1983). *Peabody Developmental Motor Scales and activity cards: a manual.* Chicago: Riverside Publishers.

Frankenburg, W.K., Dodds, J., Archer, P., Bresnick, B., Maschka, P., Edelman, N., & Shapiro, H. (1990). *Denver II Screening Manual.* Denver: Denver Developmental Materials.

Giangreco, M.F. (1986). Delivery of therapeutic services in special education programs for learners with severe handicaps. *Physical and Occupational Therapy in Pediatrics, 6,* 5.

Glass, R. & Wolf, L. (1993). Feeding and oral motor skills. In J. Case-Smith (Ed.). *Pediatric occupational therapy and early intervention* (pp. 225-288). Boston: Andover Medical Publishers.

Greenspan, S.I. (1992). *Infancy and early childhood.* Madison, CT: International Universities Press.

Greenspan, S.I. & Meisels, S. (1994). Toward a new vision for the developmental assessment of infants & young children. *Zero To Three, 14*(6), 2-41.

Hanft, B. (1989). The changing environment of early intervention services: implications for practice. In B. Hanft (Ed.). *Family-centered care: an early intervention resource manual.* Rockville, MD: American Occupational Therapy Association.

Hanson, M. & Lynch, E. (1989). *Early intervention: implementing child and family services for infants & toddlers who are at risk or disabled.* Austin, TX: Pro Ed.

Hanson, M.J. (1990). Honoring the cultural diversity of families when gathering data. *Topics in Early Childhood Special Education, 10*(1), 112-131.

Hedrick, D.L., Prather, E.M., & Tobin, A.R. (1984). *Sequenced inventory of communication development.* Seattle: University of Washington Press.

Individuals with Disabilities Education Act of 1990 (P.L. 102-119), 20 USC Secs. 1400-1485.

Jirgal, D. & Bouma, K. (1989). A sensory integration observation guide. *Sensory Integration Special Interest Newsletter.* Rockville, MD: American Occupational Therapy Association.

Johnson, L.J. (1994). Challenges facing early intervention: an overview. In L.J. Johnson, R.J. Gallagher, M.J. La Montagne, J. Jordon, J. Gallagher, P. Hutinger, & M. Karnes (Eds.). *Meeting early intervention challenges* (pp. 1-12). Baltimore: Brookes.

Johnston, M. (1980). Cultural variations in professional and parenting patterns. *Journal of Gynecological and Neonatal Nursing 9*(1), 9-13.

Kliewer, D., Bruce, W., & Trembath, J. (1977). *The Milani-Comparetti motor development screening test.* Omaha: Meyer's Children's Rehabilitation Institute Omaha: University of Nebraska Medical Center.

Knobloch, H., Stevens, F., & Malone, A. (1980) *Manual of developmental diagnosis: the administration and interpretation of the revised Gesell and Armatruda developmental and neurologic examination.* New York: Harper & Row.

Kramer, S., McGonigel, M., Kaufman, R. (1991). Developing the IFSP: outcomes, strategies, activities, and services. In M. McGonigel, R. Kaufmann, & B. Johnson (Eds.). *Guidelines and recommended practices for the Individualized Family Service Plan* (2nd ed.). Bethesda, MD: Association for the Care of Children's Health.

Linder, T.W. (1990). *Transdisciplinary play-based assessment: a functional approach to working with young children.* Baltimore: Brookes.

Linder, T.W. (1993). *Transdisciplinary play-based intervention: guidelines for developing a meaningful curriculum for young children.* Baltimore: Brookes.

Lyon, S. & Lyon, G. (1980). Team functioning and staff development: a role release approach to providing integrated educational services for severely handicapped students. *Journal of the Association for the Severely Handicapped, 5*(3), 250-263.

McLean, M. & McCormick, K. (1993). Assessment and evaluation in early intervention. In W. Brown, S.K. Thurman, & L.K. Pearl (Eds.). *Family-centered early intervention with infants and toddlers & innovative cross-disciplinary approaches.* Baltimore: Brookes.

Miller, L.J. (1994). Journey to a desirable future: a value-based model of infant & toddler assessment. *Zero To Three, 14*(6), 23-26.

Newborg, J., Stock, J.R., Wnek, L., Guidubaldi, J., & Svinicki, J. (1988). *Battelle Developmental Inventory.* Chicago: Riverside Publishers.

Orelove, F.P. & Sobsey, D. (1991). *Educating children with multiple disabilities: a transdisciplinary approach.* Baltimore: Brookes.

Ottenbacher, K. (1983). Transdisciplinary service delivery in school environment: some limitations. *Physical and Occupational Therapy in Pediatrics, 3,* 9.

Peterson, N.L. (1987). *Early intervention for handicapped and at-risk children.* Denver: Love.

Rosetti, L. (1990). *The Rosetti Infant Toddler Language Scale.* East Moline, IL: Lingui Systems.

Safer, N.D. & Hamilton, J.L. (1993). Legislative context for early intervention services. In W. Brown, S.K. Thurman, & L.F. Pearl(Eds.). *Family-centered early intervention with infants & toddlers: Innovative cross-disciplinary approaches* (pp. 1-19). Baltimore: Brookes.

Shelton, T.L., Jeppson, E.S., & Johnson, B.H. (Eds.). (1989). *Family-centered care for children with special health care needs.* Washington, DC: Association for the Care of Children's Health.

Shonkoff, J.P. & Meisels, S.J. (1990). Early childhood intervention: the evolution of a concept. In S.J. Meisels & J.P. Shonkoff (Eds.). *Handbook of early intervention* (pp. 3-31). Cambridge, MA: Cambridge University Press.

Simeonsson, R.J. & Bailey, D.B. (1990). Family dimensions in early intervention. In S.J. Meisels & J.P. Shonkoff (Eds.). *Handbook of early childhood intervention.* Cambridge, MA: Cambridge University Press.

Simons, R. (1985). *After the tears.* New York: Harcourt Brace Javonovich.

Sparrow, S., Balla, D.A., & Cicchetti, D.V. (1984). *Vineland Adaptive Behavior Scales.* Circle Pines, MN: American Guidance Service.

Stallings-Sahler, S. (1993). Sensory integration: assessment and intervention with infants. In J. Case-Smith (Ed.). *Pediatric occupational therapy and early intervention* (pp. 309-341). Boston: Andover Medical Publishers.

Teti, T.M. & Gibbs, E.D. (1990). Infant assessment: historical antecedents and contemporary issues. In E.D. Gibbs & D.M. Teti (Eds.). *Interdisciplinary assessment of infants* (pp. 3-10). Baltimore: Brookes.

Turnbull, A.P., Turnbull, H.R., & Blue-Banning, M. (1994). Enhancing inclusion of infants and toddlers with disabilities and their families: a theoretical and programmatic analysis. *Infants and Young Children, 7*(2), 1-14.

Uzgiris, I.C. & Hunt, J. McV. (1975). *Assessment in infancy.* Urbana: University of Illinois Press.

Vohs, J. (1989). Recommendations for working with families and children with special needs from diverse cultures. In J. Vohs (Ed.). Organizational resources for understanding families from diverse cultures. *Coalition Quarterly: Toward Multiculturalism, 6*(2 & 3), 23.

Wilbarger, P. & Wilbarger, J. (1991). *Sensory affective disorders: beyond tactile defensiveness.* Available from Patricia Wilbarger, 642 Island View Dr, Santa Barbara, CA 93109.

Zimmerman, I.L., Steiner, V.G., & Pond, R.E. (1992). *Preschool Language Scales—3.* San Antonio, TX: The Psychological Corp.

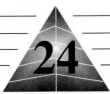

# Preschool Services

SUE ANN DUBOIS

## KEY TERMS

▲ Individuals With Disabilities Education Act
▲ Inclusion
▲ Integrated Therapy Models
▲ Supporting Classroom Activities

## CHAPTER OBJECTIVES

1. Explain the legislation and regulations that govern preschool programs.
2. Describe the developmental and functional issues with all preschool children.
3. Explain the role of the occupational therapist in the preschool classroom.
4. Explain different approaches used in occupational therapy intervention with preschool children.
5. Describe the evaluation continuum of screening through comprehensive team assessment and identify commonly used evaluation tools.
6. Explain the various models of services delivery used by occupational therapists in preschool settings.
7. Apply knowledge of therapy approaches and models of services delivery to a child with sensory integration and behavioral problems.

## WHAT ARE PRESCHOOL SERVICES?

The preschool years refer to the period of life between the ages of 3 and 5 years. Services for children 3 to 5 years of age have been available within the private and public sectors for many years as a means to support readiness skills for school entry. Occupational therapists have served this age-group through a variety of programs, in medical and educational settings, for many years. With the enactment of the 1986 Amendments to Part B of the Education for All Handicapped Act (P.L. 99-457), previously discretionary services to preschool children became required. The mandate for preschool services resulted in expansion of existing programs and opened many new opportunities for occupational therapists to work with preschool children. Children who needed occupational therapy to benefit from their special education program became "entitled to those services."

Preschool services build on the initial family-centered approach established in early intervention programming. An appreciation of the family's resources, concerns, and priorities is combined with an educational focus on readiness skills for learning in school. Collaboration with family members begins to emphasize support of the child's ability to function in community and school activities. Preschool programs and services provide the foundation for the child to move into school-related roles as well as skills to begin functioning in the community.

## LOCATION OF PRESCHOOL SERVICES

Preschool programs vary in structure and location according to the geographic region, state legislation and government, funding mechanisms, available resources, and public support for such programs. Similarly, the scope of services and use of occupational therapists in preschool settings are dependent on all these factors.

With the current trend toward inclusion of children with special needs into regular education programs, occupational therapy services are most often provided in regular preschool or day care settings. Services for preschoolers are also provided in private schools, community-based early education centers such as Head Start, community child care settings, and integrated preschool programs within a child's home school district.

## LEGISLATION THAT REGULATES PRESCHOOL SERVICES

Public health programs were the first to recognize the needs of young children. In 1935 Title V, the Social Security Act, was enacted. This Act authorized financial assistance to states to develop services that promoted the health of mothers and children of low socioeconomic status (SES) and crippled children. As a result, states developed Maternal and Child Health programs and established Bureaus for Handicapped Children (Shonkoff & Meisels, 1990). These programs continue to receive federal funds and provide health services to mothers and children. In the 1940s and 1950s occupational therapists primarily served preschoolers through nonprofit agencies such as United Cerebral Palsy and the National Easter Seal Society. In the late 1960s and early 1970s a stronger public commitment to meeting the educational and health needs of the preschool child developed. The Handicapped Children's Early Education Assistance Act of 1968 (P.L. 90-538), was enacted and provided funds for experimental programs for children up to 8 years old who had disabilities. With the enactment of the Education of the Handicapped Law (EHA) in 1975 (P.L. 94-142, Part B), services for children 3 to 5 years of age were encouraged through incentive funds that could be obtained by states if they established preschool programs.

In 1986 amendments to the EHA (P.L. 99-457) expanded the programs authorized under Part B by mandating special education services to children 3 to 5 years of age. In 1990 the EHA was reauthorized and retitled the Individuals with Disabilities Education Act (IDEA). This federal legislation has continued to support special education services for children 3 to 5 years of age and further promoted service provision in the least restrictive environment. Currently, all states mandate services to preschoolers with disabilities and their families.

Under this legislation for preschoolers, occupational therapy is identified as a "related service." Its purpose, as defined in the law, is to assist students with disabilities in benefiting from their special education program in public schools. Services for each preschool child are guided by a written plan defining goals and objectives, the Individualized Education Program (IEP), essentially the blueprint for the child's special education program. Chapter 25 provides additional information about IDEA and the federal regulations for special education.

An additional piece of legislature that affects services to preschoolers is the Americans with Disabilities Act (ADA) of 1990 (P.L. 101-336). This is a civil rights law intended to bring individuals with disabilities into the mainstream of American life (Kalscheur, 1992). Title II of this law addresses access to public services, programs, and facilities. As applied to the preschool population, segregated educational programs, recreation programs, and playgrounds administered through state and local governments for children with disabilities are prohibited (Kalscheur, 1992). Title III of the ADA requires all public accommodations and services operated by private entities to be accessible to persons with disabilities. Preschool environments in which accessibility needs to be considered include the following:

- ▲ Play environments: day care centers, playgrounds, and amusement parks
- ▲ Entertainment environments: theaters, zoos, and parks
- ▲ Sports environments: swimming pools and sports fields
- ▲ Learning environments: nursery schools, public schools, museums, and libraries
- ▲ Personal services: medical and community services offices
- ▲ Personal care environments: public bathrooms and fitting rooms

Accessibility guidelines for recreation facilities and outdoor developed areas were recently published when the Architectural and Transportation Barriers Compliance Board published its recommendations in the Federal Register (ADA 36, CFR Part 1191, September 1994). These proposed rules specify accessibility and safety requirements in the areas of places of amusement (e.g., rides and carnivals), play settings (playground equipment, sand play areas, and open areas for play), and elevated play equipment.

## EDUCATIONAL TRENDS THAT SUPPORT LEGISLATION AND AFFECT PRESCHOOL SERVICES

The emphasis of IDEA on inclusionary programming and partnerships between parents, educational professionals, and the educational process has expanded the models of service delivery and team interaction. The original multidisciplinary approaches have evolved into interdisciplinary models of collaborative teaming, integrated services, mainstreaming, and inclusion. It is important to define these trends as they relate to services for children 3 to 5 years of age.

In the educational literature, *collaboration* routinely refers to a process of problem solving by team members all having equal status who share their knowledge on behalf of a student (Rainforth, York, & MacDonald, 1992). Collaboration among the members of the preschool child's educational team (e.g., parent, teacher, occupational therapist, physical therapist, and speech-language pathologist) results in examination of performance and behavior problems from multiple perspectives. A team that works by collaborating can find creative and effective solutions to mutually defined problems. One such example of collaborative teaming with the preschool child may be the resolution of the child's difficulty taking turns and attending to the teacher during the morning circle routine. The speech therapist identifies severe delays in processing of auditory information that affect ability to follow directions and remain on task. The teacher identifies problems with the student's inability to sit for extended periods. The occupational therapist identifies difficulties in postural control of sitting and poor ability to plan and sequence motor movements. Together the team uses their information to solve the child's problem. Their joint solutions include providing more visual cues to the child to elicit responses during circle time, replacing the plastic molded chair with a beanbag chair, having the classroom assistant sit next to the child and provide touch pressure cues for orientation, and decreasing the duration of circle time. Each discipline has shared its expertise to resolve the problem.

Occupational therapy services for preschoolers are generally provided in the classroom to allow the child the opportunity to practice skills within that context. It also gives the classroom personnel opportunities to observe the occupational therapist's activities with a particular child and implement similar strategies with that child. For example, the occupational therapist works on the child's dressing skills during the daily class routine of donning and doffing outer clothing. The occupational therapist then teaches the classroom personnel specific strategies and techniques to foster development of dressing skills. Sharing the techniques with the family allows for continued work on the skill at home. Practice of the skill within the daily routine can help the child gain independence quickly.

*Mainstreaming* has been used as a program option for school-aged children for many years. This typically refers to placing students with disabilities and special education needs into the regular classrooms for academic instruction. Mainstreaming allows a child in special education placement opportunities to interact with non–special education students in one or more curriculum areas, such as physical education, art, music, and other selected academics. A preschooler may attend a local special education program for a portion of the day and attend a regular preschool or child care setting for the remainder of the day (Leister, Koonce, & Nisbet, 1993), or the child may attend two different settings on alternative days of the week. For example, the child may spend 2 days in a special education classroom and 3 days in a regular preschool (Leister et al., 1993).

*Inclusion* involves placing the preschooler in a setting where all services are provided in a community preschool program or child care facility. Inclusive schools have been referred to as *heterogeneous* schools, a term used to eliminate the perception of two systems, one of inclusion and one of exclusion (LRP, 1994a). Inclusive models are based on the least restrictive environment mandates outlined within IDEA. The use of special supports and related services are critical to meeting the individual needs of the child within inclusive preschools, for example, a child with multiple physical disabilities in a regular preschool setting with a full-time assistant to meet the child's personal care needs and occupational, physical, and speech therapy to address performance in the areas of mobility, access to the classroom materials, and communication.

In some states, systematic models of problem solving have been adopted that use site-based child study teams, preevaluation teams, or other models of educational profes-

sional teams. For example, the Heartland Area Education Agency established systematic procedures for the local teams to attempt to resolve the educational problem before the child reached the level of consideration for special education and the IEP process (Frolek Clark, 1994). Table 24-1 demonstrates the progressively more intense levels of this approach. At Level II the occupational therapist shares information and observations and at Level III provides short-

▲ Table 24-1  Problem-Solving Approach to Diversity of Learning Needs

| Level | Approach |
|---|---|
| **I**<br>Teacher/parent meeting | Collaboration may result in information sharing, strategy provision, and priority setting. |
| **II**<br>Referral to building assistance team | The previous parent-teacher collaboration and priority setting did not resolve the problem, and additional resources such as special education, occupational therapy, speech therapy, physical therapy, or psychology are accessed as supportive strategy resources. |
| **III**<br>Short-term intervention, i.e., strategies are implemented to address educational problem | With team consensus, short-term (usually 6 to 8 weeks) strategies are implemented by the supportive educational services (i.e., special education, occupational therapy, speech therapy, physical therapy, and psychology) and monitored. Progress is reported back to the team to evaluate effectiveness or need for additional intervention. |
| **IV**<br>Referral to special education and determination of eligibility | Previously implemented strategies and interventions are not effective; and evaluation by the school special education committee is recommended. Supportive educational services (i.e., special education, occupational therapy, speech therapy, physical therapy, and psychology) are requested to provide assessments. |

Modified from the Heartland Area Education Agency, Johnstown, IA.

term intervention activities for a limited time. Working with preschoolers at this critical time of readiness skill development may eliminate later difficulties with more complex skills and learning problems.

Tables 24-2, 24-3, and 24-4 provide a highlight of developmental skills relative to the ages of 3, 4, and 5 years, respectively.

## DEVELOPMENTAL PROFILE OF THE PRESCHOOL CHILD

Developmentally, the preschool years present an exciting period of growth toward competence, with play as the major occupational behavior. As internal control of behavior and sensorimotor foundations mature, the preschooler learns to master the environment, make choices, and engage in higher levels of object and social play.

## ROLE OF THE OCCUPATIONAL THERAPIST IN PRESCHOOL SERVICE

As a related service provider in special education, the occupational therapist's primary role is to "facilitate educational outcome in collaboration with other professionals who are providing services for the child and family" (AOTA, 1987). Occupational therapists implement therapeutic activities to increase independent function in play and self-care, design environments to enhance overall de-

▲ Table 24-2   Developmental Skills Profile, 3 Years

| Mobility | Eye-Hand and Arm Use | Prewriting Skills | Visual-Motor Skills | Self-Help Skills |
|---|---|---|---|---|
| Rides tricycle<br>Stands briefly on one foot<br>Jumps from step with two feet<br>Alternates feet part way walking on balance beam<br>Alternates feet walking upstairs<br>Runs with wide base | Isolates thumb from fist in imitation<br>Builds nine-block tower with 1-inch cubes<br>Catches ball with extended arms and body<br>Demonstrates preferred hand in manipulations and tool use<br>Supination emerges in grasp of spoon and fork<br>Strings ½-inch beads | Holds pencil with first two fingers and thumb with good control<br>Copies circle<br>Imitates cross<br>Traces square<br>Scribbles | Imitates 3-block bridge<br>Matches and recognizes primary colors and sizes grossly (big, little, long, and short)<br>Identifies body parts (toes, back, stomach, chin, knee, and neck)<br>Identifies front and behind | Unties bow<br>Unbuttons large and small (1-inch then ⅜-inch buttons)<br>Snaps and unsnaps<br>Unzips separating zipper<br>Zips and unzips nonseparating zipper<br>Dresses and undresses self fully with supervision; assistance needed in right and left shoe recognition and closures<br>Feeds self with little or no spillage |

▲ Table 24-3   Developmental Skills Profile, 4 Years

| Mobility | Eye-Hand and Arm Use | Prewriting Skills | Visual-Motor Skills | Self-Help Skills |
|---|---|---|---|---|
| Stands on one foot 3 to 6 seconds<br>Walks up and down steps reciprocally<br>Begins to skip, using a one-foot gallop<br>Hops on one foot 4 to 6 steps<br>Runs more controlled with feet closer together | Uses preferred hand with better coordination<br>More isolated finger movements to include finger spreading and opposition of thumb in sequence to all fingers<br>Grasps spoon and fork with fingers<br>Stacks 10 cubes<br>Threads ¼-inch beads<br>Cuts on lines<br>Throws ball overhand<br>Catches ball with arms slightly flexed | Demonstrates an open web space in tripod pencil grasp; holds distally in fingers<br>Copies cross<br>Imitates square and X<br>Colors pictures but still has difficulty remaining in lines | Identifies directionality concepts of on, under, behind, and beside in relation to body<br>Names four basic colors, shapes, and sizes<br>Builds 6-cube pyramid<br>Completes noninset puzzle of 3 to 5 pieces | Manages buttons completely<br>Zips nonseparating zipper<br>Zips separating zipper<br>Unbuckles and buckles belt or shoes<br>Unhooks pants<br>Uses napkin<br>Recognizes right shoe from left<br>Dresses with minimal supervision<br>Laces shoes |

velopment and prevent disability, and provide necessary supports (e.g., adapted equipment) for the child to benefit from special education.

In today's school settings, occupational therapists have expanded their roles with preschoolers beyond special education programs. With the emergence of civil rights legislation supporting equal access for persons with disabilities (ADA, 1990, Section 504), occupational therapists may develop roles as consultants to regular preschool programs to increase environmental access and access to basic learning curriculum. These are emerging roles that will continue to be shaped by future legislation.

Another important role for the occupational therapist is that of team member. The concept of interdisciplinary teaming clearly is inherent in the special education law and is encouraged as the best practice in the provision of occupational therapy services. The primary features of collaborative teaming include developing a unified set of student goals and making consensus decisions regarding program directions (Dennis, Edelman, & Giangreco, 1991). Isolated occupational therapy intervention without consideration of other program parameters, opportunities, and resources is not appropriate.

Occupational therapists offer a unique perspective in the educational setting. Occupational therapy programs provide carefully designed activities to expand functional capabilities and coping behaviors that enable a child to be an active learner. Neurophysiologic approaches that support functional performance are used to engage the preschooler in enriched sensory and motor experiences that serve as the foundation for higher-level functional and behavioral competencies. Occupational therapists also understand the importance of purposeful activities in daily areas of occupational performance, such as eating, playing, moving, and interacting with others to the preschooler's physical, cognitive, and psychosocial development. By adapting and structuring activities in the child's natural environment, the occupational therapist both challenges and supports the child's performance. Successes in play and self-care help the preschooler experience new levels of competency, independence, and self-worth.

Occupational therapists also support family-centered services to preschoolers. Families of preschoolers often experience stress as their child strives for more autonomy and makes the transition into the structured learning environment of school. When their child has a disability, this stress may be magnified. Along with other team members, occupational therapists help parents cope with these transitions. Interagency collaboration between service providers helps support and plan for these transitions. Occupational therapists can help parents develop and implement interactive strategies with their children and use effective coping strategies that meet the challenges of caregiving and family life (AOTA, 1989). The following sections describe the occupational therapy process of assessing the child's strengths and needs in the context of the preschool environment and curriculum, collaborative intervention planning, and strategies to promote the child's performance.

## EVALUATING FUNCTION

A referral initiates the occupational therapy evaluation process. The American Occupational Therapy Association defines *referral* as "the practice of directing initial request for service or changing the degree and direction of service" (AOTA, 1994, p. 1034). Specific to the preschooler in the educational setting, a referral initiates the process of evaluation to determine whether occupational therapy is warranted to support the student's ability to learn and function in the preschool program. The referral may be generated by the student's family, teacher, or other members of the child's educational team.

The occupational therapy evaluation includes functional abilities or capabilities and deficits or limitations in the preschooler's performance. Interpretation of performance capabilities and limitations are based on the expectations of the educational environment and the framework of typical development (AOTA, 1989). The evaluation process iden-

▲ **Table 24-4**  Developmental Skills Profile, 5 Years

| Mobility | Eye-Hand and Arm Use | Prewriting Skills | Visual-Motor Skills | Self-Help Skills |
|---|---|---|---|---|
| Stands on one foot for approximately 8 seconds with arms folded | Preferred hand used more consistent | Copies square | Matches 10 to 12 objects | Zips, unzips nonseparating back zipper |
| Skips alternating feet | Sews through holes in sewing card | Copies triangle | Counts 10 objects | Hooks pants |
| Walks on balance beam without falling off | Catches large ball using two hands | Traces diamond | Identifies body parts (shoulders and hips) | Uses knife for spreading |
| Moves rhythmically to music | Uses a mature lateral grasp of spoon or fork | Colors pictures neatly, staying within outlines | Distinguishes right and left on self | Dresses without supervision |
| | Cuts out circle | Traces letters | Builds a 6-cube step | Begins to tie shoes |
| | | Begins to copy first name | Begins to discriminate secondary colors | Brushes teeth without supervision |
| | | | Completes 12 to 15-piece puzzle | |

tifies children who demonstrate developmental delays or functional impairments or who seem to be at risk for developmental or learning problems. It provides baseline information for intervention planning, for developing the goals and objectives of the IEP, and for measuring the effects of the intervention.

The evaluation process is a continuum of data collection and analysis. Screenings in the preschool population are an initial, short-term process of data collection to determine program eligibility, need for intervention, or further in-depth assessment in a particular area of performance. The occupational therapist may independently screen the preschooler or participate in a comprehensive interdisciplinary screening. As a member of the preschool screening team, the therapist may travel to homes, agencies, and schools to complete screening procedures. In some districts, specific times of the year are dedicated to *preschool screenings*. The level of interdisciplinary teaming within each school often determines how and what procedures are used by occupational therapists in this process. Some schools rely on district-made developmental checklists with assignment of specific performance areas to be administered by specific disciplines. Others use the transdisciplinary play-based assessment (Linder, 1990) described in Chapters 8 and 23. In other school systems the occupational therapists select the screening instrument. The resulting information is then combined with the team's collection of data for a baseline picture of the child's performance.

One screening instrument specific to preschoolers is the First STEP: Screening Test for Evaluating Preschoolers (Miller, 1993). This is an individually administered, norm-referenced screening test used to identify developmental delays in children ages 2 years 9 months through 6 years 2 months. It was developed to identify preschool children who are at risk in the five domains defined by IDEA. These domains include cognition, communication, and physical, social and emotional, and adaptive functioning.

In many preschool settings, occupational therapists are not part of the initial screening team. Referrals may be generated once the child has been placed in the preschool. In some preschools, all children eligible for special educational services are eligible for occupational therapy.

As a process, the continuum of assessment is composed of various combinations of components. These components include, but are not limited to, the educational file review, skilled observations and activity analysis, interviews, checklists, and norm- and criterion-referenced tests.

## Educational File Review

The educational file review entails a review of information and data previously collected about the child. This may include medical documents, documents of services in an early intervention program, intake procedures provided by the school, or documents of the student's performance on standardized tests.

## Skilled Observations and Activity Analysis

Skilled observations and activity analysis are usually an integral part of the assessment process. Through skilled observations, combined with activity analysis and problem solving, the occupational therapist determines the types of services required to support the preschooler's function and ability to learn in a classroom. Environmental observations may be completed in the child's home or classroom, or they may be specific to a given activity. Figure 24-1 illustrates an outline format used to observe the preschooler's performance within the class environment. Each activity is analyzed, the child performance in relationship to the activity is assessed, and current environmental supports available are noted. This format can be adapted to observation of most performance areas and helps organize the assessment information and interpretation so that recommended activities and adaptations are clearly understood.

Observations of the preschoolers in the home are important to a comprehensive program and to offering family support. After observations of daily living routines (particularly dressing, grooming, and feeding), the occupational therapist can make recommendations to the family members regarding methods to support the child's independence and how to cope with difficult behaviors.

Clinical observations are often guided by the therapist's background in neurodevelopment and sensory integration. Through clinical observations the therapist develops an understanding of the components of occupational performance. Critical analysis of performance enables the therapist to identify underlying problems in sensory integration, sensorimotor output, and neuromaturation. *Clinical observations* may include assessment of (1) muscle tone, (2) reflex integration, (3) postural reactions and control, (4) range of motion, (5) movement patterns, (6) sensorimotor skills, (7) ocular motor control, (8) sensory awareness, (9) stereognosis, (10) kinesthesia and proprioception, (11) vestibular function, and (12) oral motor control.

Some standardized instruments for preschoolers also offer clinical observation formats as part of the testing procedure. In the Pediatric Examination Series (Pediatric Extended Examination at Three [PEET] and Pediatric Examination of Educational Readiness [PEER]), neuromaturational observations are included as portions of the subtests. In the Miller Assessment for Preschoolers (Miller, 1988), the Supplemental Observations Sheet provides the examiner with a structured method of recording behaviors and qualities that may influence a child's test performance. Used in conjunction with the test, the observation sheet is divided into five sections of vision, touch, speech, language, and movement.

Student: _____

Teacher: _____

Date: _____

| Activity | Performance required | Performance demonstrated |
|---|---|---|
| | | |

Classroom environment assistance:

Recommmendations presented:

_____

School Occupational Therapist

**Figure 24-1** Occupational therapy classroom observations.

## Interviews

Interviewing education staff, family, and other service providers is an integral component of assessment. Interviews provide important information about the child that the occupational therapist may not have opportunities to observe. Routinely this is done informally through discussions with teachers and service providers. Input from the parents can often be collected in person, by telephone, or through the use of a questionnaire such as that outlined in Figure 24-2. Information about the child's medical or developmental history and about his or her likes and dislikes, interests, or preferences helps provide a holistic picture of the child.

Preschooler's Name: _____

DOB: _____ Age: _____

Parent's Name: _____

Phone: Home _____ Work _____

Person filling out questionaire: _____


   The following information may be helpful to the occupational therapist in assessing your child's performance in his or her preschool program. Please try to answer each section carefully, and return to the occupational therapist at school.


**Developmental milestones:**   Have you or your physician noted any delays in reaching major age skills, i.e., moving, playing, communicating, self care?


Have you noticed differences compared with other children in the areas of play, self care, and socializing?


What does your child like?


What does your child dislike?


What would you like the occupational therapist to focus on to help you and your preschooler?


What other therapies or special education programs has your preschooler attended or is currently receiving?


Does your preschooler use any special devices at home that help him or her in their daily routine?

**Figure 24-2**   Occupational therapy parent intake.

## Checklists

Checklists are often valuable tools to assess preschoolers' performances in their educational setting. These forms typically include items for evaluating functional mobility, self-help, and manipulation of classroom materials. Often check-

lists are generated from chronologic skills profiles such as the information provided in Tables 24-2 through 24-4. Using varying combinations of this information provides occupational therapists with a quick point of reference to determine whether the preschooler demonstrates isolated or

NAME:_____

DOB:_____

PERSON COMPLETING CHECKLIST:_____

DATE:_____

Circle Y (yes) N (no) or S (sometimes) with the statement as it relates to your child

**Gross and Fine Motor Skills**

| | | | |
|---|---|---|---|
| Difficulty riding a ride-on toy with feet propelling | Y | N | S |
| Difficulty pumping self on swing | Y | N | S |
| Dislikes playing with puzzles | Y | N | S |
| Dislikes playing with small manipulatives | Y | N | S |
| Difficulty using a spoon or cup | Y | N | S |
| Seems weaker or tires more easily than others of the same age | Y | N | S |
| Appears stiff, awkward, or clumsy in movement | Y | N | S |
| Seems to have much difficulty in learning new motor tasks | Y | N | S |
| If 4 years of age or older, has difficulty dressing self | Y | N | S |
| Has messy eating habits | Y | N | S |

**Movement and Balance Skills**

| | | | |
|---|---|---|---|
| Gets car sick frequently | Y | N | S |
| Gets nauseated or vomits from other movement experiences (e.g., playground swings, merry go rounds) | Y | N | S |
| Is unable to give adequate warning about feelings of nausea | Y | N | S |
| Seeks quantities of twirling or spinning | Y | N | S |
| Seeks quantities of stimulation on amusement park rides and swings | Y | N | S |
| Hesitates to climb or play on playground equipment | Y | N | S |
| Has trouble or hesitancy in learning to climb or descend stairs | Y | N | S |
| Dislikes being lifted up and gently tossed in the air by parent | Y | N | S |
| Did not or does not like being placed on his or her stomach or back as an infant | Y | N | S |
| Rocks himself or herself when stressed | Y | N | S |
| Period of crawling was absent or very brief | Y | N | S |
| Walks on toes now or in the past | Y | N | S |

**Touch**

| | | | |
|---|---|---|---|
| Seems unaware of being touched | Y | N | S |
| Seems overly sensitive to being touched, pulls away from light touch | Y | N | S |
| Seems excessively ticklish or strongly dislikes touch | Y | N | S |
| Dislikes the feeling of certain types of clothing or material or is bothered by the tags in the back of shirts | Y | N | S |

**Figure 24-3**   Preschool sensory history for occupational therapy.

generalized skill delays. Information about sensory processing skills can also be gathered using a checklist format. Figure 24-3 illustrates a format that can be sent home with the parent or completed by team members in the school environment to gather performance information.

## Norm- and Criterion-Referenced Tests

Standardized tests are widely used in the process of preschool assessment. Used in combination with other parts of evaluation, the standardized evaluation tool can provide a comprehensive occupational therapy profile of the pre-

| | | | |
|---|---|---|---|
| Resists wearing short-sleeve shirts or short pants | Y | N | S |
| Continues to examine objects by placing them in the mouth (past age of 1½ years old) | Y | N | S |
| Dislikes being cuddled or hugged unless on child's terms | Y | N | S |
| Avoids putting hands in messy substances | Y | N | S |
| Strongly dislikes hair cutting or washing | Y | N | S |
| Strongly dislikes toe or fingernail cutting | Y | N | S |
| Pinches, bites, or otherwise hurts self | Y | N | S |
| Crawled with fisted hands | Y | N | S |
| Often unaware of bruises, cuts, or scrapes | Y | N | S |
| Seems overly sensitive to slight bumps or scrapes | Y | N | S |
| Tendency to touch things constantly | Y | N | S |
| Frequently pushes or hits other children | Y | N | S |

**Auditory and Language Skills**

| | | | |
|---|---|---|---|
| Has or has had repeated ear infections | Y | N | S |
| Particularly distracted by sounds, seeming to hear sounds that go unnoticed by others | Y | N | S |
| Often fails to listen or pay attention to what is said to him or her | Y | N | S |
| Is overly sensitive to mildly loud noises | Y | N | S |
| History of delayed speech development | Y | N | S |

**Bowel and Bladder Control**

| | | | |
|---|---|---|---|
| Late in achieving bowel and bladder control | Y | N | S |
| Occasionally has accidents during the day | Y | N | S |
| If accident occurs, does not seem to be aware ahead of time that elimination is about to occur | Y | N | S |

**Emotions**

| | | | |
|---|---|---|---|
| Does not easily accept changes in routine | Y | N | S |
| Becomes easily frustrated | Y | N | S |
| Likely to be impulsive, heedless, and accident prone | Y | N | S |
| Marked mood variation, tendency to outbursts or tantrums | Y | N | S |
| Tends to withdraw from groups; plays on outskirts | Y | N | S |

**Additional comments or observations that may be important to learning:**

**Figure 24-3, cont'd**   Preschool sensory history for occupational therapy.

schooler. Although many pediatric measures are available to assess performance (see Chapter 8), the most commonly used evaluation tools for preschoolers include the following:

*Pediatric Evaluation of Disability Inventory (PEDI)* (Haley, Coster, Ludlow, Haltiwanger, & Andrellos, 1992). The PEDI was developed to provide a compre-hensive clinical assessment of key functional capabilities and performance of functional activities in children between the ages of 6 months and 7 years. The PEDI measures three content domains: (1) self care, (2) mobility, and (3) social function. Further description of the PEDI is found in Chapter 8.

*Miller Assessment for Preschoolers (MAP)* (Miller, 1988). The MAP is designed to evaluate children from ages 2 years 9 months to 5 years 8 months. Its purposes are to identify developmentally delayed preschoolers who need further evaluation and to provide a structured clinical framework to identify the child's strengths and weaknesses. A scale of 27 test items rates performance in the areas of sensorimotor foundations, coordination, and verbal, nonverbal, and complex tasks. The MAP is designed to identify mild to moderate preacademic problems that may affect one or more areas of development and learning.

*DeGangi-Berk Test of Sensory Integration (TSI)* (Berk & DeGangi, 1983). The TSI is a diagnostic criterion-referenced tool for 3- to 5-year-old children. It is designed to measure overall sensory integrative function and focuses primarily on vestibular-based function. It has 36 items organized into three subdomains: (1) bilateral motor integration (20 items), (2) postural control (12 items), and (3) reflex integration (4 items).

*Erhardt Developmental Prehension Assessment (EPDA)* (Erhardt, 1989). The EDPA provides a scale for measuring prehension development. The criterion-referenced scale, rates involuntary arm-hand patterns; voluntary movements of approach, grasp, release, and manipulation; and prewriting skills for developmental ages 0 to 6 years. Few reliability and validity studies have been completed on the EPDA.

*Peabody Developmental Motor Scales (PDMS)* (Folio & Fewell, 1983). The PDMS is a standardized test for children from birth to 83 months. The test measures a child's ability to demonstrate fine and gross motor skills that reflect developmental milestones. The scales can be used individually to identify delays or in combination to achieve an overall motor age equivalent. The scoring system of 0, 1, or 2 provides information about the skills a child has mastered (2), those currently developing (1), and those not yet in the child's repertoire (0). Because the PDMS can produce standard scores, it is often used to determine eligibility for occupational therapy.

*Pediatric Extended Examination at Three (PEET)* (Blackman, Levine, & Markowitz, 1986). This standardized observation is a developmental assessment designed to aid in the early detection and clarification of problems with learning, attention, and behavior in children 3 to 4 years of age. Developmental performance areas addressed include gross motor, language, visual-fine motor, memory, and intersensory integration skills.

*Pediatric Examination of Educational Readiness (PEER)* (Levine & Schneider, 1985). This is a set of standardized observations that outlines empirical descriptions of the child's development and neurologic status. The PEER is designed primarily for the evaluation of children 4 to 6 years of age. Performance tasks on this evaluation include orientation, gross motor, visual-fine motor, sequential, linguistic, and preacademic learning skills.

*Bruininks-Oseretsky Test of Motor Proficiency (BOTMP)* (Bruininks, 1987). BOTMP is a standardized test of gross and fine motor skills for evaluation of children 4 years 6 months to 14 years 6 months. Eight subtests examine running speed and agility, balance, bilateral coordination, strength, upper-limb coordination, response speed, visual-motor control, upper-limb speed, and dexterity.

*Brigance Diagnostic Inventory of Early Development (IED)* (Brigance, 1978). IED is designed for children from 0 to 7 years of age. It contains items that measure gross and fine motor, self-help, communication, general knowledge and comprehension, reading, writing, and math skills. The gross motor, fine motor, and self-help checklist areas best serve the preschool performance areas addressed by the occupational therapist. Information about the publication sources for these tests is provided in Appendix 8-A of Chapter 8.

The interpretation of assessment data for the preschooler should reflect the student's strengths and weaknesses relative to educational performance, family, and team priorities. Key features of the assessment process (adapted from Struck & DuBois, 1993) are as follows:

▲ Current educational information is considered.
▲ Data have been collected in the natural environment.
▲ Evaluation tools provide interpretive findings relative to learning.
▲ Performance components relative to learning outcomes are clearly identified.
▲ Information is collected from other team members outlining student problems that impact learning.
▲ The assessment process provides information leading to program development and intervention within the learning environment.

## PROGRAM PLANNING

The occupational therapy component of the preschooler's educational plan is developed according to the IEP process outlined in the federal mandates of the IDEA. The IEP is the legal document that defines the child's program of education and related services. The process of IEP development results in a collaborative program that may include specific intervention plans by the occupational therapist (see Chapter 25).

Generating an occupational therapy plan requires the synthesis of the performance profile with home and school environments, program and curriculum outlines, and team support factors. The student profile is a picture of the student's performance strengths and weaknesses. Identifying the home and school environments where performance will be required constitutes the next step in planning. This may

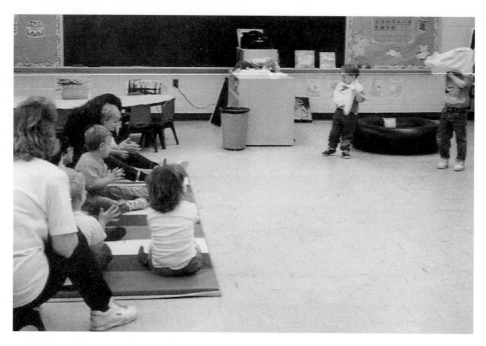

**Figure 24-4**   Support group, show and tell.

be the classroom, hallway, bathrooms, bus, or lunch room. The activities and routines demanded within the environment are then considered. What is required of the preschooler in that environment? A task analysis of the activities in the class or other environments is the next stage of planning. The therapist analyzes the steps of the activities that the teacher has planned, projects which steps will be difficult for the child, and then identifies what assistance might be given to the child so that he or she can successfully participate in the activity. Team members work together to identify what skill activities should be prioritized. In what performance area is the preschooler encountering the greatest difficulty or meeting the least success, and where should initial services focus? Planning includes identifying opportunities to work on needed skills and may include the morning toileting and toothbrushing routine, orientation circle time, snack time, or center-based activity. The key features of program planning follow, as adapted from Struck and Dubois (1993):

▲ Addresses the preschooler's needs in the least restrictive environment
▲ Enables function within the preschool and home setting
▲ Allows for mutual support through collaboration in daily routine
▲ Allows for shared decision making with other team members
▲ Supports the educational program
▲ Reflects a team approach
▲ Selects activities that support performance in home and preschool

▲ Adaptations and strategies can safely be implemented into routines with team members
▲ Allows for flexibility to meet the preschooler's changing needs.

## INTERVENTION

Delivering occupational therapy as a related service in preschool programs is a process whereby "activities, procedures and environmental modifications necessary to implement the goals and objectives of the IEP are carried out" (AOTA, 1987). A continuum of service models is outlined in much of the current literature on pediatric- and school-based services. Such terms as *direct, indirect, group monitoring, consultation, integrated therapy, collaborative consultation,* and *pull-out* are just a few of the terms used to identify service models for preschoolers. It is generally agreed that no one model of service meets the needs of all children. The assessment and program planning process must meet the individual needs of each preschooler, but a single method of delivery will not fit all.

Recent educational trends have had significant impact on intervention for preschoolers. The current focus on inclusionary practices have supported a model for integrated services. Using this model, the occupational therapist promotes the student performance in areas that the team has identified as priority goals (Rainforth et al., 1992). In integrated services, occupational therapy becomes part of the child's everyday routine and environment.

Collaborative teaming combines the design of integrated therapy with the sharing of skills and information across

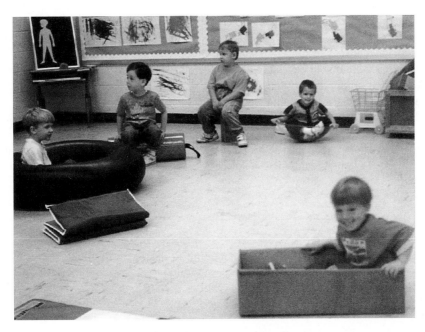

**Figure 24-5**  Support group, play.

all disciplines. It creates a child-centered rather than a discipline-focused program. Block scheduling is a program mechanism that promotes the components of integrated services and collaborative teaming (Rainforth et al., 1992). It is a strategy for scheduling time in an integrated learning environment with team members. It differs from traditional occupational therapy scheduling in that time is blocked within a certain setting for students. Instead of ½-hour "treatment times," the occupational therapist spends a block of time (e.g., 2 hours) in class. He or she is, therefore, with the children during bus-to-class transitions, orientation circle, and snack time. Other team members are also working with children in the classroom during this block of time. This proximity promotes collaboration on a child's behalf, and related service supports are provided within the performance routine. Providing services within the classroom helps reinforce the targeted skills in the natural context of performance and promotes generalization of skills into multiple classroom activities (Giangreco, 1986; Giangreco, York, & Rainforth, 1989).

## BLENDING APPROACHES FOR INTERVENTION WITH PRESCHOOLERS

The occupational therapist integrates the goals of the educational program and a selected intervention approach as these fit the individual needs of the preschooler. Supporting this unique period of development in performance areas of play, self-care, communication, and socialization requires innovation and flexibility. The following are examples of interventions that support an integrative approach.

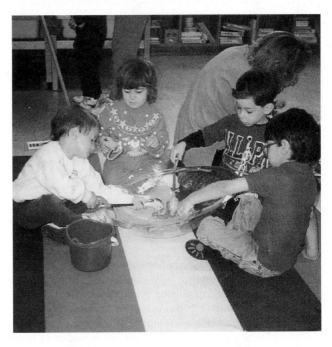

**Figure 24-6**  Support group, exploration.

## Classroom Groups

The group concept has been used in every aspect of educational programming. Often preschool teachers identify "motor time" as an integral part of their school day, with the emphasis on providing foundations for higher skill development through sensorimotor groups. Often the occupational therapist adds new perspective to activities and helps individual children participate with greater competence. Figures 24-4, 24-5, and 24-6 depict group support in the preschool setting. Collaborating with the teacher and teacher assistants and development of various performance components are supported. Parents are encouraged to attend and participate in the group as a method to develop playful and meaningful relationships at home. Parent participation may also serve as a means to introduce toys and materials not often considered by the parent, yet supportive of the preschooler's individual learning needs.

An outline of the program for preschool curriculum purposes is identified in Figure 24-7. It is important to note that any group programming in the preschool environment should not compete with other program components. It should allow the preschooler to learn and respond to natural cues in the environment and the personnel and resources in that environment.

## Adapting Classroom Activities

Another function of occupational therapists in preschools is to adapt or modify activities to promote performance. The

---

**Goals of the group activity**
1. To enhance normal development and functional adaptive responses in the 3- to 5-year-old child
2. To provide a vehicle to assist in the development of foundational sensorimotor skills that are precursors for learning and motor skill development
3. To provide a vehicle for teacher or therapist collaboration and sensorimotor principle integration in the classroom

**General structure**
The classroom teacher, occupational therapist, and classroom assistant direct and manage group activities cooperatively
The group meets twice a week for 25 to 30 minutes
Children participate with shoes removed
The occupational therapist and classroom teacher conduct sessions
Therapy sensorimotor equipment is used, but the focus is on the child's body and relativity to space rather than equipment
Materials and equipment used in group activity are often selected on the basis of their ability also to be used safely during free time in the class environment outside
Activities are designed to promote sensorimotor processing and neurodevelopmental foundational skills, necessary prerequisites for higher-level academic skills, and classroom performance.
Specific motor skills are not emphasized, however, within select activities, dressing and manipulations for dressing are emphasized in a playful manner.

**Selection of Activities**
Activities are sequenced in a developmental continuum, as outlined in the hierarchy of neurodevelopment and the sensorimotor development process:
1. Tactile: touch
2. Vestibular: movement against gravity in linear or rotary planes
3. Proprioceptive: heavy muscle work and joint position sense
4. Postural: stabilizing the trunk and large joints
5. Bilateral: incorporating two body sides
6. Motor skill development: motor sequencing and following directions
Once sensorimotor activities are provided as a precursor to function, the remaining portion of the group stresses skills for functional outcomes, such as dressing and hand skills, for classroom tool manipulation. Functional outcome emphasis is also guided by the performance skills currently emphasized in the curriculum.

**Preassessment and postassessment**
1. Child's performance on selected evaluative tools or developmental class activities, selected on the basis of the child's needs
2. Teacher's observations
3. Occupational therapist's observations
4. Parents' observations

**Figure 24-7** Preschool sensorimotor group.

occupational therapist seeks opportunities within the teacher-planned activities to help the student develop sensorimotor or perceptual performance components. Figure 24-8 illustrates an opportunity for the preschooler to work on hand strength and prehension; a project is "hung out to dry" on a line, whereby the child is required to manipulate a clothespin. In Figure 24-9, alternative positioning is suggested by the occupational therapist to support a more mature approach of the forearm and wrist during a coloring project. Typically this student would complete this project on a table top in a seated position. Asking him to color with the forearm in a pronated position is a simple and effective strategy to increase proprioceptive input and encourage wrist extension.

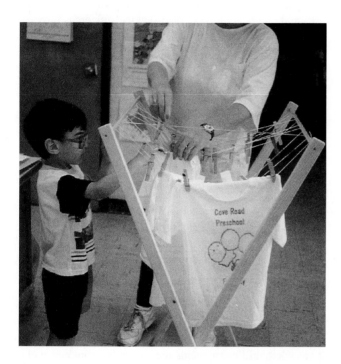

**Figure 24-8** Project is hung out to dry, thus building hand strength and prehension.

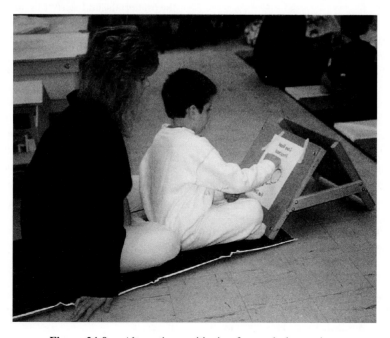

**Figure 24-9** Alternative positioning for a coloring project.

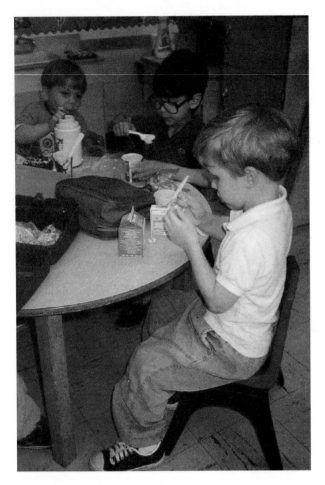

**Figure 24-10** Daily snacks offer opportunity to work on two-handed functions.

## Accessing Routines

To provide therapy in the natural contexts of the environment, the occupational therapist must become familiar with the preschool routines. Many opportunities to promote specific skill components are found in the preschool program. For example, the daily snack routine offers many opportunities for preschoolers to work on the two-handed functions of stabilizer and manipulator, fine pincer grasp, and mature use of utensils (Figure 24-10). Snack time is also ideal for working on self-feeding and social skill development. Figure 24-11 provides an outline for the occupational therapist to give to the classroom staff as a reminder for support. Letters sent home to parents identifying the focus of the snack routine are also helpful. Figure 24-12 provides parents with some ideas for snacks and packaging that may supplement the routine.

Routines for preschoolers also involve weekly assignment of jobs. One such classroom job generated by the occupational therapist and implemented in the program day is cleaning of the tables after snack time. This routine, illustrated in Figure 24-13, supports hand strength and pre-

scissor skills with the use of the spray bottle of water. Wiping the table can help increase controlled movement of the shoulder and elbow while maintaining a grasp of the cloth. It provides an opportunity for proprioceptive input, as well as a sense of participation and responsibility.

A number of strategies that support the development of children's performance components can be applied to the preschool program routine:

▲ Washing hands and arms with surgical scrub brushes and other "scrubbies" placed at the sink areas provides additional tactile input.

▲ Using floor and wall surfaces in the class when coloring requires postural stability, additional work of the arm against gravity, and different angles of wrist extension than the typical position seated at a table.

▲ Sitting on therapy balls, t-stools, and therapy cylinders during circle time helps children work on postural stability and balance.

## Support of Curricula

Many preschools adopt activity-based centers for learning. Placed in different areas of the room, the centers have themes that define their materials and activities. The centers may include a kitchen or cooking area, an office, a zoo, a sensory area, an art area, or a construction zone. Often these centers focus on manipulative tasks that support learning, and the children "rotate through" these centers on a daily basis. To use therapeutic principles and strategies during the child's play at the centers, the therapist first analyzes what skill components are naturally promoted within each center. Once the occupational therapist is familiar with the materials and activities in each center, he or she can follow the child's lead and provide support of skill performance using those materials. For example, facilitation of scissors skills can be achieved in the art center, using the strategies listed in Figure 24-14.

Many preschool programs provide outdoor time as part of their curriculum. The occupational therapist can assist the classroom teacher and staff by providing strategies for the child to access playground equipment. The playground is an ideal setting to facilitate needed sensory experiences for children with sensory integration problems.

## Supporting Parents at Home

The parents, as integral parts of the preschool team, participate at various levels; their involvement is always encouraged. Often preschool programs offer seminars or education programs for parents on a wide spectrum of topics related to their children and the curriculum. Occupational therapists become an integral part of the parent education program.

A preschool newsletter, such as that illustrated in Figure

**Please encourage these fine motor fundamentals**

1. Opening lunch boxes independently
2. Pulling outside wrappers off straws
3. Placing straws in juice boxes or milk cartons
4. Twisting off cups and lids of a thermos independently with the preferred hand "do," nonpreferred hand "hold" method (the teacher or aide may need to slightly loosen these items)
5. Pouring liquid into the cup as needed using hand-over-hand method (older children)
6. Opening snap-and-seal containers independently (preferred hand "do," non-preferred hand "hold")
7. Collecting and properly disposing of all trash
8. Placing remaining items in a box and closing the box to be put away
9. Placing items in backpack independently
10. Each day, two children clean the tables, using a sprayer and paper towels (use preferred hand's index or middle finger or thumb to spray with the trigger and use one or two hands to wipe off tables. The child should be encouraged to use pressure and good wrist extension.)
11. After snack time, encourage children to wash their hands and faces, using a mirror.

**Ms. Smith's class-specific focus**

Bobby: focus and attention, mature pinch, establish a preference, and motor plan
1. Encourage two-hand use as needed
2. Encourage use of index finger and thumb to pick up small items
3. Use firm touch pressure with hand over hand to show understanding of the action sequences to complete a task

Melissa: attention and focus, mature pinch, motor plan, and establish a preference
1. Provide hand over hand as needed to show understanding of the action sequence to complete a task
2. Left "do", right "hold"
3. Allow only one food item at a time
4. Encourage use of the index finger and thumb to pinch small items
5. If the child gets of the the seat during snack time, terminate snack time
6. Position items at child's midline

Jonathan: two-hand use, mature grasp, and motor plan
1. Encourage right "do", left "hold"
2. Encourage use of the index finger and thumb to pinch small items
3. Use hand-over-hand technique as needed, with firm touch pressure to show understanding of the action sequence to complete a task

**Figure 24-11**   Preschool snack time management program.

24-15, is useful for working parents. Providing information in this format can be helpful to parents and allows them to select the information that currently interests them. Common themes of the newsletters that the occupational therapist might write include (1) reinforcement of play as an occupational role, (2) home activities to promote manipulation skills, (3) sensory experiences that prepare the preschooler for learning, or (4) self-help skill development.

The newsletter format provides a consistent program link between parents and school. It is also a vehicle for sharing the information with other team members. The written information can strengthen the team members' understanding of the occupational therapist's role with preschoolers.

## SUMMARY

This chapter explained the effects of recent legislation and regulations that define services of preschool children with special needs. Differences between mainstreaming and inclusion were discussed. The development and functional tasks of the preschool years were defined, and the role of the occupational therapists in promoting functional performance was described. The occupational therapists works closely with the families of young children to provide them with support and information regarding caregiving and skill development. Specific strategies that characterize occupational therapy intervention within preschool programs were explained, with emphasis on integrated and ecologic models of practice.

Date

Dear Parents:

As part of your child's preschool program, Ms. Smith and I are trying to encourage fine motor skill development during snack time. We encourage many of the basic hand skills necessary for school and daily routines through independent management of snack materials.

To help us with this program, we request that you send snacks in packaging containers that support skill development. Snacks wrapped in aluminum foil, plastic wrap, or zip lock bags are great! Please avoid sending snacks in sealed containers, such as the individual fruit or applesauce cups, if your child cannot currently manage these. A nice alternative to build skills is transferring these foods into small snap and seal containers. Then we can encourage the "hold-and-do" function of the hands as they open and close the container.

In the case of sealed and wrapped packages, we may be encouraging fine pinching or scissors use to open these packages.

Thank you for your cooperation and assistance as we work together for your preschooler!

Sincerely,


School Occupational Therapist

**Figure 24-12**    Sample letter to parents.

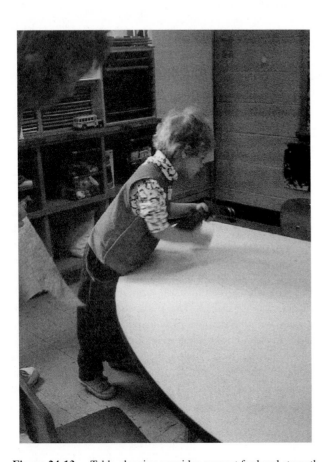

**Figure 24-13**    Table cleaning provides support for hand strength and prescissors skills.

The attached strategies and activities are provided to support the Individual Education Plan Fine Motor Goals and Objectives and support the curriculum skills array in the area of scissors skills. These include the following:

I.  Prescissors experience activities
    A. Pick up relay games as demonstrated in class
    B. Squeeze play as demonstrated in class
    C. Paper punch games
II.  Scissors positioning
    A. Correct finger and hand positioning as reviewed in class
    B. Use of sponge wedge or Koosh ball as outlined
    C. Cutting resistives, straws, and clay snakes
III.  Directionality and control activities
    A. Cut through lines
    B. Nail head worksheets
    C. Aim for the star worksheets

Considering each child's current level of functioning, the following are recommended:


Classroom:

Student_____

Strategies suggested (list):

**Figure 24-14**    Scissors skill development.

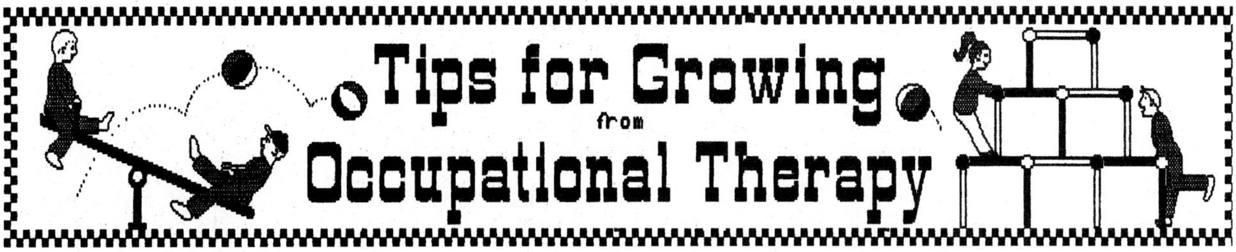

# Tips for Growing from Occupational Therapy

## May/June 1993

## Focus on Motor Planning

When we first learn a new skill we must think very carefully about how and where our movements occur. As we "learn" the movement, we find that we do not have to "think" as carefully about how the movement occurs. It becomes more "automatic." This process of motor planning is affected by the use of the sensory processes we discussed in previous newsletters. We use the systems in our body that process touch, body awareness, and sense of movement to store the memory of movements and not have to "relearn them" each time we need to call upon them. Motor planning is an important developmental consideration in young children as it forms the foundations for such things as imitation, following directions, and automatizing movements for letter formations in writing. Many of the sensory activities discussed in the previous newsletters will help develop motor planning skills. Additional activities to consider include use of constructional toys, pantomimes, follow-the-leader, catching or throwing games, and routine, simple chores at home.

## Promoting Motor Planning With Playground Equipment

With the coming summer months, hours of play can be spent out-doors. The value of good playground equipment in promoting motor planning skills can not be underestimated. I have attached some variations on standard play equipment that may provide more developmental challenges for your child. The heavy muscle work involved in negotiating playground equipment stimulates a portion of your child's brain that helps regulate balance, muscular responses, and higher challenges to the sensory systems. Encourage self-exploration. Your child will challenge his motor planning skills through the "ins and outs" and "ups and downs" of play. Explore your nearest playground or school yard or consider creating an area in your own back yard. It is exciting to see the recent offerings in modular pieces in the home center stores.

## Exciting Summer Resources

Summer can sometimes seem quite long for a young child whose attention is brief and activity level is high. You may want to consider looking at local resources to help supplement your home fun and games for the summer.

## Home Activities for the Summer

Here are some simple and inexpensive ideas that incorporate many of the sensory and muscle development exercises we have focused on all year in the newsletter.

**Magic carpet ride**
Lay a large beach blanket on the grass and have your child sit on it. Try pulling the child around on the blanket or have the child pull something on the blanket. This helps develop motor planning and stimulates body awareness and sense of movement.

**Pavement painting**
Let your child "paint" the pavement using a large utility paint brush and bucket of water. This helps develop hand, wrist, and finger control.

**Heavy hands**
Don't set large laundry containers with handles out for recycling yet. Once washed, they can be used as great containers to carry water and sand when playing at the beach. This helps to develop arm strength and control while stimulating the sensory receptors in the joints and muscles.

## Bubbling Fun

Outdoor bubble games are wonderful in the summer. They are a wonderful way to promote eye-hand coordination and motor planning skills.

**Figure 24-15** Sample newsletter for parents.

CASE STUDY #1

Melissa is a 3-year 6-month-old child who received special education services and was placed in an integrated classroom that includes preschoolers with special needs. Melissa's unusual and unmanageable behaviors in class were the basis for an occupational therapy referral. The teacher indicated Melissa was unable to engage in any of the class routines; she was easily distracted and had a high activity level. Melissa had been assigned an assistant to help her participate in the classroom routine. The referral also identified lack of communication, delayed self-care skills, limited interaction skills with peers, incidents of throwing classroom materials when angry, and constant mouthing of objects.

Her developmental history included premature birth, malnutrition, and environmental deprivation. She was recently adopted by a supportive family who became aware of services available through the school district. Evaluation procedures included a parent-teacher interview, observation, and use of a basic developmental skills checklists. She did not comply with standardized testing. The occupational therapist relied on the family to provide information through the parent intake questionnaire (see Figure 24-2) and the sensory history (see Figure 24-3). The sensory history was also collected by the teacher and the speech therapist, observing Melissa through their perspectives. Classroom observations were completed (see Figure 24-1) by the occupational therapist after spending time in the class during various routines and activities.

The assessment indicated major areas of weakness in the performance components of sensory processing, which appeared to affect all of Melissa's occupational performance. Tactile defensiveness interfered with many of her social and object interactions. Melissa's play skills were limited to repetitive actions with a few familiar toys. She rarely explored or used new toys, particularly when their sensory qualities (tactile, visual, or auditory input) were objectionable. Her primary method for exploring new toys was to mouth. She was unable to attend long enough to engage in the structured classroom activities. She was dependent in self-care, particularly feeding, dressing, and toileting.

With team collaboration, specific functional activities in class and home were targeted as priorities. These included orderly behavior when getting from the bus to the classroom, participating in the snack routine and in mealtimes at home, and decreasing mouthing behaviors. The occupational therapist began an intervention program that considered the class and home routines as opportunities to improve her sensory processing problems. The following are written recommendations that were shared among the family and team members.

## Occupational therapy classroom strategies

General considerations

When giving directions, make them short and concrete.

Use additional sensory cues such as firm touch pressure or visual cues when giving directions.

Melissa is unable to remain in a sedentary position for long periods.

Movement seems to help her to focus and orient. You may want to keep this in mind for programming.

Warm-ups for focus to an activity

Consider using deep pressure activities, (e.g., trampoline, jump on the ball, roll in the sheet on the mat, use the sit and spin, and push and pull activities) before a focused task to help in organizing the nervous system. Activities should emphasize strong, deep, or heavy input through joints and skin.

Rhythmic, repetitive activities are best.

Before hand manipulative activities, try manipulating a Koosh ball, squeezing clay, or using shaving cream. These activities help to desensitize the hands, while preparing the muscles to work.

Hand manipulatives

Use simple take-apart and put-together activities.

Try placing items in containers and closing and opening containers to facilitate functional grasp and release (e.g., snap containers or ziplock bags).

Try hand-over-hand initially to allow her to feel the sequence of movements needed for the task.

Position her in a chair with arms and foot rests so that she is posturally stable during fine motor activities.

Development of activities of daily living skills

Begin with simple dressing activities: taking on and off shoes and using oversized pullover shirts, shorts, and tube socks over her clothing. These activities should result in success and promote both her interest and skills in dressing.

When working on dressing closures, try using the large "dress-up" dolls designed for this purpose. It will be more tangible and understandable for her than the closure boards and vests.

Reducing oral stimulation behaviors

Brush her gums using the toothette each morning at the beginning of the program.

Midmorning, allow her to go to the sink and use another toothette (as behaviors decrease, this can be eliminated).

Try the techniques as outlined during the snack routine to control lip closure and develop straw drinking.

## Home activities and strategies to reduce tactile defensiveness

Strategies for communication and giving directions

When giving directions, use a firm, constant touch to help her attend to your voice. Firm pressure directly over the large joints can help her calm and organize her movements.

When giving verbal directions, face her. Use touch when speaking and a firm voice to first request her attention before giving the directives.

Avoid light brushing or intermittent light touches. This type of tactile input results in a defensive response.

Prepare Melissa for the next immediate event or situation by describing it.

These verbal cues give her an opportunity to plan and organize for that event.

Play and leisure activities

Try to provide Melissa with a full "sensory diet," using activities that emphasize joint compression (e.g., jumping and dangling or pushing and pulling). Heavy muscle work often helps reduce sensory defensiveness.

Use a variety of texture experiences on the skin; sand, rice, and packaging styrofoam are good ideas. Small toys can be hidden in a bucket of these textured materials for Melissa to find.

Use activities that provide all-over body pressure; roll paint rollers over her body surfaces or have her roll up in a sheet.

Brushes for play and in the bath tub provide different types of light touch: surgical scrub brushes, paint brushes, and nail brushes are good examples. In the tub, try using foam soaps and encourage self-bathing. Hide favorite toys in mounds of foam.

Try placing stickers on arms as a game at home, and reinforce body part identification.

Use play dough, and encourage bilateral manipulation. Build monsters with the play dough as a purposeful, nonfail activity.

When outdoors, encourage swinging on the tire or swing, on her tummy with legs pushing.

When completing puzzles and activities indoors, encourage positioning on her tummy with elbow support.

Play catch and throw with weighted materials (e.g., beanbags and heavy, padded balls).

Self-care activities

Incorporate a hand-washing routine several times a day, for example, before and after meals and after play outside. Have her use lots of liquid soap. Scrub with the surgical brush, and remind her to wash all fingers, front and back.

After washing, rub briskly with terry toweling. Choose the thick nubby type versus the thinner polyester type.

Try a lotion rub on the hands after each washing.

When choosing clothes, try some of the spandex-type clothing as undergarments, particularly on the chest. This type of clothing, found in cycling shops, can provide firm pressure to reduce the sensory defensiveness. When attending for doctor's appointments, bring the "sensory Goodie Bag" and other favorite toys. Static sitting and waiting is unreasonable to expect at this point. Select a waiting area in which it is appropriate for Melissa to be mobile. Mobility seems to be one way that she deals with new situations.

As the school year progressed and Melissa began to engage with children and activities in the classroom and home, the occupational therapist suggested that new objectives and activities were needed. The occupational therapist collaborated with Melissa's parents, teacher, and speech therapist to modify the intervention plan. Developmentally higher goals were written, and more challenging activities were planned. By the end of the school year, Melissa no longer mouthed objects and she independently fed herself, remained seated at the table for family meals, managed independent donning and doffing of clothing, and fully participated in class activities.

STUDY QUESTIONS

1. Define the developmental and functional approaches. Describe an example when the developmental approach is most appropriate. Describe an example when the functional approach is most appropriate. Give one example of intervention in which both approaches are used simultaneously.
2. Explain the various models of service delivery used by occupational therapists in preschool settings.
3. The preschool classroom may have centers where the children can explore and play in small groups. The occupational therapist may use these centers to support therapy goals for the children. Describe two activities in which the children may practice bilateral hand manipulation activities in the following centers. Describe the materials involved and the steps of the activities.
   a. An office area.
   b. A kitchen or cooking area.
   c. A construction zone.
   d. Water play area.
4. As the preschool's occupational therapist, you believe that Ted might demonstrate increased attention span if he sat on a medium-size ball during circle time. What instructions and suggestions would you give to the teacher and her assistant so that Ted's sitting on the ball is successful and will not disrupt the circle time?

## REFERENCES

American Occupational Therapy Association (1987). *Guidelines for occupational therapy services in school systems.* Rockville, MD: American Occupational Therapy Association.

American Occupational Therapy Association (1989). *Guidelines for occupational therapy services in early intervention and preschool services,* Rockville, MD: American Occupational Therapy Association.

American Occupational Therapy Association. (1994). Statement of occupational therapy referral. *American Journal of Occupational Therapy, 48,* 1034.

Americans with Disabilities Act. (1990). Public Law 101-336, 42 USC.

Berk R.A. & DeGangi, G.A. (1983). *Degangi-Berk Test of Sensory Integration.* Los Angeles: Western Psychological Services.

Blackman, J.A., Levine, M.D. & Markowitz, M., (1986). *Pediatric extended examination at three.* Cambridge, MA: Educators Publishing Service.

Brigance, A.H. (1978). *Brigance Diagnostic Inventory of Early Development.* Woburn, MA: Curriculum Associates.

Bruininks, R. (1978). *Bruininks-Oseretsky Test of Motor Proficiency.* Circle Pines, MN: American Guidance Service.

Bundy, A. (1991). Writing functional goals for evaluation. In C.B. Royeen (Ed.). *AOTA self study series: school based practice for related services.* Rockville, MD: American Occupational Therapy Association.

Dennis, R., Edelman, S., Giangreco, M. (1991). Common professional practices that interfere with integrated delivery of related services. *Remedial and Special Education, 12,* 16-24.

Education of the Handicapped Act Amendment. (1986). Public Law 99-457, 20 USC.

Erhardt, R.P. (1989). *Erhardt Developmental Prehension Assessment.* Tuscson: Therapy Skill Builders.

Folio, M.R. & Fewell, R.R. (1983). *Peabody Developmental Motor Scales.* Chicago: Riverside Publishers.

Frolek Clark, G. (August, 1994). Occupational Therapy Consultant. Johnston, IA: Heartland Area Education Agency. Personal communication.

Giangreco, M.F. (1986). Effects of integrated therapy: a pilot study. *Journal of the Association for Persons with Severe Handicaps, 11*(3), 205-208.

Giangreco, M.F., York, J., & Rainforth, B. (1989). Providing related services to learners with severe handicaps in educational settings: pursuing the least restrictive option. *Pediatric Physical Therapy, 1*(2), 55-63.

Griswald, L. (1994). Ethnographic analysis: a study of classroom environments. *The American Journal of Occupational Therapy, 48,* 397-402.

Haley, S.M., Coster, W.J., Ludlow, L.H., Haltiwanger, M.A., & Andrellos, P.J. (1992). *Pediatric Evaluation of Disability Inventory.* Boston: New England Medical Center Hospital and PEDI Research Group.

Individuals with Disabilities Education Act of 1990 (1990). Public Law 101-476, 20 USC, Chapter 33.

Kalscheur, J.A. (1992). Benefits of the Americans with disabilities act of 1990 for children and adolescents with disabilities. *American Journal of Occupational Therapy, 46,* 419-425.

Leister, C., Koonce, D., & Nisbet, S. (1993). Best practices for preschool programs: an update on inclusive settings. *Day Care and Early Education, 4,* 9-12.

Levine, M.D. & Schneider, E.A. (1985). *Pediatric Examination of Educational Readiness,* Cambridge, MA: Educators Publishing Service.

Linder, T. (1990). *Transdisciplinary play-based assessment.* Baltimore: Brookes.

LRP Publications. (1994a). Hetergenicity: strategies for accepting differences in the general classroom. *Inclusive Education Programs, 1,* 8-12.

LRP Publications. (1994b). How will IDEA reauthorization affect your program. *Early Childhood Report, 5,* 7-10.

Meyers, C.A. (1992). Therapeutic fine motor activities for preschoolers. In J. Case-Smith & C. Pehoski (Eds.). *Development of hand skills in the child* (pp. 47-59). Rockville, MD: American Occupational Therapy Association.

Miller, L.J. (1988). *Miller Assessment for Preschoolers Manual,* San Antonio, TX: Psychological Corporation.

Miller, L.J. (1993). *First STEP: screening test for evaluating preschoolers.* San Antonio, TX: Psychological Corporation.

Rainforth, B., York, J., & MacDonald, C. (1992). *Collaborative teams for students with severe disabilities.* Baltimore: Brookes.

Shonkoff, J. & Meisels, S. (1990). Early childhood intervention: the evolution of a concept. In S.J. Meisels & J.P. Shonkoff (Eds.). *Handbook of early childhood intervention.* Cambridge, MA: Cambridge University Press.

Struck, M. & DuBois, S. (1993). *Self assessment for best practice in school based occupational therapy.* Paper presented at the American Journal of Occupational Therapy Association Annual Conference. Seattle, WA.

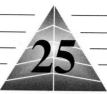

# School-Based Occupational Therapy

JAN JOHNSON

## KEY TERMS

- ▲ Individuals with Disabilities Education Act (IDEA)
- ▲ Related Services
- ▲ Inclusion
- ▲ Least Restrictive Environment
- ▲ Individual Education Program (IEP)
- ▲ Collaboration

## CHAPTER OBJECTIVES

1. Describe how educationally relevant practice differs from the traditional medical model of occupational therapy.
2. Define the roles of occupational therapy practitioners in the schools.
3. Identify levels, types, and examples of evaluations of students' functional abilities in schools.
4. Describe treatment goals and objectives of school-based occupational therapy programs for students across the age range.
5. Define direct services, monitoring, and consultation.
6. Describe management issues and strategies relevant to school-based practice.
7. Describe how occupational therapists blend different models of service delivery into a comprehensive intervention program based on the unique needs of the child.

All children are required to spend considerable time in an educational setting in preparation for adult roles in life. *Education* has been defined as "a continuous process by which individuals learn to cope with their environments" (PARC, p. 1257). The occupational therapist who works in a school setting has the unique opportunity to help students become more functional in their own environments. This chapter discusses the educational environment as it relates to the occupational therapist, as well as therapists' roles and functions in this setting.

## LEGISLATION

The role of occupational therapy in the school system has roots in the ideas of equality and civil rights that grew from monumental changes in philosophic and political thinking during the late part of the eighteenth century. Humanitarianism and moral treatment began to be part of the public consciousness, and the new democracy of the United States enacted laws that reflected this human philosophy (Hopkins, 1988). Although private institutions and organizations such as churches and hospitals addressed issues of ethical and moral decisions related to helping the less abled and powerless members of society, namely the sick, the disabled, and children, the importance of the new thinking was in the long-term pervasiveness of its impact. Over time, legislation established that public health programs were available to *all,* Social Security applied to *all* workers; vocational rehabilitation applied to *all* ages and disabilities; civil rights applied to *all* citizens; and that education was a right of *all* children, regardless of privilege or power. Rights to education began with litigation related to racial desegregation, then to integration of students with disabilities.

In the 1970s most states had statutes requiring educational services to certain children with disabilities. Although some states mandated services to all children with disabilities, inconsistencies were common across states and many children with disabilities were excluded from special education. The implementation of programs was limited because of lack of funding and bureaucratic resistance; most children with disabilities did not receive adequate levels of services through public education programs. Often the participation of parents in special education was discouraged.

When parents and educators brought concerns about the problems in the special education system to the attention of Congress, legislation was enacted to build a more cohesive system of mandated services for children with disabilities.

The Education of All Handicapped Children Act of 1975 (P.L. 94-142) and Section 504 of the Rehabilitation Act of 1973 dramatically changed the focus and availability of education for children with disabilities in the United States. Before the enactment of this federal legislation, children with disabilities were often excluded from public schools (at their parents' expense), were institutionalized, or remained at home. In 1975, when the Education of All Handicapped Children Act was enacted, approximately 1.75 million children with disabilities in the United States were receiving no education at all and 2.5 million were receiving inadequate services.

The Education of All Handicapped Children Act and its regulations had four main purposes:

1. To ensure that all children have available to them a free appropriate public education
2. To ensure that the rights of children with handicaps and their parents are protected
3. To assist states and localities to provide for the education of handicapped children
4. To assess and ensure the effectiveness of efforts to educate such handicapped children

Since that time, the law has been amended several times. In 1990 the Act was re-titled, the Individuals with Disabilities Education (IDEA), P.L. 101-476. The key provisions guaranteed by IDEA remain unchanged since the original P.L. 94-142 was enacted.

Procedural safeguards for parents and students who receive a free, appropriate, public education (FAPE) include the right to have access to student records and the right to limit access of those records to only those professionals who need to know their contents so that they may provide services. Parents have a right to written notification of program changes and must give consent for a student's initial evaluation or placement in a special education program. Parents, including appointed surrogate parents, have a right to a fair hearing to resolve disagreements regarding a child's placement and educational program; this includes the occupational therapy program for a particular child. By law, all reasonable efforts are made to include a child's parents in decisions related to the child's education.

Section 504 of the Rehabilitation Act of 1973 is a civil rights act for individuals with disabilities. It carries provisions that prohibit discrimination against persons with disabilities in all programs or activities administered by state and federal agencies. The act states that "no otherwise qualified handicapped individual . . . . shall, solely by reason of his handicap, be excluded from the participation in, be denied the benefits of, or be subjected to discrimination under any program or activities receiving federal financial assistance" (p. 22,676). This legislation also provides for a free appropriate education for children with disabilities and requires that nonacademic services and extracurricular activities be available to all students on an equal basis.

## EDUCATION ENVIRONMENT
### Systems Theory

The educational environment can be analyzed and understood in terms of systems theory. A *system* is a functional unit that consists of a structuring of events or happenings rather than physical parts; it describes a pattern of relationships. Every system is made up of a number of *subsystems*. All systems have definite boundaries, or limits, and are interdependent with surrounding systems.

The occupational therapist can be considered a subsystem interacting with other subsystems within larger systems and suprasystems. Figure 25-1 shows some of these interactions. In this example, the occupational therapist interacts with other subsystems, such as special education teachers, speech therapists, physical therapists, and the student. Because various schools have contact with one another, they represent interacting systems within the larger suprasystem—the educational organization and school administration. The suprasystem has an infinite number of contacts and interactions with other suprasystems, such as the State Board of Education, the community, and the state, local, and federal governments.

Many occupational therapists working in school settings are itinerant; they are expected to travel among several schools to provide services to children. It is important for these therapists to realize that they are moving from one system to another within the same suprasystem. Each system and subsystem has its own distinctive function, develops its own norms and values, and is characterized by its own dynamics. The effective itinerant therapist is one who recognizes the differences between systems and adapts to each unique environment.

Each occupational therapist, as an individual, can be considered a unique subsystem with different combinations of background, training, professional experience, personality, race, values, perceptions, and childhood experiences. Figure 25-2 illustrates the components of the individual as a subsystem and the interactions with other subsystems. These components are sometimes taken for granted when one individual interacts with other individuals from a similar background. When substantial differences exist, they must be examined so that interpersonal relationships can be developed for the therapist to be effective on a professional level. Some examples are the white middle-class therapist working in an inner-city black school, or an urban therapist working in a rural area.

A public school is a system made up of elements from the community reflecting the culture, traditions, and values of that community. It is a relatively open system, accepting any child within its geographic boundaries and usually encouraging participation from families and other community members. The system itself develops its own values and tra-

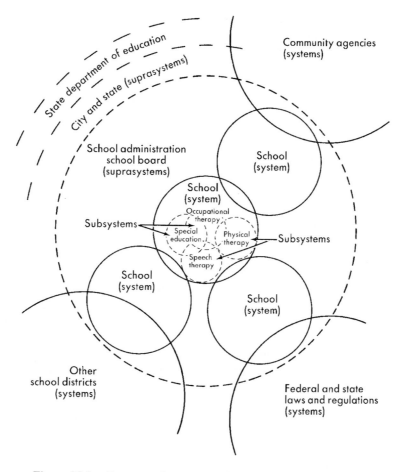

**Figure 25-1**   Systems, subsystems, and suprasystems in the schools.

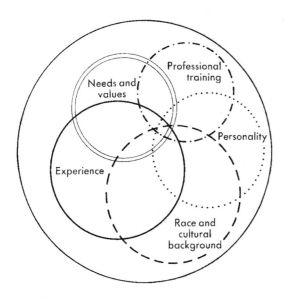

**Figure 25-2**   The occupational therapist as a subsystem.

ditions, establishes channels of communication, and bestows power on certain individuals. As a system of interacting elements with a purpose of education, the school sometimes becomes inflexible and resistant to change.

Regan (1982) described the characteristics of a rural school system and its suprasystems. Rural areas often have a high incidence of poverty, resulting in substandard housing, poor nutrition, and inadequate medical care. The rural schools are likely to have fewer funds and less modern equipment than urban schools. Rural persons often have more conservative religious and moral values and live in more homogeneous communities than do urban persons. Regan stated that "not until the population's needs and resources, as well as the school administrative structure are understood can therapists deliver their services with the cooperation and support of the community and the administrative hierarchy" (p. 88).

## Medical and Educational Models

The occupational therapist typically receives training and experience in a system referred to as the medical model. In this mode, dysfunction or disease is identified and strategies are developed to increase function and to alleviate disease and dysfunction. The occupational therapist, as a subsystem working within the medical model, interacts closely with other medical subsystems (e.g., nurses and physical therapists) under the direction of the physician. Treatment may end once the patient is considered cured or has reached a maintenance level.

The educational system is concerned primarily with the healthy child, who is expected to gain increasing skill, knowledge, and competency in moving through the system. The consumer in the educational model is the student who enters the system at a predetermined time (typically age 5 or 6) and remains within the system for a set length of time (usually 12 or 13 years).

## Occupational Therapy as a Related Service

Occupational therapy, as defined by the regulations of IDEA, is a related service that can be provided to a student to enable him or her to benefit from special education. Occupational therapists who are funded with federal monies must adhere to these guidelines by providing therapy only when the student needs it to benefit from special education. It is possible that a student may need occupational therapy in the clinic setting (medical model) but would not be eligible for services in the educational setting. "Every pediatric occupational therapist must recognize that school-based therapy services are not simply clinic therapy services delivered under the school building's roof" (Muhlenhaupt, 1985, p.20). Therapy provided within the school setting is designed to enhance the student's abilities to participate in the educational process.

The regulations that are written to enable the implementation of IDEA define occupational therapy. This definition is included here. It contains the intent and consensual definition of the profession, by the profession. *Occupational therapy,* as defined by IDEA, includes:

  (i) improving, developing, or restoring functions impaired or lost through illness, injury, or deprivation;
  (ii) improving ability to perform tasks for independent functioning when functions are impaired or lost;
  (iii) preventing or loss of function (IDEA, 1990).

If a student is able to participate in regular education and is not eligible for special education services, that student is usually not eligible for related services, despite the presence of a disability. Temporary impairments (for example, a fractured bone) usually do not make a student eligible for school-based therapy, although the student may need occupational therapy in a medical setting.

A bright first-grader had a mild left hemiparesis from cerebral palsy. This student participated in all aspects of the educational program, including physical education, with few adaptations. The disability did not interfere with the student's educational program; therefore she was not eligible for occupational therapy in school despite the fact that she did not have the full use of her left hand. In another case, a teenager suffered traumatic amputation of the left arm in an automobile accident. He returned to his high school classes and was able to participate in everything except computer lab. The occupational therapist consulted with the computer lab instructor and gave the instructor material on one-handed keyboard use but did not have to provide direct services. The student continued to receive occupational therapy services on an outpatient basis at a rehabilitation center.

To determine eligibility for a student to receive occupational therapy as a related service, the school team, including the occupational therapist, determines if the student's disability interferes with his or her education and if occupational therapy could improve the student's ability to benefit from the educational program.

### Educational Classifications

Many states are considering a change in defining which children require special education (Metzler, personal communication, October 21, 1994). At present, children are usually placed into special education programs by virtue of their primary handicapping condition: children with visual impairments are served by programs geared to their special needs, children who have learning disabilities are educated according to the curriculum designed for their particular ways of learning, and developmentally challenged students attend programs specially designed to meet the needs of their special learning problems. Future planning may reflect a move away from specific educational diagnoses and a move to *noncategorical* placement in special education, where the functional educational level of school participation determines education placement rather than the use of a diagnostic category. The philosophies of *mainstreaming* and *inclusion* outline practices for the placement of children with disabilities in the least restrictive environment (LRE) required to meet their educational needs. The continuum of learning environments ranges from education and services in the home, through a variety of special classroom settings, to a classroom of peers without disabilities.

In spite of such proposed changes that base a curriculum on educational needs rather than diagnoses, it is necessary to define current educational diagnostic categories to understand current placement practices. Many people refer to the "alphabet soup" of special education; the reason becomes clear, as these examples show. The student in an LD program has a learning disability; VH programs are for children with visual handicaps; OH, orthopedical handicaps; and DH, developmental handicaps (this includes EH, educational handicaps; MR, mental retardation; and DD, developmental delays.) Children with hearing impairments are educated in programs for HI children; which is often confused with children who have circulatory or respiratory disorders requiring special provision for the health impairments. SBH refers to children who have severe behavioral handicaps, MH refers to children who have multiple handicaps, and TBI refers to children who have had a traumatic brain injury.

The school-based occupational therapist may have the opportunity to work with children who have myriad factors interfering with their ability to benefit from education. The therapist may need to view the child's performance components as they relate to a particular medical diagnosis and blend this understanding into the student's educational challenges as viewed by the school. It is by looking and acting through this set of dual lenses that the occupational therapist identifies and delivers needed services.

## OCCUPATIONAL THERAPY PROCESS IN THE SCHOOLS

Which students need occupational therapy services to participate in their educational program? The answer to this question varies between districts and from state to state. Documents of policy and procedures, such as a state's published rules and regulations, funding sources, and the interpretation and implementation of legal mandates by a particular local education agency (LEA), often influence decisions related to the need for occupational therapy as an educationally relevant related service. Each classroom places different demands on a student. For example, a class of eight children who are taught by a special education teacher and an aide demands a different set of skills of each student than does a class of 25 students taught by one teacher who has no training in teaching disabled students. Within the frame of an educational environment, the occupational therapist, usually as a member of the educational team, makes the determination of need for occupational therapy services through a process of screening and evaluation.

### Roles of the Occupational Therapist

Service delivery in school may take a less traditional form and focus than occupational therapy in more medically based intervention settings. As a member of the interdisciplinary educational team, the occupational therapist has four primary roles:

1. *Assessment:* Assessment includes screening, evaluation, and reassessment. The multifaceted occupational therapy assessment process evaluates the student's educationally related needs, and the findings are used to develop an Individual Education Program (IEP).
2. *Program Planning:* Both the IEP and the occupational therapy intervention plan are components of program planning in school systems. The IEP contains consensus goals and objectives representing the overall educational needs of the students. The occupational therapy intervention plan reflects the specific problems that the treatment activities are addressing.
3. *Intervention:* Intervention includes all activities performed by the registered occupational therapist (OTR) and the certified occupational therapist assistant (COTA) to implement the IEP goals and objectives and the intervention plan.
4. *Management:* The management role involves the varied responsibilities required to plan, develop, implement, and evaluate the occupational therapy program.

These responsibilities include developing administrative records, reporting forms, and procedures needed to manage the program and to plan for future services (AOTA, 1989, p. 5-1).

### Screening and Referral

There are many avenues by which a student might be referred to the school-based occupational therapist. Some special education programs have policies that include screening of all children by an occupational therapist. Such policies are more frequent in programs for low-incidence handicapping conditions, such as physical and multiple disabilities, and in programs for preschool students. A student from another educational program or from a hospital discharge may come with a reference for a follow-up of previous occupational therapy services. Occupational therapists may routinely screen certain at-risk populations in routine health screenings or on admission to kindergarten programs. A teacher, psychologist, or school nurse may refer a student to occupational therapy because there is a question about the child's ability to function in the classroom. The referral process introduces the therapist and child. Once the occupational therapist has been made aware of a child's possible need for services through referral, a screening of the child's abilities and the educational requirements can be done.

Therapists use and develop a variety of methods to *screen* a student's need for occupational therapy intervention. With consideration for the child's age, background, and educational context, the therapist may do the following:

▲ Observe the child in the classroom environment
▲ Observe performance of representative key tasks required in school
▲ Talk to teachers and other school personnel about perceived functional problems the child may be experiencing
▲ Review written documentation such as information in the student's file and referral notes
▲ Administer a standardized screening tool (e.g., the Miller Assessment for Preschoolers, 1988)

During the screening process attention is on the performance areas relevant to functioning in the educational environment: *daily living skills* such as those needed at mealtimes, in the bathroom, or for dressing for recess or gym; *posture and movement* as required to participate in school activities; *work skills* such as attending to tasks, initiating responses, and following directions; and performance of specific tasks and ability to engage in *play* such as manipulating materials, following rules and directions, and interacting with others. From the information obtained in the screening process, the therapist determines whether a student should be further evaluated and if occupational therapy services are needed, and, if so, what the goals of intervention should be.

# Evaluation

In any assessment process, the occupational therapist evaluates what the client can do and how he or she does it, and what the client cannot do and why he or she is unable to do so. Once this procedure has been completed, the therapist can determine the levels and types of intervention that will help the client accomplish more and what treatment procedures are indicated. The school therapist evaluates students to determine whether and how intervention will help the student participate more fully in the school setting.

By definition, a child who receives special education services is unable to perform expected or desired activities related to physical, behavioral, or learning disabilities. The occupational therapist determines which activities of self-maintenance, play, and work interfere with school work. Limitations to performance may be in sensory, neuromuscular, motor, cognitive integration, or psychosocial component areas.

## Assessment of Task Performances

The nature of the disability is often expressed in terms of the problems encountered in performing activities. Therefore many occupational therapy assessment procedures used in working with the child with a disability are performance oriented. Therapists evaluate the child's ability to perform specific tasks. Typical assessments include the following:

1. Checklists on daily living skills of feeding, dressing, and hygiene
2. Evaluations related to skills needed to function in a particular setting, such as a classroom skills checklist, a prevocational skills checklist, or a play skills inventory
3. Developmental skill evaluations

When the therapist administers these evaluations, or checklists, the child's response in following directions to perform a specific activity is observed. The therapist determines whether the child can perform the activity and how closely the child's response meets the criteria of the test item. For example, when evaluating a child's ability to remove his coat, the therapist is not only observing whether the child can take off his coat, but also is observing and judging the quality of the action: Is the coat removed in a reasonable amount of time? Does the child use an unusual or adapted method to accomplish the task? Does the child need assistance? If so, what kind of help is needed?

Most checklists incorporate some means to record the quality of the child's response. This may be a comments section that is located by each test item or after a section or area tested or at the end of the form. Another method for grading the response is to use a letter or number that represents typical degrees of activity accomplishment. For example, a number from 0 to 3 could be used, instead of a checkmark, when recording responses: *0* could indicate that the child could not accomplish the activity; *1* could indicate difficult accomplishment only with assistance; *2* could indicate task accomplishment without assistance but with difficulty or taking an excessive amount of time; and *3* could indicate that the child accomplished the activity independently and with ease.

Although information from a recorded history or from interviews can be used to assess a child's abilities, the primary method for an occupational therapist to gather assessment information is to observe the child's actual performance of the activity. During the assessment, the therapist gains information that goes beyond the specific skills being evaluated. Causes of limitations in performance can be observed, solutions to problems can be generated, and methods for treatment may be suggested.

1. *Activities of daily living skills:* Lists of skills needed to perform self-maintenance activities are often compiled by grouping together the skills needed for one type of self-care. For example, feeding, dressing, mobility or locomotion in and around school, and grooming and hygiene are listed separately. The sections of the evaluation may also follow a developmental sequence or a simple-to-complex sequence. The occupational therapists may use assessments designed for younger children if they are more appropriate to the particular child's developmental level. The following are examples of checklists of activities of daily living skills:

   Learning Accomplishment Profile—self-help section (Sanford & Zelman, 1981)

   Functional Behavior Assessment for Children with Sensory Integration Dysfunction (Lupton & Smith, adapted by Cook, 1991)

   Functional Mobility and Self-Help Checklist (Wesley, adapted by Royeen, 1993)

   Vineland Adaptive Behavior Scale (Sparrow, Balla, & Cicchetti, 1984)

2. *School-related skills:* A child needs certain skills to function in a school setting, aside from the daily living skills previously mentioned. To work with a child, school personnel need to know which of these necessary skills a child has and which must be taught or compensated for so that the child may take advantage of the educational curriculum. Examples of evaluations of school-related skills used by occupational therapists are as follows:

   Bruininks-Oseretsky Test of Motor Proficiency (Bruininks, 1978)

   Developmental Test of Visual Perception, Second Edition (Hammill, Pearson, & Voress, 1993)

   Classroom Teachers' Intervention Checklist (Collier, 1991)

Learning Accomplishment Profile—sections on fine and gross motor skills (Sanford & Zelman, 1981)

Brigance Diagnostic Inventories (Brigance, 1978)

3. *Play skills:* The child uses play as an educational and developmental tool as well as for enjoyment. Physical and mental manipulation of objects, imagination, and social interactions are important types of play. Information regarding these skills can be gathered by observing free play, as well as by administering structured evaluation procedures. See Chapter 18 for a more detailed description of play assessment.

### Assessment of Performance Components

In addition to the documentation of specific task performance, there is frequently a need to determine the specific functional limitations that relate to performance delays. Specific information on particular performance components helps identify appropriate and effective intervention strategies, focus and set priorities among treatment goals, and give measurable criteria for assessing changes in abilities that result from the intervention program. These changes may not be evident by looking solely at the child's ability to perform a task.

1. *Sensorimotor processing and skills:* Tests and observations are used to determine the extent and degree of sensory, perceptual, neuromuscular, and motor skills that influence task performance. The following are examples of measurements of sensorimotor components of skills and tasks:

Observing and recording a child's response to various types and intensities of sensory information

DeGangi-Berk Test of Sensory Integration (Berk & DeGangi, 1983)

Sensory Integration and Praxis Tests (Ayres, 1989)

Motor Free Visual Perception Test (MVPT) (Colarusso & Hammill, 1972)

Test of Visual Motor Skills (Gardner, 1986)

Manual Muscle Tests

Measurements of range of joint motion

Bruininks-Oseretsky Test of Motor Proficiency (Bruninks, 1978)

Adaptation of Jebsen's hand function tests (Taylor, Sand, & Jebsen, 1973)

2. *Cognitive components of task performance:* Much of a school therapist's evaluation of certain cognitive processes, such as arousal level, orientation, and attention span, is done through observation of the student's responses during class or during therapy sessions. These cognitive components of activity performance are recognized as being directly related to the accomplishment of tasks; however, it seems that no standardized assessment tools are used routinely by school therapists. Instead, the occupational therapist generally analyzes cognitive components of function using evaluation reports of school psychologists, medical evaluations, observation of task performance, and interview of the teachers, parents, and other team members.

3. *Psychosocial skills and components of task performance:* In the school setting the primary method of evaluating psychosocial skills, such as initiating and making transitions between activities; social skills, such as social conduct and interpersonal skills; and self-management is through observation and behavioral data collection. The method of recording observations is by giving detailed descriptions of a particular skill and the situation in which the behavior is observed.

The more specific the assessment tools or the description of performance is, the more specific the information will be regarding areas needing remediation and the more specifically treatment goals can be stated. Treatment objectives are determined from assessment information, including (1) the reason for referral, (2) information from others about the student, (3) the results of specific evaluation procedures, (4) developmental guidelines, (5) expectations of the educational environment and the curriculum, and (6) expectations of the child's human environment (those of the teachers, parents, and other team members).

### Program Planning

In the process of moving from evaluation to intervention lies much of the *art* of therapy. The therapist first gathers information about the specific child; "weighs" that information with the classical medical picture of a disability and his or her own knowledge of growth and development and what children do in health; balances all this information with a knowledge and intuition about the needs or expectations of the child, the family, the school, or environmental setting; and formulates a recommendation for the team determination of treatment intervention. This process is scientifically based in classical occupational therapy theory and is implemented through sound clinical judgment, experience, and creativity.

The school setting is similar to other pediatric settings in determining treatment objectives by considering the following points:

1. The child's current level of functioning, which is learned from assessment, including observation and history

2. The child's expected level of performance, according to his or her age or developmental sequence

3. The environmental expectations or demands from the child's school program or family

4. The resources available to support the child's ability to function in the school environment and classroom

The areas of intervention may also be similar to those found in other clinical settings, the difference being that the focus of activities is to meet goals that enhance the student's *educational performance.*

### Goals as Related to the Individual Education Program

The IEP is a plan and a promise; it is a written statement of the educational program by which the occupational therapist and educational team members expect to help a student achieve curricular goals by participating in the most appropriate educational curriculum, and it is a promise to do so through a mutually agreed-on type and frequency of service provision (Lovitt, 1980). The parts of the IEP are clearly stated in the laws pertaining to the education of disabled students and include the following:

▲ The current level of (educational) performance
▲ Annual goals and short term objectives to meet these goals
▲ Educational and related services required
▲ Amount and type of participation in regular education
▲ Dates of implementation and review
▲ Evaluation criteria and procedures

The IEP process is similar to the occupational therapy process of intervention in other settings: there is a referral, assessment, treatment planning, treatment implementation, evaluation of the results of therapy, and documentation to account for service delivery and changes in student performance. In the educational environment, however, the goals are to be educationally relevant and clearly stated as such; the recipients of services are students, teachers, parents, and programs, rather than patients. Governance is through Boards of Education, rather than insurance companies, hospital boards, or federal health care programs such as Medicare. At the time of this writing, some school boards are billing Medicaid for reimbursement of occupational, physical, and speech therapy services given in schools. It will be interesting to follow the course of this practice.

## Intervention

Although IEP goals are stated in relation to educational performance and objectives are often stated in measurable, behavioral terms, the methods of achieving these goals, *therapeutic intervention,* follow a variety of theoretical frameworks. Both corrective and compensatory methods are used by school therapists in meeting a student's IEP goals.

### Corrective Approaches

Whenever possible, techniques are employed to improve the component abilities involved in task performances because these component skills can be generalized and used in a variety of activities. For example, increased hand strength can help the child write for extended periods, play with construction toys, manage buttons, lift a glass full of liquid, or manipulate art materials such as clay. Increasing the child's hand strength is more effective than teaching the child how to perform any one of these skills by compensating for hand weakness.

Examples of corrective approaches to treatment follow to help illustrate how different theories of treatment are applied by school therapists in meeting goals.

1. *Neurodevelopmental* approach to treatment intervention: The therapist selects an appropriate classroom chair and desk that give pelvic, trunk, and foot support and body alignment to enhance the postural control and movement needed to attend to instruction and perform classroom activities (Figure 25-3) such as paper and pencil writing tasks. To give needed control at key points, yet facilitate postural responses of balance and equilibrium, a variety of seating options with varying amounts of control need to be considered, such as the chair and less stable therapy ball and seat illustrated in Figure 25-4.

2. *Sensory integration* approach to treatment intervention. To facilitate the sensory awareness of where the child's body is in space and to enable better control and purposeful movement, the therapist selects a weighted vest and collaborates with the child's teacher on scheduled times and places for the student to wear the vest during the school day. These pictures show

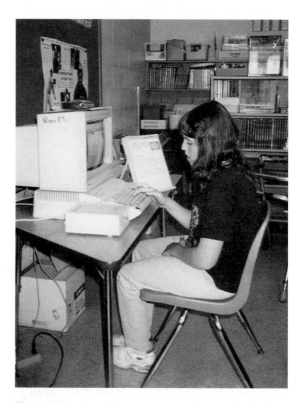

**Figure 25-3**  Appropriate chair for classroom activities.

children experiencing strong proprioceptive input in playground activities (Figure 25-5).

3. *Biomechanical* approach as applied in the school. Activities to improve muscle strength, to increase range of motion, and to improve coordination enable the student to control and use his or her body, and those improvements can be generalized and used in a variety of activities. For example, improving hand strength can enable cutting heavy paper with scissors (Figure 25-6), increasing the range of elbow extension helps the student reach within a larger work area to pick up materials or hang up outer wear on a high hook. By improving eye-hand coordination through practice of catching a ball (Figure 25-7), the student more successfully participates in playground activities.

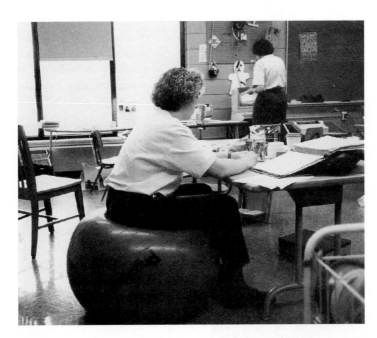

**Figure 25-4**   A therapy ball facilitates postural responses during class time.

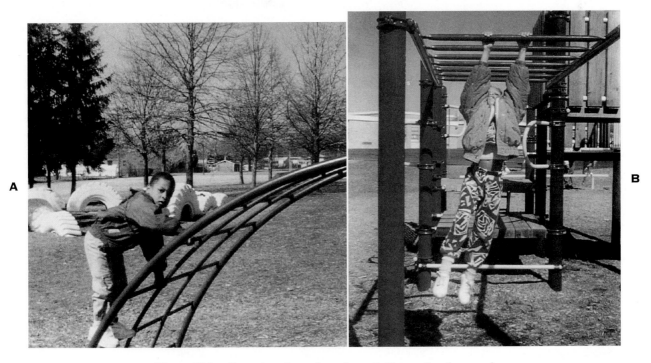

**Figure 25-5**   Examples of proprioceptive activities on the playground.

## Compensatory Approaches

When attempts to improve or enhance a child's performance ability by improving performance components are unsuccessful or inappropriate, intervention may focus instead on the student's learning to perform specific skills in whatever manner allows him or her to function as independently as possible. In such cases some adaptation or change in the skill is needed. The task is analyzed into its component parts (1) to teach the sequential parts of the skill, (2) to simplify or change the method of performing the skill, (3) to adapt the environment to accommodate for the lack of a skill, or (4) to teach the skill through the use of adaptive equipment, including assistive technology.

1. *Teaching specific skills:* A therapist may approach the skill development of a student by directly teaching the task desired, as illustrated by a student learning to open a milk carton (Figure 25-8). The task is analyzed, and intervention is focused on the mastery of specific sequential parts of the task to allow for successful accomplishment, as in learning to write (Figure 25-9). Often a *behavioral* approach, which includes a system of rewards, is used in the teaching of specific behaviors and skills. An example might be teaching a student how to manage a lunch tray without spillage to increase independence in the cafeteria.

2. *Adapting the task:* It may be more reasonable to change the way a task is performed than to teach the

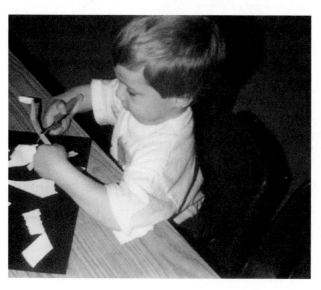

**Figure 25-6** Cutting heavy paper with scissors to improve strength.

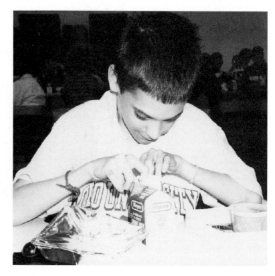

**Figure 25-8** Practicing a skill necessary for the lunchroom.

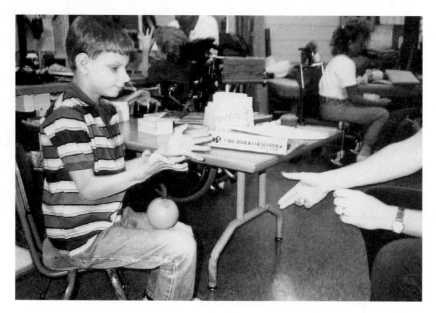

**Figure 25-7** Catching a ball improves eye-hand coordination.

traditional task performance for the student to perform the task. In Figure 25-10 a child is painting by using a sponge held by a clothespin because it is easier for him to control. Instead of assigning 20 multiplication problems, 10 well-selected problems may provide appropriate practice in a particular math skill and reduce the required amount of printing. Instead of playing baseball with a pitched ball, a "Tee" ball support can be used for the batter who cannot play to a pitched ball.

3. *Adapting the environment:* Recent changes in the Americans with Disabilities Act have made the public aware of accessibility issues and how equipment such as grab bars in a bathroom can enable functional independence in this area. Other examples in the school

are lunchroom tables or classroom desks (Figure 25-11) and playground equipment (Figures 25-12 and 25-13) that are designed to accommodate wheelchairs, classroom space that can be used for a student to calm disorganized behavior, a resilient surface under wide and low playground equipment to soften falls, seating the student closer to the board to see written directions, or increasing the light for the visually impaired student to use her remaining vision more effectively.

4. *Using adaptive equipment:* When a particular skill cannot be performed by the child following corrective therapeutic procedures or by teaching, simplifying, or adapting the activity itself, specific adaptive equipment may be necessary for the most efficient or in-

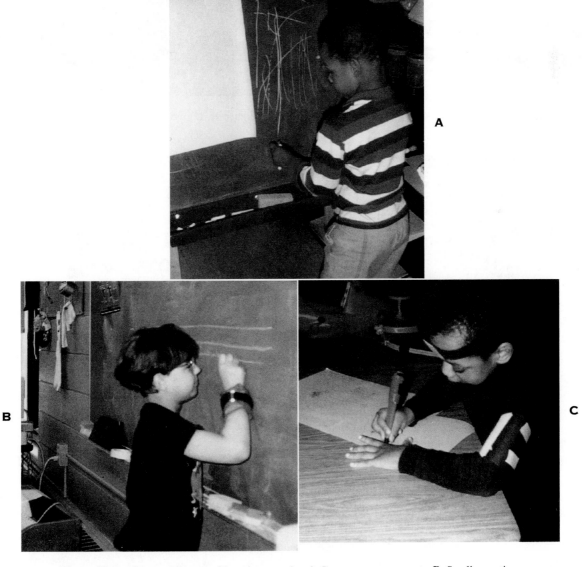

**Figure 25-9** Sequential parts of learning to write. **A,** Large arm movements. **B,** Smaller motions at the same site. **C,** Adapting to the usual medium for writing.

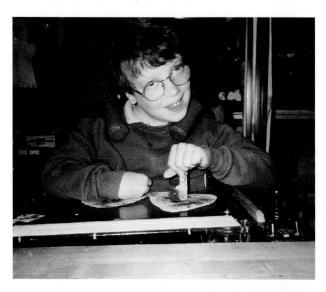

**Figure 25-10**    Painting with a sponge and clothespins.

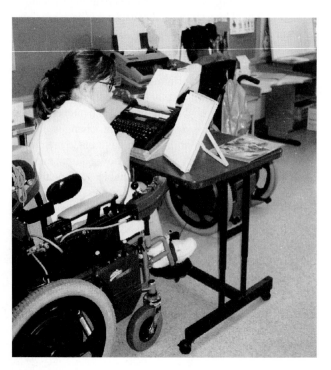

**Figure 25-11**    Adapted lunchroom table or class desk.

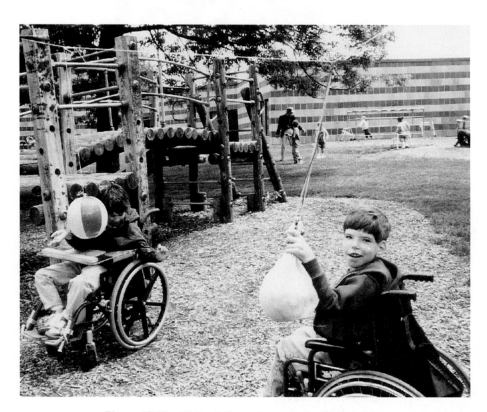

**Figure 25-12**    Tether balls are hung at wheelchair height.

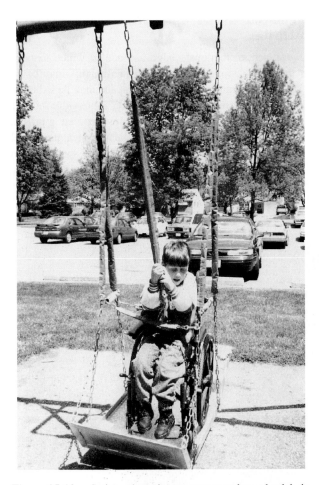

**Figure 25-13**    Swing adaptation to accommodate wheelchair.

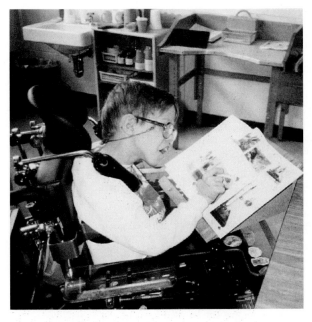

**Figure 25-14**    Child with adapted lapboard.

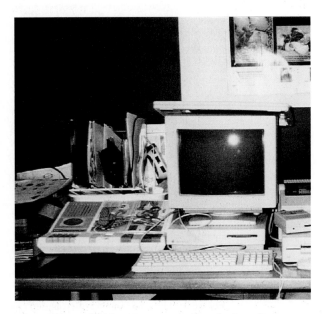

**Figure 25-15**    Computer keyboard adaptation.

dependent school performance (Figure 25-14 and 25-15). Examples of such equipment would include orthotics, illustrated here by a fabricated pointer as an aid in typing and when using a communication board (Figure 25-16), wheelchairs, and adapted feeding equipment. An occupational therapist may teach a student with muscle weakness or incoordination to do written assignments by using a word processor, may provide use of a splint to reduce muscle tone in the child's hand to allow more functional grasp, or may supply the child with a flexible straw to enable the student to drink without spilling liquid. To make a decision to use a piece of adaptive equipment; the therapist must consider the importance of the skill to be enhanced by the equipment; the acceptance of the equipment by the child, the family, and the other people in the classroom; the effort involved in its use; and the cost of acquisition and maintenance.

Assistive technology and computers may be used to enable a student to participate in educational activities by increasing, maintaining, or improving functional capabilities of individuals with disabilities. Because so much of the academic experience depends on written work, students with and without disabilities are finding the use of word processors an alternative to the physical act of writing and a tool that allows for easy editing and production of an attractive document in less time than a handwritten assignment. An abundance of software is designed to teach and reinforce early learning skills, and these are used in many classrooms. Following a sequence of steps, visually tracking a moving target, and planning solutions to visual problems can be practiced through computer interaction with programs designed for these cognitive tasks. Therefore school therapists are finding that they need to have at least a beginning knowledge of computer use and of hardware and software used for educational skill development, word processing, cognitive training, or vocational skill development. Many school therapists are on the team of specialists who select and train students in the use of augmentative communication devices (see Chapter 20). The need for assistive technology is determined by evaluation of the student and the appropriateness of that technology in meeting the IEP goals (Smith, 1993). School therapists may not have had professional training in the selection and use of technology for these students and often are involved in continuing education and on-the-job experience to develop skills in this area.

## "Pull-Out" Versus "Integrated" Therapy Activities

Some school therapists have a space in which to carry out therapy services. In a medical facility this may be referred to as a clinic; in a school this space may be a therapy room separate from the classroom, or, more often, a hallway, a corner of a classroom, an unscheduled gym, the nurses office, or a room for "special" service personnel. When the student is treated in this separate space (Figure 25-17), it is referred to as "pull-out" therapy; that is, the intervention takes place outside the classroom. The types of activities that are considered more appropriate for pull-

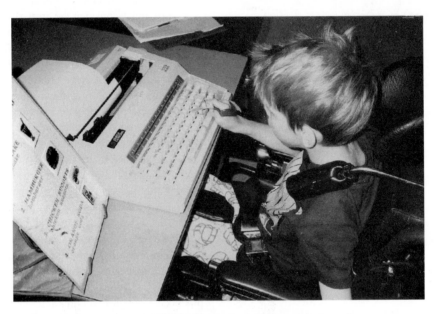

**Figure 25-16**    Child with orthotic device to assist in typing.

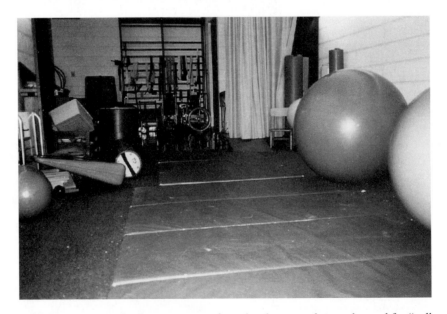

**Figure 25-17**    An example of space separate from the classroom that can be used for "pull-out" therapy.

out services are (1) those that are too distracting to the other students in the classroom to allow them to engage in their own learning activities (Figure 25-18), (2) activities in which the student is developing a particular competence, but the skill level is not mastered to the point of generalization to classroom activities, or (3) the attention and focus of the student toward the learning of a particular skill is enhanced by the one-to-one, nondistracting setting of an environment separate from the classroom.

*Integrated therapy* is that type of intervention that takes place within the classroom, bathroom, lunchroom, or playground environment along with the student's nondisabled peers. Figure 25-19 shows a child on a field trip to a farm with his class. The advantage of integrated therapy is that it provides the opportunity for the student to practice newly learned skills or try out adapted methods of performing a skill in the environment and with the other students in a normalized manner. It allows the child to follow the student role and meet the curricular demands expected of *all*

the class members. The types of activities that are used in integrated therapy are (1) activities and equipment that position the student for maximum attention and participation in the regular classroom activities, (2) adaptations to the environment that enable the child to function as independently as possible in the classroom, and (3) supervised performance of newly learned skills, such as writing or word processing, within the environment in which other students and normal classroom distractions compete for attention and ability to focus on the task at hand. Although the goal of occupational therapy is to help the child function in the classroom, it is important to determine not only activities that are appropriate for meeting the therapy goals, but also the environment that is most appropriate.

An example of an IEP goal that an occupational therapist might set for a student with motor incoordination limitations, who is integrated into a classroom of nondisabled peers, might be: "Meg will complete half the number of math problems assigned for homework." The teacher is re-

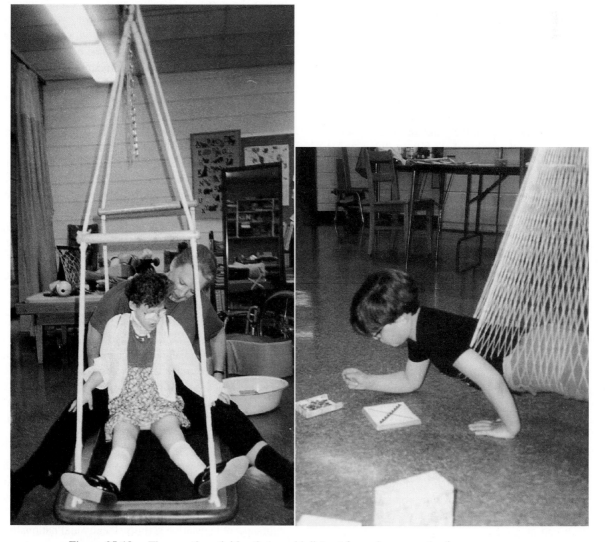

**Figure 25-18**  Therapeutic activities that would distract from classroom attention.

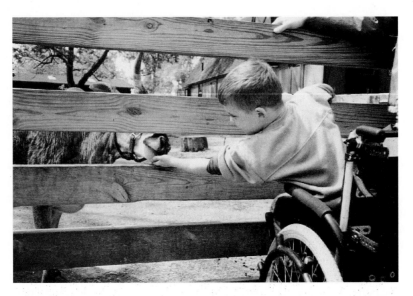

**Figure 25-19**   This child is on a field trip to a farm with his public school class.

sponsible for teaching math concepts, for selecting representative problems from the total number assigned for the class, and for grading and commenting on math performance. The occupational therapist is responsible for working with the student to determine and practice ways of accomplishing the task independently. The therapist may show a classroom aide how to enter the problems on a computer so that Meg can type and print the answers; the therapist may show Meg how to write the problems and answers on large-lined paper and monitor her skill in doing so; the therapist may "mask off" certain problems so that Meg can focus only on assigned problems. By teaching compensatory abilities, accessing technology or adapted materials, or by teaching alternative ways of accomplishing the act of writing the answers to problems, this therapist is helping the student function in as unrestricted an educational environment as possible.

## Management Considerations

There are several aspects to consider in the implementation of occupational therapy services: (1) determining the appropriate service delivery model, (2) balancing the needs of the student with available resources, (3) determining the frequency of service, and (4) determining the duration of the program, including the appropriate time to discontinue.

### Service Delivery Models

The three major models for service delivery are those of direct service, monitoring, and consultation. According to Gilfoyle (1980), *direct services* are "those related services within a student's educational program for which the occupational therapist has the primary responsibility" (p. 2). Direct service can be conducted on an individual or a group basis, but it must be implemented personally by the thera-

pist or the assistant. Weekly contact is usually considered the minimal frequency of intervention.

Monitoring programs are planned by a therapist but administered by another person. This could be a parent, teacher, or aide who is trained and supervised by the therapist for specific activities. Appropriate activities to be monitored are those specified for a particular student that do not require the presence of a qualified therapist to be carried out in a safe and effective manner. Regular and periodic contact is necessary to update programs and supervise the manner in which the programs are implemented. Examples of activities that could be monitored are handling, positioning, use of equipment, and techniques used to adhere to medical precautions.

Another type of indirect service is *consultation*. According to Dunn and Campbell (1991), consultation includes service provision such as "adapting tasks, materials, and environments; altering postural, movement, and communication requirements; and teaching adults new skills." The process of consultation may focus on the following:

1. *Case consultation:* Refers to an individual child. For example, a therapist is asked to evaluate a child's difficulties with handwriting and make recommendations related to writing tools or task modification that can be carried out in the classroom.
2. *Colleague consultation:* Refers to an educational program. For example, a therapist is asked to design sensorimotor activities appropriate for a teacher to lead during indoor recess.
3. *System consultation:* Refers to the team of adults working within the school environment. For example, an in-service training for school bus aides on safe seating on the bus (AOTA, 1987).

In current legislative activity, locally and nationally, educational and medical care are under scrutiny and possible reform. School therapists need to keep informed of these changes and how these changes might change service delivery. Therapists can be involved in these changes and influence the direction of change. Innovation and flexibility in methods of service delivery are important characteristics of occupational therapists.

## Caseloads and Time Management

Determination of an appropriate caseload and allocation of the therapist's time are subject to many variables: frequency of services needed by the child based on the therapist's evaluation, number of schools in which children are located, geographic distribution of schools, and time required for travel. Other variables are the amount of time required for meetings and staffings and the amount of consultation requested. Also to be considered are the need for community contacts, time required for documentation, number of requests for in-service programming, and availability of paraprofessionals.

The following questions might be asked in computing a reasonable caseload. The therapist must schedule each work task, allotting an appropriate amount of time to each of his or her responsibilities.

1. Do the children assigned to your caseload require direct services, monitoring, or consultation? Children who receive monitoring and consultation also need direct interaction and observation on a regular basis.
2. Do children on your caseload require a combination of services, including service coordination? Most students require a continuum of services that varies with their changing needs over the course of the school year.
3. Has sufficient time for documentation been allotted? Documentation may include written justification for equipment, reports to physicians, billing, progress notes and reports, and communication with teachers and parents.
4. Have you scheduled sufficient time for travel and allotted some time for unanticipated travel delays? Traveling time might need to be increased in the winter, during periods of snow and icy weather.
5. Is sufficient time allotted for supervision and administrative responsibilities? Supervision can require extensive amounts of time, particularly at the onset of the supervisory relationship.
6. Has time been scheduled for meetings with parents and teachers? Some time should be allotted for informal meetings. Informal interactions among team members provide opportunities to learn important information about students and to enhance continuity in each student's educational program.

Therapists need to set parameters for the number of children that they can serve based on a comprehensive overview of their responsibilities and the logisitics unique to their situations. Efficient scheduling requires time management skills; it also requires compromise and negotiation with other members of the educational team. If a child needs to be seen at lunchtime, the therapist must plan around that need. If the teacher requests that the therapist observe the child during computer lab or playground time, then the therapist should accommodate that request. Teachers often give input as to the best time for therapy based on scheduled classroom activities. The occupational therapist must also consider the student's activities. For a student to receive occupational, physical, and speech therapy back-to-back in one afternoon would not benefit the student and might limit his or her active participation in each session. The student's needs, the teacher's plans, and the schedules of the other team members all need to be considered in developing a schedule.

A number of strategies might be considered to make efficient use of the work week. Caseload management strategies may include the following:

1. Use of small groups rather than one-on-one therapy
2. Block scheduling (see Chapter 24), that is, spending 2 or 3 hours in one classroom
3. When appropriate, providing consultation and monitoring rather than direct services
4. Reducing travel time by scheduling all children at one setting at one time
5. Efficient teaming with COTAs
6. Teaching classroom aides to implement specific therapy procedures

At times a therapist may find himself or herself overscheduled, and to resolve such situations, negotiation with one's administrator and teammates becomes important. The administrator may have a limited understanding of occupational therapy services and may not appreciate the time involved in providing services. By educating administrators and supervisors about the types of activities and services provided, the time involved, and the related responsibilities associated with those services, the therapist can better negotiate for a manageable caseload. The quality of services is based on sufficient time with each student, teacher, and team member; therefore the occupational therapist must advocate for that time and set the parameters for negotiating caseload and schedule.

## Termination of Services

It is sometimes difficult to determine the appropriate duration of occupational therapy intervention for a student. It is the responsibility of the occupational therapist to make decisions regarding termination of services according to several criteria. If occupational therapy is no longer necessary for the student to benefit from special education, the student ceases to be eligible for school-based occupational therapy. It may be appropriate, however, for that student to receive occupational therapy in another setting, such as in an outpatient clinic.

In general, it is appropriate to discontinue occupational

therapy when the student no longer makes progress on established goals. Discharge plans for these students should reflect any need the student may have for continuing support services within the school system or the community. The educational planning committee needs to be involved when termination of services is considered so that smooth transitions can be made. In some cases it may be appropriate for the occupational therapist to discontinue services for a period, then resume services when the student reaches a new developmental level or must cope with new environmental demands. For example, a student with cerebral palsy functioned adequately in an elementary school environment, and occupational therapy services were terminated. However, physical growth, adolescent issues, and the stresses of a middle school environment made it necessary for the student to resume occupational therapy to cope with disability in a new environment.

### Therapist, Supervisor, and Team Member

In the school setting the occupational therapist and COTA function independently yet in collaboration with other members of the education team, including the family. Independently, the occupational therapist works one-on-one with the child to improve components of functional task performance. Collaboratively, the therapist works with the educational team, supporting their interventions and instruction and recognizing their roles and the blurring or overlap of roles.

For example, the occupational therapist's role may be to help a student achieve independent mobility about the room, efficient handling of materials, and timely completion of assignments in clear language so that the student knows what is expected and has a reference point that helps him or her stay organized. If any materials are out of the student's reach, a *classmate* is assigned to be a helper, but the student is expected to do as much as he or she can do without help. The *occupational therapist* suggests that the student sit closer to the board to more easily follow the directions. The therapist also recommends that the student sit next to the center aisle so that he or she has easy access to his or her desk and to the teacher during independent working times. The *physical therapist* may help the student make transfers between a wheelchair and a classroom chair or the floor, and back again. The physical therapist and the occupational therapist might work together on selection and placement of the student's desk for optimal movement and function in the class. The *parents* might provide notebooks and a bookbag so that the student's work is more organized, easily manipulated, and quickly accessible. Although the parents are not present in the classroom, it is helpful to the student to have reminders about homework assignments and help in gathering all school supplies for the school day in an organized way so that when at school, the student can find the homework done the previous evening.

Therapists may write collaborative IEP goals with teachers, parents, or other team members in which one goal is addressed by different professionals. A therapist may release some of this role to another who is in a position to carry out activities on a more regular basis or in a more appropriate setting, such as designing sensorimotor activities for a preschool classroom (Figure 25-20), teaching an attendant to feed a child, or showing a classroom aide how to set up computer equipment in the classroom. In such a collaborative model, teaching and follow-up inservices for those

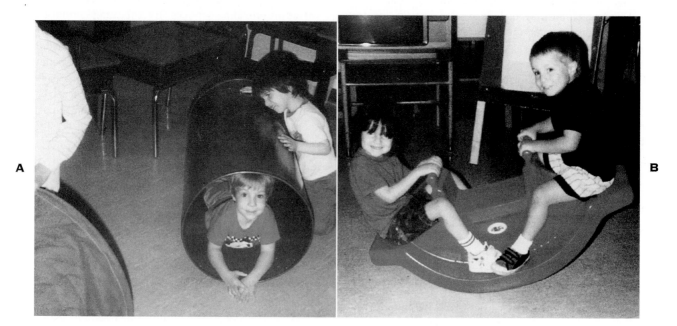

**Figure 25-20**   Sensorimotor activities designed by the consulting occupational therapist for a preschool classroom.

## Initiation of special education ·

*Parent request.* Brian, aged 5 years 6 months, entered kindergarten in an urban elementary school in January of the school year after having attended a private nursery school. Brian's mother requested staffing to explore the need for special education, and she obtained reports of recent evaluations for the in-school team to review.

*Record review.* Psychologic, medical, occupational therapy, and physical therapy evaluations had been completed on an outpatient basis at a local hospital. According to the psychologic reports, Brian had a low normal IQ, showed low self-esteem, was easily frustrated (especially with motor tasks), displayed acting-out and aggressive behaviors, and was depressed. The therapists reported these problems: crossing the midline of the body, equilibrium, fine and gross motor planning, graphic skills, prehension, and visual perception. It was reported that Brian was considerably delayed in language development and that his speech was difficult to understand. Medical reports indicated a normal physical examination with a history of ear infections and allergy. Hearing and vision were within normal limits. In addition to the services received from the hospital, the family participated in counseling sessions with a local agency.

*Initial staffing.* The in-school team, made up of the classroom teacher, speech therapist, occupational therapist, resource teachers for behavior disorders and learning disabilities, school psychologist, and Brian's parent, met on Brian's second day of school. The purpose of the meeting was to recommend evaluations and to decide on a 300-day interim placement while those evaluations were being completed. As a result of this meeting, Brian was placed in a regular kindergarten class with daily resource help from the behavior disorders teacher. Referrals were made for speech, occupational therapy, learning disabilities, and behavior disorders evaluations. Based on reports of previous evaluations and classroom observations, some goals were developed for the 30-day period; these were concerned with developing appropriate classroom behaviors and decreasing aggressiveness and fighting.

## Occupational therapy evaluation

*Preevaluation data collection.* The data collection for the occupational therapy assessment began with a review of the records, especially those of the previous occupational therapy evaluation. After consulting with the occupational therapist who had worked with Brian previously, the current therapist decided to use parent and teacher interviews, informal observation, the Sensory Integration and Praxis Tests, fine motor portion of the Peabody Developmental Motor Scales (PDMS), clinical observations, and informal assessment of play and developmental skills to evaluate Brian.

An interview conducted with Brian's mother by use of a questionnaire showed a possible tactile problem. Brian had a habit of touching everything in sight; he frequently withdrew from touch, bumped and pushed other children, and wore a coat when not needed. Brian's mother also described coordination problems, possible auditory perception problems, and slowness in reaching developmental milestones. Brian turned over at 7 months, was slow talking, and, according to the mother, had trouble walking.

The kindergarten teacher described Brian as an active, talkative child who punched and hit other children and had difficulty attending to class activities. He lagged behind his classmates in readiness skills for reading and writing. Classroom observation during show-and-tell showed that Brian sometimes watched and listened, but more often played with a toy car or wandered around the room.

## Occupational therapy evaluation

*Psychosocial skills.* In the one-to-one testing environment, Brian was lively and restless, sometimes refusing to attempt tasks presented to him. Although his behavior was often stubborn and manipulative, he appeared to have a desire to gain approval from adults. He responded well to a reward system that used a brightly colored sticker for appropriate behavior. However, in an unstructured group situation, Brian had difficulty following rules, disobeyed adults, and antagonized his peers. When observed with his mother, Brian seemed rebellious and hostile.

Although Brian appeared aggressive and rebellious, he may have been using these behaviors to hide a low self-esteem and feelings of insecurity. His refusal to attempt tasks could be a defense mechanism to avoid failure. Brian refused to draw a boy, but did finish a drawing of an incomplete man. The therapist talked to Brian about this drawing, asking, "How does he feel inside?" Brian's only response was to scribble vigorously on the stomach of the man in the drawing. When asked, "Is he happy or sad?" Brian replied, "He's angry, angry at you!"

Brian enjoyed playing with small cars and trucks, but avoided drawing, coloring, and playing with toys that required fine motor skills. His play was often destructive in nature. He made pretend bombs, destroyed towns made of blocks, or had cars and trucks engage in massive wrecks. Brian's play was usually solitary; he had not yet developed interpersonal skills needed to play cooperatively with other children.

*Developmental skills.* Gross motor skills that did not require a great deal of balance, such as jumping, hopping, and skipping, were developmentally on age level. The abilities to balance on one foot and to walk heel-to-toe were 1 to 2 years below his chronologic age. Upper-extremity gross motor planning, as measured by the Postural Praxis subtest, was above the norm.

Brian's ability to manipulate small objects was on age level, although he would not remain on task for more than a few minutes. The PDMS indicated fine motor functioning on age level. Eye-hand coordination, as measured by the Motor Accuracy Test, was above the norm for the right hand but significantly below the norm for the left. Brian is right-handed, but his left eye is dominant for sighting. He tended to use each hand on its own side of space, rather than crossing the midline of his body. Visual-motor integration, as indicated by the Design Copying Test, was significantly above the norm.

Although Brian's behaviors seem extreme, they must be viewed in light of normal emotional development. The 5½- to 6-year-old child is typically emotional, with aggressiveness and a false sense of self-confidence. Brian's emotional difficulties appear to magnify and intensify the negative aspects of normal 6-year-old children's behavior.

*Daily living skills.* Brian was independent in age-appropriate feeding, dressing, and grooming skills, although his mother described his eating as sloppy. Occupational skills needed for the classroom were, on the whole, adequate. Brian could manipulate scissors to cut straight lines; he made jerky circular cuts when cutting a circle. He was learning to print letters of his name and displayed immature, but adequate, prehension patterns with pencils and crayons. Visual perceptual tests showed average functioning.

*Sensorimotor skills.* Sitting balance was poor, with a dependence on external support. Brian was hypotonic and was unable to assume the prone extension position or maintain the flexed supine position. Brian was unstable in a quadruped position and objected to

having the therapist put her hands on his head to test for reflexes. He giggled and pulled away when he was touched and did not want his sleeves rolled up. There were indications of residuals of the symmetric tonic neck reflex and lack of integration of righting reactions.

In addition to the clinical manifestations of tactile defensiveness, Brian scored poorly on tests for graphesthesia and localizing tactile stimuli. There were irregularities in diadochokinesia, rapid thumb to finger movement, and eye tracking. He also showed deficiencies in coordinating the two sides of his body.

The occupational therapist suspected vestibular problems because of Brian's low muscle tone, lack of postural stability, eye tracking problems, and difficulty with bilateral integration. However, Brian could not maintain a sitting position on a moving nystagmus board, and overhead hanging equipment for a net hammock was unavailable at his school. Therefore duration of nystagmus could not be measured.

*Evaluation summary.* The occupational therapy evaluation indicated that Brian had a sensory integrative dysfunction in the areas of bilateral and postural integration, which could be a result of ineffective processing of the tactile system and possibly the vestibular system. There was also a disorder in psychosocial functioning in that the child displayed maladaptive methods of coping with his environment and in developing relationships with both adults and peers.

The following summary was written for the in-school team: This evaluation shows moderate sensory integrative dysfunction primarily in the areas of tactile functioning and bilateral motor integration. Significant findings are evidence of tactile defensiveness (avoidance of touch), difficulty in coordinating the two sides of the body (including avoidance of the midline and poor performance of nondominant hand), and unstable gross motor patterns. The presence of tactile defensiveness has been linked with behavioral problems in some children who display aggressiveness and hyperactivity. Brian's tendency to overreact to tactile stimuli (fight-or-flight pattern) may account for some of his behavioral problems in the classroom.

Brian's inability to stabilize large postural muscles makes his movements appear clumsy and uncoordinated. When he is seated in a chair, his motor planning with his arms is adequate, but when he is seated in a cross-legged position on the mat, he can be pushed over easily. It is important for Brian to have a chair of the proper size in the classroom so that his

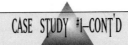

CASE STUDY #1—CONT'D

feet can be firmly on the floor. Round tables are not recommended because they do not give enough surface for arm support.

## Placement staffing

*Review of evaluation data*. The in-school team reconvened after the 30-day evaluation period to write goals and determine placement for Brian. Evaluation results were discussed. The speech therapist found no language deficits but indicated that there were some articulation errors that interfered with the intelligibility of Brian's speech. Speech therapy was recommended twice a week. Testing in the area of learning disabilities showed that Brian did not meet the state requirements for this exceptionality and therefore would not need help from the learning disabilities teacher. The behavior disorders teacher found significant deficiencies in accepting authority from adults, relating to peers, and in developing acceptable behavior patterns. The occupational therapist reported on the results of the occupational therapy assessment and recommended occupational therapy on an individual basis two times a week.

*Development of the Individual Education Plan*. All of the evaluation results were used in developing statements of present levels of performance for the Individual Education Plan (IEP). These were in the areas of academic skills, psychomotor skills, career-vocational areas, self-help skills, and physical-medical considerations. Next, goals were written for each of the identified deficit areas needing intervention from special education and support services. The occupational therapy goals were as follows:

*Annual goal:* To improve classroom coping skills through improved postural stability and decreased tactile defensiveness

*Objectives:*
1. When working on a pencil-and-paper task at the table, Brian will remain in his chair and cross the midline of his body 80% of the time without verbal reminders.
2. When touched on the arm, leg, or face without visual cues, Brian will locate the touch accurately without withdrawing four of five times.
3. Brian will play a game requiring him to balance on three extremities without falling 70% of the time.

*Special education placement*. Based on the information gathered and the needs that had been identified, the team agreed that Brian's functional status qualified him for the behavior disorders program. The next task was to decide on the most appropriate and least restrictive educational placement for Brian. The team agreed that Brian's needs could be met with placement in a regular kindergarten class with a resource class for behavior disorders 2 hours daily and itinerant services from the speech therapist and occupational therapist. All of these services were available at the current school, so no change in school placement was needed. Brian's mother agreed to this placement.

## Occupational therapy intervention

*Frequency of service*. Brian received direct and consultative occupational therapy services once a week.

*Occupational therapy activities*. A sensory integrative approach was used, with an emphasis on tactile and vestibular input. Brian participated eagerly and responded positively to the tasks presented but sometimes continued his manipulative behaviors. As a result, it was necessary to provide therapy sessions that were structured yet included opportunity for movement exploration and experimentation.

Therapy activities included numerous scooter board activities and games that challenged balance in quadruped and sitting positions. Tactile input was given by rubbing the extremities with various textures and by rolling up in a rug. Brian especially enjoyed the latter, which probably indicated a need for the moving touch-pressure stimulus it provided. A brushing program using a soft surgical scrub brush was initiated and carried out at home and in the classroom. Spinning was used cautiously, as Brian sometimes complained of nausea or headache after this stimulation. Proprioceptive input was given with activities such as the wheelbarrow walk.

Consultative service included discussions with the teacher regarding modification of his sensory experiences while in the classroom and of beneficial types of sensory input. The teacher and therapist developed methods that could be used based on Brian's changing sensory needs, including ways to help him organize his materials, diffuse his intermittent aggressiveness with peers, and self-calm when he seemed irritable or anxious.

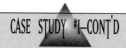

## CASE STUDY #1—CONT'D

### Review staffing

In June of the school year the in-school team met again to review goals and objectives in the IEP and to write an IEP for the next school year. The team agreed that Brian had made tremendous progress during the year. Some of the goals for improving behavior and interpersonal skills had been met, and his kindergarten teacher believed that he was ready for first grade. The occupational therapist's progress report read in part:

Brian has shown a great deal of improvement in the short time he has received occupational therapy. He is better able to tolerate tactile (touch) stimuli and has much better control of large muscle movements. Although Brian sometimes acted in a manipulative, demanding, or stubborn manner, he always responded to firm limits and completed the task. He appeared to enjoy the sessions, and on a one-to-one situation, his behavior was controllable. However, on at least one occasion he verbalized hostile, destructive feelings toward the school and adults, saying, 'I'm going to put bombs in the school,' and 'I want to shoot arrows in all the teachers.'

For the next school year, the occupational therapist recommended continuation of direct services in a group of two or three children and continued consultation. Previous goals for occupational therapy had not yet been achieved, so they were carried over to the next year's IEP. In addition, the occupational therapist and teacher agreed to work jointly to develop the appropriate goals that were added:

*Annual goal:* To improve classroom behavior and coping skills

*Objectives:*
1. When working on an activity in a group of three children, Brian will remain in his place and allow the other children to participate in the activity without interruption 70% of the time.
2. Brian will take turns while playing a game with another child without adult direction 80% of the time.
3. When frustrated with a task, Brian will ask for assistance without destroying materials four of five times.

A new IEP was completed with goals for behavior disorders, speech therapy, and occupational therapy. It is anticipated that Brian will continue to improve with these services so that eventually he can participate fully in a regular educational environment.

---

teachers, aides, parents, and others involved in helping to implement a program are emphasized more than evaluative supervision of these team members. The relationship between the occupational therapist and certified assistant is more one of a partnership than one of supervision. Accountability is monitored primarily through the therapist's adherence to appropriate IEP procedures; however, the ability to work as a team member, whether performing direct services or providing consultation, is important to be effective as a school therapist.

### Therapist as an Employee in the School System

Occupational therapists who work in school systems are hired as *employees* of the school system or they are hired for *contract services* by the school system while they are employed in another setting, such as through a private practice or a hospital. Often therapists are hired on a contract basis because there are too few children who require occupational therapy within a school system to justify a therapist position or because of the unavailability of therapists who wish to work either full- or part-time in the school setting. Contract therapists from medical settings must switch their focus from a medical model to the educational model and use different professional language and different frames

of reference. Whether a school employee or a contract employee, the therapist provides services according to the guidelines described earlier in this chapter. The therapist's direct supervisor is usually an educator rather than another therapist.

### Pros and Cons of School-Based Therapy

As in any practice setting, there are advantages and disadvantages to working in the schools. The following are some of the *advantages* of working as an occupational therapist in the schools. There is an opportunity to develop long-term relationships with the students—and families—with whom one works because intervention may last a whole school year, or longer. Children in school present a variety of problems; each student is a new challenge. Providing creative solutions to service delivery and developing programs to meet the growing needs of student populations is stimulating. The 9- or 10-month school year, including generous holidays, allows time for the therapist to meet family obligations or pursue other interests or projects. For example, school therapists may use the vacation time to work in another type of practice setting, such as private practice or a hospital setting. Summer is a time to update knowledge and

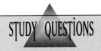

## STUDY QUESTIONS

1. How are occupational therapy services defined in the Individuals with Disabilities Education Act? What are the parameters for occupational therapy practice compared with those in a medical setting?

2. Explain what is meant by the term *least restrictive environment?* What are the implications for this mandate for occupational therapy service delivery?

3. After observing a student in a regular education classroom, the occupational therapist believes that the student would benefit from occupational therapy services; however, the student has not been categorized as eligible for special education. Describe two different actions that the occupational therapist might take to enable the child to receive services.

4. Explain three ways that an occupational therapist can manage a large caseload in the school system. Include examples of indirect service delivery, scheduling options, and supervision of others.

5. A student in third grade is having difficulty copying words from the classroom's front blackboard. It takes him twice as long to copy sentences as the other students. The occupational therapy evaluation shows that the student has difficulty in eye tracking and in keeping his place on the paper. Give one example of an activity that uses a corrective approach to improve his ability to copy from the board. Give an example of a classroom adaptation that uses a compensatory approach to this problem.

6. As the school's occupational therapist, you examine a child's wheelchair and believe that it is unsafe for transportation on the school bus. Whom would you consult with to help correct this safety issue? Explain how you would approach this issue in a way that would consider the needs of other students and personnel involved.

skills through graduate course work or through professional workshops. It is a time also for extended vacations, rest, and renewal.

There are also *disadvantages* for school therapists. There is often a large caseload of children who are served by a variety of models of intervention; meeting the needs of each of the students is a challenge. Therapists often spend a significant part of their days in travel from school to school; this is true not only in rural areas, but also in urban areas. Because therapy services are spread out over great dis-

tances, there may be no regular contact with other occupational therapists; there may be a feeling of isolation from the profession. The salary of a school therapist is often not competitive with other occupational therapy positions in the same geographic area. As with any area of practice, the therapist must decide if school-based practice is the best individual choice of employment based on personal and professional goals, values, and life-styles.

Of special note is an increasingly expressed concern among therapists that school-based practice does not allow occupational therapists to adequately deal with social-emotional aspects of student programs. Informal conversations indicate that occupational therapy services are not well used in programs for children with severe behavioral problems. Although therapists use their expertise in social-emotional components, throughout their interventions they appear to be restricted in formal acknowledgement of this.

## REFERENCES

American Occupational Therapy Association. (1987). *Guidelines for occupational therapy services in school systems.* Rockville, MD: American Occupational Therapy Association.

American Occupational Therapy Association. (1989). *Guidelines for occupational therapy services in early intervention and preschool services.* Rockville, MD: American Occupational Therapy Association.

Ayres, A.J. (1989). *Sensory Integration and Praxis Tests.* Los Angles: Western Psychological Services.

Berk, R. & DeGangi, G.(1983). *DeGangi-Berk Test of Sensory Integration.* Los Angles: Western Psychological Corporation.

Boehme, R. (1986) *Improving upper body control: an approach to assessment and treatment of tonal dysfunction.* Tucson: Therapy Skill Builders.

Brigance, A.H. (1978). *Brigance Diagnostic Inventory of Early Development.* North Bilerica, MA: Curriculum Associates.

Bruininks, R.H. (1978). *Bruininks-Oseretsky Test of Motor Proficiency.* Circle Pines, MN: American Guidance Service.

Colarusso, R.P. & Hammill, D.D. (1972). *Motor-Free Visual Perception Test (MVPT).* Novato, CA: Academic Therapy Publications.

Collier, T. (1991). The screening process. In W. Dunn (Ed.). *Pediatric occupational therapy: facilitating effective service provision.* Thorofare, NJ: Slack.

Cook, D. (1991). The assessment process. In W. Dunn (Ed.). *Pediatric occupational therapy: facilitating effective service provision.* Thorofare, NJ: Slack.

Dunn, W. (1989). Models of occupational therapy service provision in the school system. *American Journal of Occupational Therapy, 42*(11), 718-723.

Dunn, W. (1991). Consultation as a process: how, when, and why? In C. Royeen (Ed.). *AOTA self study services: school-based practice for related services.* Rockville, MD: American Occupational Therapy Association.

Dunn, W. & Campbell, P. (1991). Designing pediatric service provision. In W. Dunn (Ed.). *Pediatric occupational therapy: facilitating effective service provision.* Thorofare, NJ: Slack.

*Education for All Handicapped Children Act of 1975* (P.L. 94-142), 20 U.S.C. 1401.

Education of Handicapped Children: implementation of part B of the Education of the Handicapped Act, (1977). *Fed Reg 42*, 163.

Federal Register. (1976). (41) 252, Thursday, December 30, pp. 56966-56998.

Federal Register. (1977). (42) 163, Tuesday, August 23, pp. 42474-42518.

Federal Register. (1977). *Nondiscrimination on basis of handicap: program and activities receiving or benefitting from federal financial assistance, 42*, 86.

Gardner, M.F. (1986). *Test of Visual Motor Skills.* San Francisco: Psychological and Educational Publications.

Gardner, M.F. (1992). *Test of Visual-Perceptual Skills (non-motor).* San Francisco: Psychological and Educational Publications.

Gilfoyle, E. (1980). *Training occupational therapy educational management in schools* (Vol. 1-4). Rockville, MD: American Occupational Therapy Association.

Haley, S.M., Coster, W.J., Ludlow, L.H., Haltiwanger, M.A., & Andrellos, P.J. (1992). *Pediatric Evaluation of Disability Inventory.* Boston: New England Medical Center Hospitals and PEDI Research Group.

Hammill, D.D., Pearson, N.A., & Voress, J.K. (1993). *Developmental Test of Visual Perception* (2nd ed.). Austin, TX: Pro Ed.

Hopkins, H.L. (1988). An historical perspective on occupational therapy. In H.L. Hopkins, & H. Smith (Eds.). *Willard and Spackman's occupational therapy* (7th ed.). Philadelphia: J.B. Lippincott.

Ilg, F.L. & Ames, L.B. (1981). *The Gesell Institute's child behavior.* New York: Harper & Row.

Individuals with Disabilities Act of 1990 (P.L 101-476), 20 U.S.C., Chapter 33.

Linder, T. (1990). *Transdisciplinary play-based assessment: a functional approach to working with young children.* Baltimore: Brookes.

Lovitt, T. (1980). *Writing and implementing an IEP.* Belmont, CA: Pitman Learning.

Miller, L. (1988). *Miller Assessment for Preschoolers.* San Antonio, TX: The Psychological Corp.

Muhlenhaupt, M. (1985). *Occupational therapy in New York public schools.* Northport, NY: The Press Room at TMC.

Muhlenhaupt, M. (1992). Educationally relevant assessments: registered occupational therapist and occupational therapy assistant role delineations. In C. Royeen (Eds.). *AOTA self study series: classroom applications for school-based practice* (pp. 63-69). Rockville, MD: American Occupational Therapy Association.

*PARC v Commonwealth of Pennsylvania* (1971). 344 F Supp 1257.

Rebell, M.A. (1981). Implementation of court mandates concerning special education: the problems and the potential. *Journal of Law Education, 10*, 335.

Regan, N.N. (1982). The implementation of occupational therapy services in rural school systems. *American Journal of Occupational Therapy, 36*, 85.

Sanford, A.R. & Zelman, J.G. (1981). *Learning Accomplishment Profile* (rev. ed.). Winston-Salem, NC: Kaplan Press.

Smith, R.O. (1993). Technology. Part II. Adaptive equipment and technology. In C. Royeen (Ed.). *AOTA self study series: classroom applications for school-based practice.* Rockville, MD: American Occupational Therapy Association.

Sparrow, S.S., Balla, D.A., & Cicchetti, D.V. (1984). *Vineland Adaptive Behavior Scale.* Circle Pines, MN: American Guidance Service.

Taylor, N., Sand, P.L., & Jebsen, R.H. (1973). Evaluation of hand function in children. *Archives of Physical Medicine and Rehabilitation, 54*, 129-135.

Wesley, A.J. (1993). Functional mobility/self-help assessment. In C. Royeen (Ed.). *AOTA self study series: classroom applications for school-based practice.* (#1: pp. 35-39). Rockville, MD: American Occupational Therapy Association.

CHAPTER

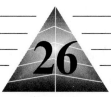

# Services for Children with Visual or Auditory Impairments

ELIZABETH SNOW

## KEY TERMS

- ▲ Conductive Hearing Loss
- ▲ Sensorineural Hearing Loss
- ▲ Mixed Hearing Loss
- ▲ Audiogram
- ▲ Decibels
- ▲ Hertz
- ▲ Hard of Hearing
- ▲ Audiometry
- ▲ Total Communication
- ▲ Speech Reading
- ▲ American Sign Language
- ▲ Legal Blindness
- ▲ Cataract
- ▲ Glaucoma
- ▲ Mobility Training
- ▲ Blindisms
- ▲ Braille
- ▲ Low Vision Training

## CHAPTER OBJECTIVES

1. Describe the role that the senses of vision and hearing play in a child's life.
2. Define terms related to visual and hearing impairment.
3. Explain the basic anatomy of the eye and ear.
4. Describe the effects of visual and hearing impairments on a child's development.
5. Identify intervention goals appropriate for children with visual and hearing impairments.
6. Describe examples of occupational therapy intervention for children with visual or hearing impairments.

Hearing and vision are the distant senses that allow us to understand what is happening in the environment outside our bodies. Those of us with normal sensory function cannot truly understand the total nature of the disability but can be helped by participating in sensory awareness activities. Eating a meal blindfolded to simulate blindness or listening to records that simulate what common songs sound like to an individual with a certain type of hearing loss are examples of sensory awareness activities. They are good exercises but do not give the total picture. Each person with normal senses has a vast wealth of visual and auditory memories to call on that people with impaired senses do not have. It is important to note that most of the children with sensory loss who are seen in occupational therapy will be congenitally impaired and therefore will have no reservoir of unimpaired information to review.

The *sense organs* (eyes, ears, skin, nose, and tongue) are all extensions of the brain. The brain's primary function is to receive information from the world for processing and coding. These sensory stimuli are integrated and associated with past experiences. Because the nature and the intensity of the stimulation to the sense organs vary greatly, one may take precedence over the others, depending on the situation. If a particular sense organ is not working properly, the others do not take over and totally compensate, but another sensory system may take precedence.

Ayres (1972) developed a *hierarchy of sensory perceptual development* that helps in the understanding of sensory impairments. The senses develop and work in an interactive manner in all everyday activities. They do not perform in isolation but develop in a building block manner. The *vestibular* system gives information about the body's position in space, movement or lack of movement through space, and direction of movement. The receptors for the vestibular system are located in the inner ear, and it is thought that the auditory system evolved out of the more

**717**

primitive vestibular system (Ayres, 1972). The vestibular and *tactile* (touch) systems are the foundations of sensation. Visual and auditory sensations are received by the brain against a constant background of tactile stimuli and the body's position in space. It is important to think about the level of alertness required by the brain for auditory and visual perceptual processes to occur. The vestibular system and the *reticular activating* system have a great influence on this level of alertness. Being either overly alert or not sufficiently alert can obviously have detrimental effects on visual and auditory perceptions.

*Vision* is the sense we use for understanding the relationships between people and objects. It puts the environment in perspective for us and precedes auditory development by building concepts and perceptual abilities. Children with visual defects often have a diminished verbal language because the relationships and associations between people and objects are not fully grasped. In discussing vision, it is important to differentiate between visual acuity, visual awareness, and visual perception. Impairment can occur at any or all levels, and the child has to be assessed accurately.

In addition to its function as the building block for speech, *audition* is the sense that conveys sound. Sound gives information on distance and direction. We can hear a dog bark and, without seeing the dog, judge where and how far away it is. Auditory perception is the attachment of meaning to sound patterns. Sound has qualities of tone and pitch that make up auditory acuity. As with vision, impairment can occur at the level of acuity, awareness, or perception. Although language development appears to be the most serious problem for a hearing-impaired child, the situation is much more complex because language is a force in the socialization and development of inner logic of the child and affects personality development (Ling, 1989; Sapir, 1966). Language is not innate; it is a product of the child's environment. As the child learns the language, he or she can exert greater control over the environment.

The problems of children with visual or hearing impairments can be enormous. Although deaf and blind children face many shared difficulties, there are also striking differences. For this reason, this chapter deals separately with the hearing impaired, the visually impaired, and the multiply impaired. It is important to point out early in the chapter that the occupational therapist is usually not the primary professional for the primary problems of the child with visual or hearing impairment but instead provides critical services for the associated functional problems incurred by these children. The occupational therapist is often employed in the role of consultant with those populations, providing services to individual children, entire classrooms, or institutions. Consultation often revolves around problems typically addressed in occupational therapy:

1. Activities of daily living, for example, feeding, dressing, and toileting
2. Fine motor coordination and dexterity
3. Sensory processing and perceptual skills
4. Gross motor and body movement skills
5. Preparation for vocational training

Consultation is given to parents, teachers, and care workers as part of the child's overall developmental and educational plan and in conjunction with those professionals primarily involved with the child who has visual or hearing impairment.

In providing occupational therapy, the importance of play cannot be overemphasized for these children. Play is the means by which the child learns how to solve problems, to cope with the environment, to face the unknown, and to adapt by changing behaviors (Gunn, 1971; Michelman, 1971). For children whose distance senses (and therefore their abilities to perceive the environment) are limited, the development of play skills, particularly active play involving use of the vestibular and proprioceptive systems, should be the highest priority.

## HEARING IMPAIRMENT
### Diagnostic Information

The estimates of children with hearing impairment vary with the criteria being applied. The prevalence of severe bilateral hearing loss in high-risk neonates ranges from 1.7% to greater than 5%, depending on the population surveyed. It is estimated that 8% to 10% of children from 5 to 14 years of age have at least a unilateral hearing loss of greater than 15 decibels (dB) (Behrman & Vaughan, 1987). Total deafness is rare and usually only happens when there is aplasia or failure of the inner ear to develop. A person with deafness is one whose hearing is so severely impaired that he or she must depend primarily on visual communication such as writing, lipreading, manual communication, or gestures. A person classified as hard-of-hearing is one whose hearing is impaired but not to the extent that he or she must depend primarily on visual communication. Almost all children who are deaf or hard-of-hearing have some residual audition that can be used for at least environmental awareness (Davis & Silverman, 1978; Newby, 1972; Northern & Downs, 1992).

To properly examine the subject of hearing loss, it is important to have a basic understanding of the nature of sound and the anatomy of the ear. Sound sets up a disturbance in the air. Air consists of more than 400 billion particles per cubic inch, and as we speak or make a sound, these particles are set in motion, hitting against each other and forming a wave of sound energy. The ear acts as a receiver, amplifier, and transmitter.

The ear is composed of three separate sections (Figure 26-1), and the type of hearing loss that a child has depends on where the damage is located. The outer ear includes the visible part *(pinna)* and the ear canal extending to the *eardrum (tympanic membrane)*. The function of the outer ear is to collect the sound or acoustic energy and channel it to

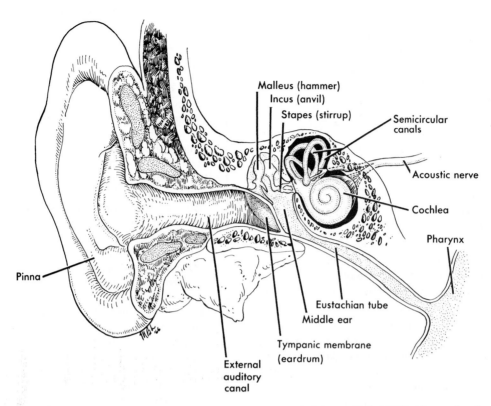

**Figure 26-1**   Cross section of the ear. (From Ingalls, A.J. & Salerno, M.C. (1983). *Maternal and child health nursing* (5th ed.). St Louis: Mosby.)

the eardrum, which vibrates with the sound wave and changes the acoustic energy to mechanical energy. The middle ear consists of the three small bones *(hammer or malleus, anvil or incus,* and *stirrup or stapes)* that conduct vibrations from the eardrum to the inner ear. The stapes is inserted into the *oval window,* beyond which is the fluid-filled vestibule of the inner ear, which, along with the *semicircular canals,* make up the organs of equilibrium. The motions of the bones of the middle ear result in an increase of the mechanical energy of sound so that by the time sound travels from the eardrum to the oval window, it has been intensified many times. The inner ear is composed of the hearing organ, *cochlea,* that coils off the vestibule and the *acoustic nerve* (eighth cranial nerve). The cochlea transforms the mechanical energy of the sound waves into neural energy for reception by the auditory nerve.

There are two types of hearing loss: conductive and sensorineural. In *conductive hearing loss* the problem lies in the sound-transmitting portions, that is, the outer or middle ear. One of the most frequent conditions causing conductive hearing loss in children is chronic otitis media (Sataloff, Sataloff, & Vassolo, 1980). Some common causes of conductive loss are wax buildup, punctured eardrum, or inability of the middle ear bones to move properly. Diagnoses with conductive hearing loss include Treacher Collins syndrome, a hereditary underdevelopment of the external canal and middle ear, and otosclerosis, a progressive condi-

tion occurring as early as late adolescence. We hear by bone conduction as well as by air conduction, and the relationship of these two functions gives diagnostic information about the location of the hearing loss. Fortunately many conductive losses can be corrected by medical-surgical means when detected early. Unfortunately, considerable impairment of the developmental process can occur before the time the child's loss is detected. Poor articulation, delayed speech development, and poor school performance can be caused by conductive hearing loss.

The *sensorineural hearing loss* or nerve loss, problem occurs in the inner ear with damage to the cochlear hair cells or nerve fibers. A nerve loss is generally not correctable by medical-surgical means, and it requires the use of amplification (hearing aids, cochlear implants, or tactile devices). This type of loss often produces problems with loudness and distortion of sound. Sensorineural hearing loss is often associated with meningitis and can be a sequela of ototoxic drugs. Several drugs used especially in early infancy to save lives can have a toxic effect on the hearing organs. Other diagnoses include tumors of the auditory nerve. These are most usually unilateral, with the exception of von Recklinghausen's disease in which they are bilateral.

It is common to have a *mixed hearing loss* with both conductive and sensorineural loss present. Obviously it is important to medically treat the conductive portion of the loss as efficiently as possible to minimize the total effect. Generally speaking, if a hearing loss is measured in the "marked loss" range, it is likely to include sensorineural components.

The occupational therapist working with a child with hearing impairment must have an understanding of the measurement of hearing loss. This includes knowledge of the severity of the loss and its practical meaning to the child. The most common measuring device for hearing loss is the *audiogram* (Figure 26-2). This uses a gridlike score sheet to record the child's response to auditory stimuli. The audiogram has a vertical axis that measures *decibels*. The decibel level is an indication of loudness or intensity of the sound or sound pressure and goes from 0 dB (the point at which sound is first perceived) to 140 dB (the point or threshold of pain).

The horizontal axis of the audiogram is the *hertz (Hz) level*. This is a measure of the frequency or number of sound vibrations per minute—the pitch or tone of sound. Pitch or frequency ranges from a low of 125 Hz to a high of 12,000 Hz on the audiogram. The range of 500 to 4000 Hz is the most important because it encompasses the majority of speech sounds. On the audiogram the scores are plotted on the graph beginning with the *hearing threshold level* (where the child first begins to hear sounds). On the audiogram of a particular child, the left and right ears are differentiated by use of colors or by the symbol of a circle for right and a cross for left.

Decibel level is related to the distance that a sound moves an air particle and is measured by a particular standard or norm such as the 1969 American National Standards Institute (ANSI). Although it varies slightly with the norm being used, a hearing level from 0 to 25 dB is considered within normal limits. Figure 26-3 details typical loss classifications according to loudness or decibel loss and their respective therapy-education effects (Anderson & Matkin, 1991). These effects as stated are general in nature and of

*Mild loss: 25 to 40 dB*
May have difficulty hearing faint or distant speech. Needs favorable seating and lighting in therapy or school settings. May need speech therapy, special attention to vocabulary, or aid in some instances.

*Moderate loss: 40 to 55 dB*
Will understand face-to-face conversational speech (at a distance of 3 to 5 feet). May miss as much as 50% of group discussion if voices are low or not in the direct line of vision. May show limited vocabulary and speech anomalies. Will need hearing aid evaluation and training, speech therapy, help in vocabulary and reading, and favorable seating and lighting. May need special class placement or lipreading training.

*Moderate to severe loss: 55 to 70 dB*
Will have increasing difficulty in group discussions. Will show limited vocabulary and is likely to have speech anomalies and be delayed in language use and comprehension. Will need special education services, speech therapy, lipreading instruction, special help with language skills, and hearing aids. Needs to be encouraged in therapy-education settings to pay attention to visual and auditory input at all times. Use of sign language may increase understanding.

*Severe loss: 70 to 90 dB*
May hear loud voices about 1 foot from ear and may be able to identify environmental sounds such as a vacuum cleaner. May have speech difficulties with some ability to discriminate vowels but not all consonants. If loss is present before 1 year of age, the child will not develop spontaneous language. Will need special education services, support services, and hearing aid. Needs a comprehensive program emphasizing language and concept development, speech, lipreading, and sign language.

*Profound loss: 90 dB and more*
May hear some loud sounds, such as an automobile horn, very close but is aware of vibrations more than tonal patterns. Will have to rely on vision as the primary means of communication, rather than on hearing. Sign language is often the primary means of communication. Speech will be deficient and will not develop spontaneously if loss is present before 1 year of age. Will need special education on a comprehensive intensive basis.

NOTE: Shouting, talking loudly or exaggerating mouth movements, and distorted speech are not helpful techniques to increase understanding.

**Figure 26-3** Therapy-education implications of typical hearing loss classifications.

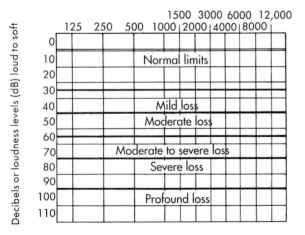

Frequency of tones (Hz) lows to highs

**Figure 26-2** Audiogram indicating typical loss classifications.

course vary somewhat for each individual child and program, but they give the occupational therapist a general idea of what to expect with a certain level of hearing loss.

Although a person with a mild hearing loss may often use a hearing aid, the greatest benefit is derived when the hearing aid is used with a loss of up to 80 dB. Beyond that point the loss is so severe that only partial help can be obtained from the use of an aid.

The hertz level also has to be examined more closely in relationship to the child and his or her particular hearing loss. The hertz level, or frequency level, is related to the number of times per second the air particle moves and produces tone. In humans the hertz level goes from 20 to 20,000 Hz. Other animals have a much broader range; for example, the porpoise's range is 150 to 150,000 Hz, and the dog's range is 15 to 50,000 Hz. A child may have limitation in frequency, and this in turn affects hearing and language development. The hair cells inside the cochlea respond best to varied levels of frequency, depending on location, with the innermost hairs responding best to the low tone frequencies. This means that, depending on the location and extent of damage, there may be high tone loss, low tone loss, or flat loss. Frequency limitations can adversely affect syllable discrimination and understanding of speech.

A *high tone loss* means that the child can hear most of the vowel sounds because they have a lower frequency but misses the consonants. This is serious because the consonant sounds carry most of the information needed to understand speech. If vowels are removed from a sentence, chances are that its contents will remain clear. However, if the consonants are deleted, understanding will be impossible. With a *low tone loss* the child misses vowels but hears many consonants. Voices sound weak and thin but understandable if the child with hearing impairment is close enough to the speaker. A *flat loss* means that all frequencies are evenly affected. Voices sound far away, and certain strong vowels like the *a* in *ate* will be heard best.

The audiogram gives information on both the decibel and the hertz loss of a particular child, but the therapist should consult with the other professionals involved with the individual child to get an accurate picture of the child's hearing loss.

## Other Services Involved

Although there may be many professionals involved with a particular child with hearing impairment, the most common ones are the following (Davis & Silverman, 1978; Newby, 1972):

*Otolaryngologist or ear, nose, and throat specialist:* A physician who specializes in the anatomy, physiology, and pathologic conditions of the head and neck, including the ears, nose, and throat, by using medical and surgical treatment techniques

*Otologist:* A physician who specializes in the anatomy, physiology, and pathologic conditions of the ear, by using medical and surgical treatment techniques

*Audiologist:* A specialist in the study of hearing who performs various hearing tests and provides rehabilitation and treatment, including hearing aids, for those whose hearing impairment cannot be improved by medical or surgical means

*Audiometrist:* A technician trained to test and measure hearing ability

## Practice Settings

The occupational therapist usually encounters children with hearing impairment in hospitals at the time of diagnosis or later in the school setting. Many are identified as "suspicious" in the neonatal unit, and others show up for developmental testing in the clinic. The percentage of children with hearing impairment going to state residential schools has decreased with the advent of more local programs, although a great number of deaf children (especially those with severe hearing losses or multiple handicaps) still do attend state schools. The occupational therapist has a strategic role in special education programs in the areas of self-help skills, socialization, fine motor, sensory integration, and perceptual motor development. The increasing number of infant programs also allows for more therapist involvement in the development of the young child with hearing impairment and intervention in the all-important parent-child interaction.

## Special Characteristics Relevant to Occupational Therapy

To the occupational therapist the most important characteristic of the hearing-impaired child is the lack of early language development and the profound effect of this on all other areas of the child's development (Furth, 1973; Liben, 1978; Myklebust, 1964). What appears at first to be a fairly simple problem becomes complicated in consideration of the importance language plays in our society. Language assists in environmental manipulation and gives the child labels for objects and concepts. It plays a critical role in socialization. The infant smiles and quiets with the sight and sounds of his or her mother. The infant with hearing impairment does not respond to his or her mother's soft voice, unless the mother is in the direct line of sight. Early intervention is imperative, but infantile deafness is often not diagnosed until later. *Babbling* is vocal play, that is, use of the vocal cords and muscles of the mouth, tongue, and larynx, and all children do this. Children who can hear get the stimulus of hearing themselves and their parents' vocalized response. Children with hearing impairment, on the other hand, get insufficient feedback so that the babbling does not continue and progress on to language development. The infant with deafness generally babbles normally up until 5 to 6 months, but then, as the typically developing infant develops a growing repertoire of sounds, the child with hearing impairment will demonstrate language delay.

Many researchers in the field (e.g., Leenenberg, 1967; Meadow, 1980) believe that if intervention is delayed until 3 or 4 years of age, the most important formative period of language development is on the decline and permanent damage is done. If the child is denied cortical stimulation by organic means because of impaired auditory stimuli, he or she will need to conceptualize by other means. Provision of organized alternative stimuli should be one of the main goals of therapy and education for the child with hearing impairment.

## Occupational Therapy Assessment Procedures

The therapist can use the general scales of child development, such as the Bayley Scales of Infant Development or the Battelle Developmental Inventory, with some modification of the language areas and by taking a known hearing loss into account when reporting any score. However, the validity of results using standardized tests must always be questioned. If the child is using a hearing aid, lipreading, or sign language, the therapist should be cognizant of the implications of these specialized techniques. There are some basic suggestions to follow, and these are covered in more detail on pp. 724 to 726. If the child uses sign language and the therapist testing the child is unable to give the commands in sign, the test results should include the information that the therapist was unable to speak the language of the child. In some instances a registered interpreter for the deaf is necessary to obtain accurate test results.

Through developmental testing, the occupational therapist frequently identifies the child with a mild problem not yet diagnosed. Often a pediatrician refers a child who is lagging for developmental testing. Part of the problem can be hearing loss. Unfortunately there are no hard and fast rules for development, and each child is an individual. However, certain findings indicate the possibility of hearing loss and suggest referral to appropriate professionals (see box at right).

In most cases the parents are the keenest observers of their infants. Special note should be taken if the mother reports that the infant does not awaken to loud noises, respond when called, or attend to noisy toys or uses gestures to indicate wants to the exclusion of words. Also notable are the mother's complaints of the child's distractability, inattention to commands, lack of feedback to the mother, or inappropriate responses to verbal stimuli. Obviously all of these difficulties could be attributable to other causes, but hearing impairment should be considered. Also, any child with a history of recurrent ear infections or upper respiratory infections could be a prime candidate for a conductive hearing loss and should be referred to the appropriate professionals.

## Findings That Indicate the Possibility of Hearing Loss

Possible hearing impairment must be considered in the following instances:

A newborn does not exhibit a startle (Moro) reflex in response to a sharp clap 3 to 6 feet away

A 3-month-old child has not developed auditory-orienting responses as indicated by not becoming alert to toys that make noise

An 8- to 12-month-old child does not turn to a whispered voice

An 8- to 12-month-old child does not turn to sounds such as a rattle 3 feet to the rear

A 1-year-old child does not understand a variety of words, such as "bye-bye" and "doggie"

A 2-year-old child is not using words

A 2-year-old child is unable to identify an object with a verbal clue alone, such as "Show me the ball"

A 3-year-old child has largely unintelligible speech

A 3-year-old child omits beginning consonants

A 3-year-old child does not use two- and three-word sentences

A 3-year-old child uses mostly vowel sounds

A child of any age speaks in a voice that is too loud, too soft, of poor quality, or of a quality that does not fit his or her age and sex

A child always sounds as if he or she has a cold

Other kinds of tests such as visual-motor, sensory integration, and self-care checklists can be administered to this population with some adaptation in instructional methods. However, written instructions should be used only if the therapist has in some way made sure that the child has the appropriate level of written comprehension. Writing is language based. Written sentences are formed in the same way oral statements are formed. Therefore in children with hearing impairments, consideration of the language demands of any written test is important to interpreting the results.

### Specialized Assessments

In the area of *psychologic testing,* several tests are used often with children with hearing impairment. The *Hiskey Nebraska Test of Learning Abilities* (Hiskey, 1983) was developed and standardized on the hearing impaired and covers ages 2 to 17. It consists of 12 subtests selected to cover a broad span of intellectual abilities without language. It includes subtests such as bead patterns, picture associations, puzzle blocks, completion of drawings, and memory for digits; it is given in an untimed fashion (Anastasi, 1989).

The *Leiter International Performance Scale* (Leiter, 1969) is a widely used individual IQ test administered without language with a range from 2 to 16 years. It is a performance test that was developed as a nonverbal counterpart to the Stanford-Binet test. It is used with children with hearing impairment as well as others, such as those who do not speak English. Directions are pantomimed, and the test is not timed. Administration begins with items below the child's estimated skill level so that the child has an opportunity to become accustomed to the testing procedure. There are numerous subtests divided into three trays for different age levels: tray 1 for children ages 2 to 7 years, tray 2 for children ages 8 to 12 years, and tray 3 for children up to 18 years. Pattern strips and blocks are used for subtests such as matching colors, number discrimination, pattern completion, similarities, classification of animals, and spatial relations (Anastasi, 1989).

*Audiologic testing* is a complicated and involved process (Newby, 1972; Pollack, 1970). The occupational therapist should consult the professional administering the test on details of testing with the individual child. The most common method of testing requires placement of the child with earphones in a soundproof testing booth. The child indicates when he or she hears a sound.

There are other forms of testing used with various types and ages of children about which the therapist should be aware. *Behavioral observation audiometry (BOA)* is often used with young children. The parent holds the child in his or her lap, and the audiologist notes different behavioral responses of the child to sounds at different levels. *Visual reinforcement audiometry (VRA)* teaches the child to orient to a sound source reinforced with light or a visual stimulus. *Tangible reinforcement operant conditioning audiometry (TROCA)* uses a token or candy for reinforcement of sounds identified. In *play audiometry* the child does a certain task, such as putting a cube in a bucket, when the sound is heard. These are all forms of behavioral observations.

Some forms of *objective observations* can be helpful in the diagnosis of hearing impairment. *Evoked response audiometry (ERA)* is often done with infants or unresponsive children. It uses an electroencephalogram-type machine hooked up to a computer. Earphones are placed on a sedated or quiet child, and a series of clicks are played into the ears. The computer records the brain wave responses to these clicks and supplies information regarding the hearing mechanism response to sound. *Tympanometry* is a procedure to assess eardrum mobility or the presence of fluid in the middle ear. This requires the placement of a probe in the ear canal and can be difficult to perform on an uncooperative child. The *acoustic reflex measurement* is tested with the same instrument as the tympanogram but measures the response of the two eardrum muscles to the presentation of sound. *Electrocochleography* measures the electric activity of the inner ear and auditory nerve, and *electroacoustic impedance* testing measures the way sound is conducted by the middle ear to the inner ear. With the advent of newer and more sophisticated technology every day, these types of testing promise much for the future.

## Objectives of Intervention and Treatment Modalities

As mentioned earlier, the occupational therapist is usually not the primary therapist who works with the child with hearing impairment. Therapy and educational goals must be coordinated with the special educator, the speech therapist, the audiologist, and others working with the child. Some typical occupational therapy objectives follow. These are by no means all-inclusive. Each child should be assessed as an individual by the therapist, and the treatment program should be fitted carefully into the child's total program. Typical goals are the following:

1. *To enhance sensory processing and stimulation.* The child with hearing impairment is denied adequate cortical stimulation by auditory channels and must learn to perceive and conceptualize by other means. The functions of the kinesthetic, tactile, and visual systems can be enhanced by the therapist with various activities and techniques. Sensory integrative techniques are useful in developing the kinesthetic system to its fullest. The tactile and proprioceptive systems are important in the use of sign language. Tactile activities such as having the child locate objects hidden in sand or identify objects behind a shield are among many that can be used. The visual system can be enhanced by tracking exercises, perceptual motor activities, and many games or crafts.

2. *To encourage age-appropriate self-maintenance behaviors.* The occupational therapist can act as a consultant to others for related activities. The parents and others around the child may need consultation regarding what is or what is not appropriate for a certain age. Also, self-maintenance skills involve many concepts that the child should be assisted with in whatever ways possible; for example, the idea of left shoe and right shoe can be shown visually with color coding.

3. *To encourage fine motor and hand coordination skills.* The movements of the hands of a fluent signer require opposition, finger and thumb flexion and extension, and finger and thumb abduction and adduction. These movements are performed by isolated digits and in total patterns but all in rapid succession and with remarkable coordination. The hand's coordination seems to be related to its sensory abilities, particularly tactile discrimination. This skill does not come naturally to a child with hearing loss but has to be learned. Occupational therapy's emphasis on hand skills can do much for the child with hearing loss in general and especially for those children who have an identified delay in these skills. Many games and activities can be incorporated in the treatment program.

4. *To encourage socialization.* This part of occupational therapy intervention cannot be done in isolation and is of utmost importance to the child with hearing im-

pairment. Socialization can be encouraged by involvement in groups for peer interaction. Developing skills of environmental adaptation and understanding the language-oriented points of behavior can be stressed. Deafness is not an easily visible disability, and therefore a child with hearing impairment can be mistaken as being rude if he or she does not answer questions or respond to social overtures when in fact the child has simply not received the correct stimuli.

## Special Techniques

The therapist working with the child with hearing impairment is intimately involved with the special techniques used with that child. The three most commonly used techniques are lipreading, sign language, and hearing aids.

*Total communication* is the use of all avenues such as oral speech, lipreading, sign language, finger spelling, gesture, and body language, simultaneously in communication. Sign language encourages communication and language development (Grinnel, Dentamore, & Lippke, 1976; Mindel & Vernon, 1971). There has been a historic battle in the field of deafness between the *oralists* (oral language only through the use of lipreading and speech therapy) and the *sign language users*. The oralists maintain that if taught sign, the child will never learn to talk. The sign language proponents argue that the deaf child needs sign language for early concept development. Fortunately today there seems to be a softening of the lines and a general acceptance of the concept of total communication.

*Speechreading (lipreading)* would seem easy at first glance. However, consider that only one third of speech sounds are visible to the speech reader. In addition, many of the sounds made in English look alike. For example, *p, m,* and *b* are all made with the same lip movement (lips together). Try looking in the mirror or at a friend and saying *ma, pa,* and *ba* without voice; the problem is readily observed. Another example of look-alike movements would be *f* and *v*, which are both formed with the teeth to the lower lip.

*Cued speech* is a system of hand signs and positions to help speech readers distinguish between things that look the same on the lips (Ling, 1989).

*Sign language* is not one easily understood entity but involves many different methods. *Finger spelling* (dactylology) in the United States is done with one hand, each configuration representing a letter in the English alphabet (Figure 26-4). Finger spelling is used by itself or in conjunction with the other forms of sign language. Although it is not too difficult for the hearing person to learn to do, it is difficult to receive. When receiving or listening, the tendency is to see the individual letter and not the words. With finger spelling it is important that the hand be close enough to the face that the person with hearing impairment can see both the lip movements and the finger spelling at the same time. For fluency and readability, the hand has to be held in a comfortable position, not stiffly.

For simplification, sign language can be divided into *American Sign Language (ASL)* and *Signing Exact English (SEE)* (Fant, 1971; Klima & Bellugi, 1978). ASL is a language in itself, and it is not directly translatable to English. Although it is not universal, ASL is the primary language of persons with prelingual deafness in the United States. It has many abbreviations and phrases contained in a single sign and does not conform to the structure of English. SEE (Gustafson, Pfetzing, & Zawalkow, 1975), however, does conform to the structure and form of the English language and thus is preferred by many educators. There are many arguments for and against both these types and other types of sign. The important thing for the occupational therapist to realize and understand is the philosophy of the particular unit or school of which the child is a part. It is equally important to become as fluent as possible in that particular system. Obviously, for many it is impossible to learn but a few of the most simple and frequently used words and phrases, but this is important to the therapy of the child. Many good texts are available. However, it is best to attend a class or practice with a friend who knows sign because it is often difficult to correctly interpret the configuration and movement patterns of the hands.

The occupational therapist is often involved in the initial stages of learning sign. It is usually best to select the first signs to be taught from those that represent familiar objects, real-life situations, and familiar actions. Begin with what is available: things to feel, handle, or do. The parent can be given a likes-dislikes checklist to help the therapist know what is appropriate for the individual child. Often a food item is used first because of its value as a reward. The adult should work at the eye level of the child, obtain eye contact, do the sign, and then physically manipulate the child's hands through the sign. Some basic suggestions for the use of total communication are listed in the box on p. 726. It is hoped that, with total communication, the child will demonstrate earlier development of linguistic skills, better interpersonal relationships, and understanding of self and environment.

The occupational therapist also is often involved in the initial stages of *hearing aid use*. Often a history shows that the child had a hearing aid but rejected it. This can sometimes be traced to the lack of professional support for the parents and child during the difficult adjustment period or to the professional's lack of familiarity with the aid. It is regrettable when an instrument that can be of help to the child is not used. One of the problems that occurs is that the aid does not cause the child to hear normally, it only amplifies the sounds in the environment. It does not restore hearing as glasses can restore vision. It does not localize sounds but instead amplifies all sounds in the environment, thus leading to distortion. The therapist can help the parents and child by clarifying realistic expectations of the aid and what it can and cannot do for the child.

One of the main problems found in children with new

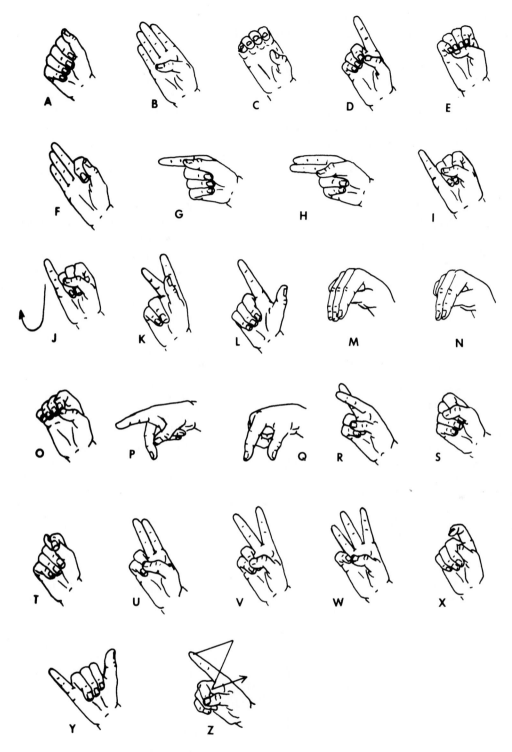

**Figure 26-4**    American one-hand manual alphabet.

aids is *tactile defensiveness*. The therapist can work on this with the parents and the child. The head is often the most sensitive portion of the body. The child must learn to think of the aid as a piece of clothing that is put on automatically in the morning along with shoes and socks. The earlier an aid is fitted to a child and put into use, the better the

chances for language development (Ling, 1989). The young infant learns much about language watching his or her mother's face while being held in her arms. The first need is to adjust to the feel of the aid. It is usually best to begin wearing the aid during a quiet activity that involves the speech of just one person. The maximal benefit from an aid is obtained in relatively quiet settings. Because the aid does not localize sounds, the following situations present difficulties: a place with a lot of background noise; a group with three to four people speaking at once; listening to reamplification such as with a television or tape recorder; and distance listening.

The hearing aid is a sensitive piece of equipment with several parts and can often be out of order. Everyone involved with the child should be aware of some of the common problems because an improperly working aid is use-less to the child. Some of the common problems are (1) dead batteries, (2) squeal—check for looseness of the cord or earmold, (3) batteries improperly placed or corroded, and (4) opening of earmold impacted with wax.

The type of hearing aid prescribed for a particular child depends on the degree and configuration of the loss (Northern & Downs, 1992). There are three major types of hearing aids. The *in the ear* aid is used only for mild losses and has no external wires. The *behind the ear* aid is usually for mild to severe losses and can be built into eyeglasses. It is a small unit made up of a microphone, amplifier, and receiver located together behind the ear and connected with a short tube to an earmold. The *body aid* is by far the type most commonly used with children. It is usually prescribed for marked to extreme losses. The microphone, amplifier, and power supply are together in a case carried in a pocket or harness worn by the child. The case is connected by small wires or earmolds seated directly in the ear. A monaural aid signifies just one aid, and binaural refers to the use of two separate aids. The parts of the body aid (Figure 26-5) are as follows:

1. *Microphone* picks up the sound waves and converts them to electric signals. It is usually behind a protective grill. The aid should always be worn with the microphone facing away from the body.
2. *Amplifier* increases the strength of the signal and is located inside the case.
3. *Battery* provides the energy source.
4. *Receiver cord* extends from the case to the ear and is the most vulnerable part of the aid.
5. *Receiver* changes the electric signals back to sound waves and is attached to the earmold.
6. *Earmold* is custom-formed of plastic to the shape of the individual's ear.

A *phonic ear* is often worn by children with hearing impairments in the classroom. The teacher wears a microphone that is directly connected to the child's phonic ear device.

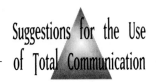

## Suggestions for the Use of Total Communication

1. Face the child squarely at eye level.
2. Position yourself so that the child can see your face and hands at the same time without strain.
3. Make sure you have the child's attention.
4. Avoid light behind you. If the child has to look into the light, he or she may be unable to clearly see your lips.
5. Use a normal tone of voice. Do not exaggerate mouth movements because this practice tends to confuse the lipreader.
6. Speak the word and give the sign at the same time, rather than in sequence.
7. Use appropriate pauses between words, especially when finger spelling is used.
8. Better results are obtained when you sit close to the child, rather than across the room.
9. Keep instructions simple and to the point.
10. Be consistent, especially with the young child.
11. Above all, *talk* to the child. He or she needs to receive the same amount of input as a hearing child, although the method may be altered.

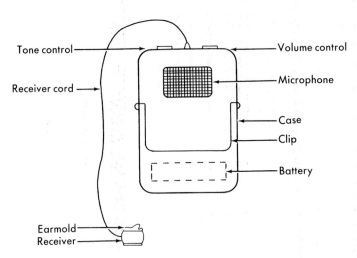

**Figure 26-5**   Diagram of a body aid.

Through this device the teacher's voice can be amplified for the students who have hearing loss without distortion of sound and for the other students in the classroom.

Cochlear implants are recently developed devices that can be surgically placed in children with profound hearing loss (Kreton & Balkany, 1991). The cochlear implant is attached to the cochlea and provides direct stimulation to the auditory nerve. This external stimulation acts as a substitute for the hair cells of the organ of Corti. The child wears four device components: a receiver buried in the temporal bone, an external microphone attached to a transmitter, a signal processor that records and electronically codes incoming sounds, and the cochlear implant. Although this technique brings state-of-the-art technology to the child's functional hearing ability, the degree of hearing improvement is variable. Therapists need to observe several precautions when working with children who have cochlear implants. The equipment is expensive, and the implant may become dislodged given certain types of physical activity. The equipment worn on the child's body (usually the chest) can easily be damaged during rough physical activity. This external equipment may also cause discomfort when the child is in certain positions, such as weight bearing on his or her chest.

### Preparation for Adulthood

The adolescent with hearing impairment must try to blend into a hearing world. Although this task is difficult, there have been many advances in social acceptance of individuals with hearing impairment. The growing technology of communication has improved future prospects. One of the important tasks of most adolescents is learning to drive a car. Most schools for the deaf have special driving training available. All students are taught by driving instructors to constantly scan the environment visually. To the student with hearing impairment, this is of utmost importance.

Another important aspect of blending into the hearing world is the use of the telephone, a daily communication device often taken for granted. The telephone companies have various forms of amplification devices available. Some hearing aids have a telephone setting. If amplification alone is not sufficient to understand conversation, the Telephone Typewriter (TTY) is available. The TTY is a communication device that uses the telephone lines with a typewriter keyboard to "talk" and a printout device to "listen," or receive, the conversation. The telephone ring is replaced with a flashing light or a fan that moves back and forth to indicate an incoming call. The obvious disadvantage is that both ends of the line need to be equipped with this system for it to work. Today technology is, however, making the system cheaper, easier to use, and more portable.

Television provides another aspect of daily life. The frequency of closed-captioned programs has increased, and in 1976 the Federal Trade Commission authorized the Public Broadcasting Service to develop more special programs for the deaf. At present, all televisions produced must provide closed-caption capability. The hearing impaired use a decoding device, a "black box," to view the same programs as the regular audience but with the addition of captions. Another approach is the use of a sign language interpreter in a cameo spot, but the disadvantage is that this is difficult to read on smaller television screens.

One medical problem of adolescents with hearing loss is of such magnitude that it should be mentioned: *Usher's syndrome*. This is a genetic disease that affects 3% to 6% of all people with congenital deafness. It is marked by the progressive blindness of *retinitis pigmentosa,* a degeneration of the retina that progresses from impaired night vision, to gradual constriction of the visual field with loss of peripheral vision, to blindness, usually by 20 to 30 years of age. There is much emphasis on early screening for this problem because of the obvious changes it would make in the education and vocational choice of the adolescent with hearing impairment.

Occupational choice has always been difficult for the deaf. Schein and Delk (1975) stated that the average worker with hearing loss earns 25% less than the average hearing worker and is usually employed in skilled manual labor. Gallaudet College in Washington, D.C., was for a long time the only place available to a deaf student for higher education. There are now many programs available where students with hearing loss are integrated with the hearing students because of the availability of special services such as interpreters and notetakers. California State University at Northridge and New York University have well-established model programs. The Americans with Disabilities Act (ADA) (1990) requires that all public education programs provide interpreters or notetakers when needed by persons with hearing impairment.

In addition to the obvious communication problem, there are three factors that adversely affect occupational choice for persons with hearing loss (Schein & Delk, 1975): (1) psychologic perception differences that affect self-perception and perception of reality, (2) restricted life space that adversely affects knowledge of areas outside of the immediate social or geographic area, and (3) limited sociocultural understanding. The occupational therapist, as part of an interdisciplinary team, can help alleviate these three blocks to fuller participation in occupation. For resources for additional study and information on hearing impairment, see the reference section of this chapter.

## VISUAL IMPAIRMENT
### Diagnostic Information

As with hearing impairment, the estimates of children with visual impairment vary with the criteria being applied. However, approximately 50 to 64 children per 100,000 have serious visual impairments, and at least another 100 chil-

## CASE STUDY #1

Ed is 2 years 3 months old. He had meningitis during the neonatal period with resultant hearing loss of a severe degree. Ed is the first and only child to date of this young couple. Both parents are employed. Ed attends a local day program for children younger than 3 with handicaps of all types. He has been assessed by use of the Gesell Developmental Scale and by subjective observation. Ed performed as follows:

*Motor area:* Ed passed all items at the 24-month level except the cube tower of six to seven, where he functioned at the 21-month level. Although he passed items such as walking up and down stairs alone, it should be noted that he often stumbled and appeared uncoordinated. However, on subjective observation, a great deal of this could be attributed to his "looking everywhere," that is, searching for visual output.

*Adaptive area:* Again Ed passed all items except for the cube tower and adaptation of form board. The item that requires repetition of three to four syllables was deleted from the testing. Distractability was noted.

*Language area:* Ed passed none of the items suitable for 24 months. He had vowel sounds and receptive total communication vocabulary of five words and no expressive vocabulary to date. He attempted to form words verbally and with sign language.

*Self-care:* Ed passed all items at the 24-month level except toileting items, communication items, and the play item of parallel play. He demonstrated domestic mimicry and would pull a person to show (21-month level).

As noted, Ed attends a day program with a teacher as the primary professional and with speech therapy, audiology, and occupational therapy as supportive services. Occupational and speech therapists are available on a half-time basis, and the audiologist is employed on a consulting basis.

**Treatment goals**

1. *Tactile desensitization* of the head and face area to promote acceptance of the hearing aid: activities such as rubbing different textures; touching different parts of face on therapist, self, dolls, and felt board (this activity also promotes body identification and sign skills); and playing dress-up with different hats.
2. *Improvement of fine motor coordination* through use of manipulative activities, with a variety of shapes, textures, and weights; eye-hand and tactile-discrimination are emphasized.
3. *Improvement of attention to activities* through activities such as mimicry games, vestibular stimulation activities such as self-regulated swinging in net and using rocker board, and use of "look" sign in gross motor playground activities.
4. *Consultation regarding toileting* to both school and home and establishment of schedule.

---

dren per 100,000 have less serious difficulties (Davidson, 1992). Total blindness is found in only a few children and is often a result of *anophthalmos* (absence of the eyeball). Hereditary causes account for approximately one half of all childhood blindness. Numerous low-incidence syndromes with eye and associated deformities are seen. *Retrolental fibroplasia* (Kinsey, 1956; Silverman, 1980) was a disease that surfaced shortly after World War II, when oxygen was used liberally to save the lives of premature infants. In the middle 1950s it was discovered that because the blood vessels of the eyes of premature infants are not fully developed, they are especially sensitive to oxygen. Raised oxygen levels cause hemorrhaging, followed by retinal detachment and the formation of a membrane behind the lens. Today, even with controlled oxygen use, *retinopathy of prematurity* (Ryan, Dawson, & Little, 1985) occurs in 25% to 30% of infants who weigh 1500 g or less at birth. Once the condition has been identified, it is difficult to determine whether the process will continue and become a major problem. It is estimated to cause an average of 550 cases of blindness yearly. The neurologic damage from *maternal substance abuse* can also cause visual deficits.

The legal definition of blindness is important to understand. In the United States it is defined as follows:

> Central visual acuity of 20/200 or less in the better eye after correction, or visual acuity of more than 20/200 if there is a field deficit in which the widest diameter of the visual field subtends to an angle distance no greater than 20 degrees (Sardegna & Paul, 1991, p. 31).

To put it more clearly for our understanding, this means that the child who is legally blind can see an object clearly at 20 feet that a child with normal vision can see at 200 feet. *Acuity* refers to central vision. The *peripheral vision*, or second part of the definition, means that the child can only see in a field of 20 degrees whereas a child with normal vision can see in a field of over 180 degrees. This peripheral vision is most important in mobility and general observation of the environment. There are some generally accepted gradations of acuity with correction (see box, p. 729). Acuity is not the

## Gradations of Acuity With Correction

| | |
|---|---|
| 20/20 to 20/70 | = Normal to slightly defective vision |
| 20/70 to 20/100 | = Mild visual limitation or good partial vision |
| 20/100 to 20/200 | = Moderate visual impairment or fair partial vision |
| 20/200 to 20/1,000 | = Legally blind with severe impairment |
| Over 20/1,000 | = 1. Finger counting ability |
| | 2. Form perception |
| | 3. Hand movement |
| | 4. Light perception (sees light and can tell where it is) |
| | 5. Light perception (sees light but cannot locate it) |

only factor in assessing vision, and two children with equal acuity can have different visual functions. Of course with many children it is difficult to know where and how a child sees. Spotty or irregular visual loss may occur in both the central and peripheral areas. The young child may use postural accommodation or head tilt to position to a focus point, or where he or she sees best.

As with the ear, it is important for the occupational therapist to have a basic understanding of the anatomy and physiology of the eye to understand visual impairment. The reader should review the anatomy of the eye on pp. 358 to 359.

Visual impairment can occur within the structures of the eyeball, at the retina, along the nerve pathway to the brain, and in the brain itself. *Refractive errors* occur when there is deviation in the course of the light rays as they pass through the eye, preventing sharp focus on the retina. The most common are the following (Ryan, Dawson, & Little, 1985):

1. *Myopia,* or *nearsightedness:* This child sees most clearly at close range and much less efficiently at a distance. The eyeball is too long or refractive power is too strong so that the focus point is in front of the retina; the child has blurred vision, possibly external strabismus when looking at a distance, and often holds printed material close to the eyes.
2. *Hyperopia,* or *farsightedness.* This child has blurred vision and may have headaches when trying to focus. The eyeball is too short and underdeveloped, the refractive power is too weak, and the focus point is behind the retina. This child sees most clearly at a distance and, with constant effort to focus at close range, becomes fatigued.

These refractive errors can usually be corrected with

lenses but can have a devastating effect on the development of the child in all areas if left undiagnosed or untreated during early school years.

*Cataracts* are often a congenital problem that give rise to poor vision. A cataract occurs when the lens of the eye changes from clear to cloudy or opaque. After removal of the lens, the child will have to wear corrective lenses. Although often the result of heredity, childhood cataracts have other common causes:

1. *Juvenile diabetes,* or other metabolic disease: Cataracts can occur as early as 3 years of age
2. *Down syndrome:* Approximately 60% of these children develop cataracts from 8 to 17 years of age
3. *Rubella,* or *German measles:* Approximately 75% of infants whose mothers contracted the disease within the first trimester will have cataracts at birth

*Glaucoma* is another visual problem that can occur in childhood. Glaucoma is an increase in the intraocular pressure of the eyeball resulting in hardening of the eye and damage to the cornea. The congenital type occurs in the first year of life, and the infantile type occurs between 6 and 12 years of age. It may be secondary to ocular inflammation or neurologic diseases.

There are many other eye conditions the occupational therapist may encounter. Some of the most important of these are listed here along with common optical terms (Perera, 1957).

*Amblyopia:* A condition of diminished visual acuity that usually cannot be relieved by lenses. The child may have depth perception problems and may tilt his or her head. Sometimes called lazy eye.

*Astigmatism:* Unequal curvature of the refractive surfaces of the eye. This may result in focusing problems because light is not sharply focused on the retina but spread over a more or less diffused area. Distorted images may result.

*Cortical blindness:* The ocular structures are intact, but the child is functionally blind because of severe insult to the visual cortex of the brain. Occurs as a result of near drowning or prolonged shock, for example.

*Coloboma:* Congenital defect of the eye because of its failure to complete growth in the part affected (usually the iris, choroid, or ciliary body).

*Microphthalmos:* An abnormally small eyeball.

*Nystagmus:* Rapid involuntary movement of the eyes. May be hereditary, and results in inability to fixate accurately and constantly. The movement is repetitive and may be lateral, vertical, rotary, or mixed.

*Optic atrophy:* Degeneration of the optic nerve fibers.

*Ptosis:* Drooping eyelid resulting from weak or absent muscle and usually does not interfere with vision.

*Retinoblastoma:* Malignant tumor of the retina and eye orbit, either unilateral or more often bilateral.

*Strabismus:* Squint or cross-eyes. Failure of the eyes to converge properly on an image, or both eyes not directed at the same point. This condition is often caused by muscle imbalance and often results in double vision. In esotropia the eye turns inward; in exotropia the eye turns outward; in vertical strabismus the eye turns up or down.

*Toxoplasmosis:* Parasitic disease that can be congenital or acquired from household pets; causes scarring, usually on retina and choroid.

Any of these conditions may affect visual acuity. Visual acuity is most often tested with the use of the *Snellen chart.* This tests central acuity with letters, numbers, or symbols in graded sizes drawn to Snellen measurements. Each size is labeled with the distance it can be seen by the normal eye. The child stands 20 feet from the chart and indicates to the examiner what he or she sees line by line. Eye report terms include *OD,* which refers to the right eye, *OS,* to the left eye, and *OU,* to both eyes.

## Other Services

Children with visual impairment often have a number of other professionals involved in their treatment. The most common are the following:

*Ophthalmologist:* A physician who specializes in the diagnosis and treatment of defects and diseases of the eye, performing surgery when necessary, and prescribing other types of treatment, including corrective lenses.

*Optometrist:* A licensed specialist in vision (OD) who is trained in the art and science of vision care. Specializes in the examination of the eyes and the preservation and restoration of vision by optometric means; measures refractive errors and eye muscle disorders.

*Optician:* A person who grinds lenses, fits them into frames, and adjusts frames to the wearer.

*Orientation and mobility specialist:* An individual specializing in orientation and mobility training of the visually impaired. *Orientation* is the process of using the remaining senses to establish one's position and relationship to all other significant objects in one's environment. *Mobility* is the ability to move safely and efficiently from one point to another in the environment.

## Practice Settings

The child with visual impairment is more likely to be identified earlier in life than the child with hearing impairment. The occupational therapist encounters these children in the neonatal and acute units of the hospital. Children with visual impairment often are referred by pediatricians to outpatient clinics for developmental testing and treatment because the effects of visual impairment are evident in the development of mobility and manipulation. Therefore these children are often identified in the first year of life and begin to receive services from local early intervention programs. The number of children with visual impairment who attend state schools has been drastically reduced in recent years with the advent of integrated community programs. The therapist is involved in both community and state school settings.

## Special Characteristics Relevant to Occupational Therapy

Children with visual impairments typically incur delays in developmental skills across domains. Children with visual impairment have to learn about the world with their hands. Children with normal sight develop eye-hand coordination early in life, but children with severe visual impairment have to wait for ear-hand coordination to come at a later stage in development. They need good tactile system performance for exploration and concept development (Lydon & McGraw, 1973). These children have to pick up a ball and feel it to tell if it is round: there is no other way to develop that concept and know what *round* means. Yet, because of their blindness these children often exhibit tactile defensiveness. They also need to learn to move their bodies to understand how they move and to understand spatial aspects of the environment. Blindness itself often results in fear of movement. The blind child has difficulty progressing through the developmental sequence of random-to-purposeful movements.

Among the limitations imposed by visual impairment, three are key to development. *Mobility* is restricted because of the child's inability to visualize the environment with its potential obstacles and dangers. *Understanding of the physical environment,* is limited, particularly in shape, form, distance, and object relationships. Finally, *communication* is often delayed because the child cannot read body language or gestures and does not see the physical cuing that accompanies speech (Lowerfeld, 1969). Behaviors and mannerisms particular to blindness can occur, and many authors trace these to early sensory deprivation (Fraiberg, 1977; Jastrzembska, 1976). Children with blindness are deprived of adequate visual stimuli and are often secondarily deprived of tactile, vestibular, kinesthetic, and proprioceptive stimuli because of the lack of mobility. Further, because of the lack of stimuli, these children are often extremely resistant to change, setting up a cycle reinforcing resistance to new stimuli. Also, as toddlers, they walk late and are not as mobile as children with normal sight. Studies of animal deprivation (Jastrzembska, 1976) clearly show that sensory deprivation during the formative periods can result in the failure of the deprived system to ever achieve maximal development. Multisensory deprivation has an even more pronounced effect.

Hendrickson (1969) discussed some of the implications of blindness for concept development. Concept development is affected by vision loss. Vision is normally used to identify the position of things in space, to recognize shapes without feeling them, and to know the length of a room without pacing it. These concepts and many more have to be acquired by the child with visual impairment by alternate means.

*Blindisms* may also develop. These include eye poking and flicking hands. Such actions appeal to children because they break up light and change what little they are able to see. However, blindisms make it impossible for them to try to use residual vision for purposeful activity. Blindisms need to be limited and activity diverted to other more productive avenues (Halliday, 1970; Thurnell & Rice, 1970).

## Developmental Considerations

Developmental differences characteristic of children with visual impairment are important for the therapist to know when planning intervention. The usual developmental scales can be used with notation as to the child's impairment. Every area of development is affected, but it still should be kept in mind that generalizations may not apply. The infant with normal sight takes hold of the world with his or her eyes in the first weeks of life (Gesell, Ilg, & Bullis, 1967). The infant has monocular fixation at first, but by the eighth week, binocular vision is dominant. The infant has sustained fixation on a nearby object (e.g., mother's face) during the first week and on more distant objects by the end of the first month. The typical infant develops eye-hand coordination by 5 months, perfecting the accuracy of visually guided reach and grasp by 12 months. This performance contrasts sharply with the infant with visual impairment, who develops *ear-hand coordination* (the ability to locate and reach for sound), but not until almost the end of the first year. This ear-hand coordination begins at about the 10- to 12-month level, (Fraiberg, 1977); but does not reach proficiency until the second year of life.

The typically developing child learns to associate visual experiences with symbolism, and although vision always retains a concrete core, the child learns to associate visual experiences with words. The absence of the association of words with visual experiences explains why, although the child with visual impairment receives the same auditory stimuli, *language development* is affected. Pronouns can be especially difficult for the young child to understand. The child with visual impairment often learns to use language for reassurance or as an attention-getting device.

*Gross motor development* is generally greatly affected by visual limitation. The infant with visual impairment clings to the parent's shoulder like the infant with normal sight but will not spontaneously turn his or her head as will the child with normal sight (Adelson & Fraiberg, 1974). The prone position without sight is not particularly interesting or comfortable. A fixed supine position is definitely preferred. The child with visual impairment learns to creep, if at all, only after the development of ear-hand coordination. Often the child prefers to scoot on the back to move around.

The child with visual loss typically demonstrates a delay in crawling of approximately 6 months. Sitting usually develops within established norms because it is a static position, but the child with visual loss may have to be positioned in sitting, demonstrating difficulty with fluid movement to and from sitting. Also, time spent in this position is limited because of the lack of the visual stimulation that motivates the child's attention. Standing is also a static position and occurs roughly within the normal age range. However, walking is a dynamic movement and may be delayed by approximately 7 months (Adelson & Fraiberg, 1974). Walking involves a self-initiated movement, and the child with visual loss needs to learn the hazards and layout of the environment. Stair climbing also is delayed and requires a great deal of guidance. The typical climbing and exploring of the 18- to 24-month-old child does not take place spontaneously.

*Fine motor development* is strongly affected by the loss of eye-hand coordination. The child with visual loss sits and manipulates toys within reach, but once out of reach, the toy disappears. The sound of a familiar noise toy is not spontaneously connected with the feel of the toy. The child develops age-appropriate object transfer and hand play at midline, but reach for and release of objects may well be delayed.

In the *social-emotional area* a delay in the development of play may be anticipated. A doll or a toy truck initially has no meaning. As miniatures of visual objects, these are difficult to perceive. Parallel play and mimicry are difficult to learn without the opportunity to see and imitate others.

Development of peer relationships can be difficult because the child cannot see the smile or the frown of playmates. The child with visual impairment may find it difficult to accurately read the feelings of others without the clues of body language and facial expressions.

Feeding may well be delayed by parental apprehension about the mess and by the child's initial difficulty in finding and prehending the food. Also, many children with vision loss have difficulty weaning away from familiar and comforting routines such as the use of the bottle. Feeding problems involve tactile sensitivity and the child's natural resistance to change. Difficulty in introducing new foods, storing food in cheeks, spitting out different textures, and finding and sorting out lumps are all common feeding behaviors.

Perceptual skill development is delayed. Discrimination of shape and space, which normally appears from 12 to 18 months, does not occur in the child with visual impairment until 24 to 36 months (Robbins, 1960). Concept development is problematic. The child with vision loss experiences difficulty learning that one word signifies many different tactile experiences. For example, a chair can have many different shapes, sizes, and textures, but all related forms are identified by that one word.

Figure 26-6 lists some critical observations in functional

*Posture:* Is the child's head up and held at midline? Often the head is down or the child displays unusual posturing. This needs to be noted because of its relation to the prevention of back problems and the promotion of social acceptance. Caution must be taken in interpreting unusual postures or head tilts as these may be natural ways for the child to try to see most effectively.

*Balance and stability:* Can the child maintain a position well? How good is his or her balance on one foot? This is important for mobility training.

*Ambulation and gait:* Is the gait stiff? Are the steps normal in size? How does the child manage on stairs or uneven surfaces?

*Strength and tone:* Is the child's tone normal, and is strength adequate for age? Such children often have low tone because of the lack of movement.

*Endurance:* Can the child pursue a gross or fine motor task for an appropriate length of time?

*Coordination:* The dexterity of children who have visual impairment can be subjectively assessed on tests, such as the Minnesota Rate of Manipulation Test (MRMT). The MRMT in particular has norms for the blind.

*Identification of body planes and body parts:* Does the child know front from back? Can he or she identify body parts at an age-appropriate level? The child who is visually impaired needs to know "boundaries of self."

*Laterality:* Can the child identify right and left on self and others and locate objects placed to either side? This is necessary in exploring the environment.

*Directionality:* Can the child tell which direction to go to reach an object or person, moving or stationary?

*Controlled isolated body movements:* Are extraneous movements present? Control is important for work and school skills, as well as social acceptance.

*Tactile discrimination:* Can the child use his or her hands and body to their fullest to explore?

*Auditory discrimination:* Can the child discriminate distances of sound and types of sound and identify different people by voice?

*Spatial orientation:* Is the child able to judge distances? This is important in mobility.

**Figure 26-6**  Observation of the child with visual impairment.

assessment of children with visual impairments (Cratty, 1971; Warner, 1984). The list is not all-inclusive and would vary according to the particular situation and the child's developmental level.

The therapist may wish to administer portions of the Sensory Integration and Praxis Test to the child. Several parts of the test do not require sight, and others can be adapted. The scores should not be strictly interpreted because the test has not been standardized for individuals with visual impairment. However, test results can give important information on the child's spatial awareness or orientation, proprioception, and tactile awareness or orientation. Parts of the

test that can be administered most readily include finger Identification, Graphesthesia, Localization of Tactile Stimuli, Standing Balance, Kinesthesia, Praxis on verbal command, and the parts of the Manual Form Perception and Standing and Walking Balance tests. Any interpretation of postrotary nystagmus responses would be difficult because children with visual impairment often have ocular nystagmus as part of their visual deficit.

### Specialized Assessments

There are several tests especially adapted or devised for use with individuals with visual impairment. One of special interest to therapists and psychologists is the *Maxfield-Buchholz Social Maturity Scale for Blind Pre-School Children* (Maxfield & Buchholz, 1995). It is an adapted version of the Vineland Social Maturity Scale and helps obtain an accurate developmental picture of an individual child. The Maxfield-Buchholz scale covers seven areas of the Vineland scale: self-help general, self-help dressing, self-help eating, communication, socialization, locomotion, and occupation. The Maxfield-Buchholz scale is designed for preschoolers to children of the 5- to 6-year level. Of the 95 items on the Maxfield-Buchholz scale, 44 are from the Vineland scale. The Maxfield-Buchholz items were all standardized with children with visual impairment and give the examiner information about how children compare with each other. It is administered exactly as the original Vineland scale: the parent or caregiver gives information about the performance of the child.

Another test of interest is the *Reynell-Zinkin Developmental Scales for Young Visually Handicapped Children* (Reynell & Zinkin, 1979). Similar to the Bayley Scales, the Reynell-Zinkin has two parts—one covering mental development and one assessing motor development. The mental scales include sections on social adaptation, sensorimotor understanding, exploration of the environment, response to sound and verbal comprehension, expressive language, and communication. The motor scales cover hand function, locomotion, and reflexes. They use a profile-type of scoring, and standard scores are not available. Age equivalents are given, however, for children 0 to 5 years old with and without visual impairment.

The *Oregon Project Developmental Checklist* (Brown, Simmons, & Mathvin, 1984) has also been developed for assessing the child with visual impairment up to 6 years of age and for writing educational and treatment objectives. It covers the areas of socialization, self-help, fine motor, cognition, language, and gross motor. This checklist also takes into account the fact that there is a vast difference in the degree of visual impairment by indicating items that are acquired at a later age or that may not be appropriate at all for children with total vision loss. Several intelligence tests have also been adapted for use with the visually impaired, including the Binet and the Wechsler. Other oral tests are easily adaptable. The American Foundation for the Blind publishes a comprehensive listing of psychologic, vocational, and educational tests appropriate for use with the visually impaired.

*Visual testing* has had many subjective and objective aspects. As with audiologic testing, it is becoming more sophisticated with increased technology. In addition to the Snellen-type acuity examinations, there are others developed to test young children and retarded children. Sheridan (1969) published a series of vision tests including such items as matching distant pictures to objects on a table. Observation of the young child's functional vision is important; the child's use of objects and toys often provides the skilled observer with more information than the actual physical examination. The subjective description of functional vision from the parent, teacher, or therapist can add greatly to the physician's assessment. Physicians use an ophthalmoscope to view the internal structure of the eye. Electroretinography (ERG) can be done under sedation for a thorough examination of the retina and fundus. A visual evoked response (VER) test may be done with the use of an electroencephalogram to assess cortical response to light stimulation. Results of these tests provide information about the function of the eye, the optic nerve, and the visual cortex.

The *Erhardt Developmental Vision Assessment (EDVA)* (Erhardt, 1989) measures development of ocular-motor skills from birth to 6 months. This assessment is divided into a section on primarily involuntary visual patterns (eyelid reflexes, pupillary reactions, and doll's eye responses) and a section on voluntary patterns (fixation, localization, ocular pursuit, and gaze shift). It can be helpful to the therapist in determining the child's developmental level of functional ocular-motor abilities.

## Objectives and Activities of Intervention

The occupational therapist may be the primary therapist for a child with visual impairment but most often works with a team that includes the special educator, the physical therapist, and the orientation and mobility specialist. Other professionals are involved as the child's needs indicate. The treatment plan is based on the individual assessment of the child. The following are some typical intervention goals for this group:

1. *To develop self-care skills at age-appropriate times.* The therapist can consult with those who work with the child about the developmental sequence of self-care skills. The therapists may physically guide the child through eating and dressing activities. If abnormal eating patterns develop and are not corrected, they usually become ingrained patterns. Good supportive seating is important to the self-feeding process. For dressing, differential tabs can be sewn on clothing to indicate front and back. The child needs practice time with buttons and zippers. Toilet train-

ing can be facilitated by (1) a consistent schedule, (2) an established route to the bathroom, (3) the familiar sounds and smells of the room, (4) consistent use of one or two words for toileting, and (5) establishing an association between changing wet clothes and going to the bathroom.

2. *To enhance sensory integration.* The child with blindisms needs considerable vestibular stimulation from tilt boards, swings, and scooters. Sensory feedback in children who are blind is interrupted and can cause distortion of movement (deQuiros, 1976). It is important, however, that safety be maintained in the use of equipment and that the child be allowed to control the movement. Excessive fear of falling, poor grasp of room layout, and inability to organize or cross midline are all indications of difficulty in sensory integration. Van Benschoter (1975) outlined a successful summer camp experience for children who are blind that stressed sensory integrative programming. Children at the camp aged 6 to 21 years were given a sensory integration treatment program that had a positive effect on the movement skills of the children involved. Baker-Nobles and Bink (1979) studied three adults who, after 6 months of sensory integration treatment, improved in areas of mobility, activities of daily living, handwriting, and behavior.

3. *To encourage movement in space.* The infant's position must be changed often early in life to counteract the resistance to movement and change. Prone positions should be encouraged. The underdevelopment of dynamic movements, such as crawling and walking, cannot be totally eliminated, but much can be done in the therapy setting to help compensate for these. Crawling over different surfaces and movements on bolsters, therapy balls, and other objects are helpful activities. A chair or wagon can be pushed to develop security in walking. Balance activities are helpful to decrease fear of movement. General strengthening is often indicated because children with visual impairment may be weak because of their lack of mobility and passivity. Resisted creeping and moving heavy objects to build an obstacle course may improve strength.

4. *To develop maximal tactile perceptual abilities.* The child with visual impairment obviously needs to maximize tactile abilities to learn about the environment and eventually read braille, if he or she will need it. Activities such as finger painting, finding and identifying objects hidden in sand or beans, and identifying gradations of textures and puzzles are among those that increase tactile awareness.

5. *To decrease tactile defensiveness.* The child with visual impairment does not see the approach of people and objects and can exhibit a defensive reaction to touch. Use of a firm touch is better than a light touch,

which can be interpreted as being aversive, such as a tickle. Techniques to decrease tactile defensiveness include activities using graded textures and exploration and play with various material, such as sand, dried lentils, beans, and rice. Activities that include vibration or proprioceptive input are often helpful.

6. *To encourage use of hands for manipulation.* At first the world has to come to the child. Toys should be maintained within reach (tied to the crib, walker, or table top). Practice of in-hand manipulation activities that involve rotation and translation of small objects can dynamically improve use of tools.

7. *To encourage knowledge of parts of the body and body planes.* The child has to know his or her own body before understanding how it moves and fits into the environment. Body image is important to mobility and social function (Cratty, 1971). Obstacle courses can teach the child how large his or her body is in relation to other objects. Touching body parts on others is helpful. Use of a vibrator may increase body awareness. Life-size dolls can also be used.

8. *To encourage laterality and directionality.* Especially for mobility skills, a child who is blind must know the concepts of right-left, up-down, and in-out. The child must develop the awareness that things outside the body have sides and must be able to measure distance and direction.

9. *To provide education and consultation to family members.* The parents and the family of the child with visual impairment should be encouraged to handle the child as they would an infant without disability. Verbal and physical interaction should be encouraged because the child may not always demand interaction. The family should be informed about the importance of early intervention and their options for services. Occupational therapists may consult with parents on ways to create a safe environment in which the child can play unsupervised. They often make recommendations for adapting the environment to optimize the independent functioning of the child.

10. *To maximize residual vision.* The therapists should always use whatever vision the child has in the treatment program activities. The more a child uses visual pathways, the better his or her vision develops (Barraga, 1964). Visual awareness and discrimination activities are important, such as color or shape recognition and matching. Activities such as use of a flashlight in a darkened room may improve visual skills.

The following goals are generally addressed by the team, of which the occupational therapist is a contributing member:

11. *To encourage socially acceptable behaviors.* The child should be encouraged to look at people when they speak, to smile appropriately, to keep the head up in midline, and to avoid posturing. He or she must learn how others are reacting based on voices rather than gestures, facial expressions, or body language. Hill (1977), in her article on intervention with preschoolers, stressed the area of parental and professional encouragement of socially acceptable behaviors in children with visual impairments.

12. *To encourage language and concept development.* The child must consciously be taught to develop cognitive schemes that the sighted child picks up in a relatively casual manner. This is done with verbalization and the use of the remaining senses. Those things that cannot be touched or heard, such as clouds, need to be explained.

13. *To strengthen cognitive skills such as object permanence, cause and effect, object recognition, and ability to match and sort.* Games and many simple craft activities can easily be used to accomplish these goals. The unique abilities and limitations of the child must be considered in addressing academic goals.

14. *To develop maximal auditory perceptual abilities.* The child with visual impairment has to learn to identify sounds and their meanings and react to them appropriately. Sounds come from three basic sources: toys, speech, and the environment. Active rather than passive listening should be emphasized. Activities such as locating a squeak toy, identifying sounds such as cars and trains, and following directions from persons and recordings are helpful.

## Special Techniques

Children with severe visual handicaps usually have to rely on braille and talking books for their education. For the person who will eventually use braille in school, the importance of early tactile perceptual training cannot be overemphasized. Braille is a system of six raised dots arranged in a cell (Figure 26-7). These dots are arranged in various configurations to represent the letters of the alphabet, numbers, and words (Rugers, 1969). Braille can be written in three levels or grades, depending on the degree of contraction used. It is read left to right with one or two hands. Usually the index finger is used with a light touch. Braille was developed by a young blind French student, Louis Braille, in 1824 and was found to be more efficient than attempting to read the raised Roman alphabet. Speeds do vary, but 104 words per minute is the average, which makes it quite useful in the educational setting. Braille is produced on a special slate or machine called a *braillewriter.*

Talking books are also available for almost any subject at any age level. The young child with visual impairment can be tuned in to listening with short storytelling sessions. The adult should carefully monitor the child's attention to promote good listening skills. Scratch-and-sniff books and

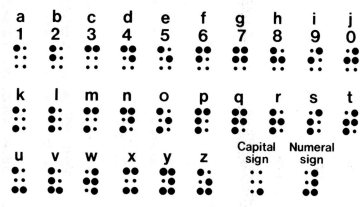

**Figure 26-7**   Braille alphabet and numbers.

tactile books are also available to help in early storytelling. Large-print books may be used by those who can discriminate a large typeface.

Various types of lenses are available for people with visual impairment, from the relatively common ones used to correct refractive errors to telescopic and microscopic lenses that are used as low vision aids with certain types of blindness. There are also projection devices and magnifying devices such as the opticon, which converts inkprint into a readable vibrating tactile form.

In *mobility training* such techniques as using the Seeing Eye dog, sighted guides, and long canes are taught (Kaarela & Widerberg, 1970; Welsh & Blasch, 1980). The techniques of echo detection, trailing, and body protection are also important. Seeing Eye dogs are specially selected and expertly trained. Sighted guides usually walk a half-step in front of the person with visual impairment, who holds the guide's arm just above the elbow with fingers inside (next to guide's body) and the thumb outside. A small child may do better holding the guide's wrist. With this use of the sighted guide, body movement on uneven surfaces and changes of direction can best be perceived. Should the person with visual impairment need to change sides, the guide gives a verbal clue and the guided person slides over, tracing a finger along the guide's waist in back of the guide, switching hands to the guide's opposite elbow. In going through a narrow passage the guide puts his other elbow behind his or her waist as a clue and the person with visual impairment falls back to a full step behind the guide with the elbow straight and more directly in back rather than to the side. For stairs, the sighted guide gives a verbal indication of stairs ahead, whether they are up or down, as well as information on rail availability and placement. One technique is for the guide to pause and turn at a right angle to the person with visual impairment and they go down one step at a time in a foot-to-step fashion with the guide one step ahead of the person who is blind. Another technique involves using the rail, if available, as the guide goes down or up, without turning, one step ahead of the guided person. Cane tech-

nique is also a specialized procedure that requires the training skills of a professional in the field.

Although as a rule the orientation and mobility specialist is the one who teaches trailing and body protection, there are certain basic principles that the occupational therapist should know. Trailing is the use of a wall as a guide for walking. The hand closest to the wall is extended at hip level until the outside of the little finger touches the wall, then the back of the fingertips are used to guide the person in walking. In the protection technique the upper arm is held at shoulder height and parallel to the floor with the palm facing out to meet any obstacle before the body does. The lower arm is extended downward and forward with the palm facing out. Another protection technique is to extend the arm palm out in front of the head while bending down to retrieve a dropped object. The child with visual impairment can search for a lost object by touching the ground to establish a beginning point and then searching in an ever-widening concentric circle pattern. A technique for exploring a room is to search the parameters of the room first, then mentally divide it into grids to be methodically searched. This is extremely helpful in introducing the child with vision loss to a new classroom or new home setup. The use of landmarks and clues, such as the grass edge of the sidewalk, are important for independent travel, as is the idea of "squaring off" or using one point of reference to locate another. Chairs can be approached from the side and checked with hands before sitting.

*Low vision training* is another specialized technique (Barraga, 1964; Fonda, 1970). Some educational personnel specialize in this method. The basic premise is that the child can be taught to use vision. Visual acuity is, by itself, not really the most important part of visual ability. Through planned stimulation, visual efficiency can be increased. Often light is used initially to increase focusing ability. Once fixation is achieved, the child can learn to discriminate global aspects of the image. When this happens, the child can move on to analyze discrete elements of the image and finally to identify form, outline, and other aspects. Obviously this method does not work with all children with visual impairment, but it does have good results with others, especially when combined with a good overall program to heighten the child's levels of perception.

*High technology* with increasing use of sophisticated electronics and miniature computers continue to result in positive results for training people with visual impairment. Schaefer and Specht (1979) discuss the use of one such device in occupational therapy—a light sensor that enables the blind to detect variable light intensities and that may be adapted to various industrial uses in rehabilitation training. Other advances that give individuals with visual impairment access to computers include voice-activated software and keys with braille. Computers can increase the quantity and quality of written output. They often provide opportunities for interactive learning with sound capabilities. Given the versatility and increasing capacities of computers, this technology holds great promise for persons with visual impairments related to school and vocational success.

### Preparation for Adulthood

The most obvious challenge for the adolescent who is blind is the choice of an appropriate occupation. Almost all textbooks are available in braille or talking books. An appropriate fit between the personality and talent areas of the adolescent can result in a successful and enduring career. Lack of exposure to many vocational options can be a problem that the occupational therapist can address through community orientation and various activities to give the child more prevocational experiences.

There are certain mannerisms that should be discussed because these behaviors often interfere with optimal social interaction. Again, these are things that the therapist and all the other professionals involved with the child should work to eliminate:

1. Standing in the personal space of others
2. Rocking the body
3. Blinking, rubbing, or rolling the eyes
4. Stamping or shuffling the feet
5. Not looking at a person when speaking

Daily living skills such as cooking, cleaning, and recreation become increasingly important as the child with visual impairment reaches adolescence. The American Foundation for the Blind puts out a comprehensive list of aids and appliances. For the kitchen there are such devices as a sugar meter that dispenses one half a teaspoon of sugar at a time and an elbow-length oven mitt to prevent accidental burning. A canned goods marking kit is available, as well as self-threading needles and tools with marking gauges. For recreational activities there are braille cards and low vision cards, as well as table games such as Scrabble and Monopoly with braille markings.

Self-care can be facilitated by careful organization of the wardrobe and tactile clues for color of clothing. Handling money and shopping can be difficult tasks and require much training and assistance.

Leisure time activities are important for well-rounded adulthood. Exercise groups, weight lifting, dance classes, and bowling are all excellent physical activities that should be encouraged because many adults who are blind lead sedentary lives. Persons with visual impairment can play ball sports with sound balls and can run or jog with minimal track guidance aids. For resources for additional study and information on visual impairment, see pp. 741 to 742.

## MULTIPLE SENSORY IMPAIRMENT (DEAF-BLIND AND MULTIPLY IMPAIRED)
### Diagnostic Information

There is one important concept to understand regarding any multiple involvement, that is, any combination of visual, hearing, cognitive, and motor disabilities: The result is not just a simple addition of the results of the handicaps, but rather a *multiplication of disability.* This combination of sensory losses with each other and with other problems presents the most devastating results, and the interaction of the problems has to be considered.

A common challenge for the occupational therapist is the child whose primary problem is a physical disability or mental retardation and who additionally has visual or hearing deficits. Whenever a developing brain incurs injuries (such as in cerebral palsy), the chances of multiple resulting impairments are great. For instance, 50% of children with cerebral palsy have some visual deficit and 13% have some form of auditory problem; the percentages of visual and auditory deficits are also high for children with mental retardation. With both of these diagnoses, accurate assessment of acuity, awareness, and perception is often difficult because these children do not always give reliable feedback to the examiner.

Another special problem encountered in the therapy setting is deaf-blindness. Many diagnoses are known to cause loss of both vision and hearing. Embryologic studies show that there is much similarity in the time-table of development of the eye and the ear (Smith, 1982). Therefore many diagnoses involve both systems, for example, cytomegalovirus infections, toxoplasmosis, congenital syphilis, Hurler's syndrome, Waardenburg's syndrome, and Goldenhar's syndrome. Meningitis is the leading cause of noncongenital deaf-blindness in children.

### Other Services

An extraordinary number of professionals may be involved with children who have multiple disabilities. Orthopedists, neurologists, and cardiologists are a few medical specialists whose expertise is often needed. As the severity of the child's disability increases, so does the chance that the occupational therapist will become involved. The occupational

## CASE STUDY #2

Bonnie is 7 years 4 months old. She had congenital cataracts removed during her first year of life. Her resultant condition is legal blindness with form perception. Bonnie is the third and last child of a couple who have divorced since her birth. The mother works while Bonnie attends a local grammar school where she is included in a regular second grade class. She has been assessed informally by the therapist, and parts of the Bruininks Oseretsky Test of Motor Proficiency have been administered. Bonnie performs as follows:

*Motor area:* Bonnie can trail in familiar settings such as home and school but needs a sighted guide for unfamiliar areas. Her gait is shuffling and hesitant, and she fears falling. Balance activities are difficult, and she can only stand on one foot momentarily. She has difficulty with motor planning. Her coordination skills, grasp, and pinch are age-appropriate.

*Language area:* On the school testing she is 1 to 2 years behind in vocabulary. She enjoys music and talking books. Her attention span is variable and auditory discrimination is poor for sound location.

*Personal-social area:* Bonnie was in an infant stimulation program before school placement and has acquired some play skills but remains shy and withdrawn especially in playground activities and physical education. She feeds herself, but her mother has a great deal of difficulty getting her to dress herself. The mother attributes this in part to her own inability to "let go."

As noted, Bonnie is in a regular second grade class. She receives occupational therapy as well as special education services three times a week. She attends regular physical education with some adaptation of requirements.

**Treatment goals**

1. *To increase balance, motor planning, and equilibrium skills* by using swing, bolster, tilt board, and scooter activities and counseling with the teacher and the physical education instructor to provide tactile input for planning motor activities.
2. *To increase dressing skills* by providing counseling to the mother regarding age-appropriate dressing skills. Practicing with the child on manipulation of fasteners and use of tactile strips for clothing identification, and home visits to observe and assist in arranging clothing for ease of identification.
3. *To increase social skills* by assisting the child plan and participating in group activities with small groups of her classmates; cooking or craft projects might be used.

**Individual education plan objectives for the present school year**

1. Bonnie will be able to stand and balance on one foot for 10 seconds.
2. Bonnie will be able to manipulate buttons, snaps, and zippers 100% of the time.
3. Bonnie will plan with the therapist four group activities during the school year.

---

therapist may be a major team member, especially with the physically involved child who has visual deficits or with the child who is both deaf and blind. Often the occupational therapist's first contact with visual or hearing impairment is through a child with multiple disabilities.

## Practice Settings

The number of children with multiple sensory handicaps is often too small to establish an effective local program. The number of residential placements tends to rise with the level of impairment. Also, as children grow older they need more specialized programming. Although most professionals favor local programs that allow children to live at home, there are definite advantages to residential programs as the child matures.

1. Continuity of program and skills training

2. Twenty-four-hour care and supervision
3. Transition for those who will always need assistance

## Special Characteristics Relevant to Occupational Therapy

Some behaviors are characteristic of children who are deaf-blind. Typically they show extreme tactile defensiveness. They do not like anything new or different, and changes of any type are not well accepted. Often the child exhibits oral defensiveness, and the change from smooth to textured foods is difficult. Neuromotor function is often affected by hypotonicity and hypermobility of the joints or by spasticity. Such children usually learn to walk but are delayed and cautious about giving up support. They can go from walking holding onto a wooden stick, then a smaller stick, then a piece of rope, then a piece of yarn, then a thread and still immediately fall if the thread is taken away. They often have had difficult infancy periods, setting up a cycle of negative reactions to parental handling that led to less and less parental handling. Stimuli may not make sense to children who are deaf-blind, so they ignore it or respond in a defensive manner (McInnes & Teffry, 1982). They can have many primitive withdrawal reactions and can seem autistic. Blindisms such as eye poking, eye rubbing, flicking hands in front of eyes, head bumping, hair twirling, and rocking are often present and can become self-abusive. Perseverative behaviors are common, as are teeth grinding and masturbation. Certainly, every child is different and may manifest these behaviors to different degrees.

With the child who has visual or hearing impairment and physical or cognitive disabilities, characteristics such as autistic-like behaviors, tactile defensiveness, and resistance to change can be noted. One of the important characteristics for the occupational therapist to keep in mind is that these children need consistent repetition to learn skills. Progress can be made but often is extremely slow. A simple task, such as learning the hand-to-mouth pattern necessary for self-feeding, may well take years of hand-over-hand practice with multiple clues and much consistency. Campbell, McInerney, and Cooper (1984) found that functional patterns of movement were achieved at faster rates when children with multiple disabilities were able to practice the desired movement patterns more frequently; therefore specific techniques were taught to school staff and parents. The therapist assesses the child and identifies specific tasks or movements to be targeted, determines the appropriate intervention strategies, and instructs others to carry out the tasks or movements with accuracy. Training of caretakers and school staff becomes extremely important. The role of the occupational therapist is often that of consultant. Consultation and monitoring to promote self-care skills such as dressing requires that the therapist develop rapport with the persons doing the training and develop the ability to encourage and reward others to help them follow the program correctly. In many cases written programs with diagrams or pictures are used, and the directions need to be clear and simple without confusing medical jargon. Monitoring entails not just observing others implement a program but doing it oneself on occasion to receive direct feedback about the child's performance. Direct service based on specific goals is also given, but the pervasive characteristics of the child who has multiple impairments necessitates involvement of all personnel in attaining developmental skills.

## Occupational Therapy Assessment Procedures

Developmental scales can be used for assessment and treatment planning for children with visual and hearing impairments. Of special interest are the prehension and tactile abilities because almost everything has to be taught in a hand-over-hand manner. The Callier-Asuza Scale (Stillman, 1973) is a checklist for use with this population. It has five areas of subscales: motor development, daily living skills, language development, perceptual abilities, and socialization. It covers developmental skills up to approximately the age of 7 and is based on observations of spontaneous behaviors in structured and unstructured situations. Each subscale is further divided; for example, the daily living skills subscale consists of dressing and undressing, personal hygiene, development of feeding skills, and toileting. The directions specify that it should be administered by an individual familiar with the child. The teacher or therapist should spend a substantial period (at least 2 weeks) working directly with the child before attempting to use the checklist. It is also suggested that aides, parents, and others be consulted about their observations of the child to obtain the most accurate picture.

A complete descriptive assessment of levels in all areas of development must be done for children who have physical or mental disabilities in addition to visual and auditory impairment. The therapist often emphasizes play and social skills, activities of daily living, arm and hand skills, and prevocational skills. According to the child's diagnosis, testing may include assessments of developmental age levels, range of motion, reflexes, tone, and noting the presence of any deformities or behaviors that interfere with function. The child should be observed in structured and unstructured settings, and significant others should be consulted about the child's skills. The therapist sorts out what part each of the contributing factors plays in the total picture of the child's difficulties.

## Objectives of Intervention and Treatment Modalities

Although the goals of treatment depends on the individual assessment of the child and identified levels of functioning, some typical treatment goals follow:

1. *To minimize tactile defensiveness and promote integration of the tactile system.* Because little can be done with these children until they are able to accept touch, this is usually a basic goal. The child should be gradually introduced to a large variety of tactile stimulation activities and encouraged to reach out and explore independently. Use of vibration and proprioceptive input may be helpful.

2. *To provide family members with support and education.* Family members need information about appropriate levels of stimulation and effective strategies for interaction with the child. Support groups or parents of children with similar disabilities can become a greatly valued resource for the parents.

3. *To provide adequate positioning.* The child with multiple disabilities often cannot or will not, because of

fear, move by himself or herself. Adequate positioning of the child to interact with the environment and to prevent contractures and deformities is extremely important. Functional positioning, so that the child can use his or her strongest sensory systems is the aim of much treatment. For those children not moving by themselves, teaching the caretakers and school staff different positions and encouraging them to change these positions often is important.

4. *To maximize movement.* The child at first needs to be moved, and later encouraged, if able, to move by himself or herself. For the child with reflex or tone problems, much effort has to be made to provide movement so that the cycle of lack of movement, contractures, and deformities is interrupted. Practice time should be allowed and new items introduced gradually. Activities with tilt boards, swings, and bolsters are useful, but most important is movement with another person, such as walking (holding on) or rocking together. Moersch (1977) detailed a treatment program that strongly emphasizes the use of meaningful activity, play, and movement in treating the child with multiple disabilities.

5. *To improve feeding skills.* Feeding is often a problem for children who have multiple disabilities. Often they have had stormy neonatal periods with long periods of tube feedings. Therapy intervention with the neonate should focus on obtaining good sucking skills (good rhythm and appropriate strength) and decreasing facial tactile defensiveness. Later, problems such as tongue thrusting, fatigue during feeding, and poor coordination of mouth movements occur. Learning to accept textured foods and chewing usually requires intervention. Physically moving the child through the movements of self-feeding and cup placement is often necessary. Tactile defensiveness and resistance to change are two major difficulties that can be intensified with the presence of increased tone and reflex patterns. Strategies need to be developed for the child who remains on a bottle or extensively drinks a food supplement such as Pediasure. The transition to drinking from a glass and eating table foods is a long process and can take several years to achieve.

6. *To improve self-maintenance skills.* As much independence as possible should be the goal for each individual child. Toileting is often a problem because of resistance to the potty chair and difficulty in understanding what is required. For the child who has physical disabilities in addition to visual or auditory impairments, the use of toilet scheduling techniques may be needed. A rapid program by Foxx and Azrin (1973) for daytime and nighttime independence has often been successful. The only prerequisite is that the child must be able to pull his or her pants up and down.

Dressing and hygiene skills are also often difficult, requiring adaptation and hand-over-hand guidance. Adaptive equipment is often required to increase independence. Examples are a large wheelchair tray with raised edges and a scooper bowl with suction cups.

As a team member, the occupational therapist may also assist with the following goals:

1. *To develop cause-and-effect relationships.* The child needs to learn to make things happen outside himself or herself. Many switch-activated toys provide sensory input that the child would perceive. For example, pressing the switch may activate a fan or a vibrator.

2. *To develop functional behaviors.* Not only must the perseverative, nonproductive behaviors be stopped, but more purposeful and functional behaviors must be substituted. Otherwise, equally undesirable behaviors are established. The child needs consistency and continuity. If tactile signs are used, they should be simple initially and consistent from one person to the next. The development of interpersonal and play skills is crucial.

## Special Techniques

Many of the specialized techniques used with these children deal with the development of some form of communication. *Clueing* is a system that was developed primarily by the mother of a rubella child in England (Freeman, 1966). It is a signal-type of language (one-way communication) between the mother and child. In this technique the daily activities of the child must be analyzed for clues or signals that can be picked up by the child. These signals tell the child what is happening or what is about to happen and form the beginning of communication. For example, the mother might rub the child's arms with a warm wet cloth before putting him into the bath.

*TADOMA* is a method of teaching speech and speech reading by placing the child's hand on the speaker's face and throat and thereby having the child pick up the vibrations that are made by sound. Children usually place the thumb on the speaker's lips and spread the fingers over cheek and neck.

Other more sophisticated communication techniques are often used by people who developed visual and hearing loss later in life. These methods include the following:

1. *Printing in the palm.* The block letters of the alphabet are traced in the palm of the person's hand.

2. *Alphabet glove.* A thin glove with the letters of the alphabet placed on different parts of the hand is worn by the person with visual and hearing impairment. The interpreter simply spells out the words.

With children with multiple disabilities and their slower pace of development, task analysis and breaking a task down into its smallest component parts can be useful in setting realistic goals for therapy and in establishing individual education plan (IEP) objectives. Task analysis can be especially useful in activities of daily living and vocational skills. The total task, such as buttering a piece of bread, is broken down into its components, and then backward or forward chaining of steps is used. In forward chaining the object is to teach the first step until it is mastered, then the second, and so on. In backward chaining the last step is taught until mastered, then the next to last, and so on. It is important to fade out assistance but still give as much as needed.

Another useful technique with children who are multiply impaired is *behavior modification.* This is a systematic approach to alter the child's behavior through environmental programming. Reinforcement is often used, and detailed records of the child's responses are kept. Often a positive trait needs to be reinforced, such as urinating when placed on the potty, or a negative trait such as eye poking needs to be extinguished. These behaviors are charted, and positive reinforcement is given for the desired behavior. Although being ignored can be a good behavioral conditioner for many children, children who are deaf-blind and have multiple disabilities are often happy to be left alone. Therefore this technique may not have the desired effect.

For the child who is severely physically and mentally involved, the therapist may decide to focus on teaching functional skills. These may often be related to survival or self-care skills that the child will benefit from even if learned in a rote manner and requiring very specific environment cues to elicit. Carryover should be sought if possible, but after weighing all factors, therapeutic judgment may support concentrating on certain splinter skills.

### Preparation for Adulthood

The child with multiple disabilities is usually prepared for workshop employment rather than for independent living. Approximately 75% of the these children need assisted living and supported employment (Smith, 1974). There are four levels of independence to consider:

1. *Custodial care:* Not capable of taking care of his or her own needs, although may have some self-help skills and may participate in recreation programs.
2. *Supported employment—assisted living:* Capable of working with close supervision and living in a group home situation with supervision and assistance in some tasks.
3. *Supported employment—semi-independent living:* Capable of working in a sheltered workshop and living with some support services available.
4. *Self-sufficient:* Employed and competent in daily living skills.

Some of the behaviors that the adolescent has to develop for more self-sufficient living are (1) communication of at least basic emergency and survival words such as *stop, eat, more, no,* and *finish;* (2) social skills; (3) self-care skills;

## CASE STUDY #3

Mary is 17 years 3 months old. She had congenital cataracts, severe hearing loss, and markedly delayed development. Mary is presently in a state residential facility for the visually impaired that has a treatment unit for individuals with visual and hearing impairment. She is gradually developing the skills to make the transition from the school program into the sheltered workshop program. She has been at the state facility since the age of 10, when her parents could no longer maintain her at home because of self-abusive behaviors and the need for constant supervision. Since her placement, she has been placed on a behavior modification program that has markedly reduced her self-abusive behaviors. She was assessed with a self-help skills checklist used by the school. She has difficulty with cup placement in eating, with fasteners in dressing, and with rigidity in walking. She understands and uses some tactile sign language and is functioning overall on a level of about a 3- to 4-year-old child.

**Treatment goals**

1. *To increase coordination and manipulative skills for workshop experience* by including activities such as sorting nails by size and shape, folding letters, and stamping envelopes.
2. *To improve eating skills* by reinforcing techniques to locate the plate and utensils and to place a cup upright with gradually fading physical assistance.
3. *To improve dressing skills* by practicing with fasteners on self, practice boards, and dolls.
4. *To promote independent exploration of the environment* by moving through space in such activities such as trampoline jumping, swimming, using a tilt board, and using a scooter board.

(4) telling time; (5) cooking and shopping skills; (6) home management; (7) travel and mobility; and (8) housekeeping. Workshop activities are manipulative for the most part and can include folding, stamping, collating, counting, gluing, bending, sorting, assembling, wrapping, stuffing, filing, measuring, stapling, and clipping.

If the child has remained at home with the family unit through school, adolescence is often the time when a move must be made to a residential facility. Both the family members and the child must be prepared for this. Also, the emerging sexuality of the child has to be dealt with at the level of the child's understanding. For resources for additional study and information on multiple sensory impairment, see the reference section of this chapter.

**STUDY QUESTIONS**

1. Children with hearing impairment may use one of four basic methods to improve communication skills. How would use of each method affect occupational therapy intervention?
2. What are common problems of children with visual impairment that would suggest the need for referral to occupational therapy? How can the occupational therapist help them with each of these problems?
3. How do the developmental motor skills of the 1-year-old child with severe visual impairment differ from those of a typical 1-year-old child?
4. How do the developmental skills of a 3-year-old child with deafness differ from a typical 3-year-old child?
5. Describe four examples of assistive technology used in occupational therapy intervention with children who have visual or hearing impairments.

## SUMMARY

This chapter has provided an overview of occupational therapy intervention with the child with visual or hearing impairment. Degrees of impairment have been investigated, as well as typical causes of impairment. Eye and ear anatomy has been reviewed to give information on the dynamics of a sensory loss. Emphasis in occupational therapy assessment has been placed on the interruption in the developmental process caused by the loss of one or both of these distance senses. General treatment goals have been given, stressing provision of activities and experiences to allow the child to develop adaptive behaviors and to develop to his or her fullest potential. Brief explanations have been given regarding specialized techniques used with these children, including the use of hearing aids, sign language, braille, and low-vision aids. It is my hope that the profession of occupational therapy will become increasingly involved with these children because of its emphases on adaptation, activity analysis, and developmental sequence.

## REFERENCES

Adelson, E. & Fraiberg, S. (1974). Gross motor development in infants blind from birth. *Child Development, 45,* 114.

Anastasi, A. (1989). *Psychological testing* (6th ed.). London: Macmillan.

Anderson, K.L. & Matkin, N.D. (1991). *Relationship of degree of longterm hearing loss to psychosocial impact and educational needs.* Los Angeles: John Tracy Clinic.

Ayres, A.J. (1972). *Sensory integration and learning disorders.* Los Angeles: Western Psychological Services.

Baker-Nobles, L. & Bink M.P. (1979). Sensory integration in the rehabilitation of blind adults. *American Journal of Occupational Therapy, 33,* 559-564.

Barraga, N. (1964). *Impaired visual behavior in low vision children.* New York: The American Foundation for the Blind.

Behrman, R.E. & Vaughan, V.C. (1987). *Nelson textbook of pediatrics* (13th ed.). Philadelphia: W.B. Saunders.

Brown, D., Simmons, V., & Mathvin, J. (1984). *The Oregon project for visually impaired and blind preschool children.* Medford, OR: Jackson County Education Service District.

Bruininks, R.H. (1978). *Bruininks-Oseretsky Test of Motor Proficiency: examiner's manual.* Circle Pines, MN: American Guidance Service.

Campbell, P.H., McInerney, W.F., & Cooper, M.A. (1984). Therapeutic programming for students with severe handicaps. *American Journal of Occupational Therapy, 38,* 594-602.

Cratty, B.J. (1971). *Movement and spatial awareness in blind youth.* Springfield, IL: Charles C. Thomas.

Davidson, P.W. (1992). Visual impairment and blindness. In M.D. Levine, W.B. Carey, & A.C. Crocker (Eds.). *Developmental-behavioral pediatrics* (2nd ed.). Philadelphia: W.B. Saunders.

Davis, H. & Silverman, S. (1978). *Hearing and deafness* (4th ed.). New York: Holt, Rinehart & Winston.

deQuiros, J. (1976). *Neuropsychological fundamentals in learning disorders.* San Rafael, CA: Academic Therapy Publications.

Erhardt, R.P. (1987). Sequential levels in the visual-motor development of a child with cerebral palsy. *American Journal of Occupational Therapy, 41,* 43-49.

Fant, L.J.(1971). *Ameslan: an introduction to American sign language.* Silver Springs, MD: The National Association for the Deaf.

Fonda, G. (1970). *Management of the patient with subnormal vision* (2nd ed.). St. Louis: Mosby.

Foxx, R.M. & Azrin, N.H. (1973). *Toilet training the retarded.* Champaign, IL: Research Press.

Fraiberg, S. (1977). *Insights from the blind: comparative studies of blind and sighted infants.* New York: Basic Books.

Freeman, P. (1966). *Parent's guide to early care of a deaf-blind child.* London: The National Association for Deaf-Blind and Rubella Children.

Furth, H.G. (1973). *Deafness and learning: a psychological approach.* Belmont, CA: Wadsworth.

Gesell, A., Ilg, F.L., & Bullis, G.E. (1967). *Vision: its development in infant and child.* New York: Hafner.

Grinnel, M.F., Dentamore, K.L., & Lippke, B.A. (1976). *Sign it successful: manual English encourages expressive communication* (p. 123). Teach Except Child, Spring Publications.

Gunn, S.L. (1971). Play as occupation: implications for the handicapped. *American Journal of Occupational Therapy, 25,* 285-290.

Gustafson, G., Pfetzing, D., & Zawalkow, E. (1975). *Signing exact English.* Silver Springs, MD: Modern Sign Press.

Halliday, C. (1970). *The visually impaired child: growth, learning, development: infancy to school age.* Louisville, KY: The American Printing House for the Blind.

Hill, L. (1977). Working with blind pre-schoolers. *American Journal of Occupational Therapy, 31,* 417-419.

Hiskey, M.S. (1983). The development, administration, scoring, and interpretation of the Hiskey-Nebraska Test of Learning Aptitude. In C.R. Reynolds & J.H. Clark (Eds.). *Assessment and programming of young children with low incidence handicaps.* New York: Plenum.

Jastrzembska, Z.S. (1976). *The effects of blindness and other impairments on early development.* New York: The American Foundation for the Blind.

Kaarela, R. & Widerberg, L. (1970). *Basic components of orientation and movement techniques.* Kalamazoo: Western Michigan University.

Kinsey, E. (1956). Retrolental fibroplasia: cooperative study of the use of oxygen and RLF, *Archives of Ophthalmology, 56,* 481.

Klima, E.S. & Bellugi, U. (1978). *The signs of language.* Cambridge, MA: Harvard University Press.

Kreton, J. & Balkany, T.J. (1991). Status of cochlear implantation in children. *Journal of Pediatrics, 118,* 1-7.

Leenenberg, E.H. (1967). *Biological foundation of language.* New York: John Wiley & Sons.

Leiter, R.G. (1969). *General instructions for the Leiter International Performance Scale.* Los Angeles: Western Psychological Services.

Liben, L.S. (1978). *Deaf children: developmental perspectives.* New York: Academic Press.

Ling, D. (1989). *Foundations of spoken language for hearing impaired children.* Washington DC: A.G. Bell Association.

Lowerfeld, B. (1969). *Our blind children.* Springfield, IL: Charles C. Thomas.

Lydon, W.T. & McGraw, L.M. (1973). *Concept development for the visually handicapped child.* New York: The American Foundation for the Blind.

Maxfield, K.E. & Buchholz, S. (1957). *A social maturity scale for blind pre-school children.* New York: The American Foundation for the Blind.

McInnes, J.M. & Teffry, J.A. (1982). *Deaf-blind infants and children.* Toronto, Canada: University of Toronto Press.

Meadow, P.M. (1980). *Deafness and child development.* Berkely: University of California Press.

Michelman, S. (1971). The importance of creative play, *American Journal of Occupational Therapy, 25,* 285-290.

Mindel, E.D. & Vernon, M. (1971). *They grow in silence: the deaf child and his family.* Silver Springs, MD: The National Association for the Deaf.

Moersch, M. (1977). Training the deaf-blind child, *American Journal of Occupational Therapy, 31,* 425-431.

Myklebust, H.R. (1964). *The psychology of deafness: sensory deprivation, learning and adjustment.* New York: Grune & Stratton.

Nelson, C. (1993). *Effective intervention for successful self-feeding.* Albuquerque: Edit Point.

Newborg, J., Stock, J., Wneck, L., Guidubaldi, J., & Svinicki, J. (1988). *Battelle Development Inventory.* Chicago: Riverside Publishers.

Newby, H. (1972). *Audiology.* New York: Appleton-Century-Crofts.

Northern, J.L. & Downs, M.P. (1992). *Hearing in children.* Baltimore: Williams & Wilkins.

Perera, C.A. (1957). *May's diseases of the eye.* Baltimore: Williams & Wilkins.

Pollack, D. (1970). *Educational audiology for the limited hearing infant.* Springfield, IL: Charles C. Thomas.

Reynell, J. & Zinkin, P. (1979). *Reynell-Zinkin Developmental Scales for young visually handicapped children.* Windsor, England: NFER.

Robbins, N. (1960). *Educational beginnings with deaf-blind children.* Watertown, MA: Perkins School for the Blind.

Rugers, C.T. (1969). *Understanding braille.* New York: The American Foundation for the Blind.

Ryan, S.J., Dawson, A.K., & Little, H.L. (1985). *Retinal diseases.* Orlando, FL: Grune & Stratton.

Sapir, R. (1966). *Culture, language, and personality.* Los Angeles: University of California Press.

Sardegna, J. & Paul, T. (1991). *The encyclopedia of blindness and vision impairment.* New York: Facts on File.

Sataloff, J., Sataloff, R.T., & Vassolo, L.A. (1980). *Hearing loss* (2nd ed.). Philadelphia: J.B. Lippincott.

Schaefer, K.J. & Specht, M.A. (1979). A light probe adapted for use in training the blind. *American Journal of Occupational Therapy, 33,* 640-643.

Schein, J.D. & Delk, M.T. (1975). *The deaf population of the United States.* Silver Springs, MD: The National Association for the Deaf.

Sheridan, M.D. (1969). *Manual for the STYCAR Vision Tests (screening tests for young children and retardates).* Berks, England: NFER.

Silverman, W.A. (1980). *Retrolental fibroplasia: a modern parable.* New York: Grune & Stratton.

Smith, D.W. (1982). *Recognizable patterns of human malformations.* Philadelphia: W.B. Saunders.

Stillman, R.D. (1973). *The Callier-Asuza Scale.* Dallas: Callier Speech and Hearing Center.

Thurnell R.J. & Rice, D.F.G. (1970). Eye rubbing in blind children: application of a sensory deprivation model. *Exceptional Child, 36,* 325.

Van Benschoter, R. (1975). A sensory integration program for blind campers, *American Journal of Occupational Therapy, 29,* 615-617.

Warner, D.H. (1984). *Blindness and early childhood development.* New York: The American Foundation for the Blind.

Welsh, R.L. & Blasch, B.B. (1980). *Foundations of orientation and mobility.* New York: The American Foundation for the Blind.

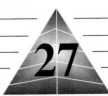

# Hospital Services

BARBARA BURRIS WAVREK

## KEY TERMS

▲ Hospital-Based Services
▲ Pediatrics
▲ Acute Care
▲ Intensive Care
▲ Outpatient
▲ Hospitalized Children
▲ Medical Teams
▲ Children with Severe Burns
▲ Bone Marrow Transplant
▲ Failure to Thrive

## CHAPTER OBJECTIVES

1. Understand characteristics of hospitals for children.
2. Explain the roles and functions of occupational therapists in pediatric hospitals.
3. Describe occupational therapy intervention in intensive care units and acute care units.
4. Explain outpatient intervention models.
5. Describe hospital-based occupational therapy services for children with burns, bone marrow transplant, and failure to thrive.

Occupational therapy intervention with children in hospitals presents the occupational therapist with a unique set of challenges. The demands of the health care system as they affect hospitals, the varied and sometimes unusual medical conditions involved, and the characteristics of hospitals as

The author gratefully acknowledges the assistance of the following individuals in the completion of this chapter: Cynthia Snyder, Teresa Canode, Pamela Carlson, Laura Farrel, Kimberly Lindsey, Elizabeth Loehr, and Heather MacLehose Pritchard.

health care institutions all have an impact on occupational therapy practice. This chapter addresses issues as they pertain to occupational therapy service provision to children in hospitals, as well as the medical model of service delivery, the scope of hospital-based services, and the roles and functions of occupational therapy personnel.

## CHARACTERISTICS OF HOSPITALS

Hospitals, by definition, are institutions where individuals who are ill or injured receive medical care designed to diagnose the presenting problem and provide treatment. Over time, however, hospitals have greatly expanded their roles in the provision of health care, offering both inpatient and outpatient services for the ill and injured, as well as prevention or wellness programs designed to decrease the need for future hospitalizations and treatment.

Hospitals may be categorized in several ways. *General hospitals* are institutions that serve patients of various ages and provide services for a broad range of diagnoses. General hospitals may have special facilities for children but are oriented toward meeting the broad range of community needs. Consequently, an occupational therapist employed in a general hospital is likely to be responsible for providing services to adults as well as children. *Specialty hospitals* are institutions whose missions define and restrict the types of diagnoses or the ages of patients to be seen, or both. *Pediatric hospitals,* which primarily serve infants, children, and adolescents, are placed in this category. Pediatric or children's hospitals tend to provide a full range of inpatient and outpatient services for children. A wider range of pediatric diagnoses are evaluated and treated, and length of stay tends to be longer than in a general hospital. Children hospitalized in pediatric facilities have access to a broad range of professionals in various specialties who have had experience in treating complex medical problems. Because of the high volume of patient activity in hospitals, hospital personnel have the opportunity not only to gain experience in evaluation and treatment of medical conditions, but also to learn to recognize individual differences in children's responses to similar medical problems.

Whether provided in a general or specialized hospital, services to children in hospitals tend to differ from the services to adults in terms of the extent of nursing care and other services. Provision of medical intervention to children in hospitals tends to be more labor intensive. "Sick children need more nursing care and therapy than sick adults, and children's care is about 30% more labor intensive. . . ." (Considine, 1994, p. 84).

Hospitals may differ in the size of their service regions. Children's hospitals, as specialized health care institutions, tend to serve a broader geographic region than general hospitals. This has several implications. First, a child may be hospitalized a significant distance from home, increasing the sense of separation from family and familiar environment. Second, the distance between home and hospital may affect the family's ability to visit the child in the hospital and remain in contact with the health personnel caring for the child. Third, the size of the service area, as well as the part of the country in which it is located, may mean greater cultural diversity and socioeconomic variation among those served by the hospital. Medical services, including occupational therapy, must be sensitive to the cultural beliefs and practices of the patient and family. Finally, the broader geographic region served by most children's hospitals usually requires hospital personnel to interact with a large number of organizations and programs in the community to plan for services after hospital discharge (Gilkerson, Gorski, & Panitz, 1990).

In addition to government-sponsored institutions, hospitals may be classified as private, nonprofit institutions or private, for-profit institutions. One trend among hospitals has been the affiliation of similar institutions, offering opportunities for consolidation of information and equipment, achievement of common goals, and program development. "Hospitals are attempting to coordinate and consolidate services to allow them to compete more aggressively, increase efficiency, and remain financially viable" (Levy, 1993, p. 365). An issue of concern facing hospitals as part of the health care delivery system is the cost of health care. Levy (1993) cited 1989 statistics from the National Center for Health Statistics that suggest that 90% of hospital expenses incurred by patients are financed by private and public insurance. Insurance plans differ in the amount of coverage they provide and the services they choose to cover. However, a common concern of all insurers is the need to contain health care costs. "Health plans are interested in providing 'appropriate' care while controlling costs to remain competitive in the marketplace" (Pontzer, 1994, p. 36). Managed care strategies designed to promote quality care while containing costs vary and may include

. . . financial incentives and management controls imposed on providers, the decision-making systems used to channel patients

to care, and the criteria used by the plan to identify efficient providers and cost-effective systems (Pontzer, 1994, p. 36).

In addition, the trend toward the development of standardized protocols for decision making regarding the most appropriate care has and will affect the provision of occupational therapy services. Strategies such as these may result in shorter hospital stays, provision of fewer services, or limited reimbursement for services provided. One result of shorter hospital stays is the increased emphasis on outpatient diagnostic and treatment services within the hospital environment (Torrance, 1993). According to Pontzer (1994),

Hospitals are moving in the direction of 'hospital systems' where they are serving their patients across the spectrum of placement options including acute, subacute, rehabilitation, outpatient, skilled nursing facilities, and home health care (p. 36).

Health care trends that have an impact on service delivery to children also have the potential to affect the occupational therapy services provided. For example, affiliating children's hospitals may compare productivity statistics and quality improvement strategies among occupational therapy departments or share program development information. Trends in managed care that may result in shorter hospital stays and limited reimbursement have the potential to restrict the occupational therapy services that may be provided or shift the emphasis to the provision of outpatient services.

Hospitals are governed by internal policies and procedures that are usually designed to assist the institution in meeting standards of external, private accrediting agencies, government agencies, and insurance providers. Organizations such as the Joint Commission for the Accreditation of Health Care Organizations (JCAHO) and the Commission for the Accreditation of Rehabilitation Facilities (CARF), as well as government agencies such as the Occupational Safety and Health Administration (OSHA), have set standards regarding hospital operations that include standards for provision of professional services, documentation of patient care activities, patient and employee safety, and quality improvement activities (1995 Comprehensive Accreditation Manual for Hospitals, 1994 CARF Standards Manual). Employee education regarding safety practices when there is risk of exposure to patient blood or body fluids or to hazardous materials is also mandated (Federal Register, 1991). Standards such as these also influence occupational therapy department policies and procedures and, therefore, occupational therapy practice.

Licensing or other credentialing of personnel of specific disciplines, including occupational therapy personnel, is also required in a hospital environment as one means of ensuring the hiring of qualified personnel and protecting the consumer. Both occupational therapists and occupational therapy assistants are subject to the requirements of the institution and, where applicable, the state in which the hospital is located.

## Scope of Hospital-Based Services

Most services in a hospital are directed toward providing medical care to the ill or injured. However, many hospitals also have teaching and research as part of their missions. The hospital, as a teaching institution, provides clinical education experiences for medical students, interns, residents, nursing students, and students from other health-related professions. As a research institution, a hospital often provides resources and opportunities for clinical research to advance medical knowledge and practice. Consequently, although the primary role of the occupational therapist in the hospital is that of a clinician, occupational therapy personnel may also assume roles in education and research. For example, occupational therapists in hospitals also serve as fieldwork supervisors for occupational therapy students and have opportunities to educate students from other health professions about issues relevant to occupational therapy. Hospital-based occupational therapists may also design and implement research pertinent to occupational therapy or assist in multidisciplinary research efforts.

Clinically, hospitals offer a range of services designed to provide medical care to children with acute or chronic illness, traumatic injury, or special needs. The method of service delivery varies according to the needs of the patient and the nature of the medical care required. Gilkerson (1990) identified the preservation of life as the most important function in a hospital and suggested that life-threatening conditions take priority in the scheme of hospital activities. *Acute care, ambulatory* or *outpatient services, rehabilitation,* and *emergency* or *trauma services* are terms often used to differentiate between the types and levels of care provided in a hospital. Occupational therapists are most likely to provide acute care, rehabilitation, and outpatient services to children (see Chapter 30).

Most patient care activity in hospitals is acute care. Acute care refers to short-term medical care provided during the acute phase of an illness or injury, when the symptoms are generally the most severe. Just as there are degrees of severity that categorize illnesses and injuries, there are also levels of acute care designed to meet these varied needs.

Critically ill patients who require continuous, close monitoring and frequent medical attention and who often need special equipment to maintain or monitor vital functions are admitted to intensive care units (ICUs) or critical care units (CCUs). Hospitals may have several intensive care units, each of which is designated for a specific patient population or purpose. Neonatal intensive care units (NICUs), pediatric intensive care units (PICUs) for older children, and surgical intensive care units (SICUs) are examples of intensive care units that may be found in hospitals. Personnel who provide care for patients in ICUs receive special training to enable them to respond quickly and effectively to meet the needs of medically unstable patients in this challenging environment.

A child whose illness or injury results in hospitalization but who does not need the continuous attention, high tech-

nology, and specialized care of an ICU, may be admitted to a medical or surgical acute care unit. Medical and surgical units also tend to be designated for specific types of patients. For example, neurosurgical patients may be served on one unit, and orthopedic patients may be served on another. In some instances, acute care units may be designated as special units for patients with a particular diagnosis who require a specific treatment protocol and environment or for patients whose medical conditions require special precautions to prevent the spread of infection to others. Three conditions that require the child to be treated in a special care unit are acute burns, infectious diseases, and bone marrow transplantation. For patients with burns or those who require bone marrow transplants, the hospital environment is designed to minimize the risk of infection to patients who are especially susceptible, while still enabling the completion of the medical protocol. Although all patients in a special care unit may share a common diagnosis, they may be at different points in their treatment and recovery. By contrast, patients with infectious conditions may have a variety of diagnoses that require treatment under isolation conditions to protect others.

Medical intervention for chronically ill patients may also be provided in hospitals that emphasize acute care. Often, chronically ill patients are admitted for an acute exacerbation of their illnesses or for treatment of complications. Diabetes, asthma, cystic fibrosis, and cancer are examples of chronic illnesses occurring in children that may require periodic hospitalization. In some instances, chronically ill patients who are medically fragile may receive long-term care in an acute hospital setting because the family is unable or unwilling to care for them at home and a special placement elsewhere in the region is not readily available. DeWitt, Jansen, Ward, and Keens (1993) found that children who required ventilator assistance often remained in the hospital for nonmedical reasons after becoming medically stable. Two factors that significantly delayed hospital discharge were difficulty arranging either out-of-home placement or financial assistance to enable care in the home.

Ambulatory or outpatient programs are designed for patients who require medical services but whose conditions do not require hospitalization. Outpatient services may include diagnostic procedures such as radiographs or laboratory tests; visits to clinics for continuity of care after discharge from the hospital, or special services, outpatient occupational therapy or physical therapy, or, in some cases, primary care.

Although many children enter and leave the hospital system at different points along this continuum of services, others experience the full range of services. A child with severe burns, for example, may initially be admitted to an ICU because of the life-threatening nature of the injury. Once the child's medical condition stabilizes, he or she may be transferred to a special unit for children with burns for continuation of treatment. When hospitalization is no longer necessary, the child may be discharged yet return for visits for occupational therapy and physical therapy or for follow-up visits with physicians, therapists, and other hospital personnel in an outpatient clinic.

## Medical Model and Team Interaction

In a hospital, care of the patient focuses on the individual's medical needs, and, to some extent, the family's needs, particularly in the ways those needs affect the child's illness, recovery, and general well-being. The composition of the medical team tends to reflect the immediate needs of the patient and family. In general, the physician is considered the leader of the medical team for a given child, although leadership may shift to other team members during the course of the child's stay (Case-Smith & Wavrek, 1993). The child's primary nurse or designate, personnel from other disciplines whose services are formally requested by the physician, and in some cases the parents form the remainder of the team responsible for the child's care. Two factors that often affect the parents' participation in the child's care are the distance between the family's home and the hospital and the parents' other obligations, including work and child care. These factors may limit the parents' visitation to the hospital and, therefore, their accessibility to health care professionals involved in the care of their child.

Another significant characteristic of medical teams is their dynamic nature. Because the actual health care disciplines involved depend on each child's needs, the medical team is continually changing (see Chapter 2). For example, a child with a feeding disorder who is failing to grow and gain weight may have a physician, nurses, an occupational therapist, a dietitian, and a social worker as members of the medical team. However, a child hospitalized with multiple injuries resulting from a motor vehicle accident may have several physicians, nurses, an occupational therapist, a physical therapist, a speech pathologist, a dietitian, a respiratory therapist, and a social worker as members of the medical team caring for him or her. As a potential member of multiple medical teams within one hospital, the occupational therapist must communicate and collaborate with professionals from many different health-related fields. Frequently, the therapist may be required to continually redefine or explain the role of the occupational therapist to other team members, as well as develop an understanding of the ways in which different team members' roles complement each other in the provision of services to children. With the trend toward "hospital systems," described previously, occupational therapists employed by hospitals may face the more complex challenges of defining their roles in several different settings within one integrated system of care and participating in interdisciplinary medical teams across the spectrum of care (Pontzer, 1994).

Communication among hospital team members is dependent on a number of factors. One significant factor is the limited availability of team members for scheduled meetings. Communication tends to occur through the formal documentation in the patient's chart and informally between two or more team members during telephone calls or chance meetings throughout the day. "What appear as unplanned interactions are actually an accepted and effective way of doing business in a setting where time is at a premium, needs are immediate, and staff schedules can change daily" (Gilkerson, Gorski, & Panitz, 1990, pp. 453 to 454). Communication with the patient or parent occurs at separate times, one-on-one, with each team member involved. Regular team meetings, although ideal, are not always feasible in a hospital setting because of the multiple demands on hospital personnel and the likelihood of schedule changes.

## Special Needs of Children in Hospitals

Hospital services, including occupational therapy, must take into consideration the child's developmental level and needs, the impact of illness or injury and hospitalization on development, and the coping strategies and needs of the family in relation to the child's medical condition. Hospitalized children are placed in a situation filled with unknowns and events over which they have little control (Gohsman, 1981). Sources of stress for the child include separation from family and the home environment, the unfamiliarity of the hospital, the increased dependency that often is associated with illness or injury and hospitalization, the unfamiliar and frequently changing hospital caregivers, and the often painful medical procedures that may be required. Realization of potential disability or disfigurement and boredom may also add to the child's stress. Anxiety, withdrawal, regression, increased demand for parental attention, and a need for behavioral management may result (Knudson-Cooper, 1982; Suhr, 1986). For very young children, this is complicated by their limited ability to understand the purpose or need for the hospitalization and the anxiety produced by separation from parents or other caregivers (Wilson & Broome, 1989). The fears provoked by hospitalization may be exacerbated by a diminished ability to cope resulting from the illness and injury (Gohsman, 1981). Consequently, the illness or injury and the stress of hospitalization may result in developmental regression or hinder developmental progress. Petrillo and Sanger (1980) suggested that successful adaptation in response to the overwhelming stresses of illness and hospitalization requires the child to achieve a sense of mastery over the situation. The occupational therapist's educational preparation in child development, knowledge of age-appropriate developmental tasks, and understanding of the importance of purposeful activity in achieving environmental mastery enables him or her to provide occupational therapy intervention within a developmental context. This enhances the child's sense of mastery in the hospital environment, helps other members of the medical team understand the developmental issues of concern, and suggests strategies to hospital caregivers and the family to help support normal development and help the child better cope with hospitalization.

## Characteristics of Hospital-Based Occupational Therapy

Many of the evaluation and treatment strategies used by occupational therapists to intervene with children in the hospital are not unique to hospital-based practice but tend to be the same approaches used with children in other settings. However, the diagnoses seen in hospitals challenge the occupational therapist to adapt intervention to meet specific, often acute, needs. Children may be referred for occupational therapy with presenting problems such as prematurity, birth defects, developmental delay, feeding disorders, orthopedic disorders, traumatic brain injury or other neurologic problems, burns, cancer, renal disease, cardiac defects, endocrine disorders, or other acute or chronic conditions. The occupational therapist must have a thorough understanding of the diagnosis, prognosis, contraindications, and other implications of the child's illness, injury, or medical treatment for occupational therapy intervention (see Chapter 7).

For most children, services are provided in a relatively brief period, requiring the occupational therapist to be highly efficient in the provision of services and to establish realistic treatment priorities appropriate for the patient's projected length of stay in the hospital (Levy, 1993). Rausch and Melvin (1986) suggested that "a target skill for the acute care therapist is the ability to integrate evaluation, treatment and patient instruction into each therapy session" (p. 321). In a children's hospital, the broad range of diagnoses requires the occupational therapy department to offer a wide range of occupational therapy assessment and treatment options. However, the need for a broad range of services does not mean a lack of specialization. "Occupational therapy services tend to be highly specialized in a pediatric facility and well-developed in specialty areas (e.g., neonatal care, upper extremity anomalies, and burns)" (Case-Smith & Wavrek, 1993, p. 129). Although occupational therapy services may tend to have a narrower focus in a general hospital that serves children, intervention still requires special skills and knowledge and an understanding of the ways that the needs of children and adults differ.

Occupational therapy services for the hospitalized child varies according to the type of facility, the child's diagnosis, and the length of stay. For a child with a short or acute stay, the emphasis of occupational therapy tends to be on assessment, with program planning, recommendations for follow-up postdischarge, and equipment provision or fabrication occurring as needed. A child hospitalized for a long time may have the benefit of receiving occupational therapy services one or two times daily, depending on the child's needs. A longer stay also provides the occupational therapist with more opportunities to interact with the family, pro-

vide parent education, and plan for discharge cooperatively with the family and other team members. Children with extended acute phases of illness or injury, such as burns, traumatic brain injury, or encephalitis, also tend to require different and possibly more comprehensive services than chronically ill children, such as those with cystic fibrosis or diabetes, who are hospitalized frequently for exacerbations of their illness.

In some instances, services for children with acute illness or injury may be limited to provision of a piece of adaptive equipment, such as a protective helmet for a neurosurgical patient or a reacher for a patient in traction with a lower-extremity fracture. For patients with chronic conditions who receive occupational therapy in the community, occupational therapy services in the hospital may focus on provision of equipment or completion of evaluations that are not readily available to the occupational therapist in the community. For example, a child with a severe developmental disability who is hospitalized with pneumonia resulting from the aspiration of food might be referred to the hospital radiology, occupational therapy, and speech pathology departments for an evaluation of feeding, which would include a videofluoroscopic swallowing study (Figure 27-1). In situations of this type, close communication between the hospital- and community-based occupational therapists is essential and can result in better total care for the child and family.

## Scope of Occupational Therapy Services

Rausch and Melvin (1986) identified four types of acute care patients referred to occupational therapy departments in hospitals. The first type is the patient with a single injury, such as a hand injury, or a single episode of illness. This type of patient tends to have a short hospital stay with a predictable course of treatment. The second type of patient is one with an acute illness or injury who requires extended rehabilitation. Traumatic brain injury and spinal cord injury are two examples of injuries that require both initial acute treatment and long-term rehabilitation. The length of the hospital stay for this type of patient during the acute phase of illness or injury tends to vary because the potential for complications is greater. The third type of patient is the chronically ill patient who is hospitalized periodically for acute episodes of an illness or complications of an illness. Children with diabetes, cancer, or cardiac conditions fall into this category. The length of hospital stay for these patients is also variable. The last type are patients hospitalized for diagnostic testing or adjustment of medications. A comparatively short hospital stay is characteristic of patients with these types of presenting problems. In each case, occupational therapy intervention may differ according to the patient's needs and the length of stay. In some instances, occupational therapy intervention may be affected by staff shortages, which result in prioritizing which patients receive

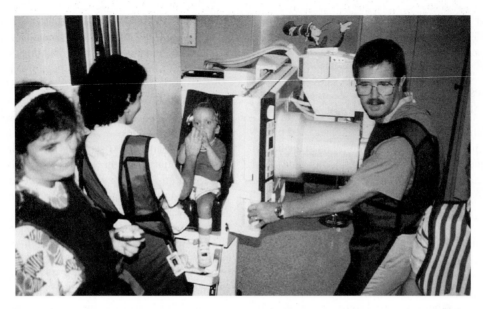

**Figure 27-1**    An interdisciplinary team uses videofluoroscopy to assess a patient's swallowing and risk for aspiration.

occupational therapy services (Rausch & Melvin, 1986; Torrance, 1993).

Occupational therapy evaluation in acute care services focuses on the child's developmental or functional status within the context of the illness or injury that has resulted in hospitalization. Completion of the assessment may present a challenge for the occupational therapist because the length of hospital stay is often short and other hospital services are competing for the patient's time.

Patients often have a multitude of diagnostic tests as well as additional services that are being provided to the patient, such as respiratory care, social service, speech pathology, physical therapy, and occupational therapy. It thus becomes extremely important that assessment is completed in a short time to maximize the time for treatment (Torrance, 1993, p. 772).

Evaluation may begin with a chart review to obtain information about the child's medical status, the current course of medical care and goals, contraindications or precautions that may have an impact on the occupational therapy services provided, and the patient's functional level before the hospitalization. Information concerning family structure, birth history, and the child's past developmental course may also contribute to the occupational therapist's understanding of the child's and family's needs. An interview with the parents, if available, is often the source of valuable information regarding the child's current status and the parents' goals for the child.

Before completing a functional or developmental evaluation, the occupational therapist must establish rapport with the child and family. This is especially important because of the stressful and frightening nature of the hospital environment to the child. A positive relationship between the child and therapist serves to decrease the child's anxiety about the evaluation process, foster cooperation, and enable the therapist to obtain results that more accurately reflect the child's actual level of function.

The choice of evaluation tools and methods depends on the child's age and needs and the protocol of the occupational therapy department. For example, a 10-year-old child with a serious hand injury might be referred for evaluation of strength, sensation, fine coordination, passive and active range of motion, independence in self-care, and the need for a splint to assist function or prevent deformity. By contrast, a 2-year-old child referred for developmental delay secondary to chronic illness may receive a developmental assessment that includes administration of a standardized test, such as the Bayley Scales of Infant Development—Revised, and evaluation of sensorimotor function (e.g., muscle tone, automatic postural responses, or sensory processing), self-care, and play skills. An evaluation of this type is often performed in collaboration or cooperation with professionals from other disciplines, such as physical therapy and speech pathology (Figure 27-2). In both instances, the occupational therapist is concerned with occupational performance areas, components, and contexts in relation to the child's age and development.

In some cases, the child's medical condition, a short length of stay, or a stressful and restrictive environment, such as an ICU, may prohibit the administration of a standardized evaluation. In these instances, the therapist's clinical observations of key functions may be the best alternative (Figure 27-3).

Finally, assessment in acute care also includes evaluation of the need for specialized equipment or splints, both for use in the hospital and for use after discharge. Specialized

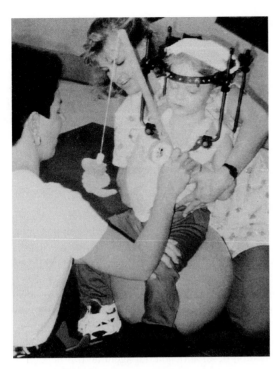

**Figure 27-2** An occupational therapist and physical therapist collaborate on a patient evaluation.

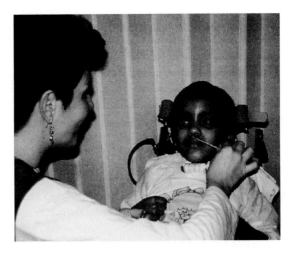

**Figure 27-3** An occupational therapist evaluates oral-motor skills before feeding a patient.

equipment may include adapted utensils for self-feeding for a patient with a spinal cord injury, an adapted bath seat for a patient with cerebral palsy, a pressure garment to prevent hypertrophic scarring for a patient with burn injuries, a protective helmet for a patient with a skull fracture, or splints for a patient with juvenile rheumatoid arthritis. In some instances, the therapist and child may need to experiment with different pieces of equipment to determine which is best for the child's use.

### Intensive Care Unit Services

Occupational therapy services may be initiated with a patient at any point during the course of hospitalization; however, they usually occur once a patient has achieved sufficient medical stability to benefit from occupational therapy. In the intensive care unit, the child must be evaluated and treated by the occupational therapist at bedside because of the critical nature of the illness or injury and the need for constant monitoring of the child's medical status. Occupational therapy intervention in intensive care supports the medical team's priorities and goals for the child. It is also essential that the occupational therapist be knowledgeable about the child's diagnosis and the implications of medical procedures, the use of life support or monitoring equipment, and contraindications for occupational therapy intervention. Constant monitoring of the child's status is also the responsibility of the occupational therapist during the time he or she is with the patient, making it imperative for the thera-

pist to understand the significance of changes in the patient's vital signs, respiratory function, appearance, or symptoms. Affleck, Lieberman, Polon, and Rohrkemper (1986) identified three problems related to the intensive care environment and child's status that affect both the child and occupational therapy intervention. These are immobility and the need for bed rest, sensory deprivation and stress, and extended mechanical ventilation.

Prolonged bed rest and immobility often occur as a result of the critical nature of the illness, the use of high-technology equipment, or the need for restraints for the child's safety and care. Wilson and Broome (1989) estimated that the average length of stay for a child in the ICU is 4 to 6 days; however, it may extend into weeks or months. The potential impact of extended immobility includes decreased endurance, generalized weakness, and poor tolerance for sitting. As part of an occupational therapy program, the use of graded activity may improve the child's endurance and strength and enhance functional performance.

Activities can be graded in terms of length of treatment time, amount and speed of active movement, level of assistance given, adaptive aids, and position and postural support. The most important parameter in grading a task is a patient's physiological response. The patient's level of activity can be upgraded only when vital signs, symptoms, and respiratory function are acceptable at the existing level of activity (Affleck et al., 1986, p. 324).

In addition to a program of graded activity, occupational therapy intervention may include positioning recommendations or splints to preserve range of motion and prevent deformity and specialized equipment to facilitate function.

Sensory deprivation and stress resulting from the intensive care environment may also complicate a child's illness and recovery. The lack of privacy, immobility, and the continuous sounds and lights of the intensive care unit provide the child with an atypical sensory experience. In addition, there are few indicators to orient the child to changes in time and day. Occupational therapy intervention may help counteract the effects of stress and sensory deprivation by fostering the establishment of a routine for the child and providing purposeful activities to facilitate cognitive, psychosocial, and motor functions (Affleck et al., 1986). Positive social interaction and the use of entertainment and play activities may be especially helpful to reduce stress and promote development of young children in the ICU.

To summarize, the occupational therapist providing services in the ICU must have a thorough understanding of the patient's condition, the purpose of intensive care, the medical priorities for the patient, and the importance of monitoring the patient's physiologic status before, during, and after occupational therapy. In general, occupational therapy goals for the intensive care patient include (1) completion of assessment procedures and identification of functional status and needs, (2) provision of graded, meaningful activities (e.g., play activities, self-care activities) to improve endurance, strength, and functional abilities (e.g., cognition, psychosocial function, and motor abilities), and (3) provision of specialized equipment, splints, and positioning recommendations as needed (Figure 27-4).

The occupational therapist providing intervention for patients on *special care units* faces some of the same challenges as the occupational therapist who provides services to ICU patients. In both instances, it is imperative that the therapist understand the purpose of the unit, the medical goals and treatment protocol for the patients, and the reasons why the child requires hospitalization on the particular unit in question. It is also important for the occupational

therapist to know the roles and functions of the other members of the medical team and to collaborate with them during the course of the child's hospitalization. In addition, the occupational therapist assigned to a special care unit often must become a specialist at assessing and treating children of all ages and at different stages of recovery with similar medical conditions. The therapist must also be aware of and use infection control procedures that must be observed to prevent infection of the patient or the transfer of infection from one patient to another.

## Burn Unit

One of the specialty ICUs found in larger hospitals is the *burn unit*. The cause of the burn injury, the depth of the burn (e.g., first degree, second degree, or third degree), the percentage of total body surface area (TBSA) affected, the location of the burn, and the age of the patient are factors considered in classifying a burn according to severity. Medical treatment for burns varies according to the severity; however, in general, burn wounds are treated with a local application of an antibacterial agent and, if needed, surgery to remove burned tissue and cover the affected area with skin grafts (Leman, 1993). The long, often painful recovery process and the potential for lasting disfigurement and disability challenge the child's and family's coping skills. For these reasons, occupational therapy with the burned child presents a special challenge.

Leman (1993) described three stages in the recovery process: the acute care stage, the surgical and postoperative stage, and the rehabilitation stage. The medical focus of the acute care stage is the replacement of lost body fluids, stabilization of the patient, and care of the burn wounds. Occupational therapy intervention during this phase may include prevention of the loss of joint mobility, strength, and endurance; self-care activities; and education of the child and family regarding the rehabilitation process (Leman, 1993).

Surgical removal of burned tissue, skin grafts, and postoperative recovery characterize the surgical and postoperative stage. Immobilization of the affected area through positioning or splints is required for approximately 3 to 7 days after surgery. In addition to the fabrication of splints and provision of positioning recommendations, the occupational therapist may need to provide adaptive devices to assist with self-care or other activities.

During the rehabilitation stage, wound healing continues. The patient is susceptible to scarring and contracture formation during this period. The rehabilitation phase begins during hospitalization; however, it often continues after discharge on an outpatient basis and through home programs until the patient's scars are mature; a process that may take up to 2 years. Scarring, especially hypertrophic scars, can significantly interfere with a patient's functional recovery. Hypertrophic scars tend to be thick, inflexible, and red and, if they cross joints, can impair joint mobility because of

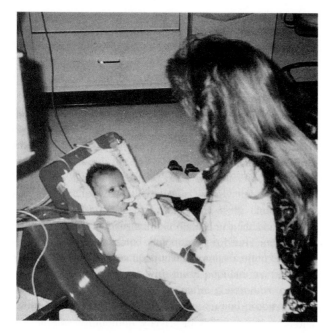

**Figure 27-4** An occupational therapist assesses oral motor and feeding abilities in a patient requiring ventilator assistance for respiration.

shortening of the skin (Leman, 1993). Occupational therapy intervention goals include the following:

1) to assist in the prevention of deformity, contracture, and hypertrophic scar formation,
2) to provide appropriate and carefully selected treatment techniques and therapeutic activities for range of motion, strength, functional coordination, and developmental skills,
3) to enable the child to return to as independent a life-style as possible and as is appropriate for the child's age,
4) to provide psychosocial therapeutic intervention for the child's emotional well-being. (Doane, 1989, p. 525).

Activities to facilitate play skills and return to school are also essential components of occupational therapy.

### Example of Intervention for Burn Injury

The following case report illustrates the complexity of intervention with a child admitted to the burn unit of a hospital.

***Presenting information.*** Sabrina is a 4-year-old white girl who presented with burn injuries to 60% to 70% TBSA. The burns were sustained during a house fire in which her mother and younger brother died. Sabrina's maternal grandmother and 6-year-old sister survived with no injuries. The fire was believed to have been started by a cigarette. Sabrina received second- and third-degree burns to all areas of her body, including face, head, hands, trunk, arms, anterior knees, and the dorsum of the feet and toes. She was referred to occupational therapy by the burn surgeon for splinting and therapeutic intervention.

***Background information.*** Sabrina was a healthy child with no disabilities before the house fire. She resided with her mother, maternal grandmother, sister, and brother and attended a Head Start preschool class.

***Occupational therapy and medical intervention.*** The burn team, consisting of the physician, occupational therapist, physical therapist, nurses, social worker, psychologist, dietitian, and child life specialist, was consulted. Initial occupational therapy involvement that began when Sabrina was admitted to the ICU, focused on providing splints and guidelines for positioning. The primary occupational therapy goal at that time was to prevent the development of contracture deformities during burn wound healing. Positioning strategies included the following: the shoulders were abducted at 90 degrees using pillows or stockinette slings tied to the head of the bed; foot drop splints were fabricated to maintain 90 degrees of ankle dorsiflexion while the patient was confined to bed and to prevent hyperextension of toes. Resting hand splints were also fabricated, placing the hands in a safe position to protect damaged extensor tendons and ligaments and to provide 90 degrees of metacarpophalangeal flexion. Once Sabrina was medically stable and transferred to the Burn Unit, the occupational therapist provided daily active range of motion exercises to improve upper body mobility and range of motion. Bilateral airplane splints were fabricated for shoulder positioning, and facial expression exercises were initiated. A figure 8 clavicle strap was used for retraction of shoulders and chest. Ongoing evalua-

tion of joint mobility and the functional limitations related to decreased joint mobility occurred throughout Sabrina's hospitalization.

The therapist used lotion to massage Sabrina's scars, particularly those on her face, one to two times per day. Stacked tongue blades were used for vertical expansion exercises to the mouth for 5 minutes before each meal. Commissure expansion was not indicated because of the location of Sabrina's burns. Pressure garments were provided for early scar management, which included elastic wrap bandages, Coban wrapping (3M Corporation, Medical-Surgical Division, St. Paul, MN) to the hands, Elastinet stockings (Jobst Company, Toledo, OH), and prefabricated pressure garments. A Polyform face mask with a silicone mold was fabricated to provide pressure on healed areas of her face.

Initially Sabrina required a Velcro strap on her feeding utensils. Later she became independent in self-feeding, using a large-handled spoon and fork. These adapted utensils were not required for feeding at the time of her discharge from the hospital. She did continue to require moderate assistance in dressing and bathing. The occupational therapist provided several simple aids to improve her independence in dressing and bathing at home and recommended types of clothing that were easy to don and were comfortable. In other performance areas, Sabrina quickly returned to her previous level of function. She used playground equipment with supervision, including her tricycle and scooter board. Although certain manipulative toys were difficult, she played with her favorite toys without assistance.

Custom pressure garments were ordered once sufficient healing had occurred, approximately 2 months postburn. Several surgeries followed, including scar excision and skin grafting to the hands, axillae, anterior chest, and face (Figure 27-5).

Sabrina was discharged to her father's and stepmother's home, where her sister also resided. She began attending kindergarten after a school reentry program in which two members of the burn

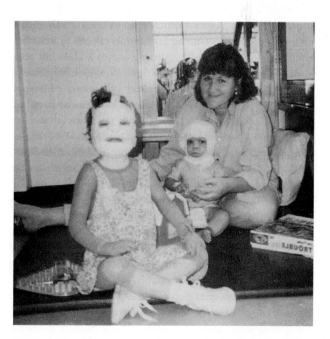

**Figure 27-5** Face masks and custom-fabricated pressure garments assist in scar management for children with severe burns.

team visited the school and educated her classmates about burns, splints, and pressure garments, especially as they related to Sabrina's injuries.

After hospital discharge, Sabrina was treated by the occupational therapist on an outpatient basis three to five times per week, with additional therapy provided through a community agency near her home until she could easily achieve normal active range of movement. Sabrina continued to be measured and fitted with new pressure garments every 2 to 3 months because of growth or wear. A clear face mask was used for scar management of the face. All pressure garments were worn 23 hours a day and were expected to be worn for up to 18 months. Sabrina continued to be followed every 2 to 3 months to monitor joint mobility and to assess pressure garment needs and effectiveness.

As is evident in the case report, the preservation of joint mobility, prevention of deformity, management of scar tissue, and promotion of independence in self-care were major occupational therapy emphases in the treatment of Sabrina. The school reentry program was designed not only to educate Sabrina's classmates about burns, but also to help make them and her more comfortable with the disfigurement and special equipment, thus making the transition easier for Sabrina as she returned to the community.

## Bone Marrow Transplant Unit

Another type of highly specialized acute care service is the bone marrow transplant unit. Bone marrow transplants are used as part of a medical treatment protocol for a number of life-threatening childhood illnesses, including leukemia, aplastic anemia, immunodeficiency syndromes, and tumors (Furman & Feldman, 1990; Williams, 1990; Williams & Safarimaryaki, 1990). The procedure for bone marrow transplant involves chemotherapy, radiation, or both before the transplant, followed by intravenous infusion of the bone marrow taken from a compatible donor or from the patient before the pretransplant regimen of chemotherapy and radiation. The intense chemotherapy or radiation before the transplant and the underlying disease processes cause severe immunosuppression in patients, making them highly susceptible to life-threatening infections until the new bone marrow is established and the patient's immunohematopoietic system is once again functioning effectively (Lenarsky, 1990; Zander & Aksamit, 1990). The immunologic compromise that occurs requires that the bone marrow transplant and resultant hospitalization occur in an environment designed to greatly reduce the risk of infection. The type of environment may vary among hospital to hospital; however, common strategies to protect bone marrow transplant patients include room isolation, reverse isolation, and laminar airflow in a clean or sterile environment (Lenarsky, 1990).

Another issue of concern is the psychosocial stress for the patient and family. Sources of stress include the child's life-threatening illness, the risks of bone marrow transplantation, the painful or uncomfortable medical procedures and extended period of isolation that the child must endure, and

concern about the cost of the treatment. In addition, the transplant may occur at a hospital distant from the family's home, creating an additional burden for family members (Williams, 1990).

The many complex needs of the patient and family emphasize the importance of a collaborative team approach. The physician, nurses, occupational therapist, physical therapist, pharmacist, clinical social worker, psychologist, dietitian, chaplain, child life specialist, and a hospital-based teacher may all serve as members of a team caring for the bone marrow transplant patient and the patient's family (Spruce, 1990).

Intervention may include a pretransplant assessment of the child's development and functional abilities, as well as identification of limitations or problems caused by the underlying disease process. After the transplant, the occupational therapist's goals may be to (1) promote normal development and age-appropriate functional skills, (2) enhance coping skills, and (3) assess for posthospital discharge needs.

This case report illustrates the role of occupational therapy in a bone marrow transplant unit. When a child has a tumor that does not involve the bone marrow, the bone marrow transplant may be used in conjunction with large doses of chemotherapy or radiation to reduce or eradicate the tumor. The toxicity of large doses of chemotherapy and radiation have the potential to inhibit the normal functions of the patient's bone marrow, resulting in a need for a bone marrow transplant. For this purpose, some of the child's own bone marrow is removed before high-dose chemotherapy and is reinfused later (Williams & Safarimaryaki, 1990).

***Presenting information.*** Katie was an 8-year-old girl who had a brain tumor. She was referred for occupational therapy by her oncologist after bone marrow transplantation. The oncologist noted that Katie exhibited decreased strength in her left arm and that she had difficulty with fine motor skills.

***Background information.*** Katie resided with her mother and older sister. Although her parents are separated, her father visited regularly. Katie attended a regular public school class before her illness and transplant. Medical history included a craniotomy and excision of a right thalamic glioma, chemotherapy and radiation, placement of a broviac catheter, placement of a right ventricular-perineal shunt secondary to hydrocephalus, a history of pneumonia, and an episode of generalized tonic clonic seizures that remained under control with medication.

***Occupational therapy intervention.*** After diagnosis and initial medical and surgical intervention for the tumor, the family and oncologist determined that chemotherapy followed by a bone marrow transplant was the most desirable course of treatment. Katie's own bone marrow was excised and harvested before her admission to the hospital. After admission, she received large doses of chemotherapy, followed by reinfusion of her previously harvested bone marrow. Katie was placed in strict isolation, progressing to modified isolation as her condition improved. Occupational therapy was provided as part of a collaborative team approach, led by the physician, which included physical therapy, dietetics, dentistry, clinical social work, child life, and other medical specialists (e.g., neurosurgeon). Daily team meetings were open to all disciplines.

Occupational therapy assessment focused on evaluation of Katie's self-care and fine motor skills. The fine motor evaluation included manual muscle testing, the nine-hole peg test, eye-hand coordination, in-hand manipulation skills, and clinical observations of the quality of movement and of endurance. Self-care was evaluated through an interview with her mother and observation of dressing and feeding. Her mother indicated that she was concerned about the impaired movement of Katie's left arm and hand and her general strength and endurance.

The fine motor evaluation results showed full active range of motion of the right arm, but limitations in end ranges noted of her left arm. Strength of her right arm was within normal limits, but was decreased in her left arm. Left-side neglect was noted. In the area of fine motor skills, Katie demonstrated decreased coordination and in-hand manipulation in the right hand. Her left hand was significantly impaired, with decreased accuracy in gross reach and grasp and an inability to pick up or manipulate small objects. Katie used her left hand primarily as an assist. Her general endurance and tolerance for activity varied and ranged from an inability to sit independently to being able to get out of bed and move to sit in a chair with minimal assistance.

Based on her mother's report and clinical observation, Katie required moderate assistance with all self-care activities. Initial occupational therapy goals focused on improving her sitting tolerance while engaged in activity, improving left upper-extremity function in bilateral tasks, improving upper-extremity strength and coordination, and promoting independence in activities of daily living. Because of isolation requirements, treatment was provided in Katie's room. Treatment equipment was limited to those items that met the criteria for prevention of infection.

In addition to medical and nursing care, Katie also received services from other members of the hospital team. Physical therapy intervention was provided for lower-extremity strength, endurance, and gait. The dietitian was concerned with caloric needs and nutritional status. The clinical social worker assessed family dynamics and reactions to Katie's illness, as well as provided supportive intervention and assisted the family with financial issues. Dentistry was concerned with the condition of Katie's teeth, mouth, and gums because dental problems may be a source of infection. The child life specialist provided activities to assist Katie with her psychosocial adjustment to hospitalization and to help her cope with the stresses of hospitalization. Physicians from other medical specialties were involved as needed for specific problems.

After discharge, Katie returned to her mother's home, where she received home-based education services as a precaution against exposure to infections. She continued to receive occupational therapy in the bone marrow transplant day treatment program at the hospital.

In this case, occupational therapy's role focused on upper-extremity strength and coordination and general strength and endurance as these variables affected functional performance. The provision of occupational therapy has influenced environmental constraints designed to protect the child from infection. Cooperative efforts by team members enabled services to be provided in a manner that offered Katie the greatest benefit while still meeting the goals of individual disciplines.

## General Acute Care Unit

General acute care units tend to be designated by medical specialty. For example, patients of various ages with different types of orthopedic conditions and treatment needs may be served on one acute care unit. Another type of unit is a general surgical unit, where patients requiring different types of surgery are admitted for preoperative and postoperative care. Designating units in this manner enables the physician and other members of the medical team to use their patient care time and equipment more efficiently and results in increased opportunities for formal and informal communication regarding each child's care.

General acute care units differ from ICUs in several ways. Patients tend to be more medically stable and less dependent on life-sustaining equipment as part of their medical treatment. The less serious nature of their medical conditions may enable them to receive greater benefit from occupational therapy and permits the children to leave the unit for occupational therapy or other services, although services may be provided at bedside if needed. Occupational therapists may be responsible for patients on one or more acute care units, requiring them to be familiar with the procedures of each unit, the types of patients admitted to the different units, and the nurses and other hospital personnel who provide services. Patients admitted directly to an acute care unit of this type also tend to have a shorter hospital stay than those who progress from ICU to another type of unit. Consequently, the occupational therapist often has less opportunity to develop a relationship with both the patient and family.

## Failure to Thrive

Children with failure to thrive (FTT) often require hospitalization for acute care. FTT is a diagnosis given to children, frequently infants and toddlers, who fail to grow or gain weight. FTT may be designated as organic, arising from a diagnosable physical cause, or as nonorganic, which denotes impaired growth without apparent physical cause (Frank, 1985). Although organic FTT can be attributed to a specific physical disorder, nonorganic FTT has been associated with psychosocial factors. Disturbances in the parent–child interaction early in life and in the development of attachment, difficult infant temperament and behavior, maternal social isolation, and financial difficulties within the family are some of the variables associated with nonorganic FTT (Bithoney & Newberger, 1987; Drotar, 1985). In some instances, FTT may be attributed to both organic and nonorganic factors.

Frank (1985) suggested that children with nonorganic FTT may still have biologic risks. She identified three categories of risk: perinatal, toxic and immunologic, and neurodevelopmental. Perinatal risk refers to the potential for FTT in infants who are considered low birth weight, possibly as a result of prematurity or intrauterine growth retardation. Toxic and immunologic risks arise from significant nutritional deficiency, which has the potential to increase vulnerability to infection and increase susceptibility to lead toxicity. Neurodevelopmental risk results from effects of inadequate nutrition on the developing nervous system. Although toxic and immunologic risks are generally reversible through medical treatment, treatment may not fully reverse the neurodevelopmental consequences.

The complexity of factors implicated in FTT emphasizes the need for a coordinated team approach that offers medical, nutritional, developmental, and psychosocial intervention. As a member of the hospital-based team, the occupational therapist may contribute to both the diagnosis and treatment of the child with FTT. A comprehensive occupational therapy assessment provides the medical team with information regarding the infant's developmental status, feeding behaviors, infant-caregiver interactions during play and feeding, and infant interactions with nonfamily members (e.g., the occupational therapist).

Denton (1986) differentiated between FTT in infants and toddlers, suggesting that the toddlers who fail to thrive present with poor feeding skills that may be the result of behavioral issues. Infant assessment emphasizes interactional issues with the caregivers; toddler assessment focuses more on the toddler's behaviors in the feeding situation and attempts to differentiate between environmental factors and neuromotor difficulties that may be affecting feeding. A developmental and feeding history obtained from the parent is a valuable component of the occupational therapy assessment with both infants and toddlers.

Occupational therapy treatment goals with a child who fails to thrive may include improving oral motor and feeding skills and facilitating development. Promoting positive parent-child interaction may also be emphasized, using strategies that help the parent understand infant behavioral cues, engage in positive, developmentally appropriate play experiences, and develop behavioral expectations consistent with the child's level of functioning.

The following case report illustrates occupational therapy intervention with FTT children.

Kevin was a 3-month 7-day-old boy transferred from a community hospital to a regional children's hospital by helicopter after suffering a seizure. He was intubated en route. Initial diagnoses included rule-out abuse, severe nonorganic FTT, anemia, rule out sepsis and bacteremia, hyponatremia, dehydration, and seizure. On examination, Kevin was noted to have bruising above both knees and over his right buttocks. He was observed to have diaper rash and wasting of the left hip and extremities. Kevin was referred to occupational therapy by the PICU attending physician on day 3 of inpatient admission because the child demonstrated poor oral feeding.

Kevin's parents brought him to the referring hospital's emergency room after a home visit by a Child Protective Services worker. He was left at the emergency room, and his parents did not visit during his 14-day hospitalization at the children's hospital. His maternal great aunt visited occasionally and expressed interest in adopting him.

Kevin was born at term weighing 5 pounds 12 ounces. He went home after a noncomplicated 48-hour hospital stay. He was hospitalized at 2 months of age for FTT, upper respiratory tract infection, and otitis media. He was discharged to his parents with home health nursing, a Child Protective Services referral, and pediatric follow-up. Kevin's parents missed all follow-up appointments until presenting him to the emergency room, leading to this hospitalization.

A pH probe showed severe gastroesophageal reflux. An upper gastrointestinal series was performed and ruled out anatomic abnormality. Stool samples were analyzed and showed malabsorption, reducing substances, increased fatty acids, and *Giardia Lamblia,* all of which combined to reduce his level of nutrient absorption and increase fluid loss. As a result, Kevin was severely underweight and lethargic. Medical treatment for the reflux included positioning on an elevated wedge, thickened feeds, and medications.

Kevin was evaluated by occupational therapy using clinical observations for his oral motor and feeding and developmental skills and the Infant Neurological International Battery (INFANIB) to assess reflexes, muscle tone, and posture. He demonstrated intact oral structures and sensation with functional oral skills for safe oral feeding. He had small sucking pads with a weak suck and fair coordination of suck-swallow-breathe. His suck and coordination improved with support at his jaw and cheeks. Kevin's developmental skills were delayed, and he demonstrated poor state control with high irritability. His score on the INFANIB indicated transient muscle tone, which is not uncommon for his age. It was the therapist's impression that Kevin's weak suck, poor feeding, and irritability were from overall weakness, malnutrition, and recent intubation rather than from a neurologic deficit.

The occupational therapist developed a bedside plan of specific facilitation techniques to be used during feeding. These included jaw and cheek support, external tongue stimulation, flexion swaddling, decreasing external stimulation, upright and well-aligned feeding positioning, limiting oral feeding to 30 minutes, and turning off the continuous pump feeding Kevin through a nasal gastric tube. After implementation of occupational therapy recommendations by nursing staff, Kevin's oral intake increased dramatically over the next 3 days, with the occupational therapist feeding him once daily to monitor progress. Once the acute feeding issues were resolved, occupational therapy focused on developmental activities to improve self-calming, visual tracking, and social skills. The therapist also made recommendations for positioning and providing normal movement opportunities. He was referred for outpatient occupational therapy and early intervention services before discharge. Children's Protective Services assumed custody of Kevin, and he was discharged to a foster home with a 2.4-pound weight increase and scheduled weekly weight checks with his pediatrician. The occupational therapist provided the foster parents with a home program including positioning, feeding, and activities to promote development.

## Outpatient Services

Outpatient services are an important component of the total spectrum of hospital care. Occupational therapy is generally provided on an outpatient basis for one of three reasons: (1) as part of a diagnostic assessment, (2) to provide needed intervention after hospital discharge, or (3) to provide occupational therapy intervention for individuals with disabilities or other chronic conditions (Figure 27-6). Occupational therapy intervention may be provided at the hospital, at a hospital satellite center, or as part of an interdisciplinary hospital-based clinic (e.g., arthritis clinic, feeding clinic, or cerebral palsy clinic).

In general, the referral base for outpatient services may extend beyond the hospital's medical staff. Patients may be referred for outpatient occupational therapy by their attending physicians in the hospital, by a community-based physician (e.g., pediatrician or family practitioner), or by a physician in a hospital-based specialty clinic. As with inpatient services, a referral from a physician determines the services to be provided.

Provision of occupational therapy services on an outpatient basis differs from provision of services to acute care patients in a number of ways. Services are usually provided to outpatients less frequently (e.g., one to three times per week) and may continue for weeks or months. The longer duration provides a greater opportunity for the occupational therapist to get to know the child's family and develop a collaborative relationship. Also, children seen on an outpatient basis are essentially well, as opposed to children who are hospitalized for an acute or transient illness. One disadvantage of outpatient therapy is the limited opportunity for

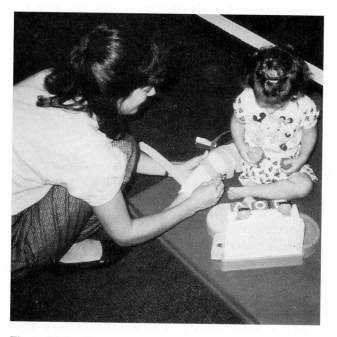

**Figure 27-6** An occupational therapist fabricates a splint for a young patient with juvenile rheumatoid arthritis.

collaboration and communication with other professionals who provide services to the child. In most cases the child served as an outpatient does not have a medical team with members who meet to discuss and coordinate services.

Outpatient services provided as part of an interdisciplinary medical clinic usually have a specific, well-defined purpose. In some instances the occupational therapist functions as a consultant, completing an assessment, then making recommendations to the physician. In other cases the occupational therapist is an integral part of the decision-making team and may be involved in patient assessment, treatment or equipment recommendations, or provision of splints and adaptive equipment. Usually, children visit specialty medical clinics infrequently, one to two times per year, for example, limiting the role of the occupational therapist in the clinic. However, children treated as patients in medical specialty clinics may also receive occupational therapy services separately, either at the hospital or in their home communities.

## DOCUMENTATION OF OCCUPATIONAL THERAPY SERVICES

Documentation of patient care is an essential and time-consuming component of occupational therapy service provision in hospitals. Occupational therapy evaluation reports, treatment plans, patient progress notes, and discharge summaries are used to communicate occupational therapy intervention to the physician, other members of the medical team, the patient and family, and reimbursement agencies.

Format and frequency of documentation are determined by the policies and procedures of the hospital and occupational therapy department. Accreditation guidelines regarding documentation are provided to institutions by agencies such as the JCAHO and the CARF. Agencies that reimburse services, such as Medicaid or private insurance, also have requirements for documentation with which occupational therapists must comply.

Documentation of services to hospitalized patients through evaluation reports with accompanying treatment plans, progress notes, and discharge summaries occurs in the patient's medical chart. Because the medical chart remains on the unit or accompanies the patient when he or she receives services elsewhere in the hospital, information is readily available to other health professionals. Documentation of occupational therapy intervention with outpatients may take a different form because reports are often sent to referring physicians or other agencies in the community. Copies of outpatient reports are retained in the patient's hospital medical record, however. Documentation of services in clinics may also follow a different format because each clinic may have a medical chart for the patient. Regardless of the format, documentation of services must meet minimum criteria established by accrediting and reimbursement agencies.

## STUDY QUESTIONS

1. Consider the child diagnosed as failure to thrive. What occupational performance components and environmental contexts should be the focus of occupational therapy evaluation and intervention with this child?

2. List three roles of the occupational therapist with the child who has received severe burns. Give examples of occupational therapy activities at each phase of recovery (i.e., acute, surgical, and rehabilitation).

3. Describe the characteristics of occupational therapy services in a medical model. Compare these characteristics with those of occupational therapy in education settings (Chapters 24 and 25). What are advantages and disadvantages of each model of service delivery?

## SUMMARY

The provision of occupational therapy services to children in hospitals is a specialized and challenging area of practice. Occupational therapists in hospitals must have a thorough understanding of the hospital's roles and characteristics in health care delivery, the numerous factors and trends that affect hospitals, and the specialized needs of hospitalized children. Occupational therapists who are employed in hospitals have the opportunity to gain expertise in assessment and treatment of children of various ages with many different diagnoses within a dynamic, fast-paced environment. As hospitals broaden their range of services in response to a changing health care system, hospital-based occupational therapists will have opportunities to broaden their areas of expertise into different inpatient and outpatient settings.

## REFERENCES

Affleck, A.T., Lieberman, S., Polon, J., & Rohrkemper, K. (1986). Providing occupational therapy in an intensive care unit. *American Journal of Occupational Therapy, 40,* 323-332.

Bithoney, W.G. & Newberger, E.H. (1987). Child and family attributes of failure-to-thrive. *Developmental and Behavioral Pediatrics, 8,* 32-36.

*1994 CARF standards manual: an interpretive guideline for organizations serving people with disabilities.* (1994). Tucson: CARF.

Case-Smith, J. & Wavrek, B.B. (1993). Models of service delivery and team interaction. In J. Case-Smith (Ed.). *Pediatric occupational therapy and early intervention* (pp. 27-159). Boston: Andover Publishers.

*1995 Comprehensive accreditation manual for hospitals.* (1994). Oakbrook Terrace, IL: Joint Commission on the Accreditation of Health Care Organizations.

Considine, W.H. (1994). Children's needs: a health care reform priority. *Hospital and Health Networks, 68,* 84.

Denton, R. (1986). An occupational therapy protocol for assessing infants and toddlers who fail to thrive. *American Journal of Occupational Therapy, 40,* 352-358.

DeWitt, P.K., Jansen, M.T., Ward, S.L., & Keens, T.G. (1993). Obstacles to discharge of ventilator-assisted children from the hospital to home. *Chest, 103,* 1560-1565.

Doane, C. (1989). Children with severe burns. In P. Pratt & A. Allen (Eds.). *Occupational therapy for children* (2nd ed.) St. Louis: Mosby.

Drotar, D. (1985). Failure to thrive and preventative mental health: knowledge gaps and research needs. In D. Drotar (Ed.). *New directions in failure to thrive* (pp. 27-44). New York: Plenum Press.

Frank, D.A. (1985). Biologic risks in "nonorganic" failure to thrive: diagnostic and therapeutic implications. In D. Drotar (Ed.). *New directions in failure to thrive* (pp. 17-26). New York: Plenum Press.

Furman, W.L. & Feldman, S. (1990). Infectious complications. In F. L. Johnson & C. Pochedly (Eds.). *Bone marrow transplantation in children* (pp. 427-450). New York: Raven Press.

Gilkerson, L. (1990). Understanding institutional functional style: a resource for hospital and early intervention collaboration. *Infants and Young Children, 2,* 22-30.

Gilkerson, L., Gorski, P., & Panitz, P. (1990). Hospital-based intervention for preterm infants and their families. In S. Meisels & J. Shonkoff (Eds.). *Handbook of early childhood intervention* (pp. 445-468). Cambridge, MA: Cambridge University Press.

Gohsman, B. (1981). The hospitalized child and the need for mastery. *Issues in Comprehensive Pediatric Nursing, 5,* 67-76.

Knudson-Cooper, M. (1982). Emotional care of the hospitalized burned child. *Journal of Burn Care and Rehabilitation, 3,* 109-115.

Leman, C.J. (1993). Burn rehabilitation. In H.L. Hopkins & H.D. Smith (Eds.). *Willard and Spackman's occupational therapy* (pp. 691-705). Philadelphia: J. B. Lippincott.

Lenarsky, C. (1990). Technique of bone marrow transplantation. In F. L. Johnson & C. Pochedly (Eds.). *Bone marrow transplantation in children* (pp. 53-67). New York: Raven Press.

Levy, L.L. (1993). Occupational therapy's place in the health care system. In H.L. Hopkins & H.D. Smith (Eds.). *Willard and Spackman's occupational therapy* (pp. 357-372). Philadelphia: J.B. Lippincott.

Occupational exposure to bloodborne pathogens; final rule, 56 Federal Register 64175-64182 (1991).

Perinchief, J.M. (1993). Service management. In H.L. Hopkins & H.D. Smith (Eds.). *Willard and Spackman's occupational therapy* (pp. 375-398). Philadelphia: J.B. Lippincott.

Petrillo, M. & Sanger, S. (1980). *Emotional care of hospitalized children.* Philadelphia: J.B. Lippincott.

Pontzer, K. (1994). Responding to managed care. *OT Week, 8,* 35-36.

Rausch, G. & Melvin, J.L. (1986). Nationally speaking: a new era in acute care. *American Journal of Occupational Therapy, 40,* 319-322.

Spruce, W.E. (1990). Supportive care in bone marrow transplantation. In F.L. Johnson & C. Pochedly, (Eds.). *Bone marrow transplantation in children* (pp. 69-86). New York: Raven Press.

Suhr, M.A. (1986). Trauma in pediatric populations. *Advances in Psychosomatic Medicine, 16,* 31-47.

Torrance, M. (1993) Acute care occupational therapy. In H.L. Hopkins & H.D. Smith (Eds.). *Willard & Spackman's occupational therapy* (pp. 771-783). Philadelphia: J.B. Lippincott.

Williams, T.E. (1990). Ethical and psychosocial issues in bone marrow transplantation in children. In F.L. Johnson & C. Pochedly (Eds.). *Bone marrow transplantation in children* (pp. 497-504). New York: Raven Press.

Williams, T.E. & Safarimaryaki, S. (1990). Bone marrow transplantation for treatment of solid tumors. In F.L. Johnson & C. Pochedly (Eds.). *Bone marrow transplantation in children* (pp. 221-242). New York: Raven Press.

Wilson, T. & Broome, M.E. (1989). Promoting the young child's development in the intensive care unit. *Heart & Lung, 18*, 274-281.

Zander, A.R. & Aksamit, I.A. (1990). Immune recovery following bone marrow transplantation. In F.L. Johnson & C. Pochedly (Eds.). *Bone marrow transplantation in children* (pp. 87-110). New York: Raven Press.

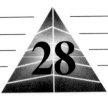

# Home-Based Intervention

JILL ANDERSON ▲ JOANNE S. SCHOELKOPF

## KEY TERMS

▲ Home-Based Service
▲ Medically Fragile Children
▲ Family Participation
▲ Cultural Sensitivity

## CHAPTER OBJECTIVES

1. Describe the types of children and family circumstances that benefit from home-based services.
2. Describe the role of the occupational therapist in home-based services.
3. Describe differences between home-based and center-based intervention.
4. Explain assets and limitations of occupational therapy evaluation and intervention in the home.
5. Identify examples of cultural values and differences to be respected and appreciated.
6. Describe issues in safety and universal precautions for home-based intervention.

There has been a significant expansion in home-based intervention for infants and children with disabilities, with concurrent increase in referrals for occupational therapy. Advances in medical care and dramatic reduction of mortality rates for very premature or low-birth-weight infants over the past 25 years have increased the number of infants at risk for developmental disabilities (Sandall, 1990). Prenatal detection of fetal problems and early surgical intervention have led to greater rates of survival among children with a variety of anomalies. Other advances in medical technology and life-sustaining equipment have resulted in extended life spans of seriously ill infants.

In addition to the increase in *number* of infants who have

or are at risk for disability, the *types and nature* of disabilities have changed in recent years. For example, the identified number of infants who sustained intrauterine exposure to cocaine and crack has increased. More infants in the drug-exposed population have been diagnosed as carriers of human immunodeficiency virus (HIV) (Parks, 1994; Russell & Free, 1991).

Recent changes in the education laws for individuals with disabilities, emphasizing intervention in the child's natural setting, have also resulted in an increase in home-based early intervention (Bailey & Simeonsson, 1988). Occupational therapy is an integral service of home-based early intervention programs. School-aged children may continue to receive home-based occupational therapy if they have serious, chronic medical conditions such as uncontrolled seizure disorders or depressed immune systems, are dependent on technology, or are acutely ill (Ahmann & Lipsi, 1991). Families may elect to supplement their child's school-based occupational therapy with private, home-based services because this form of service delivery allows greater flexibility in length and frequency of sessions and in treatment approaches. Home-based services also provide consistent, direct communication between parents and therapists.

## NATURE OF HOME-BASED SERVICES

P.L. 99-457, Part H, provides incentive funding for states to develop early intervention programs that serve developmentally delayed and at-risk infants. The law designates the home as an appropriate environment to support the social and emotional well-being of the young children and their families. Service delivery in the home environment appears to reduce the stress of frequent visits to a center-based program and to be more effective in facilitating the child's development (Hanft, 1988). Literature supports this rationale and suggests that home-based services provide an opportunity for enhanced family involvement in the child's services (Bailey & Simeonsson, 1988).

Initially, home-based services were either paid directly by private clients or were reimbursed through private insurance companies. Recently the trend shifted to public funding through Medicaid, Medicare, school systems, and state-funded agencies. Home-based services may be provided by private practitioners, home health agencies, private non-profit associations, private for-profit agencies, hospitals, schools, early intervention programs, medical personnel, social service agencies, or a combination of these.

In general, children who are referred for home-based occupational therapy services have been identified through an evaluation process as developmentally delayed or at risk for disability. Children with specific medical diagnoses, those identified as *at-risk* because of birth complications and those considered to be medically fragile, are frequently referred for home-based services on discharge from a hospital. Many of these babies have respiratory, cardiac, and feeding problems and may be dependent on cardiac monitors and oxygen, suctioning, and feeding devices. Other babies have severe, uncontrolled seizure disorders that necessitate close monitoring of heart and breathing rates during the seizure and recovery period.

A family may choose home-based services when transportation to a center-based program is complicated by the need to carry medical equipment or personnel to monitor the child's medical status. For example, the family of a 3-year-old child with severe seizure disorder, glaucoma, and significant developmental delay elected to continue home-based services even though the child was eligible for a center-based program. His mother was concerned that the bus ride and the lights and noise in the classroom might result in increased seizure activity. She also thought that it would be to the child's benefit to have therapy services at home to take advantage of his sleep and wake cycles. The home-based occupational therapist provided a program of graded sensory input that increased the child's level of alertness to his environment and decreased self-stimulatory behaviors. During the sensory activities the child's responses were carefully monitored to prevent overstimulation or induction of seizures.

Children who have acute medical conditions that require chemotherapy or those who have received organ transplants are likely to be unable to attend school for a defined period. They often need occupational therapy to provide adaptive equipment and to develop techniques to maintain independence. A young girl who required a 3-month course of chemotherapy for leukemia received home-based occupational therapy. Because chemotherapy suppressed her immune system and significantly increased the risk of infection, the physician restricted her activity to the home while on treatment. When home-based services are provided for a limited time, it is important that intervention goals and plans are coordinated with the therapists who previously provided services and those who will continue services in settings outside the home.

# ROLE OF THE OCCUPATIONAL THERAPIST

Occupational therapy in the home-based setting encompasses evaluation, direct and consultation services, and service coordination. The therapist must assess the impact of the child's disability on family-child interactions and among family members to determine how this may affect the child's development. When the evaluation process occurs in the home, the therapist can be more sensitive to family issues and the psychosocial aspects of the child's development. The home is an optimal setting for the therapist to gain an understanding of the family's interaction with the child and the effect of the environment on the child's performance.

## Direct Services

In addition to one-on-one interactions with the child, direct services include *education of and emotional support to caregivers.* Education may include explanation of the interrelationship of performance components (e.g., trunk control, shoulder stability, isolated finger use, or flexible palmar arch) and functional skills (e.g., play and self-care). Explanation of the therapy activities helps family members understand the rationale for occupational therapy goals and increases the likelihood of collaboration and follow-through of the activities. Families of children with sensory integrative dysfunction also need education and explanations of their children's behaviors. The family may be concerned with their child's high activity level and inability to pay attention. They may also describe frustrations in their daily interactions with their child. The occupational therapist can explain how sensory integrative intervention techniques lower the activity level so their child can concentrate more easily. The therapist can help the parent develop strategies to facilitate positive interactions.

When the occupational therapist is the primary health professional who has consistent contact with a family or when a family feels most comfortable with the occupational therapist, the therapist may be called on to provide emotional support and help the family deal with issues other than those resulting from the child's disability. Family functioning may be affected by other stressors such as illness of another family member, substance abuse, unemployment, or financial problems. One mother spent a session speaking with the therapist about her husband's recent unemployment and alcoholism. The therapist suggested that other professionals could help in this situation and asked if she might request that the social worker contact her.

The home setting is generally more casual and informal than a center or clinic. Often the demands of caring for a special child prevent socialization opportunities for a mother and other family members. Some parents express an interest in expanding their relationship with the therapists so that it becomes more social. When one child fell asleep during the treatment session, his mother used the time to have coffee with the therapist and discuss other aspects of her life. It appeared important for her to talk about issues other than her child. The therapist must identify each family's needs and recognize how much flexibility they can allow themselves in their relationship with the family, while continuing to provide services to the disabled child (Bryant, Lyons, & Wasik, 1990).

The extent of a therapist's role in parent education varies according to family needs or individual parent responses to therapist recommendations. When parents have limited education or are cognitively impaired, an important role of the occupational therapist is education of the parents about their child's development. He or she may help the parents select and purchase appropriate toys and facilitate appropriate caregiving at each developmental phase (e.g., suggest that the parent introduce new foods). The therapist may also help them interpret their child's behaviors; for example, the therapist may explain the causes of the irritability or hyperactivity. With these explanations, the therapist offers methods to manage behaviors and to promote development.

## Consultation

The occupational therapist often recommends specific positioning, adaptive equipment, or placement of toys and manipulatives that should be implemented by all the other professionals who work with the child. As part of the intervention program with a child with hemiparesis, the occupational therapist consulted with the educator to demonstrate how to position an activity to promote use of both sides of his body. She recommended that toys be placed on the affected side to encourage weight bearing on that side, to promote crossing the midline, and to encourage visual scanning of the visual field on that side. The educator then modified how and where she presented activities to the child to encourage the use of both upper extremities.

## Service Coordinator

The occupational therapist as service coordinator is responsible for formal documentation and communication regarding all aspects of services being provided to the family. The therapist helps families access appropriate services and helps coordinate services so that goals and recommendations are cohesive and consistent with those of the family. One mother expressed her need to learn English. She indicated that she was overwhelmed with her family's problems. The occupational therapist referred her to social work and psychology services, who were able to arrange counseling and a language class.

## INTERVENTION PROCESS
### Evaluation

In evaluation of the child in the home, the therapist must adapt to the physical environment in the home as well as the presence of family members. There may be space limitations or other activities occurring in the home, and the therapist may be called on to explain the evaluation procedures continuously throughout the process. The therapist must also be aware of the impact of these factors in the interpretation of test results. For example, a child may appear extremely distractible or hyperactive in a busy home with high activity and noise levels. Before the evaluation the therapist may ask if the child has eaten, is well rested, and is in good health to facilitate the child's best performance. Parents do not always plan ahead for the therapist's visit, nor is it always possible to ensure that a child is fed and rested. The therapist may need to explain the relationship between the child's performance and hunger, illness, or lack of sleep. He or she may decide to reschedule an evaluation if the child appears unusually tired or irritable.

## Intervention

The home environment also affects the types of intervention activities that are provided. Using selected frames of reference, such as sensory integration, may be more difficult to implement in the home (Hinojosa, Anderson, & Strauch 1988). Limitations in space or the need for large or suspended equipment may restrict the therapist's ability to carry out these techniques in the home. Therapists need to be creative in adapting techniques to use space and equipment that may be available in the home; for example, a weighted backpack may be substituted for a weighted vest in the treatment of a child with attention deficit disorder. A little red wagon and a toy flying saucer were used to provide vestibular stimulation for this child. He squeezed soft rubbery toys and a Koosh ball to decrease the tactile hypersensitivity in his palms.

Many types of intervention are easily and successfully implemented in the home. The family of a preschool-aged girl with a diagnosis of juvenile rheumatoid arthritis chose to continue private therapy in which myofacial release and craniosacral techniques were emphasized. The family arranged a quiet space with controlled lighting in which the therapist could implement the handling techniques without the time constraints imposed by a clinic or school setting. These intervention techniques are often not implemented in school-based settings because of busy schedules of therapists and the orientation toward school-based goals. The therapist also used opportunities after the intervention sessions to discuss strategies for increasing the child's independence at home and general endurance in physical activities.

## Family-Centered Services

The presence of siblings in the home can have an impact on intervention. Therapists may set limits to their involvement or include them in activities as a means to motivate the child. Siblings close in age to the child receiving services may display disruptive behavior during intervention, often because they perceive the therapy as special attention to their sibling. Parents may need reassurance that this is a normal occurrence. In one family in which the parents had marital problems and sibling behavioral problems, the therapist was unable to limit the sibling's presence in the therapy area. To limit his disruptive behaviors, the therapist provided the sibling with activities and materials during each session. This allowed the therapist to focus on the child who was receiving services. In another family the older brother held materials at the therapist's direction to encourage his sibling's ability to reach and visually search. The older brother's participation held two advantages: it freed the therapist's hands for positioning and handling, and it increased the motivation of the sibling.

The therapist must adapt to the style the parent has chosen to use in coping with the child's disability (Figure 28-1). Some families prefer that therapists provide services without their active participation in carrying out therapeutic activities, and others may prefer to learn and carry out therapeutic techniques used by each discipline. Some parents demonstrate their involvement by regularly communicating with each therapist and may be particularly eager for specific feedback regarding their child's progress. Many families become involved in organizations or political action groups for individuals with disabilities. In each of these circumstances the therapist adjusts his or her timing, style, and mode of communication so that it promotes effective therapist-family relationship. Sensitivity and responsivity to the needs of family members requires ongoing listening and communication skills (Bazyk, 1989) (see Chapter 5).

The therapist may need to help the family include and

encourage their child's participation in family activities. The therapist may concentrate on use of equipment and positioning techniques that allow the child to sit at the dinner table, watch television with siblings, or go on an outing to the mall. For example, a child with spastic diplegia who ambulated short distances in her home and in the special education setting required assistance in mobility for longer distances. The therapist helped the family select a stroller that fit in their car, was light enough to be lifted easily by all family members, and allowed them to take their child to places that required long-distance walking without worrying about the child's fatigue. Materials found in the home can also be used for positioning, particularly when financial resources are limited or when the family has difficulty accepting adaptive equipment. An 8-month-old infant, born prematurely and fed with a gastric tube, required support to maintain a side-lying or sitting position. Pillows were used to break up extensor and adductor tone in a child's lower extremities, which allowed him to sit and work on upper-extremity skills. A commercially available ring pillow, the Boppy, was purchased to provide support at the hips and pelvis, thus promoting sitting independence. Other inexpensive and cosmetically appealing products are commercially available and can be recommended for positioning or sensory input. These include molded plastic floor seats with lap trays, infant carriers that hold the baby close to the mother's chest, and cloth inserts for shopping carts that abduct the legs and support the lower trunk. Figure 28-2 shows a tumble form chair commonly used to position the child for feeding. The easy access to these products and the opportunity to demonstrate their versatility in the home setting are additional benefits.

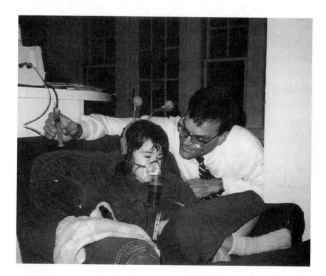

**Fig. 28-1** When the father is at home during a visit, the occupational therapist can solicit his concerns and perceptions. Discussions about the progress of the child, changes in goals, and family priorities should transpire on a regular basis.

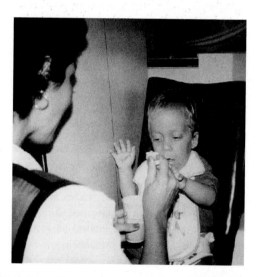

**Fig. 28-2** The therapist models feeding techniques. The home is an ideal environment to work on daily living skills such as feeding because the parent can easily replicate the positions and handling methods used by the therapist. Consistent use of handling and positioning methods by different caregivers supports the child's acquisition of new skills.

## Cultural Sensitivity

When working in the home, the therapist must be aware of and respect cultural differences. Particularly in self-help skills there are different expectations for the age of achievement of independence. In some cultures children are bottle fed for extended periods. Certain foods are acceptable at different ages in different cultures, and dietary restrictions based on religion or culture must be respected. Among some groups, children are carried even after they have learned to walk as a means of providing affection. In certain cultures the presence of a child with a disability stigmatizes the family and may influence the way they are accepted within the community. Often these families attempt to hide the presence of intervention professionals by requesting that they not bring recognizable therapy equipment, or that they park a distance from the house. These families may also find it difficult to discuss their emotional reactions to their children's disabilities with their family, community members, or with therapists providing services (Wayman, Lynch, & Hanson, 1990).

In some cultures it may be difficult for female therapists to interact with fathers because of cultural or religious dictates that limit male contact with nonrelated females. There may be styles of dress that are inappropriate to certain cultures or styles of language that are not acceptable. Modern technology such as television or electronic devices and toys related to these products may be prohibited by a culture and should not be used as a therapeutic activity. For example, in Hasidic or orthodox Jewish households only the kosher foods prepared within the home can be used for feeding. Therapists also cannot bring foods into the house for their own consumption. Religious Jewish and Muslim families observe a conservative dress code. Therapists should respect this by avoiding shorts, short skirts, and sleeveless and low-cut shirts. In both of these cultures, therapies are canceled for religious holidays, which may involve extended periods.

Families who do not speak English pose a particular challenge to the therapist. Creative strategies are needed to communicate successfully. Therapists for a child of Arab parents developed a system of communicating with gesture and

CASE STUDY #1

This case study illustrates that a well-coordinated home-based program benefits both the child and the family and may be the most appropriate mode of intervention for a child who is medically fragile.

At the time of this evaluation, Carl was 12 years old. He was diagnosed with cerebral palsy and mental retardation, with onset attributed to administration of diphtheria-tetanus-pertussis injection in infancy. He was on medication for seizure disorder and was reported by his family to have many allergies and to be susceptible to illnesses when exposed to other children. He has been educated at home, with inconsistent provision of any therapy services. The previous year the school district had insisted that Carl attend school. His parents reported that during the first week of school he had suffered a seizure and had been unattended during this episode. They were called to the school, where they found him lethargic with depressed responses. After this he never regained his previous functional level. His parents decided that they would not send him to school again for fear of further episodes. They petitioned for a full home-based program that would include all therapies in addition to the educational services.

Based on clinical assessment and interview with the family, the occupational therapist recognized the need for adaptive equipment for transportation, communication, and positioning. During the first months of intervention, after further evaluation of Carl and of the home environment, the occupational therapist recommended that the family obtain an adjustable wheelchair with environmental controls, a transportable positioner, and an augmentative communication device. She provided information regarding where and how to order the equipment and helped the family obtain funding for payment by documenting medical necessity. The equipment met the family's needs to have Carl seated in a manner they perceived as comfortable and to allow him visual contact with family members during social activities.

Because of his previous interest in music, it was important to his family that he be able to activate a tape player and the television set. Switches were provided for these purposes. A small-in-scale, lightweight wheelchair was ordered so that Carl had access to all rooms in the family's home and so that it could be put in the car easily for transport. The occupational therapist coordinated the choice of an augmentative communication device with the speech therapist so that access to the device was appropriate to Carl's visual-motor and fine motor abilities. Communication among team members and between team and family was maintained through use of a notebook. The family expressed satisfaction that home-based intervention was most appropriate for Carl's safety and met their priorities for developing his ability to participate in family life.

simple English when the mother was home alone. The father's work hours did not allow him to be present during therapy, and no interpreters could be found in the community. Written notes were left for the father to translate on his return from work. The occupational therapist, serving as service coordinator, helped locate an Arab-speaking pediatrician and neurologist so that the family could communicate more easily.

## OTHER CONSIDERATIONS IN HOME-BASED INTERVENTION

In addition to the cultural and psychosocial environment, physical, socioeconomic, and medical factors need to be considered when working in the home. Homes that are dirty or in disrepair may be unsafe settings for therapy. Thera-

pists need to carry disinfectants and personal cleansing items with them for infection control and general hygiene. In addition to observing universal precautions, which are primarily to prevent exposure to blood products, therapists must protect themselves and the children they treat from airborne diseases. Children with HIV and many other immune disorders should not be exposed to any common flu or virus because of their increased vulnerability and the complications that may result. Therapists with allergies or asthma should carry appropriate medications with them. Homes infested with cockroaches or mice necessitate taking precautions to seal equipment so as to not contaminate other homes.

The homes of families in poverty or of low socioeconomic status may have major structural problems that pose as hazards to the therapist. For examples, stairs or flooring

## CASE STUDY #2

This case study illustrates how medical, cultural, and family issues affected home-based occupational intervention for a medically fragile infant with a congenital anomaly. Peter was the youngest of five siblings in a Hasidic family. He was diagnosed at birth with Pierre-Robin syndrome associated with cleft palate and hypoplasia of the mandible. At the time services were initiated, he was 3 months old. He had a tracheostomy that required regular suctioning and a gastric tube for feeding. He had been hospitalized several times for surgeries and had 12 hours of skilled nursing care daily. Because of the closeness of the Hasidic community and involvement of extended family, there was always someone available to care for the siblings during Peter's hospitalizations. Peter's parents managed all aspects of his medical care at night but relied on the nurses for relief during the day.

The occupational therapist provided two 45-minute sessions weekly with an emphasis on positioning, handling, and sensory input to facilitate Peter's development during this period of intensive medical intervention. Because of the tracheostomy, oral-facial anomalies, and hypotonicity, Peter displayed hyperextension of his head, elevation and tightness in shoulders, and lack of reach and grasp patterns.

Peter's mother was concerned about Peter's progress and was conscientious about observing therapy and communicating with the therapist. She also requested that the nursing personnel follow through with therapeutic activities because her time to do so was limited, given the need to attend to her other children during the day and to Peter's medical needs at night. During the course of intervention, a

young member of the extended family died suddenly and unexpectedly. The family continued their daily activities and did not interrupt Peter's services, although there was a great deal of tension and sadness in the home for an extended period. His mother was comfortable enough to discuss some of her feelings of loss with the occupational therapist during home visits with Peter. It is unusual within the Hasidic community to share feelings with someone outside their culture.

Peter's 2-year-old brother initially interfered with therapy because of his demand for attention and because of the limited living space in the home, typical of many Hasidic households. The therapist adapted by bringing him in his own set of toys. Later on in Peter's therapy, his brother was included in the therapy sessions and helped motivate Peter by demonstrating and participating in motor activities.

The therapist had to select toys on the basis of their acceptability in the culture. An infant activity center with television characters and representations of dinosaurs was not appropriate for use. Use of audio tapes with children's songs and music from the Hasidic culture was particularly successful, first in calming Peter and later in developing visual regard and fine motor control.

Despite the stresses of a large family, Peter's extensive medical needs, and other family crises, Peter's mother was able to coordinate all his services and be an active participant in his intervention. At age 2, Peter was discharged from occupational therapy because his perceptual-motor and fine motor self-help skills were developmentally appropriate.

may be unsafe. Rusted nails and floors with splinters should be covered by transportable mats. The therapist and parents also might discuss ways to prevent injury to an infant who is learning to crawl on floor surfaces that are unsafe.

Service delivery in rural areas also poses particular challenges. Families may live in remote, isolated settings, with driving distances of 1 hour or more to different homes. Weather conditions, particularly in winter months, can significantly affect frequency of therapist visits to home access by unpaved roads. Similarly, there is often limited access to supplies and equipment that are readily available in densely populated areas. In addition, regional values, levels of education and income, and a variety of other support services tend to differ in rural areas and in different regions of the country. It becomes important for the therapist to know where and how to access support services within each community served.

Homes visits in urban high-crime areas may require therapists to work in teams and sometimes to make a decision to provide center-based therapy for reasons of personal safety. Therapists should also be alert in situations with a history of domestic violence, child abuse, or substance abuse so that they can protect themselves and family members.

Another consideration of practice in the home is the possibility for early identification of problems that may affect the child's and family's health and safety. For example, the therapist may believe that the living conditions are unsuit-

able for the child's well-being and contact a social worker to investigate the availability for alternative housing. In addition, specific indications of child abuse can be detected more easily in the home than in a school or clinical setting.

In most clinical and school settings, medical, transportation, and equipment emergencies are manageable because of readily available resource personnel and procedures. The therapist has easy access to closets of supplies and materials. In contrast, the home-based therapist must plan ahead for emergencies or special needs and rely on what they can successfully transport. Investment in communication technology may be a priority for the home-based therapist. Cellular telephones, beepers, and personal computers are used to facilitate communications, for personal safety and for record keeping. Table 28-1 lists equipment, toys, and supplies that occupational therapists frequently carry with them on home visits.

## SUMMARY

Home-based occupational therapy is a growing area of practice. This growth has been driven by changes in public health law and the increased survival of children with complex and severe medical problems that prevent entrance into community center-based programs. The holistic philosophy of occupational therapy makes it ideally suited to the home setting where intervention includes consideration of psychosocial issues, cultural factors, and family values as essential in intervention with the child.

The respect for family values inherent in the philosophy of occupational therapy facilitates a close relationship and enhanced communication between the therapist and family.

▲ **Table 28-1** Examples of Equipment, Toys, and Supplies for the Home-Based Occupational Therapist

| Equipment and Toys | Supplies |
|---|---|
| T-Stool | Bubbles |
| Scooterboard | Brushes |
| Vestibular board | Textured cloths |
| Spinning saucer | Puzzles |
| Small trampoline | Different-sized balls |
| Cardboard boxes and packing cases for tunnels | Coloring books and painting supplies |
| Small cuff weights | Carpet squares |
| Different sizes of plastic buckets for a small sand or water table (family's sink) | Beanbags |
| Gymnastic balls | Rice, beans, and lentils in containers (for tactile activities) |
| Laptop computer or other portable video games | Vibrators |
| Electronic toys and switch toys | Foam balls |
| Corner Chair or other small seating devices | |

Modified from Astill-Clausen, R. (1995). Pediatric services in the home. *AOTA Home Health Guidelines*. Bethesda, MD: American Occupational Therapy Association.

▲ **STUDY QUESTIONS**

1. List three examples of types of children for whom home-based intervention would be the most appropriate type of service delivery.
2. Define two family circumstances in which some level of home-based services is appropriate.
3. Compare evaluation methods and procedures in the home versus those in the clinic (refer to Chapters 27 and 30 for comparison). What are advantages and disadvantages of evaluation in the home?
4. What are two ways to appropriately elicit the participation of an older sibling in therapy sessions?
5. Explain two advantages of home-based care in the following instances:
   a. A family in poverty
   b. A family from a Mideastern country
   c. A situation of suspected child abuse

Home-based therapy may also provide parents with a greater sense of control over their child's treatment because they can set limits and define parameters of behavior in their own homes. Consideration of family needs and priorities in setting therapeutic goals and objectives adds to this sense of empowerment.

Home-based therapy requires a great deal of clinical expertise, flexibility, and adaptability. The case studies in this chapter illustrate methods for developing positive and productive relationships with families and providing effective intervention.

## REFERENCES

Ahmann, E. & Lipsi, D.A. (1991). Early intervention for technology-dependent infants and young children. *Infants and Young Children, 3*(4), 67-77.

Austill-Clausen, R. (1995). Pediatric services in the home. *AOTA Home health guidelines,* Bethesda, MD: Americation Occupational Therapy Association.

Bailey, D.B. & Simeonsson, R.J. (1988). Home based early intervention. In S. Odem & M. Karnes (Eds.). *Early intervention for infants and children with handicaps.* Baltimore: Brookes.

Bazyk, S. (1989). Changes in attitudes and beliefs regarding parent participation and home programs: an update. *American Journal of Occupational Therapy, 43*(11), 723-728.

Bryant, D.B., Lyons, D., & Wasik, B.H. (1990). Ethical issues involved in home visiting. *Topics in Early Childhood Special Education, 10* (4), 92-107.

Hanft, B. (1988). The changing environment of early intervention services: implications for practice. *American Journal of Occupational Therapy, 42*(11), 724-731.

Hinojosa, J., Anderson, J., & Strauch, C. (1988). Pediatric occupational therapy in the home. *American Journal of Occupational Therapy, 42*(1), 17-22.

Parks, R.A. (1994, November). HIV in the pediatric population: *NDTA network.* Chicago: The Neurodevelopmental Treatment Association.

Russell, F.F. & Free, T.A. (1991). Early intervention for infants and toddlers with prenatal drug exposure. *Infants and Young Children, 3*(4), 78-85.

Sandall, S.R. (1990). Developmental interventions for biologically at-risk infants at home. *Topics in Early Childhood Special Education, 10*(4), 1-13.

Wayman, K.I., Lynch, E.W., & Hanson, M.J. (1990). Home-based early childhood services: cultural sensitivity in a family system approach. *Topics in Early Childhood Special Education, 10*(4), 56-75.

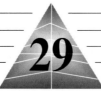

# The Dying Child

MARGARET J. BARNSTORFF

## KEY TERMS

▲ Hospice
▲ Respite Care
▲ Perception of Death
▲ Kübler-Ross Five Stages

## CHAPTER OBJECTIVES

1. Understand how children at different ages view death.
2. Recognize the impact of hospitalization on children, and their awareness of the severity of their conditions.
3. Gain insight into the feelings and attitudes of families of children who are dying; also those of the personnel who are working with them.

On a pediatric ward in a large medical center, I met two people who challenged me to learn more about death, especially children's perceptions of death.

Jan was an 11-year-old girl with a distorting facial malignancy that had been in progress for over 2 years. She had been seen periodically in various outpatient clinics, interspersed with hospital stays both in her hometown and in the regional medical center. The treatment she received, as well as the disease process, was extremely painful.

Finally, when Jan was dying in the medical center, she was in a private room that was darkened at all times. Her contacts with the outside world were few. The medical staff rarely visited her room, except to administer medications or during rounds.

Donna, a nursing student, was Jan's only meaningful contact with the outside world. Jan looked for Donna's visits, asked for her when she was not there, and allowed only Donna to spend extended periods with her. It was a relationship full of meaning for both, and it sparked my interest in the problems of dying children.

## SCOPE OF THE PROBLEM

One hundred years ago, childhood deaths were common, and many families had to learn to accept the loss of a child. Today, children's deaths are more unusual and often unexpected, even though a child may have a terminal disease. Our beliefs in the medical system and its ability to cure us leave all of us unprepared for death. Therefore children's deaths grievously affect those around the child: the family, the medical staff, and the community of friends and peers.

In the United States it is expected that tens of thousands of children die annually. The most prevalent cause of childhood deaths is accidents. This is followed by congenital abnormalities, respiratory complications, neoplasms, and acquired immunodeficiency syndrome (AIDS) (Ashby, Kosky, Laver, & Sims, 1991; Oleske et al, 1983).

When a child is terminally ill with an acute or chronic situation, various people care for that child: the family; the medical staff, consisting of the child's primary care physician and the many specialists who work together to provide diagnosis and treatment; and the nursing staff, dealing with the dying child on a daily basis, taking care of the child, administering the medications, charting the course of the disease, and providing opportunities for the child to use daily living skills. Allied health personnel also may be involved in the child's care and include the social worker, the physical therapist, the occupational therapist, the recreational therapist, the dietitian, and the medical technician.

Children who are dying also have the concern of parents, grandparents, aunts and uncles, siblings and cousins, as well as members of the community, such as teachers, classmates, and family friends. All of these individuals are affected by, and may be involved in the care of, the dying child.

It is typical for a child who is an accident victim to die in the hospital. However, children with terminal illnesses are now more often involved in home care programs (Martinson, 1986-1987) or hospice, palliative, or respite care programs, such as the Ronald McDonald Houses attached to hospitals in major cities (Dominica 1983; Pizzi, 1984; Tigges, 1983; Wilson, 1988). Here they are followed by her nurses, physical therapists, occupational therapists, aides, and volunteers. Other agencies that work with these children and their families include those that grant children's wishes, such as the "Make a Wish Foundation" and the "Sunshine Foundation," as well as those that provide familial bereavement counseling, such as the "Compassionate Friends" in Illinois or "the Candlelighters" in Washington, D.C. (Wessel, 1983).

Children with chronic diseases are often seen in outpatient clinics until they become too ill to remain at home. They are admitted to the hospital until disease remission allows them to return home. A pattern of recurrent hospitalizations is typical. In the last 10 years a trend has developed to allow the child for whom treatment fails to have the option to die at home, rather than in a hospital. This has been fostered through programs such as the hospice and individually developed programs at various medical centers (Mulhern, 1983).

## CHILDREN'S PERCEPTIONS OF DEATH

Depending on one's frame of reference for understanding children, there are either three or four stages in the development of a child's understanding of death. Nagy (1959), one of the earliest individuals to study this topic, suggested three stages: (1) from birth to 5 years the child believes that death is a reversible process in which life activities such as growing, hearing, and feeling can take place, (2) from the ages of 5 to 9 years the child personifies death as a distinct personality, and (3) from the age of 9, onward, death is understood to be a cessation of corporeal life and is a universal phenomenon.

Kane (1979) and Koocher (1973, 1979) related the development of a child's perception of death to Piaget's stages of development during the preoperational, concrete operations, and formal operations states. Their research suggested that as a child's mind matures, the cognitive stages are reflected in the child's understanding of death.

Childers and Wimmer (1971) studied children's perceptions of death, and their results indicated that differential awareness of death is a universal function of age. Among the subjects of their study, the understanding of death as being irrevocable was not demonstrated systematically until age 10.

Meliar (1973) suggested that there are four stages to the development of the concept of death: (1) the majority of 3- and 4-year-old children demonstrate a relative ignorance of the meaning of death, (2) among 4- to 7-year-old children, death is seen as a temporary state, (3) 5- to 10-year-old children appear to function in a transitional state; these children believe that death is final but that the dead function biologically, (4) to most older children death is a cessation of all biologic functioning.

## Infants

As a child matures from infancy to adulthood, his or her concepts of self, life, and eventual death parallel Erikson's and Piaget's developmental theories. The very young infant facing death reacts only physiologically, using all of his or her strength to continue living. As the child reaches the end of the period of bonding at around 6 months of age, he or she reacts to the physical process of the disease symptoms and the resulting treatment procedures. At this age the infant is capable of recognizing that he or she creates stress and conflicting emotions in others, especially his or her parents. The infant equates this with being bad. The infant may respond to treatment with anxiety and fear, which is further aggravated by separation anxiety. These reactions continue throughout the ages of 2 and 3. It is also during this period that the child learns the word *death*, but the word has little or no meaning for the toddler.

## Preschool Children

Egocentricity diminishes as the child is introduced to a world larger than the one known during the toddler years. At 4 years of age the child is beginning to conceptualize himself or herself as an individual; however, this conception is accompanied by that of "not me" as well. Feelings of being and not being must be dealt with by a preschooler. The thought of not being produces anxiety because it means separation from family and also loss of all the independence that has so far been acquired. The child focuses on the single dimension of comparing objects at a given time. Therefore the child focuses on life, which means being with others on earth as compared to death, which means separation from loved ones. Death also means that one becomes immobile, unable to move (Salladay & Royal, 1981). Thus thoughts of dying suggest dependency and loss of the self-control that a child of this age has just begun to acquire. Disease then threatens a child's very psychosocial existence.

Although children of ages 4 and 5 approach death with fantasy reasoning and magical thinking (Koocher 1973; Von Hug-Hellmuth, 1965), they begin to appreciate the meaning of a diagnosis, and this greatly influences their reactions to the world around them. Television, radio, magazines, books, and communications with others disclose many ideas. They hear words, view the responding emotions, and develop associations that can be applied to later experiences. Children begin this application process as they come to identify with others. Concurrently they develop an increased curiosity about burial, dead animals and flowers, and the accidental features of death.

For 3- to 5-year-old children, death means absence or going away and is a temporary, impermanent state (Meliar, 1973). Death is seen as a continuation of life but in a different place. Preschool children are incapable of cognitively understanding the process as being irreversible; such a concept is indicative of the ability to abstract thought. This is also true of retarded children who function cognitively at the preoperational level. Neither are these children realistic about the permanence or timing of death (Sternlicht, 1980). The most painful aspect of dying is the realization of separation. Denial is processed to overcome feelings of helplessness and the sense of loss. Narcissism develops with the threat to life and the recognition of the reality of the situation (Cook, Renshaw, & Jackson, 1973).

## School-aged Children

Children of school age come to realize that death is irreversible, it is the cessation of bodily functions as we know them, and it is universal to the species (Speece & Brent, 1984).

The prognosis and its significance are understandable to children of 5 to 7 years of age. Although children may realize that death is imminent, thoughts about this are seldom vocalized. They perceive absence and death with a sense of impending tragedy. By this time the concept of time has been mastered. School-aged children can think of an object as a whole, as well as consider its parts. With the vivid imagination that is also present at this time, the physical change and deterioration that occurs with death can be visualized. Death is specific and concrete and has both internal and external causes (Salladay & Royal, 1981). The prognosis becomes absolute and creates such anxiety that the child can no longer cope. As increasing age brings increased emotional and intellectual capability, it also brings greater meaning to a child's own death. This may lead to needing more assistance in coping.

Going to school full time adds to the child's continually changing social role and relationships within it. A 6- or 7-year-old child realizes that with death there comes a change in previously established relationships. Again, death symbolizes separation from loved ones. This breeds anxiety. The child now understands that separation cannot be avoided, and because of this knowledge, he or she learns to be a "good patient": death is not mentioned and feelings of pain and emotions are repressed. The rules of life are learned. At this time there is an emotional shift from anxiety to fear of physical injury and mutilation, operations, body intrusions, and needles (Spinetta, 1974). Often these children die lonely, pretending they will not die, even though all others around them are aware of this. They rarely ask questions related to their disease or treatment, and they tend to avoid the topic of death as if to protect their families from their approaching demise (Jeffrey & Lansdown, 1982).

From ages 5 to 9, death is personified and thought of as a contingency. Death, as a personality, is usually invisible, either having no form or going through the night so that it cannot be seen (Cook et al., 1973). This is the time of life when children may have difficulty going to bed at night in the dark for fear that they may not wake the next morning.

There is much talk at this age about the boogeyman. Death is remote; it exists outside of one's self, and through careful living, it can be kept at a distance. This is also a period of interest in animate and inanimate things, which evolves into a transition period of superstitions and rituals around death, being uncertain as to whether death is funny or fearful— "Don't step on the crack, it will break your mother's back."

It is not until children reach 8 or 9 years old that play and verbal expressions come to terms with each other. Weininger (1979) found that previous to this age, when children were told that a doll was sick and going to die, they tended to talk about the doll's death as being permanent but continued on in the play situation to have the doll return to life, recovering.

Grade-school children are also aware of their own identity. This allows them to think beyond self boundaries and to imagine. They understand about past and future concepts and fantasize about death and the idea of their own deaths. Thus they develop an alternative to death, seen in such forms as heaven, paradise, and hell. Children want their existence to continue. Through learning rules, they pattern themselves after other individuals, leading to the realization that their parents are not perfect. Children therefore seek alternative heroes, groping for something to believe in and worship. These beliefs allow them to organize their worlds methodically, including a cause and purpose behind every action. This is then followed by a reward or punishment. Death being perceived as a punishment may cause religious guilt (Lewis & Lewis, 1973). Secondary to this perception of punishment, dying children may reject the idea of heaven, which then represents only separation from family. Understanding of death increases throughout this stage, but these children tend to think that death comes suddenly and quickly. They may blot out feelings of death and in turn rely on parental authority (God, physicians, or teacher) for final protection from death.

Egocentricity is decreased in the 9- and 10-year-old child, while mature concepts of time, space, quantity, and causality are emerging. These children appreciate living and begin to understand death as the physical finality of living. Anxiety about death is characteristic in preadolescents and serves as a lead-in to adolescence (Toews, Martin, & Prosen, 1985).

## Adolescents

Adolescence is the bridge from childhood to adulthood; it is a period of transition. These transitions occur not only in the physiologic, but also in the cognitive, psychodynamic, and sociocultural aspects of development. Cognitively, adolescents move into the world of abstract thought. They learn to speculate on possibilities beyond reality and what might occur, as well as what does occur (Salladay & Royal, 1981). In this exploration adolescents will delve into the limits of life and the meaning of death.

Adolescents appreciate the reality of death (O'Brien, Johnson, & Schmink, 1978). However, personal death is not accepted (McDonald & Carroll, 1981). The adolescent tends to assume the attitude of "Everyone else but me can die." Adolescence is a period of intense present, with the immediate life situation being important and past and future being pallid. More structure is given to the past than to the future, but the past represents a period of confusion. Attitudes toward the future are subjective and distinctly negative. Often the future is viewed as being risky and devoid of any positive values (Cook et al., 1973). Even if imminent, death is thought of as remote because it distorts the importance of the present.

Adolescence represents the drive for complete independence and self-sufficiency. It is a time of group identity with peers and the development of personal ideas and behavior, usually through the peer group relationships. Guilt and vague feelings of badness are felt during rejection of parental control. This rejection bothers the adolescent. Because most deaths in this age group occur secondarily to trauma or accidents (frequently resulting from the breaking of rules), death becomes a confirmation of badness and is perceived as punishment that is meted out by the unforgiving parent. This idea leads to fear of the authority figure and eventual bitterness and resentment, deepening the adolescent's guilt and accentuating his or her depression (Eason, 1970).

In dealing with death the *adolescent* progresses through the stages outlined by Dr. Elisabeth Kübler-Ross (1969): (1) denial, (2) anger, (3) bargaining, (4) depression, and (5) acceptance. Emotions in adolescents are more likely to be expressed than in younger children. Death is representative of loneliness and passivity. Hospitalized adolescents fear being returned to the dependent role and may overtax their strength, seeking continued independence. Although they long for warmth and caring, they reject support and thus force people to withdraw from them, even while dreading loss of control. With approaching death, they become weakened and allow themselves to be loved and cared for. At this point they rationalize that control will be regained as strength is. The adolescent wants to live, but at the same time may be fascinated with the concept of death (Eason, 1970).

Death in the middle teens defeats the newly developed self-control, self-confidence, and self-direction that all led to the enjoyment of self. Older grade-school children and adolescents who know they are dying and accept death's finality prepare their families for the event. They gradually withdraw their expectations from the family and seemingly reject them. It is as if they are trying to comfort their families and ease them through the final phase of death with as little pain as possible.

Death also means rejection by their peers, as it emphasizes the vulnerability of the individual, as well as the difference between individuals. The rejection cannot be toler-

ated by an emerging independent individual. Death then becomes a function of dependency in isolation.

As the child gets older, there is an increase in expressed death anxiety in relation to illness. Before the age of 9 this anxiety is expressed in terms of separation or mutilation fears. After age 9 it is expressed in the younger patients as anxiety demonstrated through symbolization and physiologic expression. Older boys tend to act out, while older girls are prone to depression (Cook et al., 1973). This expression appears to be directly related to our society's role models and the difficulty on the part of men to actively express emotions. Anxiety may also appear as regression to an earlier stage of development.

It may be concluded that children at any age perceive their own death according to their developmental level and through the catalyst of some crisis event, such as a catastrophic illness (Table 29-1). Research also indicates that the extent of understanding that children have about their own death is difficult for their parents to accept (Weber, 1985).

## IMPACT OF HOSPITALIZATION

At some time a dying child will be hospitalized for medical intervention. Even when the child is carefully prepared, the hospital represents something fearful, simply by virtue of its difference and newness in a child's repertoire of experiences.

The *toddler* views home as the seat of security, safety, and guidance. When hospitalized, the toddler experiences separation anxiety, separated from his or her familiar surroundings, routine, and family. Compounding the strangeness of the hospital setting, the treatment personnel cause the child pain and discomfort. The child, in turn, reacts to the physical pain and his or her perceptions of his or her parents' discomfort rather than to any understanding of the end of his or her own existence (Eason, 1970).

Erikson pointed out that with increasing age, increasing independence develops. The preschool child does not separate thinking from concrete reality. Thus hospitalization is thought of as punishment for bad thoughts (Eason, 1970). The child reacts with guilt and noncomprehension of the treatment. The child is angry with the hospitalization process, and the treatment he or she receives is viewed as a form of punishment. Anger is usually directed toward the treatment team or other patients. In addition to anger and guilt, such a child also must deal with loneliness.

The awareness of self increases as children develop. They begin to think in terms of "me" and "mine" versus "not me" and "not mine." The thought of not being produces anxiety; thus children react through the process of denial. Denial allows them to deal with more tolerable and productive subjects that ultimately lessen the anxiety. These children avoid speaking of death. Often their play behavior centers around accidents and disasters as they attempt to prove to themselves that existence can be controlled just as toys

▲ Table 29-1   Developmental Stages: Children's Perception of Death Compared With Erikson's Psychosocial and Piaget's Cognitive Stages

| Erikson's Psychosocial Stages | Piaget's Cognitive Stages | Perception of Death |
|---|---|---|
| 1. *Trust vs. mistrust* (birth to 1 year)<br>  Development of the sense of trust through the pairing of the infant's actions with pleasant events<br>2. *Autonomy vs. doubt, shame* (1 to 3 years)<br>  The terrible twos. Beginning development of control over one's body, self, and environment<br>3. *Initiative vs. guilt* (3 to 5 years)<br>  Beginning exploration of the physical environment through senses and the social, physical worlds through language<br>4. *Industry vs. inferiority* (5 to adolescence)<br>  Begins to be a worker<br>  Wants to please<br>  Learns the meaning of rules and uses them<br>5. *Identity vs. role diffusion*<br>  Merging of past identity with future expectations (bodily, societal, and one's own) | 1. *Sensorimotor period* (birth to 2 years)<br>  Based on the formation of action schemas for skilled movement, language, visual perception, and object permanence<br>2. *Preoperational period* (birth to 7 years)<br>  The ability to symbolize through language, thought, drawing, and play<br>  Egocentricity<br>  Asks questions and why? Is more able to employ past events and to consider more than one aspect of an event at a time<br>3. *Concrete operations* (7 to 11 years)<br>  Time of real, concrete thought<br>  Orders, counts, and thinks in terms of cause and effect<br>  Beginning to compare own views and ideas<br>4. *Formal operations*<br>  Beginning of abstract thought and reasoning. Ability to form hypotheses and test them | 1. *Birth to 1 year*<br>  Reacts physiologically<br>  Without bonding there is little desire to live (failure to thrive)<br>2. *1 to 4 years*<br>  Responds with fear and anxiety to treatment<br>  Death has little or no meaning<br>3. *4 to 6 years*<br>  Has the concept of "me" and "not me." Fantasy reasoning with an increased curiosity about dead animals, flowers, burial, and so on<br>  Death is temporary<br>4. *6 to 8 years*<br>  Death means being separated from loved ones and causes anxiety<br>  The child learns to be a good patient<br>  Superstitions about death predominate<br>5. *8 to 11 years*<br>  Death is realized to be permanent<br>6. *Adolescence*<br>  Speculates about what occurs after death. Death is perceived in terms of loss of independence and identity |

are controlled (Eason, 1970). Frequently hospitalized children of this age also show less maturity in the level of their play, as well as less playfulness when compared with non-hospitalized children (Kielhofner, Barris, Bauer, Shoestock, & Walker, 1983).

The *school-aged child* is busy learning rules and is expected to exert some self-control and cooperation. Intellectually the child of this age is able to solve problems through thoughts, as well as by action. The child develops increased self-awareness, leading to independence from parents. Meanwhile, parental beliefs are internalized. By late grade school, the child has developed special friends, and the children play with teach, and help each other.

Studies suggest that children in this stage are aware of the seriousness of their disease, even though they may not be capable of speaking about it (Spinetta et al., 1973), and even though no one has told them how ill they are (Spinetta, 1974).

Smallness, vulnerability, and inadequacy characterize the grade-school child. Such a child deals with these feelings through the use of denial and reaction formation (Eason, 1970). For example, he or she may try to act fearless, taking unnecessary risks.

Hospitalization involves various degrees of separation from family and friends. The grade-school child may be lonely and sad, as well as fearful of the unknown. A study by Spielberger and others (Spielberger, Gorsuch, Lushene, Vagg, & Jacobs, 1972) indicated strong support for the hypothesis that terminally ill children show greater awareness of their hospital experience than do children who are chronically ill. These same children also expressed more hospital- and non–hospital-related anxiety. Homesickness, anger, frustration, and anxiety are usually expressed to the treatment staff in the form of refusing to cooperate. Some children might withdraw and become obviously depressed; however, the usual course of behavior is one of regression. They learn quickly from others and become sensitive to the feelings of the team. When involved with the hospital through the use of activities, children may become happier and their self-image tends to improve. As death approaches, they may become sad and bitter, not wanting to leave. They feel lonely from the realization that this is one trip that must be made alone. Thus comfort and security are sought.

On the whole, then, most children recognize the severity of their own illness whether or not they have been presented with the diagnosis (Spinetta et al., 1973). They react according to their stage of development, as well as their sociocultural expectations. For the most part, a terminal illness and the resulting thoughts of death are recognized by the children as the removal of independence. This and the intense feelings of separation affect their response to their own deaths.

## ASSESSING THE CHILD'S UNDERSTANDING OF DEATH

Assessing the child's understanding of death is important when working with a terminally ill child. This process helps the therapist know how to deal with the child's understanding of what is happening to him or her. Therefore it is helpful to assess what stage of Piaget's cognitive and Erikson's psychosocial development the child evidences (Table 29-1). This gives a fairly accurate assessment of the child's understanding of death. Using a general assessment of cognitive level is more appropriate than interviewing the child about death because children tend to avoid this subject with someone they have just met. Use of rating scales to assess cognitive understanding and anxiety toward death may be helpful (Prichard & Epting, 1992; Schell, 1991).

A second consideration in assessing the child's understanding is to record the parents' understanding of death and any relevant sociocultural ideas they have (Wenestam, 1989). These sociocultural aspects color a child's perception of death and may differ from the occupational therapist's. When working with terminally ill children, one should also ask what expectations the parents have, whether they are willing to have their child told that he or she is terminally ill, and what approach they are using with the child.

## OBJECTIVES FOR OCCUPATIONAL THERAPY INTERVENTION

Determining objectives for the child with a terminal illness is often difficult for the medical team. The team members realize this is a child who will not get well and who is different from the usual pediatric patient for whom they can set goals and develop long-term expectations. Therefore their objectives are mainly psychologic in nature, emphasizing quality of life, with less emphasis on physical aspects. The focus is not only on the child, but also on family members and their ability to develop adaptive responses. Their objectives are as follows:

1. Understand the origin and intensity of the child's anxiety.
2. Allow thoughts or reactions to death to come into the open.
3. Encourage expressions of grief.
4. Maintain comfort and provide support.
5. Facilitate and maintain independence.
6. Facilitate and maintain participation in activities of daily living.
7. Facilitate age-appropriate play skills.
8. Facilitate adaptive child-family relationships.

## TREATMENT MODALITIES

The underlying principle when providing occupational therapy care for children with terminal illness is to add qual-

ity to their remaining days. Two performance areas, important to occupational therapists are appropriate to address in children with terminal illness: play activities and activities of daily living.

Until the age of 5, children learn about their world exclusively through play. They learn and practice activities before incorporating them into practical application. Once they go to school, play and teaching help them learn. The more playful and interesting the subject, the more likely they are to learn. Play encourages social and emotional expression and development of coping strategies in children with terminal illness.

Activities that are appropriate for the child's developmental level, physical level (including endurance and tolerance), intellectual level, and emotional state should be chosen. Play allows the child to work through some of the feelings that he or she either has no words for or cannot express. It also allows the child to focus his or her interests on something other than himself or herself, something in the world around him or her. The occupational therapist can also suggest play activities (appropriate for the family) that involve family members.

The second performance area that should be addressed in therapy with children who have terminal illness is activities of daily living. Too often adults take away the independence that a sick child has acquired. Parents and staff often jump to perform an activity such as dressing or eating to save the child's strength. However, by doing so they take away the vestiges of independence that remain for the child. Encouraging the continuation of routine activities of daily living allows a child to look forward to consistency and to know and have some control over what is coming. As the child becomes weaker, energy conservation methods can be taught to parents and introduced to children, allowing them to remain as independent as possible in self-care. These modifications can be as simple as changing from metal to plastic utensils, using Velcro fastenings on clothing, and using pushcarts so that the child does not have to carry objects as weakness progresses. The modifications allow the child to continue functioning and to feel useful, rather than force the child to spend numerous hours on the sofa or bed watching countless television programs. The focus is not only on the child, but also on family members and their ability to develop adaptive responses.

## WORKING WITH THE FAMILY OF THE DYING CHILD

Parents must deal with the loss of their child throughout the process of the illness. They must also deal with the idea that they will continue to survive after their child's death.

Parents often suspect the severity of the child's illness and anticipate the news (Noland, 1971). Their reaction on hearing the diagnosis may range from loss of control to outward calm. Those who display a lack of affective response do so as a defense mechanism to allow themselves to deal realistically with the problems at hand. Clinical observers, as well as parents, report that it takes several days or weeks for the realization of the diagnosis to "sink in." Typically both parents are eager to hospitalize the child once it is suggested, as this renews their hope that the diagnosis is faulty and that treatment will cure their child.

With the realization of the diagnosis and the major decisions made as to treatment, the parents are then free to react to the situation. Initially the reaction appears as shock or denial contaminated by guilt (Noland, 1971). This guilt takes the form of the parents' thinking either that they are the cause of the illness or that they had not paid enough attention to the child. This, combined with questioning of the medical staff, represents an attempt to search for meaning or understanding of the situation. A problem occurs, however, if feelings of guilt become prolonged in nature and lead to overindulgence or to lack of discipline.

Denial is often part of the parents' coping strategy and may be the underlying reason for seeking other opinions. Representing the hope that the diagnosis is wrong and that the physician and medical staff have been in error. Binger and others (1969) studied 23 families of children with terminal illness and found this reaction is not usually shown by the immediate family, but rather by the grandparents and friends of the family.

Intellectualization also occurs. Parents seek information about the disease and cures, especially from other parents on the hospital ward and in support groups. Information seeking is a natural and helpful coping strategy. It gives the family an intellectual understanding of the disease to help them deal with the situation and the decisions that surround the treatment. However, the increasing numbers of questions usually indicate increasing anxiety and guilt, which are not resolved by more information and suggest that the therapist instead engage the parent in a give-and-take sharing of perceptions and feelings.

Throughout the course of the child's illness, hostility and anger are expressed by parents. Initially this reaction appears as a fight to reverse the diagnosis. Next, parents often feel resentment that they and their child should suffer in such a manner. This may be complicated by guilt over their feelings of resentment. Resentment is usually channeled outward, often directed toward the medical team. Third, anxiety of the unknown produces feelings of anger and hostility. Further, in the course of an illness, sick children often do not act sick, which reinforces the parents' denial (Eason, 1970).

Parents often want to stay with their child during the course of his or her hospitalization. Urging the parents to return home may add to feelings of distress and guilt. Often other children at home are neglected, thus increasing sibling rivalry and resentment toward the sick child. Seeking to cheer a child is a constant need felt by the parents. However, this does not acknowledge a child's true feelings.

Hospitalization promotes feelings of separation and anxiety on the part of the parent and the child. The parents are eager to hospitalize the child but are fearful to let the child go. Hospitalization represents a loss of control. No longer is the parent in charge; the authority is transferred to the medical personnel, and eventually the parents must come to depend on the strength and support of the hospital.

Resentment is increased if the physician is unable to provide a curative treatment. This is complicated by the child's feelings. The child expects his or her parents to ease the pain and make him or her well. The parents are unable to do this, and the child becomes angry. This leaves the parents confused with feelings of failure.

A remission is anticipated eagerly until the child is allowed to return home. The child's parents then realize that they are in sole care of the child, and this increases their anxieties. Overprotective behavior displayed by the parents leads to resentment by others and affects all family matters (Noland, 1971).

A relapse confronts the parents with the cold reality of the situation. They may react as if they had just learned of the diagnosis. A relapse causes great stress, and effective coping behavior is needed. There is a dynamic balance of emotional states, and transient episodes of ineffective coping are not uncommon. Successful coping behavior protects the parents from being overwhelmed by environmental and psychologic stress while they continue to function in the medical and psychologic care of their child.

Anticipatory grief is the gradual occurrence of mourning behavior, precipitated by the first acute critical phase of a terminal illness (Cook et al., 1973). It is typically characterized by somatic symptoms: apathy, weakness, preoccupation with thoughts of the ill child, sighing, occasional crying at night, and appearing depressed. At other times, there is increased motor behavior and increased talk about the child. These symptoms help to reintegrate the feelings with the gradual redirection of external energies (Friedman, 1967).

Physical complaints are gradually replaced by resignation and the desire to have the situation resolved. Parents turn their energies to other matters. Visits become a duty; the parents seem detached from their own child and more interested in the remaining children on the ward (Cook et al., 1973). This is indicative of acceptance. Mourning energies are being converted to more constructive means.

Exhaustion of treatment options accelerates the grieving. The child's parents may experience decreasing understanding and become more prone to anger.

In chronic terminal cases the parents have had time to rehearse how they will act. They usually control their expressions of grief, taking death calmly. However, if the parents have expressed denial continually throughout the course of their child's illness, death will be a shock, an experience of immediate loss. The parents often need many months before they can speak about the child without distress.

Finally, death is experienced with relief, and guilt is tinged with remorse (Lewis & Lewis, 1973). Mourning may deepen feelings of self-value through thoughts of death. Also, the love and warmth felt for the dead child may lead to a greater sense of self-worth. Three to six days after the child's death, the parents' mourning becomes less pronounced. However, there tends to be a continued interaction with the hospital staff through such things as gifts, initiation of research foundations, and library donations. After the child's death there is a tendency of the parents to reverbalize the guilt, which is bound up with the feelings of relief.

Binger et al. (1969) found that in half of the 23 families they studied, one or more members required psychiatric help after a child's death, although none had required it before. Mulhern (1983) found, in the families they worked with, 50% of the bereaved families had at least one member who had sought psychiatric or psychologic care, 70% reported serious marital discord after the child's death, and 25% to 50% of the surviving siblings experienced significant emotional, behavioral, or academic difficulties. Siblings evidenced higher levels of behavior problems and social incompetencies before and up to a year after their sibling's death (Birenbaum, Robinson, Phillips, & Stewart, 1989-1990). This finding makes it important to understand the three types of unhealthy family protective maneuvers that can occur. The first is the *conspiracy of guilt* that occurs when the parents feel the death was preventable. Communication about the lost child is shrouded and evasive to protect the living members of the family. This tends to support the idea that if the parents had acted differently, the child would still be alive. Therefore guilt is maintained, and there is no chance for the exploration of the event for fear that someone will be blamed (Krell & Rabkin, 1979). Surviving children in such a family live in a world of distrust and in constant fear of what may be in store, and they are hesitant to ask for clarification. A second unhealthy coping mechanism is the *preciousness of the survivor.* This leads to overprotection and shielding of the surviving children with fantasied attributes and expectations placed on them. This may lead to implications of specialness and good fortune placed on the survivors. Survivors may be filled with feelings of omnipotence and the desire to test fate, which limits their ability to develop practical coping mechanisms (Krell & Rabkin, 1979). The last type of unhealthy coping is the *substitution for the lost child* in one of the survivors or a new child. The chosen child is likely to be vulnerable and forced to live a dual life: one of his or her own, and one of the dead sibling's. Because of this, the child is not likely to develop a secure sense of identity (Krell & Rabkin, 1979). Unhealthy coping strategies used by families require outside intervention from mental health professionals. Even in the healthier families, as evidenced by their more adaptive coping patterns, one finds persisting guilt, sadness, and health fears that continue to be problematic after a child's death (Mulhern, 1983).

After their experiences, families of dying children have made the following suggestions to health professionals. Listening seems to be the most valuable asset of a medical staff (Noland, 1971). This is followed in importance only by offering reassurance, which often calms a parent's guilt feelings. Knowledge presented at the parents' level of understanding is calming. Questions should be answered patiently, kindly, and realistically. Families may be grateful, as well as angry. These angry feelings are dealt with best if the treatment team does not react to them as a personal insult or attack, and if the anger can be channeled productively. If information is available on support groups, the staff members should make it known to parents (Brown, 1989).

General components of good management include the following (Bergman, 1967):
1. Competence of staff
2. Availability of staff
3. Continuity of care
4. Personalized care
5. Well-prepared procedures
6. Active treatment role for the child
7. Questions encouraged
8. Supportive actions and discussions

After a child's death, the family also experiences difficulty relinquishing the ties with the health care personnel who have been involved with their child's treatment. Increasing numbers of agencies and facilities offer bereavement counseling to aid the family through the first year after the child's death. This is thought to be the average length of time for family grief to be resolved, but it may endure as long as 3 years (Powell, 1991; Wessel, 1983).

## WORKING WITH PERSONNEL CLOSE TO THE DYING CHILD

Among the personnel who treat the dying child and counsel the family, there may be a feeling of ambivalence in which compassion struggles against repulsion inherent in the threat of death. The degree of success in resolving this conflict determines the degree of success of the health care team. Therapists should be aware of this ambivalence in their colleagues and in themselves as well.

Because the primary goal of a health care professional is to help the sick child get well, a dying child prevents reaching this goal, thus causing feelings of frustration and anger. However, one cannot get angry with a sick child, so instead this situation often leads to feelings of guilt and even greater anger toward the one causing the guilt. This emotional state may become cyclic. Sack, Fritz, Krener, & Springer (1984) found that the physicians used the following coping strategies to deal with a child's death: (1) they had a tendency to try to master anxiety-provoking situations; (2) they tended to want to change the environment and not themselves; and (3) they habitually used intellect to master their anxieties.

## CASE STUDY #1

When Jan, the 11-year-old girl described at the beginning of this chapter (p. 766), first had treatment, her facial cancer was hardly noticeable. She often came down to the playroom. In the playroom, occupational therapists worked with the children, allowing them to express their feelings about the medical procedures through the use of play, for example, playing nurse and doctor with a doll and actual nonharmful medical items, and encouraging the children to play with age-appropriate toys.

After several admissions and subsequent surgery, Jan began to withdraw to her room. The staff initially tried to get her to come out, but eventually obeyed her wishes and went to her in her room. By this time, Jan preferred quieter activities, such as painting, drawing, sewing, and crafts. These activities offered recognizable end products and allowed her to feel purposeful, able to accomplish a task from the beginning to the end. As she became weaker because of the disease and the treatment for it, the activities often consisted only of talking and reading. Now Jan was being bathed primarily by the nursing staff, although she was encouraged to perform at least part of the routine. She could still feed herself most of her meals, although her intake was supplemented with intravenous feedings. She continued to refuse to leave her room. At the same time she began to draw away from the majority of the staff, as well as her parents—as if to spare them the pain of death. She allowed only a few within her realm, thus adding to her life an element of control respected by the staff. It was during this time that Donna, the nursing student, became important to her. Donna and Jan talked together as Jan grew weaker and lost her ability to perform activities. Treatment eventually failed to produce a response, and Jan grew weaker and died.

## CASE STUDY #2

Courtney is an 11-year-old youngster. As an infant and toddler, she was diagnosed with many allergies to everyday substances, which caused her to have chronic otitis media and pulmonary difficulties. Initially she entered the therapy setting for treatment of her sensory integrative difficulties. The treatment she received for her balance and praxis difficulties was considered to be successful, yet Courtney's endurance continued to be poor.

Further medical evaluation suggested that she suffered from an AIDS-like immunologic dysfunction. She had periods of good health, usually during the summers. During winter, pulmonary problems increased, and because of her immunologic problems, she was often unable to attend school with her friends. She was susceptible to communicable diseases and, because of her allergies, she could not be treated with antibiotics because she was allergic to most of them. Fatigue is a constant with Courtney. When at school, she puts on a strong front, but her mother reports that she is often in tears at home, wishing she could be "normal."

For those days she is unable to attend, she receives homebound instruction. Her occupational therapy services have emphasized energy conservation and adaptations of her home environment to accommodate her reduced energy level. They have become consultative with her mother and the school staff, suggesting ways on intervening that are less taxing to Courtney's system, but allowing her feelings of independence. Currently they have included suggestions such as using a tape recorder to record assignments and a computer to write them rather than requiring her to handwrite them. Further suggestions have been provided for word-prediction software that will predict Courtney's style of writing. At-home suggestions have been provided for organizing their multilevel home so that Courtney does not have to go up and down stairs needlessly. Time has been spent listening to her mother and providing suggestions for community resources to help. For a sick child like Courtney, the goal of occupational therapy should be to allow her to participate in the remainder of her childhood to the greatest extent possible (Gray, 1989).

## SUMMARY

In working with dying children, occupational therapists must be aware of developmental differences in the way children and their parents view death. These differences, added to the impact of hospitalization, affect children's responses to treatment and to surrounding people. Therapists can be effective with play activities and activities of daily living. It is important to understand the positive and negative emotions affecting parents, staff, and self.

**STUDY QUESTIONS**

1. Write down your feelings about working with children who are dying. How do you think these feelings are going to influence your ability to work professionally with dying children?
2. Children's understanding of death varies from age to age. How would this affect occupational therapy intervention with a preschool child, a grade-school child, and an adolescent?
3. What is the major role of the occupational therapist with the family of the dying child?
4. How does the therapist's own view of death affect his or her interactions with the family?

These patterns benefit neither the child, the family, nor the health care team involved with the child.

Reactions of the personnel toward the child are influenced by previous experiences with death. The health care personnel may take the approach of being overprotective toward the child. This overprotectiveness often leads to overt or covert reactions of anger by the child. On the other hand, the staff members may be overindulgent, and thereby put an added burden of guilt on the child; after all, what has the child done to deserve this special treatment? When both types of behaviors are shown by the staff, there is inconsistency and confusion within the child, who then may not know how to behave.

When treatment fails, workers may accuse each other of failure, thus redirecting toward each other the anger, frustration, and irritation they feel because they were unable to help.

One staff member reacted to a child's dying by hopping into his sports car and racing the highways until he had worked through his distressed feelings. This is one method of coping; however, in this case it produced anxiety in the rest of the staff until he returned. More constructive methods can channel anger and irritation into productive actions, whether oriented to motor release or to talking. Some of the methods currently used by staff members to deal with a child's death include individual counseling, team support group meetings, and case conferences where a child's course of treatment and eventual death are discussed.

Although a child's death is painful to all, it can also be a time of learning about life, love, and the appreciation of others. The best advice is often the hardest to take. Parents recommend trying to live each day as it comes, and with each day enjoying one's child (Binger et al., 1969). Occupational therapists are able to provide aid and support to these special children and their families.

## REFERENCES

Ashby, M.A., Kosky, R.J., Laver, H.T., & Sims, E.B. (1991, February 4). An inquiry into death and dying at the Adelaide Children's Hospital: a useful model. *Medical Journal of Australia, 154*(3), 165-170.

Bergman, A.B. (1967). Psychosocial aspects in the care of children with cancer. *Pediatrics, 40*(3), 492-497.

Binger, C.M., Ablin, A.R., Reuerstein, R.C., Kushner, J.H., Zoger, S., & Mikkelsen, C. (1969). Childhood leukemia: emotional impact on patients and family. *New England Journal of Medicine, 280*, 414-418.

Birenbaum, L.K., Robinson M.A., Phillips, D.S., & Stewart, B. (1989-90). The response of children to the dying and death of a sibling. *Omega Journal of Death and Dying, 20*(3), 213-28.

Brown, P.G. (1989). Families who have a child diagnosed with cancer: what the medical caregiver can do to help them and themselves. *Issues in Comprehensive Pediatric Nursing, 12*(2-3), 247-260.

Childers, P. & Wimmer, M. (1971). The concept of death in early childhood. *Child Development, 42*, 1299-1301.

Cook, S.S., Renshaw, D.C., & Jackson, E.N. (1973). *Children and dying: an exploration and a selected bibliography.* New York: Health Sciences Publishing.

Dominica, F. (1973). The dying child. *Lancet, 1*(8333), 1107.

Eason, W.M. (1970). *The dying child: the management of the child or adolescent who is dying.* Springfield, IL: Charles C. Thomas.

Friedman, S.B. (1967). Care of the family of the child with cancer. *Pediatrics, 40*, 498-507.

Gray, E. (1989). The emotional and play needs of the dying child. *Issues in Comprehensive Pediatric Nursing, 12*(2-3), 207-224.

Huffman, S.L. & Martin, L. (1994). Child nutrition, birth spacing, and child mortality. *Annuals of New York Academy of Science, 709*, 236-248.

Jeffrey, P. & Lansdown, R. (1982). The role of the special school in the care of the dying child. *Developmental Medicine and Child Neurology, 24*(5), 693-697.

Kane, B. (1979). Children's concepts of death. *Journal of General Psychology, 134*, 141-153.

Kielhofner, G., Barris, R., Bauer, D., Shoestock, B., & Walker, L. (1983). A comparison of play behavior in non-hospitalized and hospitalized children. *American Journal of Occupational Therapy, 37*(5), 305-312.

Koocher, G.P. (1973). Childhood, death, and cognitive development. *Developmental Psychology, 9*(3), 369-375.

Koocher, G.P. (1974). Talking with children about death. *American Journal of Orthopsychiatry, 44*, 404-411.

Krell, R. & Rabkin, L. (1979). The effects of sibling death on the surviving child: a family perspective. *Family Process, 18*(4), 471-477.

Kübler-Ross, E. (1969). *On death and dying.* New York: Macmillan.

Lewis, M. & Lewis, D.O. (1973). The crisis of death: a child dies. *Current Problems in Pediatrics, 3,* 1-11.

Martinson, I.M. (1986-1987). Home care for the dying child with cancer: feasibility and desirability. *Loss, Grief and Care, 1*(1-2), 97-114.

McDonnald, R.T. & Carroll, J.D. (1981). Appropriate death: college students preferences vs actuarial projections. *Journal of Clinical Psychology, 37*(1), 28-31.

Meliar, J.D. (1973). Children's conception of death. *Journal of General Psychiatry, 123,* 359-366.

Mulhern, R.K. (1983). Death of a child at home or in the hospital: subsequent psychological adjustment of the family. *Pediatrics, 71*(5), 743-747.

Nagy, M. (1959). The child's view of death. In W.H. Feifel (Ed.). *The meaning of death.* New York: McGraw-Hill.

Noland, R.L. (1971). *Counseling parents of the ill and the handicapped.* Springfield, IL: Charles C. Thomas.

O'Brien, C.R., Johnson, J.L., & Schmink, P.D. (1978). Death education: what students want and need. *Adolescence 1*(52), 729-734.

Oleske, J., Minnefor, A., Cooper, R., Thomas, K., dela Cruz, A., Ahdieh, H., Guerrero, I., Joshi, V.V., & Desposito, F. (1983). Immune deficiency syndrome in children. *Journal of the American Medical Association, 249,* 2345-2349.

Pizzi, M. (1984). Occupational therapy in hospice care. *American Journal of Occupational Therapy, 38*(4), 252-257.

Powell, M. (1991). The psychosocial impact of sudden infant death syndrome on siblings. *Irish Journal of Psychology, 12*(2), 235-247.

Prichard, S. & Epting, F. (1992). Children and death: new horizons in theory and measurement. *Omega Journal of Death and Dying, 24*(4), 271-288.

Sack, W.H., Fritz, G., Krener, P.G., & Sprunger, L. (1984). Death and the pediatric house officer revisited. *Pediatrics, 73*(5), 676-681.

Salladay, S.A. & Royal, M.E. (1981). Children and death: guidelines for grief work. *Child Psychiatry and Human Development, 11*(4), 203-212.

Schell, D. (1991). Development of death anxiety scale for children. *Omega Journal of Death and Dying, 23*(3), 227-234.

Speece, M.W. & Brent, S.R. (1984). Children's understanding of death. *Child Development, 55*(5), 1671-1686.

Spielberger, C.D., Gorsuch, R.L., Lushene, R., Vagg, P.R., & Jacobs, G.A. (1972). *Children's state-trait anxiety inventory.* Palo Alto, CA: Consulting Psychologist's Press.

Spinetta, J.J. (1974). The dying child's awareness of death: a review. *Psychology Bulletin, 81*(4), 256-260.

Spinetta, J.J., Rigler, D., & Karon, M. (1973). Anxiety in the dying child. *Pediatrics, 52*(6), 841-845.

Sternlicht, M. (1980). The concept of death in preoperational retarded children. *Journal of General Psychology, 137*(2), 157-164.

Tigges, K.N. & Sherman, L.M. (1983). The treatment of the hospice patient: from occupational history to occupational role. *American Journal of Occupational Therapy, 37*(4), 235-238.

Toews, J., Martin, R., & Prosen, H. (1985). Death anxiety: the prelude to adolescence. *Adolescent Psychiatry, 12,* 134-144.

Von Hug-Hellmuth, H. (1965). The child's concept of death. *Psychoanalysis Quarterly, 34,* 499-516.

Weber, J.A. (1985). Family support and a child's adjustment to death. *Family Relations Journal of Applied Family and Child Studies, 34*(1), 43-49.

Weininger, O. (1979). Young children's concepts of dying and dead. *Psychology Report, 44,* 395-407.

Wenestam, C.G. (1989). *Om barns tankade om doden.* (On the thoughts of children about death.). *Psykisk-Halsa, 30*(3), 229-236.

Wessel, M.A. (1983). The primary physician and the death of a child in a specialized hospital setting. *Pediatrics, 71*(3), 443-445.

Wilson, D.C. (1988). The ultimate loss: the dying child. *Loss, Grief and Care, 2*(3-4), 125-130.

## SUGGESTED READINGS

Kübler-Ross, E. (1983). *On children and death.* New York: Macmillan.

Oremland, E.K. & Oremland, J.D. (1973). *The effects of hospitalization on children.* Springfield, IL: Charles C. Thomas.

Picard, H.B. & Magno, J.B. (1982). The role of occupational therapy in hospice care. *American Journal of Occupational Therapy, 36*(9), 597, 1982.

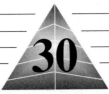

# Pediatric Rehabilitation

BRIAN J. DUDGEON

I wish to thank the children and families involved with Children's Hospital and Medical Center, Seattle, Washington, for their willingness to share their experiences. I also want to acknowledge the advice and help of Arlene Libby, Pam Horn, and Amy Lloyd from Children's Hospital and Medical Center in preparation of this chapter.

Historically, children who required pediatric rehabilitation often experienced long-term hospital stays or frequent rehospitalizations. For some children the hospital and staff nearly took on the roles of a home and family. These environments addressed medical care and rehabilitative intervention and often branched into programs addressing socialization, education, and vocation (Burkett, 1989; Edwards, 1992). Today, most pediatric therapy practice is now delivered through school systems. This shift in policy, along with advances in medical care and rehabilitation practice, has changed the role of hospital-based pediatric rehabilitation. In general, most hospital-based programs now focus on acute-onset problems and provision of specialized services for children and adolescents with disabilities that are of low occurrence but high complexity. Hospital-based programs are continuing to evolve, aiming to address known and newly identified health threats in a way that emphasizes a partnership with the child and family and resources in their local community.

This chapter describes the scope of occupational therapy services provided as part of hospital-based pediatric rehabilitation services. As a context for occupational therapy practice, the organization of rehabilitation services is outlined along with discussion of the types of children treated in these settings. Interdisciplinary care is emphasized, with the child and family as central participants in goal setting and decision making. The occupational therapist's role in family-based evaluation, goal setting, and intervention processes are reviewed and illustrated by selected case stories. This chapter stresses strategies used by occupational therapists to address activities of daily living (ADL) and the work of children, which is participation in school and other community activities. Specific techniques that reduce impairment and minimize disability are prioritized to support the child's requisite and desired performance goals within the environment they regard as home and community.

In studying pediatric rehabilitation, it is discovered that most physical medicine and rehabilitation practice has been developed to meet the needs of adults. Gans (1993) has cautioned that some rehabilitation specialists seem to think of children as if they were simply small adults. This orientation is obviously flawed. Being oriented to the developmental needs of children and having an appreciation for intensive involvement with families are critical to working within hospital-based pediatric rehabilitation programs.

A primary concept in the study of pediatric rehabilitation is the differentiation of *habilitation* and *rehabilitation*. For children, *habilitation* is the term most often used to denote attention to the child's acquisition of expected age level skill and function. *Rehabilitation* is the classic term used to reflect the process of an individual working to regain skills and functions that had been established but subsequently lost. For most practitioners in pediatrics, the term *rehabilitation* is actually used to encompass both concepts. This is true because disability, whether new or chronic, creates ongoing challenges to current function as well as future demands that evolve as part of growth and development. In this chapter the term *rehabilitation* will be used to include both concepts. Children who experience injuries, diseases or illness, and complications from chronic disorders often experience loss of existing functions for which rehabilitation of previous skills becomes the primary goal. And as expected, development of age-specific skills throughout childhood, adolescence, and young adult years necessitates frequent reappraisal and shifts in rehabilitation goals and programming.

## PURPOSE

Described in general terms, pediatric rehabilitation may be characterized as a planned approach involving any type and number of providers who specify a mission to focus on functional as well as psychosocial needs of children and their families. More formally, rehabilitation services for children and adolescents may be received within one or more levels of care that have evolved as part of the health care delivery system. Like services organized for adults, levels of rehabilitation care can be categorized as subacute, acute, and outpatient or ongoing care. Rehabilitation that occurs as part of inpatient hospital services receive primary attention here. In general, these interdisciplinary services are designed to address the management of acute disabling conditions, prevention of secondary complications, recovery or enhancement of function, and a return to home, school, and community participation. Outcomes from pediatric rehabilitation can be difficult to predict because of the complexity of factors shaping performance. Severity

of impairments and spontaneous recovery, developmental changes and maturation, use of specific rehabilitation approaches, and characteristics of families and their environments are included in influencing and appraising outcomes. Rehabilitation care should also be perceived as an ongoing process and one that is best carried out as a partnership between family, community, and school, as well as the hospital's specialized programs.

## LEVELS OF SERVICES

Levels of rehabilitation services can be described as subacute, acute, and outpatient or ongoing care. This range is best understood by reviewing typical programs of care and by contrasting different purposes within and across settings.

### Subacute Rehabilitation

The newest component of rehabilitation services is the subacute level, typically organized within skilled nursing facilities (SNFs) or other long-term care settings. Such programs are designed for children and adolescents who are too medically fragile or dependent to be cared for at home but who are not yet able to tolerate or benefit from the intensive efforts of acute rehabilitation. After initial hospitalization, children and adolescents with moderate to severe head injury, multitrauma, or other systemic illnesses may be admitted to a SNF with subacute rehabilitation services. In these settings, children may receive daily therapy to prevent secondary complications and to work toward goals of greater independent function. This interdisciplinary care often culminates in admission to an acute rehabilitation program or a planned discharge to an organized home- and community-based service system of care.

### Acute Rehabilitation

Acute pediatric rehabilitation is characterized by inpatient hospital units and services. Three types of programs are included in this category. The most common are dedicated rehabilitation units within children's hospitals. Another form of organization is the specification of beds and services for pediatric patients within a large rehabilitation hospital. A third setting involves the designation of pediatric beds in a large rehabilitation unit that is part of a comprehensive hospital system. Adolescents aged 15 years or more may also be admitted to rehabilitation units that most commonly serve adults and older adults. Children and adolescents are admitted to acute rehabilitation from other acute or transitional care medical services within the hospital, other local hospitals, or subacute rehabilitation settings. Children and adolescents who are admitted to trauma centers may be regularly screened to identify the need for transfer to children's hospitals or other rehabilitation units. Some children are also admitted to acute rehabilitation directly from community care providers or through the hospital's outpatient clinics and services.

Essential to acute rehabilitation programs is the presence of a broad range of services, including occupational therapy, and specific requirements for intensity of services to meet goals that are systematically developed. Such programs can be characterized as meeting three types of needs: (1) to organize and implement a planned approach for the management of recovery and rehabilitation of children with *rapid-onset disorders;* (2) to redirect care after onset of complications in children with *chronic disorders;* or (3) to provide an environment for *specialized medical or surgical procedures* or use of assistive technology that involves specific care regimens and protocols (see Tables 30-1, 30-2, and 30-3).

Children and youths who sustain a sudden illness or injury are the most common type of admission in acute rehabilitation. Table 30-1 indicates the most common diagnoses that affect a typically developing child who experiences an injury from accident, violence, or rapid-onset disease. Acquired injuries or diseases represent a substantial health threat to children (Moront & Eichelberger, 1994; Rodriquez & Brown, 1990). Injuries are the leading cause of death and disability among children older than 1 year of age. Traumatic brain injuries, including closed head injury, skull fracture, and penetrating brain injuries, are an increasingly recognized problem among youth because of transportation-related accidents, falls, recreational injury, and violence. Such causes are also associated with children who sustain spinal cord injury and multitrauma. Environmental hazards, accidents, and abuse are also implicated among children who experience burns, near drowning, smoke inhalation,

carbon monoxide poisoning, or drug overdose. Aside from known hazards, children also develop infections that involve the central nervous system; they may sustain cerebrovascular accidents, or they may acquire other neurologic disorders such as transverse myelitis or Guillain-Barré syndrome. Cancer and its treatment may cause children and adolescents to develop problems necessitating acute rehabilitation. All of these disorders are characterized by typical development and an acute health crisis that causes a severe loss of function, a likelihood of prolonged recovery with residual disability, and chronic health complications associated with disability. For such children and their families the purpose of rehabilitation is to prevent further deterioration or development of complications and to organize and implement an approach to initial and long-term management that optimizes function in family and community life.

Table 30-2 exemplifies the groups of children with congenital or chronic disorders who may require acute rehabilitation. Many youths with congenital disability, or those who experience chronic diseases, often have delayed or atypical patterns of functional skill development. These same children are also at risk for complications that can create a gradual or critical loss of function. Episodes of respiratory infection, bony fractures and dislocations, skin breakdown, or other systemic complications may be associated with functional deterioration. Children with cerebral palsy, myelodysplasia, or other types of congenital defects are included in this at-risk group. Likewise, children with congenital limb deficiency, arthrogryposis multiplex congeni-

▲ Table 30-1  Sudden or Rapid Onset of Disability: Accidental Injury, Violence, Disease Processes

| Type of Onset | Example |
|---|---|
| Accidental injury | Traumatic brain injury (e.g., closed head injury) |
| | Skull fracture or penetrating head injury |
| | Burns and smoke inhalation |
| | Multitrauma |
| | Near drowning |
| | Spinal cord injury |
| Violence | Multitrauma |
| | Traumatic brain injury (e.g., gunshot wound) |
| | Burns, iron burns, cigarette burns, and scalding |
| Disease processes | Central nervous system infection: encephalitis and myelitis |
| | Transverse myelitis |
| | Guillain Barré syndrome |
| | Cancer |

▲ Table 30-2  Congenital Onset, Chronic Disease With Complications

| Type | Examples |
|---|---|
| Neurologic | Myelodysplasia |
| | Cerebral palsy |
| | Multihandicapped |
| Orthopedic | Juvenile rheumatoid arthritis |
| | Congenital amelia and dwarfism |
| | Arthrogryposis multiplex congenital |
| Muscular | Muscular dystrophy |

▲ Table 30-3  Special Procedures

| Type | Examples |
|---|---|
| Clinical procedures | Selective dorsal rhizotomy |
| | Continuous intrathecal baclofin |
| | Ilizarov |
| Assistive technology | Seating and mobility |
| | Aided and augmentative communication |
| | Environmental control |

tal syndrome, or osteogenesis imperfecta may have episodes of curtailed functional gains or loss of skills necessitating an acute rehabilitation effort. Juvenile rheumatoid arthritis and related disorders may also cause children to experience rapid decline in function. For these children, the goals of rehabilitation are to limit or prevent further losses and to facilitate reacquisition of skills consistent with the pattern of functional progression that was previously shown.

The third major group of children who receive acute rehabilitation services are those who are hospitalized for treatment with special medical, surgical, or technologic procedures (Table 30-3). For children with cerebral palsy, use of new medical interventions such as selective dorsal rhizotomy, continuous intrathecal baclofen, or other neurologic techniques to reduce spasticity may involve admission to acute rehabilitation. Ilizarov procedures, the surgical technique of increasing congenital limb length or repairing severe orthopedic injury, may also be associated with acute rehabilitation (Karger, Guile, & Bowen, 1993). Children who are ventilator dependent may be admitted for acute rehabilitation to assist families in learning how to use medical technology (Richardson & Robinson, 1989). These interventions often involve the therapists in following specific evaluation and treatment protocols designed to optimize functional outcomes. Efforts to augment function beyond the child's current pattern of development is also represented by efforts to apply uses of assistive technologies. Acute rehabilitation admissions may be planned to permit intensive evaluation and trials in use of aided and augmentative communication systems, therapeutic seating, and powered mobility or other technologies that enable environmental access and control. These applications of special procedures or assistive technologies are characterized by preplanned and often short lengths of stay, and they culminate in intensive family training and transitions to prearranged outpatient follow-up in the community.

A key feature of all types of admissions to acute rehabilitation is an emphasis on the planning and facilitation of community-based care plans. Discharge planning typically begins at referral to rehabilitation. School and other community-based providers are invited to participate in discharge arrangements that ease the transition from hospital to home and school settings. Often the hospital's outpatient services or clinics are recommended to monitor care and to serve as an ongoing resource to the family and local care providers who implement the greater part of rehabilitation that takes place in home and school settings.

## Outpatient and Ongoing Rehabilitation

Another major component of pediatric rehabilitation is seen within specialized outpatient services and clinics that provide ongoing care. Typically, as part of children's hospitals or rehabilitation hospitals, interdisciplinary outpatient clin-

ics are organized to provide monitoring and interventions with children who experience particular types of chronic health risks and disabilities. Follow-up and follow-along attention is often provided to children and families after hospitalization, but most clients have never been hospitalized. Occupational therapists who work at these clinics most often focus on the child's or adolescent's health status and development, emphasizing functional progress and participation within the family, local community, and school systems. Clinic programs that most commonly involve occupational therapists are displayed in Table 30-4. Such clinic programs may be scheduled weekly, monthly, quarterly, or even annually as needed. Sometimes these programs are conducted away from the hospital facility at community sites such as schools. Often the therapists provide consultation with the family and local therapists who know the particular child well but have limited experience with a specific disorder or type of specialized intervention. For example, school personnel may have limited experience with children who have arthrogryposis, limb deficiency, or various forms of muscular dystrophy. Rapid developments in assistive technology also limits the likelihood that all schools or local programs can remain current and effective in applying new systems and approaches. Therapists who work in specialized hospital programs are provided with unique exposure to otherwise uncommon diagnoses and clinical procedures and can pass on this experience to other families and therapists as a conduit of information and new ideas.

Outpatient services are also provided in the form of in-

▲ **Table 30-4**   Outpatient Clinics and Programs Often Served by Occupational Therapists

| Clinic Title | Example of Clients or Services |
|---|---|
| Congenital defects | Myelodysplasia |
| Neuromuscular disorders | Cerebral palsy |
| Developmental disabilities | Down syndrome |
| | Fetal alcohol syndrome |
| Rheumatology | Juvenile rheumatoid arthritis |
| | Systemic lupus erythematosis |
| Craniofacial defects | Cleft lip and palate |
| Orthopedic | Traumatic hand injury |
| | Congenital limb deficiency |
| Rehabilitation | Traumatic brain injury |
| | Spinal cord injury |
| Muscular dystrophy | Duchenne's muscular dystrophy |
| | Spinal muscle atrophy |
| Limb deficiency | Congenital amelia |
| | Traumatic amputation |
| Cystic fibrosis | |
| Assistive technology | Seating and positioning |
| | Wheelchair control |
| | Augmentative communication |

dividualized therapy at the hospital or free-standing outpatient clinics. Outpatient services often occur concurrently with the child's return to school and school-based therapy, the former is organized around medical needs, whereas the latter addresses educational performance.

Another form of rehabilitation service is characterized by residential or intensive day-treatment programs. These services have most often been organized for children and adolescents with acquired brain injury. These extended care programs are geared toward direct assistance with community reentry. Simulated or actual environments become the training site for skills that enable community participation and effective performance toward goals of independent living, education, and work activities.

## Accrediting Agencies

Pediatric rehabilitation advocates and service providers have both influenced and been shaped by accreditation processes. For example, the Heath Care Financing Administration (HCFA), the agency responsible for administering Medicare and Medicaid programs in most states, designates requirements for services that are organized and paid to provide "medical rehabilitation." To meet HCFA guidelines for rehabilitation, rules are placed on such systems that mandate specific program emphasis, dedicated space and personnel, admission and discharge procedures, service intensity, goal setting, and monitoring of progress toward goals. Most rehabilitation programs also pursue voluntary accreditation by groups such as the Joint Commission on Accreditation of Health Organizations (JCAHO) and the Commission on Accreditation of Rehabilitation Facilities (CARF). These organizations prescribe additional mandates that also shape program characteristics. Such guidelines may involve procedures that assure inclusion of the patient and family in planning, integrated planning with community-based services, continuous quality improvement procedures, individualized programs and team monitoring frequency, and further specifications of dedicated space, use of other service providers, and greater intensities of service provision. Every few years, accreditation standards and procedures based on JCAHO and CARF shift emphasis and specification of essential requirements. Generally, after initial accreditation, reaccreditation visits are scheduled every 3 years and programs may be subject to periodic interim review and reporting about their overall performance.

## Reimbursement for Services

Inpatient pediatric rehabilitation services are typically funded by a combination of private insurance carriers, Medicaid, and under some circumstances by Medicare. Preadmission review and authorization are generally required. Comprehensive rehabilitation units continue to be exempt from the prospective payment funding systems that were based on diagnosis-related groups (DRGs) under current HCFA guidelines. However, new DRG equivalents called *function-related groups* specific to medical rehabilitation are currently being developed. Rehabilitation costs are generally regarded as difficult to predict, and additional work is underway to develop appropriate prospective payment systems for both inpatient and outpatient services. Occupational therapy has typically been recognized as a service that is reimbursed within inpatient medical rehabilitation, home health care, and less commonly in outpatient services. Medicare guidelines are generally universal across different states. However, each state's Medicaid rules and regulations, as well as local insurance companies, have differing provisions related to funding of occupational therapy services. Review of local regulations is necessary to assure that appropriate levels of reimbursement are available, and that families are informed about service options.

Lengths of stay for acute pediatric rehabilitation are varied, from as little as a few days, to weeks, or perhaps months. Like adult rehabilitation units and all inpatient hospitals, pressure is being applied by third-party payers and other regulators to reduce lengths of stay and transfer patients more quickly to skilled nursing facilities, home care, outpatient, or school-based services in the family's local community. Changes within and across treatment settings can be problematic, often resulting in confusion among families about entitlements and expectations for services. Case managers, who are familiar with funding rules and regulations, work with families and rehabilitation teams to coordinate services and prepare the family for transitions between care settings.

## REHABILITATION TEAM

Hospital-based rehabilitation permits the child and family to benefit from a wide range of medical care specialists and services that can be accessed as needed. Pediatric rehabilitation teams as well include a wide variety of providers with differing expertise. Such teams are most often led by physicians who are trained as pediatricians and who are credentialed in other arenas of practice such as neurology, orthopedics, or developmental medicine. In recent years, leadership in pediatric rehabilitation has come primarily from pediatricians jointly certified in the practice of physiatry (rehabilitation medicine).

An emphasis is placed on interdisciplinary teamwork, with each discipline having particular capabilities or areas of focus. Sometimes a transdisciplinary model is used so that fewer individuals work directly with a particular child or family. Specific roles for each discipline within acute rehabilitation have been described for teams consisting of physicians, nurses, occupational therapists, physical therapists, speech-language pathologists, recreational therapists, psychologists, social workers, educators, and other specialists (Blatzheim, Edberg, & Lacy, 1987; Eigsti, Aretz, & Shannon, 1990; Gardner & Workinger, 1990). In larger programs, specialty teams may develop so that the same personnel treat children grouped by diagnosis (e.g., head injury).

## Team Interaction

Interdisciplinary care within pediatric rehabilitation is common and mandated by most regulatory mechanisms. The success of such collaboration is often dependent on a shared mission that focuses the team's energy and creativity. Team panels that involve the family are characteristic. Panel meetings are held on admission, at key decision points during the hospitalization, and at discharge to assure communication and clarification of care recommendations with the family and local care providers. In addition, problem-oriented medical records (POMRs) are often used, and weekly rounds are conducted by the team to review the progress of each child and to discuss any changes in treatment plans that are designed for each problem.

The occupational therapist's holistic concerns related to health, function, and participation necessitate and are enriched by a collaborative relationship with team members of other disciplines. For example, occupational and physical therapists often take a joint interest in addressing a child's gross and fine motor skills related to positioning, transfers, wheelchair seating, and functional mobility. Feeding and swallowing, as well as augmentative communication, may be evaluated and interventions planned in cooperation with speech-language pathologists. Nursing and occupational therapy personnel typically have collaborative roles dealing with skills such as grooming, dressing, and bathing, as well as training in special care routines of toileting and skin care. Occupational therapists may work together with recreational therapists to provide adaptive play and socialization through activity and community outings. A primary concern with children is to improve their participation and performance in educational programs. Acute rehabilitation programs, as well as children's hospitals in general, typically have teachers on staff. In conjunction with the occupational therapist and other team members, these educators and developmental specialists can address skills and special needs the child will have on return to school. Psychologists and those who specialize in neuropsychology also provide suggestions for school placement and may work with occupational therapists to adapt learning strategies for the child as he or she returns to the classroom. Social workers typically address issues of adjustment and coping with the child and family. Occupational therapists, like all team members, are sensitive in working with family members as they train to assume new duties as care providers. Such planning and training should seek a realistic balance between established family roles and new responsibilities for care.

## Families

It is important to recognize that families are generally dealing with tragic events or at least unexpected complications that seriously affect their life processes. The children and adolescents are also challenged to deal with changes, and this process can be further complicated by their own cognitive or behavioral impairments (Donders, 1993). An educational model may provide a helpful perspective. Recognizing that family members have a short amount of time to learn a great deal about caring for their family member who is faced with new disabilities, rehabilitation team members also need to devote their time and attention to learning from the family about each child and the family's systems. In all cases, the normal routines of the family are severely disrupted by hospitalization (Rivara, 1993). Healthy and resilient families may show exceptional caring, open communication, balancing of family needs, and positive problem-solving abilities. Families with limited coping skills may need increased support and help in identifying resources to meet immediate needs, as well as in coping with problems they will face during transitions back to managing the child at home. In either case, the needs of families often change during the rehabilitation process, requiring ongoing attention to maintain a collaborative partnership that can achieve the best outcomes for the child.

## RESEARCH ON EFFICACY OF PEDIATRIC REHABILITATION PROGRAMS

In most hospital-based pediatric rehabilitation programs, occupational therapists are typically called on to address ADL, school-related functions, and the component skills that enable such performance. Improvements in ADL and disposition at discharge are typically the most common measures used to justify and to document the benefits of rehabilitation.

Functional outcomes and cost of care associated with various configurations of hospital-based rehabilitation services have been described as beneficial for adults from a variety of diagnostic groups, such as those with stroke or head injury (Fuhrer, 1987). Outcomes for children and adolescents undergoing rehabilitation have been less commonly reported, but evidence is mounting regarding benefits that are similar to those found for adults. Jaffe, Okamoto, and Lemire (1986) examined the experiences of 319 children who received acute rehabilitation. Over a 5-year period, acquired disability secondary to injury accounted for 42% of admissions, congenital conditions were involved in 39%, and acquired diseases accounted for 14%. Functional problems at admission included a wide range of concerns, with the greatest percentage having problems with bowel and bladder function, as well as self-care and mobility. Median length of stay was 21 days, and most were discharged to a family home.

Early referral to rehabilitation specialists is often recommended, but patterns of recovery and benefits from services vary by diagnostic group. For example, after head injury, an extended period of recovery is expected. Boyer and Edwards (1991) reviewed outcomes of 220 children and adolescents with traumatic brain injury (TBI) who were admitted to a comprehensive pediatric rehabilitation program. They reported continued progress in mobility, ADL, and education and cognition for up to 3 years after injury. Physical recovery was greatest in the first year; cognitive and language gains generally occurred later.

Complications from pediatric head injury have also been studied by following series of children identified in trauma registries. Di-Scala, Osberg, Gans, Chin, and Grant (1991) assessed functional recovery patterns of 598 children ages 8 to 19 years who had been hospitalized after TBI. Approximately 22% were judged to have disability that necessitated a period of 7 months to over 2 years for recovery. Significant motor as well as cognitive and behavioral impairments were common. Despite functional compromise, only 57% of the most severely injured were admitted to acute rehabilitation. Coster, Haley, and Baryza (1994) followed a group of children who were age 6 or younger at onset of TBI and also found patterns of dysfunction and family adjustment concerns among selected cases. The most thorough follow-up of children with head injury has been conducted by Jaffe and colleagues (Chaplin, Deitz, & Jaffe, 1993; Fay et al., 1994; Jaffe et al., 1992; Jaffe et al., 1993). In this series, which studied 72 children, an age-matched cohort was developed to provide a careful assessment of sequelae from mild, moderate, and severe classifications of TBI. Among these children who were aged 6 to 15 years at the time of injury, those with moderate and severe injury evidenced persisting and comprehensive neurocognitive, academic, and functional deficits.

Research about benefits of specific intervention strategies used with children who have brain injury are known to be lacking. In fact, throughout pediatric rehabilitation it has been difficult to conduct research that analyzes application of particular techniques of rehabilitation. Experimental research of rehabilitation effectiveness is particularly difficult to conduct because of the heterogeneity of patients and ethical conflicts encountered by suspending or withholding services to specific children. Haley, Baryza, and Webster (1992) reviewed research pertaining to rehabilitation and recovery from head injury in childhood and contend that definitive studies have yet to be reported.

More common than appraisal of rehabilitation techniques or measurement of specific outcomes, the pediatric rehabilitation literature has shown a growing attention to both inpatient and outpatient rehabilitation needs of specific populations. Massagli and Jaffe (1990) have described rehabilitation needs of children with spinal cord injury and are reporting follow-up of a series of children returning to school. Outcomes of care after spinal cord injury (SCI) from achondroplasia has also been reported (Wieting & Krach, 1994). Children with primary brain tumor who received rehabilitative care have been reported to show improved management of residual disability (Philip, Ayyangar, Vanderbilt, & Gaebler-Spira, 1994). Rehabilitative needs of other children have also been demonstrated, including burns (Herndon, Rutan, & Rutan, 1993), osteogenesis imperfecta (Binder et al., 1993), myelodysplasia (Watson, 1991), asthma (Strunk, Mascia, Lipkowitz, & Wolf, 1991), and other disorders (Heery, 1992; Russman, 1990).

In summary, the service model of inpatient rehabilitation has been well supported for adults, and comparable benefits appear to be found in similar programs designed for children. However, specific analysis of different priorities within pediatric rehabilitation, mixtures of service providers, or contrasts with less intensive subacute or outpatient services have not been reported. Routine appraisal of individual benefits and overall program effectiveness are being mandated by professional organizations, the insurance industry, and government agencies involved in regulation and reimbursement of rehabilitation programs and services. Further literature regarding measures of pediatric rehabilitation program benefits and specific analysis of common diagnostic groups seen in rehabilitation can be expected in coming years.

## OCCUPATIONAL THERAPY SERVICES
### Functions of Occupational Therapists

As suggested, the primary focus of the occupational therapist within pediatric rehabilitation is on ADL and other instrumental tasks associated with independent living, school performance, and community participation. Many frames of reference are used to develop insights about the child's function, to establish priorities for treatment, and to guide the organization of treatment goals with the child, family, and local care providers. Most commonly, a prioritization system is followed that first focuses on prevention, then resumption of the able self, and finally restoration of lost skills and functions. A key concept in rehabilitation is the recognition that therapy is learning (Schwartz, 1991). Thus therapy as teaching is designed around behavioral and cognitive learning principles as well as the interpersonal relationship inherent in a teacher-pupil relationship. A blending of the therapist's technical competency, along with personal caring and mutuality of goals and efforts with children and their families, should be emphasized.

Activity analysis is another universal strategy used by therapists to determine skill requirements of functional tasks, as well as the therapeutic activities selected to improve skills. Such analysis leads to the breakdown of tasks into specific steps that can be reorganized to modulate the sensorimotor, cognitive, and psychologic components of learning and of performance. Specific intervention techniques used to achieve prioritized goals emerge from simultaneous use of methods primarily from biomechanical, sensorimotor, and rehabilitative treatment approaches (see Chapters 11, 12, and 14).

### Prevention

*Primary prevention* is a term used to denote efforts that decrease the likelihood of accidents, violence, or disease. Secondary or tertiary prevention refers to specific interventions, arrangement of care systems, and environmental modifications to prevent onset of problems among at-risk populations. Children admitted to pediatric rehabilitation units are typically at risk for developing a number of secondary disabilities. The therapist, along with other team members, has a responsibility to be familiar with such risks. Included are concerns for safety in positioning and movement, risks of aspiration in swallowing, provision of orientation, and appropriate measures to reduce stresses experienced in an unfamiliar environment and to prevent self-injurious behaviors. The therapist must be aware of risks and avoid involving the child in ADL that would be harmful or would perpetuate impaired habits that could hamper recovery. Complications from immobilization, abnormal muscle tone, and other neuromuscular abnormalities often necessitate careful attention to maintain range of motion, strength, and general fitness (Figure 30-1). Concern for wound healing and protection of neurogenic skin are also essential to the early planning and ongoing achievement of goals, interventions, and education of the child and their family.

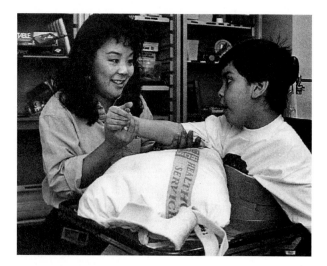

**Figure 30-1** Active assistive range of motion exercises are performed several times each day to prevent joint and muscle contractures with this boy who sustained a severe closed head injury. Stretch is also applied to existing contractures, along with other joint mobilization techniques.

### Resumption

The second level of priority for occupational therapy is a focus on resuming use of available skills and independence in easily accomplished tasks. Emphasizing the able self provides the individual child with an opportunity to resume doing tasks on their own, or at least to have a say about how they are assisted. Such an approach may be important in preventing the child or adolescent from developing dependent behaviors or learned helplessness. The latter has been commonly described in adults who are admitted to institutional-like settings where supervision is abundant and independence is poorly rewarded (Raps, Peterson, Jonas, & Seligman, 1982). Efficiency demands placed on nursing may often cause the child to become a passive recipient of care. The child should be allotted sufficient time to perform activities on his or her own. Early emphasis on allowing children opportunities to make choices about the types of assistance they receive or activities they pursue should help them redevelop a sense of their own abilities.

### Restoration

Lost skills and function follows in priority, with efforts to restore abilities. Sensorimotor, neurophysiologic, biomechanical, and rehabilitative approaches can be used individually or in combination to restore function. Such approaches may necessitate extensive retraining or complex adaptation. When performance is severely impaired, reacquisition of skill is often initiated during acute rehabilitation with continuation of training as part of outpatient and ongoing rehabilitative care.

Each prioritization level may capitalize on treatment strategies drawn from frames of references that directly address occupational performance component skills versus those that address occupational performance areas. For example, biomechanical and sensorimotor techniques are designed to improve component skills such as strength, range of motion, postural control, skilled movements, and coordination. Such approaches include use of therapeutic activities and exercise, splinting and positioning, physical handling, and use of biomedical devices like functional electric stimulation. Perceptual and cognitive difficulties can also be addressed through techniques designed to retrain or use substitution methods in performance. Practicing activities that selectively challenge component skills are often used with the expectation that skills will transfer or generalize to ADL and work performance. By contrast, rehabilitative approaches are designed as compensatory techniques that use existing skills to maintain or to restore function regardless of current or changing sensorimotor, cognitive, or psychologic skill levels. Rehabilitative approaches are characterized by instructional methods designed to teach the use of modified routines and use of assistive devices within carefully organized environments. Critical to the course of therapy is to recognize the simultaneous or complementary use of strategies addressing component skills, functional performance, and environmental influences.

## Evaluation

In nearly all instances, occupational therapy services in hospital-based pediatric rehabilitation are initiated through physician's orders. Often required by law or regulatory guidelines, therapists respond to initial orders and negotiate as necessary with the physician to add specific elements to assessment and intervention activities. Most commonly, initial orders to occupational therapy involve a focus on ADL and component skills that support function.

Multiple sources for data are available within the pediatric rehabilitation setting. Review of medical records and discussions with other providers may form the initial basis for evaluation. In general, clinical interview and observation initiate the assessment process. Observed areas of concern may necessitate more thorough evaluation through physical examination and direct observation and by use of standardized tests. Such measures help in the diagnostic process. Impairment in performance components are likely to be implicated as causes of ADL disabilities. Once such hypotheses are made and treatment plans initiated, the repeated use of clinical examination and standardized tests serve as objective measures of skill improvement. For diagnostic purposes, a child's performance is judged against normed scores, but for evaluative purposes, the child's scores on reassessment are judged against his or her previous performance. Selection of specific measures should be based on the instrument's reliability and value in diagnostic workup and the tool's sensitivity in demonstrating changes in performance.

Evaluation of ADL skills may occur before, during, or after assessment of occupational component skills and is dependent on what has been prescribed for therapy. The initial evaluation of ADL helps prioritize which components and impairments require more detailed evaluation. In contrast, if the initial assessment focuses on component skills, the findings allow the therapist to predict which ADL would be problematic and what types of adaptations should be recommended.

Assessment of ADL may be organized around checklists or other reporting tools that specify activities and methods of rating the child's or adolescent's level of skill. For example, the Functional Independence Measure (FIM) was developed as part of a Uniform Data System for Medical Rehabilitation for use in patient and program monitoring and outcome evaluation systems (Keith, Granger, Hamilton, & Sherwin, 1987). The FIM is generally designed for individuals age 7 and older. A pediatric version of this tool, called the *Wee-FIM*, has been developed for children of developmental age 6 months to 7 years (Msall, DiGaudio, & Duffy, 1993). Eighteen specific ADL tasks, including communication and social cognition, are rated for dependence based on the individual's need for adaptation and assistance

from a helper. Another tool that can be used for rating and describing function in children is the Pediatric Evaluation of Disability Inventory (PEDI) (Haley, Coster, Ludlow, Haltiwanger, & Andrellos, 1992). Based on a combination of interview and observation, the PEDI specifies discrete levels of skills in domains of self-care, mobility, and social function. Description of needs for care provider assistance and reliance on assistive devices are included with the measure. Both the FIM and PEDI are used for individualized assessment and planning; both are also used in program evaluation. Although these tools focus directly on daily functional tasks, use of additional broad-based measures that assess play- and school-related performance are also encouraged in rehabilitation settings (Johnston & Granger, 1994).

## Determining Treatment Goals

As stated throughout this text, goals for services must be explicitly stated, measurable, and functionally relevant. A goal to "increase ADL skills" is not adequate. For the child, family, and third-party payers, clearer targets for functional outcome must to be specified. Long-term goals are most often written to reflect the outcomes expected during the child's length of stay (i.e., acute rehabilitation admission). Short-term goals are specified as interim steps toward reaching long-term goals. Specific tasks that will be performed, conditions of performance, and the type and frequency of assistance needed should be described. Component skills that are being treated may be described as goals if appropriately linked to meaningful functional outcomes (e.g., achieve hand grasp and manipulation skills sufficient for desktop activities and writing at school).

Functional goals must include specification of skills as well as the level of independence that is being sought. Although *independence* is traditionally regarded as autonomy, dependence on adaptive environments and use of assistive devices is often required. In many cases, ADL goals describe how the child or adolescent will manage personal care assistants to achieve a self-managed dependence. Level of independence in ADL is often reported as degree of dependence, usually rated by use of scales that reflect either or both of the amount of physical and cognitive assistance needed as a proportion of the task (i.e., moderate assist = 50% assistance) or the amount of time required for partial task, whole task, and task transition assistance by a care provider. However, when concerned with the integration of an individual back into their home, the concept of *interdependence* among family members may be a more important consideration. Given the negative value associated with *dependence in the Anglo-American culture*, perhaps a more positive term to express shared needs between family members is one of *interreliance*.

In pediatric rehabilitation, the selection of specific ADL goals is influenced by a variety of factors. Goals based on family's priorities are likely to garner the best motivation and support. Priorities for function are individualized and may differ from those presumed by therapists. The child's or adolescent's ability to restore skills in self-care and important everyday activities help restore a sense of well-being. Selection of ADL goals are also influenced, nevertheless, by institutional and insurance directives. Reduction of dependence makes care possible in progressively less restrictive and less costly environments. Intervention goals most often focus on functional skill acquisition that enables the child to be discharged from inpatient hospital settings to services provided within long-term care, home-health care, outpatient care, and eventually to use of nonmedical community support systems.

## Intervention

### Preventing Secondary Disability and Restoring Component Skills

The prevention of secondary disability and reduction of existing complications is of the highest priority in a treatment plan. Neuromuscular and musculoskeletal complications are typically addressed by programs to maintain or regain normal passive range of motion. Through use of special handling techniques, the occupational and physical therapists carry out daily programs that can involve slow stretch and joint mobilization. Existing limitations may be corrected by a combination of these techniques as well as by use of specialized positioning and splinting. Splints may be applied for a variety of purposes, including maintaining positions (e.g., resting hand splint), correcting motions (e.g., drop-out splints, dynamic splints with spring tension forces, or serial casting), or to be used to promote function (e.g., wrist cock-up, tenodesis splints) (Figure 30-2).

Facilitation of movement and strength may be accomplished by use of activities and exercises that are most of-ten incorporated into play. For children and adolescents with musculoskeletal and lower motor neuron or motor unit disorders, use of progressive exercise and activity routines may be appropriate. For those with brain injury causing upper-motor neuron dysfunction, muscle tone and voluntary motor control are addressed. Various neurodevelopmental techniques can be used to manage muscle tone, with the goal of promoting agonist and antagonist balance as a basis for movement (see Chapters 11 and 12).

A second major concern of pediatric rehabilitation is skin care. Pressure areas from bed positioning, static sitting, and use of orthosis and splints calls for routine skin monitoring. Tolerance to new positioning strategies and to splint applications must often be developed over several days, with skin tolerance being a critical issue in decisions to change bed positions, to increase sitting time, and to use splints or other orthotic devices.

Perceptual, cognitive, and behavioral dysfunction are often experienced after brain injury. With a prevention emphasis, programs to assure safety in movement and with manipulation of objects is critical. Methods to alleviate stresses of disorientation and memory loss must also be implemented, although restricted environments and restraints may be necessary initially. However, when the child is more alert and aware of his or her surroundings, an educational approach coupled with behavioral interventions are most often used. Informing the child of unit rules, posting of such rules, and strict adherence to them are emphasized. Use of reinforcement programs structured through a team and family approach may be carried out to shape behaviors (Silver, Boake, & Cavazos, 1994). Daily orientation programs and memory books are used to ease the burden of confusion. Teaching the family about the child's perceptual and cog-

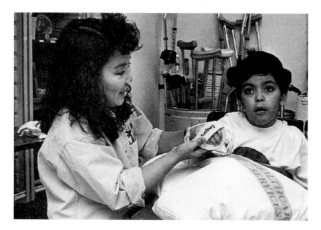

**Figure 30-2** Splints are used to prevent or to reduce contractures. Use of serial static splints requires regular monitoring and clear instructions for use to family members and other care providers.

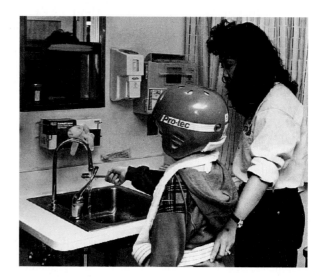

**Figure 30-3** The occupational therapist provides the child with cues and performance feedback while he carries out an adapted self-help sequence. A helmet is required to protect the head because of an open skull fracture.

nitive impairments and programs in place to assure safety and comfort are important. Managing the environment to reduce risk and placement of family pictures and other familiar items from home create a stimulating as well as more comforting environment.

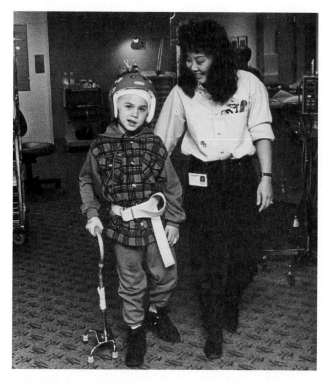

**Figure 30-4** Mobility is a fundamental part of self-help routines. After completing a morning care routine, this child walks to breakfast with assistance from the occupational therapist for safety and techique.

## Resuming and Restoring ADL and Work Performance

Once goals for ADL performance are negotiated, the therapist determines what the child needs to learn, how such learning will take place, and how training can best be organized within the clinical care setting. Schwartz (1991) described the basis of natural learning versus mediated learning. By *natural learning,* the child or adolescent may discover, in one or more sessions, simple strategies to resume activity performance. If these techniques are safe and efficient, the therapist need only guide the child in determining appropriate means to achieve consistent performance. Many times, however, the child is unable to make natural adaptations to achieve performance. Therapists then *mediate new learning* by instructing the child or adolescent and other care providers in the principles of adaptation and engage them in joint problem solving to determine the most effective methods of performance.

Once the therapist determines what needs to be learned, specific and desired routines for learning are organized. In mediated learning, some form of instruction takes place through a combination of guided activity and use of instructional aids. For initial instruction of new or adapted tasks, the therapist may demonstrate the task to be learned and have the child copy that demonstration. The therapist may also use verbal or manual guidance cues to assist learning (Figures 30-3 and 30-4). For some tasks, predetermined scripts or learning materials are available (Pedretti & Zoltan, 1990; Trombly, 1995).

When a particular task sequence has been determined, the therapist selects methods to achieve repetition, generalization, and development of new skills (Figure 30-5). For example, the child may be helped to memorize a routine so that he or she can guide his or her own performance using

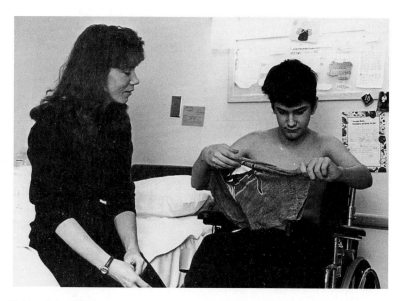

**Figure 30-5** Adapted dressing routines are developed to achieve success and to ease learning. For this boy, who has perceptual and cognitive deficits after brain injury, the occupational therapist cues him in a repetitive sequence of steps that accomplish the task.

**CASE STUDY #1**

Stephen is an 8-year-old boy from a two-parent, three-sibling home in a small coastal town. Stephen was described as energetic and well-liked. In October he was riding as a passenger on a three-wheel all-terrain vehicle when it rolled over. Stephen was not wearing a helmet and was reported to have struck his head. He was initially alert, but soon experienced diminished wakefulness and was unresponsive when paramedics arrived. At the trauma center Stephen was found to have a left basilar skull fracture, and a computed tomography scan showed bilateral frontal punctate lesions and an apparent left temporal-parietal focal lesion. Three days after injury Stephen became more responsive, demonstrating minimal movement of right arm and leg, no vocalizations, and dysphagia. He continued to show gradual improvement in his level of consciousness and was evaluated for transfer to acute rehabilitation. His injury was classified as moderate. Twelve days after the accident, Stephen was transferred to the local children's hospital.

On admission to rehabilitation he was following simple one-step commands and attempting to verbalize, but word finding was difficult. He was noted to be fatigued and difficult to engage for more than a few minutes at a time. He was also regarded as quiet and reserved, being fearful of separation from his mother, who stayed with him nearly full-time during the day and evenings. Diminished alertness, easy distraction, and disorientation to place and time were also noted. Mild, nonspastic right hemiplegia was observed, characterized by effortful movements of both upper and lower limbs. Passive range of motion was normal. In sensory testing Stephen showed impaired proprioception and localization to touch in distal portions of the arm and leg. Stephen did not ambulate but had partial weight bearing in stance with foot drop when he tried to walk. Use of a right ankle-foot orthosis (R-AFO) and cane was initiated. Little spontaneous use of his right arm was observed, and he showed characteristic synergy patterns and increased muscle tone when he attempted to grasp objects on command. Swallowing was judged to be safe from aspiration, although one-to-one supervision was needed because of Stephen's tendency to overstuff food and poorly sequence his intake of fluids and solids. During observation of grooming and dressing tasks, the occupational therapist found Stephen to be disorganized. In part because of his age, he showed poor ability to make natural adaptations to hemiplegia. Continual verbal cues were needed to initiate, set up, and proceed with grooming, dressing, and bathing tasks. Physical demonstration and cues were needed initially to teach adapted sequences. No perceptual deficits were found by observation or by use of standardized tests. Word finding difficulty, disorientation, and diminished sustained attention skills caused Stephen to become anxious. Use of an orientation board in his room, regular reminders provided by staff and his mother, written schedules, and a memory book that Stephen completed after each treatment session were initiated. Consistent routines for self-care, sequenced daily therapies, and structured play activities were planned. Familiar play items, pictures of family, his own clothes, favorite music, and art supplies were used to enhance comfort and provide memory cues and prompts for orientation. Visits by other family members and friends from school were organized and used in scheduling and memory book entries.

Stephen was scheduled for one-to-one therapy sessions twice each day. Morning self-care training and afternoon therapeutic activities were planned. In addition to structured self-care routines and orientation-memory programs, occupational therapy also engaged Stephen in selected activities to facilitate use of the right arm and to provide cognitive challenge in organizing steps, following sequences, and sustaining engagement in both familiar and novel tasks (Figure 30-6). Daily self range of motion and whole-body stretches were taught to maintain normal range and to facilitate symmetric trunk and limb use. Spontaneous use of the right arm improved, but poor recovery of his right hand resulted in Stephen attempting to perform activities using his nondominant left hand. Such attempts proved to be awkward and unsuccessful. Stephen was trained and cued to use both hands together (Figure 30-7), using the right hand as an assistor to the left hand. This strategy improved his self-care performance so that use of adaptive devices such as a button-aide and a rocker knife were discontinued after 2 weeks. Handwriting with either the right or left hand was not satisfactory for schoolwork because of illegibility and slow speed. The occupational therapists introduced a computer keyboard and initiated supplementary handwriting activities to facilitate movement and augment function. Physical management of other school-related tasks was judged to be adequate, although communication and cognitive impairments posed major challenges to Stephen's return to school.

Three weeks after admission, Stephen was ambulatory with use of an AFO. He continued to show evidence of topographic disorientation but otherwise was thought to be a safe ambulator, even on uneven surfaces and stairs. Self-care activities of grooming, dressing, and bathing were performed with supervision for initiation and safety. Stephen appropriately initiated toileting, and hygiene after bowel movements was judged by his mother to be adequate. Discharge planning included meetings with school personnel to address academic program needs and potential benefits from school-based therapy services. Eligibility for special education was determined, and planning of assessments related to an individualized educational plan were initiated. Interim school visits by the hospital neuropsychologist were scheduled to occur after Stephen's return to a half-day school program 2 weeks after discharge. A Rehabilitation Medicine Outpatient Clinic follow-up visit to include occupational therapy was scheduled in 6 weeks, with a plan for regular follow-along clinic visits at 2-month intervals during the next half-year.

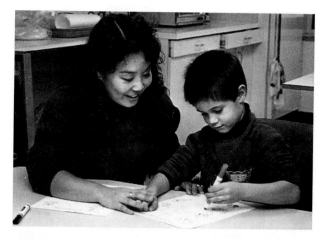

**Figure 30-6**  Use of the hemiparetic arm to hold the paper is promoted by the occupational therapist while the child carries out a drawing and writing activity.

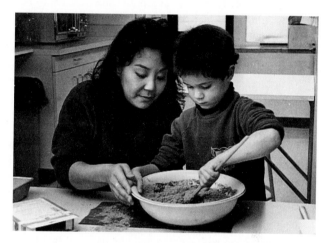

**Figure 30-7**  Guidance in using both arms is provided by the therapist while participating in a cookie-baking activity.

verbal, visual, or tactile feedback. If a routine cannot be memorized, other training tools can be used. Written instructions, pictorial step cues, and audio tapes with specific directions can be prepared. Whole-task instruction or the use of forward or reverse step sequence training are commonly suggested. Training that capitalizes on use of naturally occurring times when tasks are routinely performed can be implemented over several days (e.g., dressing in the morning and at night or before and after swimming). As training progresses, the extent of external cuing from a person or instructional aids is gradually reduced so that only a minimal amount of such support is required for safe and efficient performance. Often a planned approach to withdrawal of aides and assistance is expected to occur after discharge from the inpatient hospital setting. Such strategies form the basis of family or care provider training.

The environment used for ADL training is also important. Most agree that environments familiar to the child are preferred. However, except in home health care service delivery, environments must be simulated in hospital wards or clinics. Generalization of performance from one setting to another can be difficult because familiar settings may provide unrecognized prompts that are not present in simulated settings. Home visits with the child and family to survey and to collaborate in planning of organizational changes, equipment needs, and architectural modifications can facilitate

the necessary transition. Day or weekend home passes for the child are desirable when possible. Specific goals are often developed, and feedback from the family about the time at home can be important to prioritizing goals, equipment, and family training needs.

## Adaptations for Daily Living Skills

Basic principles apply to adapted performance of daily living skills. First, safety in performance and the avoidance of abnormal or unhealthy movements are essential. New learning is generally more difficult and more energy consuming. Principles of work simplification and joint protection are commonly used, and performance is geared toward function in the most barrier-free environment, with use of familiar conveniences. Adaptations of a routine are aimed at reducing complexity, assuring safety, and minimizing complications if errors do occur.

Lydia is a 9-year old girl with a history of cerebral palsy, developmental delay, seizure disorder, and a recent onset of viral pneumonia. Her mother brought her to the emergency room last spring because of severe pulmonary distress. She was intubated with a tracheotomy and did well for a time with medications and vigorous chest physical therapy. Extubation was performed, but she soon experienced another episode of pulmonary distress that required reintubation and use of a ventilator for about 1 week. In all, her respiratory problems dramatically altered her participation in school and her regular routines for over 6 weeks. Her mother's attempts to have Lydia resume walking resulted in refusals, with apparent swelling and pain in her left ankle. Orthopedic consultation determined that she had developed a stress fracture of her distal fibula. Her ankle was casted, but she was free to bear weight. Late in her second hospitalization she was evaluated for admission to acute rehabilitation. Transfer was thought to be necessary because of Lydia's deterioration in gross motor function, oral motor function, and ability to perform ADL compared with her baseline skills when seen through the neuromuscular clinic and from school records. A short-term rehabilitation program was planned to assure safety and adequate nutrition by oral feeding; to reattain functional short-distance ambulation with the use of bilateral plastic ankle-foot orthoses (AFOs) and a walker, with crawling up and down stairs, and with long-distance wheelchair mobility; to promote upper extremity endurance and resume a routine of assisted dressing and supervision with feeding and hygiene, and family use of adaptive equipment for safety in transfers; to improve speech intelligibility to preinfection status; and to facilitate transition back to school and an extended schoolyear program. Lydia was seen as an imaginative girl who enjoyed a variety of games and activities. She was generally cooperative and could normally express needs in short words and phrases, although picture boards for communication in self-care and therapy routines were developed. Task-specific communication boards had also been used at school. She was observed to pull her hair, bite her hands, and use her wheelchair to collide with objects; these behaviors were believed to be signs of frustration and fatigue. The therapy team chose to follow Lydia's school and home behavior routine, including short-term time-out, acknowledging her emotions and then redirecting her to a new activity.

The occupational therapist focused on Lydia's use of sequenced routines of dressing and hygiene with the nursing staff. In conjunction with speech pathology, a swallowing evaluation showed microaspirations that required a change in Lydia's foods to a dysphagia mechanical diet with thick liquids. One-to-one supervision was needed to cue for bite size and complete chewing before swallow. The speech therapist gave Lydia oral exercises to increase strength and coordination of her tongue, lips, and jaw for purposes of speech and the oral phase of feeding.

The occupational therapists emphasized strengthening her arms through therapeutic activities emphasizing aerobic tolerance. Wheelchair propulsion, wheelchair pushups for pressure relief, and crawling were also stressed to help Lydia recover her baseline abilities in use of the upper extremities. Fatigue in fine motor tasks was also noted, although skilled movements appeared similar to prepneumonia status. Endurance with tabletop tasks of writing and use of manipulatives were stressed. Lydia's mother was infrequently involved with therapy sessions because of her job responsibilities. Care provider instruction emphasized methods for making bathtub and car transfers and strategies to increase Lydia's participation in assisted routines of dressing, toileting, and hygiene. Lydia and her mother had previously developed a fast-paced care routine that allowed Lydia few opportunities to participate in or influence her care. The occupational therapists placed emphasis on having Lydia and her mother develop and follow simplified written routines, which enabled Lydia to direct more of her own care. This was thought to be important to her mother but also essential for use with other care providers like her father, with whom she stayed every other month for a weekend.

Lydia's admission to acute rehabilitation lasted 15 days. Her tolerance of bracing returned, and she was able to use a walker for up to 25 yards. She continued to need contact guarding in wheelchair-to-floor transfers and was able to crawl up and down seven carpeted steps. Manual wheelchair propulsion was limited to 100 yards on smooth and level surfaces. No complaints of arm fatigue were noted with activities of 15 minutes' duration. Lydia advanced to a regular diet, although her mother was instructed to follow precautions that included use of an upright posture while eating and drinking, a slow pace of eating, and avoidance of foods with stringy texture that were difficult for her to manage as a bolus and during the pharyngeal phase of swallowing. Plans were made with the school for an extended schoolyear program to complete the work missed during her long absence. At discharge, follow-up clinic visits were scheduled for orthopedics and pulmonary disorders in 3 weeks, and Lydia was scheduled to see her physiatrist as part of her routine neurodevelopmental clinic visit in 2 months.

## CASE STUDY #3

Kyle has a long history of involvement with rehabilitation specialists. He was born with a unique combination of limb deficiencies. His right upper-extremity amelia resulted in the equivalent of a right shoulder disarticulation, and his left upper extremity hemimelia results in a short above-elbow residual limb. His left lower extremity has femoral and tibial shortening with ankle and foot deformity. Kyle's right lower limb was comparatively normal. Multilimb abnormalities resulted in Kyle being followed for several years through a specialized clinic for children with limb deficiency. Several attempts to fit a prosthesis for his left leg proved difficult, expensive, and nonfunctional. Kyle developed good use of his right foot for prehension and used his left foot as an assist. As an early teenager, Kyle had good family support, attended school with his same-aged cohort in their hometown, and was a good student.

At this time Kyle was considered a good candidate for left leg surgery to correct a rotation deformity and to lengthen the limb by the Ilizarov procedure. Kyle's balance had begun to deteriorate with growth. His leg length discrepancy became more pronounced, causing severe problems when barefoot and not using his large shoelift, which was also viewed as unsightly. Although he could walk and run and use his lower limbs well for many daily living skills, it was believed that he would benefit from the surgical procedure, which would add approximately 6 cm of length to his left tibia. Anticipated benefits included better single-leg balance and reduced need for extensive lifts on his left shoe.

Two stages were planned for the surgical correction. The first included a left distal femoral wedge osteotomy to correct the rotation deformity of his knee and a heel cord release at the ankle. The second procedure would involve tibial lengthening with the Ilizarov technique. Kyle underwent the first part of this series with mixed results. Because of his upper limb deficiency, use of traditional crutches was not possible, and he required a lengthened period of rehabilitation to learn to walk again. He experienced several falls and had complaints of ankle pain as well. Because his running skills decreased after the first surgery, he became reticent about the second procedure. Anxiety and depressive reactions were seen and referrals made for more extensive assessment and treatment. It was determined that both Kyle and his family needed more information about the surgery and the expected course of recovery. In planning his second surgery, which was expected to have an even longer recovery time, careful assessment of rehabilitative needs were addressed. The procedure necessitated the development of a customized crutch to be used on the right side and careful planning to address concerns he and his family had regarding his independence. A prosthetist developed a crutch device that molded to the axilla for weight bearing through the ribs and the latissimus muscle and had a detachable post modified from a Loftstrand design (Mosca, Okumura, & Jaffe, 1993). Kyle learned to use the crutch quickly. During the summer he underwent the second procedure and was admitted to acute rehabilitation.

Goals after his surgery were to restore safe mobility and, before returning home, to reestablish desired independence in feeding, grooming, bathing, dressing, and written communication skills. The admission also provided an opportunity to more directly evaluate and explore options for the skills that Kyle had been inconsistent in performing. External fixation of the tibia created some difficulty in using his left foot as an assistor. He was seen in occupational therapy twice per day to address further adaptation of functional skills. Kyle participated in problem solving and willingly tried new techniques. He resumed feeding by using his regular routine of right foot over his left thigh and handling utensils to bring food to his mouth from a specially positioned plate. He continued to have difficulty opening packaged foods because of his left foot immobility. The occupational therapist introduced adaptations to his usual assistive devices that allowed him to resume independence in grooming and in bathing tasks. A dressing board similar to the one used at home was configured to allow Kyle independence in donning and doffing his clothes by use of specially placed stationary hooks. Kyle also resumed right foot writing and computer operation. Adaptive driving was also explored, and a referral to a special drivers' training program was scheduled for a time after healing and before his sixteenth birthday. Physical therapy engaged Kyle in ambulation training and specific muscle strengthening of the left lower extremity. At discharge he was able to walk with his crutch for distances up to 300 feet and bear approximately 80% of his body weight over his left leg. Transfers from seated surfaces and standing were independent, but he continued to require assistance getting up from the floor. Kyle's admission to acute rehabilitation lasted 3 weeks, with additional community-based physical therapy planned. Continued visits to the rehabilitation limb deficiency clinic program were scheduled.

# Basic Rehabilitation Strategies

A number of strategies for specific types of impairments are used by occupational therapist to adapt activities for children with functional limitations.

## MOTOR LIMITATIONS
### Limited Range of Motion

Reduced range of motion in the neck, trunk, and proximal and intermediate joints of the limbs limits ability to reach all parts of the body and objects within the immediate environment. Limitations of hand motion can reduce holding and handling of objects. To substitute for reach, extended and specially angled handles are used (e.g., long-handled spoon or fork, bath brush, dressing stick, or shoe horn) or more specialized devices such as reachers are employed. If a child is unable to use devices that extend reach, other strategies are employed to permit function. Mounting objects on the floor, wall, or table and bringing the body part to the device (e.g., boot tree for removing shoes, friction pad on floor for socks, hook on the wall to pull up or down pants, or sponges mounted in the shower to wash) prove useful. For some tasks, devices may replace any reach requirement, such as use of a bidet for hygiene after toileting or manual or electric feeders operated by microswitches to bring food to the mouth.

When motion of the hand is limited, holding and manipulation of objects is assisted by using enlarged or differently styled handles that reduce grasp requirement (e.g., T-handled cup). Holding functions may be replaced by use of universal cuff or C-shaped handles. Friction surfaces may provide more secure grasp. When forearm rotation is limited, swivel spoons or angled utensils may assist bringing food to the mouth.

Limited range of motion also reduces gross motor movements such as in bed mobility and in making elevation changes (moving from sit to stand and performing transfers in bathing and toileting). Surface levels are typically changed (i.e., raised or lowered) to limit the extent of elevation change required. The bed height may be lowered to allow ease in wheelchair transfers or raised to ease in coming up to standing from sitting. Raised chairs, toilet seats, and bath benches are employed to reduce extreme changes in elevation required in transfers.

### Decreased Strength and Endurance

Strength and endurance limitations are common among children who are acutely ill or injured. The goals of adaptation are to reduce the effects of gravity by use of lightweight objects, movements in the horizontal plane, reduced friction, and when possible the use of body mechanics for leverage and gravity to assist movement. Electrically powered devices may be suggested to meet goals of work simplification. Efficiency of movement is essential. Similar to limited range of motion, weakness can cause inability to reach body parts or to make elevation changes. Extended handles may be necessary; however, increased weight and forces required to handle and apply leverage can increase difficulty.

A major goal with activity adaptation for decreased strength is to limit the need to sustain static postures and prolonged holding. Using surfaces to support posture and proximal limb positions is accomplished in a variety of ways. Bed positioning, seating adaptations, and use of armrests and table surfaces are examples. The need for sustained holding is reduced by mounting devices or stabilizing devices with friction (e.g., Dycem or spike board) or by using an enlarged lightweight object. Universal cuffs or C-cuffs are also commonly employed to limit demands for grasp. Manipulation may be impaired and necessitate use of hooks and loops on clothing and adaptation of fasteners by use of Velcro, zippers, enlarged buttons, or elastic shoelaces. Less complex movement and reduced force is required to manipulate lever handles on faucets, doors, and appliances. Reducing movement against gravity in transfers is accomplished by changing heights of surfaces as well as by using assistive devices such as sliding boards, springs, or hydraulic lifts to aid movement.

For children with cardiac or pulmonary disorders, progression of activities of daily living (ADL) performance may be based on estimated metabolic equivalents levels or by direct monitoring. Scheduling and pacing of tasks, work simplification, and use of rest breaks within tasks are suggested.

### Incoordination

Incoordination primarily causes difficulty with manipulation skills. The extent to which incoordination influences performance is determined by the range of movement required, weight and resistance of objects being handled, and positioning of the body in relation to objects. A primary concern is to achieve proximal stability when executing movements. Stabilizing the trunk and head while making movements of the arm and hand is thought to improve skilled movements. Likewise, stabilizing the proximal segments of the limb while manipulating the hand is suggested (e.g., resting the elbow and forearm on the table while using the wrist and fingers to manipulate objects). Friction surfaces may also be suggested for stabilization of the limb, as well as containers that hold objects being manipulated. (e.g., friction pad plate or nonslip cup).

Another common strategy is to determine if increased weight dampens exaggerated movements and tremor. Heavier objects may be selected, or weight may be added to objects. A weight can be attached to the arm or resistance to movement can be applied by devices placed across joints (i.e., elastic sleeves or friction feeder) to determine if more precise movements can be achieved. When such methods are inadequate, other techniques employed are similar to those for reduced range of motion and strength. These include the mounting of devices on stable surfaces and bringing the body to these devices using gross movements.

### One-Handed Techniques

When a child has to perform most activities with one hand, the barriers to be overcome typically involve replacing the stabilization function of the other limb, improving the skills of the hand being used, and adapting tasks that require alternating movements of two hands. Generally, many tasks can be accomplished rather easily with the use of one hand. If the hand being used was not previously the preferred or dominant hand, skilled movements may take a greater amount of time to develop. For those with perceptual and cognitive impairments, learning to use one hand may be particularly difficult. For children with hemiplegia, various dressing routines have been scripted that follow the rules of dressing the affected limb first and avoiding the use of abnormal postures. The stabilization function of the impaired limb may not be entirely lost, although the child may need to learn how to assist movement in placing or positioning the limb to effectively stabilize objects. To entirely replace the stabilization function of the impaired or lost upper limb, mounting or use of friction surfaces may be used. Some two-handed tasks require the use of specially designed devices or methods. For example, cutting with a knife and fork can be adapted for by use of a rocker-knife or cutting edged fork, buttoning by use of a button hock, shoe tying by use of a special lacing technique, and typing by use of a one-handed training program.

### PERCEPTUAL AND COGNITIVE LIMITATIONS

Sensory, perceptual, and cognitive impairments alone pose a variety of challenges to ADL performance but are most often associated with other physical disorders previously described. If retraining of component skills is ineffective and impairment continues, substitution for impaired skills by using more intact sensory, perceptual, or cognitive skills is considered (e.g., using a bell on the hemiplegic arm to draw attention if being neglected tactually or visually). Compensation techniques may also be planned that modify activity sequence and environment to enable the child to accomplish the challenging task.

### Perceptual and Cognitive Deficit

Such impairments affect daily living skill routines and school performance. To compensate for perceptual or cognitive deficits, step-by-step routines with cuing systems are typically designed and repeated in training. Work simplification principles are employed, and substitution strategies are used. Children with perceptual or cognitive deficits may rely on memorizing and reciting a verbal routine or follow audiotaped instruction. They may also rely on written instructions or pictorial cues. With impaired visual perception, reliance on tactile feedback cues may need to be taught. At times, materials used in ADL are specially selected to compensate for impairments. Color-contrasted clothing, texture, or color-coding cues may be used with objects. Sometimes the use of mirrors can be encouraged to give the child feedback about his or her performance.

### Visual Impairment

Blindness or severe visual impairment requires that strategies be employed to substitute for vision by use of other sensory skills and cognitive routines. Consistent organization of the environment and storage of items is necessary. Tactile identifiers on objects such as raised letters and locations of more transient items described by a companion, using a standard technique such as analog clock location may be used. Sound feedback may be built into some items to aid orientation or search. Mobility specialists instruct individuals to use techniques such as long canes or guide dogs for ambulation or wheelchair guidance and to use a leader's arm for guidance in walking.

Adaptive methods of ADL may include the use of assistive devices (see Section III). Reliance on devices may be temporary or permanent. Early use of devices can increase safety or immediate function during recovery. Permanent use of devices is also common when there is residual disability for which no nondevice methods can be accomplished. When selecting devices, therapists often choose to adapt existing equipment that is already familiar to the child. If such adaptation is not desirable or practical, the therapist may first direct the family to try to purchase items with features more compatible with the child's or adolescent's special needs through standard shopping sources. If needs cannot be met, specialized rehabilitation devices are purchased through medical and rehabilitation equipment vendors. Assistive devices are generally designed to accommodate or substitute for skill limitations in gross movement, reach, prehension manipulation, perception, or sensation. Use of devices should reduce task difficulty and complexity, although initial learning and use may be awkward.

## SUMMARY

Hospital-based pediatric rehabilitation services play a unique role in the overall management of children with new or chronic disability. In addressing acute and chronic problems, the emphasis of practice is nearly always on function

Boyer, M.G. & Edwards, P. (1991). Outcome 1 to 3 years after severe traumatic brain injury in children and adolescents. *Injury, 22,* 315-320.

Burkett, K.W. (1989). Trends in pediatric rehabilitation. *Nursing Clinics of North America, 24,* 239-255.

Chaplin, D., Deitz, J., & Jaffe, K.M. (1993). Motor performance in children after traumatic brain injury. *Archives of Physical Medicine and Rehabilitation, 74,* 161-164.

Coster, W.J., Haley, S., & Baryza, M.J. (1994). Functional performance of young children after traumatic brain injury: a 6-month follow-up study. *American Journal of Occupational Therapy, 48,* 211-218.

Di-Scala, C., Osberg, J.S., Gans, B.M., Chin, L.J., & Grant, C.C. (1991). Children with traumatic head injury: morbidity and post-acute treatment. *Archives of Physical Medicine and Rehabilitation, 72,* 662-666.

Donders, J. (1993). Bereavement and mourning in pediatric rehabilitation settings. *Death Studies, 17,* 517-527.

Edwards, P.A. (1992). The evolution of rehabilitation facilities for children. *Rehabilitation Nursing, 17, 191-195.*

Eigsti, H., Aretz, M., & Shannon, L. (1990). Pediatric physical therapy in a rehabilitation setting. *Pediatrician, 17,* 267-277.

Fay, G.C. Jaffe, K.M., Polissar, N.L., Liao, S., Rivara, J.B., & Martin, K.M. (1994). Outcome of pediatric traumatic brain injury at three years: a cohort study. *Archives of Physical Medicine and Rehabilitation, 75,* 733-741.

Fuhrer, M.J. (1987). *Rehabilitation outcomes, analysis and measurement. Baltimore:* Brookes.

Gans, B.M. (1993). Rehabilitation of the pediatric patient. In J.A. Delisa (Ed.). *Rehabilitation medicine, principles and practice* (2nd ed.). Philadelphia: J.B. Lippincott.

Gardner, J. & Workinger, M.S. (1990). The changing role of the speech-language pathologist in pediatric rehabilitation/habilitation. *Pediatrician, 17,* 283-286.

Haley, S.M., Baryza, M.J., & Webster, H.C. (1992). Pediatric rehabilitation and recovery of children with traumatic injuries. *Pediatric Physical Therapy, 4,* 24-30.

Haley, S.M., Coster, W.J., Ludlow, L.H., Haltiwanger, J.T., & Andrellos, P.J. (1992). *Pediatric Evaluation of Disability Inventory.* Boston: New England Medical Center Hospitals.

Heery, K. (1992). Restoring childhood through rehabilitation. *Rehabilitation Nursing, 17,* 193-195.

Herndon, D.N., Rutan, R.L., & Rutan, T.C. (1993). Management of the pediatric patient with burns. *Journal of Burn Care and Rehabilitation, 14,* 3-8.

Jaffe, K.M., Fay, G.C., Polissar, N.L., Martin, K.M., Shurtleff, H., Rivara, J.B., & Winn, H.R. (1992). Severity of pediatric brain injury and early neurobehavioral outcome: a cohort study. *Archives of Physical Medicine and Rehabilitation, 73,* 540-547.

Jaffe, K.M., Fay, G.C., Polissar, N.L., Martin, K.M., Shurtleff, H., Rivara, J.B., & Winn, H.R. (1993). Severity of pediatric traumatic brain injury and neurobehavioral recovery at one year: a cohort study. *Archives of Physical Medicine and Rehabilitation, 74,* 587-595.

Jaffe, K.M., Okamoto, G.A., & Lemire, C. (1986). Inpatient pediatric rehabilitation: a five year review. *Rehabilitation Literature, 47,* 286-289.

## STUDY QUESTIONS

1. For a child with traumatic injury, suggest reasons why acute rehabilitation would be recommended. How would recommendations differ from care in subacute or outpatient rehabilitation settings? How would this differ for a child with a congenital onset disorder?
2. Considering the intensive yet comprehensive nature of acute rehabilitation, suggest types of case-specific or program outcomes that would be most meaningful to reflect on occupational therapy practice in this setting.
3. For a new admission to acute rehabilitation, describe how assessment and treatment planning would be prioritized. Consider how the family is involved in the process of setting goals and selecting treatment strategies.
4. For teaching adaptive methods that may involve use of assistive devices, suggest three alternatives for providing such instruction.
5. Short of independence, suggest long-term goals for acute rehabilitation that would be relevant to the child's function at home and in the school setting.

and participation in life's events at home, at school, and in the community. Both new and established impairments and disabilities pose risks for further complications, which necessitate a prevention prioritization through subacute, acute, and outpatient or ongoing rehabilitation interventions.

Services are medically oriented and are delivered within constraints imposed by accreditation and regulatory agencies, as well as third-party payers. Collaboration with school- and community-based services are critical to effective intervention and transition. The challenge of pediatric rehabilitation is to address the acute problems while considering the overall development of the child and the priorities of the family.

## REFERENCES

Albright, A.L. (1992). Neurosurgical treatment of spasticity: selective posterior rhizotomy and intrathecal baclofen. *Stereotactic and Functional Neurosurgery, 58,* 3-13.

Binder, H., Conway, A., Hanson, S., Gerber, L.H., Marini, J., Berry, R., & Weintraub, J. (1993). Comprehensive rehabilitation of the child with osteogenesis imperfecta. *American Journal of Medical Genetics, 45,* 265-269.

Blatzheim, L.L., Edberg, A., & Lacy, L. (1987). Operationalizing primary nursing in the pediatric rehabilitation setting. *Journal of Pediatric Nursing, 2,* 434-437.

Johnston, M.V. & Granger, C.V. (1994). Outcomes research in medical rehabilitation: a primer and introduction to a series. *American Journal of Physical Medicine and Rehabilitation, 73,* 296-303.

Karger, C., Guile, J.T., & Bowen, J.R. (1993). Lengthening of congenital lower limb deficiencies. *Clinical Orthopedics and Related Research, 291,* 236-245.

Keith, R.A., Granger, C.V., Hamilton, B.B., & Sherwin, F.S. (1987). The functional independence measure: a new tool for rehabilitation. *Advances in Clinical Rehabilitation, 1,* 6-18.

Massagli, T.L. & Jaffe, K.M. (1990). Pediatric spinal cord injury: treatment and outcome. *Pediatrician, 17,* 244-254.

Moront, M. & Eichelberger, M.R. (1994). Pediatric trauma. *Pediatrics Annals, 23,* 186-191.

Mosca, V.S., Okumura, R., & Jaffe, K.M. (1993). Prosthetic crutch for a patient with congenital bilateral, upper extremity deficiencies undergoing lower extremity lengthening by the Ilizarov method. *Journal of the Association of Children's Prosthetic-Orthotic Clinics 28,* 19-20.

Msall, M.E., DiGaudio, K.M., & Duffy, L.C. (1993). Use of functional assessment in children with developmental disabilities. *Physical Medicine and Rehabilitation Clinics of North America, 4,* 517-527.

Philip, P.A., Ayyangar, R., Vanderbilt, J., & Gaebler-Spira, D.J. (1994). Rehabilitation outcome in children after treatment of primary brain tumor. *Archives of Physical Medicine and Rehabilitation, 75,* 36-39.

Raps, C.S., Peterson, C., Janas, M., & Seligman, M.E. (1982). Patient behavior in hospitals: helplessness, reactance, or both? *Journal of Personality and Social Psychology, 42,* 1036-1041.

Richardson, C.J. & Robinson, S.S. (1989). Neonatal intensive care and pediatric rehabilitation: a joint program for care of chronically ill infants. *Journal of Perinatology, 9,* 52-55.

Rivara, J.B. (1993). Family functioning following pediatric traumatic brain injury. *Pediatric Annals, 23,* 38-43.

Rivara, J.B., Jaffe, K.M., Polissar, N.L., Fay, G.C., Martin, K.M., Shurtleff, H.A., & Liao, S. et al. (1994). Family functioning and children's academic performance and behavioral problems in the year following traumatic brain injury. *Archives of Physical Medicine and Rehabilitation, 75,* 369-379.

Rodriquez, J. & Brown, S.T. (1990). Childhood injuries in the United States, Division of Injury Control, Center for Environmental Health and Injury Control, Center for Disease Control. *American Journal of Diseases of Children, 144,* 627-646.

Russman, B.S. (1990). Rehabilitation of the pediatric patient with a neuromuscular disease. *Neurology Clinics, 8,* 727-740.

Schwartz, R.K. (1991). Educational and training strategies, therapy as learning. In C. Christiansen & C. Baum (Eds.). *Occupational therapy: overcoming human performance deficits* (pp. 664-698). Thororfare, NJ: Slack.

Silver, B.V., Boake, C., & Cavazos, D.I. (1994). Improving functional skills using behavioral procedures in a child with anoxic brain injury. *Archives of Physical Medicine and Rehabilitation, 75,* 742-745.

Strunk, R.C., Mascia, A.V., Lipkowitz, M.A., & Wolf, S.I. (1991). Rehabilitation of a patient with asthma in the outpatient setting. *Journal of Allergy and Clinical Immunology, 87*(3), 601-611.

Trombly, C.A. (1995). *Occupational therapy for physical dysfunction* (4th ed.). Baltimore: Williams & Wilkins.

Watson, D. (1991). Occupational therapy intervention guidelines for children and adolescents with spina bifida. *Child: Care, Health, and Development, 17,* 367-380.

Wieting, J.M. & Krach, L.E. (1994). Spinal cord injury rehabilitation in a pediatric achondroplastic patient: case report. *Archives of Physical Medicine and Rehabilitation, 75,* 106-108.

## SUGGESTED READINGS

Carney, J. & Gerring, J. (1990). Return to school following severe closed head injury: a critical phase in pediatric rehabilitation. *Pediatrician, 17,* 222-229.

Del Vecchio, J. (1992). Home pediatric rehabilitation. *Journal of Home Health Care Practice, 5,* 12-15.

DiCowden, M. (1990). Pediatric rehabilitation: special patients, special needs. *Journal of Rehabilitation, 56,* 13-18.

Kurtz, L.A. & Scull, S.A. (1993). Rehabilitation for developmental disabilities. *Pediatric Clinics of North America, 40,* 629-643.

Matthews, D.J., Meier, R.H., & Bartholome, W. (1990). Ethical issues encountered in pediatric rehabilitation. *Pediatrician, 17,* 108-114.

Molnar, G.E. (1988). A developmental perspective for the rehabilitation of children with physical disability. *Pediatric Annals, 17,* 766, 768-776.

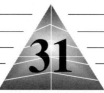

# Programs and Services for Children with Psychosocial Dysfunction

DEBORA A. DAVIDSON

## KEY TERMS

▲ Early Childhood Intervention Programs
▲ Students with Behavioral Disorders
▲ Classroom-Based Psychosocial Therapy
▲ Outpatient Mental Health Services
▲ Day Treatment Programs
▲ Residential Treatment Centers
▲ Juvenile Justice System
▲ Inpatient Psychiatric Hospitals

## CHAPTER OBJECTIVES

1. Identify the continuum of services available to children and youth with psychosocial disorders.
2. Define the roles of occupational therapists who provide services to children and youth with psychosocial disorders.
3. Explain frames of reference and intervention strategies used in psychosocial intervention.
4. Explain the variety of service delivery models used by occupational therapists in psychosocial settings.

Health care professionals who work with children and adolescents can expect to encounter clients with psychosocial problems, regardless of the setting. Research on random samples of children and adolescents in the community indicates that 15% to 22% of the general population have psychosocial problems, but only about 2% receive intervention specific to mental health concerns (National Advisory Mental Health Council, 1990; Tuma, 1989). One reason for this is that mental health services for children and adolescents have typically been sparse

and poorly funded in the United States (Knitzer, 1982; Solomon & Evans, 1992; Tuma, 1989). Another reason is the pervasive cultural bias that deters families from admitting to having and seeking help for psychosocial problems. Lastly, there can be a tendency to ignore the psychosocial needs of clients who have other more visible physical and cognitive problems such as cerebral palsy or Down syndrome, despite evidence that children with chronic health problems are at increased risk for mental health dysfunction (Offard & Fleming, 1991).

Occupational therapists are uniquely educated and positioned to provide needed psychosocial evaluation and treatment to children and adolescents in a wide variety of contexts. Despite this, occupational therapists are often limited in their ability to address mental health needs of referred children because of reimbursement regulations (Schultz, 1992). Neglect of mental health needs can range from client dissatisfaction to regression rather than progress. Any parent of a child whose developmental problems warrant professional intervention experiences strong emotions, which may range from anxiety to anger. When these feelings are ignored, a genuine therapeutic alliance cannot be formed. For example, many times school-aged children are referred to occupational therapists for handwriting problems when the real problem is that the student does not complete written work because of inattention or misbehavior. If the perceptual and motor aspects of writing are all that is addressed, the student, parent, and teacher do not receive meaningful help.

The purposes of this chapter are to describe ways in which occupational therapists may provide psychosocial intervention in a variety of settings and to inspire therapists to use all of their skills to address the full spectrum of children's needs. These goals are approached by describing a variety of treatment settings that represent a continuum of less to more psychiatrically oriented and less to more intensive and restrictive. The mission, clientele, services, frames of reference, and staffing patterns for each type of facility are described, along with traditional or potential roles for occupational therapists in each setting. Case studies synthesized from the author's clinical experiences illustrate innovative ways of providing psychosocial intervention in a variety of traditional and nontraditional settings.

Therapeutic environments to be discussed in this chapter include early childhood intervention programs, public schools, outpatient mental health centers, day treatment programs, residential treatment centers, correctional facilities, and inpatient acute care hospitals. Some of these programs are designed specifically to assist children and adolescents who have identified mental health problems; others are oriented toward meeting more general educational or developmental needs. Occupational therapists have been well established in some of these settings, and in others they are pioneers. In any case, pediatric occupational therapists have the knowledge base, skills, and opportunities to provide psychosocial intervention to children and adolescents in need, regardless of the service setting.

# EARLY CHILDHOOD INTERVENTION PROGRAMS

The primary mission of early childhood intervention (ECI) programs is the prevention and amelioration of developmental disabilities in children from birth to 3 years of age. Clients include infants and toddlers who are diagnosed as having developmental delay, those considered to be at risk for developmental problems, and their families (Individuals with Disabilities Act [IDEA], 1990). Although infants and toddlers are primarily referred to early intervention for evaluation and treatment of neurologic and physical conditions, children may be referred when development is at risk because of parental psychosocial problems. Such problems include chemical dependency, domestic violence, parental depression, or psychiatric disorder. Occasionally the identified child may have a diagnosed mental health disorder, such as nonorganic failure to thrive or pervasive developmental disorder (American Psychological Association, 1994; Hunter & Powell, 1990).

Professionals working in ECI programs are likely to use developmental, neurodevelopmental, rehabilitation, behavioral, interactional, and family systems as frames of reference (Table 31-1) (Dunn, Campbell, Oetter, Hall, & Berger,

▲ Table 31-1  Settings for Psychosocial Treatment of Children and Adolescents

|  | Early Childhood Intervention Programs | School Systems | Outpatient and Day Treatment Programs | Residential Treatment Centers | Correctional Facilities | Inpatient Hospitals |
|---|---|---|---|---|---|---|
| Frames of reference | Developmental Neurodevelopmental Rehabilitation Behavioral Family systems | Educational Developmental Behavioral | Behavioral Cognitive Developmental Psychodynamic Family systems Neurobehavioral | Behavioral Developmental Milieu | Behavioral Educational | Developmental Neurobehavioral Behavioral Cognitive Psychodynamic Family systems |
| Clientele | Families of children aged 0 to 3 years who are diagnosed with developmental delay or are at risk for delay | Children and adolescents 2 to 18 years of age | Children and adolescents 5 to 18 years of age and their families | Children and adolescents 5 to 10 years of age, sometimes families | Children and adolescents 10 to 18 years of age | Children and adolescents 3 to 18 years of age |
| Staffing* | 2 and 3 Special educators Speech-language pathologists Audiologists Occupational therapists Physical therapists Social workers Psychologists Nurses Nutritionists | 1 and 2 Educators Special educators Speech-language pathologists Occupational therapists Physical therapists Counselors Psychologists Administrators | 1, 2, and 3 Psychiatrists Psychologists Social workers Nurses Counselors Occupational therapists Art therapists Recreational therapists Music therapists | 2 and 3 Houseparents Psychologists Social workers Educators | 1 and 2 Guards Police officers Parole officers Lawyers Psychologists Psychiatrists Social workers Educators Counselors Occupational therapists | 1 and 2 Psychiatrists Nurses Unit Staff Psychologists Social workers Occupational therapists Recreational therapists Music therapists Art therapists |

*Dominant team style: *1*, Multidisciplinary; *2*, interdisciplinary; *3*, transdisciplinary.

1989). Infants and toddlers whose environment is characterized by abuse, emotional neglect, or deprivation are at increased risk for developing psychosocial dysfunction. Such situations are likely to occur when the parents have personality or conduct disorders, severe depression, or substance abuse problems (Constantino, 1993). Poverty, social isolation, and cultural acceptance of harsh or neglectful parenting practices also engender abuse, neglect, and deprivation (Davidson, 1995).

Occupational therapists, educated to recognize and treat persons with mental illness, contribute significantly to the ECI team's effectiveness with high-risk families. By addressing some of the key factors contributing to a family's distress, the entire family system can achieve a healthier state. For example, if the parent of a child with medical complications reports that the family is having difficulty following through with the child's care because of unemployment and marital stress, the ECI case manager is in a position to refer the parents for financial assistance, work placement, and counseling services. Once these concerns are resolved, parents have more energy available for child care.

## PUBLIC SCHOOL SYSTEMS

The primary mission of public education is academic and social preparation for future education and work roles. Prevalence studies have indicated that approximately 30% of students display school adjustment problems, with an even higher rate of occurrence among urban children (Kellam, Branch, Agrawal, & Ensinger, 1975; Rubin & Balow, 1978). Children and adolescents with moderate to severe behavioral problems are unable to fully avail themselves of education, and experience repeated academic and social failure. The long-term outcomes of such failure include delinquency and crime, dropping out of school, and economic dependency. Lifelong feelings of inadequacy and economic underachievement may result. The public schools represent an arena where occupational therapists have an as-yet unrealized opportunity to make a tremendous impact on the lives of children with psychosocial problems.

Students whose special needs are primarily of a psychosocial nature may be identified by the school system as *seriously emotionally disturbed*. Federal regulations define this special education classification as

. . . a condition exhibiting one or more of the following characteristics over a long period of time and to a marked degree, which adversely affects educational performance:
   (A) An inability to learn that cannot be explained by intellectual, sensory, or health factors;
   (B) An inability to build or maintain satisfactory interpersonal relationships with peers or teachers;
   (C) Inappropriate types of behavior or feelings under normal circumstances;
   (D) A general pervasive mood of unhappiness or depression; or

   (E) A tendency to develop physical symptoms or fears associated with personal or school problems (Individuals with Disabilities Education Act of 1990).

Children who exhibit thought disorders are included under the classification "seriously emotionally disturbed." This category does not include children who demonstrate socially maladjusted behavior (e.g., delinquency, school truancy, or conduct disorder) in the absence of the problems listed previously. Other categories in which psychosocial problems and behavioral disorders often present are pervasive developmental disorders, mental retardation, and traumatic brain injuries (IDEA, 1990).

A variety of school settings serve special education students with behavioral problems, depending on the school districts' and individual schools' philosophies, individual students' needs, and parents' preferences. Before the increased emphasis on inclusion, students with severe psychosocial disabilities were typically designated as behaviorally disturbed or emotionally disturbed and placed in a self-contained classroom. Self-contained classroom arrangements allow students whose behavior is frequently disruptive or otherwise inappropriate to receive intensive behavioral intervention while being educated in a small group setting. However, students in such classrooms are segregated from peers and role models and suffer the stigma of being identified as different. The current trend is toward the inclusion of special education students in regular education settings as much as possible. In this model, students attend regular education classrooms with support services that may include a resource room for specific subjects, classroom aides, crisis intervention, and counseling services. Benefits of this approach include regular exposure to a normal school environment, opportunities to interact with typically developing peers, and positive experiences that reinforce learning of social skills. Problems can arise with this approach when the teachers have large numbers of students and little training in preventing or managing disruptive behaviors. Teachers and students then feel inadequate and frustrated.

Many schools incorporate social skills training programs into their regular curricula, which are taught by the classroom teachers. These programs are suitable for all children, and they address areas such as communication skills (Gresham & Elliot, 1993), social problem solving (Shure & Spivak, 1982; Weissburg, 1985; Weissberg, Caplan, & Bennetto, 1988), and drug abuse prevention (Cohen, Brennan, & Sexton, 1984). Such educational programs can provide an excellent means of developing prosocial thinking and behavior in typical children. However, these programs do not provide the intensive guidance required by children and adolescents who have psychosocial dysfunction affecting performance in these areas.

School-based therapeutic intervention is directed toward enhancing students' academic and future vocational performance, with an emphasis on both scholastic and social de-

CASE STUDY #1

Vanessa, who is 16 years old, and her 4-month-old daughter Nicole, live independently in a subsidized housing development. Nicole was referred to an early childhood intervention (ECI) program by her pediatrician, who was concerned about the possibility of developmental delay related to her low birth weight and probable fetal alcohol effects. Nicole was evaluated by the center's interdisciplinary team and was found to be a passive baby who rarely interacted with people or the environment, had low muscle tone, and was slow to drink from a bottle. Vanessa decided that, because of transportation problems, she would prefer home-based intervention. The team agreed that the occupational therapist would provide therapeutic and case management services. The therapist worked with Nicole and Vanessa individually and together. To coordinate care, she established communication with two outside agencies that were also providing services to the family.

The work with Nicole was focused toward increasing her arousal level and responsiveness to the social and physical environment, improving her efficiency in eating, and increasing movement. Neurodevelopmental and sensory integrative therapy techniques were applied to these goals. The therapist provided a selection of toys each week and encouraged Vanessa to give Nicole opportunities to move and explore the environment.

Vanessa was initially shy and guarded with the therapist but became increasingly comfortable after several weeks. The therapeutic relationship was forged when the occupational therapist and Vanessa worked together to assemble a colorful mobile for the baby's crib. During that session, Vanessa confided that she was living in fear of Nicole's father, who had beaten Vanessa repeatedly during her pregnancy and was threatening her life if she did not agree to let him move into the apartment. The occupational therapist assisted Vanessa in contacting a battered women's service organization, which offered support groups, crisis shelter, legal services, and adult education programs. She also helped Vanessa identify family members who might be able to assist with child care and

help with occasional transportation needs. During the course of their relationship, the occupational therapist continued to listen to Vanessa's concerns and encouraged her to pursue the resources that were available to her. She also monitored the home situation for potential violence toward Nicole, in case a referral to Child Protective Services was needed. Additionally, she maintained regular communication with the referring pediatrician, who assisted with monitoring Nicole's health and the family's progress.

Although Vanessa consistently expressed strong feelings of affection and the desire to be a good mother to Nicole, the therapist observed that the mother-infant interactions were often poorly synchronized, resulting in frustration for both. The occupational therapist taught Vanessa to recognize Nicole's changing states of arousal and to time her attempts to engage the baby in social play when Nicole was calm and alert. Vanessa learned to involve Nicole in developmentally appropriate interactive activities such as peek-a-boo, gentle tickling, and "so big." She also learned the importance of providing Nicole with a variety of sensory, motor, and language experiences.

After 6 months of therapy, Vanessa was attending educational and support activities sponsored by the women's shelter three afternoons per week. She planned to enroll in a vocational training program once the occupational therapist, as the family's service coordinator, completed arrangements for Nicole to attend day care. Nicole had become appropriately active and sociable, and she and her mother interacted warmly in a manner that bespoke their mutual emotional development and attachment. Nicole's motor development was in the low-average range.

The therapist in this example helped the family address key psychosocial needs through direct intervention and community referral. The ECI team carried out its mission by providing direct assistance and coordinating the provision of services among various agencies. As with most young families, the psychosocial and physical needs of the infant could only be fully met when those of the primary caretaker were also met.

velopment. Traditionally the school psychologist, counselor, or social worker assumes responsibility for evaluating psychosocial needs and may work with students in individual or small group sessions. Frames of reference usually include behavioral, cognitive, and developmental approaches (see Table 31-1).

Many leaders in education and occupational therapy believe that the services provided to behaviorally disturbed students are inadequate in quantity and quality (Florey, 1989; Schultz, 1992). Teachers express despair as they find themselves sacrificing creative educational methods to attend to behavioral crises. Parents of students with behavioral disorders are frustrated by the paucity of services to address their children's particular needs. All parents are concerned about their children's safety and social education while they are at school.

Two notable models for providing psychosocial occupational therapy services in the school systems have been recently described in the literature. Agrin (1987) described an occupational therapy group for fourth and fifth grade boys who attended a self-contained classroom for emotionally disturbed children. The students attended a 45-minute group each week. Craft and cooking activities were used to increase self-awareness, personal responsibility, communication skills, peer interaction, and relationships with adult authority figures. The therapist worked closely with special educators, the school psychologist, and the principal. The program gained support from these colleagues as the boys made visible improvements in their social behaviors. Although not all of the students generalized their improvements beyond the confines of the group, Agrin suggested that students' future success in regular education settings could be predicted by observing how well established their new social skills had become in the therapy group.

Another model for providing occupational therapy to students with behavioral disorders was proposed by Schultz (1992), who recommended that groups meet two to five times weekly. Schultz pointed out that most special education students with psychosocial dysfunction are socially isolated in the classroom and prevented from engaging in typical extracurricular activities that provide social experience. The primary focus of occupational therapy for these children and adolescents is to facilitate and guide the development of peer social interaction skills. Motivating activities help students develop competencies in daily living skills while practicing adaptive responses to interpersonal challenges. Schultz suggested meal planning and preparation, newspaper production, theatrical productions, and furniture refinishing as examples of therapeutic activities. She concluded that,

> Occupational Activity Grouping may provide the setting for the student not only to develop the skills essential to benefit from special education but also to reinforce, in a naturalistic environment, those competencies acquired in special education (p. 195).

Occupational therapists may also provide psychosocial therapy within the context of the regular classroom. For example, a sixth grader with poor peer and teacher relationships because of inadequate communication skills was referred to occupational therapy. Rather than providing direct services to this child outside the classroom, the occupational therapist led the entire class in a role-play game that involved learning and practicing effective ways of dealing with peer conflict, accepting responsibility for mistakes, and expressing feelings assertively. The teacher worked with the therapist to develop visual and verbal cues to help her class remember key principles of effective communication and to reinforce efforts to use them. Such an approach benefits everyone and establishes a powerful system of peer modeling.

Students who are referred for occupational therapy services to address fine motor, perceptual, or orthopedic problems may also have social and emotional needs that impair academic performance. The case study on p. 801 exemplifies how one student's multiple needs were addressed.

The idea of school-based occupational therapists providing psychosocially oriented therapy is innovative. Based on a review of the special education literature, Schultz (1992) thought that teachers would welcome the kind of assistance that occupational therapists can provide in improving students' social skills. School administrators who appreciate the shortage of therapists to meet even the traditional referrals may initially be less encouraging. School-based therapists who are committed to providing holistic services need to educate and persuade colleagues regarding the potential effectiveness of occupational therapy approaches to help students meet central academic goals by developing essential psychosocial skills. This may be approached directly through inservices and program proposals and indirectly by incorporating psychosocial goals into students' individual education plans. Trends in integrated programming and inclusion for students with behavioral problems have created an atmosphere in which occupational therapy leadership in comprehensive holistic intervention approaches should be welcomed.

## OUTPATIENT MENTAL HEALTH SERVICES

Children and adolescents who seek help from mental health facilities usually have significant behavioral disturbances. Typically the young person's problems have caused moderate to severe levels of disturbance for family, school, or community members by the time mental health care commences. The primary goals of outpatient mental health services are the diagnosis and management of mental health problems to improve functioning within the community and the prevention of crises necessitating hospitalization.

The child's initial contact with an outpatient mental health facility usually consists of an intake interview exploring the nature and severity of the child's and family's problems. Responses to the interview form the basis for decisions regarding appropriate evaluation and intervention. Often the intake interviewer is a social worker or a paraprofessional who is trained in mental health screening. Possible dispositions include outpatient evaluation at a later date or crisis evaluation with immediate short-term intervention.

Outpatient mental health services may be provided through free-standing clinics, hospital-based programs, community mental health centers, and private practice offices. Funding sources may include clients' families, private insurance, Medicaid, federal grants, and state monies

CASE STUDY #2

Darnell was an 8-year-old second grader who was referred for an occupational therapy assessment because his handwriting was slow and illegible. The teacher completed a Preassessment Checklist (Figure 31-1), indicating that Darnell often exhibited problems with incomplete and careless work, disorganized work habits, and peer relations characterized by teasing and rejection, as well as the handwriting difficulty that precipitated the referral. During the evaluation session Darnell was polite and compliant. His affect was generally sad, and he made frequent self-disparaging comments, such as, "I'm not good at this." When motor testing was completed, the occupational therapist asked about Darnell's feelings about school this year and whether he had anyone in his class whom he played with on a regular basis. He reported feeling "OK" about school in general, but said, "I don't have any friends at school. They all say I'm fat and dumb." Darnell's fine motor skills were significantly below average.

He was enrolled in 30 minutes per week of occupational therapy with two other second graders. The group worked on developing writing and cutting skills by making group collages with themes such as, "I can be a friend by . . .", and "The five best things about me"; drawing pictures of what they would like to be doing 20 years into the future, and writing and illustrating collective stories. Group members discussed their ideas and, with guidance and encouragement from the therapist, began to listen to one another, express their ideas, and give and accept positive feedback. The boys shared ideas about how to make friends and cope with teasing and rejection. Darnell and another boy developed a friendship that continued outside of the sessions. The group members voted to name themselves "The Tuesday Club," adding to their sense of belonging. Additionally, the therapist worked with Darnell's teacher regarding adaptations that would facilitate improved organization, handwriting performance, and social interactions. Together they designed a behavioral reward system to increase all students' timely completion of written work. Finally, the occupational therapist advised the parents regarding recreational opportunities, such as YMCA day camp and Boy Scouts, that would further enhance Darnell's social and motor skills.

After one semester of occupational therapy, Darnell's grades improved significantly. His mother reported that he no longer resisted attending school on most days, and Darnell reported satisfaction with his school performance and social life. The teacher was pleased both with Darnell's progress and with her success in using a behavior charting system. At that point the occupational therapist reduced her intervention to biweekly monitoring and occasional consultation to the teacher.

The therapist in this example met the concerns of the referring teacher, who could not read the student's writing, and the concerns of the student, who felt isolated and anxious at school. Both problems significantly impaired the student's academic progress and were effectively and efficiently addressed through a combination of direct service and consultation.

(Manderscheid & Sonnenschein, 1992). The agency's sources of funding influence the types of clientele served and the types of services provided. For example, private for-profit services are generally affordable only by upper-income families with generous insurance plans. These programs may offer special services such as yoga or academic tutoring, in addition to the traditional interventions. Middle- and lower-income families usually seek services that are partially publicly funded and therefore more basic (Tuma, 1989).

The Diagnostic and Statistical Manual of Mental Disorders, Fourth Edition (DSM-IV) (APA, 1994) is used to classify clinical problems into diagnostic categories. Children and adolescents seek services from community and outpatient mental health services for help with problems ranging from attention deficit disorder to major depression. Service provision often begins with screening and crisis interven-

tion. Comprehensive evaluation of the child and family may consist of interviews, play sessions, and standardized psychologic or developmental testing. Therapy may be provided for the individual child or parent, couples, groups, and families. Parent education groups, pharmacotherapy, and case management may also be available. Some mental health centers offer primary prevention services such as public education and wellness programs and consultation to public schools. Other services include vocational training, respite care, and day care services (Homonoff & Maltz, 1991).

Frames of reference used in outpatient programs vary with the philosophies of the specific facilities, but they commonly draw from cognitive, behavioral, family systems, neurobiologic, and psychodynamic theories (see Table 31-1). Treatment approaches are most commonly goal focused, time limited, and involve the family and school. Clients

NAME:_____AGE:_____DOB:_____GRADE:_____

SCHOOL:_____TEACHER:_____

Thank you for your referral to OT services. Your completion of the following will help us to effectively plan evaluation and intervention.

| Difficulties Observed in Pupil Behavior | never | seldom | occasionally | often | always |
|---|---|---|---|---|---|
| Has trouble following directions | | | | | |
| Cries easily | | | | | |
| Has difficulty with balancing (climbing steps) | | | | | |
| Fatigues easily | | | | | |
| Has difficulty with matching shapes (3-5 yr.) | | | | | |
| Has difficulty identifying letters & numbers (5+ yr.) | | | | | |
| Has reading problems (6+ yr.) | | | | | |
| Has poor awareness of self in space; bumps into children, desks, and walls | | | | | |
| Seems "nervous" or anxious | | | | | |
| Easily frustrated, gives up quickly | | | | | |
| Confuses directional concepts (up and down, in and out, before and behind) | | | | | |
| Has poor understanding of spatial concepts | | | | | |
| Over-reacts to unexpected touch and/or sound | | | | | |
| Dislikes removing outer garments or standing close to classmates | | | | | |
| Unable to control distractibility | | | | | |
| Unable to control over-activity | | | | | |
| Has difficulty in independent work habits | | | | | |
| Disorganized in manner of working, inexact, careless | | | | | |
| Does not participate in classroom and playground activities; "withdrawn" | | | | | |
| Does not automatically hold paper while writing | | | | | |
| Ignores or cannot use one side of body in gross motor activities | | | | | |
| Aggressive behavior | | | | | |
| Disregards the feelings of others | | | | | |
| Makes decisions impulsively | | | | | |
| Is teased or rejected by peers | | | | | |
| Is socially immature | | | | | |

**Figure 31-1**   Preassessment checklist for occupational therapy services in public schools.

generally attend one or two 1-hour sessions per week for a specified period. In publicly funded mental health centers, payment for services is based on the individual's income. Third-party payers have variable levels of coverage for mental health care. Therapeutic modalities commonly include play therapy (for young children), talking, expressive art, therapeutic board games, group discussions, and family discussions. Staffing patterns may take the form of multidisciplinary, interdisciplinary, or transdisciplinary models

and typically include psychologists, social workers, and psychiatrists, with some combination of psychiatric nurses, licensed counselors, and trained paraprofessionals (Manderscheid & Sonnenschein, 1992).

The number of occupational therapists who currently work with children and adolescents in community-based mental health practice is relatively small. In 1990 approximately 9.2% of all practicing occupational therapists currently specialized in mental health, and only 14.8% of these worked with clients younger than 19 years of age (AOTA Member Survey, 1990). Work with children and adolescents who have significant emotional and behavioral problems is extremely challenging. A well-developed understanding of developmental and biopsychosocial theories and their occupational therapy applications, as well as excellent communication and behavioral management skills, are required. Personal maturity and comfort with role sharing are needed. Empathy and the ability to relate to troubled children and their families must coexist with the knowledge that often the clients' values and behaviors run counter to those of the therapist. However, many communities that lack social resources such as work training and social activities may not be able to provide comprehensive programs for these children and families.

With the challenges inherent in community-based mental health practice come some compelling rewards. Children and adolescents bring a sense of spontaneity and energy to treatment that is less often found in adult clients. The crafts, games, and daily living activities that are so much a part of occupational therapy are extremely motivating and developmentally appropriate for most young people. The therapeutic relationships formed with many young clients can be powerful in their capacity to facilitate positive change, giving therapists a tremendous sense of accomplishment. Working with clients within the context of their families, schools, and communities affords the greatest opportunities for carry-over of therapeutic effects into everyday living. Additionally, occupational therapists have a unique combination of skills, for example, expertise in developmental evaluation, sensory integration evaluation and therapy, and activities-based therapy, that is highly valued by intervention teams (Case-Smith, 1994). Client and public education regarding issues such as parenting, stress reduction, and child development are needed services that occupational therapists can provide. Teaching child care workers, educators, and vocational trainers ways of promoting effective social and work-related behavior is a valuable consultation service. Service coordination and interfacing with other service agencies are also important roles well suited to occupational therapists (Adams, 1990). Program planning and administration are areas of mental health practice in which occupational therapists can excel (Nielson, 1993). Such services may be provided in clinical or community settings, including the public schools or clients homes.

A promising new development is the Child and Adolescent Service System Program (CASSP), an initiative that was launched by the National Institute of Mental Health in 1983. The goal of CASSP is to help states develop comprehensive, coordinated systems of care by providing grant money for demonstration projects and guidance for the development of needs assessments, program planning, interagency collaboration, constituency building, technical training, and system development (Stroul, 1985). One of the outcomes of CASSP is the emergence of day treatment programs for children and adolescents. This service model allows an array of intensive interventions to be provided while maintaining the client in the home and community.

*Day treatment programs* are offered in a variety of settings, including psychiatric hospitals, community mental health facilities, and schools for special needs students (Pruitt & Kiser, 1991). Such programs provide a middle step between outpatient intervention and hospitalization and are becoming popular for clinical and economic reasons (Erker, Searight, Amant, & White, 1993). Clients attend programming 4 to 6 hours per day, 5 days per week, and are at home during evenings and weekends (Block & Lefkovitz, 1992).

Day treatment may facilitate a child's transition from the hospital back to the home and community, provide crisis stabilization, allow comprehensive evaluation, or serve as an intensive therapeutic alternative to outpatient or inpatient treatment (Pruitt & Kiser, 1991). Programming often follows a psychoeducational model and may include vocational evaluation and training for adolescents (Nelson & Condrin, 1987). Treatment teams are typically led by a psychiatrist or psychologist who specializes in child and adolescent mental health. Other team members are listed in Table 31-1 and very often include occupational therapists.

Occupational therapy activities are selected to motivate and facilitate self-awareness and communication skills, develop grooming and etiquette habits, and teach life skills such as cooking and community mobility. Crafts, role-playing exercises, cooperative action games, and therapeutic board games are popular modalities in such occupational therapy programs. Transition from intensive day treatment programs to the community and public school can be facilitated by working with the client's parents, child care providers, teachers, job coach, or school-based occupational therapist to enhance the carry-over of interventions and goals. The family may also benefit from assistance with locating and securing social and leisure resources. The case study on p. 804 describes how a consultative model of intervention may be used to assist with transitioning a client from day treatment back into full community involvement. The focus in this example is on educating and problem solving with personnel from another agency.

## RESIDENTIAL TREATMENT CENTERS

The number of residential treatment centers in the United States for children and adolescents increased from 261 in 1970 to 440 in 1988 (Manderscheid & Sonnenschein, 1992). Lengths of stay in residential treatment vary considerably and are influenced by funding constraints, the facility's philosophy, and the needs of the client and family. Placement may last from weeks to years (Durrant, 1993). Approximately 15% of residential treatment centers serve children with severe chronic disabilities such as severe mental retardation and autism (Tuma, 1989). Program philosophies range from highly structured and intensively therapeutic to

## CASE STUDY #3

Mario was 17 years old and had diagnoses of mild mental retardation, anxiety disorder, and impulse control disorder. He had a lifelong history of poor socialization with nonfamily members, separation anxiety, and occasional temper tantrums. Mario was admitted to day treatment after a series of explosive episodes during which he broke furniture and a window. He attended the program for 4 weeks of evaluation and treatment, with excellent results. Mario, his family, and the treatment team decided that he would begin a job training program on discharge from day treatment. It was determined that the occupational therapist would serve as the liaison between the treatment and a job training program. The administrators at the job training site expressed both interest and a little trepidation at the notion of working with a client who had a history of psychiatric disturbance with aggressive behavior.

To facilitate his transition, the occupational therapist accompanied Mario and his mother to Mario's first appointment at the job training program. As the job trainer and Mario discussed the program's operations, the therapist made suggestions to increase Mario's chances of success. One suggestion was for Mario to write the program schedule into his pocket calendar and to negotiate with the job trainer any times needed for psychiatric or medical appointments. Another was for the job trainer to provide Mario with a written list of basic expectations for participation in the program, such as arriving on time, wearing appropriate clothing, and bringing a sack lunch. Mario's mental health problems were discussed, and the thera

pist was able to clarify the nature of the disorder and the behavioral cues that had been effective in therapy.

Once Mario began the job training program, the occupational therapist remained available on an as-needed basis. Things progressed smoothly until Mario graduated from the sheltered training site into competitive employment with a job coach. At this point Mario began to evidence anxiety and occasionally became verbally threatening to his supervisor and coworkers. The job coach called the occupational therapist, who helped to analyze the process. It was learned that Mario was acting out when he was given what he perceived as conflicting directives from different supervisors. The therapist met with Mario, the coach, and the supervisors to negotiate a plan, and it was decided to (1) assign Mario routine tasks that needed to be performed the same way each time, as much as possible, (2) limit Mario's supervision to one person at a time, and (3) encourage Mario to verbalize his feelings of confusion, anxiety, and frustration to his supervisor before he felt overwhelmed. The therapist assisted Mario and his supervisor in writing and signing a behavioral contract that outlined consequences for behavioral outbursts: a 30-minute break after the first outburst, and suspension without pay for the remainder of the day if there was a second outburst. Finally, the therapist spent some time in the company lunchroom helping Mario meet and find some commonalities with his coworkers. Once Mario was integrated with his colleagues and supervisor, he was able to demonstrate his full potential as a reliable and capable worker.

more naturalistic and homelike environments. Facilities vary in size from a few to hundreds of residents. Children and adolescents who require residential treatment are usually troubled by combinations of psychosocial, behavioral, and family problems that are severe and chronic enough to warrant extended periods of care and respite. However, residential treatment does not offer the security and staffing to manage clients who are actively aggressive, suicidal, or psychotic (Tuma, 1989).

The primary goals of most residential treatment facilities are to provide safe and nurturing living environments while preparing the children and adolescents for successful return to the community and their families, foster homes, or independent living arrangements. The staffing reflects the facilities' philosophies and target populations. Most programs are largely staffed by trained paraprofessionals (sometimes

called houseparents) who provide around-the-clock care. Psychotherapists and administrators, who may be social workers, psychologists, or psychiatrists, provide supervision. Educational services for the children may be provided onsite, or through the local public school system.

Traditionally occupational therapists are not full-time staff. Some residential treatment facilities may contract for services that include consultation to house staff regarding the residents' developmental needs and limitations, ways to organize and guide household responsibilities to include the residents, and ways to teach self-care and community living skills. Direct intervention with the children and adolescents could include many of the goals and approaches outlined in the discussion of occupational therapy in day treatment programs.

A small but growing area of occupational therapy psy-

CASE STUDY #4

One common goal of psychiatric treatment with adolescents is to facilitate a youth's identification with the peer group. This developmentally appropriate goal may be met counterproductively, such as when the patients group together to perform antisocial activities like smuggling alcohol into the unit or assisting a peer in running away from the hospital. This type of dynamic occurred in the adolescent psychiatric unit of a large teaching hospital about twice per year, usually soon after a large influx of new patients entered the unit. The traditional manner of response to such group behavior was unit restriction, during which time the regular schedule of therapies, school, and passes was suspended. During unit restriction the patients, nurses, and therapists gathered several times daily to try to facilitate the adolescents' understanding of the group process and their individual roles in contributing to the negative behaviors. Often this was a lengthy and painful process because of the adolescents' limited comfort and skills in communicating their feelings and concerns. Meetings were characterized by periods of silence and blaming and often ended in frustration on all sides.

The occupational therapist hypothesized that the group meetings would be more productive if the patients had a fund of basic communication skills and a better sense of their own values and feelings. She met with the program director and proposed incorporating daily self-awareness and assertiveness groups into the unit restriction protocol in an effort to catalyze the unit restriction process. The director approved the idea and suggested presenting it to the rest of the team for feedback. Other team members were less enthusiastic because they viewed occupational therapy as fun and rewarding to the patients. They thought that this would undermine the punitive aspects of unit restriction. The occupational therapist explained that the

highly structured activities would develop skills that are foundational to the verbal processing that was needed. Inappropriate behavior would lead to suspension from the session. The team agreed to a trial of occupational therapy during unit restriction with the provision that if the misbehavior increased, the sessions would discontinue. Unit nurses and staff were invited to observe or join the sessions, at their discretion.

The adolescents, many of whom felt bored, isolated, and confused by the unit restriction, immediately welcomed the occupational therapy sessions. Initial sessions facilitated learning and applying words to express feelings about being hospitalized, being a part of the patient group, and the causes and effects of unit restriction. Subsequent sessions were devoted to teaching concepts and skills related to assertive communication.

The incidence of group behavior was significantly decreased, and as a result the unit staff had to cope with fewer disciplinary problems. Most importantly, the patients discussed pertinent issues during process meetings. They were able to explore and understand the group's responsibility to the progress of each member and each individual's responsibility to the betterment of the group. The ensuing maturation led to the development of a positive peer group culture in which individuals' antisocial behaviors were discouraged by the majority.

The unit staff were pleasantly surprised to observe that the occupational therapy sessions were clearly related to the goals of the unit restriction, and they expressed their support by direct feedback and by helping to prepare the room and gather the patients for sessions. Additionally, the occupational therapist believed that her treatment philosophy and skills were better understood by the rest of the team, resulting in greater job satisfaction.

---

chosocial practice is the *juvenile justice system.* Juvenile justice and mental health service systems have always worked closely together to evaluate and rehabilitate young offenders (Mulvey, 1984). Children and adolescents who steal, vandalize property, or assault others may enter either the mental health or the correctional system, depending on whether the behavior is interpreted as a symptom of conduct disorder or a violation of the law (Tuma, 1989). Occupational therapists are increasingly involved in the comprehensive psychiatric evaluations of children and adolescents who are under consideration for psychiatric commitment or to be tried as adults. Youth offenders who are

enrolled in diversional programs or who are being treated in state or other psychiatric facilities may also receive occupational therapy.

## INPATIENT PSYCHIATRIC HOSPITALS

Inpatient psychiatric hospitalization provides the most restrictive, intensive, and costly therapeutic intervention. It is generally reserved for children and adolescents whose symptoms pose a safety risk to themselves or others, who have complicating medical conditions, whose families are unable to safely manage them, or who are considered to have poor prognoses if treated as outpatients (Mabe, Riley, & Sunde, 1989). Inpatient psychiatric units may be found in general hospitals, state psychiatric hospitals, and private psychiatric hospitals. There was a burgeoning of inpatient facilities from the mid-1970s through the 1980s, when reimbursement for such care was abundant. This trend ended and reversed with the advent of managed mental health care and increased controls by third-party payers on admissions and lengths of stay (Dalton & Forman, 1992). Despite such shifts in service availability, there will always be a need for the rapid diagnosis and stabilization that such specialized facilities provide.

Child and adolescent inpatient psychiatric units are usually locked facilities that are staffed by nurses and paraprofessionals who are trained in the care and management of severely impaired patients (Dalton & Forman, 1992). Very often patients are hospitalized when in crisis, such as after a suicide attempt, an assault, or a psychotic episode. Sometimes patients are admitted for comprehensive psychologic and medical evaluation of complex chronic problems. In most cases the length of stay is limited to days or weeks, with the goal being rapid discharge to less costly and restrictive treatment alternatives.

The treatment team is interdisciplinary and may include psychiatrists, nurses, paraprofessional direct care staff, social workers, recreational therapists, psychologists, special educators, and music therapists, as well as occupational therapists (see Table 31-1). Trainees representing these professions may also circulate through the team. Frames of reference reflect a variety of psychosocial theories, with behavioral and neurobiologic approaches among the most commonly used (Dalton & Forman, 1992).

Occupational therapists who work with children and adolescents who are experiencing acute psychiatric problems have an important role in diagnosis and disposition. Activities within a locked hospital unit are typically quite structured, limiting opportunities for individual choices and decisions. Often the occupational therapist's evaluation of hospitalized children includes observation of the patient performing activities that are optimally motivating and require the cognitive, social, and adaptive skills needed at home and school. Additionally, occupational therapists evaluate the child's performance levels as they compare with developmental norms. This evaluation information allows the team to reasonably predict how the youth performs when coping with the demands of community settings.

It is essential for members of any interdisciplinary team to combine their unique perspectives on each patient's needs into a cohesive and coherent plan that is mutually agreeable. This cohesion is especially important when working with patients who are challenging and often volatile. The case study on p. 805 illustrates how an occupational therapist recognized a programmatic need and worked with an administrator and interdisciplinary team to implement changes.

## STUDY QUESTIONS

1. What are three ways that a therapist can help prevent or ameliorate an early childhood intervention of a client's psychosocial problems?
2. Contrast the advantages and disadvantages of including students with psychosocial dysfunction in regular classrooms.
3. List three ways that an occupational therapist can help public schools better educate students with behavioral and emotional problems.
4. If a child or adolescent does not pose an immediate danger to himself or herself, but is too behaviorally uncontrolled for a public school program, where would he or she best seek intervention? What is the occupational therapist's role in this type of setting?
5. An occupational therapist has learned of a new residential treatment center that specializes in adolescents with moderately severe mental illness. Describe how he or she could approach the facility's program director with the goal of being hired to provide consultative services.
6. What is the most restrictive setting for the treatment of psychosocial dysfunction in children and adolescents? When is such a setting required?
7. What are two unique roles of the occupational therapist in an acute inpatient psychiatric setting?

## SUMMARY

Children and adolescents with emotional, cognitive, and behavioral problems are unable to participate satisfactorily in home, school, and community life. Social problems such as poverty, family sociopathy, and cultural violence have been linked with increased incidence of psychosocial dysfunction in young people (Constantino, 1993; Wolfner & Gelles, 1993). Such social problems are increasing steadily in our country, while mental health services for young people continue to be inadequate in quantity and quality. Occupational therapists who work with young people have the knowledge and skills to help improve their clients' psychosocial functioning through individual and group therapy, program development, and consultation. Pediatric occupational therapists in all settings need to become psychosocial practitioners to help meet the urgent and growing needs of young people.

## REFERENCES

Adams, R. (1990). The role of occupational therapists in community mental health. *Mental Health Special Interest Newsletter, 13*(1), 1-2.

Agrin, A. (1987). Occupational therapy with emotionally disturbed children in a public school. *American Journal of Occupational Therapy, 7,* 105-114.

American Occupational Therapy Association (1990). *Member Data Survey.* Rockville, MD: American Occupational Therapy Association.

American Psychiatric Association (1994). *Diagnostic and statistical manual of mental disorders* (4th ed.). Washington, DC: American Psychiatric Association.

Block, B. & Lefkovitz, P. (1992). *Standards and guidelines for partial hospitalization.* Alexandria, VA: American Association for Partial Hospitalization.

Case-Smith, J. (1994). Defining the specialization of pediatric occupational therapy. *American Journal of Occupational Therapy, 48,* 791-802.

Cohen, J., Brennan, C., & Sexton, B. (1984). A social cognitive approach to the prevention of adolescent substance abuse. *Intervention I: sixth grade. (a manual).* New Haven, CT: Yale University School of Medicine, The Consultation Center.

Constantino, J. (1993). Parents, mental illness, and primary health care of infants and young children. *Zero to Three, 13*(5), 1-10.

Dalton, R. & Forman, M. (1992). *Psychiatric hospitalization of school-age children.* Washington, DC: American Psychiatric Press.

Davidson, D. (1995). Physical abuse of preschoolers: identification and intervention through occupational therapy. *American Journal of Occupational Therapy, 49,* 235-243.

Dunn, W., Campbell, P., Oetter, P., Hall, S., & Berger, E. (1989). *Guidelines for occupational therapy services in early intervention and preschool services.* Rockville, MD: The American Occupational Therapy Association.

Durrant, M. (1993). *Residential treatment: a cooperative, competency-based approach to therapy and program design.* New York: W.W. Norton.

Erker, G., Searight, H.R., Amant, E., & White, P. (1993). Residential versus day treatment for children: a long-term follow-up study. *Child Psychiatry and Human Development, 24,* 31-39.

Florey, L. (1989). Nationally speaking: treating the whole child: rhetoric or reality? *American Journal of Occupational Therapy, 43,* 365-368.

Gresham, F. & Elliot, S. (1993). Social skills intervention guide: systematic approaches to social skills training. *Special Services in the Schools, 8,* 137-158.

Homonoff, E. & Maltz, P. (1991). Developing and maintaining a coordinated system of community-based services to children. *Community Mental Health Journal, 27,* 347-358.

Hunter, J. & Powell, G. (1990). Failure to thrive. In C. Semmler & J. Hunter (Eds.). *Early occupational therapy intervention.* Gaithersburg, MD: Aspen Publications.

Individuals with Disabilities Education Act of 1990 (Public Law 101-476), 20 U.S.C. 1401(a)(17).

Kellam, S., Branch, J., Agrawal, D., & Ensinger, M. (1975). *Mental health and going to school: the Woodlawn program of assessment, early intervention, and evaluation.* Chicago: University of Chicago Press.

Knitzer, J. (1982). *Unclaimed children.* Washington, DC: Children's Defense Fund.

Mabe, P., Riley, W., & Sunde, E. (1989). Survey of admission policies for child and adolescent inpatient services: a national sample. *Child Psychiatry and Human Development, 20,* 99-111.

Manderscheid, R. & Sonnenschein, M. (Eds.). (1992). *Mental health, United States, 1992.* Rockville, MD: U.S. Department of Health and Human Services.

Mulvey, E. (1984). Judging amenability to treatment in juvenile offenders: theory and practice. In R. Price & J. Monahan, (Eds.). *Children, mental health, and the law.* Beverly Hills, CA: Sage Publications.

National Advisory Mental Health Council. (1990). *National plan for research on child and adolescent mental disorders.* Washington, DC: National Institute of Mental Health.

Nelson, R. & Condrin, J. (1987). A vocational readiness and independent living skills program for psychiatrically impaired adolescents. *Occupational Therapy in Mental Health, 7,* 105-113.

Nielson, C. (1993). Occupational therapy and community mental health: a new and unprecedented turn. *Mental Health Special Interest Newsletter, 16*(3), 1-2.

Offard, D. & Fleming, J. (1991). Epidemiology. In M. Lewis (Ed.). *Child and adolescent psychiatry: a comprehensive textbook.* Baltimore: Williams & Wilkins.

Pruitt, D. & Kiser, L. (1991). Day treatment: past, present, and future. In M. Lewis (Ed.). *Child and adolescent psychiatry: a comprehensive textbook.* Baltimore: Williams & Wilkins.

Rubin, R. & Balow, B. (1978). Prevalence of teacher identified behavior problems: a longitudinal study. *Exceptional Children, 45,* 102-111.

Schultz, S. (1992). School-based occupational therapy for students with behavioral disorders. *Occupational Therapy in Health Care, 8,* 173-196.

Shure, M. & Spivack, G. (1982). Interpersonal problem-solving in young children: a cognitive approach to prevention. *American Journal of Community Psychology, 10,* 341-356.

Solomon, P. & Evans, D. (1992). Service needs of youths released from a state psychiatric facility as perceived by service providers and families. *Community Mental Health Journal, 28,* 305-315.

Stroul, B. (1985). *Child and adolescent service system program (CASSP) system change strategies: a workbook for states.* National Institute of Mental Health Office of State and Community Liason.

Tuma, J. (1989). Mental health services for children: the state of the art. *American Psychologist, 44,* 188-199.

United States Department of Education. (1987). Fifteenth annual report to Congress on implementation of Public Law 94-142: the Education of All Handicapped Children Act. Washington, DC: United States Government Printing Office.

Weissberg, R., Caplan, M., & Bennetto, L. (1988). *The Yale-New Haven problem solving (SPS) program for young adolescents.* New Haven, CT: Yale University.

Weissberg, R. (1985). Developing effective social problem-solving programs for the classroom. In B. Schneider, K.H. Rubin, & J. Ledingham (Eds.). *Peer relationships and social skills in childhood,* (Vol. 2). New York: Springer-Verlag.

Wolfner, G. & Gelles, R. (1993). A profile of violence toward children: a national study. *Child Abuse and Neglect, 17,* 197-212.

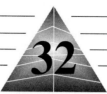

# Transition Services: From School to Adult Life

KAREN C. SPENCER

## KEY TERMS

- ▲ Legal Mandates
- ▲ Collaborative Teaming
- ▲ Ecologic Curriculum
- ▲ Community-Referenced Assessment
- ▲ Interagency Linkages
- ▲ Models of Service Delivery

## CHAPTER OBJECTIVES

1. Define transition services for youth and young adults with disabilities.
2. Describe the mandate for transition services based on federal legislation.
3. Describe collaborative teamwork as it applies to the school-to-adult life transition process.
4. Describe an ecologic curriculum model as it relates to transition-age students.
5. Describe interagency linkages needed for effective transition services.
6. Identify the role of occupational therapy in the transition process, including assessment, service planning, and service delivery.
7. Compare alternative models of service delivery, including direct service, consultation, monitoring, and service coordination.

Individuals with disabilities may spend 12 to 18 years receiving some form of education. Education is seen as a way to transmit or promote the knowledge, skills, and experiences needed to assume productive adult roles. These adult roles can include pursuing postsecondary education, main-

taining paid employment, volunteering, living in the community, and maintaining meaningful relationships.

Occupational therapists have valuable contributions to make to the transition process as individuals with disabilities move from school to a variety of adult roles, activities, and environments. With a focus on promoting human performance of essential occupations in a variety of natural environments, occupational therapy personnel can help design and implement effective transition services. These services may be characterized as a cooperative venture between the occupational therapist, the student, his or her family, and other members of the educational team.

This chapter discusses federal legislation as it relates to mandated transition services, describes "best practice" models for the delivery of transition-related services, and presents specific roles for occupational therapy personnel in the transition process for youth with disabilities.

## LEGISLATIVE BACKGROUND

Since passage of Public Law 94-142, The Education for All Handicapped Children Act of 1975 (EHA), special education and related services have been made available through the public education system to the nation's children and youth with disabilities. Occupational therapy is defined in the EHA as a "related service." Related services were included in the federal law to complement and extend the efforts of teachers by helping children and youth with disabilities to more fully participate in, and obtain maximum benefit from, educational activities.

The EHA and its subsequent amendments guaranteed a free and appropriate education for all children with disabilities. An appropriate education was believed to be one in which children with disabilities would acquire, to the maximum extent possible, skills, knowledge, and behaviors that would ultimately help them function successfully as adults. After passage of EHA, several major benefits related to the initial intent of the law were realized:

1. Formal mechanisms were established to identify and bring children with disabilities into the public education process
2. All identified children were provided with Individualized Education Programs (IEPs) developed by an educational team that included the student's parents or guardian
3. Parents and guardians were identified as essential members of the educational team and provided with legal rights related to their child's education

These features of EHA related primarily to the *process* of delivering specialized education to children and youth with disabilities. The law did not really speak to the *content* of the education program except to say that each child's program should be individualized and based on documented needs and goals.

As with many public laws and policies, the full intent of EHA has not been realized. The shortcomings are evidenced in large part by the negative postschool outcomes reported for many youths with disabilities. For the majority of these individuals, the benefits of a free public education have not consistently translated into community living, gainful employment, income, social connectedness, and quality of life. Follow-up studies of young adults who had completed special education showed that life after high school was far less than optimal (Edgar, Levine, & Maddox, 1986; Hasazi, Gordon, & Roe, 1985; Wagner, 1989). These studies identified that a large percentage of individuals who completed the special education system would enter adult lives characterized by segregation, dependency, and nonproductivity. People with disabilities, despite the availability of special education and related services, experienced 50% to 75% unemployment and high levels of dependency on public entitlement programs (Halloran, 1992). This dependency with its associated human and economic costs helped spur the passage of EHA amendments in 1990. The amendments directly specified what was thought to be the appropriate content of transition-related services for youths with disabilities. The EHA was retitled *Individuals with Disabilities Education Act of 1990* (IDEA) (P.L. 101-476) to reflect the commitment of the federal government to use respectful, nonstigmatizing language when referring to people with disabilities.

The focus on the school-to-adult life transition processes and the mandate for transition services represent significant changes for the special education systems. Schools are now required to provide comprehensive transition services for all special education students on entrance into high school (or its equivalent). Transition services typically begin when students are 14 to 16 years old but may begin at earlier ages, when it is anticipated that the student needs more time to achieve needed transition skills and experiences or when the student is at risk for dropping out of school. Transition services are defined in the law as follows:

. . . a coordinated set of activities for a student, designed with an outcome-oriented process, which promotes movement from school to post-school activities, including post-secondary education, vocational training, integrated employment (including supported employment), continuing and adult education, adult services, independent living, or community participation. The coordinated set of activities shall be based on the individual student's needs, taking into account the student's preferences and interests, and shall include instruction, community experiences, the development of employment and other post-school adult living objectives, and, when appropriate, acquisition of daily living skills and functional vocational evaluation (P.L. 101-476, 1990, pp. 1103-1104).

Transition services, mandated by IDEA, reflect the major performance areas that are typically addressed by occupational therapy: work or education, independent living (including activities of daily living), and community participation, which may include community mobility and transportation, access to community services and activities, recreation and leisure, and socialization and relationships. Additionally, the law states that educational activities in the community may constitute appropriate transition services.

It is now well understood that for many students, learning must take place in highly relevant and realistic environments if skills are to be retained and used. Education and training that occur exclusively in school buildings or in simulated environments have been determined to be ineffective for many students who are unable to transfer or generalize learning to real-life situations (Brown, Nietupski, & Hamre-Nietupski, 1976; Rainforth, York, & Macdonald, 1992). The law's provision for community experience translates into education and related services being delivered in a variety of environments beyond the school. These environments include the home, work site, community recreation facilities, and a variety of other relevant community settings. Occupational therapy personnel are well prepared to actively participate in community-based service delivery by (1) using environmentally referenced (contextual) or situational assessment, (2) directly teaching and practicing needed skills in context, (3) altering or selecting a new environment to enable the individual to perform with his or her current skills, and (4) adapting or changing contextual features and task demands to support performance in context (Dunn, Brown, & McGuigan, 1994). Occupational therapy, therefore, can help students with disabilities to perform essential roles and activities in real-life settings and situations.

Each student's IEP has been identified as the vehicle for transition planning. The IEP process includes a meeting of the team to discuss the student's needs, abilities, and goals, followed by the development of an individualized program of education and related services. Each student's IEP, therefore, is unique and serves as that student's personal curriculum. As a part of the IEP meeting, a written document is generated to capture the team's decisions and to delegate responsibility for implementation of the IEP among team members. The written IEP is a legal document that is intended to provide assurances and accountability for the delivery of appropriate education and related services.

The composition of the IEP team was expanded with passage of IDEA. In addition to school personnel (administrators, teachers, related services, and others as needed) and the student's parents or guardian, the student must now be included on the team. The law's formal inclusion of the transition-age student as a member of his or her education team is significant. Although it may seem obvious that students should participate in any planning activities related to their own lives, student attendance and participation in the IEP has been the exception rather than the rule. The student's presence at the IEP meeting requires other team members to pay close attention to effective communication and to create a comfortable environment that respects the student and allows him or her to participate to the maximum extent possible. Student presence at the IEP meeting requires professionals to abandon jargon and negative labeling to focus on the student's strengths and abilities. It is hoped that a positive outcome from increased student participation in the IEP process will be the gradual empowerment of students to participate in and make decisions that affect their own lives. If the ability to make informed decisions, take risks, and evaluate consequences is the ultimate goal of education (Halloran, 1992; Ward, 1992), students *must* participate in the IEP process.

## "BEST PRACTICE" FOR TRANSITION

Transition services clearly emphasize an outcome-driven process. This means that IEPs are specifically developed with the student's eventual school-to-adult life transition in mind. The student's educational program, therefore, must prepare him or her to perform desired and necessary adult roles in a variety of current and anticipated community environments. Effective transition services are evaluated, based on the extent to which graduated students and young adults actually achieve meaningful work roles, live in the community, engage in chosen recreation activities, and have ongoing positive social relationships. Being accountable for these types of outcomes has significant implications for how teachers and related service personnel provide transition-related services. A description of the "best practices" related to the design and delivery of transition services follows. For the purposes of this introductory chapter, the best practices related to the school-to-adult life transition process include three major features:

1. Use of *collaborative teaming* among professionals, agencies, the student, and family members (NICHCY, 1993; Rainforth et al., 1992; Wehman, 1992).
2. Use of an *ecologic curriculum* that focuses on the in-

teractions between the student and his or her environments (Brown et al., 1979; Sample, Spencer & Bean, 1990).
3. Establishment and use of *interagency linkages* to facilitate the smooth transfer of support and training services from the school to adult and community agencies when the student exits public schools (Everson & McNulty, 1992; Halloran, 1992; NICHCY, 1993).

## Collaborative Teaming

Rainforth and colleagues (1992) stated that ". . . the essence of collaborative teamwork is work accomplished jointly by a group of people in a spirit of willingness and mutual reward" (p. 11). For transition-age students, collaboration is seen as an effective way for a team to help the student achieve his or her goals related to future adult living. The primary team member is the student. Other team members may include family, the student's friends and classmates, teachers, related service professionals, representatives of adult service agencies, and others as appropriate. The collaborators on the team must have a shared sense of purpose that is driven by the student and the student's unique interests, abilities, and needs. Central to effective collaborative team work is each team member's ability to share responsibility for student outcomes and not work solely from their discipline's perspective. For example, the occupational therapist, teacher, and paraprofessional may all work with a student who has significant motor limitations on her goal of completing written classroom assignments. This would be an appropriate transition goal because it is based on the student's anticipated need for literacy as an adult and her aspirations for postsecondary education. The occupational therapist may oversee and coordinate an assessment of the student's technology-related needs and abilities followed by the selection of specific hardware and software for adapted computing. With the technology in place, the occupational therapist may then spend time working with the student, teacher, and paraprofessional who will be involved in the day-to-day use of the technology in the classroom. A collaborative working relationship, therefore, is established, with the team sharing responsibility for meeting the *student's* goal of completing written work.

Collaboration requires a commitment on the part of the different team members to teach each other and to learn from each other across traditional discipline or professional boundaries (Lyon & Lyon, 1980). Collaboration also requires services to be delivered in functional, real-life situations (Rainforth et al., 1992). In the previous example, the occupational therapist would be working in the student's classroom on the use of assistive technology for educational purposes. Occupational therapy services would not be provided in a separate location isolated from the real-life demands of the student's classroom, where other students are also engaged in written work.

In addition to the need for collaboration among the team members at the student's school, there is a need for collaboration by the school and other community agencies related to transition (NICHCY, 1993). As students with disabilities approach the end of their school career, many need ongoing supports or services. These services may be needed to help the young adult obtain and maintain community employment, live in the community, and participate in social and recreational activities. To achieve a smooth transition from the supports and services of the schools to the supports and services of other external community agencies requires extensive communication, cooperation, and collaboration. It is therefore considered the best practice to include community agencies in the transition planning process. These agencies are also potential providers of some transition services, even while the student is still enrolled in school (Everson & McNulty, 1992). A word of caution, however, is in order: Members of collaborative, interagency transition teams must create or identify services or supports based on each individual student's needs. They must refrain from simply matching students with available "slots" in existing programs or agencies (Mount, 1987). This requires time and effort on the part of all members of the team to maintain clear communication and to conduct planning and services that are truly in the best interests of any student who is making the difficult transition from familiar education environments to an array of separate community services and settings.

Collaborative teamwork can clearly benefit transition-age students when the diverse perspectives, backgrounds, and skills of team members can be brought together to create effective services and solve challenging problems. A second benefit can be realized by the team members themselves because collaboration promotes the establishment of cooperative and caring relationships among team members characterized by communication, shared responsibility, and mutual support (Rainforth et al., 1992). Members of collaborative teams have a sense of belonging and do not have a strong need to compete with other team members for status or authority.

## Ecologic Curriculum

For the purposes of this chapter, curricula are viewed as carefully selected and sequenced activities and learning materials used primarily by teachers to guide classroom teaching. Curricula may be commercially developed and purchased by a school, or they may be locally designed and developed by the education professionals who hope to use them. Regardless of the source, curricula are widely viewed as structured guides for teaching groups of children. For students enrolled in special education, however, curricula look quite different.

The IEP represents a uniquely developed curriculum for a particular student. The IEP, as conceived in federal law, is seen as a blueprint guiding the implementation of each student's educational program. Theoretically, no two students enrolled in special education should have the same curriculum, or IEP. Each student's individual interests, needs, abilities, goals, and anticipated performance environments are used to guide IEP development.

The student's IEP, or personal curriculum, exists within the broader context of the school and a larger, overarching curriculum model. For students with disabilities, this overarching curriculum model provides broad guidelines for the delivery of transition-related education. Brown et al. (1979) first described a broad curriculum model for students with significant disabilities that addressed student performance in essential life domains: domestic (home), vocational, community, and leisure. These domains were later expanded to include school (York & Vandercook, 1991), where children and youth spend a great deal of time. This domain-based curriculum model is highly relevant for transition-age students because it focuses the efforts of teachers and related service personnel on enhancing student performance in areas that are essential for productive and meaningful adult life (Spencer & Sample, 1993; York & Vandercook, 1991). It considers each student as a unique individual who must function in a variety of contexts both while in school and more so as an adult.

A domain-based curriculum for transition-age youth specifies to some extent *how* and *where* transition services should be delivered. The *how* aspect of service delivery relates to collaborative teaming among members of the education team and the use of highly relevant learning materials and activities. The *where* aspect of service delivery relates to the team's use of highly relevant teaching and learning environments to include the home, school, and assorted community environments. Taken together, the *how* and *where* aspects of a transition curriculum may be termed *ecologic,* focusing on the interaction between the student and the environments in which he or she participates (Rainforth et al., 1992). The use of ecologic curriculum models is considered to be best practice for students with significant disabilities (Rainforth et al., 1992; Williams, Fox, Thousand, & Fox, 1990), including those students who are approaching the transition from school to adult life.

An effective ecologic curriculum model is built on some core principles that must be embraced by all members of a student's educational team, including the occupational therapist. These principles include the following:

1. Age-appropriate placement of the student with chronologic age peers with and without disabilities
2. Integration of education and related services
3. Use of community-referenced, ecologic assessment
4. Active involvement of the student in planning and decision making
5. Instruction in a variety of relevant school and community environments
6. Evaluation of the extent to which students are achieving targeted transition outcomes

*Age-appropriate placement* of students with disabilities in educational activities alongside their chronologic age peers, with and without disabilities, has been deemed the best practice (Williams et al., 1990). The inclusion of students who have disabilities in typical educational activities and environments is believed to promote student performance, offer rich opportunities for learning, provide age-appropriate role modeling, increase awareness among all students of diverse learning styles and abilities, and provide opportunities for relationship building that is so important during adolescent development. Age-appropriate placement does not mean that students with disabilities are simply placed in a typical class or at a community job site. These placements must be accompanied by appropriate support services and resources that facilitate the student's full inclusion and maximum participation in the environment.

Total responsibility for meeting the needs of students with disabilities cannot fall on the teacher. It must be shared among different members of the student's education team such as the occupational therapist who may be identified as an essential support person for a given student. The occupational therapist may work in the classroom or on a job site directly with a student, consult with the teacher or employer on how to best adapt activities to accommodate student abilities, or train a paraprofessional to implement specific occupational therapy recommendations throughout the course of the student's day.

*Integrating education and related services* brings members of the team together to address a student's goals. An integrated approach is best explained using an example.

Amelia is an 18-year-old student who wants to live in the community after she completes high school. At her IEP meeting a transition goal to use neighborhood services was developed. Amelia has significant cognitive, communication, and mobility limitations that currently interfere with her ability to access and use services and businesses in her neighborhood. To meet her transition goal, the team identified a need for Amelia to begin to actively participate in purchasing needed food and personal items at her neighborhood grocery store. An integrated approach was developed involving the teacher, speech-language pathologist, and occupational therapist. Amelia's special education teacher developed strategies with Amelia that allowed her to shop from a picture list of items. Amelia's speech-language pathologist worked with Amelia at the grocery store teaching her to initiate a transaction and functionally communicate with grocery store employees. The occupational therapist, also addressing the same goal, worked at the grocery store with Amelia to devise a way for her to carry grocery items and move safely around the store. In addition to their own specific responsibilities, each professional worked with Amelia in the grocery store environment and communicated what occurred to the other team members so that efforts were overlapping, complementary, and reinforcing.

*Community-referenced assessment (ecologic assessment)* is considered an essential feature of the best transition-related practice with youth and young adults (Spencer, Mur-phy, Bean, & Schelly, 1991; Spencer & Sample, 1993; Woolcock, Stodden, & Bisconer, 1992). The purpose of a community-referenced or ecologic approach is to identify student performance needs and abilities in the environments that he or she is expected to use as an adult. For example, if the team seeks to identify the student's interests, needs, and abilities as they relate to future employment, the assessment must take place to a large extent in actual employment settings. Systematic and careful observation of the student's performance during real work tasks are completed to identify discrepancies between the demands of the job and the student's current performance level. Services are subsequently designed to reduce these discrepancies as the student acquires context-specific work skills.

Because of the highly individual nature of transition planning, services, and environments for any given student, formal or standardized approaches to assessment often do not provide the information needed (Rainforth et al., 1992). This is particularly true for students with significant or severe disabilities. Formal assessments of student performance, therefore, are not generally recommended for transition-age youth.

The *active involvement of the student in planning and decision making* is considered one of the most important aspects of effective transition services (P.L. 101-476, Halloran, 1992; Ward, 1992). The ultimate goal of education according to Ward (1992) is for students to actively participate in and fully manage their own lives.

Professionals can facilitate the development of self-determination skills by involving youth with disabilities in the transition planning process. . . . The goal is for students to assume control (with appropriate levels of support) over their transition program and identify and manage its various components (p. 389).

Active involvement of the student in planning and decision making related to his or her transition requires the thoughtful attention of the professional members of the educational team. The format of the IEP meeting may need to be adjusted to facilitate student involvement. For example, the student (with or without support) may prepare the agenda, introduce team members, or chair the meeting. To assume these functions, it is likely that the student would need help preparing for the meeting ahead of time. This preparation should include some discussion of possible transition goals, activities, and timeliness. During the IEP meeting, the attending professionals must accept the student's lead and keep discussions constructive by focusing primarily on the student's strengths and abilities.

Effective transition services require the delivery of *instruction in a variety of relevant school and community environments* (Brown et al., 1979; Rainforth et al., 1992; Udvari-Solner, Jorgenson, & Courchane, 1992). Students with disabilities, particularly those with severe disabilities, often have difficulty learning needed skills. This, combined with the associated challenge of identifying optimal learning styles and teaching approaches, requires the attention of both education and related service professionals. In addition to difficulty with learning, students with significant disabilities may not be able to readily transfer or generalize learning to new environments or situations. For these reasons, it is best to provide education and related services in the actual environments the student will be using. This allows for explicit teaching to the real-life demands of a particular environment and eliminates the need for the student to transfer skills. For example, if a student is learning to prepare simple meals to eat at his or her home, it is best to provide meal preparation training in that home environment. Meal preparation in a different kitchen environment may not promote acquisition of skills that transfer to the home.

Implementation of an ecologic curriculum requires periodic *evaluation of the extent to which students are achieving targeted transition outcomes* (Hasazi, Hock, & Cravedi-Cheng, 1992). Given the focus of an ecologic curriculum on preparing students to function in five major life domains (domestic, school, community, leisure, and vocational), best practice would suggest the need for ongoing evaluations of the extent and quality of performance in each domain. Without periodic evaluation of the overall effectiveness of transition services, decisions about local educational practices and policies cannot be well informed. Accountability for the expenditure of public resources on transition services also requires such an evaluation.

Outcomes that may be tracked by school districts include the extent to which students are (1) employed in the community, (2) living in the community, (3) satisfied with their lives, (4) using community services, (5) socially connected, and (6) participating in chosen leisure activities. These outcome data can be helpful to the members of the educational team who have responsibility for designing and implementing individualized transition services. Occupational therapists, as members of educational transition teams, can specifically benefit from feedback regarding the efficacy of occupational therapy services.

## Interagency Linkages

Although transition services, as mandated in IDEA (P.L. 101-476), are to be initiated by the school on behalf of students with disabilities, Congress did not intend for schools to have total responsibility for the entire transition process. The need for *interagency linkages* became a part of the law, indicating the need for shared responsibility between local education agencies and adult or community service agencies such as state vocational rehabilitation agencies (NICHCY, 1993). The interagency linkages envisioned by Congress included shared financial responsibility for the cost of needed transition services, including the sharing of personnel resources and expertise.

Implementing Congress' vision of interagency linkages and shared resources is, without a doubt, challenging. This task is viewed as an administrative responsibility that should not fall solely on already overextended teachers and related-service personnel (NICHCY, 1993). Education and related-service personnel responsible for the implementation of transition services must know, however, who the other transition "players" and agencies are and be prepared to invite them to fully participate in the transition process. The potential benefits of clear interagency linkages, however difficult to implement, are many.

Establishing such interagency linkages can be of enormous benefit to students planning for transition. This is because, as students with disabilities leave the public education system, their entitlement to educational, vocational, and other services ends. In the place of one relatively organized service provider (the school system), there may now be a confusing array of many service providers (i.e., the local vocational rehabilitation agency, the state department of mental health, developmental disability councils, community service boards, the federal social security system, and so on). Individuals with disabilities who have left school become solely responsible for identifying where to obtain the services they need and for demonstrating their eligibility to receive the services. Therefore, for many students with disabilities, identifying relevant adult service providers, establishing eligibility to receive adult services, and having interagency responsibilities and linkages stated in the IEP, all while in school, will be necessary to ensure a smooth transition from school to adult life (NICHCY, 1993, p. 7).

Linking the resources of different agencies can greatly facilitate the smooth transition of students with disabilities from school to an array of other services. Failure to initiate and formalize these connections while the student is still in school can result in the student being left out of services, sitting for extended periods on waiting lists, or losing skills because of the lost opportunity to participate in active learning. The importance of strong interagency linkages cannot be overstated.

## OCCUPATIONAL THERAPY'S ROLE IN TRANSITION

The focus of transition services is on helping students with disabilities acquire essential skills needed for meaningful and productive adult life. This is consistent with occupational therapy's focus on promoting individual performance of essential life occupations including participation in activities of daily living, work (and school), and leisure. Occupational therapists also consider the context within which a person is functioning (AOTA, 1993). Dunn et al. (1994) have presented a framework for considering the effect of context in occupational therapy. An understanding of context and environment in the design and delivery of transition services is essential and represents one of occupational therapy's unique contributions to the transition process for students with disabilities. Context includes temporal and environmental aspects. Temporal aspects may relate to an individual's age, level of maturation, life stage, status along a continuum of ability and disability, and the time it takes to accomplish a given task. Environmental aspects of context include both the nonhuman and human (social) characteristics of context. Objects, tools, and buildings are examples of nonhuman contextual variables. Human or social characteristics of a given context may include friends and family members, social roles and expectations, and cultural features such as values, beliefs, and customs.

Occupational therapy is most effective when it is imbedded in real life. If occupational therapists evaluate individual performance without considering the context of the performance, there is a great risk of interpreting the behavior inappropriately (Dunn et al., 1994, p. 602).

Three main areas for occupational therapy involvement in transition are presented and include (1) evaluation, (2) service planning, and (3) the actual delivery of transition-related services.

## Evaluation

Evaluation using an ecologic model requires that the student, family, occupational therapist, and other members of the educational team, envision a desirable future for the student (Mount, 1987; Mount & Zwernik, 1988; Rainforth et al., 1992). This requires thinking about the student in the five major performance domains: domestic, school, vocational, community, and leisure. In general, the student and the team envision a future that includes a home in the community, use of assorted community services and amenities, some sort of job or productive activity, ongoing relationships, and participation in chosen recreational or leisure activities. These are the types of things most people, with or without disabilities, envision for themselves.

In addition to clarifying a positive vision for the future, the team must also discuss the types of and long-term needs for resources and supports the student may need to achieve the vision. For example, a young adult with significant disabilities may require long-term job support in the form of a job coach who provides on-the-job training and other supports needed to maintain employment (Spencer, 1989). Another individual may require short- or long-term in-home support with personal hygiene, dressing, meal preparation, and eating to live in the community.

Evaluation follows the establishment of a vision of a quality life in the community *and* the team's identification of areas where the student is likely to need support. The occupational therapist and other members of the collaborative team must assess the extent to which the student can currently achieve this vision based on existing skills and experience. The team also identifies discrepancies between where the student needs to be functioning for a successful transition and his or her current level of performance. Evaluation, therefore, must include observation of student

performance in the actual situations and environments he or she is likely to encounter as a young adult. To conduct an ecologic transition evaluation, the team must do the following:

1. Specify environments in which the student will participate (domestic, school, vocational, community, and in leisure)
2. Prioritize, as a team, the performance environments considered to be most essential in the short term and those that will become more important over time
3. Identify activities that naturally occur in the selected, prioritized environments. The student's actual performance of relevant activities in relevant environments provides essential information from which the team can plan and make decisions
4. Divide responsibility for conducting different parts of the assessment across members of the educational team. Family members as well as professionals may participate in the assessment process
5. Conduct the assessment by actually observing student performance during activities in the selected environments. Based on careful observation, discrepancies between the environment and activity demands and the student's ability to perform are noted. This type of *discrepancy analysis* forms the heart of the assessment and guides planning and decision making
6. Record evaluation findings for the purposes of communicating with all members of the educational team, including the student and his or her parents. It is recommended that a consistent recording format be used such as the one presented in Figure 32-1
7. Present findings to the team during the IEP meeting. With all the needed information before them, the team can proceed with planning transition services using an ecologic model

An example of a transition-related assessment completed by an occupational therapist is presented here.

Ron is 16 years old and enrolled in his neighborhood high school. He is about to attend his first IEP meeting for transition, and his team has already discussed what a desirable future for Ron would look like. Ron's desired future includes living in the community with other people that he chooses, using his neighborhood grocery store, and having a few ongoing and close friendships. Ron is very social, enjoys music, communicates with a combination of sign language and words, and walks slowly with a walker. Ron has cerebral palsy and severe mental retardation.

In preparation for the IEP, members of the team have been assigned to gather information about Ron's current performance in domestic, vocational, school, community, and recreational domains. An ecologic assessment format was chosen, with different members of the team coordinating assessment activities in each domain. The occupational therapist, with specific skills in assessing activities of daily living in the home environment, coordinated assessment of the domestic domain. This involved a trip to Ron's home, an interview with Ron and his mother, and direct observation of Ron during dressing, meal preparation, and eating activities. Evaluation findings are presented, in part, in Figure 32-2.

Student: _____

Date and time of assessment: _____

Persons involved and roles: _____

Domain: ___ Domestic
         ___ School
         ___ Vocational
         ___ Community
         ___ Recreation

Environment observed (describe general environment along with physical, social, and cultural attributes):

Activities observed in this environment:
1.
2.
3.

STUDENT PERFORMANCE

| Strengths/interests | Supports needed/barriers |
|---|---|
| Activity: | |
| add pages as needed | |

Summary:

**Figure 32-1** Ecologic assessment. (Modified from Spencer, K., Murphy, M., Bean, G., and Schelly, C. (1991). Vocational needs assessment: a functional, community-referenced approach. In K. Spencer (Ed.). *From school to adult life: the role of occupational therapy in the transition process* (pp. 185-213). Fort Collins, CO: Office of Transition Services Department of Occupational Therapy, Colorado State University.)

The occupational therapist also collaborated with the teacher to evaluate Ron's use of public transportation. While the teacher evaluated Ron's ability to follow a bus schedule, identify correct stops, pay, and communicate with the bus driver, the occupational therapist focused on the physical barriers that interfered with Ron's ability to ride the bus. This type of shared responsibility for an aspect of the assessment reflects collaborative teamwork.

## Transition Service Planning

The mechanism for planning transition services is the IEP. Members of the team come together with assessment findings and meet to discuss the students identified abilities, interests, and needs. A useful way to approach the development of an IEP for transition has been clearly laid out by

Student: <u>Ron Hunt</u>

Date and time of assessment: <u>October 3, 1994, 7:30AM-9:00AM</u>

Persons involved and roles: <u>Ron Hunt, student; Marie Hunt, mother; Sara Clark, occupational therapist</u>

Domain:    <u>X</u>  Domestic
              ___ School
              ___ Vocational
              ___ Community
              ___ Recreation

Environment observed (describe general environment along with physical, social, and cultural attributes):

The assessment took place at Ron's home, which is located in a quiet, older residential neighborhood with large trees and off-street sidewalks. The single-level, three bedroom house has five steps up to the entrance. Ron lives with his mother and a younger sister who is 13 years old. Assessment activities took place in the well-equipped kitchen and in Ron's bedroom and bathroom.

Activities observed in this environment:
1. Clothing selection, dressing, grooming
2. Breakfast preparation and eating
3. Lunch preparation/packing

## STUDENT PERFORMANCE

| Strengths/interests | Supports needed/barriers |
|---|---|
| Activity: Clothing selection, dressing, grooming. | |
| Ron selected a matching shirt and pants from his closet that were appropriate for the cool season. | Ron's mother, Marie, does Ron's clothes shopping and buys clothes in basic colors and styles that can be mixed and matched. |
| | Clothes are washed and hung in the closet by Marie. |
| Ron located socks and shoes, which he put on independently while sitting down. | Ron's shoes have velcro closures. |
| Ron combed his hair while looking in the mirror in the bathroom. | Marie verbally directed Ron to comb his hair. She also "touched up" his hair combing job. |
| | Marie schedules Ron's haircuts with the local barber. |
| Ron located his toothbrush and opened and squeezed a small amount of toothpaste onto his toothbrush. He brushed his teeth while receiving verbal guidance from his mother. | Marie verbally reminded Ron to brush his teeth. During the activity she verbally cued him to "brush the back teeth, top teeth," etc. |
| Ron independently located his wallet and pocket comb and put these in his rear pants pocket. | |
| Ron and Marie "talked" about plans for the day as Ron got ready. Ron used gestures, basic sign language, and "yes" and "no" to communicate. Ron initiated communication by saying "Mom!" loudly. | Marie communicates primarily by asking Ron "yes" and "no" questions, or she asks Ron to "show me." |

**Figure 32-2**   Example of ecologic assessment.

Sample, Spencer, and Bean (1990). Specifically, an IEP meeting is held and attended by the student and team members who know the student well and who have information to contribute to the planning effort. One member of the team facilitates the meeting and guides discussion around five questions:

1. What are the dreams for the student when he or she leaves school?

   The team records these dreams as *Transition Goals.*

2. What is the student able to do now?

   The team records current student abilities as *Current Levels of Function.*

3. What does the student need?

   Needs relate to the discrepancies between what the student is able to do now in all five performance domains (domestic, school, vocational, community, and leisure) and the level of performance needed for an effective transition. *Student needs* also encompass the types of services and supports needed by the student to maximize performance in the different transition domains.

4. What is the student going to do this year?

   The team records this year's plan as *Annual Goals.*

5. Who, what, when, where, and how?

   Responsibility for implementation of the transition plan is assigned to members of the team and recorded as *Characteristics of Services.* In addition to the delegation of responsibility, the nature of services are determined and must be consistent with an ecologic curriculum approach.

A useful way to organize and summarize transition planning during the IEP meeting is to write main points on a blackboard or flip chart for all team members to see. The five questions previously listed serve as headings (Figure 32-3). This type of recording allows all members of the

team to follow the process and actively participate in decisions.

The role of the occupational therapist during transition service planning is to contribute information (based on evaluation results) and share ideas for service delivery (goals, learning activities, and learning environments) that will help the student ultimately achieve his or her transition goals. The occupational therapist may contribute information about the student in all domains or may focus on one or two domains, depending on the areas evaluated and on how the team has divided up responsibilities. It is important to remember that transition and annual goals belong to the student and not to members of the educational team. Effective transition planning requires that the team work in a collaborative manner, respecting the input of the student, family members, teachers, and related service personnel.

## Implementation

The delivery of occupational therapy services in the schools requires close collaboration between the occupational therapists and the entire team. An ecologic approach is also required for transition-related occupational therapy services to be considered *best practice.* The specific focus of occupational therapy intervention for transition-age students is to maximize student performance of essential roles and activities in real-life situations and environments.

Effective occupational therapy services are driven by the student's IEP for transition, specifically the student's long-term transition goals and shorter-term annual goals. These services may be delivered in a number of ways based on the needs of the student and the resources of the team:

1. *Direct service* provided by the occupational therapist to the student
2. *Consultation with the student's core educational team,*

| Question #1 | Question #2 | Question #3 | | Question #4 | Question #5 |
|---|---|---|---|---|---|
| Transition goals | Current levels of function | Student learning needs | Support/ training needs | Annual goals | Characteristics of services |
| | | | | | |

**Figure 32-3** Individual Education Plan for transition.

including the student, family members, and other school personnel

3. *Consultation with community agencies* that share responsibility for the implementation of transition-related services

4. *Monitoring* of services designed by the occupational therapist but delivered primarily by other team members

5. *Service coordination* or management of a particular student's overall transition program

To illustrate direct service approaches for transition-age students, some examples are useful. Consider a student with limited joint range of motion caused by severe and persistent spasticity. Direct occupational therapy services for this student may include evaluating, designing, and testing a wheelchair positioning device that allows him or her to maintain an upright seating position needed to complete school assignments and to work in the community. Direct occupational therapy services could include teaching the student how to use an electronic environmental control system that increases the student's ability to independently manage and control the home environment. For example, the occupational therapist may directly teach a student who has limited mobility to use wheelchair-mounted switches to operate a phone, unlock and open doors, turn lights on and off, and turn a television or radio on and off.

Direct occupational therapy services may occur in a variety of environments. If the student's needs relate to home management and community living, it is best for direct services to take place in the student's home (e.g., teaching adapted techniques for dressing and grooming). If the needs are vocational, services are most appropriately delivered in the relevant community or job settings (e.g., teaching the student how to safely enter and exit a public bus when balance problems exist). For many students, transition-related needs are present in the area of school performance. In this situation, the occupational therapist may deliver direct services to the student in his or her classroom (e.g., modifying assignments and writing methods), during lunch period (eating with the use of adaptive equipment), or during extracurricular school activities (learning how to function effectively in a locker room). The occupational therapist must, however, be *sensitive* to the stigma that any type of "special" or "different" services can have on a teenager or young adult. If the direct services involve unusual equipment, activities, or additional adults nearby to help, the student may strongly resist participating. If this is the case, direct service may result in resistance and other intervention strategies should be considered.

*Consultation with the student's core educational team* is a frequently used service model for transition-age youth. It requires excellent listening, observing, and communication skills on the part of the consulting occupational therapist. Consultation fits well within a collaborative team framework where information is readily shared among team members and where no one team member is viewed as having ultimate "authority" or decision-making responsibility. Although all team members have unique knowledge, experience, and perspectives, these are blended within a collaborative team. The consulting occupational therapist is invited into the team because he or she is viewed as having needed expertise that can be combined with the expertise of other team members to address a student's transition-related needs. This occupational therapy expertise may be conveyed through discussion, joint problem-solving sessions with the student and other members of the team, demonstrations, or training.

Unlike direct services, consultation requires communication and problem solving with many other players. It is incumbent on the consulting occupational therapist to effectively listen and communicate in a way that helps other team members evaluate alternatives and make decisions. Accountability for those decisions is shared by the consultant and the other members of the team. On occasion, the team may choose not to accept the consulting occupational therapist's suggestions. This may happen for a myriad of reasons, two of which are mentioned here. Ineffective consulting may be attributable to a failure on the part of the occupational therapist to effectively listen and interpret the team's needs. In this situation the occupational therapist may carry his or her own agenda into the consulting situation, rendering him or her unable to listen to or hear what other team members are requesting. The result is an occupational therapist advocating and making recommendations that do not match what the team perceives as needs or priorities. A second reason that consultation may not be well received is the team's perception that they lack the expertise, time, or resources to carry out the occupational therapist's recommendations. The recommendations are sound, but team members perceive that they do not have the resources and time to implement them. The consultation effort, therefore, remains incomplete unless the occupational therapist stays involved and helps the team identify implementation alternatives.

To increase the likelihood of effective occupational therapy consultation with the team, it is strongly recommended that the occupational therapist maintain involvement with the student and his or her team over time. This continuing contact makes it possible for the occupational therapist to evaluate the extent to which information has been received, understood, and acted on by team members. It also allows for new information to be gathered and for further clarification or modification of recommendations. Effective consultation, therefore, is more than a one-time event. Ideally, it is an ongoing "conversation" between the consultant and other team members.

From the school district's perspective, occupational therapy consultation with the student's core educational team is often viewed as a way for the occupational therapist to have a greater impact on the educational environment than can be achieved through direct service. A strong relationship between the occupational therapist and a core educational team can clearly benefit individual students and families, as well as an interdisciplinary group of professionals. The benefits to the team include identifying solutions that may help more than one student, learning to interactively solve problems, and gaining a better awareness of the expertise and roles of different team members. The ultimate goal of consultation is to enable the person or persons seeking the consultation to solve current and future problems in a more skillful way (Dunn, 1988).

Consider a 16-year-old student who was working on community job skills as a part of his transition program. The student had a work-study position at the local hospital in the laundry area. The teacher, paraprofessional, job coach, and speech pathologist had recognized that the student could not perform some of the required job tasks despite his strong motivation to work. To address the student's difficulties on the job, the team requested consultation from the school's occupational therapist. After an assessment of the student's current performance at the job and interviews with the employer, the student, and the job coach, the occupational therapist met with the team for discussion and joint problem solving. It was determined that the student lacked the coordination and strength to safely push the heavily loaded laundry carts and was unable to manipulate and simultaneously load up to six bedsheets into the large presser. Additionally, the student lost track of the number of towels he had folded and frequently overstocked the clean laundry carts, causing clean linens to fall onto the floor. On the positive side, the student was skillful at folding towels and small linens, locating supplies, asking for help, and interacting with coworkers in a friendly way. During one consultation session, the occupational therapist and the team identified the need to revise the student's job description to include more towel folding and linen cart stocking, which would replace pushing the large carts and pressing sheets. As this was being negotiated with the employer, the team continued to meet to discuss ways to facilitate accurate counting of towels and other items that get stocked onto the clean linen carts. The team devised a *jig* that was built by the paraprofessional to eliminate the student's need for counting. The jig was a work station adaptation resembling a box that was carefully sized to hold exactly eight folded towels. When the jig was full, the student moved the stack to the cart, making each stack on the cart exactly the right size. A third consultation session occurred at the job site between the occupational therapist, student, job coach, and employer. During this time, the jig was tested, modified, and determined to be effective. The jig idea was then extended to other items that go onto the clean laundry carts. A final consultation session was held about 2 weeks after the student had begun using the jigs at work. The purpose of this session was to evaluate the student's progress on the job and the effectiveness of the recent job modifications. When it was determined that the student was performing well, the occupational therapy consultation ended.

*Consultation with community agencies* represents another type of consultation that can benefit transition-age students with disabilities. Although similar to the consultation that occurs between the occupational therapist and other members of the student's core educational team, consultation with community agencies tends to be short term and specific. Because a student's entitlement to public education services ends when he or she exits high school (typically between the ages of 18 and 21), it is important for members of the educational team to work with the community agencies and employers who are likely to be involved with the student after high school. For this reason, the occupational therapist may find himself or herself consulting with prospective community employers, community job placement agencies, local residential service providers, and others to create and maintain opportunities for the student to participate in meaningful adult roles and activities after exiting the public school system.

An example of occupational therapist involvement with a community employer may illustrate the nature of consultation with community agencies.

Renee is a 19-year-old student who sustained a brain injury when she was a sophomore in high school. She is now working part-time at a local sporting goods store and hopes to continue her job after she completes high school. The employer has reported that Renee has difficultly following through with assigned tasks, even though she seems to understand the task. The occupational therapist, who is familiar with the student and the job tasks, offers to consult with the employer. The purpose of the consultation is to identify strategies that will help Renee perform her job more effectively. The consulting occupational therapist visited the job site while Renee is working and spent time observing her job performance, characteristics of the job environment, and the student's interactions with her job coach and the employer. Based on these observations, the occupational therapist recommended the following:

1. The employer shows the student what to do rather than telling her
2. The student's job coach develops a small, inconspicuous notebook that lists routine job tasks and materials. The student is then asked to carry the notebook and use it as a guide when she is unsure about how to proceed
3. The employer provides the student with daily, positive feedback in the quiet of the office as she punches out for the day
4. The materials used on the job are modified to accommodate the student's need to use one hand for most tasks. This includes locating a wheeled cart that the student can use to conveniently transport cleaning supplies and merchandise for restocking

These recommendations were shared with Renee, her employer, and her job coach at an informal meeting at the job site. After some discussion, they were modified slightly and resources were identified to obtain and adapt a wheeled cart for Renee. The occupational therapist then followed up within a week to check on Renee's progress and the employer's satisfaction. A few additional adjustments were made to Renee's cart during this visit. A second follow-up visit was made by the occupational therapist after another 2 weeks to be sure that Renee was maintaining adequate job performance. When the occupational therapist determined that Renee and her employer were both pleased, the consultation ended. The occupational therapist, however, made it clear that if new needs should come up, she would be available to reenter the job site to help solve problems.

*Monitoring of services* that are designed by the occupational therapist but delivered primarily by other members of the team represents a fourth model for occupational therapy service provision. Monitoring requires the occupational therapist to be involved in assessing the student's performance and needs, intervening for a short period, and then turning over responsibility for ongoing intervention to other members of the team. When responsibility for actual service delivery is turned over to other team members, the occupational therapist begins a monitoring role. Although similar to consultation, monitoring differs in the sense that the occupational therapist continues to maintain primary responsibility for student outcomes and must continue regular contact (at least twice a month) with the student for the duration of the intervention (AOTA, 1987). Responsibility on the part of the occupational therapist continues despite the fact that he or she has delegated the day-to-day implementation of the program to another person. This person may be a teacher, a paraprofessional, or others who have regular, daily contact with the student.

Before monitoring is selected as the approach, it must be determined that the persons identified to implement the services are sufficiently skilled and available to carry out the program. Training and supervision must be provided by the occupational therapist to assure that the services being delivered are those that are needed (AOTA, 1994).

Monitoring can be an effective approach to service delivery for a student who is learning to use an adapted computer to communicate and complete school assignments. After a thorough assessment of the student's assistive technology needs and the acquisition of an adapted computer, the occupational therapist may design services to teach the student to become an independent computer user. These services may involve student use of alternative computer access methods such as a head-mounted switch with specific software. The occupational therapist teaches the student, teacher, and paraprofessional how to set up and use the equipment. Once the teacher and paraprofessional demonstrate proficiency with the assistive technology and in teaching the student, the occupational therapist would then reduce involvement to occasional but regular visits for monitoring purposes. Should the student fail to make expected progress toward independent computer use, the occupational therapist would evaluate and redesign the intervention.

Monitoring can be an effective way to deliver transition-related services. It requires an intensive, up-front investment of time followed by decreased involvement from the occupational therapist. When monitoring is effective, the people who work most frequently with the student acquire the skills needed to implement occupational therapy recommendations throughout the student's day. This infusion of occupational therapy into the student's overall education program can significantly increase the impact of occupational therapy (Giangreco, 1986).

*Service coordination* refers to the efforts of one member of a student's transition team to assist the student and his or her family with coordination and management of the many details associated with transition-related services. Service coordination has also been termed *case management*.

As students approach the school-to-adult life transition they experience changes in their day-to-day activities and the accompanying support services and resources. Students who need ongoing, transition-related support beyond high school may need assistance identifying resources to assist with community employment, living, recreation, or postsecondary education. These supports and services do not come from the schools but from an array of adult and community service agencies. To assure the student's smooth transition from the familiar surroundings of the school to new and unfamiliar adult roles, service coordination may be essential if needed supports and services are to be in place *before* the student exits the public school system. Proactive coordination of transition-related services can prevent gaps in service and unnecessary "down-time" for the student.

Serving as a transition services coordinator requires skill in working directly with the family and student so that their choices and interests are reflected in any and all planning activities. The service coordinator also needs to know, understand, and communicate effectively with other team members including teachers, related service personnel, and adult service agencies. Maintaining a broad view of the student's current performance and performance needs across all domains (domestic, school, vocational, community, and leisure) constitutes a third skill of a transition service coordinator.

The occupational therapist has an understanding of human performance needs in different environments as well as training and skill in communication, group process, individualized assessment, and service delivery. The occupational therapist is, therefore, well suited to work as a transition service coordinator. This role requires keeping the interests, preferences, and abilities of the student foremost in mind while working with available resources to identify or create needed services. The service coordinator then facilitates the transition process by supporting (and gently prodding) other team members to complete their assessment or service responsibilities, managing a transition timeline, linking resources and services, and most importantly, helping the student participate to the maximum extent possible in all decisions related to his or her transition services.

## SUMMARY

What happens to people with disabilities after they complete 12 to 18 years of public education? This question has received a great deal of attention from legislators, researchers, teachers, and related service personnel (including oc-

1. Consider the school-to-adult life transition process for a student with significant disabilities. How would this be similar or different from your own transition from high school to new and different adult roles?

2. What does an occupational therapist bring to the transition process for students with disabilities? How would you describe the occupational therapist role to a high school teacher? A transition-age student? A transition-age student's parent?

3. What skills do you have that will help you work as a collaborative team member? What skills do you think you will need to develop?

4. What would an ecologic assessment have looked like for you during your initial transition from high school to the adult world?

cupational therapists) over the years. Public education is often viewed as an "investment" in the future of our society and specifically in youth. As with all investments, there is a desire to obtain a positive and profitable return on the investment. The return on the education investment for children and youth with disabilities relates to their eventual and successful transition from school to productive and meaningful adult life.

Responsibility for the delivery of transition services clearly rests with all members of the IEP team, including occupational therapy personnel (Brollier, Shepherd, & Flick Markley, 1994; Dunn, 1991; Spencer & Sample, 1993). The ability of occupational therapists and certified occupational therapy assistants to focus on the needs of youth in the context of their approaching adult roles and performance environments adds strength to an educational team charged with designing and implementing transition services. Occupational therapy assessment and intervention related to activities of daily living, work, and recreation are consistent with the transition services mandated in federal law and are essential components of effective transition planning and service delivery. Occupational therapy personnel may assume roles in consulting, providing direct service, monitoring occupational therapy programs, or coordinating transition service. Each role requires an understanding of the overall transition process for students with disabilities along with an understanding of each student's unique abilities, interests, and needs.

## REFERENCES

American Occupational Therapy Association. (1987). *Guidelines for occupational therapy services in school systems.* Rockville, MD: American Occupational Therapy Association.

American Occupational Therapy Association. (1994). Uniform terminology for occupational therapy (3rd ed.). *Journal of American Occupational Therapy 48,* 1047-1054.

Brollier, C., Shepherd, J., & Flick Markley, K. (1994). Transition from school to community living. *American Journal of Occupational Therapy, 48,* 346-353.

Brown, L., Branston-McLean, M.B., Baumgart, D., Vincent, L., Falvey, M., & Schroeder, J. (1979). Using the characteristics of current and future least restrictive environments in the development of curricular content for severely handicapped students. *American Association for Education of the Severe and Profound Handicapped Review, 4*(4), 407-424.

Brown, L., Nietupski, J., & Hamre-Nietupski, S. (1976). Criterion of ultimate functioning. In M.A. Thomas (Ed.). *Hey, don't forget about me!* (pp. 2-15). Reston, VA: Council for Exceptional Children.

Dunn, W. (1988). Models of occupational therapy service provision in the school system. *American Journal of Occupational Therapy, 42*(11), 718-722.

Dunn, W. (Ed.) (1991). *Pediatric occupational therapy: facilitation of effective service provision.* Thorofare, NJ: Slack.

Dunn, W., Brown, C., & McGuigan, A. (1994). The ecology of human performance: a framework for considering the effect of context. *The American Journal of Occupational Therapy, 48*(7), 595-607.

Edgar, E., Levine, P., & Maddox, M. (1986). *Statewide follow-up studies of secondary special education students in transition.* Working Paper of the Networking and Evaluation Team. Seattle: University of Washington.

Education of All Handicapped Children Act (Public Law 94-142). (1975). 20 U.S.C., 1401.

Everson, J. & McNulty, K. (1992). Interagency teams: building local transition programs through parental and professional partnerships. In F. Rusch, L. Destefano, J. Chadsey-Rusch, L.A. Phelps, & E. Szymanski (Eds.). *Transition from school to adult life: models, linkages, and policy* (pp. 342-351). Pacific Grove, CA: Brooks/Cole.

Giangreco, M. (1986). Effects of integrated therapy: a pilot study. *Journal of the Association for Persons with Severe Handicaps, 11*(3), 205-208.

Giangreco, M., York, J., & Rainforth, B. (1989). Providing related services to learners with severe handicaps in educational settings: pursuing the least restrictive option. *Pediatric Physical Therapy, 1*(2), 55-63.

Halloran, W. (1992). *Transition services requirement: issues, implications, challenge.* Washington, D.C.: United States Department of Education.

Hamre-Nietupski, S., Nietupski, J., Sandvig, R., Sandvig, M.B., & Ayres, B. (1984). Leisure skills instruction in a community residential setting with young adults who are deaf/blind severely handicapped. *The Journal of the Association for Persons with Severe Handicaps, 9*(1), 49-54.

Hasazi, S., Gordon, L., & Roe, C. (1985). Factors associated with the employment status of handicapped youth exiting high school from 1973-1983. *Exceptional Children, 51,* 455-469.

Hasazi, S., Hock, M., & Cravedi-Cheng, L. (1992). Vermont's postschool indicators: using satisfaction and post-school outcome data for program improvement. In F. Rusch, L. Destefano, J. Chadsey-Rusch, L.A. Phelps, & E. Szymanski (Eds.). *Transition from school to adult life: models, linkages, and policy* (pp. 485-506). Pacific Grove, CA: Brooks/Cole.

Individuals with Disabilities Education Act (Public Law 101-476). (1990). 20 U.S.C., 1401.

Lyon, S. & Lyon, G. (1980). Team functioning and staff development: a role release approach to providing integrated educational services for severely handicapped students. *Journal of The Association for the Severely Handicapped, 5*(3), 250-263.

Mount, B. (1987). *Personal futures planning: finding directions for change.* Unpublished doctoral dissertation, University of Georgia.

Mount, B. & Zwernik, K. (1988). *It's never too early, it's never too late: a booklet about personal futures planning.* St. Paul: Metropolitan Council.

NICHCY: National Information Center for Children and Youth with Disabilities. (1993). Transition summary. *NICHCY, 3*(1), 1-19.

Rainforth, B. & York, J. (1987). Integrating related services in community instruction. *Journal of the Association for Persons with Severe Handicaps, 12,* 190-198.

Rainforth, B., York, J., & Macdonald, C. (1992). *Collaborative teams for students with severe disabilities: integrating therapy with educational services.* Baltimore: Brookes.

Sample, P., Spencer, K., & Bean, G. (1990). *Transition planning: creating a positive future for students with disabilities.* Fort Collins, CO: Office of Transition Services, Department of Occupational Therapy, Colorado State University.

Spencer, K. (1989). The transition from school to adult life. In S. Hertfelder & C. Gwin (Eds.). *Work in progress: occupational therapy in work programs.* Rockville, MD: American Occupational Therapy Association.

Spencer, K., Murphy, M., Bean, G., & Schelly, C. (1991). Vocational needs assessment: a functional, community-referenced approach. In K. Spencer (Ed.). *From school to adult life: the role of occupational therapy in the transition process* (pp. 185-213). Fort Collins, CO: Office of Transition Services Department of Occupational Therapy, Colorado State University.

Spencer, K. & Sample, P. (1993). Transition planning and services. In C. Royeen (Ed.). *Classroom applications for school-based practice* (pp. 6-48). Rockville, MD: American Occupational Therapy Association.

Udvari-Solner, A., Jorgenson, J., & Courchane, G. (1992). Longitudinal vocational curriculum: the foundation for effective transition. In F. Rusch, L. Destefano, J. Chadsey-Rusch, L.A. Phelps, & E. Szymanski (Eds.). *Transition from school to adult life: models, linkages, and policy* (pp 285-320). Pacific Grove, CA: Brooks/Cole.

Wagner, M. (1989). *The transition experiences of youth with disabilities: a report from the national longitudinal transition study.* Menlo Park, CA: SRI International.

Ward, M. (1992). Introduction to secondary special education and transition issues. In F. Rusch, L. Destefano, J. Chadsey-Rusch, L.A. Phelps, & E. Szymanski (Eds.). *Transition from school to adult life: models, linkages, and policy* (pp. 387-389). Pacific Grove, CA: Brooks/Cole.

Wehman, P. (1992). *Life beyond the classroom: transition strategies for young people with disabilities.* Baltimore: Brookes.

Williams, W., Fox, T.J., Thousand, J., & Fox, W. (1990). Level of acceptance and implementation of best practices in the education of students with severe handicaps in Vermont. *Education and Training in Mental Retardation, 25*(2), 120-131.

Woolcock, W., Stodden, R., & Bisconer, S. (1992). Process- and outcome-focused decision making. In F. Rusch, L. Destefano, J. Chadsey-Rusch, L.A. Phelps, & E. Szymanski (Eds.). *Transition from school to adult life: models, linkages, and policy* (pp. 219-244). Pacific Grove, CA: Brooks/Cole.

York, J. & Vandercook, T. (1991). Designing an integrated education for learners with severe disabilities through the IEP process. *Teaching Exceptional Children, 23*(2), 22-28.

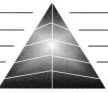

# Index

Page numbers in italics indicate illustrations; *t* indicates tables..

Coloboma, 729
Comminuted fractures, 126
Commission on Accreditation of Rehabilitation
    Facilities (CARF), 781
    standards for hospital operations, 744
Communication
    augmentative and alternative; *see*
        Augmentative and alternative
        communication (AAC)
    defined, 545
    early intervention assessment and, 658
    impairments; *see* Communication
        impairments
    for self care/IADL, 488
    teams and, 239-240
    of test results, 219
    between therapists and families, 87-90
    total, 724, 726
    written; *see* Written communication
Communication Aids Manufacturers
    Association (CAMA), 561
Communication impairments
    AT services for, 549-551
    evaluation of, 549
    intervention for, 550
Community activities
    mobility for, 492
    skills for, 492
Community teams, 19
Compensatory skills
    approach to self care/IADL, 471-472
    developing in school-based occupational
        therapy, 702-706
    developing in sensory integrative
        intervention, 338-339
Competency, of examiners, 217-219
Competency behavior, 505
Comprehensive evaluation, 171
Computers
    adapted, 553
        in school-based occupational therapy,
            705-706
    visual perception intervention and, 382
Concepts of Left and Right Test, for
    visual-cognitive assessment, 373
Concrete operational period, of Piaget's
    cognitive theory, 34
Concurrent validity, 213-214
Conditional reasoning, 233
Conditioning, operant, 37
Conduct disorders, 399
Conduction disturbances, 116
Conductive hearing loss, 719
Confidence intervals, 212
Confidentiality, standardized tests and, 219
Conflict resolution, by teams, 240-241
Congenital defects
    cardiac, 113-116, 646-647
    clubfoot, 121-122
    clubhand, 122
    of hands and feet, 123
    herpes, 151
    hip dislocation, 122
    of limbs, 122-124
    in metabolism, 146-147
    syphilis, 150

Congenital disorders
    musculoskeletal, 120-122
    need for rehabilitation and, 779
Congenital heart disease, 113-116, 646
Congenital muscular dystrophy (CMD), 134
Congenital obstructive hydrocephalus,
        implications for neonatal occupational
        therapy, 642*t*
Consciousness, levels of, 29-30
Construct-related validity, 213
Consultation
    collaborative, as service delivery model, 239
    home-based intervention and, 760
    in school-based occupational therapy,
        708-709
    sensory integrative intervention and,
        340-341
    in transition services, 818-819
Content-related validity, 213
Contingencies of behavior, Skinner and, 37
Continuum of function-dysfunction; *see*
    Function-dysfunction continua
Continuum of sensory responsivity, 324
Contract services, in school-based occupational
        therapy, 714
Contracts, performance, 424
Contusions, 125
Convergence, 360
Coping
    families with disabled children and, 81-83
    frames of reference, 42
Coping Inventory, 197
    for assessment of cognitive and psychosocial
        skills, 167
Coping model, *234*
    case studies, 236-238
    for intervention plans, 233-234
Correctional facilities, psychosocial
        intervention and, 797*t*, 805
Correlation coefficients
    between PDMS and BSID-II, 214*t*
    of standardized tests, 209-210
Cortical blindness, 729
Cost-effectiveness, of pediatric occupational
        therapy, 15
Coxa plana, 127
CP; *see* Cerebral palsy (CP)
CPS; *see* Children's Playfulness Scale (CPS)
Crawling; *see* Creeping
Creeping, sensorimotor development and, 49*t*,
    51
CRF; *see* Chronic renal failure (CRF)
*Cri du chat* syndrome, 146
Criterion-referenced tests, 184; *see also*
        Standardized tests
    for preschool children, 679-681
    *vs.* norm-referenced tests, 206*t*
Criterion-related validity, 213-214
Critical care units (CCU), 745
Critical periods, readiness and, 27
Crohn's disease, 159
Crush injuries, 125
CSF; *see* Cerebrospinal fluid (CSF)
CTG; *see* Closing the Gap (CTG)
Cued speech, 724
Cultural bias, standardized tests and, 219

Cultural diversity, early intervention and, 661
Culture; *see also* Environment
    effect on families with disabled children, 85*t*
    effect on hand skills, 270
    as performance context, 7
    sensitivity to in home-based intervention,
        762-763
Curricula; *see also* School activities
    ecologic, as best practice for transition
        services, 811-813
    integration of preschool services with, 686,
        *687, 688*
Cursive style, of handwriting, 533
Curvature, of spine, 127-128
Cylindrical grasp, 275, *276*
Cystic fibrosis (CF), 117-118
Cytomegalovirus, 151

**D**

Dactylology, 724, *725*
Day treatment centers, as setting for
        psychosocial intervention, 797*t*, 803
DDST; *see* Denver Developmental Screening
        Test (DDST)
Deaf-blind; *see* Multiple sensory impairments
Death; *see also* Terminal illnesses
    adolescents' perception of, 768-769
    children's perception of, 767-769, 770*t*
        assessing, 771
    instincts, 29
Decibels, 720-721
Decision by consensus, 240
Decision-making
    families with disabled children and, 87
    by teams, 240-242
Decoding, problems in reading, 379
Decubiti, 478
Dedicated systems, for AAC, 553
Defense mechanisms, 29
Deformities
    caused by fractures, *125*
    positional, 594, 598
    torsional, 126-127
DeGangi-Berk Test of Sensory Integration
        (TSI), 197, 256
    for evaluation of preschool children, 681
Dental hygiene, 487
Denver Developmental Screening Test
        (DDST), 107, 170, 197, 655
Denver Handwriting Analysis, 530, 542
Depressive disorders, major, 400, 402*t*
Descriptive statistics, standardized tests and,
        207-208
Desensitization, oral, 437-438
Despair, *vs.* integrity, 32
Development; *see also* Growth
    adolescent period of, 62-64
    biologic, 26
    cognitive; *see* Cognitive development
    defined, 26
    dimensions of, 26
    early childhood period of, 57-61
    feeding and, 453
    fetal/neonatal effects on, 147
    impact of visual impairments on, 731-732
    infancy period of, 48-57